T0189307

Lecture Notes in Computer Science   11492

Commenced Publication in 1973
Founding and Former Series Editors:
Gerhard Goos, Juris Hartmanis, and Jan van Leeuwen

More information about this series at http://www.springer.com/series/7412

Albert C. S. Chung · James C. Gee ·
Paul A. Yushkevich · Siqi Bao (Eds.)

Information Processing in Medical Imaging

26th International Conference, IPMI 2019
Hong Kong, China, June 2–7, 2019
Proceedings

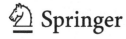 Springer

Editors
Albert C. S. Chung ⓘ
Department of Computer Science
and Engineering
The Hong Kong University of Science
and Technology
Hong Kong, China

Paul A. Yushkevich ⓘ
Department of Radiology
University of Pennsylvania
Philadelphia, PA, USA

James C. Gee ⓘ
Department of Radiology
University of Pennsylvania
Philadelphia, PA, USA

Siqi Bao ⓘ
Department of Natural Language Processing
Baidu Inc.
Shenzhen, China

ISSN 0302-9743   ISSN 1611-3349   (electronic)
Lecture Notes in Computer Science
ISBN 978-3-030-20350-4   ISBN 978-3-030-20351-1   (eBook)
https://doi.org/10.1007/978-3-030-20351-1

LNCS Sublibrary: SL6 – Image Processing, Computer Vision, Pattern Recognition, and Graphics

This Springer imprint is published by the registered company Springer Nature Switzerland AG
The registered company address is: Gewerbestrasse 11, 6330 Cham, Switzerland

Preface

The 26th biennial international conference on Information Processing in Medical Imaging (IPMI) was held during June 2–7, 2019, at The Hong Kong University of Science and Technology, Hong Kong. The first IPMI meeting in 1969 took place in Brussels, organized by a group of young researchers who worked on the use of computers in nuclear medicine. In 1973, IPMI crossed the Atlantic to Boston (Cambridge), and the meeting's site has since alternated between Europe and the United States. IPMI 2019 broke new ground as the conference's first appearance in Asia, a continent that is ascendant on the global stage and is already a primary source of the young talent whose careers and development IPMI specifically strives to foster. This edition of the meeting also celebrated the 50th year of IPMI conference and its enduring impact on the field.

This year, 229 full paper submissions were received. Of these, 25 papers were accepted as oral presentations and 43 papers were selected for posters, resulting in an acceptance rate of 30%. Submissions underwent a double-blind review by three members of the Scientific Committee, who evaluated the clarity, novelty, methodological development, quality of evaluation, and clinical relevance of each paper. The Paper Selection Committee met in February to select papers for the scientific program based on the reviewers' detailed comments, rankings, and recommendations, and its independent judgment of the merits of each paper. A total of 68 papers were accepted and divided into 13 single-track oral and two poster presentation sessions, respectively. The breadth of the topics covered in IPMI 2019 reveals a diverse spectrum of exciting developments in medical imaging, including reconstruction, segmentation, registration, connectivity, disease modeling and prediction, shape analysis, functional and white matter imaging, computer-aided diagnosis, and other related topics.

IPMI meetings are renowned for cultivating a vibrant atmosphere in which in-depth academic exchange and community spirit are fostered. This year, the conference was attended by 141 participants, all of whom contributed to small study groups. Now a hallmark feature of IPMI, study groups are assigned and discuss papers selected for oral presentation, then help lead the discussion of the work at its presentation. Each talk was allotted a nominal amount of time on the schedule but discussion length was unrestricted and at the discretion of the session chair. The poster presentation sessions were also programmed to offer ample opportunity for interactive and in-depth discussion. Conference attendees enjoyed both social and sporting activities—including the Dragon's Back hike, Peak Circle Walk, a boat trip to Sharp Island, competitive athletic games, and the beloved IPMI choir—during the afternoons of conference day 3 and 4.

The keynote session featured two presentations: the first led by Drs. Stephen Pizer, Kenan Professor at the University of North Carolina at Chapel Hill, and James Duncan, Ebenezer K. Hunt Professor at Yale University, who celebrated the 50th year of IPMI by reviewing its illustrious past (including the third and 15th meetings organized by Steve and Jim, respectively); and the second by Dr. Xiaodong Tao, CEO of iFLYTEK

Health, who provided a glimpse of the meeting's future as represented by one country's ambitions, namely, China, in medical imaging artificial intelligence. The François Erbsmann Prize is awarded to a young scientist of age 35 or below, who is the first author of a paper, giving his/her first oral preparation at IPMI. This year, 22 of the 25 oral presenters were eligible for the prize. Once again, scholarships were offered to promote participation from minorities, women, and other underrepresented groups.

The meeting would not have been possible without the significant contributions and generous support from our dedicated colleagues at universities, foundations, and industry. We are particularly grateful for the financial sponsorship provided by the following organizations:

The Hong Kong University of Science and Technology
University of Pennsylvania
Croucher Foundation
K. C. Wong Education Foundation
National Institute of Biomedical Imaging and Bioengineering
National Institutes of Health
United Imaging Intelligence
Imsight Medical Technology Company Limited
Springer Nature
International Business Machines

The IPMI 2019 chairs would like to thank the Scientific Committee members for their essential reviewing work, the Paper Selection Committee members for their critical role in forming the meeting's scientific program, previous IPMI organizers, especially Martin Styner and Marc Niethammer, for sharing their experiences, Sharon Chiu for her invaluable administrative support, and our research group members (Jierong Wang, Tony Mok, Ziyi He, Yongxiang Huang, Han Zhang, Yishuo Zhang, Rongzhao Zhang, Pei Wang, and Colin Tsang) for their dedicated assistance in every aspect of the meeting.

By strengthening the connection of IPMI to the research community in Asia, the 2019 meeting in Hong Kong represented an exciting new chapter for the conference. We are delighted to have organized and served as hosts of IPMI 2019, and applaud the excellence of all of the work that appeared at the meeting and is documented in this volume.

June 2019

Albert Chung
James Gee
Paul Yushkevich

Organization

Conference Chairs

Albert C. S. Chung   The Hong Kong University of Science
and Technology, Hong Kong, China
James C. Gee   University of Pennsylvania, USA

Paper Submission and Reviewing Chair

Paul A. Yushkevich   University of Pennsylvania, USA

Local Organizing Committee

Jierong Wang   The Hong Kong University of Science
and Technology, Hong Kong, China
Tony C. W. Mok   The Hong Kong University of Science
and Technology, Hong Kong, China

Proceedings Chair

Siqi Bao   Baidu, China

Paper Selection Committee

Aasa Feragen   University of Copenhagen, Denmark
Ender Konukoglu   ETH Zürich, Switzerland
Marc Niethammer   The University of North Carolina at Chapel Hill, USA
Jerry L. Prince   Johns Hopkins University, USA
Anqi Qiu   National University of Singapore, Singapore
Simon K. Warfield   Harvard Medical School and Boston Children's
Hospital, USA
Paul A. Yushkevich   University of Pennsylvania, USA

Scientific Committee

Purang Abolmaesumi   The University of British Columbia, Canada
Daniel Alexander   University College London, UK
Stéphanie Allassonnière   École Polytechnique, France
Elsa D. Angelini   Columbia University, USA
Alexis Arnaudon   Imperial College London, UK
John Ashburner   University College London, UK
Suyash P. Awate   Indian Institute of Technology (IIT) Bombay, India

Ulas Bagci	University of Central Florida, USA
Christian Barillot	IRISA-CNRS, Rennes, France
Kayhan Batmanghelich	University of Pittsburgh, USA/Carnegie Mellon University, USA
Pierre-Louis Bazin	Netherlands Institute for Neuroscience, The Netherlands
Sylvain Bouix	Harvard Medical School and Brigham and Women's Hospital, USA
J. Micheal Brady	University of Oxford, UK
M. Jorge Cardoso	University College London, UK
Chao Chen	Stony Brook University, USA
Gary E. Christensen	University of Iowa, USA
Albert C. S. Chung	The Hong Kong University of Science and Technology, Hong Kong, China
Moo Chung	University of Wisconsin at Madison, USA
Olivier Commowick	Inria, France
Tim Cootes	Manchester University, UK
Claire Cury	Inria, France
Adrian V. Dalca	Massachusetts Institute of Technology, USA
Sune Darkner	University of Copenhagen, Denmark
Benoit Dawant	Vanderbilt University, USA
Marleen de Bruijne	Erasmus MC Rotterdam, The Netherlands/University of Copenhagen, Denmark
Karen Drukker	University of Chicago, USA
Lei Du	Northwestern Polytechnical University, China
James S. Duncan	Yale University, USA
Shireen Elhabian	Scientific Computing and Imaging Institute, University of Utah, USA
Yong Fan	University of Pennsylvania, USA
Aasa Feragen	University of Copenhagen, Denmark
Tom Fletcher	University of Utah, USA
Alejandro F. Frangi	University of Leeds, UK
Mona K. Garvin	The University of Iowa, USA
James C. Gee	University of Pennsylvania, USA
Guido Gerig	New York University, USA
Polina Golland	Massachusetts Institute of Technology, USA
Miguel A. González Ballester	Pompeu Fabra University, Spain
Ali Gooya	University of Leeds, UK
Horst Hahn	Fraunhofer MEVIS, Germany
Justin Haldar	University of Southern California, USA
Ghassan Hamarneh	Simon Fraser University, Canada
Tobias Heimann	Siemens AG, Germany
Mattias Heinrich	University of Lübeck, Germany
Yi Hong	University of Georgia, USA

Anand Joshi   Signal and Image Processing Institute at University
                                of Southern California, USA
Konstantinos Kamnitsas   Imperial College London, UK
Boklye Kim   University of Michigan, USA
Andrew King   King's College London, UK
Stefan Klein   Erasmus MC Rotterdam, The Netherlands
Frithjof Kruggel   University of California, Irvine, USA
Elizabeth A. Krupinski   University of Arizona, USA
Sebastian Kurtek   Ohio State University, USA
Roland Kwitt   University of Salzburg, Austria
Jan Kybic   Czech Technical University in Prague, Czech Republic
Bennett A. Landman   Vanderbilt University, USA
Georg Langs   Medical University of Vienna, Austria
Boudewijn Lelieveldt   Leiden University Medical Center, The Netherlands
Shuo Li   University of Western Ontario, Canada
Wenqi Li   King's College London, UK
Tianming Liu   University of Georgia, USA
Hervé Lombaert   ÉTS Montréal, Canada
Cristian Lorenz   Philips Research, Germany
Marco Lorenzi   Inria Sophia Antipolis, France
Razvan V. Marinescu   University College London, UK
Bjoern Menze   Technical University of Munich, Germany
Marc Modat   University College London, UK
Jan Modersitzki   University of Lübeck, Germany
Bernard Ng   The University of British Columbia, Canada
Marc Niethammer   The University of North Carolina at Chapel Hill, USA
J. Alison Noble   University of Oxford, UK
Xenophon Papademetris   Yale University, USA
Xavier Pennec   Inria Sophia Antipolis, France
Dzung Pham   National Institutes of Health, USA
Stephen M. Pizer   The University of North Carolina at Chapel Hill, USA
Kilian Pohl   SRI, USA
Jerry L. Prince   Johns Hopkins University, USA
Jinyi Qi   University of California, Davis, USA
Gwenolé Quellec   LaTIM, Inserm, UMR 1101, France
Yogesh Rathi   Harvard Medical School and Brigham and Women's
                                Hospital, USA
Hariharan Ravishankar   GE Global Research, India
Joseph Reinhardt   University of Iowa, USA
Islem Rekik   Istanbul Technical University, Turkey
Laurent Risser   French National Center for Scientific Research, France
Karl Rohr   German Cancer Research Center, Germany
Daniel Rueckert   Imperial College London, UK
Olivier Salvado   Australian e-Health Research Centre, Australia
Benoit Scherrer   Harvard Medical School and Boston Children's
                                Hospital, USA

IPMI 2019 Board

Christian Barillot	IRISA-CNRS, Rennes, France
Randy Brill	Vanderbilt University, USA
Marleen de Bruijne	Erasmus MC Rotterdam, The Netherlands/University of Copenhagen, Denmark
Gary E. Christensen	University of Iowa, USA
Albert C. S. Chung	The Hong Kong University of Science and Technology, Hong Kong, China
James S. Duncan	Yale University, USA
Polina Golland	Massachusetts Institute of Technology, USA
Richard M. Leahy	University of Southern California, USA
J. Alison Noble	Oxford University, UK
Sebastien Ourselin	King's College London, UK
Stephen M. Pizer	The University of North Carolina at Chapel Hill, USA
Jerry L. Prince	Johns Hopkins University, USA
Martin Styner	The University of North Carolina at Chapel Hill, USA
Gábor Székely	ETH Zürich, Switzerland
Chris Taylor	University of Manchester, UK
Andrew Todd-Pokropek	University College, London, UK
William M. Wells III	Harvard Medical School and Brigham and Women's Hospital, USA

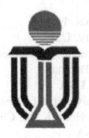

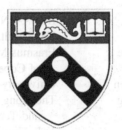

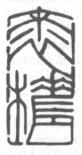

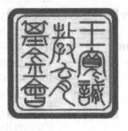

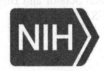

National Institute of
Biomedical Imaging
and Bioengineering

National Institutes
of Health

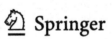

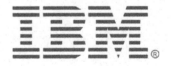

Contents

Reconstruction

Disease Modeling

Shape

Registration

Learning Motion

Functional Imaging

White Matter Imaging

Posters

Segmentation

A Bayesian Neural Net to Segment Images with Uncertainty Estimates and Good Calibration

Rohit Jena and Suyash P. Awate[✉]

Computer Science and Engineering, Indian Institute of Technology Bombay,
Mumbai, India
`suyash@cse.iitb.ac.in`

Abstract. We propose a novel *Bayesian decision theoretic deep-neural-network* (DNN) framework for image segmentation, enabling us to define a principled measure of *uncertainty* associated with label probabilities. Our framework *estimates uncertainty analytically* at test time, unlike the state of the art that relies on approximate and expensive algorithms using sampling or multiple passes. Moreover, our framework leads to a novel *Bayesian interpretation of the softmax* layer. We propose a novel method to improve DNN *calibration*. Results on three large datasets show that our framework improves segmentation quality and calibration, and provides more realistic uncertainty estimates, over existing methods.

Keywords: Image segmentation · Deep neural network ·
Bayesian decision theory · Generative model · Bayesian utility ·
Uncertainty · Calibration

1 Introduction

Deep neural networks (DNNs) have been successful at *image segmentation* in radiology and digital pathology [2,3,9,10,14–17]. Typical DNN methods propose new architectures, e.g., dual-path convolutional [10] or skip connected [3,16,17], or new loss functions, e.g., based on weighted cross entropy [14] or the Dice similarity coefficient (DSC) [15,17], to improve performance.

For clinical decision support relying on automated image segmentation, e.g., radiotherapy and neurosurgery, exposing the *uncertainty* in segmentation [4,13] can lead to better informed decisions or better outcomes. It can also improve reliability in scientific studies. In DNN-based segmentation, the per-voxel label probabilities can be unreliable because of, e.g., poor quality of the data due to low contrast or high noise, high variability in the object structure, etc. In such cases, a clear unique "answer", i.e., label probabilities, at a voxel, fails to

S. P. Awate—Supported by: Wadhwani Research Centre for Bioengineering (WRCB) IIT Bombay, Department of Biotechnology (DBT) Govt. of India BT/INF/22/ SP23026/2017; Nvidia GPU Grant Program; Whiterabbit.ai Inc.; Aira Matrix.

© Springer Nature Switzerland AG 2019
A. C. S. Chung et al. (Eds.): IPMI 2019, LNCS 11492, pp. 3–15, 2019.
https://doi.org/10.1007/978-3-030-20351-1_1

exist, but rather multiple answers are almost equally likely. We propose a novel *Bayesian decision theoretic DNN* framework that leads to sound interpretations of the DNN architecture and outputs, and, in turn, enables us to define and efficiently infer the variability/uncertainty over label probabilities per voxel.

A DNN classifier is well *calibrated* [8] if, for the subset of the data for which the DNN assigns the probability of being in (some) class C to be within the interval $(p - \delta, p + \delta)$ (termed "confidence"), the empirical fraction of the data actually being in class C (termed "accuracy") equals p. In practice, typical DNN classifiers are poorly calibrated [8], producing class probabilities that are significantly overestimated (near 1) or underestimated (near 0), even when the data around that voxel is very ambiguous. In the literature on DNN frameworks for image segmentation, miscalibration has been largely ignored. In our Bayesian framework, we propose a novel method to improve calibration for segmentation.

This paper makes several contributions. We propose a novel DNN framework for image segmentation rooted in *generative modeling* and *Bayesian decision theory*, which leads to a Bayesian interpretation of the DNN's architecture and outputs, including novel interpretation of the *softmax* layer. Furthermore, our Bayesian DNN framework enables a sound definition and efficient inference of the *uncertainty* in per-voxel label probabilities. We propose a novel method to improve DNN *calibration*, while improving segmentation quality. Evaluation on 3 large datasets, qualitatively and with a variety of quantitative measures, shows that our framework outperforms the state of the art in improving segmentation quality and calibration, and providing realistic uncertainty estimates.

2   Related Work

Typical works in DNN-based image segmentation propose modifications to the DNN architecture or loss functions heuristically or without a statistical interpretation. Such approaches make it difficult to define a sound measure of uncertainty of the resulting DNN outputs. In contrast, our novel Bayesian decision theoretic framework allows a clear statistical interpretation of label probabilities and the associated uncertainties, at each voxel. Moreover, our framework (i) provides a *Bayesian interpretation* of the popular *softmax* layer in DNNs and (ii) includes DSC based optimization through the principle of Bayesian utility.

In non-DNN based segmentation methods, to estimation uncertainty, while [4] uses traditional MCMC to sample nonparametric curves, [13] uses a Gaussian-process approximation for label distributions. [18] performs uncertainty estimation in superresolution by formulating it as a patchwise regression problem and using variational dropout. Recently, [7] proposes perfect MCMC in probabilistic graphical models to estimate uncertainty, while [1] model expected segmentation per-voxel error in ensembles. On the other hand, this paper focuses on DNN frameworks for image segmentation.

A recent DNN-based method [11] provides uncertainty estimates using a sampling-based approach, but their approach primarily focuses on continuous-valued regression tasks where they assume a Gaussian probability

density function (PDF) on the DNN outputs, which can be a poor approximation for discrete labels or label-probability vectors in segmentation tasks. For
classification tasks, they append a softmax layer to the DNN and sample the
resulting outputs. However, unlike their regression framework, their classification framework (i) entails estimating twice the number of parameters in the
last layer and (ii) does *not* penalize small variances explicitly, thereby risking
DNN overfitting or miscalibration. In contrast, we rely on a generative model
that models DNN outputs as parameters that *exactly* model a multivariate PDF
on the label-probability vectors. The mean and covariance of this PDF give
us label probabilities and their uncertainty analytically, without needing any
Monte Carlo approximations at test time. Another DNN approach estimates
(epistemic) uncertainty based on dropout [5] that suffers from poor calibration,
which can be improved by parameter tuning after a continuous relaxation of
the discrete Bernoulli-distribution dropout scheme [6]. However, dropout-based
approaches focus on epistemic uncertainty (that can be reduced using larger
training sets), instead of aleatoric uncertainty (stemming from noise and artifacts in the test datum) that we retain focus on. Also, dropout-based methods
require MCMC approximation with multiple forward passes through the DNN
at *test time*, unlike our approach that infers uncertainty analytically after a single forward pass. Furthermore, unlike the theoretical frameworks in [5,6,11], our
Bayesian formulation mathematically derives the softmax layer as part of the
DNN architecture.

A simple way of calibrating a DNN regressor is temperature scaling [8]. While
the literature on DNN-based image segmentation largely ignores the issue of
miscalibration, we propose a novel scheme to improve calibration in our Bayesian
framework by introducing an additional utility function.

3   Methods

Our formulation for DNN training and inference for image segmentation (i) relies
on utility maximization in Bayesian decision theory, (ii) gives a mathematically
sound interpretation to DNN outputs to estimate uncertainty in per-voxel label
probabilities, and (iii) introduces a utility-based scheme to improve calibration.

3.1   Our Bayesian DNN Framework: Modeling and Formulation

The random field X models an *acquired intensity image* comprising V voxels.
The random field Z models an *expert-labeled discrete segmentation* indicating
the presence of one of K objects at each voxel. At voxel v, we represent the presence of the k-th object using a K-length vector Z_v having its k-th component
Z_{vk} as 1 and all other components as 0. Any single expert-rated segmentation
Z is typically imperfect because of intra-rater and inter-rater variability stemming from imaging artifacts and human errors in the labeling. Thus, our framework theoretically allows for multiple expert segmentations associated with each
acquired image X. The random field Y models the *true discrete segmentation*

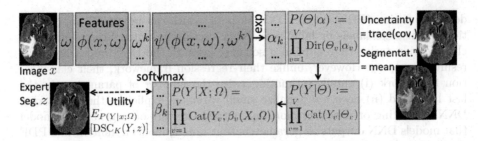

Fig. 1. Our Bayesian decision theoretic DNN framework to estimate uncertainty with segmentation. DNN components $\phi(\cdot)$ and $\psi(\cdot)$ are generic. Green boxes $\equiv$ our novel theoretical analysis to estimate per-voxel uncertainty. (Color figure online)

that is *unknown*. The joint distribution $P(X, Y; \Omega)$ models statistical dependencies between acquired images X and their true segmentations Y, where Ω is the set of real-valued DNN parameters. We formulate a novel Bayesian DNN framework that, for a given x, outputs *distributions on the label-probability images* and, in turn, the true segmentations Y. The *training set* $\{(x^n, z^n)\}_{n=1}^N$ has N image pairs (x^n, z^n), one pair for every x and each of its expert segmentations z (Fig. 1).

Learning to Maximize Bayesian Utility. For DNN training, we propose the Bayesian decision strategy of maximizing utility. For an acquired image x, its true segmentation y should be close to its expert segmentation(s) z. We measure the *utility* of an estimated segmentation y by the multi-label DSC $\mathrm{DSC}_K(y, z)$ between y and z. If the training set provides multiple expert segmentations z for a single x, then our formulation would effectively add such utilities over all available z. The multi-label DSC is $\mathrm{DSC}_K(Y, Z) := \sum_{k=1}^K \mathrm{DSC}(Y_k, Z_k)$, where Y_k and Z_k are binary label images indicating the k-th object. For gradient-based training, we use the differentiable DSC as $\mathrm{DSC}(Y_k, Z_k) := (2\sum_{v=1}^V Y_{vk}Z_{vk} + \epsilon)/(\sum_{v=1}^V Y_{vk} + \sum_{v=1}^V Z_{vk} + \epsilon)$ [15], with a fixed small $\epsilon \in \mathbb{R}_{\geq 0}$ for numerical stability; we set $\epsilon = 1$. Because our DNN output indicates a *distribution* $P(Y|x; \Omega)$ of true segmentations, we define an *expected utility* with respect to z as $E_{P(Y|x;\Omega)}[\mathrm{DSC}_K(Y, z)]$. We train the DNN by optimizing parameters Ω to maximize the *empirical expected utility* over the training set as

$$\arg\max_{\Omega} \sum_{n=1}^N E_{P(Y|x^n;\Omega)}[\mathrm{DSC}_K(Y, z^n)]. \tag{1}$$

Bayesian DNN Model, Formulation, and Architecture. We formulate a novel DNN framework that produces, at each voxel v, a *PDF on label-probability vectors* $\Theta_v \in \mathbb{R}^K$, where each component $\Theta_{vk} \in (0, 1)$ and $\sum_{k=1}^K \Theta_{vk} = 1$. This PDF indicates the *variability* in the probability-vector outputs Θ_v at each voxel v, as a function of the acquired image X and the DNN parameters Ω. A small variability indicates a lower *uncertainty* on the label probabilities.

We propose to model the PDF on Θ_v, at each voxel v, by a *Dirichlet* PDF parametrized by the positive concentration vector $\alpha_v \in \mathbb{R}^K_{>0}$. The per-voxel Dirichlet PDF is $P(\Theta_v | \alpha_v) := \prod_{k=1}^{K} (\Theta_{vk})^{\alpha_{vk}-1} / B(\alpha_v)$, where the Beta function $B(\alpha_v) := \prod_{k=1}^{K} \Gamma(\alpha_{vk}) / \Gamma(\sum_{k=1}^{K} \alpha_{vk})$ with $\Gamma(\cdot)$ as the gamma function. Subsequently, we propose the measure of uncertainty in the per-voxel label-probability vector Θ_v as the square root of the trace of the covariance matrix, which evaluates to the square root of $(\alpha_{v0}^2 - \sum_{k=1}^{K} \alpha_{vk}^2) / (\alpha_{v0}^2 (1 + \alpha_{v0}))$, where $\alpha_{v0} := \sum_{k=1}^{K} \alpha_{vk}$.

We model our DNN framework to output the values α_k as a combination of two parts in sequence. The first part is modeled by a set of real-valued parameters w, underlying the deep architecture, and represents a nonlinear transformation $\phi(X, \omega)$ that performs *feature extraction* on the acquired intensity image X. The subsequent part takes the features $\phi(x, \omega)$ and produces K images, where the k-th image is the same size as the acquired image x and is modeled by the transformation $\psi(\cdot, \omega^k)$ using real-valued parameters ω^k. Let the DNN parameters $\Omega := \{w, \{\omega^k\}_{k=1}^{K}\}$. Let $[\psi(\phi(x, \omega), \omega^k)]_v$ denote the v-th voxel in the k-th transformed image. At voxel v, we model the Dirichlet PDF $\text{Dir}(\Theta_v | \alpha_v)$ with parameters $\alpha_{vk} := \exp([\psi(\phi(x, \omega), \omega^k)]_v)$, ensuring $\alpha_{vk} > 0$. This gives

$$P(\Theta | \alpha) := \prod_{v=1}^{V} P(\Theta_v | \alpha_v) := \prod_{v=1}^{V} \text{Dir}(\Theta_v | \alpha_v) = \prod_{v=1}^{V} \frac{1}{B(\alpha_v)} \prod_{k=1}^{K} (\Theta_{vk})^{\alpha_{vk}-1}. \quad (2)$$

The PDF $P(\Theta_v | \alpha_v)$ generates label-probability vectors θ_v that, in turn, generate discrete labels y_v, at voxel v. We model $P(Y_v | \Theta_v)$ as a *categorical* distribution $\text{Cat}(Y_v | \Theta_v)$, parametrized by the probability vector Θ_v, on the one-hot vector Y_v that indicates the the true (latent) segmentation at voxel v. Thus,

$$P(Y | \Theta) := \prod_{v=1}^{V} P(Y_v | \Theta_v) := \prod_{v=1}^{V} \text{Cat}(Y_v | \Theta_v) = \prod_{v=1}^{V} \prod_{k=1}^{K} (\Theta_{vk})^{Y_{vk}}. \quad (3)$$

We have a *generative model* for the true segmentation Y starting from the acquired image X, i.e., (i) map X to α, (ii) then draw $\theta \sim P(\Theta | \alpha(X, \Omega))$, and (iii) then draw $y \sim P(Y | \theta)$. We propose to model $P(Y | X)$ by treating Θ as a *hidden random variable* and marginalizing it out. Thus, we simplify $P(Y | X) = P(Y | \alpha(X, \Omega)) = \int_\theta P(Y | \theta) P(\theta | \alpha(X, \Omega)) d\theta$. $P(\Theta | \alpha)$ factors into per-voxel Dirichlet PDFs that are *conjugate* "priors" to the categorical distribution factors in $P(Y | \Theta)$. Thus, we can model per-voxel "posterior" factors $P(Y_v | \alpha_v) =$

$$\int_{\theta_v} P(Y_v | \theta_v) P(\theta_v | \alpha_v) d\theta_v = \int_{\theta_v} \frac{\prod_{k=1}^{K} (\theta_{vk})^{\alpha_{vk}+Y_{vk}-1} d\theta_v}{B(\alpha_v)} = \frac{B(\alpha_v + Y_v)}{B(\alpha_v)}. \quad (4)$$

This makes $P(Y_v = [1, 0, \cdots, 0] | \alpha_v) = \alpha_{v1} / \sum_{k=1}^{K} \alpha_{vk}$ that equals the *softmax* value $\exp([\psi(\phi(x, \omega), \omega^1)]_v) / \sum_{k=1}^{K} \exp([\psi(\phi(x, \omega), \omega^k)]_v)$. For other one-hot vectors Y_v, similar expressions hold, which are the outputs of the softmax function applied to the DNN layer giving $[\psi(\phi(x,\omega),\omega^k)]_v$ at voxel v. Thus, we derive

$$P(Y|X;\Omega) = \prod_{v=1}^{V} P(Y_v|\alpha_v(X,\Omega)) = \prod_{v=1}^{V} \text{Cat}(Y_v;\beta_v(X,\Omega)), \quad (5)$$

where β_v is a (softmax) label-probability K-vector with $\beta_{vk} := \alpha_{vk}/\sum_{k=1}^{K}\alpha_{vk}$.

3.2   Our Bayesian DNN Training

DNN training optimizes parameters Ω to maximize empirical expected utility:

$$\max_{\Omega} \sum_{n=1}^{N} E_{P(Y|x^n;\Omega)}[\text{DSC}_K(Y,z^n)] \approx \max_{\Omega} \sum_{n=1}^{N}\sum_{s=1}^{S} \text{DSC}_K(\widetilde{y}^{ns}(x^n,\Omega),z^n), \quad (6)$$

where we evaluate the intractable expectation by Monte-Carlo integration sampling discrete segmentations $\widetilde{y}^{ns}$ drawn (easily) from $\prod_{v=1}^{V}\text{Cat}(Y_v|\beta_v(x^n,\Omega))$. To use gradient-based optimization for the DNN parameters Ω, we need an appropriate representation of the sampled segmentations $\widetilde{y}^{ns}$ involving the acquired image x^n and parameters Ω. We can sample exactly from a categorical distribution with parameters $\{\beta_{vk} \in \mathbb{R}_{>0}^{K}\}_{k=1}^{K}$ by (i) drawing $\{g_{vk}\}_{k=1}^{K}$ independently from a Gumbel PDF with location 0 and scale 1, and then (ii) taking $\arg\max_k(\log\beta_{vk} + g_{vk})$ [12]. Further, we can approximate the non-differentiable $\arg\max_k(\cdot)$ function by the softmax function to give a K-length representation of the categorical variable whose k-th component equals $\exp((\log\beta_{vk} + g_{vk})/\tau)/(\sum_{k=1}^{K}\exp((\log\beta_{vk} + g_{vk})/\tau))$, where $\tau \in \mathbb{R}_{>0}$ is a free parameter that balances the fidelity of the approximation with the ease of differentiability. The aforementioned softmax fraction equals $\exp(([\psi(\phi(x^n,\omega),\omega^k)]_v + g_{vk})/\tau)/\sum_{k=1}^{K}\exp(([\psi(\phi(x^n,\omega),\omega^k)]_v + g_{vk})/\tau)$. So, our training formulation is

$$\arg\max_{\Omega} \sum_{n=1}^{N}\sum_{s=1}^{S} \text{DSC}_K(\widetilde{y}^{ns}(x^n,\Omega),z^n), \text{ where}$$

$$\forall v,k : \widetilde{y}_{vk}^{ns} := \frac{\exp(([\psi(\phi(x^n,\omega),\omega^k)]_v + g_{vk}^{ns})/\tau)}{\sum_{k=1}^{K}\exp(([\psi(\phi(x^n,\omega),\omega^k)]_v + g_{vk}^{ns})/\tau)}; g_{vk}^{ns} \sim \text{Gum}(0,1). \quad (7)$$

We tune τ using annealing. We start training to optimize Ω with a larger τ that makes the objective function smoother. Subsequently, we decrease τ, initialize Ω with the solution obtained in the previous step, and again optimize for Ω. A few annealing iterations suffice in practice. In our experiments, we start with $\tau = 10$ and linearly decrease it to $\tau = 0.1$ during training.

Training to Improve Calibration. To make our DNN well calibrated, during optimization of the parameters Ω, we introduce another utility function focusing on the intermediate-layer DNN outputs $[\psi(\phi(x,\omega),\omega^k)]_v$, to prevent these values from having large magnitudes. Larger magnitudes of these intermediate-layer outputs typically lead to larger discrepancies between magnitudes of the

Dirichlet parameters α_{vk}, which, in turn, lead to generated probability vectors θ_{vk} that severely overestimate or underestimate class probabilities at voxel v, causing miscalibration. We propose to measure the utility of the DNN parameters/model by (i) *not* only being able to lead to high DSCs with the expert segmentations, but also (ii) being well calibrated. Thus, in addition to $\mathrm{DSC}_K(y(x, \Omega), z)$, we introduce an additional utility term on the DNN model, i.e., $\lambda \sum_{v=1}^{V} \sum_{k=1}^{K} ([\psi(\phi(x, \omega), \omega^k)]_v)^2$, to improve calibration, where the weighting factor $\lambda \in \mathbb{R}_{>0}$ is a free parameter that we tune by cross validation. A value of λ ranging from 5×10^{-4} to 5×10^{-3} were sufficient to provide good calibration results on the validation set without hampering the other scores. Section 4 shows that the augmented utility in the objective function improves calibration without reducing DSC between the predicted and expert segmentations.

3.3 Our Bayesian DNN Inference

After training our DNN model to optimize Ω, we apply the DNN on a new acquired image x^0 to estimate (i) its probabilistic segmentation and (ii) the uncertainty associated with the probabilistic segmentation. Given x^0, we compute the Dirichlet parameters $\alpha_{vk} := \exp([\psi(\phi(x^0, \omega), \omega^k)]_v)$ that model the distribution on probability vectors Θ_v as $\mathrm{Dir}(\Theta_v; \alpha_v)$. This Dirichlet distribution leads, at each voxel v, to (i) the *label-probability estimate* that is the Dirichlet PDF's mean vector, i.e., the vector whose k-th component equals $\alpha_{vk} / \sum_{k=1}^{K} \alpha_{vk}$ that is the same as the softmax output β_{vk}, and (ii) the *uncertainty estimate* that is the square-root of the trace of the covariance matrix for Dirichlet PDF on Θ_v.

4   Results and Discussion

We compare our framework with a recent DNN-based uncertainty estimation method [11] as the *baseline*. We evaluate our framework, quantitatively and qualitatively, on 3 large publicly available datasets: (i) brain tumor segmentation (BraTS 2017) in 3D magnetic resonance images (MRI) (braintumorsegmentation.org) with $K = 2$ classes (background versus whole tumor) on both high-grade and low-grade glioma subjects, (ii) organ segmentation in 2D chest radiographs (db.jsrt.or.jp/eng.php) with $K = 6$ classes, and (iii) cell membrane segmentation in 2D transmission electron microscopy images (brainiac2.mit.edu/isbi_challenge) with $K = 2$ classes. We partition the available data, i.e., images and their segmentations, as follows: (i) 55% into a training set, (ii) 10% into a validation set, to tune the DNN free parameters, and (iii) 35% into a test set. We use a spectrum of 14 quantitative measures to evaluate performance: (i) 11 to evaluate the *quality of discrete segmentations* obtained by assigning a voxel to the segment with the maximum probability, i.e., DSC (on soft segmentations), Jaccard, Hausdorff distance between predicted and expert-labeled segment boundaries, negative log likelihood (NLL), NLL-weighted (NLLw) that introduces weights to re-balance varying fractions

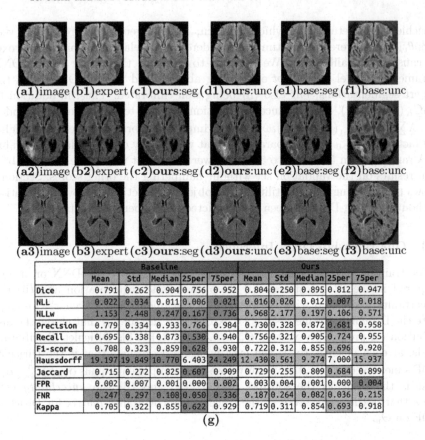

Fig. 2. Results: brain MRI tumor segmentation. (a1)–(a3) Test image. (b1)–(b3) Expert segmentation. (c1)–(c3) Our segmentation. (d1)–(d3) Our uncertainty (e1)–(e3) Baseline segmentation [11]. (f1)–(f3) Baseline uncertainty [11]. (g) Quantitative measures with mean, standard deviation (std), median, 25-th percentile (25per), 75-th percentile (75per) across test set; green entry indicates significant improvement (≥10%) over other method, red entry indicates opposite, white entry indicates both methods give perform equally well. (Color figure online)

of voxels in classes, precision, recall, F1-score (on binary segmentations), false positive rate (FPR), false negative rate (FNR), Cohen's kappa coefficient; and (ii) 3 to evaluate *calibration performance*, i.e., expected calibration error (ECE), maximum calibration error (MCE), and average calibration error (ACE) [8], which we compute as one scalar over the entire test set, to ensure sufficient sample sizes in each bin of the confidence-accuracy plot. We evaluate uncertainty estimates qualitatively. We choose the same DNN architecture for modeling $\psi(\cdot)$ and $\phi(\cdot)$ for both methods. Both methods use the Adam optimizer with learning rate 10^{-3}, with a small batch size of 4 and instance normalization, with 2000 iterations for the chest and cell datasets and 8000 iterations for the brain dataset.

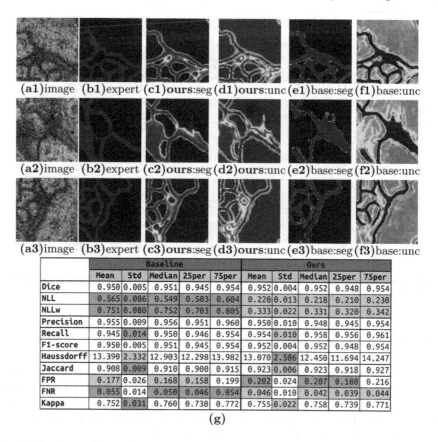

	Baseline					Ours				
	Mean	Std	Median	25per	75per	Mean	Std	Median	25per	75per
Dice	0.950	0.005	0.951	0.945	0.954	0.952	0.004	0.952	0.948	0.954
NLL	0.565	0.086	0.549	0.503	0.604	0.220	0.013	0.218	0.210	0.230
NLLw	0.751	0.080	0.752	0.703	0.805	0.333	0.022	0.331	0.320	0.342
Precision	0.955	0.009	0.956	0.951	0.960	0.950	0.010	0.948	0.945	0.954
Recall	0.945	0.014	0.950	0.946	0.954	0.954	0.010	0.958	0.956	0.961
F1-score	0.950	0.005	0.951	0.945	0.954	0.952	0.004	0.952	0.948	0.954
Haussdorff	13.390	2.332	12.903	12.298	13.982	13.070	2.586	12.450	11.694	14.247
Jaccard	0.908	0.009	0.910	0.900	0.915	0.923	0.006	0.923	0.918	0.927
FPR	0.177	0.026	0.168	0.158	0.199	0.202	0.024	0.207	0.180	0.216
FNR	0.055	0.014	0.050	0.046	0.054	0.046	0.010	0.042	0.039	0.044
Kappa	0.752	0.031	0.760	0.738	0.772	0.755	0.022	0.758	0.739	0.771

(g)

Fig. 3. Results: cell membrane microscopy segmentation. (a)–(g) Analogous to the descriptions in Fig. 2(a)–(g). Images are zoomed-into regions.

Brain MRI Tumor Segmentation. We use the Wnet architecture for $\psi(\cdot)$ and $\phi(\cdot)$, training on a 3D block of 19 axial slices as in [19]. The results (Fig. 2) show that our method, with its principled Bayesian design producing analytical estimates of uncertainty and a novel utility improving calibration, outperforms the baseline in estimating *not* only uncertainty, but also segmentations. The baseline, overall, significantly overestimates the uncertainty, and incorrectly/undesirably indicate high uncertainty in regions far from the tumor (Fig. 2(f1)–(f3)), whereas our method correctly exhibits uncertainty (i) near object boundaries and (ii) ambiguous regions (Fig. 2(d2)) where the expert segmentation (Fig. 2(b2)) seems to mismatch with the image data (Fig. 2(a2)) in the region that likely exhibits partial voluming of cerebrospinal fluid and tumor. The baseline also misses big parts of some tumors (Fig. 2(e1)–(e3)). Our method clearly improves segmentation quality, over the baseline, quantitatively (Fig. 2(g)). Improved uncertainty estimates of our method are closely related to significantly improved quantitative calibration measures (Fig. 6).

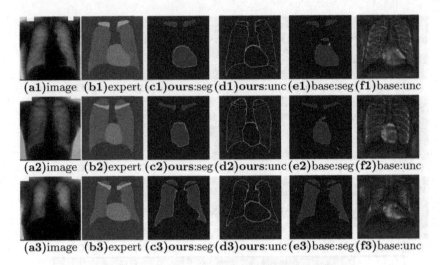

(a1)image (b1)expert (c1)ours:seg (d1)ours:unc (e1)base:seg (f1)base:unc

(a1)image (b1)expert (c1)ours:seg (d1)ours:unc (e1)base:seg (f1)base:unc

(a2)image (b2)expert (c2)ours:seg (d2)ours:unc (e2)base:seg (f2)base:unc

(a3)image (b3)expert (c3)ours:seg (d3)ours:unc (e3)base:seg (f3)base:unc

Fig. 4. Results: chest radiographs organ segmentation. (a)–(f) Analogous to the descriptions in Fig. 2(a)–(f).

Cell Membrane Microscopy Segmentation. We use Unet to model $\psi(\cdot)$ and $\phi(\cdot)$. Our uncertainty estimates (Fig. 3(d1)–(d3)) are far more realistic in regions where the cell membrane location is clearly ambiguous, whereas the baseline underestimates the uncertainty (Fig. 3(f1)–(f3)). Our segmentations (Fig. 3(c1)–(c3)) have fewer false positives and false negatives. Quantitatively, our method performs significantly better for many more segmentation-quality measures (Fig. 3(g)) and all calibration measures (Fig. 6).

Chest Radiographs Organ Segmentation. We use a modified Wnet for 2D images to model $\psi(\cdot)$ and $\phi(\cdot)$. Unlike our method that gives high uncertainty around organ boundaries, the baseline gives high uncertainty inside organs, e.g., inside lungs showing the rib structure. When our method makes segmentation errors (Fig. 4(c3); left lung), our uncertainty is also high in that region; however, when the baseline makes segmentation errors (Fig. 4(e1), (e2); heart), the uncertainty dangerously stays low. The baseline performs worse quantitatively on overall segmentation quality (Fig. 5) and calibration (Fig. 6).

Calibration. Our method's confidence and accuracy values have far less discrepancy (Fig. 6(a2)–(c2)), unlike the baseline. Our lower calibration errors (Fig. 6(d)) agree with our visually better uncertainty maps shown before.

Conclusion. We proposed a novel *Bayesian DNN framework* to segment images, enabling us to define a principled measure of *uncertainty*, associated with the label probabilities. We *estimate uncertainty analytically* at test time, without needing approximate or expensive algorithms. Our framework naturally derives

	Baseline					Ours				
	Mean	Std	Median	25per	75per	Mean	Std	Median	25per	75per
Dice	0.969	0.013	0.973	0.968	0.977	0.972	0.012	0.975	0.970	0.979
NLL	0.304	0.194	0.257	0.190	0.350	0.102	0.051	0.090	0.073	0.115
NLLw	0.427	0.261	0.354	0.264	0.491	0.157	0.083	0.139	0.100	0.182
Precision	0.953	0.004	0.953	0.953	0.953	0.964	0.005	0.965	0.965	0.966
Recall	0.968	0.002	0.968	0.967	0.968	0.961	0.002	0.960	0.960	0.961
F1-score	0.960	0.003	0.960	0.960	0.961	0.962	0.003	0.963	0.963	0.963
Haussdorff	42.960	31.826	31.224	17.692	63.387	27.793	23.992	19.723	16.132	27.134
Jaccard	0.940	0.024	0.948	0.937	0.955	0.946	0.022	0.951	0.942	0.958
FPR	0.007	0.001	0.007	0.007	0.008	0.006	0.001	0.005	0.005	0.006
FNR	0.032	0.002	0.032	0.032	0.033	0.039	0.002	0.040	0.039	0.040
Kappa	0.954	0.003	0.954	0.954	0.954	0.956	0.004	0.957	0.957	0.957

(g1) Lungs

	Baseline					Ours				
	Mean	Std	Median	25per	75per	Mean	Std	Median	25per	75per
Dice	0.934	0.035	0.942	0.922	0.956	0.937	0.031	0.944	0.923	0.958
NLL	0.304	0.194	0.257	0.190	0.350	0.102	0.051	0.090	0.073	0.115
NLLw	0.427	0.261	0.354	0.264	0.491	0.157	0.083	0.139	0.100	0.182
Precision	0.953	0.003	0.953	0.953	0.953	0.964	0.005	0.965	0.964	0.966
Recall	0.967	0.003	0.968	0.967	0.968	0.960	0.002	0.960	0.960	0.961
F1-score	0.960	0.003	0.960	0.960	0.961	0.962	0.003	0.963	0.962	0.963
Haussdorff	42.528	57.187	21.000	14.866	38.800	27.561	32.472	19.013	13.601	27.554
Jaccard	0.879	0.058	0.890	0.855	0.916	0.883	0.053	0.894	0.857	0.920
FPR	0.007	0.001	0.007	0.007	0.008	0.006	0.001	0.005	0.005	0.006
FNR	0.033	0.003	0.032	0.032	0.033	0.040	0.002	0.040	0.039	0.040
Kappa	0.954	0.004	0.954	0.954	0.954	0.956	0.004	0.957	0.957	0.957

(g2) Heart

	Baseline					Ours				
	Mean	Std	Median	25per	75per	Mean	Std	Median	25per	75per
Dice	0.923	0.031	0.930	0.912	0.942	0.926	0.027	0.933	0.916	0.944
NLL	0.304	0.194	0.257	0.190	0.350	0.102	0.051	0.090	0.073	0.115
NLLw	0.427	0.261	0.354	0.264	0.491	0.157	0.083	0.139	0.100	0.182
Precision	0.953	0.003	0.953	0.953	0.953	0.964	0.005	0.965	0.964	0.965
Recall	0.967	0.003	0.968	0.967	0.968	0.960	0.002	0.960	0.960	0.961
F1-score	0.960	0.003	0.960	0.960	0.961	0.962	0.003	0.963	0.962	0.963
Haussdorff	34.342	69.007	10.535	7.616	16.093	13.924	28.267	8.062	6.325	10.735
Jaccard	0.858	0.051	0.869	0.839	0.890	0.864	0.045	0.874	0.845	0.894
FPR	0.007	0.000	0.007	0.007	0.007	0.006	0.001	0.005	0.005	0.006
FNR	0.033	0.003	0.032	0.032	0.033	0.040	0.002	0.040	0.039	0.040
Kappa	0.954	0.003	0.954	0.954	0.954	0.956	0.004	0.957	0.957	0.957

(g3) Clavicles

Fig. 5. Results: chest radiographs segmentation. (g1)–(g3) Analogous to the descriptions in Fig. 2(g), for the lung, heart, and clavicles, respectively.

the need for a *softmax* layer. We propose a novel method to improve *calibration* of the segmentation. Results show that our framework improves segmentation quality and calibration, and provides more realistic uncertainty estimates.

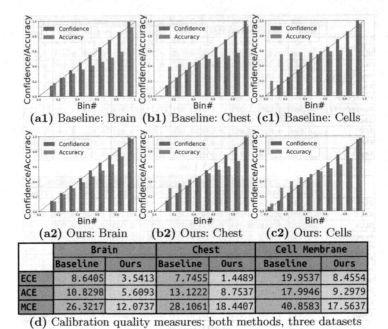

(a1) Baseline: Brain (b1) Baseline: Chest (c1) Baseline: Cells

(a2) Ours: Brain (b2) Ours: Chest (c2) Ours: Cells

	Brain		Chest		Cell Membrane	
	Baseline	Ours	Baseline	Ours	Baseline	Ours
ECE	8.6405	3.5413	7.7455	1.4489	19.9537	8.4554
ACE	10.8298	5.6093	13.1222	8.7537	17.9946	9.2979
MCE	26.3217	12.0737	28.1061	18.4407	40.8583	17.5637

(d) Calibration quality measures: both methods, three datasets

Fig. 6. Results: calibration performance. Confidence-accuracy plots for baseline and our methods, respectively, for (a1)–(a2) brain, (b1)–(b2) chest, and (c1)–(c2) cell datasets. (d) Calibration quality measures.

References

1. Awate, S.P., Whitaker, R.: Multiatlas segmentation as nonparametric regression. IEEE Trans. Med. Imag. **33**(9), 1803–1817 (2014)
2. Brosch, T., Yoo, Y., Tang, L.Y.W., Li, D.K.B., Traboulsee, A., Tam, R.: Deep convolutional encoder networks for multiple sclerosis lesion segmentation. In: Navab, N., Hornegger, J., Wells, W.M., Frangi, A.F. (eds.) MICCAI 2015. LNCS, vol. 9351, pp. 3–11. Springer, Cham (2015). https://doi.org/10.1007/978-3-319-24574-4_1
3. Drozdzal, M., Vorontsov, E., Chartrand, G., Kadoury, S., Pal, C.: The importance of skip connections in biomedical image segmentation. In: Carneiro, G., et al. (eds.) LABELS/DLMIA -2016. LNCS, vol. 10008, pp. 179–187. Springer, Cham (2016). https://doi.org/10.1007/978-3-319-46976-8_19
4. Fan, A.C., Fisher, J.W., Wells, W.M., Levitt, J.J., Willsky, A.S.: MCMC curve sampling for image segmentation. In: Ayache, N., Ourselin, S., Maeder, A. (eds.) MICCAI 2007. LNCS, vol. 4792, pp. 477–485. Springer, Heidelberg (2007). https://doi.org/10.1007/978-3-540-75759-7_58
5. Gal, Y., Ghahramani, Z.: Dropout as a Bayesian approximation: representing model uncertainty in deep learning. In: Advances in Neural Information Processing Systems (2016)
6. Gal, Y., Hron, J., Kendall, A.: Concrete dropout. In: Advances in Neural Information Processing Systems, pp. 3584–3593 (2017)

7. Garg, S., Awate, S.P.: Perfect MCMC sampling in Bayesian MRFs for uncertainty estimation in segmentation. In: Frangi, A.F., Schnabel, J.A., Davatzikos, C., Alberola-López, C., Fichtinger, G. (eds.) MICCAI 2018. LNCS, vol. 11070, pp. 673–681. Springer, Cham (2018). https://doi.org/10.1007/978-3-030-00928-1_76
8. Guo, C., Pleiss, G., Sun, Y., Weinberger, K.: On calibration of modern neural networks. In: International Conference on Machine Learning, pp. 1321–1330 (2017)
9. Chen, H., Qi, X., Yu, L., Heng, P.A.: DCAN: deep contour-aware networks for accurate gland segmentation. In: IEEE Computer Vision and Pattern Recognition, pp. 2487–2496 (2016)
10. Havaei, M., et al.: Brain tumor segmentation with deep neural networks. Med. Imag. Anal. **35**, 18–31 (2017)
11. Kendall, A., Gal, Y.: What uncertainties do we need in Bayesian deep learning for computer vision? In: Advances in Neural Information Processing Systems, pp. 5580–5590 (2017)
12. Kingma, D., Welling, M.: Auto-encoding variational Bayes. arXiv:1312.6114 (2013)
13. Le, M., Unkelbach, J., Ayache, N., Delingette, H.: Sampling image segmentations for uncertainty quantification. Med. Imag. Anal. **34**, 42–51 (2016)
14. Lin, T., Goyal, P., Girshick, R., He, K., Dollár, P.: Focal loss for dense object detection. In: International Conference on Computer Vision (2017)
15. Milletari, F., Navab, N., Ahmadi, S.: V-net: fully convolutional neural networks for volumetric medical image segmentation. In: International Conference on 3D Vision, pp. 565–571 (2016)
16. Ronneberger, O., Fischer, P., Brox, T.: U-net: convolutional networks for biomedical image segmentation. In: Navab, N., Hornegger, J., Wells, W.M., Frangi, A.F. (eds.) MICCAI 2015. LNCS, vol. 9351, pp. 234–241. Springer, Cham (2015). https://doi.org/10.1007/978-3-319-24574-4_28
17. Shah, M.P., Merchant, S.N., Awate, S.P.: MS-net: mixed-supervision fully-convolutional networks for full-resolution segmentation. In: Frangi, A.F., Schnabel, J.A., Davatzikos, C., Alberola-López, C., Fichtinger, G. (eds.) MICCAI 2018. LNCS, vol. 11073, pp. 379–387. Springer, Cham (2018). https://doi.org/10.1007/978-3-030-00937-3_44
18. Tanno, R., et al.: Bayesian image quality transfer with CNNs: exploring uncertainty in dMRI super-resolution. In: Descoteaux, M., Maier-Hein, L., Franz, A., Jannin, P., Collins, D.L., Duchesne, S. (eds.) MICCAI 2017. LNCS, vol. 10433, pp. 611–619. Springer, Cham (2017). https://doi.org/10.1007/978-3-319-66182-7_70
19. Wang, G., Li, W., Ourselin, S., Vercauteren, T.: Automatic brain tumor segmentation using cascaded anisotropic convolutional neural networks. In: Crimi, A., Bakas, S., Kuijf, H., Menze, B., Reyes, M. (eds.) BrainLes 2017. LNCS, vol. 10670, pp. 178–190. Springer, Cham (2018). https://doi.org/10.1007/978-3-319-75238-9_16

Explicit Topological Priors for Deep-Learning Based Image Segmentation Using Persistent Homology

James R. Clough[✉], Ilkay Oksuz, Nicholas Byrne, Julia A. Schnabel,
and Andrew P. King

School of Biomedical Engineering and Imaging Sciences, King's College London,
London, UK
james.clough@kcl.ac.uk

Abstract. We present a novel method to explicitly incorporate topological prior knowledge into deep learning based segmentation, which is, to our knowledge, the first work to do so. Our method uses the concept of persistent homology, a tool from topological data analysis, to capture high-level topological characteristics of segmentation results in a way which is differentiable with respect to the pixelwise probability of being assigned to a given class. The topological prior knowledge consists of the sequence of desired Betti numbers of the segmentation. As a proof-of-concept we demonstrate our approach by applying it to the problem of left-ventricle segmentation of cardiac MR images of subjects from the UK Biobank dataset, where we show that it improves segmentation performance in terms of topological correctness without sacrificing pixelwise accuracy.

Keywords: Segmentation · Topology · Persistent homology · Cardiac MRI · Topological data analysis

1 Introduction

Image segmentation, the task of assigning a class label to each pixel in an image, is a key problem in computer vision and medical image analysis. The most successful segmentation algorithms now use deep convolutional neural networks (CNN), with recent progress made in combining fine-grained local features with coarse-grained global features, such as in the popular U-net architecture [18]. Such methods allow information from a large spatial neighbourhood to be used

A.P. King—This work was supported by an EPSRC programme Grant (EP/P001009/1) and the Wellcome EPSRC Centre for Medical Engineering at School of Biomedical Engineering and Imaging Sciences, King's College London (WT 203148/Z/16/Z). This research has been conducted using the UK Biobank Resource under Application Number 40119. We would like to thank Nvidia for kindly donating the Quadro P6000 GPU used in this research.

A. C. S. Chung et al. (Eds.): IPMI 2019, LNCS 11492, pp. 16–28, 2019.
https://doi.org/10.1007/978-3-030-20351-1_2

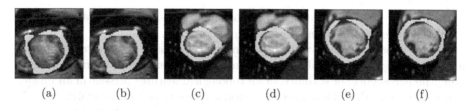

(a)　　　　(b)　　　　(c)　　　　(d)　　　　(e)　　　　(f)

Fig. 1. Three typical clinically acquired MRI images of the short-axis view of the heart. The estimated segmentations produced by a U-net model trained with $N_s = 100$ supervised cases (a, c, e) show topological errors. The segmentations for the same model trained with our topological prior (b, d, f) have the correct topology.

in classifying each pixel. However, the loss function is usually one which considers each pixel individually rather than considering higher-level structures collectively.

In many applications it is important to correctly capture the topological characteristics of the anatomy in a segmentation result. For example, detecting and counting distinct cells in electron microscopy images requires that neighbouring cells are correctly distinguished. Even very small pixelwise errors such as incorrectly labelling one pixel in a thin boundary between cells can cause two distinct cells to appear to merge. In this way significant topological errors can be caused by small pixelwise errors that have little effect on the loss function during training but may have large effects on downstream tasks. Another example is the modelling of blood flow in vessels, which requires accurate determination of vessel connectivity. In this case, small pixelwise errors can have a significant impact on the subsequent modelling task. Finally, when imaging subjects who may have congenital heart defects, the presence or absence of small holes in the walls between two chambers is diagnostically important and can be identified from images, but using current techniques it is difficult to incorporate this relevant information into a segmentation algorithm. For downstream tasks it is important that these holes are correctly segmented but they are frequently missed by current segmentation algorithms as they are insufficiently penalised during training. See Fig. 1 for examples of topologically correct and incorrect segmentations of cardiac magnetic resonance images (MRI).

There has been some recent interest in introducing topological features into the training of CNNs, and this literature is reviewed in Sect. 2 below. However, such approaches have generally involved detecting the presence or absence of topological features *implicitly* in order to quantify them in a differentiable way that can be incorporated into the training of the segmentation network. The weakness of this approach is that it is hard to know exactly which topological features are being learned. Instead, it would be desirable to explicitly specify the presence or absence of certain topological features directly in a loss function. This would enable us to designate, for example, that the segmentation result should have one connected component which has one hole in it. This is challenging due to the inherently discrete nature of topological features, making it hard to create a differentiable loss function which accounts for them.

In this paper we demonstrate that persistent homology (PH), a tool from the field of topological data analysis, can be used to address this problem by quantifying the persistence, or stability, of all topological features present in an image. Our method uses these high-level structural features to provide a pixelwise gradient that increases or decreases the persistence of desired or undesired topological features in a segmentation. These gradients can then be back-propagated through the weights of any segmentation network and combined with any other pixelwise loss function. In this way, the desired topological features of a segmentation can be used to help train a network even in the absence of a ground truth, and without the need for those features to be implicitly learned from a large amount of training data, which is not always available. This topologically driven gradient can be incorporated into supervised learning or used in a semi-supervised learning scenario, which is our focus here.

Our main contribution is the presentation of, to the best of our knowledge, the first method to explicitly incorporate topological prior information into deep-learning based segmentation. The explicit topological prior is the sequence of desired Betti numbers of the segmentations and our method provides a gradient calculated such that the network learns to produce segmentations with the correct topology. We begin by reviewing literature related to introducing topology into deep learning in Sect. 2. In Sect. 3 we cover the theory of PH and introduce the relevant notation. In Sect. 4 we then describe in detail our approach for integrating PH and deep learning for image segmentation, and then demonstrate the method in a case study on cardiac MRI in Sect. 5.

2 Related Work

The need for topologically aware methods for image processing is becoming increasingly recognised in the literature. In [13] the task of detecting curvilinear structures was addressed by supplementing a conventional U-net [18] architecture with a secondary loss function designed to capture topological features. This was calculated by passing both the ground truth and the predicted segmentations through a pre-trained VGG network [19] and comparing the feature maps at intermediate layers. These feature maps appeared to capture some topological features such as the presence of small connected components and including this loss function improved performance in the task at hand. However, it is unclear exactly which topological features were relevant, and how the presence or absence of particular structures were weighted, since they were only captured by the distributed and hard-to-interpret representation of activations in the hidden layers. Depending on the dataset on which the VGG network was trained, there may be important topological features which were ignored entirely and non-topological features may also contribute to this loss function. This loss function also still requires ground truth masks, and so cannot be used in a semi-supervised context. The work of [14] used a similar approach in that the output of a second network, in this case an autoencoder, was used to define a loss function which identified global structural features, in order to enforce anatomical constraints, but again, this can only implicitly match the desired topological features and still requires a ground truth segmentation for comparison. Other approaches have involved encouraging the correct adjacencies of various object classes, whether they were learned from the data as in [7] or provided as a prior as in [8]. Such methods allow the introduction of this simple topological feature into a loss function when performing image segmentation but cannot be easily generalised to any other kinds of higher-order feature such as the presence of holes, handles or voids.

The recent work of [4] introduced a topological regulariser for classification problems by considering the stability of connected components of the classification boundary and can be extended to higher-order topological features. It also provided a differentiable loss function which can be incorporated in the training of a neural network. This approach differs from ours in that firstly, it imposes topological constraints on the shape of the classification boundary in the feature space of inputs to the network, rather than topological constraints in the space of the pixels in the image, and secondly it aims only to reduce overall topological complexity. Our approach aims to fit the desired absence or presence of certain features and so complex features can be penalised or rewarded, as is appropriate for the task at hand.

PH has previously been applied to the problem of semantic segmentation, such as in [2,9,17], and has been used to extract topological features from data which can then used as inputs to deep neural networks [11]. The important distinction between our method and these previous works is that they apply PH to the input data to extract features, which are then used as inputs to some other algorithm for training. Such approaches can capture complex features of the input images but require those topological features to be directly extractable from the raw image data. Our approach instead processes the image with a CNN and it is the output of the CNN, representing the pixelwise likelihood of the structure we want to segment, which has PH applied to it.

3 Theory

PH is an algebraic tool developed as part of the growing mathematical field of topological data analysis, which involves computing topological features of shapes and data. We give a brief overview of PH here, but direct the reader to [5,6,15] for a more thorough background of the subject. PH most commonly considers *simplicial complexes* due to their generality but for the analysis of images and volumes consisting of pixels and voxels, *cubical complexes* are considerably more convenient and so we introduce them, and their theory of PH here.

3.1 Cubical Complexes

A cubical complex is a set consisting of points, unit line segments, and unit squares, cubes, hypercubes, and so on. Following the notation of [12] its fundamental building blocks are *elementary intervals* which are each a closed subset of the real line of the form $I = [z, z+1]$ for $z \in \mathbb{Z}$. These represent unit line segments. Points are represented by *degenerate intervals* $I = [z, z]$. From these, we can define *elementary cubes*, Q as the product of elementary intervals,

$$Q = I_1 \times I_2 \times ... \times I_d, \quad Q \subset \mathbb{R}^d. \tag{1}$$

By setting up the theory in this way, we are restricting the class of objects we can talk about to unit cubes, which will represent pixels in the images we will consider. From hereon we will describe the two-dimensional case, but our approach is generalisable.

Consider an array, S, of $N \times N$ pixels, where the pixel in row i and column j has a value $S_{[i,j]} \in [0,1]$. In terms of the cubical complex each pixel covers a unit square described by the elementary cube $Q_{i,j} = [i, i+1] \times [j, j+1]$. We then consider filtrations of this cubical complex. For each value of a threshold $p \in [0,1]$, we can find the cubical complex $B(p)$ given by

$$B(p) = \bigcup_{i,j=0}^{N-1} Q_{i,j} : S_{[i,j]} \geq (1-p). \tag{2}$$

In the context of an image, $B(p)$ represents a binarised image made by setting pixels with a value above $1-p$ to 1, and below $1-p$ to 0. By considering these sets for various values of p we obtain a the key object of PH, the sequence

$$B(0) \subseteq B(p_1) \subseteq B(p_2) \subseteq ... \subseteq B(1). \tag{3}$$

3.2   Persistent Homology

PH measures the lifetimes of topological features within a filtration such as the sequence above. The premise is that those features with long lifetimes, in terms of the filtration value p, are significant features of the data. We consider the topology of each $B(p)$ by calculating[1] its Betti numbers, β_n. These numbers are topological invariants which, informally speaking, count the number of d-dimensional holes in an object. β_0 counts the number of connected components, β_1 counts the number of loops, and, although not relevant to the 2D case we consider here, β_2 counts the number of hollow cavities, and so on. As the filtration value p increases, more pixels join the cubical complex and topological features in the binarised image are created and destroyed.

A useful way of visualising the PH of a dataset is to use a *barcode diagram*, an example of which is given in Fig. 2. This diagram plots the lifespans of all topological features in the data, where each feature is represented by one bar, and with different colour bars representing different Betti numbers. The Betti numbers of $B(p^*)$ are given by the number of bars present at the x-coordinate $x = p^*$. A key feature of the barcode diagram is that it is stable in the presence

---

[1] We avoid the details of how the Betti numbers are computed here. In our experiments we used the implementation from the Python library Gudhi [1].

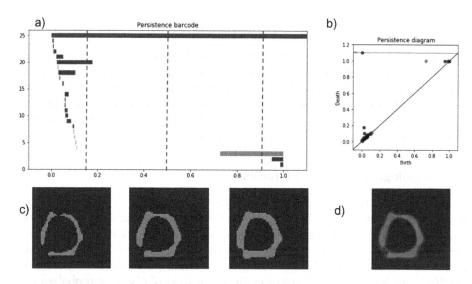

Fig. 2. The barcode diagram for the predicted mask shown in (d). As the filtration value is increased, moving left to right on the barcode diagram (a), more pixels join the cubical complex, and topological features are created and destroyed. 0-dimensional features (i.e. connected components) are shown by red bars, and 1-dimensional features (i.e. closed cycles) by green bars. The pixels in the cubical complex for three filtration values (corresponding to the vertical dashed lines on the barcode diagram) are shown here in (c). In the first complex, there are two connected components, corresponding to the two red bars crossing the first dashed line. In the second, there is only one connected component (and so one red bar). In the third, one connected component and one closed cycle (and so one red, and one green bar) are present. The persistence diagram showing the lifespans of these topological features is shown in (b). (Color figure online)

of noise, and there are theoretical guarantees that small changes to the original data can only make small changes to the positions and lengths of the bars [10]. For an array of input data S, we will describe its PH by denoting each bar in the barcode diagram as $H_d^\ell(S) = (p_{\text{birth}}, p_{\text{death}})$ which is an ordered pair of the birth and death filtration values of the ℓth longest bar of dimension d, where $\ell \geq 1$ and $d \geq 0$.

Our method will use these barcode diagrams as a description of the topological features in a predicted segmentation mask. In the case we consider below, we begin with the prior knowledge that the object being segmented should contain one hole (i.e. $\beta_1 = 1$) and so aim to extend the length of the bar corresponding to the most persistent 1-dimensional feature. It is important to note both that our method can be applied generally to encourage the presence or absence of topological features of any number or dimension, but also that this prior information must be specified for the task at hand.

4   Method

Throughout this paper we consider only the problem of binary segmentation, that is, assigning a value between 0 and 1 to each pixel in an image which represents the probability of it being classified as part of a particular structure. Our approach does generalise to multi-class segmentation (inasmuch as it can be described as several binary segmentation problems) but, for convenience and simplicity, we will discuss only the binary case here.

4.1   Topological Pixelwise Gradient

In our approach the desired topology of the segmentation mask needs to be specified in the form of its Betti numbers. For ease of explanation we consider the case in which $\beta_1 = 1$ is specified, corresponding to the prior knowledge that the segmentation mask should contain exactly one closed cycle. Given a neural network f which performs binary segmentation and is parameterised by a set of weights ω, an $N \times N$ image X produces an $N \times N$ array of pixelwise probabilities, $S = f(X; \omega)$. In the supervised learning setting, a pixelwise gradient is calculated by, for example, calculating the binary cross-entropy or Dice loss between S and some ground-truth labels Y.

We additionally calculate a pixelwise gradient for a topological loss as follows. Firstly the PH of S is calculated, producing a set of lifetimes of topological features H_d^ℓ, such as that shown in Fig. 2a. For each desired feature, the longest bars (and so the most persistent features) of the corresponding dimension are identified. In our case the presence of a closed cycle corresponds to the longest green bar in the barcode diagram, denoted by $H_1^1(S)$. In order to make this feature more persistent we need to identify the pixels which, if assigned a higher/lower probability of appearing in the segmentation, will extend the length of this bar in the barcode diagram, and therefore increase the persistence of that topological feature. These pixels are identified by an iterative process which begins at the pixels with the filtration values at precisely the ends of the relevant bar, which are $H_1^1(S) = (p_{\text{birth}}^*, p_{\text{death}}^*)$ for the left and right ends of the bar respectively. For each of k iterations, where k is an integer parameter which can be freely chosen, the pixels with these extremal filtration values are filled in (with a 1 and 0 respectively), extending the bar in the barcode, and these pixels have a gradient of ∓1 applied to them. The PH is recomputed, and another pixel chosen for each end of the bar. These pixels are also filled in, and more chosen, and so on, until k pixels have been identified for each end of the bar. These are now the $2k$ pixels which, if their filtration values are adjusted, will result in the most significant change in the persistence of the relevant topological object, and it is these $2k$ pixels which will have a gradient applied to them. Algorithm 1 shows pseudo-code for the $\beta_1 = 1$ example[2].

---

[2] Our implementation will be made publicly available upon publication.

Algorithm 1. Topological loss gradient $\beta_1 = 1$

Input

S: Array of real numbers - pixelwise segmentation probabilities

k: Integer - number of pixels to apply gradient to

ϵ: Real number > 0 - threshold to avoid modifying already persistent features

Output

G: Array of real numbers - pixelwise gradients

1: **procedure** TOPOGRAD(S, k, ϵ)
2:      $t \leftarrow 0$
3:      G is initialised as an $N \times N$ array of 0
4:      **while** $t < k$ **do**
5:          $H_d^\ell(S) \leftarrow$ PersistentHomology(S) $\triangleright$ Calculate Barcode Diagram of S
6:          $(p_{\text{birth}}^*, p_{\text{death}}^*) \leftarrow H_1^1(S)$ $\triangleright$ Longest bar for 1-dimensional features
7:          **for** pixel [i,j] in array S **do**
8:             **if** $p_{\text{birth}}^* > \epsilon$ **then** $\triangleright$ Skip if bar already begins close to $p = 0$
9:               **if** $S_{[i,j]} = 1 - p_{\text{birth}}^*$ **then**
10:                 $S_{[i,j]} \leftarrow 1$ $\triangleright$ Set the pixel with value $1 - p_{\text{birth}}^*$ to 1
11:                 $G_{[i,j]} \leftarrow -1$ $\triangleright$ Set its gradient to -1
12:             **if** $p_{\text{death}}^* < (1 - \epsilon)$ **then** $\triangleright$ Skip if bar already ends close to $p = 1$
13:               **if** $S_{[i,j]} = 1 - p_{\text{death}}^*$ **then**
14:                 $S_{[i,j]} \leftarrow 0$ $\triangleright$ Set the pixel with value $1 - p_{\text{death}}^*$ to 0
15:                 $G_{[i,j]} \leftarrow +1$ $\triangleright$ Set its gradient to $+1$
16:          $t \leftarrow t + 1$
17:      **return** G $\triangleright$ Return the pixelwise gradient array

---

4.2 Semi-supervised Learning

We incorporate the topological prior into a semi-supervised learning scheme as follows. In each training batch, firstly the binary cross-entropy loss from the N_ℓ labelled cases is calculated. Next the pixelwise gradients, G, for the N_u unlabelled cases are calculated as in Algorithm 1 and multiplied by a positive constant λ, which weights this term. The gradient from the cross-entropy loss and the topological gradient are then summed. In our experiments we set $k = 5$, $\epsilon = 0.01$ (chosen by manual tuning rather than optimisation over a separate validation set), and experiment with a choice of λ. Note that the method in general does not need to be applied in this semi-supervised context, and can also be applied to labelled cases. We avoid doing so here to make clearer that this topologically derived gradient is useful even in the absence of a label.

5 Experiments and Results

We demonstrate our approach on real data with the task of myocardial segmentation of cardiac MRI. We use a subset of the UK Biobank dataset [16,20], which consists of the mid-slice of the short-axis view of the heart. Example images and segmentations from this dataset are shown in Fig. 3. We use one end-systole image from each of 1500 subjects, each of which has a gold-standard left-ventricle segmentation provided. The images were cropped to a 64x64 square centred around the left ventricle. Since the UK Biobank dataset contains high-quality images compared to a typical clinical acquisition we made the task more challenging, degrading the images by removing k-space lines in order to lower image quality and create artefacts. For each image in the dataset we compute the Fourier transform, and k-space lines outside of a central band of 8 lines are removed with 3/4 probability and zero-filled. The degraded image is then reconstructed by performing the inverse Fourier transform, and it is these images which are used for both training and testing. Examples of original and degraded images are shown in Fig. 3. In the semi-supervised setting each experiment has a small number of labelled cases, N_ℓ, and $N_u = 400$ unlabelled cases are used. As a baseline we evaluated a fully supervised method using just the labelled cases, and also post-processed the supervised results using image processing tools commonly used to correct small topological errors. We used the binary closure morphology operator with a circular structuring element with a radius of 3 pixels. Additionally, we compared our method to an iterative semi-supervised approach similar to [3]. In this method the predicted segmentations from unlabelled cases were used as labels for training such that the network's weights and the predicted segmentations of unlabelled cases are iteratively improved. In our experiments, as in [3] we use 3 iterations of 100 epochs after the initial supervised training.

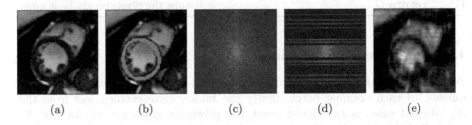

(a)   (b)   (c)   (d)   (e)

Fig. 3. An example image (a) and segmentation (b) from the UK Biobank dataset. We degrade images by transforming them to k-space (c) and randomly removing non-central k-space lines (d), making the task of myocardial segmentation more challenging by causing blurring and aliasing artefacts (e).

Each of these methods was evaluated with the same network architecture. We used a simple U-net-like network [18] but with 3 levels of spatial resolution (with 16, 32, and 64 feature maps in each, and spatial downsampling by a factor of 2) and with 3 3×3 convolution plus ReLU operations before each upsampling or downsampling step, with the final layer having an additional 1×1 convolution followed by a sigmoidal activation. This results in 16 convolutional layers in total. All models were trained using the Adam optimiser with a learning rate of 10^{-4} and the supervised part of the model was trained with the Dice loss. The trained networks were then evaluated against a held-out test set of $N_\text{test} = 500$ cases. To evaluate our approach we measured the Dice score of the predicted segmentations, as a quantifier of their pixelwise accuracy, and the proportion of segmentations with the correct topology when thresholded at $p = 0.5$.

Table 1 shows the mean results over the test cases averaged over 20 experiments. For each experiment images were randomly allocated to the labelled and unlabelled training sets, and the test set, from a dataset of 1500 images in total (each from a different subject). The image degradation was also randomised for each experiment. Our method provides a significant reduction in the proportion of incorrect topologies of the segmentations compared to the baseline supervised learning scenario. Notably, this can occur without significantly sacrificing the pixelwise metrics of segmentation quality demonstrating that an increase in topological accuracy does not need to come at a cost to pixelwise accuracy. In Fig. 1 we show a typical clinically acquired short-axis image and its estimated segmentations with and without our method. This image has not been artificially degraded as in our experiment above and is shown to illustrate that clinically acquired scans are often of a low quality compared to the UK Biobank dataset on which we demonstrate our method, and so are challenging to segment. Qualitatively observing these cases we see that a topological prior is beneficial in this realistic scenario.

Table 1. Comparison of supervised learning (SL), supervised learning with binary closure (SL + BC), the semi-supervised approach of [3] (SSL) and our semi-supervised learning (Ours) with a topological prior, averaged over the 20 training/testing runs. Bolded results are those which are statistically significantly better than all three benchmark methods. Starred results are statistically significantly worse than at least one benchmark method. Significance was determined by $p < 0.01$ when tested with a paired t-test.

N_ℓ	Dice score					Percentage of correct topologies				
	20	40	100	200	400	20	40	100	200	400
SL	0.739	0.762	0.802	0.824	0.842	69.1%	78.1%	89.0%	92.8%	96.2%
SL + BC	0.739	0.762	0.802	0.823	0.841	70.2%	78.9%	89.3%	92.8%	95.6%
SSL	0.740	0.763	0.801	0.826	0.842	71.4%	79.2%	89.7%	93.6%	95.4%
Ours $\lambda = 1$	0.742	0.762	0.803	0.825	0.843	**77.4%**	**84.4%**	**91.8%**	**94.0%**	**96.4%**
Ours $\lambda = 3$	0.730*	0.749*	0.792	0.824	0.844	**82.9%**	**89.8%**	**95.5%**	**94.9%**	**96.7%**

6   Discussion

Although we have only demonstrated our approach for the segmentation of 2D images here, in the often challenging task of 3D segmentation, the ability to impose a topological loss function could be of significant use as the number of connected components, handles, and cavities may be specified. Our future work will investigate this generalisation and its utility in challenging tasks such as the 3D segmentation of cardiac MRI volumes of subjects with congenital conditions causing atypical connections between chambers of the heart. We will also investigate extending our approach to incorporate first learning the topology of a structure from the image, and then incorporating that knowledge into the segmentation, which would allow our approach to be applicable to cases such as cell segmentation where the number of components in the desired segmentation is not known *a priori* but can be deduced from the image.

In our experiments we found that setting $\lambda = 1$ meant that our method had no significant difference in Dice score to the other methods but an improved topological accuracy. As seen in Table 1 a higher λ results in even better performance according to the segmentation topology, but pixelwise accuracy begins to drop. We found that changing λ allows one to trade off the pixelwise and topological accuracies and in future work we will also investigate the extent to which this trade-off can be managed so as to learn the optimal value of λ for a given objective.

The dominant computational cost in our method is the repeated PH calculation which occurs k times when calculating the pixelwise gradients for each image. Computing the PH for a cubical complex containing V pixels/voxels in d dimensions can be achieved in $\Theta(3^d V + d2^d V)$ time, and $\Theta(d2^d V)$ memory (see [21]) and so scales linearly with respect to the number of pixels/voxels in an image. We found that, using 64×64 pixel 2D images, the PH for one image was calculated in approximately 0.01 s on a desktop PC. Consequently, when using $k = 5$ and a batch of 100 images for semi-supervised learning, one batch took about 5 s to process. On large 3D volumes this cost could become prohibitive. However, the implementation of PH that we use is not optimised for our task and our algorithm allows for parallel computation of the PH of each predicted segmentation in the batch of semi-supervised images. With a GPU implementation for calculating the PH of a cubical complex, many parallel calculations could allow for significant improvements in overall run-time. Finally we acknowledge that our approach of directly calculating a modification to the gradient updating the network's weights is harder to interpret or be sure of convergence than approaches which explicitly minimise a loss function. In future work we hope to develop a loss-minimising framework for our method, and compare with a wider range of approaches, especially those with hard topological constraints.

7   Conclusions

We have presented the first work to incorporate explicit topological priors into deep-learning based image segmentation, and demonstrated our approach in the 2D case using cardiac MRI data. We found that including prior information about the segmentation topology in a semi-supervised setting improved performance in terms of topological correctness on a challenging segmentation task with small amounts of labelled data.

References

1. GUDHI User and Reference Manual (2015). http://gudhi.gforge.inria.fr
2. Assaf, R., Goupil, A., Vrabie, V., Kacim, M.: Homology functionality for grayscale image segmentation. J. Inf. Math. Sci. **8**(4), 281–286 (2016)
3. Bai, W., et al.: Semi-supervised Learning for network-based cardiac MR image segmentation. In: Descoteaux, M., Maier-Hein, L., Franz, A., Jannin, P., Collins, D.L., Duchesne, S. (eds.) MICCAI 2017. LNCS, vol. 10434, pp. 253–260. Springer, Cham (2017). https://doi.org/10.1007/978-3-319-66185-8_29
4. Chen, C., Ni, X., Bai, Q., Wang, Y.: TopoReg: a topological regularizer for classifiers. arXiv 1806.10714 (2018)
5. Edelsbrunner, H., Harer, J.: Persistent homology-a survey. Contemp. Math. **453**, 257–282 (2008)
6. Edelsbrunner, H., Letscher, D., Zomorodian, A.: Topological persistence and simplification. In: Foundations of Computer Science, pp. 454–463. IEEE (2000)
7. Funke, J., Hamprecht, F.A., Zhang, C.: Learning to segment: training hierarchical segmentation under a topological loss. In: Navab, N., Hornegger, J., Wells, W.M., Frangi, A.F. (eds.) MICCAI 2015. LNCS, vol. 9351, pp. 268–275. Springer, Cham (2015). https://doi.org/10.1007/978-3-319-24574-4_32
8. Ganaye, P.-A., Sdika, M., Benoit-Cattin, H.: Semi-supervised learning for segmentation under semantic constraint. In: Frangi, A.F., Schnabel, J.A., Davatzikos, C., Alberola-López, C., Fichtinger, G. (eds.) MICCAI 2018. LNCS, vol. 11072, pp. 595–602. Springer, Cham (2018). https://doi.org/10.1007/978-3-030-00931-1_68
9. Gao, M., Chen, C., Zhang, S., Qian, Z., Metaxas, D., Axel, L.: Segmenting the papillary muscles and the trabeculae from high resolution cardiac CT through restoration of topological handles. In: Gee, J.C., Joshi, S., Pohl, K.M., Wells, W.M., Zöllei, L. (eds.) IPMI 2013. LNCS, vol. 7917, pp. 184–195. Springer, Heidelberg (2013). https://doi.org/10.1007/978-3-642-38868-2_16
10. Ghrist, R.: Barcodes: the persistent topology of data. Bull. Am. Math. Soc. **45**(1), 61–75 (2008)
11. Hofer, C., Kwitt, R., Niethammer, M., Uhl, A.: Deep learning with topological signatures. In: Advances in Neural Information Processing Systems, pp. 1634–1644 (2017)
12. Kaczynski, T., Mischaikow, K., Mrozek, M.: Computational Homology, vol. 157. Springer, Heidelberg (2006)
13. Mosinska, A., Marquez-Neila, P., Kozinski, M., Fua, P.: Beyond the pixel-wise loss for topology-aware delineation. In: CVPR (2018)
14. Oktay, O., et al.: Anatomically constrained neural networks (ACNNs). IEEE Trans. Med. Imag. **37**(2), 384–395 (2018)
15. Otter, N., Porter, M.A., Tillmann, U., Grindrod, P., Harrington, H.A.: A roadmap for the computation of persistent homology. EPJ Data Sci. **6**(1), 17 (2017)
16. Petersen, S.E., et al.: UK biobank's cardiovascular magnetic resonance protocol. J. Cardiovasc. Magn. Resonan. **18**(1), 8 (2015)
17. Qaiser, T., Sirinukunwattana, K., Nakane, K., Tsang, Y.W., Epstein, D., Rajpoot, N.: Persistent homology for fast tumor segmentation in whole slide histology images. Proc. Comput. Sci. **90**, 119–124 (2016)
18. Ronneberger, O., Fischer, P., Brox, T.: U-net: convolutional networks for biomedical image segmentation. In: Navab, N., Hornegger, J., Wells, W.M., Frangi, A.F. (eds.) MICCAI 2015. LNCS, vol. 9351, pp. 234–241. Springer, Cham (2015). https://doi.org/10.1007/978-3-319-24574-4_28

19. Simonyan, K., Zisserman, A.: Very deep convolutional networks for large-scale image recognition. arXiv preprint arXiv:1409.1556 (2014)
20. Sudlow, C., et al.: UK biobank: an open access resource for identifying the causes of a wide range of complex diseases of middle and old age. PLoS Med. **12**(3), e1001779 (2015)
21. Wagner, H., Chen, C., Vuçini, E.: Efficient computation of persistent homology for cubical data. In: Peikert, R., Hauser, H., Carr, H., Fuchs, R. (eds.) Topological Methods in Data Analysis and Visualization II, pp. 91–106. Springer, Heidelberg (2012). https://doi.org/10.1007/978-3-642-23175-9_7

Semi-supervised and Task-Driven Data Augmentation

Krishna Chaitanya[1]([✉]), Neerav Karani[1], Christian F. Baumgartner[1], Anton Becker[2], Olivio Donati[2], and Ender Konukoglu[1]

[1] Computer Vision Lab, ETH Zurich, Zürich, Switzerland
krishna.chaitanya@vision.ee.ethz.ch
[2] University Hospital of Zurich, Zurich, Switzerland

Abstract. Supervised deep learning methods for segmentation require large amounts of labelled training data, without which they are prone to overfitting, not generalizing well to unseen images. In practice, obtaining a large number of annotations from clinical experts is expensive and time-consuming. One way to address scarcity of annotated examples is data augmentation using random spatial and intensity transformations. Recently, it has been proposed to use generative models to synthesize realistic training examples, complementing the random augmentation. So far, these methods have yielded limited gains over the random augmentation. However, there is potential to improve the approach by (i) explicitly modeling deformation fields (non-affine spatial transformation) and intensity transformations and (ii) leveraging unlabelled data during the generative process. With this motivation, we propose a novel task-driven data augmentation method where to synthesize new training examples, a generative network explicitly models and applies deformation fields and additive intensity masks on existing labelled data, modeling shape and intensity variations, respectively. Crucially, the generative model is optimized to be conducive to the task, in this case segmentation, and constrained to match the distribution of images observed from labelled and unlabelled samples. Furthermore, explicit modeling of deformation fields allows synthesizing segmentation masks and images in exact correspondence by simply applying the generated transformation to an input image and the corresponding annotation. Our experiments on cardiac magnetic resonance images (MRI) showed that, for the task of segmentation in small training data scenarios, the proposed method substantially outperforms conventional augmentation techniques.

1 Introduction

Precise segmentation of anatomical structures is crucial for several clinical applications. Recent advances in deep neural networks yielded automatic segmentation algorithms with unprecedented accuracy. However, such methods heavily rely on large annotated training datasets. In this work, we consider the problem of medical image segmentation in the setting of small training datasets.

© Springer Nature Switzerland AG 2019
A. C. S. Chung et al. (Eds.): IPMI 2019, LNCS 11492, pp. 29–41, 2019.
https://doi.org/10.1007/978-3-030-20351-1_3

Let us first consider the question: *why is a large training dataset necessary for the success of deep learning methods?* One hypothesis is that a large training dataset exposes a neural network to sufficient variations in factors, such as shape, intensity and texture, thereby allowing it to learn a robust image to segmentation mask mapping. In medical images, such variations may arise from subject specific shape differences in anatomy or lesions. Image intensity and contrast characteristics may differ substantially according to the image acquisition protocol or even between scanners for the same acquisition protocol. When the training dataset is small, deep learning methods are susceptible to faring poorly on unseen test images either due to not identifying such variations or because the test images appear to have been drawn from a distribution different to the training images.

We conjecture that one way to train a segmentation network on a small training dataset more robustly could be to incorporate into the training dataset, intensity and anatomical shape variations observed from a large pool of unlabelled images. Specifically, we propose to generate synthetic image-label pairs by learning generative models of deformation fields and intensity transformations that map the available labelled training images to the distribution of the entire pool of available images, including labelled as well as unlabelled. Additionally, we explicitly encourage the synthesized image-label pairs to be conducive to the task at hand. We carried out extensive evaluation of the proposed method, in which the method showed substantial improvements over existing data augmentation as well as semi-supervised learning techniques for segmentation of cardiac MRIs.

Related Work: Due to the high cost of obtaining large amount of expert annotations, robust training of machine learning methods in the small training dataset setting has been widely studied in the literature. Focusing on the methods that are most relevant to the proposed method, we broadly classify the related works into two categories:

Data augmentation is a technique wherein the training dataset is enlarged with artificially synthesized image-label pairs. The main idea is to transform training images in such a way that the corresponding labels are either unchanged or get transformed in the same way. Some commonly used data augmentation methods are affine transformations [6] (such as translation, rotation, scaling, flipping, cropping, etc.) and random elastic deformations [15,17]. Leveraging recent advances in generative image modelling [9], several works proposed to map randomly sampled vectors from a simple distribution to realistic image-label pairs as augmented data for medical image segmentation problems [4,7,16]. Such methods are typically trained on already labelled data, with the objective of interpolating within the training dataset. In an alternative direction, [19] proposed to synthesize data for augmentation by simply linearly interpolating the available images and the corresponding labels. Surprisingly, despite employing clearly unrealistic images, this method led to substantial improvements in medical image segmentation [8] when the available training dataset is very small. None of these data augmentation methods use unlabelled images that may be more readily available and all of them, except for those based on generative models, are hand-crafted rather than optimized based on data.

Semi-supervised learning (SSL) methods are another class of techniques that are suitable in the setting of learning with small labelled training datasets. The main idea of these methods is to regularize the learning process by employing unlabelled images. Approaches based on self-training [2] alternately train a network with labelled images, estimate labels for the unlabelled images using the network and update the network with both the available true image-label pairs and the estimated labels for the unlabelled images. [20] propose a SSL method based on adversarial learning, where the joint distribution of unlabelled image-estimated labels pairs is matched to that of the true labelled images-label pairs. Interestingly, [13] show that many SSL methods fail to provide substantial gains over the supervised baseline that is trained with data augmentation and regularization.

Weakly-supervised learning tackles the issue of expensive pixel-wise annotations by training on weaker labels, such as scribbles [5] and image-wide labels [1]. Finally, other regularization methods that do not necessarily leverage unlabelled images may also aid in preventing over-fitting to small training datasets.

2   Methods

In a supervised learning setup, an objective function $L_S(\{X_L, Y_L\})$ that measures discrepancy between ground truth labels, Y_L, and predictions of a network S on training images, X_L, is minimized with respect to a set of learnable parameters w_S of the network, i.e.

$$\min_{w_S} \Big(L_S(\{X_L, Y_L\}) \Big) \tag{1}$$

When data augmentation is employed in the supervised learning setup, Eq. 2 is minimized with respect to w_S.

$$\min_{w_S} \Big(L_S(\{X_L, Y_L\} \cup \{X_G, Y_G\}) \Big) \tag{2}$$

Here, X_G and Y_G refer to generated images and labels obtained by affine or elastic transformations of X_L, Y_L or by using methods such as Mixup [19]. The set $\{\{X_L, Y_L\} \cup \{X_G, Y_G\}\}$ is referred to as the augmented training set. In augmentation methods based on generative models [4], the parameters of S are still optimized according to Eq. 2, but the generative process for X_G and Y_G involves two other networks: a generator G and a discriminator D. The corresponding parameters w_G and w_D are estimated according to the generative adversarial learning (GAN) [9] framework by optimizing:

$$\min_{w_G} \max_{w_D} \mathbb{E}_{x,y \sim p(x_L, y_L)}[\log D(x, y)] + \mathbb{E}_{z \sim p_z(z)}[\log(1 - D(G(z)))] \tag{3}$$

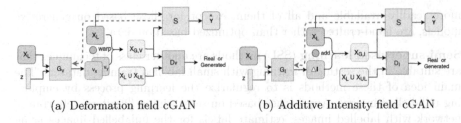

(a) Deformation field cGAN   (b) Additive Intensity field cGAN

Fig. 1. Modules for task-driven and semi-supervised data augmentation.

G takes as input a vector z sampled from a known distribution $p_z(z)$ and maps that to a $\{X_G, Y_G\}$ pair. D is optimized to distinguish between outputs of G and real $\{X_L, Y_L\}$ pairs, while G is optimized to generate $\{X_G, Y_G\}$ pairs such that D responds to them similarly as to $\{X_L, Y_L\}$. Thus, $\{X_G, Y_G\}$ are encouraged to be "realistic" in the sense that they cannot be distinguished by D.

2.1 Semi-supervised and Task-Driven Data Augmentation

Instead of solving the optimization given in Eq. 3 for generating the augmentation image-label pairs $\{X_G, Y_G\}$, we propose solving Eq. 4:

$$\min_{w_G} \left(\min_{w_S} L_S(\{X_L, Y_L\} \cup \{X_G, Y_G\}) + L_{reg, w_G}(\{X_L\} \cup \{X_{UL}\}) \right) \quad (4)$$

This incorporates two ideas. The first term dictates that $\{X_G, Y_G\}$ be such that they are beneficial for minimizing the segmentation loss L_S. Secondly, note that L_{reg, w_G} depends not only on the labelled images $\{X_L\}$ (as in Eq. 3), but also on the unlabelled images $\{X_{UL}\}$. It is a regularization term based on an adversarial loss, which incorporates information about the image distribution that can be extracted from both $\{X_L\}$ and $\{X_{UL}\}$. This is achieved by synthesizing $\{X_G\}$ as $G_C(\{X_L\})$, where G_C denotes a conditional generative model. G_C is modelled in two different ways: one for deformation field (non-affine spatial transformations) and one for intensity transformations. In both cases, the formulation is such that as a certain labelled image is mapped to an augmentation image, the mapping to obtain the corresponding augmentation label readily follows.

Deformation Field Generator: The deformation field generator, $G_C = G_V$, is trained to create samples from the distribution of deformation fields that can potentially map elements from $\{X_L\}$ to those in the combined set $\{X_L\} \cup \{X_{UL}\}$. G_V takes as input an image from $\{X_L\}$ and a vector z, sampled from a unit Gaussian distribution, and outputs a dense per-pixel deformation field, $\mathbf{v}$. The input image and its corresponding label (in 1-hot encoding) are warped using bilinear interpolation according to $\mathbf{v}$ to produce $X_{G,V}$ and $Y_{G,V}$ respectively.

Additive Intensity Field Generator: The intensity field generator, $G_C = G_I$, is trained to draw random samples from the distribution of additive intensity fields that can potentially map elements from $\{X_L\}$ to those in $\{X_L\} \cup \{X_{UL}\}$. G_I, takes as input an element of $\{X_L\}$ and a noise vector and outputs an intensity mask, ΔI. ΔI is added to the input image to give the transformed image $X_{G,I}$, while its segmentation mask $Y_{G,I}$ remains the same as that of the input image.

Regularization Loss: For both the conditional generators, the regularization term, L_{reg,w_G}, in Eq. 4 is formulated as in Eq. 5. The corresponding discriminator networks D_C are trained to minimize the usual adversarial objective (Eq. 6).

$$L_{reg,w_{G_C}} = \lambda_{adv}\mathbb{E}_{z \sim p_z(z)}[\log(1 - D_C(G_C(z, X_L)))] + \lambda_{big}L_{G_C,big} \quad (5)$$

$$L_{D_C} = -\mathbb{E}_{x \sim p(x)}[\log D_C(x)] - \mathbb{E}_{z \sim p_z(z)}[\log(1 - D_C(G_C(z, X_L)))] \quad (6)$$

The generated images are obtained as $G_V(z, X_L) = \mathbf{v} \circ X_L$ and $G_I(z, X_L) = \Delta I + X_L$, where $\circ$ denotes a bilinear warping operation. In our experiments, we observe that with only the adversarial loss term in $L_{reg,w_{G_C}}$, the generators tend to create only the identity mapping. So, we introduce the $L_{G_C,big}$ term to incentivize non-trivial transformations. We formulate $L_{G_V,big}$ and $L_{G_I,big}$ as $-||\mathbf{v}||_1$ and $-||\Delta I||_1$ respectively.

Optimization Sequence: The method starts by learning the optimal data augmentation for the segmentation task. Thus, all networks S, G_C and D_C are optimized according to Eq. 4. The generative models for the deformation fields and the intensity fields are trained separately. Once this is complete, both G_V and G_I are fixed and the parameters of S are re-initialized. Now, S is trained again according to Eq. 2, using the original labelled training data $\{X_L, Y_L\}$ and augmentation data $\{X_G, Y_G\}$ generated using the trained G_V or G_I or both.

3   Dataset and Network Details

3.1   Dataset Details

We used a publicly available dataset hosted as part of MICCAI'17 ACDC challenge [3][1]. It comprises of short-axis cardiac cine-MRIs of 100 subjects from 5 groups - 20 normal controls and 20 each with 4 different cardiac abnormalities. The in-plane and through-plane resolutions of the images range from 0.70×0.70 mm to 1.92×1.92 mm and 5 mm to 10 mm respectively. Expert annotations are provided for left ventricle (LV), myocardium (Myo) and right ventricle (RV) for both end-systole (ES) and end-diastole (ED) phases of each subject. For our experiments, we only used the ES images.

---

[1] https://www.creatis.insa-lyon.fr/Challenge/acdc.

3.2 Pre-processing

We apply the following pre-processing steps to all images of the dataset: (i) bias correction using N4 [18] algorithm, (ii) normalization of each 3D image by linearly re-scaling the intensities as: $(x - x_2)/(x_{98} - x_2)$, where x_2 and x_{98} are the 2nd and 98th percentile in the bias corrected 3D image, (iii) re-sample each slice of each 3D image and the corresponding labels to an in-plane resolution of 1.367×1.367 mm using bi-linear and nearest neighbour interpolation respectively and crop or pad them to a fixed size of 224×224.

3.3 Network Architectures

There are three types of networks in the proposed method (see Fig. 1): a segmentation network S, a generator network G and a discriminator network D. In this sub-section, we describe their architectures. Expect for the last layer of G, the same architecture is used for the G_V and G_I networks used for modelling both the deformation fields and the intensity transformations.

Generator: G takes as input an image from $\{X_L\}$ and a noise vector z of dimension 100, which are both first passed through separate sub-networks, $G_{subnet,X}$ and $G_{subnet,z}$. $G_{subnet,X}$, consists of 2 convolutional layers, while $G_{subnet,z}$, consists of a fully-connected layer, followed by reshaping of the output, followed by 5 convolutional layers, interleaved with bilinear upsampling layers. The outputs of the two sub-networks are of the same dimensions. They are concatenated and passed through a common sub-network, $G_{subnet,common}$, consisting of 4 convolutional layers, the last of which is different for G_V and G_I. The final convolutional layer for G_V outputs two feature maps corresponding to the 2-dimensional deformation field $\mathbf{v}$, while that for G_I outputs a single feature map corresponding to the intensity mask ΔI. The final layer of G_I employs the tanh activation to cap the range of the intensity mask. All other layers use the ReLU activation. All convolutional layers have 3×3 kernels except for the final ones in both G_V and G_I and are followed by batch-normalization layers before the activation.

Discriminator: D consists of 5 convolutional layers with kernel size of 5×5 and stride 2. The convolutions are followed by batch normalization layers and leaky ReLU activations with the negative slope of the leak set to 0.2. After the convolutional layers, the output is reshaped and passed through 3 fully-connected layers, with the final layer having an output size of 2.

Segmentation Network: We use a U-net [15] like architecture for S. It has an encoding and a decoding path. In the encoder, there are 4 convolutional blocks, each consisting of 2 3×3 convolutions, followed by a max-pooling layer. The decoder consists of 4 convolutional blocks, each made of a concatenation with the corresponding features of the encoder, followed by 2 3×3 convolutions, followed by bi-linear upsampling with factor 2. Batch normalization and ReLU activation are employed in all layers, except the last one.

3.4 Training Details

Weighted cross-entropy is used as the segmentation loss, L_S. We empirically set the weights of the 4 output labels to 0.1 (background) and 0.3 (each of the 3 foreground labels). The background loss is considered while learning the augmentations, but not while learning the segmentation task alone. We empirically set λ_{adv} and λ_{big} to 1 and 10^{-3} respectively. The batch size is set to 20 and each training is run for 10000 iterations. The model parameters that provide the best dice score on the validation set are chosen for evaluation. Adam optimizer is used for all networks with an initial learning rate of 10^{-3}, $\beta_1 = 0.9$ and $\beta_2 = 0.999$.

4 Experiments

We divide the dataset into test (X_{ts}), validation (X_{vl}), labelled training (X_L) and unlabelled training (X_{UL}) sets which consist of 20, 2, N_L and 25 3D images respectively. As we are interested in the few labelled training images scenario, we run all our experiments in two settings: with N_L set to 1 and 3. X_{ts}, X_{vl} and X_{UL} are selected randomly a-priori and fixed for all experiments. X_{ts} and X_{UL} are chosen such that they consist of equal number of images from each group (see Sect. 3.1) of the dataset. A separate set of 10 images (2 from each group), $X_{L,total}$, is selected randomly. Each experiment is run 5 times with X_L as N_L images randomly selected from $X_{L,total}$. When N_L is 3, it is ensured that the images in X_L come from different groups. Further, each of the 5 runs with different X_L is run thrice in order to account for variations in convergence of the networks. Thus, overall, we have 15 runs for each experiment.

The following experiments were done thrice for each choice of $X_{tr,L}$:

- **No data augmentation (Aug$_{none}$):** S is trained without data augmentation.
- **Affine data augmentation (Aug$_A$):** S is trained with data augmentation comprising of affine transformations. These consist of rotation (randomly chosen between $-15°$ and $+15°$), scaling (with a factor randomly chosen uniformly between 0.9 and 1.1), another possible rotation that is multiple of $45°$ (angle = $45° * N$ where N is randomly chosen between 0 to 8), and flipping along x-axis. For each slice in a batch, a random number between 0 and 5 is uniformly sampled and accordingly, either the slice is left as it is or is transformed by one of the 4 stated transformations.

All the following data augmentation methods, each training batch (batch size = bs) is first applied affine transformations as explained above. The batch used for training consists of half of these images along with bs/2 augmentation images obtained according to the particular augmentation method.

- **Random elastic deformations (Aug$_{A,RD}$):** Elastic augmentations are modelled as in [15], where a deformation field is created by sampling each element of a $3 \times 3 \times 2$ matrix from a Gaussian distribution with mean 0 and standard deviation 10 and upscaling it to the image dimensions using bi-cubic interpolation.

- **Random contrast and brightness fluctuations** [11,14] (**Aug$_{A,RI}$**): This comprises of an image contrast adjustment step: $x = (x - \bar{x}) * c + \bar{x}$, followed by a brightness adjustment step: $x = x + b$. We sample c and b uniformly in [0.8, 1.2] and [−0.1, 0.1] respectively.
- **Deformation field transformations** (**Aug$_{A,GD}$**): Augmentation data is generated from the trained deformation field generator G_V.
- **Intensity field transformations** (**Aug$_{A,GI}$**): Augmentation data is generated from the trained intensity field generator G_I.
- **Both deformation and intensity field transformations** (**Aug$_{A,GD,GI}$**): In this experiment, we sample data from G_V and G_I to obtain transformed images X_V and X_I respectively. We also get an additional set of images which contain both deformation and intensity transformations X_{VI}. These are obtained by conditioning G_I on spatially transformed images X_V. The augmentation data comprises of all these images $\{X_V, X_I, X_{VI}\}$.
- **MixUp** [19] (**Aug$_{A,Mixup}$**): Augmentation data ($\{X_G, Y_G\}$) is generated using the original annotated images X_L and their linear combinations using the Mixup formulation as stated in Eq. 7.

$$X_G = \lambda X_{Li} + (1 - \lambda)X_{Lj}, \quad Y_G = \lambda Y_{Li} + (1 - \lambda)Y_{Lj} \qquad (7)$$

where λ is sampled from beta distribution Beta(α, α) with $\alpha \in (0, \infty)$ and $\lambda \in [0, 1)$ which controls the ratio to mix the image-label pairs (X_{Li}, Y_{Li}), (X_{Lj}, Y_{Lj}) selected randomly from the set of labelled training images.
- **Mixup over deformation and intensity field transformations** (**Aug$_{A,GD,GI,Mixup}$**): Mixup is applied over different pairs of available images: original data (X_L), their affine transformations and the images generated using deformation and intensity field generators $\{X_V, X_I, X_{VI}\}$.
- **Adversarial Training (Adv Tr)**: Here, we investigate the benefit of the method proposed in [20] on our dataset (explained in Sect. 1), in both supervised (SL) [12] and semi-supervised (SSL) [20] settings.

Evaluation: The segmentation performance of each method is evaluated using the Dice similarity coefficient (DSC) over 20 test subjects for three foreground structures: left ventricle (LV), myocardium (Myo) and right ventricle (RV).

5   Results and Discussion

Table 1 presents quantitative results of our experiments. The reported numbers are the mean dice scores over the 15 runs for each experiments as described in Sect. 4. It can be observed that the proposed method provides substantial improvements over other data augmentation methods as well as the semi-supervised adversarial learning method, especially in the case where only 1 3D volume is used for training. The improvements can also be visually observed in Fig. 2. In the rest of this section, we discuss the results of specific experiments.

Perhaps unsurprisingly, the lowest performance occurs when neither data augmentation nor semi-supervised training is used. Data augmentation with

Table 1. Average Dice score (DSC) results over 15 runs of 20 test subjects for the proposed method and relevant works. $*, \dagger, \star$ denotes statistical significance over $\text{Aug}_{A,RD}$, $\text{Aug}_{A,RI}$ and $\text{Aug}_{A,Mixup}$ respectively. (Wilcoxon signed rank test with threshold p value of 0.05).

Method	Number of 3D training volumes used					
	1			3		
	RV	Myo	LV	RV	Myo	LV
Aug_{none}	0.259	0.291	0.446	0.589	0.631	0.805
Aug_A	0.373	0.484	0.644	0.733	0.744	0.885
$\text{Aug}_{A,RD}$	0.397	0.503	0.663	0.756	0.763	0.897
$\text{Aug}_{A,GD}$ $(\lambda_{adv} = 1, \lambda_{big} = 10^{-3})$	0.487^*	0.560^*	0.717^*	0.782^*	0.791^*	0.908^*
$\text{Aug}_{A,GD}$ $(\lambda_{adv} = 0, \lambda_{big} = 0)$	0.394	0.531^*	0.694^*	0.756	0.776^*	0.908^*
$\text{Aug}_{A,RI}$	0.429	0.554	0.742	0.744	0.759	0.896
$\text{Aug}_{A,GI}$ $(\lambda_{adv} = 1, \lambda_{big} = 10^{-3})$	$0.517^\dagger$	$0.579^\dagger$	$0.773^\dagger$	$0.803^\dagger$	$0.791^\dagger$	0.912
$\text{Aug}_{A,GI}$ $(\lambda_{adv} = 0, \lambda_{big} = 0)$	$0.500^\dagger$	$0.583^\dagger$	$0.765^\dagger$	$0.766^\dagger$	$0.748^\dagger$	0.893
$\text{Aug}_{A,GD,GI}$ $(\lambda_{adv} = 1, \lambda_{big} = 10^{-3})$	$\underline{0.651}^\star$	$\underline{0.710}^\star$	$\underline{0.834}^\star$	$\underline{0.832}^\star$	$\underline{0.823}^\star$	$\underline{0.922}^\star$
$\text{Aug}_{A,Mixup}$ [19]	0.581	0.599	0.774	0.818	0.791	0.915
$\text{Aug}_{A,GD,GI,Mixup}$	**0.679**	**0.713**	**0.849**	**0.844**	**0.825**	**0.924**
Adv Tr SL [12]	0.417	0.507	0.698	0.731	0.753	0.891
Adv Tr SSL [20]	0.409	0.506	0.692	0.692	0.719	0.874

affine transformations already provides remarkable gains in performance. Both random elastic deformations and random intensity fluctuations further improve accuracy.

The proposed augmentations based on learned deformation fields improve performance as compared to random elastic augmentations. These results show the benefit of encouraging the deformations to span the geometric variations present in entire population (labelled as well as unlabelled images), while still generating images that are conducive to the training of the segmentation network. Some examples of the generated deformed images are shown in Fig. 3. Interestingly, the anatomical shapes in these images are not always realistic. While this may appear to be counter-intuitive, perhaps preserving realistic shapes of anatomical structures in not essential to obtaining the best segmentation neural network.

Similar observations can be made about the proposed augmentations based on learned additive intensity masks as compared to random intensity fluctuations. Again, the improvements may be attributed to encouraging the intensity transformations to span the intensity statistics present in the population, while being beneficial for the segmentation task. Qualitatively, also as before, the generated intensity masks (Fig. 3) do not necessarily lead to realistic images.

(a)   (b)   (c)   (d)   (e)   (f)   (g)

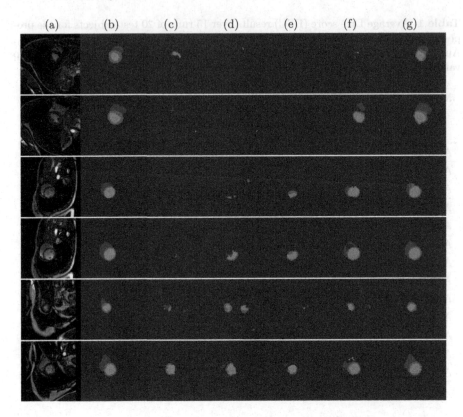

Fig. 2. Qualitative comparison of the proposed method with other approaches: (a) input image, (b) ground truth, (c) Aug_A, (d) $Aug_{A,RD}$, (e) Adv Tr SL [12], (f) $Aug_{A,Mixup}$ [19], (g) $Aug_{A,GD,GI}$

As both G_V and G_I are designed to capture different characteristics of the entire dataset, using both the augmentations together may be expected to provide a higher benefit than employing either one in isolation. Indeed, we observe a substantial improvement in dice scores with our experiments.

As an additional experiment, we investigated the effect of excluding the regularization term from the training of the generators, G_V and G_I ($\lambda_{adv} = \lambda_{big} = 0$). While the resulting augmentations still resulted in better performance than random deformations or intensity fluctuations, their benefits were lesser than that from the ones that were trained with the regularization. This shows that although the adversarial loss does not ensure the generation of realistic images, it is still advantageous to include unlabelled images in the learning of the augmentations.

Augmentations obtained from the Mixup [19] method also lead to a substantial improvement in performance as compared to using affine transformations, random elastic transformations or random intensity fluctuations. Interestingly, this benefit also occurs despite the augmented images being not realistic looking at all. One reason for this behaviour might be that the Mixup

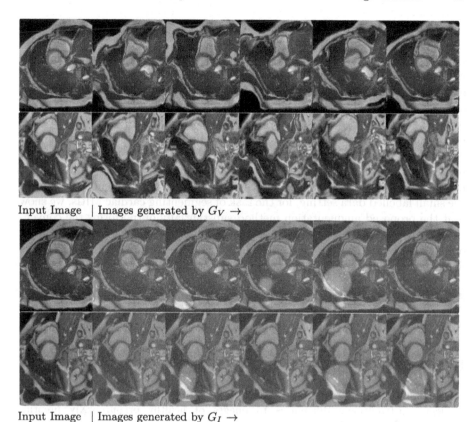

Input Image | Images generated by G_V →

Input Image | Images generated by G_I →

Fig. 3. Generated augmentation images from the deformation field generator G_V (top) and the intensity field generator G_I (bottom).

augmentation method provides soft probability labels for the augmented images - such soft targets have been hypothesized to aid optimization by providing more task information per training sample [10]. Even so, Mixup can only generate augmented images that are linear combinations of the available labelled images and it is not immediately clear how to extend this method to use unlabelled images. Finally, we see that Mixup provides a marginal improvement when applied over the original images together with the augmentations obtained from the trained generators G_V and G_I. This demonstrates the complementary benefits of the two approaches.

While semi-supervised adversarial learning provides improvement in performance as compared to training with no data augmentation, these benefits are only as much as those obtained with simple affine augmentation. This observation seems to be in line with works such as [13].

6 Conclusion

One of the challenging requirements for the success of deep learning methods in medical image analysis problems is that of assembling large-scale annotated datasets. In this work, we propose a semi-supervised and task-driven data augmentation approach to tackle the problem of robust image segmentation in the setting of training datasets consisting of as few as 1 to 3 labelled 3D images. This is achieved via two novel contributions: (i) learning conditional generative models of mappings between labelled and unlabelled images, in a formulation that also readily enables the corresponding segmentation annotations to be appropriately mapped and (ii) guiding these generative models with task-dependent losses. In the small labelled data setting, for the task of segmenting cardiac MRIs, we show that the proposed augmentation method substantially outperforms the conventional data augmentation techniques. Interestingly, we observe that in order to obtain improved segmentation performance, the generated augmentation images do not necessarily need to be visually hyper-realistic.

Acknowledgements. This work has been partially funded by the Swiss Data Science Center (project DeepMicroIA) and the Clinical Research Priority Program Grant on Artificial Intelligence in Oncological Imaging Network from University of Zurich.

References

1. Andermatt, S., Horváth, A., Pezold, S., Cattin, P.: Pathology segmentation using distributional differences to images of healthy origin. arXiv preprint arXiv:1805.10344 (2018)
2. Bai, W., et al.: Semi-supervised learning for network-based cardiac MR image segmentation. In: Descoteaux, M., Maier-Hein, L., Franz, A., Jannin, P., Collins, D.L., Duchesne, S. (eds.) MICCAI 2017. LNCS, vol. 10434, pp. 253–260. Springer, Cham (2017). https://doi.org/10.1007/978-3-319-66185-8_29
3. Bernard, O., et al.: Deep learningtechniques for automatic MRI cardiac multi-structures segmentation anddiagnosis: is the problem solved? IEEE Trans. Med. Imag. **37**, 2514–2525 (2018)
4. Bowles, C., et al.: GAN augmentation: augmenting training data using generative adversarial networks. arXiv preprint arXiv:1810.10863 (2018)
5. Can, Y., Chaitanya, K., Mustafa, B., Koch, L., Konukoglu, E., Baumgartner, C.: Learning to segment medical images with scribble-supervision alone. arXiv preprint arXiv:1807.04668v1 (2018)
6. Cireşan, D.C., Meier, U., Masci, J., Gambardella, L.M., Schmidhuber, J.: High-performance neural networks for visual object classification. arXiv preprint arXiv:1102.0183 (2011)
7. Costa, P., et al.: End-to-end adversarial retinal image synthesis. IEEE Trans. Med. Imag. **37**(3), 781–791 (2018)
8. Eaton-Rosen, Z., Bragman, F., Ourselin, S., Cardoso, M.J.: Improving data augmentation for medical image segmentation. In: International Conference on Medical Imaging with Deep Learning (2018)
9. Goodfellow, I., et al.: Generative adversarial nets. In: Advances in Neural Information Processing Systems, pp. 2672–2680 (2014)

10. Hinton, G., Vinyals, O., Dean, J.: Distilling the knowledge in a neural network. arXiv preprint arXiv:1503.02531 (2015)
11. Hong, J., Park, B.y., Park, H.: Convolutional neural network classifier for distinguishing Barrett's esophagus and neoplasia endomicroscopy images. In: 2017 39th Annual International Conference of the IEEE Engineering in Medicine and Biology Society, EMBC, pp. 2892–2895. IEEE (2017)
12. Luc, P., Couprie, C., Chintala, S., Verbeek, J.: Semantic segmentation using adversarial networks. arXiv preprint arXiv:1611.08408 (2016)
13. Oliver, A., Odena, A., Raffel, C., Cubuk, E.D., Goodfellow, I.J.: Realistic evaluation of deep semi-supervised learning algorithms. arXiv preprint arXiv:1804.09170 (2018)
14. Perez, F., Vasconcelos, C., Avila, S., Valle, E.: Data augmentation for skin lesion analysis. In: Stoyanov, D., et al. (eds.) CARE/CLIP/OR 2.0/ISIC-2018. LNCS, vol. 11041, pp. 303–311. Springer, Cham (2018). https://doi.org/10.1007/978-3-030-01201-4_33
15. Ronneberger, O., Fischer, P., Brox, T.: U-net: convolutional networks for biomedical image segmentation. In: Navab, N., Hornegger, J., Wells, W.M., Frangi, A.F. (eds.) MICCAI 2015. LNCS, vol. 9351, pp. 234–241. Springer, Cham (2015). https://doi.org/10.1007/978-3-319-24574-4_28
16. Shin, H.-C., et al.: Medical image synthesis for data augmentation and anonymization using generative adversarial networks. In: Gooya, A., Goksel, O., Oguz, I., Burgos, N. (eds.) SASHIMI 2018. LNCS, vol. 11037, pp. 1–11. Springer, Cham (2018). https://doi.org/10.1007/978-3-030-00536-8_1
17. Simard, P.Y., Steinkraus, D., Platt, J.C.: Best practices for convolutional neural networks applied to visual document analysis. In: Seventh International Conference on Document Analysis and Recognition (ICDAR), vol. 2, pp. 958–963 (2003)
18. Tustison, N.J., et al.: N4ITK: improved N3 bias correction. IEEE Trans. Med. Imag. **29**(6), 1310–1320 (2010)
19. Zhang, H., Cisse, M., Dauphin, Y.N., Lopez-Paz, D.: mixup: beyond empirical risk minimization. arXiv preprint arXiv:1710.09412 (2017)
20. Zhang, Y., Yang, L., Chen, J., Fredericksen, M., Hughes, D.P., Chen, D.Z.: Deep adversarial networks for biomedical image segmentation utilizing unannotated images. In: Descoteaux, M., Maier-Hein, L., Franz, A., Jannin, P., Collins, D.L., Duchesne, S. (eds.) MICCAI 2017. LNCS, vol. 10435, pp. 408–416. Springer, Cham (2017). https://doi.org/10.1007/978-3-319-66179-7_47

Classification and Inference

Analyzing Brain Morphology on the Bag-of-Features Manifold

Laurent Chauvin[1]($\boxtimes$), Kuldeep Kumar[1], Christian Desrosiers[1],
Jacques De Guise[1], William Wells III[2,3], and Matthew Toews[1]

[1] École de Technologie Supérieure, Montreal, Canada
laurent.chauvin0@gmail.com
[2] Brigham and Women's Hospital, Harvard Medical School, Boston, USA
[3] Computer Science and Artificial Intelligence Laboratory,
Massachusetts Institute of Technology, Boston, USA

Abstract. We propose a novel distance measure between variable-sized sets of image features, i.e. the bag-of-features image representation, for quantifying brain morphology similarity based on local neuroanatomical structures. Our measure generalizes the Jaccard distance metric to account for probabilistic or soft set equivalence (SSE), via a novel adaptive kernel density framework accounting for probabilistic uncertainty in both feature appearance and geometry. The method is based on highly efficient keypoint feature indexing and is suitable for identifying pairwise relationships in arbitrarily large data sets. Experiments use the Human Connectome Project (HCP) dataset consisting of 1010 subjects, including pairs of siblings and twins, where neuroanatomy is modeled as a set of scale-invariant keypoints extracted from T1-weighted MRI data. The Jaccard distance based on (SSE) is shown to outperform standard hard set equivalence (HSE) in predicting the immediate family graph structure and genetic links such as racial origin and sex from MRI data, providing a useful tool for data-driven, high-throughput genome wide heritability analysis.

1 Introduction

Health treatment is increasingly personalized, where treatment decisions are increasingly conditioned on patient-specific information in addition to knowledge regarding the general population, i.e. personalized medicine [7]. Modern genetic testing allows us to cheaply predict patient-specific characteristics, including immediate family relationships, and also characteristics shared across the population including racial origin, sex, hereditary disease status, etc. [1], based on a large library of human DNA samples. The brain, the root of cognition, is a complex organ tightly coupled to the genetic evolution of animals and in particular that of the human species. To what degree is the human brain phenotype coupled to the underlying genotype? How does the brain image manifold vary locally with genotype, i.e. immediate relatives sharing 50–100% of their genes,

© Springer Nature Switzerland AG 2019
A. C. S. Chung et al. (Eds.): IPMI 2019, LNCS 11492, pp. 45–56, 2019.
https://doi.org/10.1007/978-3-030-20351-1_4

or between wider sub-populations defined by more subtle genetic factors such as racial original or sex?

Large, publicly available databases allow us investigate these questions with large samples of coupled MRI and genetic data i.e. 1000+ subjects [23]. Brain shape has been modeled as lying on a smooth manifold in high dimensional MRI data space [2,6], where phenotype can be described as a smooth deformation conditioned on developmental factors determined by the environment. However the brain is naturally described as a rich collection of spatially localized neuroanatomical structures, including common structures such the basal ganglia shared across the population, and also intricate cortical folding patterns [15] or pathology only observable in subsets of the population.

An intuitively appealing representation for such phenomena is the bag-of-feature (BoF) model, where the image is described as a set of localized, conditionally independent descriptors identified at image keypoints, i.e. 3D SIFT-Rank features [21]. Bags-of-features can be viewed as existing on a high-dimensional manifold, and medical imaging applications such as regression or classification can be formulated in terms of a suitable geodesic distance metric between BoFs. As BoFs are variable sized sets, typical metrics based on fixed-length vectors such as L-norms [2,6] do not readily apply. The Jaccard distance metric [10] has proven effective in recent studies investigating genetics and brain MRI [8,22]. For example, by defining hard set equivalence (HSE) in terms of binary k-Nearest Neighbor (kNN) correspondences between keypoint image descriptors, the Jaccard distance metric can be used to approximate the genetic structure of brain MRIs, predicting family relationships including twins and siblings with high accuracy. The disadvantage of the Jaccard metric is that binary equivalence of feature descriptors is crude approximation given probabilistic uncertainty inherent to natural image structure, and is ill-defined for variable sized datasets where the number of relevant kNN correspondences may be unknown a-priori or variable.

Our primary contribution is to introduce a new Jaccard-like measure between BoFs, modeling probabilistic or soft set equivalence (SSE) [5] between elements. This is achieved via an adaptive kernel density estimator (KDE) [19] accounting for uncertainty in both local feature appearance and geometry, automatically adapting to the quantity of available feature data. A novel kernel is introduced that normalizes variability in pairwise feature displacement by the geometrical mean of feature scales, accounting for localization uncertainty in scale-space. This work extends approaches to analyzing neuroimaging data via local features [8,22], where the Jaccard distance based on binary or hard set equivalence (HSE) is defined by kNN correspondences.

2   Related Work

The BoF data model was initially used to categorize text documents from locally orderless collections of words [12], then adapted to categorize images [4] following the development of robust image keypoint detectors, e.g. the scale-invariant

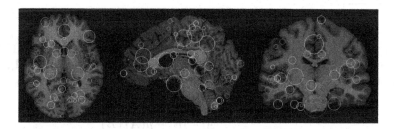

Fig. 1. Illustrating a BoF of 3D SIFT-Rank features [21] extracted from a T1w image from the Human Connectome Project dataset [23]. Circles represent feature location and scale, color also indicates scale. (Color figure online)

feature transform (SIFT) [11]. The keypoint representation serves as a highly robust and efficient basis for medical image analysis applications [21,25], and continues to be a research focus in deep learning [16] (Fig. 1).

Experimentally, our work is most closely related to neuro fingerprinting methods [3,8,9,22,24], which can be used to investigate the relationship between genotype and phenotype from magnetic resonance images (MRI) of the human brain from increasingly large, publicly available neuroimaging datasets [18,23]. The local feature framework is highly robust and requires minimal data preprocessing and scales gracefully to arbitrarily large data sets, as robust, approximate nearest neighbor (NN) correspondences can be identified in $O(log\ N)$ complexity given a dataset of N subjects via efficient KD-tree data structures [13]. This allows evaluating all $N(N-1)/2$ pairwise relationships between subjects in $O(N\ log\ N)$ computational complexity, and has resulted in highest reported accuracy in predicting genetic sibling relationships from structural MRI [8], to our knowledge. Here we compare our SSE Jaccard measure to the standard HSE-based measure used in [8,22], showing a significant improvement in prediction accuracy.

3   Method

Our method is based on bag-of-features (BoF) representation, where each image is represented as a set of local 3D scale invariant features $\{f_i\}$ automatically extracted from the image as described in [21], primarily for the purpose of highly efficient and robust feature indexing operations. We seek a pairwise distance measure between BoFs $A = \{f_i\}$ and $B = \{f_j\}$ which can be used to estimate proximity and thus genetic relationships between subjects. Previous work has adopted the Jaccard distance metric [10] $d_J(A, B)$ defined as:

$$d_J(A, B) = 1 - J_{HSE}(A, B) = 1 - \frac{|A \cap B|}{|A| + |B| - |A \cup B|} \qquad (1)$$

where $J_{HSE}(A, B)$ is the Jaccard index based on binary equivalence relationships, e.g. hard kNN feature correspondences [22]. We seek a measure based on soft set equivalence in order to more accurately model probabilistic similarity between local features extracted from natural image data. We do this in a manner similar to [5] by redefining hard set intersection $|A \cap B|$ in Eq. (1) by a suitable equivalent $\mu(A \cap B)$, where $0 \leq \mu(A \cap B) \leq |A \cap B| \leq min\{|A|, |B|\}$, leading to a Jaccard-like measure based on soft set equivalence:

$$J_{SSE}(A, B) = \frac{\mu(A \cap B)}{|A| + |B| - \mu(A \cap B)} \tag{2}$$

Defining $\mu(A \cap B)$: We begin with a generative model of the conditional probability $p(A|B)$ of set A given set B:

$$p(A|B) = \prod_i^{|A|} p(f_i|B) = \prod_i^{|A|} \left(\eta + \sum_j^{|B|} p(f_i|f_j) \right) \tag{3}$$

$$\approx \prod_i^{|A|} \left(\eta + \max_{f_j \in B}\{p(f_i|f_j)\} \right) \tag{4}$$

where the first equality in Eq. (3) is due to the assumption of conditionally IID feature samples $f_i \in A$ and the second from a mixture density model of $p(f_i|B)$ consisting of kernel components $p(f_i|f_j)$ parameterized by $f_j \in B$ and a uniform background component η accounting spurious, noisy features. The approximation in Eq. (4) can be used when a distinctive invariant feature f_i typically arises from at most a single mixture component, i.e. a unique image-to-image correspondence. Assuming an exponential kernel function $0 \leq p(f_i|f_j) \leq 1$, the logarithm of Eq. (4) is bounded as

$$0 \leq \log p(A|B) = \sum_i^{|A|} \log \left(\eta + \max_{f_j \in B}\{p(f_i|f_j)\} \right) \leq |A| \log(\eta + 1) \tag{5}$$

We define soft set intersection as follows, and show an upper bound:

$$0 \leq \mu(A \cap B) = \min \left\{ \frac{\log p(A|B)}{\log(\eta + 1)}, \frac{\log p(B|A)}{\log(\eta + 1)} \right\} \leq |A \cap B| \tag{6}$$

Defining $p(f_i|f_j)$: Finally we define the form of the kernel function $p(f_i|f_j)$ used. A scale invariant feature $f_i = \{a_i, g_i\}$ is defined by geometry g_i and an appearance descriptor a_i. Feature geometry $g_i = \{x_i, \sigma_i\}$, consists of 3D location x_i and scale σ_i. Appearance a_i is a vector of local image information, i.e. a rank-ordered histogram of oriented gradients (HOG) [21]. The kernel $p(f_i|f_j)$ is factored as

$$p(f_i|f_j) = p(a_i|a_j)p(g_i|g_j) = p(a_i|a_j)p(x_i|\sigma_i, g_j)p(\sigma_i|g_j). \tag{7}$$

In Eq. (7), the first equality expresses conditional independence between variables of appearance a_i and geometry g_i due to the use of geometrical invariant appearance descriptors. The second equality factors location $\boldsymbol{x}_i$ and scale σ_i using the chain rule of probability. Factors $p(\boldsymbol{a}_i|\boldsymbol{a}_j)$, $p(\boldsymbol{x}_i|\sigma_i, \boldsymbol{g}_j)$ and $p(\sigma_i|\boldsymbol{g}_j)$ are defined as follow:

$$p(\boldsymbol{a}_i|\boldsymbol{a}_j) = \exp\left(-\frac{\|\boldsymbol{a}_i - \boldsymbol{a}_j\|_2^2}{\alpha^2}\right) \tag{8}$$

$$p(\boldsymbol{x}_i|\sigma_i, \boldsymbol{g}_j) = \exp\left(-\frac{\|\boldsymbol{x}_i - \boldsymbol{x}_j\|_2^2}{\sigma_i^2\sigma_j^2}\right) \tag{9}$$

$$p(\sigma_i|\boldsymbol{g}_j) = \exp\left(-\log^2\left(\frac{\sigma_i}{\sigma_j}\right)\right) \tag{10}$$

Kernel $p(\boldsymbol{a}_i|\boldsymbol{a}_j)$ in Eq. (8) penalizes differences in appearance descriptors, where α is an adaptive bandwidth of the KDE, defined as

$$\alpha = \min_{f_j \in \Omega}(d(\boldsymbol{a}_i, \boldsymbol{a}_j)), \ \ s.t. \ d(\boldsymbol{a}_i, \boldsymbol{a}_j) > 0 \tag{11}$$

with $d(\boldsymbol{a}_i, \boldsymbol{a}_j)$ is the minimum Euclidean distance between appearance descriptors $\boldsymbol{a}_i$ and $\boldsymbol{a}_j$ across the entire dataset. This allows the kernel to adapt to arbitrarily data set sizes, shrinking as the number of data grows large. Kernel $p(\boldsymbol{x}_i|\sigma_i, \boldsymbol{g}_j)$ in Eq. (9) is a novel formulation penalizing distance between features in normalized image space, where the variance is proportional to the product of feature scales $\sigma_i^2\sigma_j^2$. This variance embodies uncertainty in feature localization due to scale, and is reminiscent of mass in Newton's gravitation or electric charge magnitude in Coulomb's law. Finally, Kernel $p(\sigma_i|\boldsymbol{g}_j)$ in Eq. (10) penalizes multiplicative difference in feature scale in normalized image space.

4   Experiments

The experiments aim to investigate the link between genetics and phenotypical neuroanatomical structure [20] by comparing the proximity graph structure induced by the Jaccard distance measure $d_J(A, B) = -\log J_{SSE}(A, B)$ between pairs of subjects (A, B) from MRI (BoF) observations vs. known genetic relationships. Unless mentioned otherwise, $d_J(A, B)$ will refer to the Jaccard distance with soft set equivalence (SSE).

We compare the set intersection $A \cap B$ defined by standard hard set equivalence (HSE) as in Eq. (1) vs. our soft set equivalence (SSE) definition in Eqs. (2) and (6), with a background distribution η empirically set to 1. We consider the cases of (1) close genetic links between immediate family members sharing 50–100% of their genes and (2) broad genetic links between unrelated non-siblings sharing nominal genetic information due to common racial origin, sex, etc.

Our test set consists of MRI scans of $N = 1010$ unique subjects with genetic ground truth from the Human Connectome Project Q4 release [23], aged 22–36 years (mean 29 years), 468 males and 542 females. There are thus $N(N-1)/2 = 1,020,100$ pairwise relationships, where each pair of subjects is related by one of four possible relationship labels $L = \{MZ, DZ, FS, UR\}$ for monozygotic twins (MZ), dizygotic twins (DZ), full non-twin siblings (FS) and unrelated non-siblings (UR). Note that evaluating the similarity of $N(N-1)/2$ pairwise relationships via brute force image registration, e.g. optimizing cross-correlation, quickly becomes computationally intractable as N grows large.

MRI data used consist of skull-stripped T1w images with 0.7 mm isotropic voxels, registered to a common reference frame, however the method generally applies to other scalar image modalites (e.g. T2w, FA). Generic 3D SIFT-Rank features are extracted from MRI data, where geometry g_i is identified as extrema of an difference-of-Gaussian scale-space [11] an local appearance is encoded as a 64-dimensional SIFT-Rank [21] appearance descriptor a_i. Feature extraction requires approximately 20 s/per image and results in an average of 1,400 features per image, for a total of 1,488,065 features. Approximate kNN correspondences between appearance descriptors are identified across the entire database using KD-tree indexing [13], lookup requires 0.8 s/subject for k = 200 on an i7-5600@2.60 GHz machine with 16 GB RAM (1.64 GB used).

4.1   Close Genetic Proximity: Siblings

The Jaccard distance quantifies the whole-brain dissimilarity between brain pairs. As the percentage of genes shared is 100% for MZ pairs, on average 50% for DZ and FS pairs, and a nominally low percentage for UR pairs, we hypothesize that the pairwise distances will respect the same ordering on the BoF manifold. Figure 2 shows distributions of all pairwise Jaccard distances conditional on labels, showing that this is indeed the case, with MZ pairs closest, DZ and FS pairs further, and finally UR pairs the farthest.

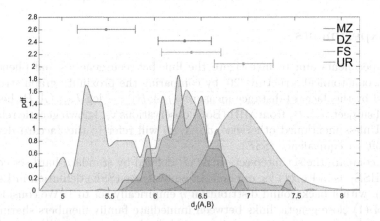

Fig. 2. Distributions of conditional Jaccard distances $p(d_J(A, B)|L)$ conditioned on pairwise labels $L = \{MZ, DZ, FS, UR\}$. $d_J(A, B)$ is evaluated with SSE and NN = 200. Multiple peaks in MZ, DZ and FS distributions result from sampling sparsity.

As sibling pairs (MZ, DZ, FS) exhibit significantly lower manifold distance than UR pairs, we investigate the degree to which siblings can be distinguished from unrelated pairs based on distance. Figure 3 shows the Receiver Operating Characteristic (ROC) curves for MZ, DZ and FS relationships based on their proximity on the bag-of-feature manifold, comparing Jaccard distances for hard (HSE) and soft set equivalence (SSE) for various numbers of nearest neighbors (20, 100, 200). Several observations can be made. First, the Jaccard measure we propose for soft set equivalence is always superior to hard set equivalence in terms of classification accuracy. HSE is noticeably sensitive to the number of nearest neighbor (NN) feature correspondences, and the classification performance generally decreases with an increase in the number of NNs. In contrast, the SSE is relatively stable and increases with the number of NNs used. Intuitively, this is because the number NN correspondences above the number of sibling pairs in the data will generally only contribute noise in HSE distance measurements, but these are down-weighted in the SSE based feature proximity. The area under the ROC curve (AUC) values in Table 1 quantify the improvement of SSE vs HSE, where the highest AUC values are obtained for SSE with 200 NN correspondences. The results for HSE are consistent with the work of [8], and our SSE results can thus be considered the state-of-the-art for sibling retrieval from structure MRI.

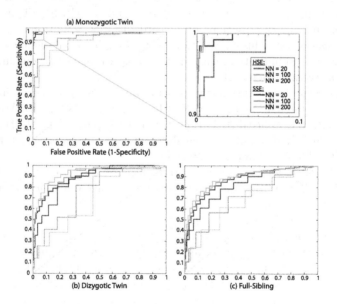

Fig. 3. ROC curves for sibling identification based on Jaccard distance for (a) MZ, (b) DZ and (c) FS pairs. Curves compare hard set equivalence (HSE) vs. the proposed soft set equivalence (SSE) for three values of nearest neighbor (NN) keypoint correspondences (NN = 20, 100, 200).

Table 1. Area Under the Curve (AUC) for monozygotic (MZ), dizygotic (DZ) and full-sibling (FS) classification with HSE and SSE methods for 20, 100 and 200 nearest neighbors (NN). SSE method consistently perform better, with an accuracy increasing with the number of nearest neighbors.

Label	NN = 20		NN = 100		NN = 200	
	HSE	SSE	HSE	SSE	HSE	SSE
Monozygotic	0.9983	**0.9996**	0.9544	**0.9998**	0.9272	**0.9999**
Dizygotic	0.8922	**0.9044**	0.8018	**0.9250**	0.7541	**0.9391**
Full-Sibling	0.8423	**0.8753**	0.7611	**0.8888**	0.7358	**0.8989**

4.2   Distant Genetic Proximity: Unrelated Subjects

As compared to siblings, unrelated (UR) subject pairs exhibit a much lower genetic overlap, with subtle similarities due to factors such as common racial original and sex, and accordingly higher Jaccard distance. We thus expect subtle variations in whole-brain Jaccard distance, with lowest distance for UR pairs of the same race and sex (R, S), medium distance for either same race (R, $\overline{S}$) or sex ($\overline{R}$, S), and highest distance for different race and sex ($\overline{R}$, $\overline{S}$). Figure 4a shows that the conditional distributions of Jaccard distance conditional on race and sex are consistent with this expectation. Note that the mean distance for ($\overline{R}$, S) is lower than (R, $\overline{S}$) indicating, that sex may be a stronger determinant of whole brain similarity than racial origin.

We investigate more closely the relationship between whole brain distance and pairwise combinations of male/female sex labels in Fig. 4(b). We see that while the Jaccard distance distributions for same sex pairs (F-F, M-M) are highly similar in terms of mean and variance, different sex pairs (F-M) generally exhibit a significantly larger distance, as expected.

A potential confound in whole brain Jaccard distance is age difference. Figure 5 plots the variation in Jaccard distance vs. age difference. Distance distributions are virtually identical across the HCP subject age range spanning 22–36 years of age, indicating that age difference is not a major confound in this relatively young HCP cohort where brain morphology is relatively stable. We expect a greater impact age ranges associated with morphological changes, i.e. neurodevelopment in young subjects (e.g. infants) and neurodegeneration in older subjects (e.g. due to natural aging). This will be investigated in future work.

4.3   Sex Prediction

While lower whole-brain Jaccard distance is generally associated with common genetic traits, e.g. same-sex MRI pairs, however it is insufficient for predicting the sex of a brain MRI. We investigate whether the Jaccard distance can be modified to predict the sex of a brain MRI, by evaluating the distances between a subject BoF A and BoFs compiled *all Males* $d_J(A, Males)$ and *all Females* $d_J(A, Females)$. These distances are combined in a basic linear classifier with

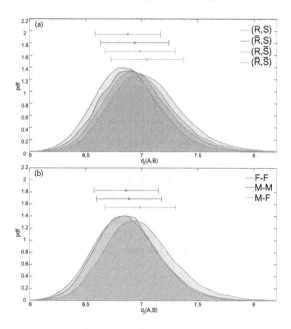

Fig. 4. (a) Distributions of Jaccard distances with SSE (NN = 200) for unrelated subjects (UR) and: same race, same sex (blue); different race, same sex (red); same race, different sex (green), and different race, different sex (yellow). Based on a two-sample Kolmogorov-Smirnov test, $p < 1.34e^{-145}$ for all pairs of distributions. (b) Distributions of Jaccard distances with SSE (NN = 200) for unrelated subjects (UR) from the same race between: Female-Female (blue), Male-Male (red), Male-Female of Female-Male (green). M-M and F-F distributions are highly similar, and both are significantly different from M-F ($p < 2.83e^{-270}$) based on a two-sample Kolmogorov-Smirnov test. (Color figure online)

a single threshold parameter τ to adjust for differences in the numbers of male and female subjects and features (12):

$$Class(A) = \begin{cases} Female & \text{if } d_J(A, Females) - d_J(A, Males) + \tau > 0 \\ Male & \text{otherwise.} \end{cases} \tag{12}$$

Figure 6 shows ROCs curves for sex classification obtained by varying τ over the range $[-\infty, \infty]$, again comparing Jaccard overlap computed via HSE and SSE. The AUC = 0.97 for SSE is significantly higher than AUC = 0.91 for HSE. SSE achieves an error accuracy rate of 91%, is slightly higher than 89% obtained using a voxel-wise support vector machine with single and multi-site MRI data reported in a recent work [14]. In comparison, our classification approach is on-the-fly and can be used to classify arbitrary subject groups with no explicit training procedure.

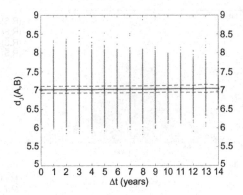

Fig. 5. Conditional distributions of Jaccard distance $p(d_J(A, B)|\Delta t)$ between unrelated subject pairs (A, B) given age difference Δt. The mean (plain red line) and standard deviation (dashed red lines) are plotted for each Δt. (Color figure online)

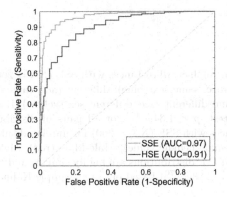

Fig. 6. ROC curves and AUC for sex classification based on Jaccard distances with HSE (red) and SSE (green) methods. AUC is noticeably higher for our SSE method. (Color figure online)

5   Discussion

We presented a novel generalization of the Jaccard distance metric to consider probabilistic set equivalence, for the purpose of evaluating distance or dissimilarity between bag-of-feature image representation. We also develop a novel kernel density estimator based on feature geometry. The method is applied to recovering the proximity graph structure between MRI brain scans of 1010 genetically related subjects, including siblings and twins, where both contributions result in significant improvement in recall rates for all sibling types. To our knowledge, these are the highest recall rates for T1w brain scans present in the literature, note that monozygotic twins can be identified with virtually perfect accuracy. Furthermore, a minor modification allows the Jaccard distance to predict subject-specific traits such as sex with high accuracy.

Our method is based on highly efficient algorithms for feature extraction and correspondence, and can be applied to arbitrarily large datasets with minimal preprocessing. It should be noted that the low number of samples per label (i.e. family members) makes it difficult to use recent Convolutional Neural Networks (CNN) approaches, which generally require large numbers of training data. We have found it to be particularly effective at automatically identifying brain scans of the same subject, and we have applied the method to several large medical image datasets to identify previously unknown, incorrectly labeled duplicate subjects. Future work will investigate the method in other image modalities and alternative anatomies, e.g. full body scans. Generic 3D SIFT-Rank features are used here, tuning parameters such as patch size could potentially be optimized for brain MRI data. The relatively frequencies of correspondences across the brain may prove useful in understanding links between genotype and phenotypical variation, potentially in the context of genome wide heritability studies [17]. All code for this work is available upon request.

Acknowledgement. This work was supported by NIH grant P41EB015902 (NAC) and a Canadian National Sciences and Research Council (NSERC) Discovery Grant.

References

1. Annas, G.J., Elias, S.: 23andMe and the FDA. N. Engl. J. Med. **370**(11), 985–988 (2014)
2. Brosch, T., Tam, R.: Manifold learning of brain MRIs by deep learning. In: Mori, K., Sakuma, I., Sato, Y., Barillot, C., Navab, N. (eds.) MICCAI 2013. LNCS, vol. 8150, pp. 633–640. Springer, Heidelberg (2013). https://doi.org/10.1007/978-3-642-40763-5_78
3. Colclough, G.L., et al.: The heritability of multi-modal connectivity in human brain activity. eLife **6**, e20178 (2017)
4. Csurka, G., Dance, C., Fan, L., Willamowski, J., Bray, C.: Visual categorization with bags of keypoints. In: Workshop on Statistical Learning in Computer Vision, ECCV, Prague, vol. 1, pp. 1–2 (2004)
5. Gardner, A., Kanno, J., Duncan, C.A., Selmic, R.: Measuring distance between unordered sets of different sizes. In: Proceedings of the IEEE Conference on Computer Vision and Pattern Recognition, pp. 137–143 (2014)
6. Gerber, S., Tasdizen, T., Fletcher, P.T., Joshi, S., Whitaker, R., Alzheimers Disease Neuroimaging Initiative, et al.: Manifold modeling for brain population analysis. Med. Image Anal. **14**(5), 643–653 (2010)
7. Hamburg, M.A., Collins, F.S.: The path to personalized medicine. N. Engl. J. Med. **363**(4), 301–304 (2010)
8. Kumar, K., Chauvin, L., Toews, M., Colliot, O., Desrosiers, C.: Multi-modal brain fingerprinting: a manifold approximation based framework. bioRxiv (2018)
9. Kumar, K., Desrosiers, C., Siddiqi, K., Colliot, O., Toews, M.: Fiberprint: a subject fingerprint based on sparse code pooling for white matter fiber analysis. NeuroImage **158**, 242–259 (2017)
10. Levandowsky, M., Winter, D.: Distance between Sets. Nature **234**(5323), 34–35 (1971)

11. Lowe, D.G.: Distinctive image features from scale-invariant keypoints. Int. J. Comput. Vis. **60**(2), 91–110 (2004)
12. McCallum, A., Nigam, K., et al.: A comparison of event models for naive Bayes text classification. In: Workshop on Learning for Text Categorization, AAAI 1998, vol. 752, pp. 41–48. Citeseer (1998)
13. Muja, M., Lowe, D.G.: Scalable nearest neighbor algorithms for high dimensional data. IEEE Trans. Pattern Anal. Mach. Intell. **36**(11), 2227–2240 (2014)
14. Nieuwenhuis, M., et al.: Multi-center mri prediction models: predicting sex and illness course in first episode psychosis patients. NeuroImage **145**, 246–253 (2017)
15. Ono, M., Kubik, S., Abernathey, C.: Atlas of the Cerebral Sulci (1990)
16. Ono, Y., Trulls, E., Fua, P., Yi, K.M.: LF-Net: learning local features from images. arXiv preprint arXiv:1805.09662 (2018)
17. Sabuncu, M.R., et al.: Morphometricity as a measure of the neuroanatomical signature of a trait. Proc. Natl. Acad. Sci. **113**(39), E5749–E5756 (2016)
18. Sudlow, C., et al.: UK biobank: an open access resource for identifying the causes of a wide range of complex diseases of middle and old age. PLoS Med. **12**(3), e1001779 (2015)
19. Terrell, G.R., Scott, D.W.: Variable kernel density estimation. Ann. Stat. **20**, 1236–1265 (1992)
20. Thompson, P.M., et al.: Genetic influences on brain structure. Nat. Neurosci. **4**(12), 1253–1258 (2001)
21. Toews, M., Wells, W.M.: Efficient and robust model-to-image alignment using 3D scale-invariant features. Med. Image Anal. **17**(3), 271–282 (2013)
22. Toews, M., Wells, W.M.: How are siblings similar? How similar are siblings? Large-scale imaging genetics using local image features. In: 2016 IEEE 13th International Symposium on Biomedical Imaging, ISBI, pp. 847–850. IEEE, April 2016
23. Van Essen, D., et al.: The Human Connectome Project: a data acquisition perspective. NeuroImage **62**(4), 2222–2231 (2012)
24. Wachinger, C., Golland, P., Kremen, W., Fischl, B., Reuter, M.: BrainPrint: a discriminative characterization of brain morphology. NeuroImage **109**, 232–248 (2015)
25. Wachinger, C., Toews, M., Langs, G., Wells, W., Golland, P.: Keypoint transfer for fast whole-body segmentation. IEEE Trans. Med. Imag. (2018)

Modeling and Inference of Spatio-Temporal Protein Dynamics Across Brain Networks

Sara Garbarino$^{(\boxtimes)}$ and Marco Lorenzi

for the Alzheimer's Disease Neuroimaging Initiative

Université Côte d'Azur, INRIA Sophia Antipolis, EPIONE project-team,
Sophia Antipolis, France
{sara.garbarino,marco.lorenzi}@inria.fr

Abstract. Models of misfolded proteins (MP) aim at discovering the bio-mechanical propagation properties of neurological diseases (ND) by identifying plausible associated dynamical systems. Solving these systems along the full disease trajectory is usually challenging, due to the lack of a well defined time axis for the pathology. This issue is addressed by disease progression models (DPM) where long-term progression trajectories are estimated via time reparametrization of individual observations. However, due to their loose assumptions on the dynamics, DPM do not provide insights on the bio-mechanical properties of MP propagation. Here we propose a unified model of spatio-temporal protein dynamics based on the joint estimation of long-term MP dynamics and time reparameterization of individuals observations. The model is expressed within a Gaussian Process (GP) regression setting, where constraints on the MP dynamics are imposed through non-linear dynamical systems. We use stochastic variational inference on both GP and dynamical system parameters for scalable inference and uncertainty quantification of the trajectories. Experiments on simulated data show that our model accurately recovers prescribed rates along graph dynamics and precisely reconstructs the underlying progression. When applied to brain imaging data our model allows the bio-mechanical interpretation of amyloid deposition in Alzheimer's disease, leading to plausible simulations of MP propagation, and achieving accurate predictions of individual MP deposition in unseen data.

Keywords: Bayesian non-parametric model · Protein propagation ·
Alzheimer's disease · Gaussian Process · Dynamical systems ·
Spatio-temporal model · Disease progression model

Data used in preparation of this article were obtained from the Alzheimer's Disease Neuroimaging Initiative (ADNI) database (adni.loni.usc.edu). As such, the investigators within the ADNI contributed to the design and implementation of ADNI and/or provided data but did not participate in analysis or writing of this report.

Electronic supplementary material The online version of this chapter (https://doi.org/10.1007/978-3-030-20351-1_5) contains supplementary material, which is available to authorized users.

© Springer Nature Switzerland AG 2019
A. C. S. Chung et al. (Eds.): IPMI 2019, LNCS 11492, pp. 57–69, 2019.
https://doi.org/10.1007/978-3-030-20351-1_5

1   Introduction

A peculiarity of neurodegenerative diseases (NDs) is the misfolding and sub-sequent accumulation of pathological proteins in the brain, leading to cellular dysfunction, loss of synaptic connections, and neuronal loss [1]. Misfolded pro-tein (MP) aggregates can self-propagate and spread the pathology across cells and tissues, along functional or structural brain networks [2].

With the aim of describing such processes, a variety of mathematical mod-els has been proposed for providing better insight into the microscopic kinetic dynamics governing the processes of proteins propagation [3]. Complementar-ily, another class of models relies on macroscopic measurements from molecu-lar and structural imaging for describing the effects of MP propagation along brain networks [4–8]. Such MP kinetics models are of strategic relevance, as they may provide new understanding of the mechanisms involved in NDs, and thus allow identification of novel strategies for treatment and diagnosis. These mod-els usually define the propagation dynamics through diffusion equations. This modelling choice allows to reduce the number of parameters to be estimated, but comes at the expenses of an oversimplification of the dynamics governing the MP process. First, while the pathological kinetics may be assimilated to dif-fusive processes in short term observations, the long term evolution of NDs are unlikely to have diffusive properties. For example, the asymptotically constant behaviour of NDs may not be described by the stationary and constant rate of change specified by diffusion equations. Second, such models require a precise definition of the time axis, which is typically not well defined in clinical data sets. To address this issue, several alternative disease progression models (DPM) have been proposed [9–12]. These approaches allow to reconstruct biomarkers trajec-tories along the long term disease progression by "stitching" together short term individual measurements. Each subject is characterized by specific time param-eters quantifying their pathological stage with respect to the estimated global group-wise evolution. However, these models provide an "apparent" description of biomarkers dynamics, without in fact elucidating the kinetics and relation-ships across biomarkers.

To date, no modelling framework allows for joint MP kinetics modelling and reconstruction of the biomarkers dynamics across the whole disease long term evolution. The problem is challenging since it requires to simultaneously account for short term observations to reconstruct the long term disease progression, and to estimate group-wise dynamics parameters specified by high-dimensional dynamical systems.

In this paper we solve this problem by formulating a model for the dynam-ics of MP accumulation, clearance and propagation (ACP) across structural brain networks, which includes data-driven estimates of the long term protein trajectories from short term data. Figure 1 shows a schematic representation of our framework. The ACP model is formulated as a constrained regression problem in a Bayesian non-parametric setting, where the MP progression is modelled by a Gaussian Process (GP), and constraints on the MP dynamics are imposed through systems of non linear ordinary differential equations (ODEs).

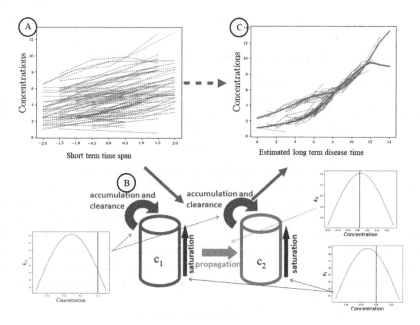

Fig. 1. Schematic representation of our framework. Here we have two brain regions whose MP concentrations c_1 and c_2 are collected for many subjects over a short term time span (A). The dynamics of such concentrations is described in terms of the accumulation, clearance and propagation processes, with unknown parameters (B). The proposed Bayesian framework estimates the distribution of such parameters (here plotted against their ground truth values - the vertical black lines in the distributions plots), and the long term trajectories with respect to the estimated disease time axis (C).

The Bayesian setting allows for uncertainty quantification of the MP dynamics while, to achieve tractability, the inference problem is solved via stochastic variational inference. The constrained regression framework provides a complete description of the MP dynamics, which can be subsequently used for simulating and predicting MP changes over time through forward integration of the estimated dynamical systems. The estimated MP dynamics also provide an instrument to investigate different hypotheses of MP propagation.

We test our framework against synthetic data and compare its performances in recovering the simulated evolution and the time reparameterization as compared to standard disease progression models based on monotonic constraints. Finally, we demonstrate our framework on AV45-PET data of Alzheimer's Disease (AD) subjects from the ADNI data set. We show that it allows to compare different hypothesis of MP kinetics: diffusive vs non-linear and time-varying dynamics properties (ACP). We show that the ACP model outperforms diffusive ones in terms of prediction of amyloid deposition in unseen follow-up data.

2   Methods

2.1   Non-linear and Time-Varying MP Kinetics Model

We consider the brain as a system of N interconnected regions, where each region i $(i = 1, \ldots, N)$ is characterized by its concentration $c_i(t)$ of MP proteins along time. Standard MP kinetics models are based on the definition of dynamical systems of the form

$$\dot{c}(t) = \beta A c(t), \tag{1}$$

where $c(t)$ is the vector of concentrations of MP across brain regions, A is a diffusion matrix and β is the parameter describing MP propagation. The operator A is usually defined as the graph Laplacian of the brain connectome, while β is typically assumed to be constant throughout the whole disease progression [4].

Here we introduce an extension of this paradigm which accounts for the dynamics characterized by the time-varying and non-linear parameters of MP accumulation, brain response via MP clearance, and long term propagation across neighbouring neuronal cells: the ACP model. Within this setting, Eq. (1) is reformulated as

$$\dot{c}(t) = M_{ACP}(c(t))c(t), \tag{2}$$

where the matrix M_{ACP} is decomposed into (dependence on t is omitted but implied): $M_{ACP}(c) = M_{AC}(c) - M_{out}(c) + M_{in}(c)$. Here, $M_{AC}(c)$ accounts for the total aggregation of MP plaques, i.e. sum of accumulation and clearance, while the remaining two matrices describe long-range propagation from $(M_{out}(c))$ or to $(M_{in}(c))$ for each region. Our assumptions on the MP dynamics are the following:

- no aggregation nor propagation occur in healthy conditions. MP plaques aggregation develops when the accumulation-clearance equilibrium breaks. This can be modelled with the assumption that $\bar{k}_a - \bar{k}_c > 0$, where $\bar{k}.$ are the maximum rates of accumulation and clearance and are assumed to be constant across regions. We define $\bar{k}_t := \bar{k}_a - \bar{k}_c$ as the maximum rate of total aggregation.
- We hypothesize a region-dependent critical threshold η_i above which the aggregation process reaches a plateau. This is modelled by a sigmoid function

$$k_t(c_i) = \frac{\bar{k}_t}{1 + e^{l_2(c_i - \eta_i)}}. \tag{3}$$

- When passing a critical threshold γ_j the MP concentration in each region j saturates and triggers propagation towards the connected regions. Also, it reaches a plateau when passing a threshold η_j. Again this can be modelled by a function asymptotically dropping to zero:

$$k_{ij}(c_j) = \frac{\bar{k}_{ij}}{\left(1 + e^{-l_1(c_j - \gamma_j)}\right)\left(1 + e^{l_2(c_j - \eta_j)}\right)}, \tag{4}$$

representing the non-linear rate of propagation from region j to region i. Here $\bar{k}_{ij}$ is the maximum rate of propagation between the two regions, and we assume $\bar{k}_{ij} = \bar{k}_{ji}$. We combine the propagation coefficients in a matrix describing the global brain-scale propagation process: $K(c) = (k_{ij}(c_j))_{ij}$.

- The substrate for propagation is the structural connectome, here represented by the symmetric and normalized adjacency matrix of connections between brain regions $A = (\alpha_{ij})$.

Such assumptions are formalized into the following functionals:

$$(M_{AC}(\mathbf{c}))_{ij} = \begin{cases} k_t(\mathbf{c}) & \text{if } i = j \\ 0 & \text{otherwise;} \end{cases} \tag{5}$$

$$M_{in}(\mathbf{c}) = K(\mathbf{c}) \odot A; \tag{6}$$

$$(M_{out}(\mathbf{c}))_{ij} = \begin{cases} \sum_j (K(\mathbf{c})_{ij} \odot A_{ij}) & \text{if } i = j \\ 0 & \text{otherwise.} \end{cases} \tag{7}$$

Overall, the ACP model depends on $1 + 2N + \frac{N^2 - N}{2}$ parameters: $\boldsymbol{\theta} = (\bar{k}_t, \eta_i, \gamma_i, \bar{k}_{ij})$ for $i, j = 1, \dots, N$.

2.2 Extending MP Dynamics Modelling to Account for Time Reparametrization

Once defined our dynamical system as the one described in (2), we need to incorporate it within a regression framework for short term data. Let us assume to have S subjects for which we have measurements of MP concentrations $\mathbf{C}$ in N brain regions at different time-points, encoded in a vector $\mathbf{t}$: $\mathbf{C}$ is therefore the realization of $c(t)$ at times $\mathbf{t}$. For notation simplicity we assume here $\mathbf{t}$ to be the same for every subject, but computations extend easily to more general cases.

The observations $\mathbf{C}$ for subject k at a time points $\mathbf{t}$ can be modelled as a random sample from the following generative model [10]:

$$\mathbf{C}^k(t) = \mathbf{f}(\boldsymbol{\tau}^k(t)) + \boldsymbol{\nu}^k + \epsilon. \tag{8}$$

Here $\mathbf{f}$ is the fixed effect function modeling the concentrations' longitudinal evolution and is modelled as a GP; $\boldsymbol{\tau}^k(t)$ is the individual time reparametrization with respect to the global group-wise evolution, and is modelled as a linear shift $\tau_l^k = t_l^k + d^k$ for each time point t_l^k; $\boldsymbol{\nu}^k$ is the individual random effect, assumed to be Gaussian correlated perturbations $\mathcal{N}(0, \phi_N^k)$; ϵ is the observational noise. We introduce constraints on the dynamics of the model $\mathbf{f}$ enforcing the concentrations' evolution to the ACP model. This means specifying a family of admissible functions whose derivatives evaluated at the inputs $\mathbf{t}$ satisfy the ACP constraint:

$$\mathcal{A} = \{\mathbf{f}(t) : \dot{\mathbf{f}}(t) = M_{ACP}(\mathbf{f}(t))\mathbf{f}(t)\}. \tag{9}$$

We note that the constraints are imposed only on the group-wise dynamics f and not on the random-effects. This is done to reduce complexity and the model's parameters. Relaxing the constraints at individual level is also meaningful, as some subjects may be characterized by potentially different dynamics due to specific clinical conditions.

2.3   The Inference Scheme

We define as F^k the realization of f at $\tau^k(t)$, and as $\dot{F}^k$ the set of realizations of f and of its derivatives at $\tau^k(t)$. We also indicate by F, ν, and $\dot{F}$ the collections of F^k, ν^k, and $\dot{F}^k$ for all the subjects ($k = 1, \ldots, S$). Similarly, we define τ as the collections of τ^k. We denote by θ the set of parameters for the MP dynamics, and by ϕ_N the parameters associated to ν. Our framework is formulated as the constrained regression defined through two likelihood elements: a data fidelity term $p(C|F, \phi_N, \tau, \epsilon)$ and a constraint term $p(\mathcal{A}|\dot{F}, \theta, \tau, \zeta)$, where ϵ and ζ are the associated noise parameters.

Following [13] we solve the constrained regression problem by determining a lower bound for the marginal function

$$
p(C, \mathcal{A}|\phi_N, \tau, t, \epsilon, \zeta) = \int p(C|F, \phi_N, \tau, t, \epsilon) p(\mathcal{A}|\dot{F}, \theta, \tau, t, \zeta) \\
p(F, \dot{F}|\phi_N, \tau, t) dF d\dot{F} d\theta,
\tag{10}
$$

where

$$
p(F, \dot{F}|\phi_N, \tau, t) = p(\dot{F}|F) p(F|\phi_N, \tau, t). \tag{11}
$$

We assume the likelihood for data and constraints to be respectively Gaussian and Student-t with parameters ϵ and ζ [13], and we approximate the GP via random features expansion, as shown in [14]. Specifically, the GP realizations can be expressed as $F \approx h(t\Omega)W$, where Ω is a linear projection of the input t into the random feature space specified by the trigonometric activation functions $h(\cdot) = (\cos(\cdot), \sin(\cdot))$, and W are the regression parameters. Such approximation extends to the derivatives of the GP thanks to the chain rule [13]. As a result, the GP function and its derivatives can be both identified by the parameters W and Ω.

Solving (10) amounts at doing inference on F, which in this setting means inference on W and Ω. Following [14], we optimize (10) through variational inference of W and θ, while Ω is assumed to be sampled from the prior [13]. This leads to the optimization of the evidence lower bound (ELBO):

$$
\log(p(C, \mathcal{A}|\phi_N, \tau, t, \epsilon, \zeta)) \geq E_{q(W)} \left[\log(p(C|\Omega, W, \phi_N, \tau, t, \epsilon)) \right] \\
+ E_{q(W)q(\theta)} \left[\log(p(\mathcal{A}|\Omega, W, \theta, \tau, t, \zeta)) \right] \\
- DKL(q(W)|p(W)) - DKL(q(\theta)|p(\theta)).
\tag{12}
$$

Here $DKL(q|p)$ is the Kullback Leibler divergence between p and its variational approximation q; we assume $q(W)$ and $q(\theta)$ to be Gaussian. Details on the implementation setting are in Supplementary Material (Supp. Mat.).

3   Simulation Results

We test the ability of our framework in reconstructing the long term trajectories of the ACP dynamical system from noisy samples of short term data (Fig. 2). Results are compared to the ones obtained by using the GP Progression Model [10], which includes a monotonicity constraints on the trajectories. We also test the model with data generated from a single subject and with known time-axis. Results of such simulation are in the Supp. Mat. Synthetic data are generated according to the parameters specified in Table 1. Figure 2(B)-top shows the reconstructed MP trajectories from short-term data in Fig. 2(A), for a two-dimensional test set. We run synthetic tests varying the initial values of the MP parameters, the noise and the number of regions. Then, we compared our estimates of the GP and time-shift parameters with results obtained using the GP Progression Model in [10]. Table 2 shows results in terms of distributions of root

Table 1. Synthetic data generation parameters.

N subjects	N regions	time interval	time–points per subject	noise
50	$\{2, 3, 11, 42\}$	$[0, 15]$	$\{1, 2, 3, 4\}$	$\mathcal{N}(0, \sigma),\ 0.2 \le \sigma \le 0.4$

$\bar{k}_{ij}$	$\bar{k}_t$	γ	η
$\mathcal{U}(0, 1)$	$\mathcal{U}(0, 1/2)$	$\mathcal{U}(1, \max(\frac{C}{2}))$	$\mathcal{U}(\max(\frac{C}{2}), \max(C))$

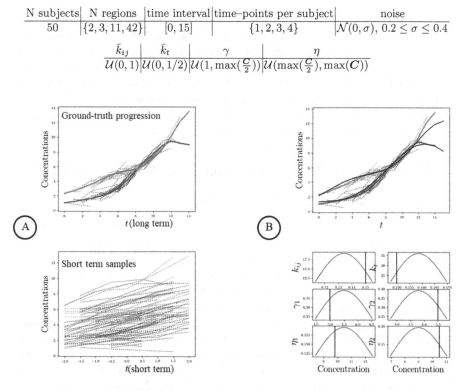

Fig. 2. Results for a 2D example data. (A) ground truth GP progressions and associated short term data used for benchmarking. (B) ground truth and reconstructed (average) long term trajectories, and reconstructed MP parameters distributions, whose ground truth values are indicated by vertical bars.

Table 2. RMSE results for GP fit, time-shifts estimates and dynamical parameters for both the GP Progression Model with monotonicity (GP) and the ACP model. The error for the dynamical parameters is expressed, in percentage, relatively to the ground truth parameters.

		N = 2	N = 3	N = 11	N = 42
Data fit					
RMSE	ACP GP	1.17(0.77)	0.93(0.37)	1.52(0.25)	1.07(0.64)
	Monotonic GP	1.32(0.68)	1.08(0.52)	1.60(0.29)	1.20(0.72)
Time-shift					
RMSE	ACP time-shift	1.67(0.49)	1.92(0.64)	1.53(0.42)	1.19(0.39)
	Monotonic time-shift	1.87(0.44)	1.97(0.58)	1.62(0.42)	1.20(0.41)
Dynamical parameters					
Relative error	ACP GP	6.3%	9.6%	11.4%	21.9%
	Monotonic GP	–	–	–	–

mean squared errors (RMSE), for increasing number of regions. Distributions of RMSE were obtained by sampling 200 times from the estimated distributions. The ACP model generally provides better estimates for the reconstruction of the long term trajectories, as well as for the estimation of the individual time-shift as compared to the standard DPM provided by the monotonic GP. Moreover, while our framework allows the identification of the prescribed dynamical system parameters with high degree of accuracy (Table 2, last row), the monotonic DPM does not allow the estimation of these quantities.

4   Modeling Amyloid Deposition from Imaging Data

4.1   Data Acquisition and Preprocessing

ADNI Data. This study used data from 1091 individuals from ADNI, with a total of 2380 longitudinal measurements. We collected clinical, demographic and AV45-PET SUVr data. All the subjects with either "Dementia", "Mild Cognitive Impairment" or "Cognitively Normal" clinical diagnosis were selected. We controlled for covariates (age, gender, APOE4 genotype, education) and selected 11 macro-regions, i.e. frontal, temporal, parietal, cingulate, thalamus, caudate, putamen, pallidum, hippocampus, amygdala, accumbens, and averaged together all the values of ROIs mapped to the same macro-region, after cerebellum normalization. The macro-region definition was done to reduce computational expenses and aid interpretability of the resulting MP parameters. Demographic and clinical details are in Supp. Mat. We split the data set in two parts: the D1 data set contains all the longitudinal data for each subject up to the second-to-last time points. The remaining time-points were included in a second data set D2. Subjects with one measurement only were included in D1. Data set D1 includes 1651 longitudinal data of 1091 subjects; D2 contains

731 cross-sectional data. We run the models on D1, estimating MP dynamics, GP parameters and individual time-shifts, and used D2 to validate model predictions.

HCP Data. Data used in the preparation of this work were obtained from the MGH-USC Human Connectome Project database. We collected 3D T1w and DTI of 24 age and gender-matched subjects. The pipeline for structural connectome generation is described in [5]. We averaged the 24 connectomes together and obtained an average young, healthy connectome. Finally, we averaged together the regions belonging to the same lobe or subcortical area (to obtain 11 macroregion) and we set to 0 all the weights below the average weights across nodes, and to 1 the weight above. This last step was performed in order to remove the weak connections.

4.2 Estimated Long Term Dynamics

We analyzed the AV45-PET data with two different models of MP kinetics: the ACP model of Eq. (2) - which has non-linear and time-varying dynamics, and a full diffusive model. The diffusion dynamics were prescribed by the system $\dot{c}(t) = Bc(t)$, where the coefficients b_{ij} of B are estimated (along with individual time parameters) with our framework. Figure 3(A) shows the long term trajectories estimated with both models, for four regions. Figure 3(B) shows the time associated to each regional trajectory at which maximal separation between "Cognitively Normal" and "Alzheimer's disease" subjects was measured. The time distribution is inferred from the trajectory distribution associated to each region. The dynamics and orderings of ACP and diffusion provide plausible description of the pathological evolution of amyloid deposition, compatible with previous findings in histo pathological and imaging studies in AD [15,16].

4.3 Predictions Performances of the Models

Figure 3(C) shows the estimated vector fields for the relative dynamics of the frontal and parietal lobes. This vector field is obtained by integrating the dynamical system estimated for respectively ACP and diffusion models. Therefore it does not correspond to extrapolation of the curves in Fig. 3(A). Here the other biomarkers are set constant to their mean values. We can appreciate the nonlinear dynamics of the ACP model, as well as the linear dynamics of the diffusive model. The resulting vector fields provide a tool for interpreting and comparing mechanistic hypotheses. Indeed, Fig. 3(C) shows that the ACP model estimates an initial fast propagation, which slows down with time. The opposite behaviour is observed by analyzing the dynamics of the diffusion model, with an acceleration in the propagation along with the progression. This behaviour is unlikely to reproduce real-case scenarios, where amyloid aggregation eventually slows down and does not accumulates indefinitely. This result points to the higher biological

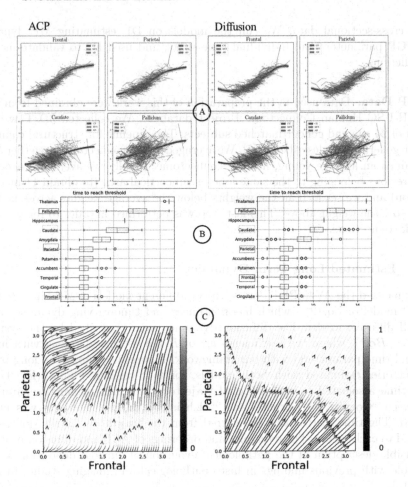

Fig. 3. (A) estimated long term trajectories and individual short term measurements for 4 regions of interest: frontal lobe, parietal lobe, caudate and pallidum, for the two models. (B) ordering derived from the trajectories. Regions visualized in (A) are highlighted. (C) streamlines of the 2D fields in the {Frontal, Parietal} plane.

plausibility of the proposed ACP model. For each subject in D1 with follow-up measurements in D2, we computed the streamline associated with their individual dynamics (in the whole 11-D space), and estimated the values of each biomarker at the corresponding follow-up time. We computed the RMSE for each estimate, and bootstrapped over the MP dynamic parameters 200 times, obtaining RMSE distributions (Table 3).

Table 3. RMSE (mean, sd) for the ACP and the diffusion models estimates. The ACP model generally provides predictions closer to the observed follow-up values.

	frontal	temporal	parietal	cingulate		
ACP	0.21(0.16)	0.18(0.14)	0.20(0.16)	0.20(0.15)		
diffusion	0.25(0.18)	0.25(0.17)	0.22(0.19)	0.24(0.18)		

	thalamus	caudate	putamen	pallidum	hippo	amygdala	accumbens
ACP	0.12(0.09)	0.16(0.12)	0.16(0.13)	0.13(0.10)	0.12(0.09)	0.12(0.10)	0.21(0.15)
diffusion	0.11(0.08)	0.17(0.13)	0.17(0.13)	0.17(0.13)	0.12(0.09)	0.11(0.09)	0.24(0.19)

4.4 Misfolded Proteins Propagation Pathways

Figure 4 shows the connectomes where the edges' colors are set to be proportional to the values of the estimated MP parameters for the ACP model (plot on the left hemisphere), or to the values of the propagation parameters for the diffusive model (plot on the right hemisphere). The parameters have been normalized to $[0, 1]$ to aid comparison. The paths appear to be different for the two models and the ACP model seems to better describe the frontal-posterior pathway known to characterize amyloid deposition in AD [15,16].

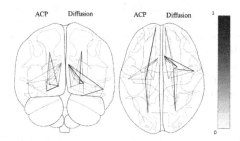

Fig. 4. Coronal and axial views of connectomes with edges' colors proportional to the values of the estimated propagation parameters for either the ACP model (left hemisphere) and the diffusion model (right hemisphere). (Color figure online)

5 Discussion

We presented a spatio-temporal model of MP dynamics over brain networks. The model is based on the joint estimation of long term MP dynamics and time reparametrization of individuals observations, and is expressed within a GP regression setting, where constraints on the MP dynamics are imposed through non-linear dynamical systems, which account for accumulation, clearance and propagation of MP. Experiments on simulated data show that our model accurately recovers prescribed rates along graph dynamics and precisely reconstructs the underlying progression. When applied to AV45-PET brain imaging data our model allows the bio-mechanical interpretation of amyloid deposition in Alzheimer's disease, leading to plausible simulations of MP propagation, and achieving accurate predictions of individual MP deposition in unseen data.

The method has some limitations: first of all, structural connectome estimation using tractography is known to be prone to false positive and negative connections. Nevertheless, here we take an average connectome over multiple young and healthy subjects, which we believe works a reasonable anatomical reference. Another limitation of the model is that it assumes that all subjects follow the same disease progression pattern, which might not be the case in heterogeneous data sets such as ADNI.

The ideas we propose here extend to a much larger range of diseases and alternative models of propagation, such as propagation via functional networks [6,8], or different kind of tractography to represent intra- and extra-axonal propagation [5,7].

References

1. Soto, C., Pritzkow, S.: Protein misfolding, aggregation, and conformational strains in neurodegenerative diseases. Nat. Neurosci. **21**(10), 1332–1340 (2018)
2. Jucker, M., Walker, L.C.: Self-propagation of pathogenic protein aggregates in neurodegenerative diseases. Nature **501**(7465), 45 (2013)
3. Carbonell, F., Iturria-Medina, Y., Evans, A.C.: Mathematical modeling of protein misfolding mechanisms in neurological diseases: a historical overview. Front. Neurol. **9**, 37 (2018)
4. Raj, A., Kuceyeski, A., Weiner, M.: A network diffusion model of disease progression in dementia. Neuron **73**(6), 1204–1215 (2012)
5. Oxtoby, N.P., et al.: Data-driven sequence of changes to anatomical brain connectivity in sporadic Alzheimer's disease. Front. Neurol. **8**, 580 (2017)
6. Zhou, J., Gennatas, E.D., Kramer, J.H., Miller, B.L., Seeley, W.W.: Predicting regional neurodegeneration from the healthy brain functional connectome. Neuron **73**(6), 1216–1227 (2012)
7. Iturria-Medina, Y., Carbonell, F.M., Sotero, R.C., Chouinard-Decorte, F., Evans, A.C.: Multifactorial causal model of brain (dis)organization and therapeutic intervention: application to Alzheimer's disease. Neuroimage **152**, 60–77 (2017)
8. Cauda, F., et al.: Brain structural alterations are distributed following functional, anatomic and genetic connectivity. Brain **141**(11), 3211–3232 (2018)
9. Young, A.L., et al.: A data-driven model of biomarker changes in sporadic Alzheimer's disease. Brain **137**(9), 2564–2577 (2014)
10. Lorenzi, M., Filippone, M., Frisoni, G.B., Alexander, D.C., Ourselin, S., Alzheimer's Disease Neuroimaging Initiative: Probabilistic disease progression modeling to characterize diagnostic uncertainty: application to staging and prediction in Alzheimer's disease. Neuroimage **190**, 56–68 (2019)
11. Schiratti, J.B., Allassonnière, S., Colliot, O., Durrleman, S.: A Bayesian mixed-effects model to learn trajectories of changes from repeated manifold-valued observations. J. Mach. Learn. Res. **18**(1), 4840–4872 (2017)
12. Donohue, M.C., et al.: Estimating long-term multivariate progression from short-term data. Alzheimer's Dementia **10**(5), S400–S410 (2014)

13. Lorenzi, M., Filippone, M.: Constraining the dynamics of deep probabilistic models. In: Proceedings of the 35th International Conference on Machine Learning, vol. 80, pp. 3233–3242 (2018)
14. Cutajar, K., Bonilla, E. V., Michiardi, P., Filippone, M.: Random feature expansions for deep Gaussian processes. In: Proceedings of the 34th International Conference on Machine Learning, vol. 70, pp. 884–893 (2017)
15. Thal, D.R., Rub, U., Orantes, M., Braak, H.: Phases of Aβ-deposition in the human brain and its relevance for the development of AD. Neurology **58**(12), 1791–1800 (2002)
16. Irvine, G.B., El-Agnaf, O.M., Shankar, G.M., Walsh, D.M.: Protein aggregation in the brain: the molecular basis for Alzheimer's and Parkinson's diseases. Mol. Med. **14**(7–8), 451–464 (2008)

Deep Learning

InceptionGCN: Receptive Field Aware Graph Convolutional Network for Disease Prediction

Anees Kazi[1]([✉]), Shayan Shekarforoush[2], S. Arvind Krishna[3],
Hendrik Burwinkel[1], Gerome Vivar[1,4], Karsten Kortüm[5],
Seyed-Ahmad Ahmadi[4], Shadi Albarqouni[1], and Nassir Navab[1,6]

[1] Computer Aided Medical Procedures (CAMP), Technical University of Munich,
Munich, Germany
anees.kazi@tum.de
[2] Sharif University of Technology, Tehran, Iran
[3] Department of Computer Science and Engineering,
National Institute of Technology Tiruchirappalli, Tiruchirappalli, India
[4] German Center for Vertigo and Balance Disorders,
Ludwig Maximilians Universität München, Munich, Germany
[5] Augenklinik der Universität, Klinikum der Universität München, Munich, Germany
[6] Whiting School of Engineering, Johns Hopkins University, Baltimore, USA

Abstract. Geometric deep learning provides a principled and versatile manner for integration of imaging and non-imaging modalities in the medical domain. Graph Convolutional Networks (GCNs) in particular have been explored on a wide variety of problems such as disease prediction, segmentation, and matrix completion by leveraging large, multimodal datasets. In this paper, we introduce a new spectral domain architecture for deep learning on graphs for disease prediction. The novelty lies in defining geometric 'inception modules' which are capable of capturing intra- and inter-graph structural heterogeneity during convolutions. We design filters with different kernel sizes to build our architecture. We show our disease prediction results on two publicly available datasets. Further, we provide insights on the behaviour of regular GCNs and our proposed model under varying input scenarios on simulated data.

1 Introduction

There is an increasing focus on applying deep learning on unstructured data in the medical domain, especially using Graph Convolutional Networks (GCNs) [1]. Multiple applications have been demonstrated so far, including Autism Spectrum Disorder prediction with manifold learning to distinguish between diseased and healthy brains [2], matrix completion to predict the missing values in medical data [3], and finding drug similarity using graph auto encoders [4]. In this paper, we study the task of Alzheimer and Autism disease prediction with complementary imaging and non-imaging multi-modal data.

© Springer Nature Switzerland AG 2019
A. C. S. Chung et al. (Eds.): IPMI 2019, LNCS 11492, pp. 73–85, 2019.
https://doi.org/10.1007/978-3-030-20351-1_6

In above works, GCNs had a remarkable impact on the usage of multi-modal medical data. One key difference to previous learning-based methods is to set patients in relation to each other with a neighborhood graph, often by associating them through non-imaging data like gender, age, clinical scores or other meta-information. On this graph, patients can be considered as nodes, patient similarities are represented as edge weights and features from e.g. imaging modalities are incorporated through graph signal processing. GCNs then provide a principled manner for learning optimal graph filters that minimize a objective. Here, we use node-level classification for our disease prediction task.

A simple analogy to node-based classification of the population is image segmentation with CNNs, where each pixel is a node and the image grid is the graph. In such domains, filters with a constant size can manage to acquire semantic features over the whole grid domain, given convolutions over a constant number of equidistant neighbors. In the case of irregular graphs, the number of neighbors and their distance from each other leads to heterogeneous density and local structure. Applying filters with constant kernel size over the whole grid domain might not produce semantic and comparable features.

In medical datasets, graphs defined on patient's data observe similar heterogeneity, as each patient may have a distinct combination of non-imaging data and different number of neighbors. A concrete example is shown in Fig. 1 (left), which depicts a population graph of 150 subjects for Alzheimer's disease classification, who are arranged in clusters of varying density and local topology (regions a, b and c). Such heterogeneity in the graph structure should be considered to learn cluster-specific features. A model capable of producing similar intra-cluster and different inter-cluster features can be designed by applying multi-sized kernels on the same input. To this end, we propose InceptionGCN, inspired by the successful inception [5] architecture for CNNs. Our model leverages spectral convolutions with different kernel sizes and chooses optimal features to solve the classification problem.

To the best of our knowledge, there is not much related literature that focuses on receptive fields of GCN filters. Earlier works [1,6] use GCNs with constant filter size for the node-based classification task and show the superiority of GCN but do not address the problem of heterogeneity of the graph. In [7], a method is proposed that determines a receptive path for each node rather than a field for performing the convolutions for representation learning. Irrespective of nearest neighbors, the aim is to perform convolutions with selective nodes in the receptive field. In [8], a DenseNet-like architecture [9] is proposed, in which outputs from consecutive layers are concatenated. Here, the receptive field is addressed in an indirect way since the output features of successive layers depend on multiple previous layers through skip connections. Another work [10] uses features that are either fixed, hand-designed or based on aggregator-functions. Moreover, the method needs a pre-defined order of nodes which is difficult to obtain.

In this paper we show that InceptionGCN is an improvement in terms of performance and convergence. Our contributions are: (1) we analyze the interdependence of graph structure and filter sizes on one artificial and two public medical datasets and in doing so, we motivate the need for multiple kernel size. (2) We propose our novel InceptionGCN model with multiple filter kernel sizes. We validate it on artificial and clinical data and the show improved performance over regular GCN architectures. (3) We demonstrate the robustness of our model towards different approaches for constructing graph adjacency from non-imaging data.

2   Methodology

Traditional models [11] use a constant filter size throughout all layers, which forces the features of every node to be learned using neighbors at a fixed number of hops away without consideration of cluster size and shape. Our proposed InceptionGCN model overcomes this limitation by varying the filters' size across the GC-layers in order to produce class separable output features. This property of our model is highly desirable when each class distribution has distinct variance and/or when the classes are heavily overlapping. Utilizing this setting, we target to solve the disease classification task by incorporating semantics of varied associations coming from different graphs within the population. We provide a detailed description of the model starting from the affinity graph construction followed by the mathematical background and a discussion of the proposed model architecture.

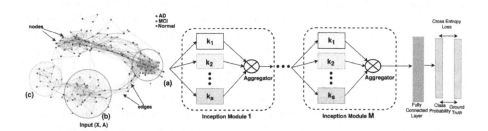

Fig. 1. Left: Affinity graph with clusters for TADPOLE dataset, different cluster sizes are depicted at points (a), (b) and (c). Right: Setup of InceptionGCN, feature matrix X is processed by several GC-layers with considered neighborhood $k_1, \cdots, k_S$ in each inception module. The output of each layer is used in the aggregator function.

2.1   Affinity Graph Construction

The construction of an affinity graph is crucial to accurately model the interactions among the patients and should be designed carefully. The affinity graph $G = (V, E, W)$ is constructed on the entire population (including training and testing samples) of the patients, where $|V| = $ N vertices, E are the edge connections of the graph and W are the weights of the edges. Considering each patient as a node n_i in the graph, G incorporates the similarities between the patients with respect to the non-imaging data η. The features $x_i \in \mathbb{R}^N$ at every node n_i are fetched from imaging data. First, we construct a binarized edge graph $E \in \mathbb{R}^{N \times N}$ representing the connections. Mathematically, E can be defined as

$$E_{i,j} = \begin{cases} 1 \; if \; |\eta_i - \eta_j| < \beta \\ 0 \quad otherwise \end{cases} \tag{1}$$

where η_i and η_j are the values of the non-imaging element for nodes i and j and β is the threshold for that element. The weight matrix $W \in \mathbb{R}^{N \times N}$ weights the edges based on the correlation distance between the features at every node. The weight matrix elements are defined as $W_{i,j} = Sim(x_i, x_j)$, where $Sim(x_i, x_j) = exp(-\frac{[\rho(x_i, x_j)]^2}{2\sigma^2})$ with ρ being the 'correlation distance' and σ being the width of the kernel. This weight computation and value of β is identical to the procedure described in [11], to provide equal grounds for comparison. The final affinity matrix A is constructed as $A = W \circ E$ with $\circ$ being the Hadamard product.

2.2 Mathematical Background of Spectral Convolution and Localization of Filters for Inception Modules

Let $L = I_N - D^{-\frac{1}{2}}AD^{-\frac{1}{2}}$ be the normalized version of the graph Laplacian of G including self loops. D is the diagonal matrix with $D_{ii} = \sum_j A_{ij}$, $I_N \in \mathbb{R}^{N \times N}$ being the identity matrix. Since L is real positive and semi-definite, it is diagonalizable by its eigen vectors $U \in \mathbb{R}^{N \times N}$ such that $L = U\Lambda U^T$, where $\Lambda = diag(\lambda_0, \lambda_1, \ldots \lambda_{N-1}) \in \mathbb{R}^{N \times N}$ are the corresponding eigen values. The graph Fourier Transform of a signal x at each node is defined as $\widehat{x} = U^T x \in \mathbb{R}^N$, the inverse Fourier Transform as $x = U\widehat{x} \in \mathbb{R}^N$. With this information, the spectral convolution can be defined as a multiplication of the signal x with a learnable filter $g_\theta = diag(\theta)$ in the Fourier domain, which results in $y = U g_\theta(\Lambda) U^T x = g_\theta(U\Lambda U^T) x = g_\theta(L) x$ interpreting g_θ as a function of the eigenvalues Λ [6]. In order to prevent the computationally prohibitive matrix multiplication necessary to perform the Fourier Transform of signal x, we redefine g_θ using the Chebyshev polynomial parameterization of the filter $g_\theta(\Lambda) = \sum_{r=0}^k \theta_r T_r(\Lambda)$, where $\theta \in \mathbb{R}^k$ is a vector of Chebyshev coefficients with degree k [1,6]. Since $L^k = (U\Lambda U^T)^k = U\Lambda^k U^T$, we can write $g_\theta(\Lambda)$ as a function of $g_\theta(L)$. Therefore, we can perform the spectral filtering on a signal x with $g_\theta * x = \sum_{r=0}^k \theta_r T_r(L)x$. The value of vertex j of the filter g_θ centered at vertex i is given by

$$(g_\theta(L)\delta_i)_j = (g_\theta(L))_{ij} = \sum_k \theta_k (L^k)_{ij} \tag{2}$$

where δ_i is Kronecker delta function. Inspired by [12], here we explain how the filters of specific receptive fields can be derived. Let G be a weighted graph, L be the graph Laplacian (normalized or unnormalized), and $k > 0$ be an integer (here k stands for the kth hop neighbor), then for any two vertices i and j:

$$(L^k)_{ij} = \begin{cases} \Omega \; d_G(i,j) \leq k \\ 0 \quad otherwise \end{cases} \tag{3}$$

where $d_G(i,j)$ is the shortest path distance between x_i and x_j and Ω is the sum of all edge weights on the shortest path from x_i to x_j. Therefore from Eq. 2 the spectral filters represented by k^{th} order polynomial of the Laplacian are exactly k-hop localized.

2.3   Inception Modules

The localization of a filter is defined by taking all the neighbors at a distance of k hops into account for the spectral convolution with a signal x. A filter s with a fixed k_s used on the full dataset X can be defined as $y_s = \sum_{r=1}^{k_s} T_r(L)X\theta_{r,s}$. Here, y_s describes the output of a filter with neighborhood in k_s-hop distance. To account for different sizes and variances of clusters and structure in the data, instead of using one filter we now use S filters with varying neighborhood k_s. These combined filters s are the centerpiece of the inception module as they simultaneously consider the close proximity of a signal x and the broader neighborhood situation. Every filter of the module has its own parameter vector θ_s and performs a convolution on the dataset X for returning an output vector y_s. The outputs of each filter are merged in an aggregator-function Ψ to determine the output y of the inception module as $y = \Psi(y_1, \cdots, y_S)$ where every $\theta_s \in \mathbb{R}^{k_s}$ with entries $\theta_{r,s}$ is the learnable parameter vector for each filter of the inception module. To merge the output of each inception module we propose two aggregators Ψ, (1) concatenation and (2) max-pooling. Our model architecture is illustrated in Fig. 1. It is built with M inception modules. Each inception module consist of S_m GC-layers in parallel with filters of different $k_{s,m}$. We apply ReLU at the output of each GC-layer. For the training set, a labelled subset of graph nodes is chosen, for which the loss is computed and gradients are back-propagated. We apply cross-entropy loss as the optimization function. Due to the graph connections, the training process on the labelled data is transferred to the unlabeled data by signal diffusion which corresponds to the behavior of a standard GCN.

3   Experiments and Results

In this section, we provide two main experimental setups to show (1) the sensitivity of spectral convolutions to different graphs and kernel sizes of the filters and (2) superiority of the InceptionGCN to other baseline methods. We show our results on two multi-modal medical datasets and thoroughly analyze both the baseline [11] and the proposed model. At last, we provide insights into generalized design choices for building a data and task-specific model.

3.1   Datasets

TADPOLE [13]: This dataset is a subset of the Alzheimer's Disease Neuroimaging Initiative (adni.loni.usc.edu), consisting of 557 patients with 354 multi-modal features per patient. The target is to classify each patient into one of the three classes (Cognitively Normal (CN), Mild Cognitive Impairments (MCI) or Alzheimer's Disease (AD). Features are extracted from MR and PET imaging, cognitive tests, CSF and clinical assessments. The protein class APOE constitutes another factor assisting in patient classification. Testing this gene status provides a risk factor of developing AD. FDG-PET imaging measures the brain cell metabolism, where cells affected by AD show reduced metabolism. Furthermore, demographics are provided (age, gender). We construct a binarized graph with each element of demographic data, APOE status and FDG PET measures. We choose $\beta = 2$ for age and $\beta = 0$ for the rest of the three respectively. The edges are based on the $Sim(x_i, x_j)$ i.e. the feature similarity measure. We construct the 'Mixed' affinity graph by averaging all the graphs weighted with W and'Mixed (noSim)' without weighting.

ABIDE [14]: The Autism Brain Imaging Data Exchange (ABIDE) aggregates data from 20 different sites and openly shares 1112 existing resting-state functional magnetic resonance imaging (R-fMRI) datasets with corresponding phenotypic elements (gender) for 2 classes normal and with Autism Spectrum Disorder (ASD). We choose 871 subjects divided into normal (468) and ASD diseased (403) subjects. For fair comparison, we follow the same pre-processing step as performed in the baseline method [11]. We construct two affinity graphs for non-imaging elements, gender and site, by choosing $\beta = 0$ for both graphs.

3.2   Experiments on Medical Datasets

In this subsection we present both the experimental setups mentioned above and discuss our findings on the medical datasets.

Effect of Different Kernel Size on Spectral Convolution: Our first set of experiments is designed to investigate the optimal kernel size of the filter required for each graph. The baseline model [11] with two GC-layers in sequence is used to find out the required graph specific filter sizes (i.e. value of k). We investigate the performance of the model with the same input (features and graph) and k_1 and $k_2 \in [1, 6]$. Here $k=1$ and $k=6$ indicate the kernel size of one-hop (smallest) and six-hop neighbors (largest) respectively. We select the value of two k corresponding to the best performance in the heatmap and incorporate them to our proposed InceptionGCN model as different kernel sizes. Like this, it is guaranteed that the sequential GCN is performing at its optimum when compared to our method. We discuss the validity of this setting in the later section.

Results: Figure 2 shows the corresponding results in terms of heatmaps. Smaller k learn local features and larger k learn global features. The performance differs with the change in k_1 and k_2 by a margin of 8% on average. It indicates that spectral convolution models are sensitive to the selection of k. The accuracy increases with the value of k, but becomes consistent with further increase. For most of the graphs $k_1 > k_2$ is the best combination, since the initial layer filters

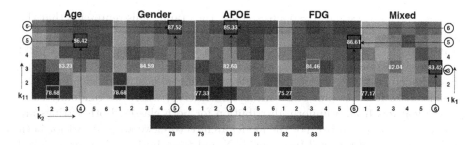

Fig. 2. Heat maps for representing the performance of GCN on the TADPOLE dataset with varying kernel size of the filters. Each heat map comes from the distinct graph mentioned above. The highest and lowest performing combination of k_1 and k_2 are highlighted with a black box and the corresponding k-values are shown.

look at global features. Each affinity graph shows a different structure over the same vertices and shows varied results over the same combination of the two k. A similar trend is seen for ABIDE, which reassures the concept of sensitivity towards k.

Comparison of InceptionGCN Against Sequential GCN Approaches: We show the comparison with four baselines. Parisot et al. [11] is the traditional GCN with $k_1 = k_2 = 3$. We modify the same architecture of [11] with the best combination of the two k mentioned as baseline $[k_1, k_2]$. We evaluate our aggregator-function Ψ for a proper selection of activations from all the individual GC-layers of the inception module by comparing them to the baseline $[k_1, k_1]$ and $[k_2, k_2]$. This comparison shows that Ψ is not biased towards any particular kernel size. With such setting for all methods, each graph yields a different performance, showing the effect of the different neighborhood affinity as shown in Table 2. Our model outperforms the baselines [11] by an average margin of 4.12% for TADPOLE dataset.

The comparative results for ABIDE are given in Table 3. Our model performs comparable to the baseline [11], but is not able to outperform it. Interestingly, the mixed graph with feature-based edge weighting performs worse than the weighting case. This confirms the non-discriminative nature of the features. Images collected from different sites make it harder for the model to learn class-discriminative features.

3.3   Experiments on Simulated Data

Seeing the contradictory performance on the two datasets, we investigate the model in detail for better understanding of the spectral model and to interpret better design choices for user-specific tasks. These experiments are specifically designed to investigate only the choice of the kernel size of the filters.

We generate two 2-dimensional clusters C_1 and C_2 having normal Gaussian distributions with 300 points each in Euclidean domain, each distribution representing one class. We construct the graph based on Euclidean distance between the features and $\beta = 0.5$ to sparsify the graph. This represents that the graph is highly correlated to the labels. In order to keep the experiment easy to interpret, we set means $[m_1, m_2] = [-1, 1]$ for C_1 and C_2 respectively and vary the corresponding variances v_1 and v_2. For features we show two settings: **class-discriminative**, where the (x, y)-values of the location of each point are considered as features and **class-indiscriminative**, where we randomly sample the features from a uniform distribution for both classes. Both settings are shown in Fig. 3(a) and (b). For the model architecture, we keep $M = 1$ for both the baseline model [11] and InceptionGCN and train both the networks at 200 epochs, with learning rate = 0.2.

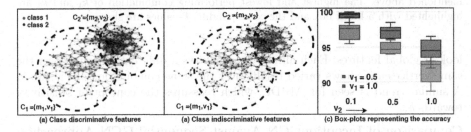

(a) Class discriminative features   (a) Class indiscriminative features   (c) Box-plots representing the accuracy

Fig. 3. (a) Represents the scenario of simulated data, where we change variances v_1 and v_2, (b) shows the scenario where the features are sampled from random distribution, (c) shows the variation in the performance in terms of accuracy for all the combinations of v_1 and v_2 for scenario (a).

Results and Interpretation: The results of this experiment are illustrated with boxplots in Fig. 3(c). Each box shows the accuracy of the classification for different values of k ranging from 1 to 10 for the baseline model for class-discriminative features. Keeping $v_1 = 0.5$, we vary v_2 for [0.1, 0.5, 1.0]. We repeat the experiments with $v_1 = 1.0$. It can be interpreted that when two clusters are clearly separable, the model is less sensitive to the value of k. Also it can be seen from the last two boxplots that with higher variance, the model becomes sensitive to k. Similar trends are observed when the value of v_1 is changed to 1.0, however a consistent drop in accuracy is observed with $v_1 = 1.0$. If there is large variance in the data, filters with larger receptive field will produce generalized global features.

Further, we apply our model to the simulated data with only one Inception module incorporating two GC-layers with different $[k_1, k_2] = [1, 10]$. We compare the results of a single-layered GCN with $k = [1, 5, 10]$ with the one layered inception module for four different settings. The superiority of our model is seen mainly in the challenging scenarios, where the variance of both classes is quite high (i.e. $v_1 = 1.0$ and $v_2 = 1.0$, cf. Table 1). Here, we report the results for class indiscriminative features, where the performance drastically drops when features are totally random for all the models. InceptionGCN outperforms the baseline in most of the cases.

4   Discussion and Conclusion

In this work we have introduced InceptionGCN, a novel architecture that captures the local and global context of heterogeneous graph structures with multiple kernel sizes. The validation included an investigation of spectral convolution parameters and the behaviour of the proposed model given varying input data, in comparison to a recently proposed baseline method [11]. Our findings show that applying different sized filters on the same input features and graph improves the process of feature learning at multi-scale levels. Such rich and heterogeneous features help the model to learn better filters for classification. We tested the method on two publicly available medical datasets for Alzheimer's and Autism disease prediction, in order to analyze the robustness of the model towards different features, graph affinities and tasks. Our results show that both the spectral convolution and the proposed model obtained high classification accuracies for TADPOLE (cf. Table 2), with a clear margin of InceptionGCN

Table 1. The performance of the model in terms of accuracy is represented in the table. v_1 and v_2 represent the variances of 2 classes of the simulated 2D Gaussian data. (a) In these cases the graph and corresponding features are highly correlated to the classes, whereas in (b) only the graph is correlated to the classes.

$v_1 = 0.5$				$v_1 = 1.0$	
	k	$v_2 = 0.1$	$v_2 = 1.0$	$v_2 = 0.1$	$v_2 = 1.0$
(a)	1	**98.50 ± 01.38**	94.50 ± 01.83	**95.67 ± 02.49**	92.50 ± 02.61
	10	**99.00 ± 01.11**	93.67 ± 04.93	**95.50 ± 07.98**	91.00 ± 04.42
	Inception-GCN (1 layer [k1, k2] = [1, 10])	94.83 ± 03.02	**97.00 ± 02.56**	92.00 ± 03.56	**94.33 ± 03.56**
(b)	1	49.33 ± 06.84	50.33 ± 07.48	49.50 ± 04.60	50.00 ± 06.28
	10	60.33 ± 16.78	53.50 ± 10.99	**50.83 ± 06.02**	55.33 ± 14.79
	Inception-GCN (1 layer [k1, k2] = [1, 10])	**66.50 ± 17.12**	**64.00 ± 17.95**	48.00 ± 07.88	**69.00 ± 24.79**

Table 2. Depicts the mean accuracies from stratified k-fold cross validation for all the setups of experiments for TADPOLE. The values of the chosen $[k_1, k_2]$ for the graphs are highlighted in the Fig. 2.

Affinity	Age	Gender	APOE	FDG	Mixed	Mixed (noSim)
Parisot et al. [11]	82.55 ± 04.78	84.59 ± 04.82	82.68 ± 05.70	84.46 ± 05.46	82.04 ± 05.71	82.11 ± 04.94
Baselines						
$[k_1, k_2]$	86.42 ± 03.95	87.52 ± 03.51	85.33 ± 04.75	86.61 ± 04.53	83.42 ± 05.93	81.95 ± 05.92
$[k_1, k_1]$	85.46 ± 05.6	86.19 ± 04.91	85.08 ± 05.21	86.55 ± 04.55	81.85 ± 06.28	81.36 ± 05.98
$[k_2, k_2]$	86.42 ± 03.98	84.59 ± 04.82	78.75 ± 04.45	84.46 ± 05.46	80.86 ± 05.69	80.99 ± 04.71
InceptionGCN						
Concat	**88.35 ± 03.03**	**88.06 ± 04.39**	**88.14 ± 03.20**	**86.99 ± 03.98**	**84.35 ± 06.97**	**83.62 ± 06.09**
Max-pool	**88.53 ± 03.27**	**88.19 ± 03.83**	**88.49 ± 03.05**	**87.65 ± 05.11**	**84.11 ± 04.50**	**83.87 ± 05.07**

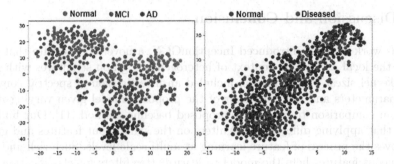

Fig. 4. TSNE embedding in 2-dimensional space visualized on raw features for TAD-POLE (left) and ABIDE (right) datasets.

Table 3. Depicts the mean accuracy from stratified k-fold Cross Validation for all the setups of experiments for ABIDE. The baseline values of $[k_1, k_2]$ are [4, 5], [6, 5] and [4, 4] for Gender, Site and Mixed, Mixed (noSim) respectively.

Affinity	Gender	Site	Mixed	Mixed (noSim)
Parisot et al. [11]	67.39 ± 04.76	67.39 ± 01.49	67.85 ± 00.63	69.80 ± 04.35
Baselines				
$[k_1, k_2]$	$\mathbf{68.19 \pm 05.38}$	$\mathbf{69.00 \pm 04.07}$	$\mathbf{70.26 \pm 03.70}$	$\mathbf{70.26 \pm 04.58}$
$[k_1, k_1]$	66.70 ± 06.90	68.65 ± 04.31	69.91 ± 07.50	69.80 ± 03.90
$[k_2, k_2]$	65.78 ± 06.50	68.65 ± 04.31	69.00 ± 03.80	69.46 ± 04.69
Inception-GCN				
Concat	66.36 ± 05.66	67.97 ± 04.43	66.70 ± 06.27	69.23 ± 06.66
Max-pool	67.05 ± 05.47	67.39 ± 05.80	66.02 ± 05.92	69.11 ± 06.68

over the baselines. In the case of the ABIDE dataset, however, both methods had comparable performance, which was considerably lower than on TADPOLE (cf. Table 3). To investigate the different performances of both models, we utilized simulated data with (i) different degrees of class overlap in the feature space and (ii) entirely random features, forcing the GCN models to rely on connectivity alone (Table 1). It can be concluded that while both GCN models are very sensitive to variance of data, our model shows the superiority in case of having large variances and overlapping of class clusters. The main factors affecting the performance of GCN are features, graph and filters. With all the experiments we discuss all the factors in detail.

Influence of the Graph: For the ABIDE dataset, images are collected from 20 different sites and imaging conditions, which adds considerable heterogeneity to the data. Consequently, the affinity graph based on site information consists of 20 disjoint clusters. Building a graph based on site information allows only the neighbors (i.e. samples from the same site) to contribute to the feature learning. This has less clinical relevance to the classification task, whereas for TADPOLE, the risk factors and demographics are clinically relevant. Such relevance of the graph can be determined using the graphs' energy function provided in [15]. Next, the mixed affinity graph performs worst overall in terms of accuracy (cf. Tables 2 and 3) and Standard Deviation (SD) (cf. Table 3). This indicates that a straightforward creation of the mixed affinity graph by averaging impairs the inherent structure of each graph, and important clinical semantics from individual graphs may get lost. This is confirmed by the unequal performance observed for each affinity graph, which may even indicate a ranking of relevance of each non-imaging element to the objective. A more elegant way to combine all the affinity graphs is by ranking them while training [16].

Influence of the Features: The importance of a proper feature choice becomes clear in the tests on simulated data. When using randomly sampled features for every node (cf. Table 1) the overall performance drops drastically. A large standard deviation in the performance shows that filters are not learned properly and the model does not converge. The same behavior can be seen for the TAD-POLE and ABIDE dataset when comparing the mixed and mixed (noSim) (cf. Tables 2 and 3). Since the features of the ABIDE dataset are not distinguishing the nodes into different clusters compared to the TADPOLE dataset (Fig. 4), the performance of the models drops for ABIDE when using the feature similarity (Sim), which is used for graph construction. At the same time, the models receive a performance boost when the meaningful features of TADPOLE are included into the graph generation process.

Influence of the Kernel Size: We investigated the effect of features and heterogeneity of the graph towards the choice of k. Our results show that in case of class separable features, a larger value of k will give more compact features. From Table 3, it is clear that InceptionGCN performs better in case that the classes have large and different variances. In such a case, InceptionGCN with multiple k_s manages to capture the class discriminative features for the nodes. If the clusters are compact ($v = 0.1$) the choice of k does not matter. From Fig. 3(c), we see that the model is not sensitive to k if the clusters are compact, whereas it becomes sensitive when the variance increases. In case of class indiscriminative features and a less relevant graph (as is the case of ABIDE) a larger kernel size helps to learn global class discriminative feature.

Sequential Model vs. InceptionGCN: Choosing the values of the two k from sequential model (GCN) for a parallel setting might seem ambiguous. In Table 2, the role of the aggregator-function is clearly visible in the performance, since the baselines are all the possible combinations that the final output of our model can get. Furthermore, our proposed model converges 1.63 times faster in terms of epochs compared to the baseline method when trained with early stopping criteria with window size of 25 due to a better feature learning process.

Future Scope: Potential improvements of the InceptionGCN model include out-of-sample inference (i.e. inductive learning), which will highly improve the usability of the model. Another area of investigation is the integration of multiple affinity graphs into one model. Furthermore, the InceptionGCN model structure itself can also be optimized, first by using a learnable pre-processing step to obtain the neighborhood values k, and second, by analyzing the number of hidden units in each GC-layer and the overall number of inception modules necessary.

Acknowledgement. The authors would like to thank Dr. Benedikt Westler for his help and support in understanding the TADPOLE dataset. The study was carried out with financial support of Freunde und Förderer der Augenklinik, München, Germany, Carl Zeiss Meditec AG, Oberkochen, Germany and the German Federal Ministry of Education and Research (BMBF) in connection with the foundation of the German Center for Vertigo and Balance Disorders (DSGZ) (grant number 01 EO 0901).

References

1. Defferrard, M., Bresson, X., Vandergheynst, P.: Convolutional neural networks on graphs with fast localized spectral filtering. In: Advances in Neural Information Processing Systems, pp. 3844–3852 (2016)
2. Ktena, S.I., et al.: Metric learning with spectral graph convolutions on brain connectivity networks. NeuroImage **169**, 431–442 (2018)
3. Vivar, G., Zwergal, A., Navab, N., Ahmadi, S.-A.: Multi-modal disease classification in incomplete datasets using geometric matrix completion. In: Stoyanov, D., et al. (eds.) GRAIL/Beyond MIC-2018. LNCS, vol. 11044, pp. 24–31. Springer, Cham (2018). https://doi.org/10.1007/978-3-030-00689-1_3
4. Ma, T., Xiao, C., Zhou, J., Wang, F.: Drug similarity integration through attentive multi-view graph auto-encoders. arXiv preprint arXiv:1804.10850 (2018)
5. Szegedy, C., et al.: Going deeper with convolutions. In: Proceedings of the IEEE Conference on CVPR, pp. 1–9 (2015)
6. Kipf, T.N., Welling, M.: Semi-supervised classification with graph convolutional networks. arXiv preprint arXiv:1609.02907 (2016)
7. Liu, Z., Chen, C., Li, L., Zhou, J., Li, X., Song, L.: GeniePath: graph neural networks with adaptive receptive paths. arXiv preprint arXiv:1802.00910 (2018)
8. Xu, K., Li, C., Tian, Y., Sonobe, T., Kawarabayashi, K.-I., Jegelka, S.: Representation learning on graphs with jumping knowledge networks. arXiv preprint arXiv:1806.03536 (2018)
9. Huang, G., Liu, Z., Van Der Maaten, L., Weinberger, K.Q.: Densely connected convolutional networks. In: CVPR, vol. 1, p. 3 (2017)
10. Hamilton, W., Ying, Z., Leskovec, J.: Inductive representation learning on large graphs. In: Advances in Neural Information Processing Systems, pp. 1024–1034 (2017)
11. Parisot, S., et al.: Spectral graph convolutions for population-based disease prediction. In: Descoteaux, M., Maier-Hein, L., Franz, A., Jannin, P., Collins, D.L., Duchesne, S. (eds.) MICCAI 2017. LNCS, vol. 10435, pp. 177–185. Springer, Cham (2017). https://doi.org/10.1007/978-3-319-66179-7_21
12. Hammond, D.K., Vandergheynst, P., Gribonval, R.: Wavelets on graphs via spectral graph theory. Appl. Comput. Harmonic Anal. **30**(2), 129–150 (2011)
13. Marinescu, R.V., et al.: TADPOLE challenge: prediction of longitudinal evolution in Alzheimer's disease. arXiv preprint arXiv:1805.03909 (2018)
14. Abraham, A., et al.: Deriving reproducible biomarkers from multi-site resting-state data: an autism-based example. NeuroImage **147**, 736–745 (2017)

15. Gansner, E.R., Hu, Y., Krishnan, S.: COAST: a convex optimization approach to stress-based embedding. In: Wismath, S., Wolff, A. (eds.) GD 2013. LNCS, vol. 8242, pp. 268–279. Springer, Cham (2013). https://doi.org/10.1007/978-3-319-03841-4_24

16. Kazi, A., Albarqouni, S., Kortuem, K., Navab, N.: Multi layered-parallel graph convolutional network (ML-PGCN) for disease prediction. arXiv preprint arXiv:1804.10776 (2018)

Adaptive Graph Convolution Pooling
for Brain Surface Analysis

Karthik Gopinath$^{(\boxtimes)}$, Christian Desrosiers, and Herve Lombaert

ETS Montreal, Montreal, Canada
`karthik.gopinath.1@etsmtl.net`

Abstract. Learning surface data is fundamental to neuroscience. Recent advances has enabled the use of graph convolution filters directly within neural network frameworks. These filters are, however, constrained to a single fixed-graph structure. A pooling strategy remains yet to be defined for learning graph-node data in non-predefined graph structures. This lack of flexibility in graph convolutional architectures currently limits applications on brain surfaces. Graph structures and number of mesh nodes, indeed, highly vary across brain geometries. This paper proposes a new general graph-based pooling method for processing full-sized surface-valued data, as input layers of graph neural networks, towards predicting subject-based variables, as output information. This novel method learns an intrinsic aggregation of input graph nodes based on the geometry of the input graph. This is leveraged using recent advances in spectral graph alignment where the surface parameterization becomes common across multiple brain geometries. These novel adaptive intrinsic pooling layers enable the exploration of entirely new architectures of graph neural networks, which were previously constrained to one single fixed structure in a dataset. We demonstrate the flexibility of the new pooling strategy in two proof-of-concept applications, namely, the classification of disease stages and regression of subject's ages using directly the surface data from varying mesh geometries.

1 Introduction

The analysis of brain surface data is essential for understanding the underlying mechanisms of cognition and perception. This surface has, however, a complex geometry. Its complex folding notably hinders current computational approaches for analyzing brain imaging data. Existing methods [1] are either volumetric or surface-based. On the one hand, volumetric approaches [2] operates over the whole brain, which is ideal for studying the brain fiber structure within the brain. The volumetric representation of imaging data, however, mostly ignore the geometry of the brain surface. Neighboring voxels in a volume may be quite far apart on the surface of a brain (see Fig. 1), posing a challenge for analyzing surface data. On the other hand, surface-based approaches [3,4] often over simplify the brain geometry to a sphere. Although topologically equivalent, the

© Springer Nature Switzerland AG 2019
A. C. S. Chung et al. (Eds.): IPMI 2019, LNCS 11492, pp. 86–98, 2019.
https://doi.org/10.1007/978-3-030-20351-1_7

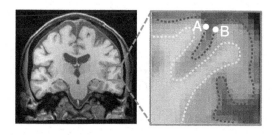

Fig. 1. Complex geometry of the cerebral cortex. As illustrated, two nearby points in the volume may in fact be far apart on the cortical surface.

important metric distortions, between a brain surface and a sphere, severely burden computations. For instance, FreeSurfer [3], a widely popular framework for brain analysis, requires several hours to inflate a brain into a sphere and parcellate its surface. Spherical harmonics approaches [5] also fundamentally rely on a spherical simplification of the brain.

Machine learning approaches has made recent breakthroughs in computer vision. In particular, convolutional neural networks [6] offer a computational advantage in terms of speed and accuracy over conventional approaches. They are, for instance, used in brain imaging for image segmentation [7,8]. However, they were limited to grid-structured data, such as images or volumes organized in a lattice. Recent advances [9–12] enable convolution operations over graphs by exploiting spectral analysis where convolutions translates into multiplications in a Fourier space. Convolutions are manipulated with eigenfunctions of graph Laplacian operators [13], approximated with Chebyshev [11] or Cayley polynomials [14]. These learned convolution filters are expressed in terms of mixtures of Gaussians [12] or splines [15]. These methods are, however, limited to a fixed graph structure, inadequate for brain imaging. Brain surfaces have, indeed, varying geometries with non-fixed degrees of nodes and edges across meshes. These variabilities pose a geometrical challenge [16] since the values of a Laplacian eigenfunction can drastically differ between brains with different surface geometries. To this effect, a learned synchronization [17] corrects for changes in eigenfunctions. An alignment of eigenbases [18] similarly provides a common parameterization of brain surfaces. Such aligned eigenbases enabled the direct learning of surface data across multiple brain geometries [19]. The architecture of these graph convolutional neural networks are, however, limited to use fixed sizes across hidden layers since pooling strategies remain to be defined on graph neural networks. Currently, heuristics are often used to mimic max pooling strategies [9,11,20]. They include varying the number of feature dimensions across layers [9] while retaining fixed sizes of layers, or relying on binary trees [11] or Graclus clustering methods [20] to coarsen the initial graph. They usually constrain choices of sizes in hidden layers or, more generally, architectural flexibility in pooling operations. This limits graph convolutional networks to fixed

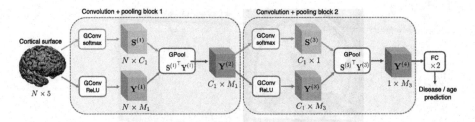

Fig. 2. An overview of the proposed graph convolutional network for subject-specific cortical surface analysis.

architectures or point-wise operations [12], such as node classification [21]. This limitation prevents, for instance, whole subject classification of diseases under graphs of varying sizes.

This paper proposes a new geometric, adaptive pooling strategy for graph convolutional networks. Its flexibility enables arbitrary architectures in graph neural networks for extracting global subject-wise information from node-wise surface data in varying brain geometries. To do so, the novel pooling strategy learns node associations between layers from the surface data. The leverage of spectral node coordinates [18] enables a precise localization of prominent associations between hidden layers. This, for instance, contrasts with hierarchical approaches [22] where nodes lack intrinsic localization within a graph. The flexibility of the new pooling strategy is demonstrated in two proof-of-concept applications, with the classification of disease stages and the regression of subject ages directly from node-wise surface data. Both are shown to improve recent state-of-the-art on the ADNI dataset [23]. This is, to the best of our knowledge, the first application of graph convolutional networks with pooling layers for classifying or regressing subject-wise information from full-sized surface-valued data using varying brain geometries.

2   Method

We start by explaining how standard convolutions can be extended to non-rigid geometries such as surfaces. We describe next our end-to-end learnable pooling strategy which provides subject-specific aggregation of cortical features. Subsequently, we present how our proposed graph convolutional neural network operates with pooling layers to predict subject-based information such as stage of disease or brain age, directly from surface-valued data.

2.1   Geometric Convolutions on Surfaces

In a standard CNN, the input of the network is given as a set of features observed over a regular grid of points, such as pixels in 2D or voxels in 3D. The network processes information from input to output predictions with a cascade of convolutional layers, typically composed of a convolution operation followed by a non-linear activation function, typically a sigmoid or ReLU. This can be formalized as follows. Let $\mathbf{Y}^{(l)} \in \mathbb{R}^{N \times M_l}$ be the input feature map at convolution layer l, such that $y_{iq}^{(l)}$ is the q-th feature of the i-th input node. The input feature map consists of N input nodes, each with M_l dimensions. Assuming a 1D grid for simplicity, the output feature map of layer l, convoluted with one kernel of size K_l, is given by $y_{ip}^{(l+1)} = f(z_{ip}^{(l)})$, where

$$
z_{ip}^{(l)} = \sum_{q=1}^{M_l} \sum_{k=1}^{K_l} w_{pqk}^{(l)} \cdot y_{i+k,\,q}^{(l)} + b_p^{(l)}. \tag{1}
$$

In this formulation, $w_{pqk}^{(l)}$ are the convolution kernel weights; $b_p^{(l)}$, the bias weights of the layer; and f, the activation function.

In the case of a general surface, points are not necessarily defined on a regular grid and can lie anywhere in a 3D Euclidean space. Such surface can conveniently be represented as a mesh graph $\mathcal{G} = \{\mathcal{V}, \mathcal{E}\}$, where $\mathcal{V}$ is the set of nodes corresponding to points and $\mathcal{E}$ is the set of edges between the graph nodes. Given a node $i \in \mathcal{V}$, we denote as $\mathcal{N}_i = \{j \mid (i, j) \in \mathcal{E}\}$ the set of nodes connected to i, called neighbors. We extend the concept of convolution to arbitrary graphs using the more general definition of geometric convolution [12,15,19]:

$$
z_{ip}^{(l)} = \sum_{j \in \mathcal{N}_i} \sum_{q=1}^{M_l} \sum_{k=1}^{K_l} w_{pqk}^{(l)} \cdot y_{jq}^{(l)} \cdot \varphi_{ij}(\boldsymbol{\theta}_k^{(l)}) + b_p^{(l)}, \tag{2}
$$

Here, φ_{ij} is a symmetric kernel parameterized by $\boldsymbol{\theta}_k$, relating the relative position of neighboring nodes j to nodes i when computing the convolutions. In [12], φ_{ij} is defined as a Gaussian kernel with learnable parameters $\boldsymbol{\theta}_k = \{\boldsymbol{\mu}_k, \boldsymbol{\Sigma}_k\}$ on the local polar coordinate $\mathbf{u}_{ij} = (\phi_{ij}, \theta_{ij})$ from node i to j:

$$
\varphi_{ij}(\boldsymbol{\theta}_k) = \exp\big(-\tfrac{1}{2}(\mathbf{u}_{ij} - \boldsymbol{\mu}_k)^\top \boldsymbol{\Sigma}_k^{-1}(\mathbf{u}_{ij} - \boldsymbol{\mu}_k)\big). \tag{3}
$$

Figure 3 illustrates the relationship between conventional and geometrical convolutions. The standard convolution (left) can in fact be seen as a special case of a geometric convolution (right), for which nodes are placed on a regular grid and kernels are unit impulses placed at the grid position of neighbor nodes, effectively spherical Gaussian kernels with zero variance.

2.2   Extension to Multiple Complex Surfaces

An important limitation of the geometric convolution model presented above is its inability to process surfaces which are aligned differently. Since local coordinates $\mathbf{u}_{ij}$ are determined using a fixed coordinate system, any rotation or scaling of the surface mesh will produce a different response for a given set of kernels. Additionally, as illustrated in Fig. 1, geometric convolutions in a Euclidean space is not well suited for complex surfaces such as the highly folded brain, where

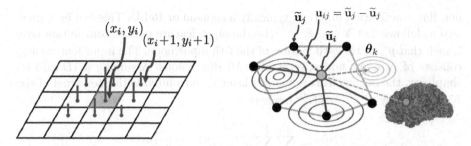

Fig. 3. Illustration of standard grid-based 2D convolutions (left) and geometric graph convolution (right). The challenge is to exploit kernels on arbitrary graph structures, and to add pooling operations over convolutional layers of graph nodes.

nearby points in space may actually be far apart on the surface in terms of geodesic distance.

We address the issues of inter-surface alignment and intra-surface distance using a graph spectral embedding approach. Specifically, we map a surface graph $\mathcal{G}$ to a low-dimensional subspace using the eigencomponents of its normalized Laplacian $\mathbf{L} = \mathbf{I} - \mathbf{D}^{-\frac{1}{2}}\mathbf{A}\mathbf{D}^{-\frac{1}{2}}$, where $\mathbf{A}$ is the weighted adjacency matrix and $\mathbf{D}$ is the diagonal degree matrix with $\mathbf{D}_{ii} = \sum_j \mathbf{D}_{ij}$. While binary adjacency values could be used in $\mathbf{A}$, we instead define the weight between two adjacent nodes as the inverse of their Euclidean distance. Denoting as $\mathbf{U}\mathbf{\Lambda}\mathbf{U}^\top$ the eigen-decomposition of $\mathbf{L}$, we compute the normalized spectral coordinates of nodes as the rows of matrix $\widehat{\mathbf{U}} = \mathbf{\Lambda}^{-\frac{1}{2}}\mathbf{U}$. Because the most relevant characteristics of the embedded graph are captured by the principal spectral components of $\mathbf{L}$, as in [24], we limit the decomposition to the $d = 3$ first smallest non-zero eigenvalues of $\mathbf{L}$. The use of a low number of main spectral components is also computationally efficient.

Since the spectral embedding of $\mathbf{L}$ is only defined up to an orthogonal transformation, we must align spectral representations of different surface graphs to a common reference. Let $\widehat{\mathbf{U}}^{(0)}$ be the normalized spectral embedding of this reference. We align an embedding $\widehat{\mathbf{U}}$ to $\widehat{\mathbf{U}}^{(0)}$ with an iterative closest point (ICP) method [18]. In this method, each node $i \in \mathcal{V}$ is mapped to its nearest reference node $\pi(i) \in \mathcal{V}^{(0)}$ in the embedding space. The transformation $\mathbf{R}$ between corresponding nodes is found by approximating $\mathbf{R} = (\widehat{\mathbf{U}}^\top\widehat{\mathbf{U}})^{-1}(\widehat{\mathbf{U}}^\top\widehat{\mathbf{U}}^{(0)})$. Denote as $\widehat{\mathbf{u}}_i$ the normalized spectral coordinates of node i, the overall alignment process can be expressed as

$$\arg\min_{\pi,\mathbf{R}} \sum_{i=1}^{N} \|\widehat{\mathbf{u}}_i\,\mathbf{R} - \widehat{\mathbf{u}}_{\pi(i)}^{(0)}\|_2^2. \tag{4}$$

This optimization is solved by updating the node correspondence mapping π and the transformation matrix $\mathbf{R}$ as described above, until convergence [18].

We use the aligned spectral embedding $\widetilde{\mathbf{U}} = \widehat{\mathbf{U}}\mathbf{R}$ to define the local coordinates corresponding to an edge $(i,j) \in \mathcal{E}$: $\mathbf{u}_{ij} = \widetilde{\mathbf{u}}_j - \widetilde{\mathbf{u}}_i$. As on Fig. 3 (right), and based on Eq. (2), the convolution at node i therefore considers kernel responses $\varphi_{ij}(\boldsymbol{\theta}_k^{(l)})$ for neighbor nodes j, *with respect to* the spectral coordinates of i.

2.3 Adaptive Graph Convolution Pooling

In standard CNNs, pooling is typically carried out by aggregating values inside non-overlapping sub-regions of features maps. In graph convolutional networks [9–12], this approach is not applicable for several reasons. First, nodes are not laid out on a regular grid. This prevents aggregation of features in pre-defined regions. Second, the density of points may spatially vary in the embedding space. Pooling regions of fixed size or fixed shape are, therefore, not suitable for graphs with different geometries. Lastly, and more importantly, input surface graphs may have a different number of nodes, while the output may have a fixed size. This is the case when predicting a fixed number of class probabilities from different brain geometries.

The limitations of traditional pooling techniques for graph convolutional networks can be addressed using different strategies. A first strategy is to aggregate features across all nodes in a *global* pooling step, typically after the last convolutional layer. A major problem with this strategy is the loss of all geometric and structural information during pooling. Another strategy, proposed by Wang et al. [25], performs a hierarchical clustering of nodes using their spectral coordinates, with a subsequent pooling of node features within each cluster. While this approach considers the graph structure, it is restricted by the chosen number of clusters. Furthermore, clusters are defined based only on node proximity in the embedding space, and the values to predict are ignored. Consequently, this unsupervised pooling strategy may not be optimal for the classification or regression task at hand.

In this work, we propose an end-to-end learnable pooling strategy for the subject-specific aggregation of cortical features. Inspired by the recently-proposed differential pooling technique of Ying et al. [22], this method splits the network in two separate paths, one for computing latent features for each node of the input graph, and another for predicting the node clusters by which the features are aggregated. This two-path architecture is shown in Fig. 2. The feature encoding path is similar to a conventional CNN, and produces a sequence of convolutional feature maps $\{\mathbf{Y}^{(1)}, \dots, \mathbf{Y}^{(l)}\}$ with $\mathbf{Y}^{(l)} \in \mathbb{R}^{N \times M_l}$. The clustering path consists of sequential convolutional blocks, but replaces the activation function of the last block with a node-wise softmax. The output of this last block, $\mathbf{S} \in [0,1]^{N \times C}$, gives for each node i the probability s_{ic} that i belongs to cluster c. Pooled features $\mathbf{Y}^{\text{pool}} \in \mathbb{R}^{C \times M_l}$ are computed as the expected sum of convolutional features in each cluster:

$$y_{cp}^{\text{pool}} = \sum_{i=1}^{N} s_{ic} \cdot y_{ip}^{(l)}, \qquad \mathbf{Y}^{\text{pool}} = \mathbf{S}^{\top} \mathbf{Y}^{(l)} \tag{5}$$

At this stage, nodes are now replaced by clusters. The convolutions of node features, downstream the pooling operation, requires computing the adjacency matrix of node clusters, $\mathbf{A}^{\text{pool}}$. The adjacency weights between pooling clusters c and d are defined as

$$a_{cd}^{\text{pool}} = \sum_{i=1}^{N} \sum_{j=1}^{N} s_{ic} \cdot s_{jd} \cdot a_{ij}, \quad \mathbf{A}^{\text{pool}} = \mathbf{S}^{\top} \mathbf{A} \mathbf{S}. \tag{6}$$

As described in [22], the bilinear formulation of Eq. (5) faces a challenging optimization problem with several local minima. To facilitate the learning process and obtain spatially smooth clusters, our approach adds the following regularization term:

$$\mathcal{L}_{\text{reg}}(\mathbf{S}) = \sum_{i=1}^{N} \sum_{j=1}^{N} a_{ij} \cdot \|\mathbf{s}_i - \mathbf{s}_j\|^2 = \text{tr}(\mathbf{S}\mathbf{L}\mathbf{S}^{\top}), \tag{7}$$

where $\mathbf{s}_i$ denotes the cluster probability vector of node i.

2.4 Architecture Details

The overall architecture of the proposed graph convolution network is shown in Fig. 2. As input to the network, we give the cortical surface features $\mathbf{x}_i$ and aligned spectral coordinates $\widetilde{\mathbf{u}}_i$ of each node i. Although various features could be considered to model the local geometry of the cortical surface [3], we used sulcal depth and cortical thickness, since the first one helps delineate anatomical brain regions [26] and the latter is related to ageing [27] and neurodegenerative diseases such as Alzheimer's [28].

The network is composed of two cascaded convolution-pooling blocks, followed by two fully-connected (FC) layers. The first block generates an $N \times 8$ feature map and an $N \times 16$ cluster assignment matrix, in two separate paths, and combines them using the pooling formulation of Eq. (5) to obtain a pooled feature map of 16×8. In the second block, pooled features are used to produce a 16×16 map of features, pooled in a single cluster. Hence, the second pooling step acts as an attention module selecting the features of most relevant clusters. The resulting 1×16 representation is converted to a 1×8 vector using the first FC layer, and then to a $1 \times$ nb.outputs vector with the second FC layer.

Except for the cluster probabilities and network output, all layers employ the Leaky ReLU as activation function: $y_{ip}^{(l)} = \max(0.01 z_{ip}^{(l)}, z_{ip}^{(l)})$. Moreover, for the graph convolution kernel φ_{ij} of Eq. (2), we used the B-spline kernels proposed by Fey et al. [15]. Compare to Gaussian kernels [12], this kernel has the advantage of making computation time independent from the kernel size.

For training, the loss function combines the output prediction loss and cluster regularization loss on the convolution-pooling block:

$$\mathcal{L}(\boldsymbol{\theta}) = \mathcal{L}_{\text{out}}(\boldsymbol{\theta}) + \alpha \mathcal{L}_{\text{reg}}(\mathbf{S}^{(1)}(\boldsymbol{\theta})), \tag{8}$$

where α is a parameter controlling the amount of regularization. For classification tasks (i.e., disease prediction), $\mathcal{L}_{\text{out}}$ is set as the cross-entropy between one-hot encoded ground-truth labels and output class probabilities. In the case of

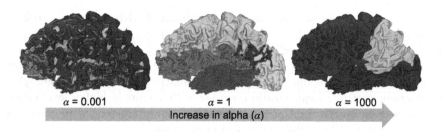

Fig. 4. Effect of α on clustering: The clusters learned with different strength of α. Smaller values of α produces multiple (10) spatially inconsistent clusters (left). Anatomically meaningful regions (middle) are learned with $\alpha = 1$ with 5 different clusters. $\alpha = 1000$ (right) results mimicking global pooling with 3 clusters. Nodes are color-coded to highlight the clustering. (Color figure online)

regression (i.e., brain age prediction), we use mean squared error (MSE) for this loss. Network parameters are optimized with stochastic gradient descent (SGD) using the Adam optimizer. Experiments were carried out on an i7 desktop computer with 16 GB of RAM and a Nvidia Titan X GPU. The model takes less than a second for disease classification or age regression.

3   Results

We now validate our adaptive pooling approach. As a benchmark, we perform a disease classification and a brain age prediction using the ADNI dataset [29]. We use all available 731 brain surfaces, generated by FreeSurfer and manually labeled as normal cognition (NC), mild cognitive impairment (MCI), and Alzheimer's disease (AD). Each surface includes pointwise cortical thickness and sulcal depth. Meshes have a varying number of vertices and different triangulation. In a first experiment, we evaluate the influence of the regularization parameters α on the clustering of our learning framework. In a second experiment, we highlight the advantages of working in the spectral domain for disease classification (NC *vs* AD, MCI *vs* AD, and NC *vs* MCI). Finally, learning performance is measured when regressing the brain age operating directly in a spectral domain.

3.1   Effect of Regularization on Clustering

In practice, we use the Laplacian regularization $\mathcal{L}_{\text{reg}}$ within the loss function to avoid early spurious local minima when training for clustering. We have a hyper-parameter in our formulation α controlling regularization. We randomly split the ADNI dataset into a 70-10-20% ratio for training, validation and testing.

To evaluate the effect of α, we first set $C_1 = 16$ in the pooling path as a maximum number of possible clusters in a pooling layer. The goal of this experiment is to study how the spatial consistency of clusters varies with an increasing regularization. Figure 4 shows the change in cluster assignments when increasing α in the NC *vs* AD classification task.

The spatial consistency of the clusters obtained with lower $\alpha = 0.0001$, enforcing a lower regularization, results in highly scattered regions, as seen on the left of Fig. 4. Equal weighting of $\mathcal{L}_{out}$ and $\mathcal{L}_{reg}$, with $\alpha = 1$, results in consistent clustered regions in the pooling layer. The middle of Fig. 4 shows clustered regions corresponding to prominent anatomical regions on the surface of the brain. A strong regularization, with $\alpha \geq 10$, results in higher level pooled regions, as seen on the right of Fig. 4. There are fewer clusters, with consistent regions that may relate with anatomical brain lobes.

3.2   Disease Classification

Our method is now evaluated in a classification problem. To do so, we validate the performance of our algorithm on the ADNI dataset for NC *vs* AD, MCI *vs* AD and NC *vs* MCI binary classification problem, using all available 731 brain surfaces, generated by FreeSurfer. We compare our method with a random forest-based approach [30]. This baseline processes similar surface-based information, such as cortical thickness and sulcal depth, using the same dataset.

One of our contributions is to provide pooling operations in a geometry-aware domain. This is enabled by aligning spectral embeddings of brain surfaces across various mesh geometries. We first illustrate the current limitations of learning pooling operations without local spectral features. Models are trained models with only cortical thickness and sulcal depth. We also evaluate the improvement of our model performance by adding geometric information as spectral coordinates to the graph learning framework. We train three independents models to classify NC *vs* AD, MCI *vs* AD, or NC *vs* MCI. We use the same random split using the same architecture described earlier for each of our three models.

The performance on classification task is reported in Table 1. The accuracy for NC *vs* MCI is 76% without the use of geometric information. Our graph convolution network with spectral information indicates an accuracy of 89.33% for the same task. This is a 13.33% improvement. This gain in performance illustrates the advantage of using geometric information when processing surface data. Improvements are also observed when classifying MCI *vs* AD and NC *vs* MCI, with an increase of 2.89% and 6.20% respectively.

Table 1. Evaluation of the proposed work: Average accuracy of disease classification, in %, with standard deviation over the complete ADNI dataset. First row shows performance of a random forest with multiple cortical-based features [30]. Second row shows performance of our graph convolutional model without geometrical information (spectral). Last row indicates the results of our model with spectral shape information.

Input	NC vs AD	MCI vs AD	NC vs MCI
Random forest (Cortical-based) [30]	80 ± 5	65 ± 6	63 ± 4
Ours (Thick. + Depth)	76.00 ± 6.06	74.03 ± 8.63	63.71 ± 5.72
Ours (Spectral + Thick. + Depth)	89.33 ± 4.30	76.92 ± 4.78	70.79 ± 6.40

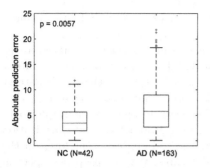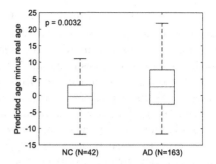

Fig. 5. Distribution of absolute prediction error (left) and predicted minus real age (right), for NC and AD test subjects. Our adaptive pooling strategy yielded graph models that could correctly capture age discrepancies between real and geometry-based ages, as expected between subjects with NC and AD.

3.3   Brain Age Prediction

In this experiment, our method is demonstrated in a regression problem where the brain age is predicted using pointwise surface-based measurements. We train our model on NC brains to regress brain ages. A model is learned with mean square error between real and predicted age with $\mathcal{L}_{\text{out}}$ as regularization. The graph convolution model uses cortical thickness, sulcal depth and spectral information as input. The model trained only on NC brain surfaces is then used to predict the real age of NC and AD subjects. Finally, we assess improvement due to the use of spectral coordinates, by comparing a model trained with and without geometric information.

The network architecture is illustrated in Fig. 2. The mean absolute error for the model predicting the real age on the NC subject is 4.35 ± 3.19 years. However, when the model is tested on the AD subjects, the prediction mean absolute error increases to 6.80 ± 6 years. The brain age calculated as the difference between prediction of our model and real age for NC and AD subjects indicate a statistically significance with a p-value of 0.0032. The real versus predicted ages over NC and AD is shown in Fig. 5.

4   Conclusion

We presented a novel strategy that enables pooling operations on graph convolutional networks of arbitrary graph structures. The ability to learn pooling patterns among graph nodes offers the possibility of exploring new graph-based neural network architectures. This new flexibility in designing network architectures is highly relevant for brain surface analysis. Subject-based prediction is, indeed, often drawn from surface-based values that resides on heterogeneous geometries.

Our experiments explore two different applications. In a first evaluation, the stage of Alzheimer's disease is learned from surface data, including cortical thickness and sulcal depth. Our results show that point-wise surface values can be efficiently aggregated into a fixed number of class probabilities using a simple network architecture. The classification accuracy in recent state-of-the-art approaches exploiting directly *surface-based* features, such as cortical areas, thickness and other measurements [30], indicates that our graph pooling strategy provides an increase in accuracy from 63–80% to 70–89% on the ADNI dataset (Table 1). This is an 11% improvement. A closer evaluation also reveals that most of the performance gain occurs when spectral localization of graph nodes is used in the learning of pooling patterns. This indicates that node localization is essential to learn pooling strategies. Our method enables, therefore, on the one hand, new graph neural network architectures, via our proposed spectral pooling strategy, and on the other hand, a novel spatially varying learning of pooling patterns, via the spectral localization of probable graph patterns. In a second evaluation, the age of subjects are predicted using the geometry of their brains with point-wise surface data. Whole subject-based values, in this case, the subject's age, is regressed using our flexible pooling strategy. The architecture of the graph convolutional neural network can combine pooled layers of decreasing sizes, from full-sized cortical feature vectors to a single output for the predicted age. This experiment indicates that such new architectures can yield graph-based regressor of subject's characteristics directly from surface-based features lying on diverse brain geometries. The results shows that our graph networks could correctly capture the age discrepancies between the real age of a subject and its predicted geometry-based age. As expected, subjects with Alzheimer's have higher discrepancies than subjects with normal cognition (Fig. 5).

To summarize, our pooling strategy enables the exploration of a new family of architectures for graph convolutional neural networks. However, the proposed method depends on having datasets of comparable brain geometries. The spectral decomposition of graph Laplacian, indeed, assumes that shapes are topologically equivalent. Heterogeneity in holes and cuts in datasets of surfaces remains challenging to exploit since they may produce incompatible sets of Laplacian eigenvectors. This method is consequently inadequate for applications where major geometrical changes exist, such as when tumors are ablated. Nevertheless, our proposed pooling strategy remains highly relevant for a wide range of applications where surface data needs to be pooled sequentially in layers from full-size surface-valued vectors to single whole-subject characteristics.

Acknowledgment. This work is supported by the Research Council of Canada (NSERC), NVIDIA Corp. with the donation of a Titan Xp GPU. Data were obtained from the Alzheimer's Disease Neuroimaging Initiative (ADNI) database.

References

1. Arbabshirani, M.R., Plis, S., Sui, J., Calhoun, V.D.: Single subject prediction of brain disorders in neuroimaging: promises and pitfalls. NeuroImage **145**, 137–165 (2017)
2. Hua, X., et al.: Unbiased tensor-based morphometry: improved robustness and sample size estimates for Alzheimer's disease clinical trials. NeuroImage **66**, 648–661 (2013)

3. Fischl, B., et al.: Automatically parcellating the cortex. Cereb. Cortex **14**, 11–22 (2004)
4. Yeo, B.T., Sabuncu, M.R., Vercauteren, T., Ayache, N., Fischl, B., Golland, P.: Spherical demons: fast diffeomorphic surface registration. TMI **29**, 650–668 (2010)
5. Styner, M., et al.: Framework for the statistical shape analysis of brain structures using SPHARM-PDM. Insight J. (2006)
6. Lecun, Y., Bottou, L., Bengio, Y., Haffner, P.: Gradient-based learning applied to document recognition. ISP **86**, 2278–2324 (1998)
7. Ronneberger, O., Fischer, P., Brox, T.: U-net: convolutional networks for biomedical image segmentation. In: Navab, N., Hornegger, J., Wells, W.M., Frangi, A.F. (eds.) MICCAI 2015. LNCS, vol. 9351, pp. 234–241. Springer, Cham (2015). https://doi.org/10.1007/978-3-319-24574-4_28
8. Kamnitsas, K., et al.: Efficient multi-scale 3D CNN with fully connected CRF for accurate brain lesion segmentation. MedIA **36**, 61–78 (2017)
9. Bruna, J., Zaremba, W., Szlam, A., LeCun, Y.: Spectral networks and locally connected networks on graphs. In: ICLR (2014)
10. Kipf, T.N., Welling, M.: Semi-Supervised classification with graph convolutional networks. In: ICLR (2017)
11. Defferrard, M., Bresson, X., Vandergheynst, P.: Convolutional neural networks on graphs with fast localized spectral filtering. In: NIPS (2016)
12. Monti, F., Boscaini, D., Masci, J., Rodolà, E., Svoboda, J., Bronstein, M.M.: Geometric deep learning on graphs and manifolds using CNNs. In: CVPR (2017)
13. Xu, Y., Fan, T., Xu, M., Zeng, L., Qia, Y.: SpiderCNN: deep learning on point sets with parameterized convolutional filters. In: ECCV (2018)
14. Levie, R., Monti, F., Bresson, X., Bronstein, M.M.: CayleyNets: graph convolutional neural networks with complex rational spectral filters. In: ICLR (2018)
15. Fey, M., Lenssen, J.E., Weichert, F., Müller, H.: SplineCNN: fast geometric deep learning with continuous B-Spline kernels. In: CVPR (2018)
16. Ovsjanikov, M., Ben-Chen, M., Solomon, J., Butscher, A., Guibas, L.: Functional maps: a flexible representation of maps between shapes. In: SIGGRAPH (2012)
17. Yi, L., Su, H., Guo, X., Guibas, L.J.: SyncSpecCNN: synchronized spectral CNN for 3D shape segmentation. In: CVPR (2017)
18. Lombaert, H., Arcaro, M., Ayache, N.: Brain transfer: spectral analysis of cortical surfaces and functional maps. In: Ourselin, S., Alexander, D.C., Westin, C.-F., Cardoso, M.J. (eds.) IPMI 2015. LNCS, vol. 9123, pp. 474–487. Springer, Cham (2015). https://doi.org/10.1007/978-3-319-19992-4_37
19. Gopinath, K., Desrosiers, C., Lombaert, H.: Graph convolutions on spectral embeddings: learning of cortical surface data. In: arXiv preprint arXiv:1803.10336 (2018)
20. Dhillon, I.S., Guan, Y., Kulis, B.: Weighted graph cuts without eigenvectors a multilevel approach. PAMI **29**, 1944–1957 (2007)
21. Parisot, S., et al.: Spectral graph convolutions for population-based disease prediction. In: Descoteaux, M., Maier-Hein, L., Franz, A., Jannin, P., Collins, D.L., Duchesne, S. (eds.) MICCAI 2017. LNCS, vol. 10435, pp. 177–185. Springer, Cham (2017). https://doi.org/10.1007/978-3-319-66179-7_21
22. Ying, R., et al.: Hierarchical graph representation learning with differentiable pooling. arXiv arXiv:1806.08804 (2018)
23. Bron, E., et al.: The CADDementia challenge. Neuroimage (2015)
24. Lombaert, H., Criminisi, A., Ayache, N.: Spectral forests: learning of surface data, application to cortical parcellation. In: Navab, N., Hornegger, J., Wells, W.M., Frangi, A.F. (eds.) MICCAI 2015. LNCS, vol. 9349, pp. 547–555. Springer, Cham (2015). https://doi.org/10.1007/978-3-319-24553-9_67

25. Wang, C., Samari, B., Siddiqi, K.: Local spectral graph convolution for point set feature learning. In: ECCV (2018)
26. Destrieux, C., et al.: A sulcal depth parcellation of the cortex. NeuroImage (2009)
27. Sowell, E.R., et al.: Longitudinal mapping of cortical thickness and brain growth in normal children. J. Neurosci. **24**, 8223–8231 (2004)
28. Lerch, J.P., et al.: Focal decline of cortical thickness in Alzheimer's disease identified by computational neuroanatomy. Cereb. Cortex **15**, 995–1001 (2004)
29. Jack, C.R., et al.: ADNI: MRI methods. JMRI **27**, 685–691 (2008)
30. Ledig, C., et al.: Alzheimer's state classification using volumetry, thickness and intensity. In: MICCAI (2014)

On Training Deep 3D CNN Models with Dependent Samples in Neuroimaging

Yunyang Xiong[1]([✉]), Hyunwoo J. Kim[2], Bhargav Tangirala[1], Ronak Mehta[1], Sterling C. Johnson[1], and Vikas Singh[1]

[1] University of Wisconsin Madison, Madison, WI 53706, USA
{yxiong43,btangirala}@wisc.edu, ronakrm@cs.wisc.edu,
scj@medicine.wisc.edu, vsingh@biostat.wisc.edu
[2] Korea University, Seoul 02841, Korea
hyunwoojkim@korea.ac.kr

Abstract. There is much interest in developing algorithms based on 3D convolutional neural networks (CNNs) for performing regression and classification with brain imaging data and more generally, with biomedical imaging data. A standard assumption in learning is that the training samples are independently drawn from the underlying distribution. In computer vision, where we have millions of training examples, this assumption is violated but the empirical performance may remain satisfactory. But in many biomedical studies with just a few hundred training examples, one often has multiple samples per participant and/or data may be curated by pooling datasets from a few different institutions. Here, the violation of the independent samples assumption turns out to be more significant, especially in small-to-medium sized datasets. Motivated by this need, we show how 3D CNNs can be modified to deal with dependent samples. We show that even with standard 3D CNNs, there is value in augmenting the network to exploit information regarding dependent samples. We present empirical results for predicting cognitive trajectories (slope and intercept) from morphometric change images derived from multiple time points. With terms which encode dependency between samples in the model, we get consistent improvements over a strong baseline which ignores such knowledge.

1 Introduction

The use of machine learning methods to perform classification or regression tasks with brain imaging data, in the last decade or so, has demonstrated that the clinical manifestation of various diseases such as Alzheimer's disease (AD) and Parkinson's disease (PD) can be reliably identified and predictive features obtained from such models are consistent with scientific hypotheses based on

---

Supported by UW CPCP AI117924, R01 EB022883 and R01 AG062336. Partial support also provided by R01 AG040396, R01 AG021155, UW ADRC (AG033514), UW ICTR (1UL1RR025011) and NSF CAREER award RI 1252725. We also thank Nagesh Adluru for his help during data processing.

© Springer Nature Switzerland AG 2019
A. C. S. Chung et al. (Eds.): IPMI 2019, LNCS 11492, pp. 99–111, 2019.
https://doi.org/10.1007/978-3-030-20351-1_8

post-mortem studies [8]. In the last five years, following the broad adoption of convolutional neural networks for learning tasks in vision, we have seen the deployment of such architectures for brain imaging data as well [7]. While the diagnosis of various diseases using brain images remains important within brain image analysis, many scientific questions such as understanding brain development, evaluating normal aging trends or assessing the course of disease progression requires moving beyond *cross-sectional* analysis [17]. In other words, instead of one scan per participant, answering a number of key questions involves studies that need multiple scans per person. While sometimes, the setting may be longitudinal (gap between scans is 1–2 years), in other cases, the temporal relation between the scans may not be important. What is relevant, however, is that when each subject in a study provides *more than one scan* (or sample), the samples are **no longer i.i.d.** – instead, scans from each person are **dependent**.

Consider a simple regression task using brain imaging data, motivated by applications in Alzheimer's disease (AD) research. Let us assume that structural magnetic resonance (MR) images are the predictor variables $\mathcal{X}$. In AD research, cognitive trends are an important outcome variable. So, the slope and intercept (calculated over multiple years) of an appropriate measure of cognition, say the Auditory Verbal Learning Test (AVLT) [14], can be the response variable $\mathcal{Y}$. This is a simple regression model which seeks to estimate $f : \boldsymbol{x} \in \mathbf{R}^p \rightarrow \boldsymbol{y} \in \mathbf{R}^2$, where $\boldsymbol{x}$ denotes the brain image and $\boldsymbol{y}$ is the multi-valued response: AVLT cognition intercept together with its slope over multiple years. The task of estimating the parameters that map the independent variable $x \in \mathcal{X}$ to the dependent variables $y \in \mathcal{Y}$ can be approached via deep methods. If one were to use recent deep learning advances, one choice could be convolutional neural networks.

Notice that most regression models in vision and machine learning, including standard CNNs, assume that the samples are independent and identically distributed (i.i.d.). This usually allows a relatively simple model derivation that does not need to take the dependency between the samples into account. We know how to analyze the behavior of such models and tractable inference schemes are also available. Under the i.i.d assumption, standard regression techniques have *one model for a dataset* which maps all the samples in the same way. These models are called *fixed effects models* [18]. For instance, a linear regression as well as non-linear (or deep) regression models involve a set of fixed coefficients for the full set of examples. However, in the applications with *dependent* measurements, the i.i.d. assumption does *not* hold and fixed effects models are often suboptimal. For instance, longitudinal data or any study with multiple samples for a subject involve data that are dependent and affected by certain subject-specific terms. This is called a *random effect*. In such situations, to accurately model global trends, the random effects should be properly utilized.

Dependent samples in regression are modeled using mixed effects models [18]. Mixed effects models handle the fixed effects and random effects by explicitly leveraging the "group" (dependent samples) information to handle the inherent non-independence in the data. Many brain imaging studies have repeated measurements and non-independence with a hierarchical structure of data. We know that CNNs have been shown to be highly effective in a variety of medical imaging problems [2]. But CNNs for non-i.i.d samples are far less explored. This paper studies how CNNs can be modified to incorporate terms that account for dependent samples, motivated by neuroimaging applications.

The main goal of our work is to use random effects within 3D convolutional neural networks, and use this 3D CNN model to predict cognitive performance on multiple brain image scans per subject with visual interpretation. Our main **contributions** are: **(1)** We use random effects within 3D convolutional neural networks (RE-CNN) built on inverted residual blocks. **(2)** We show that our proposed RE-CNN works well for brain imaging datasets with dependent samples and outperforms a strong baseline (which does not incorporate random effects) by significant margins. **(3)** We provide a module for visual interpretation of voxels that are relevant for the prediction task. Experiments suggest that regions identified are consistent with existing hypotheses (i.e., cognitive performance affected by gross brain atrophy).

Related Work: Various approaches have been proposed to analyze repeated measurements. A model with RE-EM tree was presented in [15] to combine mixed effects models for longitudinal and clustered data with the flexibility of tree-based estimation methods. In [6], mixed-effects random forest was developed to analyze clustered data consisting of individuals nested within groups. Riemannian nonlinear mixed effects models are developed in [9] for longitudinal brain data analysis. In [1], non-linear mixed effects statistical model was proposed to estimate alteration of the shape of the hippocampus during the course of Alzheimer's disease. Separately, visual interpretation methods are developed to help understand and indicate the spatial attention of convolutional neural network when making predictions. [20] shows that the visualization genuinely corresponds to the image structure that stimulates that feature map by performing occlusion sensitivity. [16] proposed the visualization of deep convolutional neural network based on computing the gradient of the class score with respect to the input image. In [5], a perturbation scheme was developed to find where highly complicated neural networks look in an image for evidence. Class Activation Mapping (CAM) in [21] is developed to visualize the linear combination of a late layer's activation and class-specific weights.

2   Preliminaries

In this section, we briefly review the basic concepts and properties of linear mixed-effects models and nonlinear mixed-effects model to setup the rest of our presentation for AVLT cognition prediction. For simplicity, we introduce models with a univariate response variable (also called labels or dependent variable).

Fixed effect models can be considered as a linear or non-linear global model. An example for fixed effect models is a standard linear regression model,

$$y = \boldsymbol{x}^T \boldsymbol{\beta} + \epsilon, \ \ \epsilon \sim \mathcal{N}(0, \boldsymbol{\Sigma}) \tag{1}$$

where $y \in \mathbf{R}$ is the response, $\boldsymbol{x} = [1, x_1, x_2, \ldots, x_p]^T \in \mathbf{R}^{p+1}$ are the covariates, $\boldsymbol{\beta} = [\beta_0, \ldots, \beta_p]^T \in \mathbf{R}^{p+1}$ are fixed effects coefficients shared over all subjects.

Mixed effect models explicitly incorporates subject information by introducing a set of parameters for each subject (or group) to yield subject-specific adjustments. Recall that AVLT cognition prediction for AD research is a function fitting problem, mapping a single input brain image to AVLT cognition. We observe from (1) that all subjects have the exactly same estimation function to map an input 3D brain image to AVLT cognition output and the noise permitted in the estimation function also comes from a distribution identical to every subject. However, with multiple measurements from each subject, these 3D brain image scans are not independent and each subject may have a slightly different estimation function. Therefore, our goal is to use fixed effects for a global model but also incorporate random effects for flexible specific-subject adjustments, yielding slightly different mapping function of AVLT cognition prediction. By adding random effects to (1) for each participant, the linear mixed effects (LME) model can be written as,

$$y = \boldsymbol{x}^T \boldsymbol{\beta} + \mathbf{z}^T \mathbf{b}_i + \epsilon_i, \mathbf{b}_i \sim \mathcal{N}(0, \boldsymbol{D}) \text{ and } \epsilon_i \sim \mathcal{N}(0, \boldsymbol{\Sigma}_{\epsilon_i}), i = 1, 2, \ldots, N \quad (2)$$

where N is the number of subjects, $\boldsymbol{\beta} = [\beta_0, \ldots, \beta_p] \in \mathbf{R}^{p+1}$ are the fixed effects (population parameters) shared over the entire population and $\mathbf{b}_i = [b_0^i, \ldots, b_q^i] \in \mathbf{R}^{q+1}$ are the subject-specific random effects (individual parameters) for i^{th} subject for subject-specific adjustment, $\boldsymbol{x}$ and $\mathbf{z}$ are the associated fixed effects and random effects covariates, $\boldsymbol{D}$ and $\boldsymbol{\Sigma}_{\epsilon_i}, i = 1, 2, \ldots, N$, are the variance components of linear mixed effects model, ϵ_i is the measurement error, drawn from a *subject-specific* unknown zero mean Gaussian distribution with covariance structure, $\mathcal{N}(0, \boldsymbol{\Sigma}_{\epsilon_i})$, for dealing with the non-i.i.d. nature. When covariance matrices, $\boldsymbol{D}$ and $\boldsymbol{\Sigma}_{\epsilon_i}$, are unknown, no closed form solution for estimation of fixed and random effects is available and EM algorithms are proposed for estimation [18].

Nonlinear mixed effects models (NLME) [18] is a generalization of a LME model. Given a nonlinear link function η, the NLME model is,

$$y = \eta(\boldsymbol{x}, \boldsymbol{\beta}, \mathbf{z}, \mathbf{b}_i) + \epsilon_i, \mathbf{b}_i \sim \mathcal{N}(0, \boldsymbol{D}), \epsilon_i \sim \mathcal{N}(0, \boldsymbol{\Sigma}_{\epsilon_i}), i = 1, 2, \ldots, N \quad (3)$$

where $\boldsymbol{\beta}$ are fixed effects vector and $\mathbf{b}_i$ are random effects vector for i^{th} subject.

3   Random Effects 3D Convolutional Neural Networks

Linear mixed effects model assumes a linear parametric form, and sometimes, this assumption might be too restrictive. Assuming a linear model may not be the best option when the parametric form is unknown. Further, when the number of covariates are large (e.g., 3D brain image), including all of the attributes may lead to overfitting and poor predictions. Therefore, we generalize linear mixed effects model to nonlinear mixed effects model using convolutional neural networks: we will learn the mapping from the input 3D brain image to AVLT cognition intercept and slope while being cognizant to individual level differences

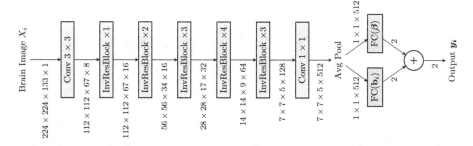

Fig. 1. An overview of 3D convolutional neural network structure incorporating linear mixed effects model, RE-CNN. InvResBlock denotes adapted 3D inverted residual block from 2D MobileNetV2 and it can be seen in Fig. 2. InvResBlock ×1/2/3/4 means the number of repeated layers within InvResBlock. The output of average pooling is denoted as $h(\boldsymbol{x})$, which is the input for the mixed effects models, $f_{\text{fix}}(\boldsymbol{x}) = h(\boldsymbol{x})\boldsymbol{\beta}$ for fixed effects estimation and $f_{\text{random}} = h(\boldsymbol{x})\mathbf{b}_i$ is for random effects estimation. The output of the network is a 2D vector, the sum of fixed effects estimation and random effects estimation.

of the subjects, denoted as random effects 3D convolutional neural network (RE-CNN). The cognition slope and intercept may be provided for each sample, or may be the same for all samples for a participant. To specify nonlinear mixed effects models, we write the model as a sum of fixed and random components,

$$\eta = f_{\text{fix}}(\boldsymbol{x}, \boldsymbol{\beta}) + f_{\text{rnd}}(\mathbf{z}, \mathbf{b}_i) \tag{4}$$

where f_{fix} is a nonlinear link function for fixed effects and f_{random} is a nonlinear link function for random effects. Generalized from the random intercept and random slope model [4], individually varying subject-specific intercept and slope, we define our nonlinear mixed effects model as

$$\eta = h(\boldsymbol{x})\boldsymbol{\beta} + h(\boldsymbol{x})\mathbf{b}_i \tag{5}$$

where h is a nonlinear link function, $h(\boldsymbol{x})\boldsymbol{\beta}$ represents the fixed component and $h(\boldsymbol{x})\mathbf{b}_i$ represents the random component. Here, (5) can be considered in the following way: we apply a nonlinear transformation $h(\cdot)$ first and then learn the fixed effects and random effects on top of the output features from h.

3.1   Architecture of RE-CNN

Our model is based on the efficient MobileNetV2 architecture and a sequence of inverted residual blocks, to represent nonlinear transformation h. To predict AVLT cognition prediction from 3D brain images, our model uses an adapted 3D MobileNetV2 architecture (see Fig. 1) for h, followed by a linear mixed regression loss after average pooling (Avg Pool).

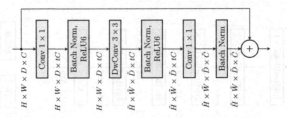

Fig. 2. The 3D inverted residual block is adapted from 2D inverted residual block of MobileNetV2. Similarly, if the output resolution of the block differs from the input resolution, the residual connection of the block is skipped.

RE-CNN can be viewed as a linear mixed effects regression for AVLT cognition prediction on the average pooling layer, $h(\cdot)$, output from 3D MobileNetV2. In Fig. 1, we can see that the top network learns the nonlinear fixed effects component, $h(\cdot)\boldsymbol{\beta}$, and the bottom network learns the nonlinear random component, $h(\cdot)\mathbf{b}_i$. Therefore, learning the nonlinear mixed effects model (see (4)) represented by RE-CNN (see Fig. 1) can be considered as an optimization where we train the network with the loss,

$$\min_{f_{\text{fix}}, f_{\text{rnd}}} \sum_{\boldsymbol{x}} loss(y, f_{\text{fix}}(\boldsymbol{x}) + f_{\text{rnd}}(\boldsymbol{x})) = \sum_{\boldsymbol{x}} ||y - f_{\text{fix}}(\boldsymbol{x}) - f_{\text{rnd}}(\boldsymbol{x})||^2, \quad (6)$$

where $f_{\text{fix}}(\boldsymbol{x}) = h(\boldsymbol{x})\boldsymbol{\beta}$ and $f_{\text{rnd}}(\boldsymbol{x}) = h(\boldsymbol{x})\mathbf{b}_i$.

3.2　Parameter Estimation of RE-CNN

Given N subjects, each subject with n_i ($\sum_{i=1}^{N} n_i = n$) observations, our goal is to estimate the parameters of our nonlinear mixed effects regression model.

$$\boldsymbol{y}_i = h(\boldsymbol{X}_i)\boldsymbol{\beta} + h(\boldsymbol{X}_i)\mathbf{b}_i + \boldsymbol{\epsilon}_i,$$
$$\mathbf{b}_i \sim \mathcal{N}(0, \boldsymbol{D}) \text{ and } \boldsymbol{\epsilon}_i \sim \mathcal{N}(0, \boldsymbol{\Sigma}_{\epsilon_i}), i = 1, 2, \ldots, N \quad (7)$$

where $\boldsymbol{y}_i = [y_{i1}, \ldots, y_{in_i}]^T$ is a $n_i \times 1$ vector of observations of the ith subject, $\boldsymbol{X}_i = [\boldsymbol{x}_{i1}, \ldots, \boldsymbol{x}_{in_i}]^T$ is a $n_i \times p$ covariates matrix, $h(\boldsymbol{X}_i) = [h(\boldsymbol{x}_{i1}), \ldots, h(\boldsymbol{x}_{in_i})]^T$, and $\boldsymbol{\epsilon}_i = [\epsilon_{(i1)}, \ldots, \epsilon_{(in_i)}]^T$ is a $n_i \times 1$ measurements error vector.

When the variance components of (7), $\boldsymbol{D}$ and $\boldsymbol{\Sigma}_{\epsilon_i}$, $i = 1, 2, \ldots, N$, and the nonlinear transformation, h, are known, the estimates of fixed effects parameters $\boldsymbol{\beta}$ and random effects parameters $\mathbf{b}_i, i = 1, 2, \ldots, N$ can be solved by minimizing the following generalized log-likelihood loss function [18],

$$loss(\boldsymbol{\beta}, \mathbf{b}_i | \boldsymbol{y}) = \sum_{i=1}^{N} [(\boldsymbol{y}_i - h(\boldsymbol{X}_i)\boldsymbol{\beta} - h(\boldsymbol{X}_i)\mathbf{b}_i)^T \boldsymbol{\Sigma}_{\epsilon_i}^{-1} \quad (8)$$
$$(\boldsymbol{y}_i - h(\boldsymbol{X}_i)\boldsymbol{\beta} - h(\boldsymbol{X}_i)\mathbf{b}_i) + \mathbf{b}_i^T \boldsymbol{D}^{-1}\mathbf{b}_i + \log|\boldsymbol{D}| + \log|\boldsymbol{\Sigma}_{\epsilon_i}|]$$

The minimization of the loss in (8) can be performed by solving the so-called mixed model equation [13] with known D, Σ_{ϵ_i} and h,

$$\begin{bmatrix} h(X)^T \Sigma_\epsilon^{-1} h(X) & h(X)^T \Sigma_\epsilon^{-1} h(X) \\ h(X)^T \Sigma_\epsilon^{-1} h(X) & h(X)^T \Sigma_\epsilon^{-1} h(X) + D_{\cdot}^{-1} \end{bmatrix} \begin{bmatrix} \beta \\ b \end{bmatrix} = \begin{bmatrix} h(X)^T \Sigma_\epsilon^{-1} y \\ h(X)^T \Sigma_\epsilon^{-1} y \end{bmatrix}. \quad (9)$$

where $y = [y_1^T, \cdots, y_N^T]^T$, $h(X) = [h(X_1)^T, \cdots, h(X_N)^T]^T$, $b = [b_1^T, \cdots, b_N^T]^T$, $D_c = diag(D, \cdots, D)$, $\Sigma_\epsilon = diag(\Sigma_{\epsilon_1}, \cdots, \Sigma_{\epsilon_N})$.

Since the covariance matrices, D and $\Sigma_{\epsilon_i}, i = 1, \cdots, N$, are unknown, we need to estimate them for solving (9). Similar to [18], we maximize the following log-likelihood function for estimating these matrices,

$$\log L(D_c, \Sigma_\epsilon | y) = -\frac{1}{2}[n \log 2\pi - \log |V| - (y - h(X)\beta)^T V^{-1}(y - h(X)\beta)] \quad (10)$$

where $V_i = h(X_i)Dh(X_i)^T + \Sigma_{\epsilon_i}, i = 1, \cdots, N$ and $V = diag(V_1, \cdots, V_N)$.

Based on (9) and (10), the last step in parameter estimation for our model (7) is to estimate the nonlinear transformation h, represented by a 3D MobileNetV2 (see Fig. 1). Stochastic gradient algorithm (SGD) is a popular scheme to optimize neural networks. We thus directly apply SGD for training h.

When the covariance matrices are replaced by the current available values, their updated values can be obtained by (9) and (10). Therefore, we use an EM algorithm for parameter estimation for our RE-CNN, denoted as RE-EM. Assume $\Sigma_{\epsilon_i} = \sigma^2 I_{n_i}, i = 1, \cdots, N$. Let t index the number of iterations and $\hat{\beta}^{\{t\}}$, $\hat{b}_i^{\{t\}}$, $h^{\{t\}}$, $\hat{\sigma}^{2\{t\}}$ and $\hat{D}^{\{t\}}$ be the estimates of β, b_i, h, σ^2 and D at t^{th} iteration. The major update equations in our RE-EM procedure are,

1. Solving (9),

$$\hat{b}_i^{\{t\}} = \hat{D}^{\{t-1\}} \hat{h}^{\{t\}}(X_i)^T \hat{V}_i^{-1\{t-1\}}(y_i - \hat{h}^{\{t\}}(X_i)\hat{\beta}^{\{t\}}) \quad (11)$$

$$\hat{\epsilon}_i^{\{t\}} = y_i - h^{\{t\}}(X_i)\hat{\beta}^{\{t\}} - h^{\{t\}}(X_i)\hat{b}_i^{\{t\}}$$

where $\hat{V}_i^{\{t-1\}} = h^{\{t\}}(X_i)\hat{D}^{\{t-1\}}h^{\{t\}}(X_i)^T + \hat{\sigma}^{2\{t-1\}}I_{n_i}$.

2. Solving (10),

$$\hat{\sigma}^{2\{t\}} = \frac{1}{n}\sum_{i=1}^{N}[\hat{\epsilon}_i^{T\{t\}}\hat{\epsilon}_i^{\{t\}} + \hat{\sigma}^{2\{t-1\}}(n_i - \hat{\sigma}^{2\{t-1\}}\text{trace}(\hat{V}_i^{\{t-1\}}))] \quad (12)$$

$$\hat{D}^{\{t\}} = \frac{1}{N}\sum_{i=1}^{N}[\hat{b}_i^{\{t\}}\hat{b}_i^{T\{t\}} + (\hat{D}^{\{t-1\}} - \hat{D}^{\{t-1\}}\hat{h}^{\{t\}}(X_i)^T \hat{V}_i^{-1\{t-1\}}\hat{h}^{\{t\}}(X_i)\hat{D}^{\{t-1\}})]$$

Then, the RE-EM algorithm for our regression task can be written formally in Algorithm 1. When the training of Algorithm 1 has been completed, we can fix h and learn a fully connected layer, g, based on the hidden representation of h to approximate $\hat{f}_{\text{rnd}}(x)$ only based on input 3D brain image without knowing the subject "id" for cognition measures estimate (AVLT slope or intercept).

Algorithm 1. Parameters estimation of RE-CNN for AVLT cognition prediction

---

0: **procedure** RE-CNN Training

1: #iter $t = 0$, Let $\hat{\mathbf{b}}_i^{\{0\}} = 0, \hat{\sigma}^{2\{0\}} = 1, \hat{\boldsymbol{D}}^{\{0\}} = I_p$, and denote $\boldsymbol{X}_i, i = 1, \cdots, N$, the input 3D brain samples for training RE-CNN.

2: #iter $t = t + 1$, SGD algorithm for training the top network (see Fig. 1) with 3D training samples, $(\boldsymbol{X}_i, \boldsymbol{y}_i'^{\{t\}} = \boldsymbol{y}_i - \hat{h}^{\{t\}}(\boldsymbol{X}_i)\hat{\mathbf{b}}_i^{\{t-1\}}), i = 1, \cdots, N$, to estimate $\hat{\beta}^{\{t\}}, \hat{h}^{\{t\}}$.

3: Update $\hat{\mathbf{b}}_i^{\{t\}}$ and $\hat{\boldsymbol{\epsilon}}_i^{\{t\}}$ using expressions 11.

4: Update variance $\hat{\sigma}^{2\{t\}}$ and $\hat{\boldsymbol{D}}^{\{t\}}$ using expressions 12.

5: Repeating steps 2, 3, and 4 until convergence.

5: **procedure** RE-CNN AVLT cognition Prediction

6: For an input 3D brain scan, $\boldsymbol{x}$, taking the sum of corresponding fixed part RE-CNN AVLT cognition prediction and predicted random part RE-CNN AVLT cognition prediction, $\hat{h}(\boldsymbol{x})\hat{\beta} + \hat{g}(\hat{h}(\boldsymbol{x}))$

---

4 Experiments

In this section, we discuss the task of predicting AVLT cognition prediction (intercept and slope) using brain images and evaluate the effectiveness of our RE-CNN model. First, we briefly review a representation that measures local morphometric changes of brains over time for each subject. Using this representation as input, we compare our model with various schemes and evaluate generalization power on unseen subjects. Further, we demonstrate how to interpret the learned model showing activation maps in the image space by a visual explanation approach [21], which allows identifying brain regions that are correlated with cognitive trajectories.

4.1 RE-CNN on Longitudinal CDT Images for Cognition Prediction

Our model uses longitudinal brain images and cognitive scores. In our experiments, morphometric change maps are used as input to the network architecture – these maps are obtained using multiple registration steps.

Morphometric change maps (given by determinant of Cauchy Deformation Tensor) brain images are subject-specific warps derived from a longitudinal neuroimaging study. In this paper, they are derived from a pre-clinical Alzheimer's disease (AD) cohort at Wisconsin. The longitudinal warps (or deformations) are *with-in* subject registrations of T_1-weighted images between two consecutive time points, $\Phi_{i,j} : \mathcal{I}_{i,j} \rightarrow \mathcal{I}_{i,j+1}$. At each voxel, a CDT Det is a determinant of Cauchy-Deformation Tensor derived from the spatial derivatives $\nabla\Phi_{i,j}(vox)$ of the deformation field, i.e., $det(\sqrt{\nabla\Phi_{i,j}(vox)^T \nabla\Phi_{i,j}(vox)})$. For downstream analysis, CDT calculation should be spatio-temporally unbiased and registered in a common coordinate system for voxel-wise analysis. Our pipeline is as follows. First, we estimate an unbiased global template space. Following [9], we estimate a temporally unbiased subject-specific average for each subject and then use the averages to generate the global template space. The averages are obtained by Advanced Normalization Tools (ANTS) [3]. Within-subject deformations (longitudinal changes) are transported to the global template space by the parallel transport of stationary velocity fields (SVFs) by Lorenzi and Pennec [11], Specifically, all brain images are registered in the global template space by a rigid transformation and then nonlinear symmetric diffeomorphic deformations are obtained by [10]. Thus brain images registered pairwise between two consecutive time points lead to a SVF, representing a longitudinal morphometric change between visits $i + 1$ and i. In our cohort, 88 subjects had at least three visits (CDT Dets brain image computed from scans at two time points, see Fig. 3) and a total of 202 samples (CDT Det images) are generated. Some subjects had two visits whereas a few had four visits.

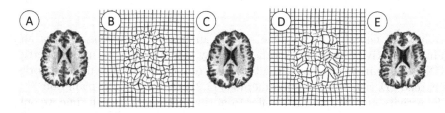

Fig. 3. Examples of input brain images and warps in AVLT cognition prediction. (A, C, E) the brain images are collected at three time points for one participant. (B) Warped spatial grid to move (A) to (C), (D) Warped spatial grid to move (C) to (E). Our CDT Det features are derived from the Jacobian of the deformations (C, E).

RE-CNN on Longitudinal CDT Dets. We now discuss how to use morphometric change maps (multiple images per subject) to predict cognition slope and intercept, i.e., subjects' multiple morphometric maps $\rightarrow$ their cognition intercept and slope. Here $x_{ij} \in \mathbf{R}^{H \times W \times C}$ represents the CDT determinant brain image between two consecutive visits of each subject and $y_{ij} \in \mathbf{R}^2$. Given the small sample size, we split the data with 8 subjects/split and perform 11-fold cross validation. Then, Algorithm 1 is used for training RE-CNN. Table 1 summarizes the comparisons of our RE-CNN and other baseline methods. Our model achieved the lowest root mean squared error. It shows that even if the subject id (group information) is not available at test time, our method leads to a more accurate fixed effects model by controlling for random effects during training. Our model performs better against a standard 3D CNN architecture for cognition slope and intercept prediction.

4.2 Visual Interpretation of RE-CNN on Brain Image

In this subsection, we describe our methods for explaining the predictions of RE-CNN in detail and then visually check heatmaps generated by a visual explanation method. There are two major ways to explain the predictions of 2D deep

Table 1. Comparison of RE-CNN and other baseline methods for AVLT cognition slope and intercept prediction. Our approach offers the smallest Root Mean Squared Error (RMSE) and the highest Pearson correlation score between AVLT cognition intercept and the predicted cognition intercept >0.6 and the highest Pearson correlation score between AVLT cognition slope and the predicted cognition slope >0.6. It means our model predicts more accurately than other baselines. Surprisingly, without any group information at test time, RE-CNN achieves better results than standard 3D CNNs that are not trained with group information. Even only using fixed effects part of RE-CNN, RE-CNN$_{\text{fix}}$ performs better than standard 3D CNN. It empirically shows that modeling random effects during training using group information may help learn better fixed effects models and leads to better generalization on unseen subjects.

Method	RE-CNN	RE-CNN$_{\text{fix}}$	3D CNN	GPR [12]	SVR
RMSE	**2.7**	**2.9**	3.1	4.8	5.2

convolutional neural network. One scheme applies perturbations to data and conducts sensitivity analysis. Another strategy is to use architectural properties of CNNs to heuristically track the attention of convolutional neural networks. We extend 2D visual explanation methods [5,21] to 3D visual explanation.

Sensitivity analysis methods suffer from the problem that each time we only get an output change for one voxel, which makes this extremely computationally intensive for a brain image of size $224 \times 224 \times 133$. To avoid the issues of one-at-a-time sensitivity analysis, we focus on a method based on the architectural properties of our 3D CNN, visualizing the activation map of convolutional layers directly when predictions are made [19,21]. We extend 2D activation mapping to 3D using the idea that the last convolution layer of the CNN contains spatial information indicating discriminative regions for making prediction. Thus, the activation mapping creates a spatial heatmap out of the activations from the last convolutional layer for visualizing discriminative parts. Assume we are given a 3D CNN, e.g., RE-CNN, and one brain image V and denote $f_u(x, y, z)$ to be the activation of unit u in the last convolutional layer at location (x, y, z). The global average pooling for unit u is $G_u = \frac{1}{N} \sum_{x,y,z} f_u(x, y, z)$, where N is the number of voxels in the corresponding convolutional layer. Notice that our RE-CNN is trained for regressing on AVLT cognition intercept and slope and the global average pooling layer is directly connected to the output layer, we extend the AVLT cognition intercept score as,

$$\text{Score(INT)} = \sum_u w_u^{\text{INT}} G_u = \frac{1}{N} \sum_{x,y,z} \sum_u w_u^{\text{INT}} f_u(x, y, z) \qquad (13)$$

where $\sum_u w_u^{\text{INT}} f_u(x, y, z)$ is defined for every spatial location (x, y, z) and their sum is proportional to the AVLT cognition intercept score. With the intercept score, we define our regression activation mapping (RAM) for AVLT cognition intercept as $\text{RAM}_{x,y,z}(\text{INT}) = |\sum_u w_u^{\text{INT}} f_u(x, y, z)|$, where $|\cdot|$ is the absolute value. The activation mapping for AVLT cognition intercept can be taken as a heatmap of weighted sum of activations in every location (x, y, z) and can

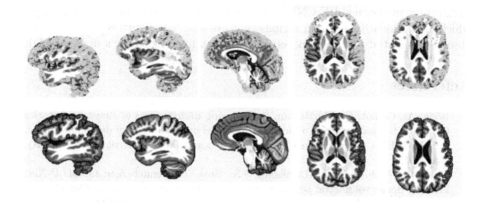

Fig. 4. Visual explanation heatmaps of brain images. RE-CNN takes CDT Dets images to associate the morphometric change of brain images with AVLT cognition scores. The regions which have relatively large morphometric change are highlighted in green in Row 1. The red highlights in Row 2 represent the activation map learned RE-CNN computed by RAM visual approach. Its activation shows the relevant regions for predicting AVLT cognition slope and intercept for each subject. (Color figure online)

be computed by one forward pass given one brain image. Similarly, we can define the regression activation mapping (RAM) for AVLT cognition slope as $\text{RAM}_{x,y,z}(\text{SLOPE}) = |\sum_u w_u^{\text{SLOPE}} f_u(x,y,z)|$. The regression activation mapping (RAM) for AVLT total cognition can be defined as,

$$\text{RAM}_{x,y,z}(\text{TOT}) = |\sum_u (w_u^{\text{INT}} + w_u^{\text{SLOPE}}) f_u(x,y,z)| \tag{14}$$

Our goal is to obtain visual explanations for highlighting brain regions important for cognition prediction. In our experiments, we take the morphometric change brain images from the test set for visual explanation/interpretation analysis and generate the heatmap from the horizontal, sagittal, and coronal sections. We present the highlighted regions which indicate that overall brain atrophy is associated with cognitive slope and intercept. The regression activation mapping heatmaps of RE-CNN are presented in Fig. 4.

5 Conclusion

This paper proposes a 3D convolutional neural network that is able to handle dependent brain imaging data (multiple samples per subject) for predicting cognitive measures. By respecting the dependencies, we present a 3D MobileNetV2 based architecture with random effects terms, RE-CNN, to exploit the representation power of 3D CNNs but systematically deal with dependencies in the samples. We develop a RE-EM algorithm for parameter estimation. Experimentally, our RE-CNN achieves promising results. We applied visual explanations to interpret the learned RE-CNN model by assessing regression activation maps, which allows identifying brain regions that are associated with cognition in this observational study focused on better understanding Alzheimer's disease (AD).

References

1. Bône, A., Colliot, O., Durrleman, S.: Learning distributions of shape trajectories from longitudinal datasets: a hierarchical model on a manifold of diffeomorphisms. In: The IEEE Conference on Computer Vision and Pattern Recognition (CVPR), June 2018
2. Çiçek, Ö., Abdulkadir, A., Lienkamp, S.S., Brox, T., Ronneberger, O.: 3D U-Net: learning dense volumetric segmentation from sparse annotation. In: Ourselin, S., Joskowicz, L., Sabuncu, M.R., Unal, G., Wells, W. (eds.) MICCAI 2016. LNCS, vol. 9901, pp. 424–432. Springer, Cham (2016). https://doi.org/10.1007/978-3-319-46723-8_49
3. Elhamifar, E., Vidal, R.: Sparse manifold clustering and embedding. In: Advances in Neural Information Processing Systems, pp. 55–63 (2011)
4. Fahrmeir, L., Tutz, G.: Multivariate Statistical Modelling Based on Generalized Linear Models. Springer, Heidelberg (2013)
5. Fong, R.C., Vedaldi, A.: Interpretable explanations of black boxes by meaningful perturbation
6. Hajjem, A., Bellavance, F., Larocque, D.: Mixed-effects random forest for clustered data. J. Stat. Comput. Simul. **84**(6), 1313–1328 (2014)
7. Ithapu, V.K., Singh, V., Okonkwo, O., Johnson, S.C.: Randomized denoising autoencoders for smaller and efficient imaging based AD clinical trials. In: Golland, P., Hata, N., Barillot, C., Hornegger, J., Howe, R. (eds.) MICCAI 2014. LNCS, vol. 8674, pp. 470–478. Springer, Cham (2014). https://doi.org/10.1007/978-3-319-10470-6_59
8. Kehagia, A.A., Barker, R.A., Robbins, T.W.: Neuropsychological and clinical heterogeneity of cognitive impairment and dementia in patients with Parkinson's disease. Lancet Neurol. **9**(12), 1200–1213 (2010)
9. Kim, H.J., Adluru, N., et al.: Riemannian nonlinear mixed effects models: analyzing longitudinal deformations in neuroimaging
10. Lorenzi, M., Ayache, N., et al.: LCC-Demons: a robust and accurate symmetric diffeomorphic registration algorithm. NeuroImage **81**, 470–483 (2013)
11. Lorenzi, M., Pennec, X.: Efficient parallel transport of deformations in time series of images: from schild's to pole ladder. JMIG **50**(1–2), 5–17 (2014)
12. Quiñonero-Candela, J., Rasmussen, C.E.: A unifying view of sparse approximate Gaussian process regression. JMLR **6**(Dec), 1939–1959 (2005)
13. Robinson, G.K.: That BLUP is a good thing: the estimation of random effects. Stat. Sci. **6**, 15–32 (1991)
14. Schmidt, M., et al.: Rey Auditory Verbal Learning Test: A Handbook. Western Psychological Services, Los Angeles (1996)
15. Sela, R.J., Simonoff, J.S.: RE-EM trees: a data mining approach for longitudinal and clustered data. Mach. Learn. **86**(2), 169–207 (2012)
16. Simonyan, K., Zisserman, A.: Very deep convolutional networks for large-scale image recognition. arXiv preprint arXiv:1409.1556 (2014)
17. Smyser, C.D., et al.: Longitudinal analysis of neural network development in preterm infants. Cereb. Cortex **20**, 2852–2862 (2010)

18. Wu, H., Zhang, J.T.: Nonparametric Regression Methods for Longitudinal Data Analysis: Mixed-Effects Modeling Approaches, vol. 515. Wiley, Hoboken (2006)
19. Yang, C., et al.: Visual explanations from deep 3D CNNs for Alzheimer's disease classification. arXiv:1803.02544 (2018)
20. Zeiler, M.D., Fergus, R.: Visualizing and understanding convolutional networks. In: Fleet, D., Pajdla, T., Schiele, B., Tuytelaars, T. (eds.) ECCV 2014. LNCS, vol. 8689, pp. 818–833. Springer, Cham (2014). https://doi.org/10.1007/978-3-319-10590-1_53
21. Zhou, B., Khosla, A., Lapedriza, A., Oliva, A., Torralba, A.: Learning deep features for discriminative localization. In: CVPR (2016)

A Deep Neural Network
for Manifold-Valued Data
with Applications to Neuroimaging

Rudrasis Chakraborty[1], Jose Bouza[2], Jonathan Manton[3],
and Baba C. Vemuri[2(✉)]

[1] University of California, Berkeley, Berkeley, USA
[2] University of Florida, Gainesville, USA
vemuri@ufl.edu
[3] University of Melbourne, Melbourne, Australia

Abstract. Developing deep neural networks (DNNs) for manifold-valued data sets has gained significant interest of late in the deep learning research community. Examples of manifold-valued data in the medical imaging domain include (but are not limited to) diffusion magnetic resonance imaging, tensor-based morphometry, shape analysis and more. In this paper we present a novel theoretical framework for DNNs to cope with manifold-valued data inputs, taking inspiration from the convolutional neural network (CNN) architecture. We call our network the ManifoldNet.

Analogous to vector spaces where convolutions are equivalent to computing weighted means, manifold-valued data convolutions can be defined using the weighted Fréchet Mean (wFM). To this end, we present a provably convergent recursive algorithm for computation of the wFM of the given data, where the weights are to be learned. Further, we prove that the proposed wFM layer achieves a contraction mapping and hence the ManifoldNet need not have additional non-linear ReLU units used in standard CNNs to achieve a contraction mapping.

Analogous to the equivariance of convolution in Euclidean space to translations, we prove that the wFM is equivariant to the action of the group of isometries admitted by the Riemannian manifold on which the data reside. This equivariance property facilitates weight sharing within the network. We present experiments using the ManifoldNet framework to achieve regression between diffusion MRI scans of Parkinson Disease (PD) patients and clinical information such as their Movement Disorder Society's Unified Parkinson's Disease Rating Scale (MDS-UPDRS) scores. In another experiment, we present results of finding group differences based on brain connectivity at the fiber bundle level between PD and controls.

This research was in part funded by the NSF grants IIS-1525431 and IIS-1724174.

Electronic supplementary material The online version of this chapter (https://doi.org/10.1007/978-3-030-20351-1_9) contains supplementary material, which is available to authorized users.

© Springer Nature Switzerland AG 2019
A. C. S. Chung et al. (Eds.): IPMI 2019, LNCS 11492, pp. 112–124, 2019.
https://doi.org/10.1007/978-3-030-20351-1_9

1   Introduction

CNNs pioneered by [16] have gained much popularity since their significant success on Imagenet data reported in [15]. In the past few years there has been a growing interest in generalizing CNNs and deep networks in general to data that reside on smooth non-Euclidean spaces. In this context, at the outset, it would be useful to categorize problems into (1) those that involve data as samples of real-valued functions defined on a manifold and (2) those that are simply manifold-valued and hence are sample points on a manifold. In this paper we will consider the second problem, namely, when the input data are sample points on known Riemannian manifolds for example, the manifold of symmetric positive definite (SPD) matrices, $SPD(n)$, the special orthogonal group, $SO(n)$, the n-sphere, $\mathbf{S}^n$, the Grassmannian, $Gr(p, n)$, and others. To be precise, the domain of interest is an n-dimensional field of points sampled from a Riemannian manifold. There is very little prior work that we are aware of on DNNs that can cope with input data samples residing on these manifolds with the exception of [12,13]. In [13], authors presented a deep network architecture for classification of hand-crafted features residing on a Grassmann manifold that form the input to the network. In [12], authors presented a deep network architecture for data on $SPD(n)$. In both of these works, the architecture does not involve the use of any convolution or equivalent operations on $Gr(p, n)$ or $SPD(n)$. Further, it does not use the natural invariant metric or intrinsic operations on the Grassmannian or the $SPD(n)$ in the network blocks. Using intrinsic operations within the layers guarantees that the result remains on the manifold and hence does not require any projection (extrinsic) operations to ensure the result lies in the same space. Further, using extrinsic operations can yield results that are susceptible to significant inaccuracies when the data variance is large [22]. Moreover, since there are no convolution type operations defined for data on these manifolds in their network, it can not be considered a generalization to the CNN and as a consequence does not consider the equivariance property to the action of the group of isometries denoted by $I(\mathcal{M})$, admitted by the manifold $\mathcal{M}$.

In this paper, we present a novel DNN framework called the ManifoldNet. This is a potential analog of a CNN that can cope with input data sampled from a Riemannian manifold. The intuition in defining the analog relies on the equivariance property. Note that convolution of functions in vector spaces are equivariant to translations in the input domain. Further, it is easy to show that traditional convolutions of functions are equivalent to computing the weighted mean [10]. Hence, for the case of manifold-valued data, we can define the analogous operation of a weighted Fréchet mean (wFM) and prove that it is equivariant to the action of $I(\mathcal{M})$. This will be presented in a subsequent section. Our key contributions in this work (**presented in Sect.** 2) are (i) we define the analog of convolution operations for manifold-valued data to be one of estimating the wFM for which we present a provably convergent, efficient and recursive estimator. (ii) A proof of equivariance of wFM to the action of $I(\mathcal{M})$. This equivariance allows the network to share weights within the layers. (iii) A novel deep architecture involving the Riemannian counterparts to the conventional CNN units (**presented in Sect.** 3). (iv) Two real data experiments, (a) regression between changes in diffusional structure – captured in the Cauchy deformation tensor obtained via nonrigid registration of the ensemble average propagator (EAP) field computed from the patient scan to the EAP control atlas – and function in movement disorder patients. (b) An experiment on finding group differences based on brain connectivity at the fiber bundle level specifically, the motor sensory area (M1) tract in both the brain hemispheres.

2   Group Action Equivariant Network for Manifold-Valued Data

In this section, we will define the equivalent of a convolution operation on Riemannian manifolds. As mentioned in the introduction, the domain of interest is an n-dimensional field of manifold valued points. Before formally defining such an operation and building the ManifoldNet, we first present some relevant concepts from differential geometry that will be used in the rest of the paper.

Preliminaries. Let $(\mathcal{M}, g^{\mathcal{M}})$ be a orientable complete Riemannian manifold with a Riemannian metric $g^{\mathcal{M}}$, i.e., $(\forall x \in \mathcal{M})\, g_x^{\mathcal{M}} : T_x\mathcal{M} \times T_x\mathcal{M} \to \mathbf{R}$ is a bi-linear symmetric positive definite map, where $T_x\mathcal{M}$ is the tangent space of $\mathcal{M}$ at $x \in \mathcal{M}$. Let $d : \mathcal{M} \times \mathcal{M} \to [0, \infty)$ be the metric (distance) induced by the Riemannian metric $g^{\mathcal{M}}$. With a slight abuse of notation we will denote a Riemannian manifold $(\mathcal{M}, g^{\mathcal{M}})$ by $\mathcal{M}$ unless specified otherwise. Let Δ be the supremum of the sectional curvatures of $\mathcal{M}$.

Definition 1. *Let $p \in \mathcal{M}$, $r > 0$. Define $\mathcal{B}_r(p) = \{q \in \mathcal{M} | d(p, q) < r\}$ to be a open ball at p of radius r.*

Definition 2. *[11]   The local injectivity radius at $p \in \mathcal{M}$, $r_{inj}(p)$, is defined as $r_{inj}(p) = \sup\{r | Exp_p : (\mathcal{B}_r(0) \subset T_p\mathcal{M}) \to \mathcal{M}$ is defined and is a diffeomorphism onto its image$\}$. The injectivity radius [19] of $\mathcal{M}$ is defined as $r_{inj}(\mathcal{M}) = \inf_{p \in \mathcal{M}}\{r_{inj}(p)\}$.*

Within $\mathcal{B}_r(p)$, where $r \leq r_{inj}(\mathcal{M})$, the mapping $Exp_p^{-1} : \mathcal{B}_r(p) \to \mathcal{U} \subset T_p\mathcal{M}$, is called the inverse Exponential/Log map.

Definition 3. *[14]   An open ball $\mathcal{B}_r(p)$ is a regular geodesic ball if $r < r_{inj}(p)$ and $r < \pi/(2\Delta^{1/2})$.*

In Definition 3 and below, we interpret $1/\Delta^{1/2}$ as ∞ if $\Delta \leq 0$. It is well known that, if p and q are two points in a regular geodesic ball $\mathcal{B}_r(p)$, then they are joined by a unique geodesic within $\mathcal{B}_r(p)$ [14].

Definition 4. *[7] $\mathcal{U} \subset \mathcal{M}$ is strongly convex if for all $p, q \in \mathcal{U}$, there exists a unique length minimizing geodesic segment between p and q and the geodesic segment lies entirely in $\mathcal{U}$.*

Definition 5. *[11] Let $p \in \mathcal{M}$. The local convexity radius at p, $r_{cvx}(p)$, is defined as $r_{cvx}(p) = \sup \{r \leq r_{inj}(p) | \mathcal{B}_r(p)$ is strongly convex$\}$. The convexity radius of $\mathcal{M}$ is defined as $r_{cvx}(\mathcal{M}) = \inf_{p \in \mathcal{M}} \{r_{cvx}(p)\}$.*

For the rest of the paper, we will assume that the samples on $\mathcal{M}$ lie inside an open ball $U = \mathcal{B}_r(p)$ where $r = \min \{r_{cvx}(\mathcal{M}), r_{inj}(\mathcal{M})\}$, for some $p \in \mathcal{M}$, unless mentioned otherwise. Now, we are ready to define the operations necessary to develop the ManifoldNet architecture.

2.1 wFM on $\mathcal{M}$ as a Generalization of Convolution

We will begin by defining a convolution type operation on points sampled from $\mathcal{M}$. This convolution operation will perform an averaging over a moving window, where weighted sums are replaced with weighted intrinsic averages. Let $\{X_i\}_{i=1}^N$ be the manifold-valued samples on $\mathcal{M}$. We define the convolution type operation on $\mathcal{M}$ as the weighted Fréchet mean (wFM) [20] of the samples $\{X_i\}_{i=1}^N$. Also, by the aforementioned condition on the samples, the existence and uniqueness of the FM is guaranteed [1]. As mentioned earlier, it is easy to show (see [10]) that convolution $\psi^* = b \star a$ of two functions $a : X \subset \mathbf{R}^n \to \mathbf{R}$ and $b : X \subset \mathbf{R}^n \to \mathbf{R}$ can be formulated as computation of the weighted mean $\psi^* = argmin_\psi \int a(\mathbf{u})(\psi - \tilde{b}_\mathbf{u})^2 d\mathbf{u}$, where, $\forall \mathbf{x} \in X, \tilde{b}_\mathbf{u}(\mathbf{x}) = b(\mathbf{u} + \mathbf{x})$ and $\int a(\mathbf{x}) d\mathbf{x} = 1$. Here, f^2 for any function f is defined pointwise. Further, the defining property of convolutions in vector spaces is the linear translation equivariance in both the domain and the range of the image. Since weighted mean in vector spaces can be generalized to wFM on manifolds and further, wFM can be shown (see below) to be equivariant to group actions admitted by the manifold, we claim that wFM is a generalization of convolution operations to manifold-valued data.

Let $\{w_i\}_{i=1}^N$ be the weights such that they satisfy the convexity constraint, i.e., $\forall i, w_i > 0$ and $\sum_i w_i = 1$, then wFM, wFM $(\{X_i\}, \{w_i\})$ is defined as:

$$\text{wFM}\left(\{X_i\}, \{w_i\}\right) = \underset{M \in \mathcal{M}}{argmin} \sum_{i=1}^N w_i d^2\left(X_i, M\right) \tag{1}$$

Analogous to the equivariance property of convolution to translations in vector spaces, we will now show that the wFM is equivariant under the action of the group of isometries of $\mathcal{M}$. We will first formally define the group of isometries of $\mathcal{M}$ (let us denote it by G) and then define the equivariance property and show that wFM is G-equivariant.

Definition 6 (Group of isometries of $\mathcal{M}$ ($I(\mathcal{M})$)). *A diffeomorphism $\phi : \mathcal{M} \to \mathcal{M}$ is an isometry if it preserves distance, i.e., $d(\phi(x), \phi(y)) = d(x, y)$. The set $I(\mathcal{M})$ of all isometries of $\mathcal{M}$ forms a group with respect to function composition. Rather than write an isometry as a function ϕ, we will write it as a group action. Henceforth, let G denote the group $I(\mathcal{M})$, and for $g \in G$, and $x \in \mathcal{M}$, let $g.x$ denote the result of applying the isometry g to point x.*

Clearly $\mathcal{M}$ is a G set (see [9] for the definition of a G set). We will now define equivariance and show that wFM is G-equivariant.

Definition 7 (Equivariance). *Let X and Y be G sets. Then, $F : X \to Y$ is said to be G-equivariant if $\forall g \in G$, $\forall x \in X$, $F(g.x) = g.F(x)$.*

Let $U \subset \mathcal{M}$ be an open ball inside which FM exists and is unique, let P be the set of all possible finite subsets of U.

Theorem 1. *Given $\{w_i\}$ satisfying the convex constraint, let $F : P \to U$ be a function defined by $\{X_i\} \mapsto$ wFM$(\{X_i\}, \{w_i\})$. Then, F is G-equivariant.*

Proof. Let $g \in G$ and $\{X_i\}_{i=1}^N \in P$, now, let $M^* =$ wFM$(\{X_i\}, \{w_i\})$, as $g.F(\{X_i\}) = g.M^*$, it suffices to show $g.M^*$ is wFM$(\{g.X_i\}, \{w_i\})$ (assuming the existence and uniqueness of wFM$(\{g.X_i\}, \{w_i\})$ which is stated in the following claim).

Claim: Let $U = \mathcal{B}_r(p)$ for some $r > 0$ and $p \in \mathcal{M}$. Then, $\{g.X_i\} \subset \mathcal{B}_r(g.p)$ and hence wFM$(\{g.X_i\}, \{w_i\})$ exists and is unique.

Let $\widetilde{M}$ be wFM$(\{g.X_i\}, \{w_i\})$. Then, $\sum_{i=1}^N w_i d^2\left(g.X_i, \widetilde{M}\right) = \sum_{i=1}^N w_i d^2(X_i, \ g^{-1}.\widetilde{M})$. Since, $M^* =$ wFM$(\{X_i\}, \{w_i\})$, hence, $M^* = g^{-1}.\widetilde{M}$, i.e., $\widetilde{M} = g.M^*$. Thus, $g.M^* =$ wFM$(\{g.X_i\}, \{w_i\})$, which implies F is G-equivariant.

A class of Riemannian manifolds on which G acts transitively are called Riemannian homogeneous spaces. We can see that on a Riemannian homogeneous space $\mathcal{M}$, wFM is G-equivariant. Equipped with a G-equivariant operator on $\mathcal{M}$, we can claim that the wFM (defined above) is a valid convolution operator since group equivariance is a unique defining property of a convolution operator.

The rest of this subsection will be devoted to developing an efficient way to compute wFM. The strategy is to cast the weighted FM computation as an unweighted FM computation, and then use efficient FM estimators. Let $\omega^{\mathcal{M}} > 0$ be the Riemannian volume form.

Let $p_{\mathbf{X}}$ be the probability density of a U-valued random variable $\mathbf{X}$ with respect to $\omega^{\mathcal{M}}$ on $U \subset \mathcal{M}$, so that $\Pr(X \in \mathfrak{A}) = \int_{\mathfrak{A}} p_X(Y)\omega^{\mathcal{M}}(Y)$ for any Borel-measurable subset $\mathfrak{A}$ of U. Let $Y \in U$, we can define the expectation of the real valued random variable $d^2(, Y) : U \to \mathbf{R}$ by $E\left[d^2(, Y)\right] = \int_U d^2(X, Y) p_{\mathbf{X}}(X)\omega^{\mathcal{M}}(X)$. Now, let $w : U \to (0, \infty)$ be an integrable function where $\int_U w(X)\omega^{\mathcal{M}}(X) = 1$.

Let $\widetilde{p}_X$ be the probability density corresponding to the probability measure $\widetilde{\Pr}$ defined by $\widetilde{\Pr}(X \in \mathfrak{X}) = \int_{\mathfrak{X}} \widetilde{p}_X(Y)\omega^{\mathcal{M}}(Y) := \int_{\mathfrak{X}} \frac{1}{C} p_X(Y)w(Y)\omega^{\mathcal{M}}(Y)$, where, $\mathfrak{X}$ lies in the Borel σ-algebra over U and let $C = \int_U p_X(Y)w(Y)\omega^{\mathcal{M}}(Y)$. Note that the constant $C > 0$, since p_X is a probability density, $w > 0$ and $\mathcal{M}$ is orientable.

Now, we will state and prove the following proposition.

Proposition 1. *Using the notation from above we have:* **(i)** *supp$(p_X) =$ supp$(\widetilde{p}_X)$.* **(ii)** *wFE$(X, w) =$ FE$\left(\widetilde{X}\right)$.*

Proof. Let $X \in \text{supp}(p_X)$, then, $p_X(X) > 0$. Since, $w(X) > 0$, hence, $\widetilde{p}_X(X) > 0$ and thus, $X \in \text{supp}(\widetilde{p}_X)$. On the other hand, assume $\widetilde{X}$ to be a sample drawn from $\widetilde{p}_X$. Then, either $p_X\left(\widetilde{X}\right) = 0$ or $p_X\left(\widetilde{X}\right) > 0$. If, $p_X\left(\widetilde{X}\right) = 0$, then, $\widetilde{p}_X\left(\widetilde{X}\right) = 0$ which contradicts our assumption. Hence, $p_X\left(\widetilde{X}\right) > 0$, i.e., $\widetilde{X} \in \text{supp}(p_X)$. This concludes the proof of part (i).

Let X and $\widetilde{X}$ be the $\mathcal{M}$ valued random variable following p_X and $\widetilde{p}_X$ respectively. We define the weighted Fréchet expectation (wFE) of X as $\text{wFE}(X, w) = \text{argmin}_{Y \in \mathcal{M}} \int_{\mathcal{M}} w(X)d^2(X, Y)p_X(X)\omega^{\mathcal{M}}(X)$.

Observe, $E_w\left[d^2(,Y)\right] := \int_U w(X)d^2(X,Y)p_X(X)\,\omega^{\mathcal{M}}(X) = C \int_U d^2(X,Y)$ $\widetilde{p}_X(X)\,\omega^{\mathcal{M}}(X) = C\,\widetilde{E}\left[d^2(,Y)\right]$ .. Hence, we get $\text{FE}\left(\widetilde{X}\right) = \text{wFE}(X, w)$, as C is independent of the choice of Y, which concludes the proof of part (ii).

Now let $\{X_i\}_{i=1}^N$ be samples drawn from p_X and $\left\{\widetilde{X}_i\right\}_{i=1}^N$ be samples drawn from $\widetilde{p}_X$. In order to compute wFM, we will now present an online algorithm (inductive FM Estimator – dubbed iFME). Note that in [6,17,22], authors present recursive algorithms for FM computation on the hyper-sphere, Stiefel and $SPD(n)$ manifolds respectively. These specific algorithms are distinct from our work here since the wFM approach is applicable to any Riemannian manifold.

iFME wFM Estimator: Given, $\{X_i\}_{i=1}^N \subset U$ and $\{w_i := w(X_i)\}_{i=1}^N$ such that $\forall i, w_i > 0$, the nth estimate, M_n of $\text{wFM}(\{X_i\}, \{w_i\})$ is given by the following recursion:

$$M_1 = X_1 \qquad\qquad M_n = \Gamma_{M_{n-1}}^{X_n}\left(\frac{w_n}{\sum_{j=1}^n w_j}\right). \qquad (2)$$

In the above equation, $\Gamma_X^Y : [0,1] \to U$ is the shortest geodesic curve from X to Y. Observe that, in general wFM is defined with $\sum_{i=1}^N w_i = 1$, but in above definition, $\sum_{i=1}^N w_i \neq 1$. We can normalize $\{w_i\}$ to get $\{\widetilde{w}_i\}$ by $\widetilde{w}_i = w_i/(\sum_i w_i)$, but then Eq. 2 will not change as $\widetilde{w}_n/\left(\sum_{j=1}^n \widetilde{w}_j\right) = w_n/\left(\sum_{j=1}^n w_j\right)$. This gives us an efficient inductive/recursive way to define convolution operation on $\mathcal{M}$. We now show that the proposed wFM estimator is consistent in the following proposition (the proof is in supplementary section).

Proposition 2. *Using the above notations and assumptions, let $\{X_i\}_{i=1}^N$ be i.i.d. samples drawn from p_X on $\mathcal{M}$. Let the wFE be finite. Then, M_N converges a.s. to wFE as $N \to \infty$.*

2.2   Nonlinear Operation Between wFM-layers for $\mathcal{M}$-valued Data

In the traditional CNN model, we need an intermediate nonlinear function between convolutional layers (e.g. ReLU). As argued in [18], any nonlinear function used in CNNs is basically a contraction mapping. Formally, let F be a nonlinear mapping from U to V. Assume U and V are metric spaces equipped with metrics d_U and d_V respectively. Then F is a contraction mapping *iff* $\exists c < 1$ such that $d_V\left(F(x), F(y)\right) \leq c\ d_U(x, y)$. F is a non-expansive mapping [18] *iff* $d_V\left(F(x), F(y)\right) \leq d_U(x, y)$.

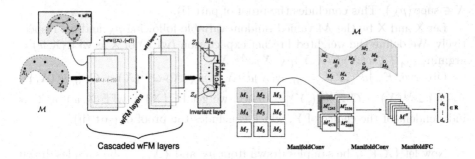

Fig. 1. *Left-Right* (a) Schematic diagram of ManifoldNet (b) 2×2 ManifoldNet conv. example

One can easily see that the popular choices for nonlinear operations like ReLU, sigmoid are indeed non-expansive mappings. We will now show that the function wFM as defined in 1, is a contraction mapping for any non-trivial choice of weights. Let $\{X_i\}_{i=1}^N$ and $\{Y_j\}_{j=1}^M$ be the two set of samples on $\mathcal{M}$. Without loss of generality assume $N \leq M$. We consider the set $\mathcal{U}^M = \underbrace{U \times \cdots \times U}_{M \text{ times}}$. Clearly $\{Y_j\}_{j=1}^M \in \mathcal{U}^M$ and we embed $\{X_i\}_{i=1}^N$ in $\mathcal{U}^M$ as follows: we construct $\left\{\widetilde{X}_i\right\}_{i=1}^M$ from $\{X_i\}_{i=1}^N$ by defining $\widetilde{X}_i = X_{(i-1) \bmod N + 1}$. Let us denote the embedding by ι. Now, define the distance on $\mathcal{U}^M$ as $d\left(\left\{\widetilde{X}_i\right\}_{i=1}^M, \{Y_j\}_{j=1}^M\right) = \max_{i,j} d(X_i, Y_j)$. We say the choice of weights for wFM is trivial if one of the weights is 1 (hence all others are 0).

Proposition 3. *For all nontrivial choices of $\{\alpha_i\}_{i=1}^N$ and $\{\beta_j\}_{j=1}^M$ satisfying the convexity constraint, $\exists c < 1$ such that,*

$$d\left(\mathsf{wFM}\left(\{X_i\}_{i=1}^N, \{\alpha_i\}_{i=1}^N\right), \mathsf{wFM}\left(\{Y_j\}_{i=1}^M, \{\beta_j\}_{i=1}^M\right)\right)$$
$$\leq c\ d\left(\iota\left(\{X_i\}_{i=1}^N\right), \{Y_j\}_{j=1}^M\right) \tag{3}$$

2.3   The Invariant (last) Layer

We will form a deep network by cascading multiple sliding wFM windows each of which acts as a convolution-type layer. Each convolutional-type layer is equivariant to the group action, and hence at the end of the cascaded convolutional layers, the output is equivariant to the group action applied to the input of the network. Let d be the number of output channels each of which outputs a wFM, hence each of the channels is equivariant to the group action. However, in order to build a network that yields an output which is *invariant* to the group action we would like the last layer (i.e., the analogue to a linear classifier) to be invariant to the group action. The last layer is thus constructed as follows: Let $\{Z_1, \cdots, Z_d\} \subset \mathcal{M}$ be the output of d channels and $M_u = \mathsf{FM}\left(\{Z_i\}_{i=1}^d\right)$

$= \mathsf{wFM}\left(\{Z_i\}_{i=1}^d, \{1/d\}_1^d\right)$ be the unweighted FM of the outputs $\{Z_i\}_{i=1}^d$. Then, we construct a layer with d outputs whose i^{th} output $o_i = d\left(M_u, Z_i\right)$. Let c be the number of classes for the classification task, then, a fully connected (FC) layer with inputs $\{o_i\}$ and c output nodes is used. Finally, a softmax operation is then used at the c output nodes to obtain the outputs $\{y_i\}_{i=1}^c$. In the following proposition we claim that this last layer with $\{Z_i\}_{i=1}^d$ inputs and $\{y_i\}_{i=1}^c$ outputs is group invariant.

Proposition 4. *The last layer with $\{Z_i\}_{i=1}^d$ inputs and $\{y_i\}_{i=1}^c$ outputs is group invariant.*

Proof. Using the above construction, let $W \in \mathbf{R}^{c \times d}$ and $\mathbf{b} \in \mathbf{R}^c$ be the weight matrix and bias respectively of the FC layer. Then,

$$\mathbf{y} = F\left(W^T \mathbf{o} + \mathbf{b}\right) = F\left(W^T d\left(M_u, Z\right) + \mathbf{b}\right), \tag{4}$$

where, F is the softmax function. In the above equation, we treat $d\left(M_u, Z\right)$ as the vector $[d\left(M_u, Z_1\right), \cdots, d\left(M_u, Z_d\right)]^t$. Observe that, $g.M_u = \mathsf{FM}\left(\{g.Z_i\}_{i=1}^d\right)$. As each of the d channels is group equivariant, Z_i becomes $g.Z_i$. Because of the property of the distance under group action, $d\left(g.M_u, g.Z_i\right) = d\left(M_u, Z_i\right)$. Hence, one can see that if we change the inputs $\{Z_i\}$ to $\{g.Z_i\}$, the output $\mathbf{y}$ will remain invariant.

In Fig. 1 we present a schematic of ManifoldNet depicting the different layers of processing the manifold-valued data as described above in Sects. 2.1, 2.2 and 2.3.

Unlike standard Euclidean CNN, note that, here we do not need a nonlinearity between two convolution layers as argued in Subsect. 2.2. Note that, in standard CNN, without the presence of non-linearity one can collapse a deep network into a shallow one. This raises the following question *Can Manifold-Net be collapsed to it's shallow counterpart as there is no non-linearity between layers?* In order to answer this question, we will show that for manifolds with non-constant sectional curvatures, we can not collapse the ManifoldNet into a shallow network.

Here we present a proof (via a counter example) to show that a multi-layer ManifoldNet can not be collapsed to a single layer ManifoldNet when $\mathcal{M} = SPD(n)$, which is a manifold with non-constant curvature.

Theorem 2. *The multi-layer ManifoldNet is not equivalent to the single layer Manifold-Net for data on Riemannian manifolds with non-constant sectional curvature.*

Proof. This is a proof by counter example. Let us suppose we are given 4 SPD matrices, $A = \begin{bmatrix} 0.9593 & 0.3429 \\ 0.3429 & 0.1493 \end{bmatrix}$, $B = \begin{bmatrix} 1.2575 & 0.5475 \\ 0.5475 & 1.8143 \end{bmatrix}$, $C = \begin{bmatrix} 1.2435 & 0.6396 \\ 0.6396 & 1.1966 \end{bmatrix}$, $D = \begin{bmatrix} 1.2511 & 0.5446 \\ 0.5447 & 1.3517 \end{bmatrix}$, whose wFM we want to compute. Let us consider two sequences $S1 = \{A, B, C, D\}$ and $S2 = \{A, C, B, D\}$. Consider a one layer ManifoldNet for computing the wFM of these four matrices. For simplicity of exposition, suppose this one layer network learns equal weights ($= 0.25$) for all matrices and hence yields the wFM $M = \begin{bmatrix} 1.1640 & 0.4667 \\ 0.4667 & 0.6388 \end{bmatrix}$ as the solution for both sequences $S1$ and $S2$ respectively. To compute the wFM, we use a gradient descent applied to the weighted sum of square geodesic distances between the unknown wFM and the sample points.

Now, let us consider a two layer wFM. For $S1$, the first layer computes wFM of $\{A, B\}$ and $\{C, D\}$ respectively and returns $M1$ and $M2$ as the wFMs. Then, the second layer takes $M1$ and $M2$ as inputs and returns their wFM say, $M3$. Analogously for the sequence $S2$, the first layer computes wFM of $\{A, C\}$ and $\{B, D\}$ and returns $\bar{M}1$ and $\bar{M}2$. Then the second layer takes as input, $\bar{M}1$ and $\bar{M}2$ and returns $\bar{M}3$ as their wFM.

It can be verified that for the first layer if we use equal weights, we need the weights for the second layer to be 0.4980 and 0.5050 for $S1$ and $S2$ respectively such that both $M3 = M$ and $\bar{M}3 = M$. This counter example shows that the weights are dependent on the input data matrices, which means that in general a multi-layer ManifoldNet can not be collapsed to a single layer ManifoldNet.

3   Experiments

We now present the basic ManifoldNet architecture and evaluate its performance on two medical imaging tasks: (1) Diffusion Tensor field hypothesis testing and (2) nonlinear regression. We remark that although the ManifoldNet architecture is perfectly capable of tackling the classification of manifold-valued data, in the medical imaging domain, procuring a very large population of such data is either prohibitively expensive or unavailable via public access repositories. Hence, we chose to demonstrate the efficacy of the ManifoldNet on other challenging applications such as regression and group testing that do not require tens of thousands of images for training and testing.

We now describe in detail how to use the basic layers defined and analyzed in Sect. 2 to create multilayer ManifoldNet architectures comparable to deep CNNs. Note that the input to ManifoldNet is always an N-dimensional field of points sampled from a Riemannian manifold. For expository purposes we will consider the case of a *manifold-valued image*, i.e., the input to any layer of the ManifoldNet architecture is, $(B \times W \times H \times C)$ points on a Riemannian manifold. Here, B the batch size, W the image width, H is the image height and C is the number of input channels.

Analogous to traditional convolution layers, we now define the **Manifold-Conv** layer, which slides a small window of weights along the spatial dimensions (W and H) of the input, but instead of weighted sums we now compute the weighted FM in each window as described in Sect. 2.1. As in the traditional CNNs, we can do this for several different weight tensors to generate multiple output channels. So the **ManifoldConv** layer transforms the original tensor of manifold valued points to a size ($B \times W' \times H' \times C'$) tensor of manifold valued points. Important properties of the **ManifoldConv** layers are:

- Traditional convolution layers are **ManifoldConv** with $\mathcal{M} = \mathbf{R}$, so **ManifoldConv** generalizes traditional convolution layers.
- The **ManifoldConv** generalization preserves the key property that has made convolutional layers among the most successful building blocks of deep network architectures: equivariance to isometric transformations of the input data. This property is preserved by wFM, and therefore also by the **ManifoldConv** layer.
- Since we have shown that the wFM operation is both a contraction mapping and, atleast in the case of non-constant curvature manifolds, non-collapsible, it follows that the same properties hold for the **ManifoldConv** layer. Therefore the stacking of such layers without an intermediate non-linearity is justified for non-constant curvature manifolds.
- The weights for a wFM computation should satisfy the convexity constraint, which can be imposed by squaring the weight matrix to be positive and then normalizing to sum to 1. This allows us to use regular backpropagation through the **ManifoldConv** layer.

After stacking several **ManifoldConv** layers we may require a vector valued output for classification purposes, and we would like this vector to be *invariant* to the natural group isometries admitted by the manifold on which the input data reside. To generate this vector we use the invariant final layer from Sect. 2.3. We henceforth call this layer the **ManifoldFC** layer, since it is an analogue to the traditional fully connected layers.

Using these two layers we can build general classifiers of non-constant curvature manifold valued data using an architecture of the form

$$\mathbf{ManifoldConv} \rightarrow \mathbf{ManifoldConv} \rightarrow \cdots \rightarrow \mathbf{ManifoldConv} \rightarrow \mathbf{ManifoldFC}$$

And for other tasks such as manifold regression we can remove the **ManifoldFC** layer. This architecture can be trained end-to-end using traditional backpropagation since the weights are real valued.

Group Testing on Movement Disorder Patients: Diffusion MRI is a commonly used modality for diagnosing and studying neurological disorders. In this experiment we use a dataset consisting of scans from a control group of 44 patients and a group of 50 Parkinsons patients (see Fig. 2). All scans were performed using a $3.0T$ Philips Achieva scanner with a 32-channel volume head coil. The parameters of the diffusion imaging acquisition sequence were as follows: gradient directions = 64, b-values = 0/1000 s/mm^2, repetition time = 7748 ms, echo time $= 86$ ms, flip angle $= 90$, field of view $= 224 \times 224$ mm, matrix size $= 112 \times 112$, number of contiguous axial slices $= 60$ and SENSE factor $P = 2$ for parameters of image acquisition. Sensory motor area tracts called M1 fiber tracts are first extracted from the scans using FSL software [2] from both the left ('LM1') and right hemispheres ('RM1') respectively. We then use the FSL software [4] to extract $SPD(3)$ diffusion tensors from each tract. Note that the space $SPD(3)$ of (3×3) SPD matrices is a homogeneous Riemannian manifold with the isometry group being $GL(n)$.

Following [5] closely, we fit a 3 layer ManifoldNet model to both the control group and the Parkinsons group data. Using the method from [23] we compute the distance between these two models, denoted by $\mathbf{d}$. Now we permute the class labels between the classes, retrain the two models and compute the network distance d_j. If there are significant differences between the classes we should expect that $\mathbf{d} > d_j$. We repeat this experiment for $j = 1, \ldots, 1000$ and let p be the proportion of experiments for which $\mathbf{d} \leq d_j$. This is a permutation test of the null hypothesis "there is no significant difference between the tract models learned from the two different classes." We can compare this to the performance of the similar dMRI architecture SPD-SRU and the baseline methods from [5]. We found that our ManifoldNet architecture achieved an 'LM1' p-value of 0.029 and an 'RM1' p-value of 0.024. The baseline method gave an 'LM1' and 'RM1' p-value of 0.17 and 0.34 respectively, while the SPD-SRU architecture gave p-values of 0.01 and 0.032 respectively. We can conclude that using ManifoldNet we can reject the null hypothesis with 95% confidence, which is competitive with SPD-SRU.

Nonlinear Regression Between Structure and Function: This dataset contains high angular resolution diffusion image (HARDI) scans from, (1) healthy controls, (2) patients with essential tremor (ET) and (3) Parkinson's disease (PD) patients. This data pool contains scans from 25 controls, 15 ET and 26 PD patients. This HARDI data was acquired using the same parameters as before. The dimension of each image is $(112 \times 112 \times 60)$. From each of these images, we identify the region of interest (ROI) (40 voxels in size) containing the Substantia Nigra (a neuroanatomical structure known to be affected most by PD and ET).

In morphometric analysis, it is common to use the Cauchy deformation tensor (CDT) field to capture changes in a patient scan with respect to a reference template/atlas. Thus, in order to capture changes in patient HARDI scans with respect to the control atlas, we first nonrigidly register each of the EAP (ensemble average propagator) fields estimated from the input HARDI scan to the computed EAP atlas and obtain the CDT at each voxel in the ROI, given by $\sqrt{J^T J}$, where, J is the Jacobian of the non-rigid transformation [8]. The CDT is an SPD matrix of dimension (3×3) in this case. Hence, for each patient we extract a CDT field of dimension $(3 \times 3 \times 40)$. In this experiment, we seek to find the relationship between structural information in the form of CDT and clinical measures such as the MDS-UPDRS (Movement Disorder Society's revision of the Unified Parkinson's Disease Rating Scale) [21].

The MDS-UPDRS score is widely used to follow the longitudinal course of PD. These scores are obtained via interviews and clinical observations by an expert. In this experiment, available to us are the MDS-UPDRS scores for all the 58 subjects in the population under consideration. This score is a nonnegative natural number, with smaller values indicating normality.

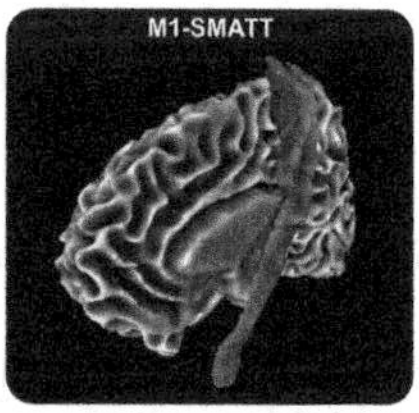

For these 58 patients, we used a 3 layer ManifoldNet to find the relation between CDT field and MDS-UPDRS scores. We used an MSE loss and obtained an R^2 statistic of 0.93. This R^2 statistic value is similar to the one reported in [3].

Fig. 2. M1-SMATT template

4   Conclusions

In this paper, we presented a novel deep network called ManifoldNet suited for processing manifold-valued data sets. Inputs to the ManifoldNet are manifold-valued and not real or complex-valued functions defined on non-Euclidean domains. Our key contributions are: (i) A novel deep network to be perceived as a generalization of the CNN to manifold-valued data inputs using purely intrinsic operations on the data manifold. (ii) Analogous to convolutions in vector spaces – which can be computed using the weighted mean – we present wFM operations on the manifold and prove the equivariance of the wFM to natural group actions admitted by the manifold. This equivariance allows us to share the learned weights within a layer of the ManifoldNet. (iii) An efficient recursive wFM estimator that is provably convergent. (iv) Experimental results demonstrating the efficacy of the ManifoldNet for, (a) regression between dMRI scans of PD patients and clinical MDS-UPDRS scores and (b) finding group differences between PD and Controls based on brain connectivity at the fiber bundle level.

References

1. Afsari, B.: Riemannian L^p center of mass: existence, uniqueness, and convexity. Proc. Am. Math. Soc. **139**(02), 655 (2011). https://doi.org/10.1090/S0002-9939-2010-10541-5, http://www.ams.org/jourcgi/jour-getitem?pii=S0002-9939-2010-10541-5

2. Archer, D., Vaillancourt, D., Coombes, S.: A template and probabilistic atlas of the human sensorimotor tracts using diffusion MRI. Cereb. Cortex **28**, 1–15 (2017). https://doi.org/10.1093/cercor/bhx066

3. Banerjee, M., Chakraborty, R., Ofori, E., Okun, M.S., Viallancourt, D.E., Vemuri, B.C.: A nonlinear regression technique for manifold valued data with applications to medical image analysis. In: Proceedings of the IEEE Conference on Computer Vision and Pattern Recognition, pp. 4424–4432 (2016)

4. Behrens, T., Berg, H.J., Jbabdi, S., Rushworth, M., Woolrich, M.: Probabilistic diffusion tractography with multiple fibre orientations: what can we gain? NeuroImage **34**(1), 144–155 (2007). https://doi.org/10.1016/j.neuroimage.2006.09.018, http://www.sciencedirect.com/science/article/pii/S1053811906009360

5. Chakraborty, R., et al.: Statistical Recurrent Models on Manifold valued Data. ArXiv e-prints, May 2018
6. Chakraborty, R., Vemuri, B.C., et al.: Statistics on the Stiefel manifold: theory and applications. Ann. Stat. **47**(1), 415–438 (2019)
7. Chavel, I.: Riemannian Geometry: A Modern Introduction, vol. 98. Cambridge University Press, Cambridge (2006)
8. Cheng, G., Vemuri, B.C., Carney, P.R., Mareci, T.H.: Non-rigid registration of high angular resolution diffusion images represented by Gaussian mixture fields. In: Yang, G.-Z., Hawkes, D., Rueckert, D., Noble, A., Taylor, C. (eds.) MICCAI 2009. LNCS, vol. 5761, pp. 190–197. Springer, Heidelberg (2009). https://doi.org/10.1007/978-3-642-04268-3_24
9. Dummit, D.S., Foote, R.M.: Abstract Algebra, vol. 3. Wiley, Hoboken (2004)
10. Goh, A., Lenglet, C., Thompson, P.M., Vidal, R.: A nonparametric Riemannian framework for processing high angular resolution diffusion images and its applications to ODF-based morphometry. NeuroImage **56**(3), 1181–1201 (2011)
11. Groisser, D.: Newton's method, zeroes of vector fields, and the Riemannian center of mass. Adv. Appl. Math. **33**(1), 95–135 (2004). https://doi.org/10.1016/j.aam.2003.08.003
12. Huang, Z., Van Gool, L.J.: A Riemannian network for SPD matrix learning. In: AAAI, vol. 1, p. 3 (2017)
13. Huang, Z., Wu, J., Van Gool, L.: Building deep networks on Grassmann manifolds. arXiv preprint arXiv:1611.05742 (2016)
14. Kendall, W.S.: Probability, convexity, and harmonic maps with small image. I. Uniqueness and finite existence. Proc. London Math. Soc. **3**(2), 371–406 (1990)
15. Krizhevsky, A., Sutskever, I., Hinton, G.E.: ImageNet classification with deep convolutional neural networks. In: Advances in Neural Information Processing Systems (2012). https://doi.org/10.1016/j.protcy.2014.09.007
16. LeCun, Y., Bottou, L., Bengio, Y., Haffner, P.: Gradient-based learning applied to document recognition. Proc. IEEE (1998). https://doi.org/10.1109/5.726791
17. Lim, Y., Pálfia, M.: Weighted inductive means. Linear Algebra Appl. **453**, 59–83 (2014)
18. Mallat, S.: Understanding deep convolutional networks. Philos. Trans. A **374**, 20150203 (2016). https://doi.org/10.1098/rsta.2015.0203, http://arxiv.org/abs/1601.04920
19. Manton, J.H.: A globally convergent numerical algorithm for computing the centre of mass on compact lie groups. In: 8th Control, Automation, Robotics and Vision Conference, ICARCV 2004, vol. 3, pp. 2211–2216. IEEE (2004)
20. Fréchet, M.: Les éléments aléatoires de nature quelconque dans un espace distancié. Annales de l'I. H. P. **10**(4), 215–310 (1948)
21. Ramaker, C., Marinus, J., Stiggelbout, A.M., Van Hilten, B.J.: Systematic evaluation of rating scales for impairment and disability in Parkinson's disease. Mov. Disorders: official J. Mov. Disorder Soc. **17**(5), 867–876 (2002)
22. Salehian, H., Chakraborty, R., Ofori, E., Vaillancourt, D., Vemuri, B.C.: An efficient recursive estimator of the Fréchet mean on a hypersphere with applications to medical image analysis. Mathematical Foundations of Computational Anatomy (2015)
23. Triacca, U.: Measuring the distance between sets of ARMA models. Econometrics **4**, 32 (2016). https://doi.org/10.3390/econometrics4030032

Improved Disease Classification in Chest X-Rays with Transferred Features from Report Generation

Yuan Xue and Xiaolei Huang$^{(\boxtimes)}$

College of Information Sciences and Technology, Penn State University,
University Park, PA, USA
suh972@psu.edu

Abstract. Radiology includes using medical images for detection and diagnosis of diseases as well as guiding further interventions. Chest X-rays are commonly used radiological examinations to help spot thoracic abnormalities or diseases, especially lung-related diseases. However, the reporting of chest x-rays requires experienced radiologists who are often in shortage in many regions of the world. In this paper, we first develop an automatic radiology report generation system. Due to the lack of large annotated radiology report datasets and the difficulty of evaluating the generated reports, the clinical value of such systems is often limited. To this end, we train our report generation network on the small IU Chest X-ray dataset then transfer the learned visual features to classification networks trained on the large ChestX-ray14 dataset and use a novel attention guided feature fusion strategy to improve the detection performance of 14 common thoracic diseases. Through learning the correspondences between different types of feature representations, common features learned by both the report generation and the classification model are assigned with higher attention weights and the weighted visual features boost the performance of state-of-the-art baseline thoracic disease classification networks without altering any learned features. Our work not only offers a new way to evaluate the effectiveness of the learned radiology report generation network, but also proves the possibility of transferring different types of visual representations learned on a small dataset for one task to complement features learned on another large dataset for a different task and improve the model performance.

1 Introduction

Deep learning has shown its strength in various types of computer vision tasks such as classification and detection in the last decade. With the rapid development of advanced algorithms and the availability of more annotated datasets, potential applications of deep learning in radiology have become possible and desired by the public. Among such applications, the report generation networks [11,14,26] and the disease classification networks [19,23,24,27] are two popular trends. An automated or computer-aided radiology reporting system

© Springer Nature Switzerland AG 2019
A. C. S. Chung et al. (Eds.): IPMI 2019, LNCS 11492, pp. 125–138, 2019.
https://doi.org/10.1007/978-3-030-20351-1_10

can provide preliminary findings to radiologists to assist with report writing; A disease classification network can help detect potential abnormalities and diseases shown in the examinations. Both systems can help reduce the workload of expert radiologists as well as make up for staff shortage.

Current report generation methods mainly follow the encoder-decoder architecture which has been widely used for image captioning [17,22,25]. In the radiology report, the *Impression* and the *Findings* can be generated based on the interpretation of images without prior examinations or patient history, which makes the generation tasks a perfect fit for deep learning models. Impression can be a single-sentence conclusion or diagnosis, and findings can be a coherent paragraph containing multiple sentences that describe the radiologist's observations and findings regarding both normal and abnormal features in the images. While the impression generation can often be handled by an image captioning algorithm, a findings paragraph consists of multiple sentences thus traditional captioning algorithms designed for generating single-sentence description no longer apply. For findings generation, state-of-the-art radiology report generation models use either a hierarchical architecture [11,14] to generate different sentences based on different topic vectors, or a recurrent architecture [26] to generate one sentence at a time whereby the following sentence is conditioned upon the content of its preceding sentence. Combining the merits of both, we propose a modified recurrent attention model where a succeeding sentence is generated based upon both the prior sentence and a global topic vector encoded by the generated impression. The recurrent attention mechanism guarantees the model to generate diverse and coherent sentences, where the global topic vector forces the model to produce sentences supporting the conclusion or diagnosis.

Although some accomplishments have been made in radiology report generation, there are still several issues remaining unsolved. First, training a general and robust report generation system on a small training set is impractical, as the ground truth report provided in the training set can be biased towards the radiologist's personal style. Even for the same image, different radiologists can produce entirely different written reports as they only provide information that they think might be important to the potential referees. More importantly, evaluation of the generated report is difficult. Any automatic metrics based on the overlap between the prediction and ground truth cannot capture the words describing negation and uncertainty and lack measurement of semantic similarity, while human evaluation requires extra efforts by human experts and can be error-prone. While the generated report learned by the decoder model can be biased towards the training data, the learned visual features from the encoder model are expected to be more general and robust. Otherwise they are not able to provide enough information to the decoder model to produce diverse sentences describing different regions. Therefore, we introduce a novel evaluation of the trained chest X-ray report generation network, where we only take the encoder part of the model as a visual feature extractor, and transfer these learned features to be used in another large chest X-ray dataset and evaluate their performance for thoracic disease classification.

Traditional transfer learning benefits from training with a large-scale dataset then transferring the learned knowledge or model weights to another dataset that is typically much smaller for better initialization and faster convergence. However, transfers from a small dataset to a large dataset with cross-task generalization are under-investigated, but such transfers have great research and clinical value since some annotations like complete radiology reports are expensive to obtain due to the difficulty of labeling or privacy concerns. In this work, taking the learned image encoder from the report generation model, we apply the extracted visual features to another chest X-ray dataset for disease classification. We combine the features from the report generator and the features extracted by a well-trained disease classification network to form an attention map, where common features learned by both networks are emphasized with higher weights. Then we apply the attention map to the original feature learned by the classification network and re-train the transition layer for new predictions. The transferred visual features along with the attention guided feature fusion shows considerable improvements over a baseline classification network, and even achieve further improvements over the state-of-the-art CheXNet [19] without changing any visual features. Our work not only offers a new way to evaluate the effectiveness of learned radiology report generation network, but also proves the possibility of transferring different types of visual representation learned on a small dataset for one task to complement features learned on another large dataset for a different task and improve the model performance.

2   Related Work

Radiology Report Generation. As a joint application of Computer Vision (CV) and Nature Language Processing (NLP) in healthcare, the automatic radiology report generation task has recently attracted considerable attention. Following the encoder-decoder architecture and attention mechanism in image captioning [17,22,25], several report generation works have been proposed. To generate long and coherent reports, previous works [11,14] use a hierarchical architecture [1,13] to generate a sequence of encoded topic vectors, then each sentence in the report is generated conditioned on the topic vector; Xue et al. [26] utilizes a recurrent attention model and brings the contextual information into the loop when predicting next words and sentences. Li et al. [14] combines a retrieval module and a generation module to either select a phrase from the template database or generate a new sentence. However, such models still suffer from the bias of training set, and automatic evaluation cannot capture the words describing negation and uncertainty in the predicted report. Taking the merits of previous methods, we modify the recurrent attention model [26] and introduce a global topic vector to guide the generation of findings. Instead of only evaluating the predicted report, we transfer the learned visual features to the ChestX-ray14 dataset and use an attention guided feature fusion scheme to help improve the disease classification performance.

Thoracic Disease Classification. Wang *et al.* [23] introduced the ChestX-ray14 dataset which is currently the largest public repository of radiographs. They also reported a weakly supervised multi-label thoracic disease classification and localization framework in their paper. Yao *et al.* [27] leveraged inter-dependencies among different pathology labels in chest X-rays via LSTMs to improve the disease classification performance. In [19], state-of-the-art disease classification result is reported using a DenseNet-121 [10] backbone; their trained model gets impressive results and exceeds the average radiologist performance on the pneumonia detection task.

A different approach for thoracic disease classification trains the model with multiple tasks to improve classification result. Li *et al.* [15] presents a unified network that simultaneously improves classification and localization with the help of extra bounding boxes indicating disease location. Wang *et al.* [24] uses a CNN-RNN model to generate a radiology report and encodes the generated report directly to improve the classification result. Different from our model, their report generation and classification models are trained on the same dataset where the ground truth disease labels and reports are inherently correlated since the labels are text-mined from the original report. Since there is no large dataset with annotated radiology report available to the public, it is hard to extend their framework to other domains and tasks.

Transfer Learning for Medical Imaging. While multi-task learning can benefit from sharing features between different tasks to get more general features, transfer learning can leverage the learned features from a source domain to improve the performance in a target domain. Traditional transfer learning use knowledge or model weights learned from tasks for which a large amount of annotated data is available in tasks where only a limited amount of labeled data is available. The large dataset can help generalize the model as training on small datasets can lead to overfitting. Transfer learning has been widely adopted in deep learning such as initializing models with weights pre-trained on ImageNet [4] and has shown performance improvements for medical image classification [9, 20].

However, in medical applications, the amount of labeled data is typically low so using features learned from other medical domains directly is often impractical. To evaluate the visual features learned by our report generator and explore the possibility of transferring visual features learned from a small set to a larger set and improving the cross-task generalization, we propose an attention based feature fusion scheme to modify the already trained classification model. Instead of averaging features in all regions as average pooling in standard models [7,10], our transfer learning model assigns more weights to the features coexisting in both original feature space and transferred feature space through an attention guided feature fusion mechanism. In this way, features learned in a small set can also help generalize the model for another domain or task.

3   Methodology

3.1   Radiology Report Generator

In our report generation model, the estimated probability of generating the i-th sentence with length T is

$$\hat{\mathbb{P}}(S_i = w_1, w_2, ...w_T | V, I; \theta) =$$
$$\mathbb{P}(S_1|V,I) \prod_{j=2}^{i-1} \mathbb{P}(S_j|V,I,S_{j-1})\mathbb{P}(w_1|V,I,S_{i-1}) \prod_{t=2}^{T} \mathbb{P}(w_t|V,I,S_{i-1},w_1,...w_{t-1}). \tag{1}$$

where V is the given frontal view image, I is the impression topic and θ is the model parameter (we omit the θ in the right hand side), S_i represents the i-th sentence and w_t is the t-th token in the i-th sentence. In other words, each succeeding sentence is conditioned upon multimodal inputs including its preceding sentence, the global impression topic and the original image.

The training is done by Maximum Log-likelihood Estimate (MLE) and minimizing the cross entropy loss as

$$\theta^* = \underset{\theta}{\text{argmax}} \sum_{i=1}^{L} \log \hat{\mathbb{P}}(S_i = G_i | V, I; \theta), \tag{2}$$

where G_i is the ground truth for the i-th sentence in the findings paragraph.

The overall architecture of our framework that takes frontal image views as input and generates a radiology report with impression and findings is shown in the lower part of Fig. 1. The report generator first takes the frontal view image as input and generates an impression sentence via a CNN-RNN model, then a Bi-directional Long Short-Term Memory (Bi-LSTM) [6] with mean-pooling over the sequence length is used as a topic encoder to produce a global topic vector. The generation of the first sentence in the findings paragraph is conditioned upon both the image input and the topic vector. Then the decoder model recurrently takes the multimodal inputs of visual features from the image encoder, semantic representation of the preceding sentence from the sentence encoder, and the global topic vector of the impression from the topic encoder and generates the next sentence. The report decoding model can be regarded as a combination of the hierarchical model and the recurrent model. More details are shown in the following subsections.

Image Encoder. Similar to [26], a Convolutional Neural Network (CNN) based image encoder is first applied to extract both global and regional visual features from the input images. To get a better initialization, the image encoder is built upon the pre-trained ResNet-152 [7] network pre-trained on ImageNet [4]. We resize the input images to 224×224 to be consistent with the pre-trained ResNet-152 image encoder. To get a better attention map, the local feature matrix $f \in \mathbb{R}^{2048 \times 49}$ (reshaped from $2048 \times 7 \times 7$) is extracted from the last convolution layer of ResNet-152. Each column of f is one regional feature vector. Thus each

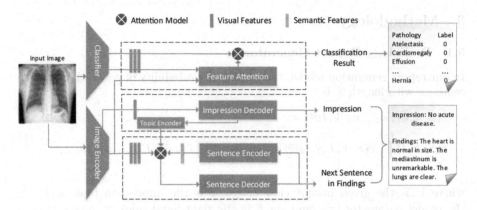

Fig. 1. The architecture of our model. Lower part is the proposed generative model for radiology reports. Upper part is the attention guided feature fusion model for improved thoracic disease classification. Best viewed in color. (Color figure online)

image has $k = 49$ sub-regions. Meanwhile, we extract the global feature vector $f \in \mathbb{R}^{2048}$ from the last average pooling layer of ResNet-152. The image encoder is fine tuned on the frontal view chest X-rays so that the learned visual features can be transferred to another classification task.

Report Decoder. The decoder network is responsible for generating both the impression and the findings paragraph. The impression decoder first takes the global visual features learned by the image encoder as input and a single layer Long Short-Term Memory (LSTM) [8] is used for sentence decoding. Following [2], we adopt a Bi-LSTM that reads the generated impression in two opposite directions along with a mean pooling over each dimension of the hidden units to get a global topic vector. The sentence decoder takes regional visual features and the topic vector to generate the first sentence. After that, each sentence is generated by taking regional visual features, the previously generated sentence and the topic vector as a multimodal input. The sentence decoder is a stacked 2-layer LSTM. All hidden and embedding dimensions are fixed to 512 for all of the LSTM models discussed herein. Both regional and global visual features are converted into channel dimension 512 to match the embedding size before being fed into any LSTMs. The regional visual features are converted as input to the sentence decoder. The global topic vector is used as the initialization of the sentence decoder, while the learned encoding of the preceding sentence is combined with the visual representations to generate an attention map. The attention weights for the regional visual features are computed as follows:

$$a = W_{\text{att}}([v; s1^k]) + b_{\text{att}}, \tag{3}$$

where $v \in \mathbb{R}^{512 \times 49}$ are the regional visual features learned by the image encoder, $s \in \mathbb{R}^{512 \times 1}$ represents the encoding of the preceding sentence, $1^k \in \mathbb{R}^{1 \times 49}$ is a vector with all ones. v and $s1^k$ are concatenated along the embedding dimension as the input to the attention network. $W_{\text{att}} \in \mathbb{R}^{1 \times 1024}$, and $b_{\text{att}} \in \mathbb{R}^{1 \times 49}$

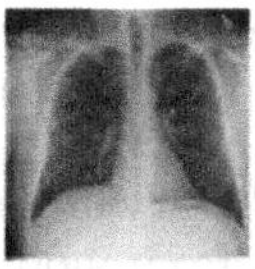

Input Image   **Predicted Report**   **Original Report**

Findings: The cardiac contours are normal. The lungs are clear. There is no pleural effusion or pneumothorax. There is no focal air space opacity to suggest a pneumonia. **Degenerative changes of the thoracic spine.**
Impression: No acute cardiopulmonary finding.

Findings: Heart size and mediastinal contour normal. Lungs are clear. Pulmonary vascularity normal. No pleural effusions or pneumothoraces. Minimal **degenerative changes thoracic spine.**
Impression: No acute cardiopulmonary process.

Fig. 2. An example report generated by our model in comparison with the original written report provided by the radiologist. The notable words in bold font in the findings indicate that our model is capable of capturing some of the abnormalities in the input image.

are parameters of the attention network. Then the weights are normalized over all regions to get the attention distribution and applied to the original visual representation as:

$$v_{\text{att}} = \sum_{i=1}^{k} \frac{\exp(a_i)}{\sum_i \exp(a_i)} v_i, \tag{4}$$

where i refers to the i-th region in the regional visual representation.

The generation process is repeated until an empty sentence is generated or a maximum number of sentences is reached, which indicates the end of the paragraph. Our model combines the recurrent and hierarchical architecture in the decoder network. While the recurrent attention mechanism forces the model to focus on different regions of the input image to generate more diverse sentences and keep intra-paragraph coherence, the global topic vector adds an additional constraint so that the generated sentences can support the theme of the entire report. An example of the generated report by our report generator is shown in Fig. 2.

Our proposed report generator is trained by the Adam optimizer [12]. The initial learning rate is set to be 1e−4, and learning rate decay is 0.5 for every 5 epochs. The batchsize is 32 for training. During inference, the greedy search is adopted for generating words and sentences in every timestep. The maximum number of sentences is set to be 7. Although the impression decoder and the findings decoder can be trained jointly, we separate the training process to get more diverse results. The final model transferred to the classification model for feature fusion is trained on all training data. Although the generated report can be biased towards the training data, we believe that the learned visual features should be more general than the semantic features and can be transferred to other domains.

3.2 Thoracic Disease Classifier and Attention Guided Feature Fusion

The basic thoracic disease classification network is a CNN that takes frontal view radiographs as input and generates multiple disease labels. We first train two different baseline classification models to get the visual features. We start from the ResNet-18 model and later move to the DenseNet-121 model with more layers. For the ResNet baseline, the final fully connected layer is replaced with one that has 14 outputs for 14 disease categories, after which we apply a sigmoid nonlinearity as in [19]. The training is done by minimizing the binary cross entropy loss. The weights of the network are initialized with weights from models pre-trained on ImageNet [4]. We pick the model with the lowest validation loss as the final model. After the training is completed, we discard the transition block including the final pooling layer, the final fully connected layer and the sigmoid nonlinearity to keep only the local visual features. Then, we run the image encoder of our report generator on the classification dataset. The extracted local visual features serve as a high-level linguistic abstract of the input images here. Both the local visual features from the classification network and the report generation network with $k = 49$ sub-regions are then fed into the feature attention module. The feature attention module can be interpreted as:

$$a^{'} = W^{'}_{\text{att}}([v^r; v^c]) + b^{'}_{\text{att}}, \tag{5}$$

where v^r are the regional visual features from the report generator, v^c are the visual features from the original classification network. v^r and v^c are concatenated along the channel/embedding dimension as the input to the feature attention network. W_{att} and b_{att} are parameters of the attention network. Then the modified visual representation is computed as:

$$v^c_{\text{att}} = \sum_{i=1}^{k} \frac{\exp(a^{'}_i)}{\sum_i \exp(a^{'}_i)} v^c_i, \tag{6}$$

where i refers to the i-th region in the regional visual representation. The detailed process is shown in the upper part of Fig. 1. Local features from the image encoder and the classification model are concatenated and fed into the feature attention module. After calculating an attention map over all regions, we apply the attention weights to the original visual features learned from the classification network. We fix the visual features and re-train the transition block to get a new classification prediction. While visual features remain unchanged, the feature attention module can discover the correspondences between features trained on two separate domains and tasks, and emphasize more on the features that coexist in both representations. We replace the average pooling operation in the original classification model with learned attention weights for feature fusion. Compared with average pooling, the attention guided feature fusion can achieve better generalization and get potentially higher classification accuracy without re-training the feature extraction model or changing any learned visual features.

To better illustrate the strength of our feature attention module, we also apply the attention guided feature fusion on the state-of-the-art CheXNet [19] which uses a DenseNet-121 backbone model. The training process is similar to the ResNet-18 baseline model; the only difference is that the output channel dimension in DenseNet-121 is 1024 while it is 512 in ResNet-18. Since the CheXNet is the state-of-the-art model and already gets very high accuracy on the ChestX-ray14 [23] dataset, it is hard to get further improvements. We did experiments that performed a naive concatenation of the two feature representations, but failed to get any significant improvements over the original classification model. Using our attention guided feature fusion mechanism, however, we are able to achieve improvements (as shown in Table 2) with the help of visual features learned on a small report generation dataset and thus demonstrate the effectiveness of our model. More details are explained in Sect. 4.

4   Experiments

Our report generator is trained on the Indiana University Chest X-Ray Collection [3]. The IU X-ray dataset contains 3,955 radiology reports from 2 large hospital systems within the Indiana Network for Patient Care database, and 7,470 associated chest X-rays from the hospitals' picture archiving systems. Each report is associated with a pair of images which are the frontal and lateral views, and contains comparison, indication, findings, and impression sections. Since the transferred visual features will be utilized in the ChestX-ray14 dataset containing only frontal view X-rays, we further filter out reports without frontal view images or without complete sections of findings and impression, resulting in 3,331 reports with associated frontal view images.

For data preprocessing, we tokenize and lowercase all the words that appear more than twice in the findings and impression sections of all reports and obtain 1,357 unique words. To mitigate the small size of the dataset and generalize our model, dropout of 0.2 is added in both the encoder and decoder networks. Moreover, considering that images in the IU X-ray and ChestX-ray14 datasets can look different, we further resize the original input images to size 256×256 then randomly crop them to size 224×224 and randomly change the brightness, contrast and saturation of input images with rate 0.1 for data augmentation. All images are normalized based on the mean and standard deviation of images in the ImageNet training set. To provide some insights to the performance of our report generator, we report BLEU [18], METEOR [5], ROUGE [16] and CIDEr [21] scores as for image captioning tasks and in previous works [11,14,26]. The automatic evaluation results reported in Table 1 are done on the test set with 300 randomly picked reports. We tokenize and lowercase all words in both the predicted report and the ground truth report, and all punctuation are considered as independent tokens. We compare with baseline model [26] on both the findings generation and the combination of findings and impression. The result of [14] is from the original paper and they use different train/test split only for findings generation; baseline model of [26] is re-trained using our train/test split with only frontal view radiographs. During the evaluation, we observe that higher scores do not necessarily indicate better generation performance and reports with more sentences describing normal findings typically get higher scores but may miss more crucial abnormalities. The combination results of findings and impression always get higher scores since most impression sentences are normal such as "no acute cardiopulmonary findings". Due to the small size of the training

Table 1. Evaluation of generated reports on our test set using BLEU, METEOR, ROUGE and CIDEr metrics. For findings generation, we compare our model with two baseline models [14, 26]. We also provide a comparison with one baseline model [26] for the impression and findings generation.

Data	Method	BLEU1	BLEU2	BLEU3	BLEU4	METEOR	ROUGE	CIDEr
Findings	Recurrent-Attn [26]	0.441	0.320	0.231	0.181	0.220	0.366	0.243
	HRGR-Agent [14]	0.438	0.298	0.208	0.151	-	0.322	**0.343**
	Ours	**0.477**	**0.332**	**0.243**	**0.189**	**0.223**	**0.380**	0.320
Findings + Impression	Recurrent-Attn [26]	0.465	0.332	0.244	0.190	0.224	**0.480**	0.495
	Ours	**0.489**	**0.340**	**0.252**	**0.195**	**0.230**	0.478	**0.565**

dataset and the nature of the radiology report generation problem, we believe that metrics designed for image captioning are not appropriate evaluations for report generation, as they cannot capture the words describing negation and uncertainty in the report. Even for the CIDEr [21] which has shown a better correlation with human judgments than other metrics for captioning tasks, it is based on term frequency-inverse document frequency (TF-IDF). However, the corpus of radiology reports is very different from other text corpora so CIDEr may not work as well as in other tasks. Thus, our goal is not to evaluate our model with these metrics and compare directly with other models. Rather, the results are only illustrated to show that our report generation model is among the state-of-the-arts and should be able to learn meaningful features by the image encoder. The learned visual features are formally evaluated on the ChestX-ray14 dataset via feature transferring and feature fusion.

ChestX-ray14 [23] is currently the largest public repository of radiographs containing 112,120 frontal view chest X-rays of 30,805 unique patients. Each image is annotated with up to 14 different thoracic pathology labels text-mined from the associated report. The labels are expected to have accuracy higher than 90%. The dataset is randomly split into training (70%), validation (10%), and test (20%) sets as in previous work on ChestX-ray14 [19,23,27]. The data pre-processing is the same as in the report generation model, including the random crop and color jitter for data augmentation and consistent with the training of the report generator. Training of both classification models and the feature fusion are done via the Adam optimizer [12] and minimizing the binary cross entropy (BCE) loss. The initial learning rate is also set to be 1e–4, and learning rate decay is 0.5 every time the validation loss has not been decreased for 5 epochs. The batchsize is 32 for training. We first train two baseline classification networks: ResNet-18 [7] and CheXNet [19] using a DenseNet-121 [10] backbone, then evaluate the disease classification performance of the feature fusion, using the area under ROC curve (AUC) score for 14 different diseases. During feature fusion, all visual features learned by the image encoder of report generator and by the original classification model are fixed to ensure the improvements are not from the re-training of the model. Table 2 illustrates the per-class and average AUCs comparison of 14 diseases on the test set. Unlike [19], random horizontal flipping is not implemented as we believe the input frontal view chest X-rays are

Table 2. Comparison of AUCs of ROC curve for classification of 14 disease categories in ChestX-ray14 test set. R18 and D121 represent the ResNet-18 and the DenseNet-121 baseline models, respectively. TF denotes the model with transferred features and attention guided feature fusion. Note that the state-of-the-art baseline model of CheXNet [19] with DenseNet-121 backbone is re-implemented and re-trained since we use different data preprocessing.

Pathology	[23]	[24]	[27]	[15]	R18	R18-TF	D121 [19]*	D121-TF
Atelectasis	0.716	0.732	0.772	0.80	0.797	0.819	0.814	**0.822**
Cardiomegaly	0.807	0.844	0.904	0.81	0.895	0.884	**0.902**	0.892
Effusion	0.784	0.793	0.859	0.87	0.874	0.875	0.878	**0.881**
Infiltration	0.609	0.666	0.695	0.70	0.694	0.709	0.706	**0.710**
Mass	0.706	0.725	0.792	0.83	0.817	0.813	0.838	**0.841**
Nodule	0.671	0.685	0.717	0.75	0.732	0.789	0.782	**0.794**
Pneumonia	0.633	0.72	0.713	0.67	0.766	**0.770**	0.774	0.767
Pneumothorax	0.806	0.847	0.841	0.87	0.857	0.852	0.845	**0.870**
Consolidation	0.708	0.701	0.788	0.80	0.795	0.810	0.806	**0.813**
Edema	0.835	0.829	0.882	0.88	0.89	0.898	0.895	**0.898**
Emphysema	0.815	0.865	0.829	0.91	0.883	0.905	0.910	**0.922**
Fibrosis	0.769	0.796	0.767	0.78	0.821	0.844	0.838	**0.851**
Pleural thickening	0.708	0.735	0.79	0.772	0.763	0.780	0.779	**0.788**
Hernia	0.767	0.876	0.914	0.77	0.923	0.929	**0.951**	0.946
Average	0.738	0.772	0.802	0.80	0.822	0.834	0.837	**0.842**

not symmetrical (e.g., cardiac abnormalities always appear in the left side of the chest) and it is not reasonable to flip the input images. For baseline classification models, we change the last fully connected layer accordingly to fit the number of categories which is 14 for the ChestX-ray14 dataset.

As we can see in Table 2, the ResNet-18 model with transferred features and attention guided feature fusion outperforms the baseline ResNet-18 classification model considerably on almost all diseases except for Mass. Remind that we do not re-train any of the visual features learned by the original classification network and the performance boost comes from better utilization of the learned features. To better illustrate the effectiveness of feature transferring and the attention guided feature fusion, we also apply our model to the state-of-the-art CheXNet [19]. With different data preprocessing, we re-train the CheXNet with a DenseNet-121 backbone as a baseline model. After feature fusion, we observe clear improvements on 12 diseases except for Cardiomegaly and Hernia, without altering any visual features learned by the original CheXNet. Moreover, our DenseNet-121 model with transferred features achieves highest AUC scores on 11 out of 14 classes, and has the highest average AUC score among all methods. The experimental results show that the image encoder in the report generator indeed learned meaningful features during training, and the attention guided feature fusion is capable of improving the classification result through a better utilization of features and an emphasis on features that generalize across tasks.

5 Conclusion

In summary, we have proposed an improved recurrent attention model for radiology report generation along with an attention guided feature transfer and feature fusion model for thoracic disease classification. The report generation model is first trained on a small chest X-ray dataset with written reports provided by radiologists, then the learned visual representations including some high-level abstract of the input radiographs are transferred to a larger chest X-ray dataset with multiple disease labels. The features are combined under the guidance of a feature attention module. After applying the attention weights to the features extracted by the original classification model, we successfully improve the disease classification result without changing any visual features on the state-of-the-art baseline classification network. The experimental results on ChestX-ray14 dataset demonstrate that the proposed transferring of visual representations learned for different tasks on different datasets and the attention guided feature fusion can improve the model performance even on a large dataset. We believe that, by utilizing feature representations from different domains or tasks in a complementary manner, such feature transfer and fusion models have great potential and can be extended to other medical imaging applications where training data are limited so as to generalize the original model and enhance performance.

References

1. Chatterjee, M., Schwing, A.G.: Diverse and coherent paragraph generation from images. arXiv preprint arXiv:1809.00681 2 (2018)
2. Conneau, A., Kiela, D., Schwenk, H., Barrault, L., Bordes, A.: Supervised learning of universal sentence representations from natural language inference data. arXiv preprint arXiv:1705.02364 (2017)
3. Demner-Fushman, D., et al.: Preparing a collection of radiology examinations for distribution and retrieval. J. Am. Med. Inform. Assoc. **23**(2), 304–310 (2015)
4. Deng, J., Dong, W., Socher, R., Li, L.J., Li, K., Fei-Fei, L.: Imagenet: a large-scale hierarchical image database. In: IEEE Conference on Computer Vision and Pattern Recognition, CVPR 2009, pp. 248–255. IEEE (2009)
5. Denkowski, M., Lavie, A.: Meteor universal: language specific translation evaluation for any target language. In: Proceedings of the Ninth Workshop on Statistical Machine Translation, pp. 376–380 (2014)
6. Graves, A., Schmidhuber, J.: Framewise phoneme classification with bidirectional LSTM and other neural network architectures. Neural Netw. **18**(5–6), 602–610 (2005)
7. He, K., Zhang, X., Ren, S., Sun, J.: Deep residual learning for image recognition. In: 2016 IEEE Conference on Computer Vision and Pattern Recognition (CVPR), pp. 770–778. IEEE (2016)

8. Hochreiter, S., Schmidhuber, J.: Long short-term memory. Neural Comput. **9**(8), 1735–1780 (1997)
9. Hoo-Chang, S., et al.: Deep convolutional neural networks for computer-aided detection: CNN architectures, dataset characteristics and transfer learning. IEEE Trans. Med. Imaging **35**(5), 1285 (2016)
10. Huang, G., Liu, Z., van der Maaten, L., Weinberger, K.Q.: Densely connected convolutional networks. In: 2017 IEEE Conference on Computer Vision and Pattern Recognition (CVPR), pp. 2261–2269. IEEE (2017)
11. Jing, B., Xie, P., Xing, E.: On the automatic generation of medical imaging reports. arXiv preprint arXiv:1711.08195 (2017)
12. Kingma, D.P., Ba, J.: Adam: A method for stochastic optimization. arXiv preprint arXiv:1412.6980 (2014)
13. Krause, J., Johnson, J., Krishna, R., Fei-Fei, L.: A hierarchical approach for generating descriptive image paragraphs. In: 2017 IEEE Conference on Computer Vision and Pattern Recognition (CVPR), pp. 3337–3345. IEEE (2017)
14. Li, C.Y., Liang, X., Hu, Z., Xing, E.P.: Hybrid retrieval-generation reinforced agent for medical image report generation. arXiv preprint arXiv:1805.08298 (2018)
15. Li, Z., et al.: Thoracic disease identification and localization with limited supervision. arXiv preprint arXiv:1711.06373 (2017)
16. Lin, C.Y.: Rouge: a package for automatic evaluation of summaries. In: Text Summarization Branches Out (2004)
17. Lu, J., Xiong, C., Parikh, D., Socher, R.: Knowing when to look: adaptive attention via a visual sentinel for image captioning. In: 2017 IEEE Conference on Computer Vision and Pattern Recognition (CVPR), pp. 3242–3250. IEEE (2017)
18. Papineni, K., Roukos, S., Ward, T., Zhu, W.J.: Bleu: a method for automatic evaluation of machine translation. In: Proceedings of the 40th Annual Meeting on Association for Computational Linguistics, pp. 311–318. Association for Computational Linguistics (2002)
19. Rajpurkar, P., et al.: Chexnet: Radiologist-level pneumonia detection on chest X-rays with deep learning. arXiv preprint arXiv:1711.05225 (2017)
20. Tajbakhsh, N., et al.: Convolutional neural networks for medical image analysis: full training or fine tuning? IEEE Trans. Med. Imaging **35**(5), 1299–1312 (2016)
21. Vedantam, R., Zitnick, C.L., Parikh, D.: Cider: consensus-based image description evaluation. In: 2015 IEEE Conference on Computer Vision and Pattern Recognition (CVPR), pp. 4566–4575. IEEE (2015)
22. Vinyals, O., Toshev, A., Bengio, S., Erhan, D.: Show and tell: a neural image caption generator. In: 2015 IEEE Conference on Computer Vision and Pattern Recognition (CVPR), pp. 3156–3164. IEEE (2015)
23. Wang, X., Peng, Y., Lu, L., Lu, Z., Bagheri, M., Summers, R.M.: Chestx-ray8: hospital-scale chest X-ray database and benchmarks on weakly-supervised classification and localization of common thorax diseases. In: 2017 IEEE Conference on Computer Vision and Pattern Recognition (CVPR), pp. 3462–3471. IEEE (2017)
24. Wang, X., Peng, Y., Lu, L., Lu, Z., Summers, R.M.: Tienet: text-image embedding network for common thorax disease classification and reporting in chest X-rays. In: Proceedings of the IEEE Conference on Computer Vision and Pattern Recognition, pp. 9049–9058 (2018)

25. Xu, K., et al.: Show, attend and tell: neural image caption generation with visual attention. In: International Conference on Machine Learning, pp. 2048–2057 (2015)
26. Xue, Y., et al.: Multimodal recurrent model with attention for automated radiology report generation. In: Frangi, A.F., Schnabel, J.A., Davatzikos, C., Alberola-López, C., Fichtinger, G. (eds.) MICCAI 2018. LNCS, vol. 11070, pp. 457–466. Springer, Cham (2018). https://doi.org/10.1007/978-3-030-00928-1_52
27. Yao, L., Poblenz, E., Dagunts, D., Covington, B., Bernard, D., Lyman, K.: Learning to diagnose from scratch by exploiting dependencies among labels. arXiv preprint arXiv:1710.10501 (2017)

Reconstruction

Limited Angle Tomography Reconstruction: Synthetic Reconstruction via Unsupervised Sinogram Adaptation

Bo Zhou[1]([✉]), Xunyu Lin[1], and Brendan Eck[2]

[1] Robotics Institute, School of Computer Science, Carnegie Mellon University, Pittsburgh, USA
bzhou2@cs.cmu.edu
[2] Department of Biomedical Engineering, Case Western Reserve University, Cleveland, USA

Abstract. Computed Tomography (CT) is commonly used in clinical procedures and limited angle tomography reconstruction has important applications in diagnostic CT, breast tomography, dental tomography, etc. However, CT images reconstructed from limited angle acquisitions suffer from severe artifacts due to incomplete sinogram data. Although existing iterative reconstruction methods improve image quality relative to filtered back projection, these methods require extensive computation and still often provide unsatisfactory images. Supervised deep learning methods have been proposed to further improve the image quality of limited angle reconstructions. However, a key limitation in supervised deep learning for this application is the lack of large-scale real sinogram-reconstruction pairs for training. Given the large number of CT images available in the wild, we can create a large number of simulated sinogram-reconstruction pairs. Thus the requirement for real paired sinogram-reconstruction data can be alleviated if simulated sinograms (e.g. monochromatic) are able to train a reconstruction network for real sinograms (e.g. polychromatic source, scattering, beam hardening). In this paper, we propose an end-to-end limited angle tomography reconstruction adversarial network (Tomo-GAN) via unsupervised sinogram adaptation without having real sinogram-reconstruction pairs. Tomo-GAN is trained by using (1) unpaired sinograms from the simulation and real domains, and (2) large-scale reconstruction images from only the simulation domain. Tomo-GAN is built based upon a cycle consistent network with similarity constrained for sinogram adaptation and a multi-scale conditional reconstruction network. Experimental results on a public dataset with a limited angle setting demonstrated a consistent improvement over previous methods while significantly reducing the reconstruction computation time.

Keywords: Limited angle CT reconstruction ·
Sinogram domain adaptation · Generative adversarial learning ·
Sinogram simulation

© Springer Nature Switzerland AG 2019
A. C. S. Chung et al. (Eds.): IPMI 2019, LNCS 11492, pp. 141–152, 2019.
https://doi.org/10.1007/978-3-030-20351-1_11

1   Introduction

Computed Tomography (CT) is one of the most common imaging modalities used in healthcare and industrial applications today. In CT, x-ray attenuation measurements are obtained from different viewing angles creating a sinogram which is then used to produce cross-sectional image stacks of 3D objects [1]. In the traditional CT setting, one assumes access to measurements collected from the full range of views of an object, i.e. $\theta \in [0, 180]$, but recent techniques are increasingly being developed that can recover images when a portion of the sinogram views is missing, i.e. when $\theta \in [0, \theta_{max}]$ with $\theta_{max} < 180$. These are referred to as limited angle projections, and reconstruction in such cases is highly ill-posed, as evidenced by the inferior performance of existing methods.

Limited angle CT scans can provide a number of benefits as compared to full scans. Firstly, scan time can be drastically reduced by restricting the physical movement of the scan arc. In clinical practice, CT is used to study highly dynamic organs such as the heart and lung. High temporal resolution is paramount; even a slightly longer scan time can lead to appreciable motion blur in the image [2,3]. Secondly, the limited angle setting can help limit the area of the scan only to a region of interest for applications such as breast tomography [4], and dental tomography [5]. It can also support applications involving objects that have physical constraints restricting the angles from which they can be scanned, for example in electron cryo-tomography [6,7].

Previous works attempted to solve the limited angle reconstruction problem via a variety of formulations, such as sinogram regression from limited view to full-view [8], reduction of artifacts obtained from Filter Back Projection (FBP) [9], and using convolutional neural networks to refine initialized reconstructions from FBP [10]. However, these techniques only use simple datasets with little variability or rely on supervised training which requires large-scale real sinogram-reconstruction CT pairs. In computer vision, the limited angle reconstruction can be formulated as reconstruction of scenes when the object of interest is partially occluded. Data-driven approaches have made significant contributions in solving similarly challenging image recovery problems [11], such as image completion [12] and super-resolution imaging [13]. These methods leverage the availability of large-scale datasets and the expressive power of deep learning to impose implicit constraints to the data recovery problem. However, limited angle CT reconstruction has several additional major challenges. Firstly, CT images of patients with diverse diseases in different organs can be very complex with no efficient low dimensional structure. In this case, training a network directly to predict the reconstructed image from a given sinogram can be very challenging even if the full-scan sinogram is available. This problem becomes more challenging due to the fact that collecting a large-scale real sinogram-reconstruction dataset is unrealistic because of limited access to both patient data and CT scanner projection data. As a result, most of the current methods still rely on FBP [10] or iterative methods such as Algebraic Reconstruction Technique (ART) [14] and Simultaneous Iterative Reconstruction Technique (SIRT) [15].

In this paper, we addressed the challenging lack of large-scale real sinogram-reconstruction pairs for training a deep model by proposing an end-to-end sinogram domain adaptation and reconstruction generative adversarial network, called Tomo-GAN. Tomo-GAN leverages a large-scale CT image dataset collected in the wild and their corresponding simulated projections/sinograms, generated by our sinogram simulation engine, to predict real CT reconstruction. Tomo-GAN consists of two parts: a sinogram adaptation subnet (Sino-GAN) and a reconstruction subnet (Recon-GAN). Sino-GAN is built based upon a cycle consistent adversarial network [16] with content consistent regularization to transfer the sinogram from the simulation domain to the real domain. Recon-GAN consists of a recurrent neural network (RNN) for encoding the limited angle sinogram and a convolutional neural network (CNN) for encoding the corresponding reconstruction as an initial guide. A multi-scale CNN decoder coupled with conditional adversarial training is used to recover the full CT reconstruction. Tomo-GAN is trained by unpaired simulated and real sinograms with ground truth reconstruction available only in the simulated sinogram domain. All sinograms contain 0–120° viewing angles at a 1° interval. To evaluate the reconstruction performance of the proposed Tomo-GAN, we use a publicly available CT projection dataset which consisted of 5436 sinograms along with ground truth full-scan reconstruction. We demonstrate state-of-the-art limited angle CT reconstruction as compared to previous methods.

Contributions: The proposed method alleviates the need for real sinogram-reconstruction pairs for training the reconstruction deep model by taking the advantage of cross-domain sinogram synthesis learning. Our methodological contributions are three-fold:

- We propose a sinogram domain adaptation adversarial scheme that transfers the simulated sinogram domain into the real sinogram domain which helps account for real-world factors such as scattering, beam hardening, etc., while keeping the general attenuation profile.
- We proposed a CT reconstruction generative adversarial network that utilizes both a limited-angle sinogram and the corresponding initial FBP reconstruction to predict full-scan CT images.
- We integrate the sinogram adaptation network with the reconstruction network in an end-to-end adversarial network, Tomo-GAN, such that it can jointly optimize the sinogram adaptation and image reconstruction.

2   Method

We proposed a novel unsupervised learning scheme to overcome the challenges from limited angle reconstruction problem and lack of real-world sinogram-reconstruction pairs. We obtain pairs of real CT images and simulated sinograms, generated from a sinogram simulation engine (described in Sect. 3.1). We apply an adaption stage to adapt simulated sinograms from simulation domain to synthetic sinogram in real domain. Then the synthetic sinograms are reconstructed back to the paired CT images of simulated sinograms. The adaptation stage can be trained with unpaired real and simulated sinograms. Thus, our method does not require supervision from real-world sinogram-reconstruction pairs. We designed Tomo-GAN to achieve this goal and the network design is shown in Fig. 2.1. In the following sections, we explain the proposed Tomo-GAN network in Sect. 2.1 and training/inference strategies in Sect. 2.2, respectively.

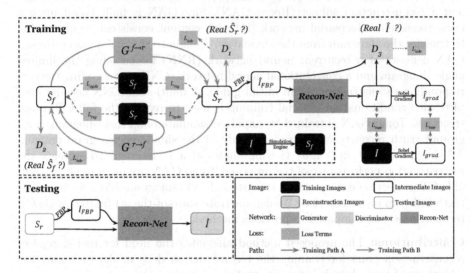

Fig. 1. Illustration of the Tomo-GAN network design. The top panel shows the network structure of Tomo-GAN during the training stages. The left portion is the Sino-GAN for sinogram domain adaptation, where S_f is the sinogram in the simulation sinogram domain and S_r is the sinogram in the real sinogram domain. Simulated sinograms S_f are adapted to synthetic sinograms $\hat{S}_r$ in the real sinogram domain, which are then used for reconstruction. The right portion is the Recon-GAN for end-to-end reconstruction training. Six loss functions are used to jointly optimize the two portions of Tomo-GAN. The lower panel shows the extracted network structure of our Tomo-GAN during the test stage. Only the trained Recon-Net is used to predict the reconstruction image from real limited angle sinograms S_r.

2.1   Tomo-GAN

We developed an end-to-end training network that can learn to reconstruct CT images from limited angle sinograms given no real-world sinogram-reconstruction pairs. To achieve this, we introduced two sub-networks in Tomo-GAN: (1) a sinogram adaptation sub-network, called Sino-GAN, that adapts sinograms between two domains i.e. simulation domain and real domain; (2) a reconstruction sub-network, called Recon-GAN, that reconstructs CT images using the sinograms from the real domain. The two sub-networks are joined together to train end-to-end in an unsupervised manner.

Sinogram Adaptation Subnet. Sino-GAN is based on a well-established cycle consistent adversarial network for domain adaptation [16] with the addition of content consistent regularization. Sino-GAN adapts sinograms between two different domains: the simulated sinogram domain $\mathbb{F}$ and the real sinogram domain $\mathbb{R}$. An illustration of Sino-GAN is shown in Fig. 1. Sino-GAN contains four networks, including two generators and two discriminators: generator $G^{f \to r}$ adapts sinograms from the simulated domain to the real domain; generator $G^{r \to f}$ works the other way around. Discriminator D_{S_r} identifies real sinograms or the adapted ones from $G^{f \to r}$; discriminator D_{S_f} identifies simulated sinograms or the adapted ones from $G^{r \to f}$. There are two training paths in Sino-GAN: path A first adapts sinograms S_r in the real domain to adapted sinograms $\hat{S}_f$ in the simulated domain through $G^{r \to f}$; then $\hat{S}_f$ is adapted back to the real domain as $\hat{S}_r$ through $G^{f \to r}$; path B first adapts sinograms S_f in the simulated domain to adapted sinograms $\hat{S}_r$ in the real domain through $G^{f \to r}$; then $\hat{S}_r$ is adapted back to the simulated domain as $\hat{S}_f$ through $G^{r \to f}$. Supervision of Sino-GAN comes from three sources:

(1) adversarial losses L_{adv} that apply discriminators to identify sinograms with or without adaptation. The adversarial objective is formed in a way such that the generators are encouraged to generate sinograms which are indistinguishable to the discriminators. Two adversarial losses are introduced to optimize two generators and discriminators:

$$
\begin{aligned}
L_{adv}(G^{r \to f}, D_{S_f}, S_f, \hat{S}_f) &= \mathbb{E}_{S_f \sim \mathbb{F}} \left[\log D_{S_f}(S_f) \right] \\
&+ \mathbb{E}_{S_r \sim \mathbb{R}} \left[\log \left(1 - D_{S_f}(G_{r \to f}(S_r)) \right) \right]
\end{aligned}
\tag{1}
$$

$$
\begin{aligned}
L_{adv}(G^{f \to r}, D_{S_r}, S_r, \hat{S}_r) &= \mathbb{E}_{S_r \sim \mathbb{R}} \left[\log D_{S_r}(S_r) \right] \\
&+ \mathbb{E}_{S_f \sim \mathbb{F}} \left[\log \left(1 - D_{S_r}(G_{f \to r}(S_f)) \right) \right]
\end{aligned}
\tag{2}
$$

(2) two cycle-consistency losses L_{cycle} act as regularization terms to ensure that sinograms will return to the original domain after passing through two generators, namely a compound of two generators should be an identity mapping:

$$
L_{cycle}(G^{r \to f}, G^{f \to r}, S_r) = \mathbb{E}_{S_r \sim \mathbb{R}} \left[\| G^{f \to r}(G^{r \to f}(S_r)) - S_r \|_1 \right]
\tag{3}
$$

$$
L_{cycle}(G^{f \to r}, G^{r \to f}, S_f) = \mathbb{E}_{S_f \sim \mathbb{F}} \left[\| G^{r \to f}(G^{f \to r}(S_f)) - S_f \|_1 \right]
\tag{4}
$$

(3) two additional regularization terms L_{reg} enforce that the similarity of the general sinogram profiles before and after adaptation is preserved. We propose to use the correlation coefficient to enforce this constraint.

$$
L_{reg}(G^{r \to f}, S_r) = \mathbb{E}_{S_r \sim \mathbb{R}} \left[\frac{Cov(G^{r \to f}(S_r), S_r)}{\sigma_{G^{r \to f}(S_r)} \, \sigma_{S_r}} \right]
\tag{5}
$$

$$
L_{reg}(G^{f \to r}, S_f) = \mathbb{E}_{S_f \sim \mathbb{F}} \left[\frac{Cov(G^{f \to r}(S_f), S_f)}{\sigma_{G^{f \to r}(S_f)} \, \sigma_{S_f}} \right]
\tag{6}
$$

For Sino-GAN, the final loss term L_{sino} is a weighted combination of all the six loss terms above:

$$L_{sino} = \lambda_1 L_{adv}(G^{r \to f}, D_{S_f}, S_f, \hat{S}_f) + \lambda_1 L_{adv}(G^{f \to r}, D_{S_r}, S_r, \hat{S}_r)$$
$$+ \lambda_2 L_{cycle}(G^{r \to f}, G^{f \to r}, S_r) + \lambda_2 L_{cycle}(G^{f \to r}, G^{r \to f}, S_f)$$
$$+ \lambda_3 L_{reg}(G^{r \to f}, S_r) + \lambda_3 L_{reg}(G^{f \to r}, S_f) \tag{7}$$

We use $\lambda_1 = 1.0$, $\lambda_2 = 0.1$ and $\lambda_3 = 0.25$ in our Sino-GAN training.

Reconstruction Subnet. Recon-GAN is built upon a multi-scale conditional GAN [17] which synthesizes a high resolution image based on multi-scale supervisions and adversarial training in the gradient domain. Recon-GAN is illustrated in Fig. 2. Both the sinogram from the real domain and its corresponding initial FBP reconstruction are used as network inputs. We model sinograms as sequential data and use Long-Short-Term-Memory (LSTM) to extract features from a sequence of projections at different angles. Recon-GAN embeds the limited angle sinogram and the initial FBP reconstruction into a latent space. The concatenated embeddings are decoded in multiple scales to generate reconstruction images. Two losses are used in Recon-GAN to generate a sharp reconstruction image, including the standard mean squared error (MSE) and conditional adversarial loss.

$$L_{mse} = \lambda_4||I - \hat{I}||^2 + \lambda_5(||I_{g_x} - \hat{I}_{g_x}||^2 + ||I_{g_y} - \hat{I}_{g_y}||^2) \tag{8}$$

$$L_{adv} = \log D_{rec}(I, I_{g_x}, I_{g_y}|I_{FBP}) + \log(1 - D_{rec}(G_{rec}(\hat{S}_r), \hat{I}_{g_x}, \hat{I}_{g_y}|I_{FBP})) \tag{9}$$

where I, I_{g_x}, I_{g_y} is the ground truth reconstruction and corresponding x, y directional gradient. I_{FBP} is the initial reconstruction from limited angle sinogram. The final loss for reconstruction generator is hence obtained as $L_{rec} = L_{mse} + L_{adv}$. We found $\lambda_4 = 1000$ and $\lambda_5 = 500$ to be a suitable choice in Recon-GAN that gives good-quality reconstruction.

2.2 Training Strategy and Reconstruction Inference

Training: Training data consisted of two parts. Firstly, we obtained pairs of original CT images and their corresponding simulated sinograms (S_f, I). Simulated sinograms were obtained by converting the HU values in the CT image to corresponding 100 keV mass-attenuation coefficients [18] and then using a forward projector to compute the sinogram values. Then, the unpaired simulated sinograms and real sinograms (S_r, S_f) were used to pre-train the Sino-GAN before full end-to-end training. After Sino-GAN converges, we jointly trained Sino-GAN together with Recon-GAN. The inputs for Recon-GAN are sinogram $\hat{S}_r$ adapted from S_f and the FBP reconstruction of $\hat{S}_r$. The ground truth reconstruction of $\hat{S}_r$ is the paired original CT image of S_f, namely I. During joint training, Recon-GAN is trained with loss L_{rec} described in Sect. 2.1 while the loss function for Sino-GAN differs from the one described in Sect. 2.1; Besides

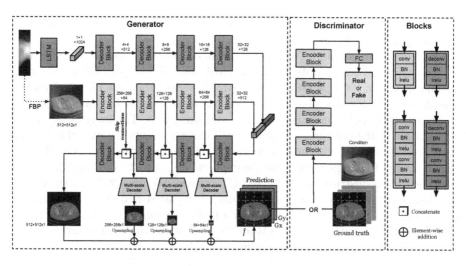

Fig. 2. Illustration of the Recon-GAN architecture. Left panel: the multi-scale generator generates a reconstruction CT image using a limited angle sinogram along with the corresponding FBP reconstruction; Middle panel: the conditional patch discriminator distinguishes real and generated reconstructed images by looking at the gradient patch and conditioning on the initial FBP image patch; Right panel: network details in blocks.

L_{sino}, Sino-GAN now also receives backpropagation from L_{mse}. Sino-GAN is further fine-tuned to produce better adapted sinograms in the real sinogram domain with loss L_{sino}^{joint}.

$$L_{sino}^{joint} = L_{sino} + \lambda_6 L_{mse} \tag{10}$$

λ_6 was chosen as 0.2 in our experiment. The parameters for every generator and discriminator are updated simultaneously at every iteration during training.

Inference: During the inference stage as demonstrated in Fig. 1, we only use Recon-GAN that takes sinograms S_r as input from the real sinogram domain and its initial FBP reconstruction to generate the reconstructed CT images $\hat{I}$.

3 Experiment and Result

3.1 Data and Setup

We collected data from both the real sinogram domain and simulation sinogram domain for our model training. In the real domain, we used 10 sets of real projection data from the AAPM Low Dose CT Grand Challenge. The provided projection data were acquired in helical CT, so we first rebinned the projection data from helical CT to 360° angular scan fan-beam CT. Then, we rebinned the projection data from fan-beam to parallel beam, such that every sinogram is geometrically normalized to parallel-beam sinogram format. There were 5935 real sinograms for experiments. In the simulation domain, we collected 232,228 CT images from a large-scale CT dataset generated from 4427 unique patients [19].

We performed 360° parallel-beam forward projection of each CT image with a monochromatic 100 keV x-ray beam onto a line detector with 729 pixel width. The size of each detector pixel is 1×1 mm^2 and the angular increment between every projection is 1, consistent with the real sinograms. The image was placed in the origin of the coordinate system which also represents the axis of rotation. Each pixel is assigned with an attenuation coefficient according to their HU values. In the limited angle reconstruction experiments, only 0°–120° angular scans were used to reconstruct limited-angle CT images. We used 232,228 simulated sinogram-image pairs with a small amount of unpaired real sinogram data for model training. We trained the model on a machine equipped with two NVIDIA Pascal 1080 Titan with 32 GB RAM for 2 epochs with batch size 6 and learning rate 0.0002. Each epoch took approximately 24 h.

3.2   Evaluation Metrics

Three metrics, commonly applied in computer vision, were used to analyze the quality of the reconstructed images. The metrics are structural similarity (SSIM), normalized mutual information (NMI), and root mean square error (RMSE). SSIM combines luminance, contrast, and structure measurements, and it is computed over a multi-scale representation of the volumes and averaged to produce a final score. NMI evaluates the similarity between images by computing the information gain between them, providing a high-level similarity metrics. RMSE measures the intensity/HU difference between ground truth and predicted images. All three metrics were used for reconstruction evaluation.

3.3   Experimental Results

After training, we extracted the Recon-Net for reconstruction of limited angle sinograms. Several qualitative examples of our reconstruction results are shown in Fig. 3. Important pathological features have been faithfully recovered, such as lung nodules as well as aortic calcification. We compared our reconstruction results with FBP [20], Gridrec [21], ART [14], and SIRT [15]. The latter two, ART and SIRT, are iterative reconstruction methods which took a relatively long computation time depending on number of iterations. The qualitative comparison of Recon-GAN to previous methods for 120° scanning are shown in Fig. 4.

As observed from Fig. 4, FBP and iterative methods suffered from severe artifacts and the internal structures are either incorrectly recovered or excessively blurred, especially in the top-left and bottom-right regions. Among the iterative methods, SIRT performed better than the others, but requires relatively longer inference time due to the iterative process. The proposed Tomo-GAN appears to reconstruct high-quality images and effectively suppresses artifacts as compared to the other methods. Comparing the entire images, the global artifacts are eliminated and the structure boundary, especially the missing boundary on

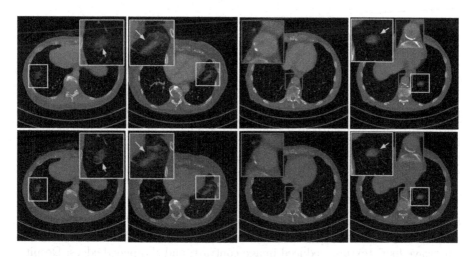

Fig. 3. Qualitative comparison of reconstructed images is demonstrated shown by comparing the ground truth CT images (top row) and the limited angle reconstruction images from Tomo-GAN (bottom row). Different pathological events are zoomed in and indicated by arrows. The lung tumor (yellow) and aortic calcification (red) is clearly visualized via our Tomo-GAN reconstruction using only 120° scan setting. (Color figure online)

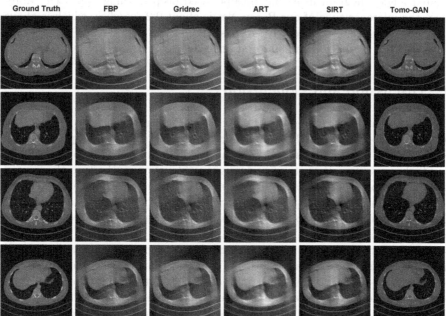

Fig. 4. Qualitative comparison of existing reconstruction methods and Recon-GAN. Please notice all methods, including Recon-GAN, are unsupervised reconstruction methods that do not use any real sinogram-reconstruction pairs.

Table 1. Quantitative evaluation of limited angle tomography reconstruction methods. Best results are marked in red and second best results are marked in blue.

	FBP	Gridrec	ART	SIRT	**Ours**
Median RMSE	392	444	395	186	24
Mean(std) RMSE	393.4(74.4)	442.7(83.2)	397.2(69.3)	190.6(54.3)	27.3(19.3)
Median SSIM	0.484	0.475	0.473	0.479	0.783
Mean(std) SSIM	0.485(0.086)	0.476(0.074)	0.473(0.086)	0.482(0.068)	0.773(0.062)
Median MI	0.554	0.552	0.551	0.572	0.803
Mean(std) MI	0.553(0.006)	0.551(0.005)	0.550(0.007)	0.571(0.008)	0.797(0.012)

the top-left/bottom-right is clearly recovered via our method. However, residual artifacts are present in Tomo-GAN as compared to the ground truth images, such as a "wave-like" texture, reduced image contrast, and sharpened edges. Despite residual artifacts, Tomo-GAN produced the highest-quality images according to SSIM, NMI, and RMSE (Table 1). Since Tomo-GAN does not rely on real sinogram-reconstruction training pairs, all 5,935 real sinograms were used for this evaluation. Tomo-GAN achieved the highest value in SSIM and NMI, and the lowest value in RMSE, indicating superior image reconstruction quality from limited angle sinogram using our unsupervised deep learning approach. Moreover, the inference time of our Recon-Net is about 0.2 sec/slice, which is about 20 times faster than the iterative reconstruction method, such as SIRT which takes about 4 sec/slice with 200 iterations.

4   Discussion and Conclusion

Tomo-GAN enables training of a limited angle CT reconstruction deep neural network without having real sinogram-reconstruction pairs. The proposed Tomo-GAN method produced images with substantially suppressed global artifacts and higher quality metrics than previous reconstruction methods in the limited angle CT reconstruction task. Without using full-scan sinograms for numerical reconstruction or real sinogram-reconstruction pairs for training a model, the Tomo-GAN predicted comparable reconstruction as the full-scan reconstruction results.

One major limitation of deep learning based reconstruction is the limited number of training data. One solution is to spend effort in collecting large-scale real sinogram-reconstruction pairs. However, the system level projection data and corresponding reconstruction is resource intensive to collect. Therefore, it is desirable and appealing to utilize large-scale simulation dataset from available CT images in the wild and invert the process to generate sinograms for training a deep model, as in the proposed Tomo-GAN. Moreover, the sinogram from simulation domain and real domain were not restricted to paired ones, which means Tomo-GAN is not limited by the number of real sinograms available.

Although the proposed deep learning reconstruction algorithm outperformed the other tested methods in terms of the evaluation metrics, there are a number of considerations for its future development. We observed small changes to the Tomo-GAN images as compared to the ground truth including image texture, edge enhancement, and alteration of contrast. A better parameter selection between intensity supervision and gradient supervision may be a target for further improvements. Despite these differences from ground truth, lung nodules and calcifications were clearly visualized which suggests that Tomo-GAN may be preferable to existing algorithms for low-dose lung screening or detection of calcifications. Task-based image quality evaluations should be performed prior to clinical deployment in order to ensure that Tomo-GAN reconstructed images are of sufficient quality for a given clinical application. Such task-based image quality evaluations of deep learning based CT reconstruction would follow in the footsteps of those used for model-based iterative reconstruction algorithms which often have substantially different image texture than convention FBP but enable tremendous radiation dose reduction [22]. Another consideration is the variability in CT data which stems from a number of factors including acquisition geometry, the emitted and detected x-ray spectrum, and more, which can limit the quality of the sinogram synthesis and reconstruction networks. Such variability highlights the need for large-scale data to train generalizable deep learning reconstruction algorithms.

In summary, we developed a novel end-to-end limited angle CT reconstruction deep model that does not rely on real sinogram-reconstruction pairs. The proposed unsupervised reconstruction method produced significantly improved images as compared to previous methods, particularly considering the global artifacts from limited angle acquisitions, and produced high-quality images which are potentially useful for a range of clinical applications.

References

1. Kak, A.C., Slaney, M.: Principles of Computerized Tomographic Imaging. IEEE Press, New York (1988)
2. Cho, J.H., Fessler, J.A.: Motion-compensated image reconstruction for cardiac CT with sinogram-based motion estimation. In: 2013 IEEE Nuclear Science Symposium and Medical Imaging Conference (NSS/MIC), pp. 1–5. IEEE (2013)
3. Mohan, K.A., et al.: TIMBIR: a method for time-space reconstruction from interlaced views. IEEE Trans. Comput. Imaging $1(2)$, 96–111 (2015)
4. Niklason, L.T., et al.: Digital tomosynthesis in breast imaging. Radiology $205(2)$, 399–406 (1997)
5. Hyvönen, N., Kalke, M., Lassas, M., Setälä, H., Siltanen, S.: Three-dimensional dental X-ray imaging by combination of panoramic and projection data. Inverse Probl. Imaging $4(2)$, 257–271 (2010)
6. Zhou, B., Guo, Q., Zeng, X., Xu, M.: Feature decomposition based saliency detection in electron cryo-tomograms. arXiv preprint arXiv:1801.10562 (2018)

7. Guo, J., Zhou, B., Zeng, X., Freyberg, Z., Xu, M.: Model compression for faster structural separation of macromolecules captured by cellular electron cryo-tomography. In: Campilho, A., Karray, F., ter Haar Romeny, B. (eds.) ICIAR 2018. LNCS, vol. 10882, pp. 144–152. Springer, Cham (2018). https://doi.org/10.1007/978-3-319-93000-8_17

8. Huang, Y., et al.: Restoration of missing data in limited angle tomography based on Helgason-Ludwig consistency conditions. Biomed. Phys. Eng. Express **3**(3), 035015 (2017)

9. Frikel, J., Quinto, E.T.: Characterization and reduction of artifacts in limited angle tomography. Inverse Probl. **29**(12), 125007 (2013)

10. Zhang, H., et al.: Image prediction for limited-angle tomography via deep learning with convolutional neural network. arXiv preprint arXiv:1607.08707 (2016)

11. Rick Chang, J.-H., Li, C.-L., Poczos, B., Vijaya Kumar, B.V.K., Sankaranarayanan, A.C.: One network to solve them all-solving linear inverse problems using deep projection models. In: ICCV, pp. 5889–5898 (2017)

12. Pathak, D., Krahenbuhl, P., Donahue, J., Darrell, T., Efros, A.A.: Context encoders: feature learning by inpainting. In: Proceedings of the IEEE Conference on Computer Vision and Pattern Recognition, pp. 2536–2544 (2016)

13. Ledig, C., et al.: Photo-realistic single image super-resolution using a generative adversarial network. In: CVPR, vol. 2, p. 4 (2017)

14. Gordon, R., Bender, R., Herman, G.T.: Algebraic reconstruction techniques (art) for three-dimensional electron microscopy and X-ray photography. J. Theoret. Biol. **29**(3), 471–481 (1970)

15. Trampert, J., Leveque, J.-J.: Simultaneous iterative reconstruction technique: physical interpretation based on the generalized least squares solution. J. Geophys. Res.: Solid Earth **95**(B8), 12553–12559 (1990)

16. Zhu, J.-Y., Park, T., Isola, P., Efros, A.A.: Unpaired image-to-image translation using cycle-consistent adversarial networks. In: Proceedings of the IEEE International Conference on Computer Vision, pp. 2223–2232 (2017)

17. Zhou, B., Lin, X., Eck, B., Hou, J., Wilson, D.: Generation of virtual dual energy images from standard single-shot radiographs using multi-scale and conditional adversarial network. arXiv preprint arXiv:1810.09354 (2018)

18. Hubbell, J.H., Seltzer, S.M.: Tables of X-ray mass attenuation coefficients and mass energy-absorption coefficients 1 kev to 20 mev for elements z= 1 to 92 and 48 additional substances of dosimetric interest. Technical report, National Institute of Standards and Technology-PL, Gaithersburg, MD (1995)

19. Yan, K., Wang, X., Lu, L., Summers, R.M.: Deeplesion: automated mining of large-scale lesion annotations and universal lesion detection with deep learning. J. Med. Imaging **5**(3), 036501 (2018)

20. Mersereau, R.M., Oppenheim, A.V.: Digital reconstruction of multidimensional signals from their projections. Proc. IEEE **62**(10), 1319–1338 (1974)

21. Rivers, M.L.: tomoRecon: high-speed tomography reconstruction on workstations using multi-threading. In: Developments in X-Ray Tomography VIII, vol. 8506, p. 85060U. International Society for Optics and Photonics (2012)

22. Eck, B.L., et al.: Computational and human observer image quality evaluation of low dose, knowledge-based CT iterative reconstruction. Med. Phys. **42**(10), 6098–6111 (2015)

Improving Generalization of Deep Networks for Inverse Reconstruction of Image Sequences

Sandesh Ghimire[1]([envelope]), Prashnna Kumar Gyawali[1], Jwala Dhamala[1], John L. Sapp[2], Milan Horacek[2], and Linwei Wang[1]

[1] Rochester Institute of Technology, Rochester, NY 14623, USA
sg9872@rit.edu
[2] Dalhousie University, Halifax, NS, Canada
http://www.sandeshgh.com

Abstract. Deep learning networks have shown state-of-the-art performance in many image reconstruction problems. However, it is not well understood what properties of representation and learning may improve the generalization ability of the network. In this paper, we propose that the generalization ability of an encoder-decoder network for inverse reconstruction can be improved in two means. First, drawing from analytical learning theory, we theoretically show that a stochastic latent space will improve the ability of a network to generalize to test data outside the training distribution. Second, following the information bottleneck principle, we show that a latent representation minimally informative of the input data will help a network generalize to unseen input variations that are irrelevant to the output reconstruction. Therefore, we present a sequence image reconstruction network optimized by a variational approximation of the information bottleneck principle with stochastic latent space. In the application setting of reconstructing the sequence of cardiac transmembrane potential from body-surface potential, we assess the two types of generalization abilities of the presented network against its deterministic counterpart. The results demonstrate that the generalization ability of an inverse reconstruction network can be improved by stochasticity as well as the information bottleneck.

Keywords: Information bottleneck · Generalization · Learning theory · Inverse problem · Electrophysiological imaging · Sequence encoder-decoder

1 Introduction

There has been an upsurge of deep learning approaches for traditional image reconstruction problems in computer vision and medical imaging [11]. Examples include image denoising [13], inpainting [14], and medical image reconstructions across a variety of modalities such as magnetic resonance imaging [19] and computed tomography [6]. Despite state-of-the-art performances brought by these

© Springer Nature Switzerland AG 2019
A. C. S. Chung et al. (Eds.): IPMI 2019, LNCS 11492, pp. 153–166, 2019.
https://doi.org/10.1007/978-3-030-20351-1_12

deep neural networks, their ability to reconstruct from data not seen in the training distribution is not well understood. To date, very limited work has investigated the generalization ability of these image reconstruction networks from a theoretical perspective, or provided insights into what aspects of representation and learning may improve the ability of these networks to generalize outside the training data.

In this paper, we take an information theoretic perspective – along with analytical learning theory – to investigate and improve the generalization ability of deep image reconstruction networks. Let x be the original image and y be the measurement obtained from x by some transformation process. To reconstruct x from y, we adopt a common deep encoder-decoder architecture [14,19] where a latent representation w is first inferred from y before being used for the reconstruction of x. Our objective is to learn transformations that are general, possibly learning the underlying generative process rather than focusing on every detail in training examples. To this end, we propose that the generalization ability of a deep reconstruction network can be improved from two means: (1) the ability to generalize to data y that are generated from x (and thereby w) outside the training distribution; and (2) the ability to generalize to unseen variations in data y that are introduced during the measurement process but irrelevant to x.

For the first type of generalization ability, we hypothesize that it can be improved by using stochastic instead of deterministic latent representations. We support this hypothesis by the analytical learning theory [8], showing that stochastic latent space helps to learn a decoder that is less sensitive to perturbations in the latent space and thereby leads to better generalization. For the second type of generalization ability, we hypothesize that it can be improved if the encoder compresses the input measurement into a minimal latent representation (*codes* in information theory), containing only the necessary information for x to be reconstructed. To obtain a minimal representation from y that is maximally informative of x, we adopt the information bottleneck theory formulated in [17] to maximize the mutual information between the latent code w and x, $I(x, w)$, while putting a constraint on the mutual information between y and w such that $I(w, y) < I_0$. This can be achieved by minimizing the following objective:

$$loss_{IB} = -I(x; w) + \beta I(w; y) \qquad (1)$$

where β is the Lagrange multiplier. Based on these two primary hypotheses, we present a deep image reconstruction network optimized by a variational approximation of the information bottleneck principle with stochastic latent space.

While the presented network applies for general reconstruction problems, we test it on the sequence reconstruction of cardiac transmembrane potential (TMP) from high-density body-surface electrocardiograms (ECGs) [18]. Given the sequential nature of the problem, we use long short-term memory (LSTM) networks in both the encoder and decoder, with two alternative architectures to compress the temporal information into vector latent space. We tackle two specific challenges regarding the generalization of the reconstruction. First, because the problem is ill-posed, it has been important to constrain the reconstruction with prior physiological knowledge of TMP dynamics [4,5,18]. This however made it difficult to generalize to physiological conditions outside those specified by the prior knowledge. By using the stochastic latent space, we demonstrate the ability of the presented method to generalize outside the physiological knowledge provided in the training data. Second, because the generation of ECGs depends on heart-torso geometry, it has been difficult for existing methods to generalize beyond a patient-specific setting. By the use of the information bottleneck principle, we demonstrate the robustness of the presented network to geometrical variations in ECG data and therefore a unique ability to generalize to unseen subjects. These generalization abilities are tested in two controlled synthetic datasets as well as a real-data feasibility study. We hope that these findings may initiate more theoretical and systematic investigations of the generalization ability of deep networks in image reconstruction problems.

2   Related Work

Deep neural networks have become popular in medical image reconstructions across different modalities such as computed tomography [6], magnetic resonance imaging [19], and ultrasound [12]. Some of these inverse reconstruction networks are based on an encoder-decoder structure [6,19], similar to that investigated in this paper. Among these, the presented work is the closest to Automap [19] in that the output image is reconstructed directly from the input measurements without any intermediate domain-specific transformations. However, these existing works have not investigated either the use of stochastic architectures or the information bottleneck principle to improve the ability of the network to generalize outside the training distributions.

The presented theoretical analysis of stochasticity in generalization utilizes analytical learning theory [8], which is fundamentally different from classic statistical learning theory in that it is strongly instance-dependent. While statistical learning theory deals with data-independent generalization bounds or data-dependent bounds for certain hypothesis space, analytical learning theory provides the bound on how well a model learned from a dataset should perform on true (unknown) measures of variable of interest. This makes it aptly suitable for measuring the generalization ability of stochastic latent space for the given problem and data.

The presented variational formulation of the information bottleneck principle is closely related to that presented in [1]. However, our work differs in three primary aspects. First, we investigate image reconstruction tasks in which the role of information bottleneck has not been clearly understood. Second, we define generalization ability in two different categories, and provide theoretical as well as empirical evidence on how stochastic latent space can improve the network's generalization ability in a way different from the information bottleneck. Finally, we extend the setting of static image classification to image sequences, in which the latent representation needs to be compressed from temporal information within the whole sequence.

To learn temporal relationship in ECG/TMP sequences, we consider two sequence encoder-decoder architectures. One is commonly used in language translation [16], where the code from the last unit of the last LSTM encoder layer is used as the latent vector representation to reconstruct x. We also present a second architecture where fully connected layers are used to compress all the hidden codes of the last LSTM layer into a latent vector representation. This is in concept similar to the attention mechanism [3] to selectively use information from all the hidden LSTM codes for decoding. We experimentally compare the generalization ability of using stochastic versus deterministic latent vectors in both architectures, which has not been studied before.

In the application area of cardiac TMP reconstruction, most related to this paper are works constraining the reconstruction with prior temporal knowledge in the form of physics-based simulation models of TMP [18] and, more recently, generative models learned from physics-based TMP simulation [4]. This however to our knowledge is the first work that investigated the use of deep learning for the direct inference of TMP from ECG. This method will also have the unique potential to generalize outside the patient-specific settings and outside pathological conditions included in the prior knowledge.

3   Methodology

Body-surface electrical potential is produced by TMP in the heart. Their mathematical relation is defined by the quasi-static approximation of electromagnetic theory [15] and, when solved on patient-specific heart-torso geometry, can be derived as: $y(t) = Hx(t)$, where $y(t)$ denotes the time-varying body-surface potential map, $x(t)$ the time-varying TMP map over the 3D heart muscle, and H the measurement matrix specific to the heart-torso geometry of a subject [18]. The inverse reconstruction of x from y at each time instant is ill-posed, and a popular approach is to reconstruct TMP time sequence constrained by prior physiological knowledge of its dynamics [4,5,18]. This is the setting considered in this study, in which the deep network learns to reconstruct with prior knowledge from pairs of $x(t)$ and $y(t)$ generated by physics-based simulation. Note that it is not possible to obtain real TMP data for training, which further highlights the importance of the network to generalize. In what follows, we use x and y to represent sequence matrices with each column denoting the potential map at one time instant.

Given the joint distribution of TMP and ECG as $p(x, y)$, the encoder gives us a conditional distribution $p(w|y)$. These together defines a joint distribution of (x, y, w):

$$p(x, y, w) = p(x)p(y|x)p(w|x, y) = p(x, y)p(w|y) \tag{2}$$

The first term in $loss_{IB}$ in Eq. (1) is given by

$$I(x; w) = \int p(x, w) \log(\frac{p(x|w)}{p(x)}) dx dw = H(x) + \int p(x, w) \log(p(x|w)) dx dw$$

where $p(\boldsymbol{x}|\boldsymbol{w}) = \int \frac{p(\boldsymbol{x},\boldsymbol{w},\boldsymbol{y})}{p(\boldsymbol{w})} d\boldsymbol{y} = \int \frac{p(\boldsymbol{x},\boldsymbol{y})p(\boldsymbol{w}|\boldsymbol{y})}{p(\boldsymbol{w})} d\boldsymbol{y}$ is intractable. Letting $q(\boldsymbol{x}|\boldsymbol{w})$ to be the variational approximation of $p(\boldsymbol{x}|\boldsymbol{w})$, we have:

$$
\int p(\boldsymbol{x},\boldsymbol{w})\log(p(\boldsymbol{x}|\boldsymbol{w}))d\boldsymbol{x}d\boldsymbol{w} = \int p(\boldsymbol{w})[p(\boldsymbol{x}|\boldsymbol{w})\log\frac{p(\boldsymbol{x}|\boldsymbol{w})}{q(\boldsymbol{x}|\boldsymbol{w})} + p(\boldsymbol{x}|\boldsymbol{w})\log q(\boldsymbol{x}|\boldsymbol{w})]d\boldsymbol{x}d\boldsymbol{w}
$$

$$
= \int p(\boldsymbol{w})D_{KL}(p(\boldsymbol{x}|\boldsymbol{w})\|q(\boldsymbol{x}|\boldsymbol{w}))d\boldsymbol{w} + \int p(\boldsymbol{x},\boldsymbol{w})\log q(\boldsymbol{x}|\boldsymbol{w})d\boldsymbol{x}d\boldsymbol{w} \quad (3)
$$

where the KL divergence in the first term is non-negative. This gives us:

$$
I(\boldsymbol{x};\boldsymbol{w}) \geq \int p(\boldsymbol{x},\boldsymbol{y},\boldsymbol{w})[\log q(\boldsymbol{x}|\boldsymbol{w})]d\boldsymbol{x}d\boldsymbol{y}d\boldsymbol{w} = E_{p(\boldsymbol{x},\boldsymbol{y})}[E_{p(\boldsymbol{w}|\boldsymbol{y})}[\log q(\boldsymbol{x}|\boldsymbol{w})]] \quad (4)
$$

The second term in $loss_{IB}$ in Eq. (1) is given by

$$
I(\boldsymbol{y};\boldsymbol{w}) = \int p(\boldsymbol{y},\boldsymbol{w})\log(\frac{p(\boldsymbol{w}|\boldsymbol{y})}{p(\boldsymbol{w})})d\boldsymbol{y}d\boldsymbol{w} = \int p(\boldsymbol{y},\boldsymbol{w})\log[\frac{p(\boldsymbol{w}|\boldsymbol{y})r(\boldsymbol{w})}{r(\boldsymbol{w})p(\boldsymbol{w})}]d\boldsymbol{y}d\boldsymbol{w}
$$

$$
= \int p(\boldsymbol{y})p(\boldsymbol{w}|\boldsymbol{y})\log(\frac{p(\boldsymbol{w}|\boldsymbol{y})}{r(\boldsymbol{w})})d\boldsymbol{y}d\boldsymbol{w} - D_{KL}(p(\boldsymbol{w})\|r(\boldsymbol{w})) \quad (5)
$$

$$
\leq \int p(\boldsymbol{y})p(\boldsymbol{w}|\boldsymbol{y})\log(\frac{p(\boldsymbol{w}|\boldsymbol{y})}{r(\boldsymbol{w})})d\boldsymbol{y}d\boldsymbol{w} = E_{p(\boldsymbol{y})}[D_{KL}(p(\boldsymbol{w}|\boldsymbol{y})\|r(\boldsymbol{w}))] \quad (6)
$$

Combining Eqs. (4) and (6), we have

$$
loss_{IB} \leq E_{p(\boldsymbol{x},\boldsymbol{y})}[-E_{p(\boldsymbol{w}|\boldsymbol{y})}[\log q(\boldsymbol{x}|\boldsymbol{w})] + \beta D_{KL}(p(\boldsymbol{w}|\boldsymbol{y})\|r(\boldsymbol{w}))] = \mathcal{L}_{IB} \quad (7)
$$

which gives us $\mathcal{L}_{IB}$ to be minimized as an upper bound of the information bottleneck objective $loss_{IB}$ formulated in Eq. (1).

Parameterization with Neural Network: We model both the encoder, $p(\boldsymbol{w}|\boldsymbol{y})$ and the decoder, $q(\boldsymbol{x}|\boldsymbol{w})$ as Gaussian distributions, with mean and variance parameterized by neural networks:

$$
p_{\theta_1}(\boldsymbol{w}|\boldsymbol{y}) = \mathcal{N}(\boldsymbol{w}|t_{\theta_1}(y),\sigma_t^2(y)) \quad q_{\theta_2}(\boldsymbol{x}|\boldsymbol{w}) = \mathcal{N}(\boldsymbol{x}|g_{\theta_2}(\boldsymbol{w}),\sigma_x^2(\boldsymbol{w})) \quad (8)
$$

where σ_x^2 denotes a matrix that consists of the variance of each corresponding element in matrix $\boldsymbol{x}$. This is based on the implicit assumption that each elements in $\boldsymbol{x}$ is independent and Gaussian, and similarly for $\boldsymbol{w}$. This gives us:

$$
\mathcal{L}_{IB}(\boldsymbol{\theta}) = E_{p(\boldsymbol{x},\boldsymbol{y})}[-E_{p_{\theta_1}(\boldsymbol{w}|\boldsymbol{y})}[\log q_{\theta_2}(\boldsymbol{x}|\boldsymbol{w})] + \beta.D_{KL}(p_{\theta_1}(\boldsymbol{w}|\boldsymbol{y})\|r(\boldsymbol{w}))]
$$

where $\boldsymbol{\theta} = \{\theta_1,\theta_2\}$. We use reparameterization $\boldsymbol{w} = \boldsymbol{t} + \sigma_t \odot \epsilon$ as described in [10] to compute the inner expectation in the first term. The KL divergence in the second term is analytically available for two Gaussian distributions. We obtain:

$$
\mathcal{L}_{IB}(\boldsymbol{\theta}) = E_{p(\boldsymbol{x},\boldsymbol{y})}\Big[E_{\epsilon\sim\mathcal{N}(0,I)}\Big(\sum_i \frac{1}{\sigma_{xi}^2}(x_i - g_i(\boldsymbol{t} + \sigma_t \odot \epsilon))^2 + \log\sigma_{xi}^2\Big)
$$

$$
+ \beta.D_{KL}(p_{\theta_1}(\boldsymbol{w}|\boldsymbol{y})\|\mathcal{N}(\boldsymbol{w}|\boldsymbol{0},\boldsymbol{I}))\Big] \quad (9)
$$

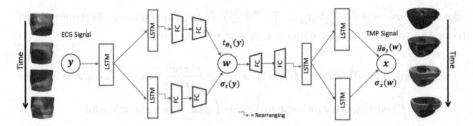

Fig. 1. Illustration of the presented *svs stochastic* architecture, where both the encoder and the decoder consists of mean and variance networks. On the left, we show high density ECG on the body torso simulated from cardiac TMP as described in experiment section.

where g_i is the ith function mapping latent variable to the ith element of mean of x, such that $g_{\theta_2} = [g_1, g_2 ... g_U]$. The deep network is trained to minimize $\mathcal{L}_{IB}(\theta)$ in Eq. (9) with respect to network parameters θ.

Network Architectures: The sequence reconstruction network is realized using long short-term memory (LSTM) neural networks in both the encoder and decoder. To compress the time sequence into a latent vector representation, we experiment with two alternative architectures. First, based on the commonly-used sequence-to-sequence language translation model [16],we consider a *svs-L* architecture that employs the hidden code of the last unit in the last encoding LSTM layer as the latent vector representation for reconstructing TMP sequences. Second, we propose a *svs* architecture where two fully connected layers are used to compress all the hidden codes of the last LSTM layer into a vector representation. In the decoder, this latent representation is expanded by two fully-connected layers before being fed into LSTM layers as shown in Fig. 1.

4   Encoder-Decoder Learning from the Perspective of Analytical Learning Theory

In this section we look at the encoder-decoder inverse reconstructions using analytical learning theory [8]. We start with a general framework and then show that having a stochastic latent space with regularization helps in generalization.

Let $z = (y, x)$ be an input-output pair, and let $D_n = \{z^{(1)}, z^{(2)}, ..., z^{(n)}\}$ denote the total set of training and validation data where $Z_m \subset D_n$ be the validation set. During training, a neural network learns the parameter θ by using an algorithm $\mathcal{A}$ and dataset D_n, at the end of which we have a mapping $h_{\mathcal{A}(D_n)}(\cdot)$ from y to x. Typically, we stop training when the model performs well in the validation set. To evaluate this performance, we define a prediction error function, $\ell(x, h_{\mathcal{A}(D_n)}(y))$ based on our notion of the goodness of prediction. The average validation error is given by $E_{Z_m} \ell(x, h_{\mathcal{A}(D_n)}(y))$. However, there exists a

so-called generalization gap between how well the model performs in the validation set versus in the true distribution of the input-output pair. To be precise, let
$(\mathcal{Z}, \mathcal{S}, \mu)$ be a measure space with μ being a measure on $(\mathcal{Z}, \mathcal{S})$. Here, $\mathcal{Z} = \mathcal{Y} \times \mathcal{X}$
denotes the input-output space of all the observations and inverse solutions. The
generalization gap is given by $\Delta_g = E_\mu \ell(\boldsymbol{x}, h_{\mathcal{A}(D_n)}(\boldsymbol{y})) - E_{Z_m} \ell(\boldsymbol{x}, h_{\mathcal{A}(D_n)}(\boldsymbol{y}))$.
Theorem 1 in [8] provides an upper bound on the generalization gap Δ_g in terms
of data distribution in the latent space and properties of the decoder.

Theorem 1 ([8]). *For any ℓ, let $(\mathcal{T}, f)$ be a pair such that $\mathcal{T} : (\mathcal{Z}, \mathcal{S}) \to ([0,1]^d,$
$\mathcal{B}([0,1]^d))$ is a measurable function, $f : ([0,1]^d, \mathcal{B}([0,1]^d)) \to (\mathbb{R}, \mathcal{B}(\mathbb{R}))$ is of
bounded variation as $V[f] < \infty$, and $\ell(\boldsymbol{x}, h(\boldsymbol{y})) = (f \circ \mathcal{T})(\boldsymbol{z}) \forall \boldsymbol{z} \in \mathcal{Z}$, where $\mathcal{B}(A)$
indicates the Borel σ- algebra on A. Then for any dataset pair (D_n, Z_m) and
any $\ell(\boldsymbol{x}, h_{\mathcal{A}(D_n)}(\boldsymbol{y}))$,*

$$\Delta_g = E_\mu \ell(\boldsymbol{x}, h_{\mathcal{A}(D_n)}(\boldsymbol{y})) - E_{Z_m} \ell(\boldsymbol{x}, h_{\mathcal{A}(D_n)}(\boldsymbol{y})) \leq V[f] \mathcal{D}^*[\mathcal{T}_* \mu, \mathcal{T}(Z_m)]$$

where $\mathcal{T}_* \mu$ is pushforward measure of μ under the map $\mathcal{T}$.

For an encoder-decoder setup, $\mathcal{T}$ is the encoder that maps the observation to the latent space and f becomes the composition of loss function and
decoder that maps the latent representation to the reconstruction loss. Theorem 1 provides two ways to decrease the generalization gap in our problem:
by decreasing the variation $V[f]$ or the discrepancy $\mathcal{D}^*[\mathcal{T}_* \mu, \mathcal{T}(Z_m)]$. Here, we
show that stochasticity of the latent space helps decrease the variation $V[f]$.
The variation of f on $[0,1]^d$ in the sense of Hardy and Krause [7] is defined
as: $V[f] = \sum_{k=1}^d \sum_{1 \leq j_1 < ... < j_k \leq d} V^k[f_{j_1...j_k}]$ where $V^k[f_{j_1...j_k}]$ is defined with
following proposition.

Proposition 1 ([8]). *Suppose that $f_{j_1,..j_k}$ is a function for which $\partial_{1,...k} f_{j_1,..j_k}$
exists on $[0,1]^k$. Then, $V^k[f_{j_1...j_k}] \leq \sup\limits_{t_{j_1},...,t_{j_k} \in [0,1]^k} |\partial_{1,...k} f_{j_1,..j_k}(t_{j_1}, .., t_{j_k})|.$
If $\partial_{1,...k} f_{j_1,..j_k}$ is also continuous on $[0,1]^k$, $V^k[f_{j_1...j_k}] = \int_{[0,1]^k} |\partial_{1,...k} f_{j_1,..j_k}$
$(t_{j_1}, .., t_{j_k})| dt_{j_1} .. dt_{j_k}.$*

In our case, f is the prediction error ℓ as a function of latent representations $\boldsymbol{t}$:

$$\ell(\boldsymbol{x}, h(\boldsymbol{y})) = ||\boldsymbol{x} - \boldsymbol{g}_{\theta_2}(\boldsymbol{t})||_F^2 = \sum_i (\boldsymbol{x}_i - g_i(\boldsymbol{t}))^2 = \sum_i \ell_i \tag{10}$$

where $||\boldsymbol{a}||_F$ denotes the Frobenius norm of matrix $\boldsymbol{a}$, and $\boldsymbol{g}_{\theta_2}$ maps the latent
space to the estimated $\bar{\boldsymbol{x}}$. Theorem 1 and Proposition 1 implies that if the cross
partial derivative of the loss with respect to the latent vector at all order is low
in all directions throughout the latent space, then the approximated validation
loss would be closer to the actual loss over the true unknown distribution of the
dataset. Intuitively, we want the loss curve as a function of latent representation
to be flat if we want a good generalization.

Using Stochastic Latent Space: In our formulation, the latent vector is stochastic with the cost function given by Eq. (9). Using reparameterization $\eta = \sigma_t \odot \epsilon$, the inner expectation of the first term in the loss function $\mathcal{L}_{IB}$ is given by

$$T_1 = E_{\epsilon \sim \mathcal{N}(0,I)}[\sum_i \frac{1}{\sigma_{xi}^2}(x_i - g_i(t + \sigma_t \odot \epsilon))^2]$$

$$= \sum_i \frac{1}{\sigma_{xi}^2}(x_i - g_i(t + \eta))^2 = \sum_i \frac{1}{\sigma_{xi}^2} E_\epsilon[\ell_i(x_i, t + \eta)]$$

Result 1

$$T_1 = \sum_i \frac{1}{\sigma_{xi}^2}\Big[\ell_i(x_i, t) + \langle \sigma_t \odot E_\epsilon[\epsilon], \frac{\partial}{\partial t}\ell_i(x_i, t)\rangle$$

$$+ \frac{1}{2}\langle[\sigma_t \otimes \sigma_t] \odot E_\epsilon[\epsilon \otimes \epsilon], \Big[\frac{\partial^2}{\partial t_{j_1}, \partial t_{j_2}}\ell_i(x_i, t)\Big]\rangle$$

$$+ .. + \frac{1}{k!}\langle[\sigma_t \otimes^k \sigma_t] \odot E_\epsilon[\epsilon \otimes^k \epsilon], \Big[\frac{\partial^k}{\partial t_{j_1}, .., \partial t_{j_k}}\ell_i(x_i, t)\Big]\rangle + ..\Big]$$

where $[\sigma_t \otimes^k \sigma_t]$ denotes k order tensor product of a vector σ_t by itself.

Proof. Using Taylor series expansion for $\ell_i(x_i, t + \eta)$,

$$E_\epsilon[\ell_i(x_i, t + \eta)] = E_\epsilon\Big[\ell_i(x_i, t) + \langle \eta, \frac{\partial}{\partial t}\ell_i(x_i, t)\rangle + \frac{1}{2}\langle[\eta \otimes \eta], \Big[\frac{\partial^2}{\partial t_{j_1}, \partial t_{j_2}}\ell_i(x_i, t)\Big]\rangle$$

$$+ ... + \frac{1}{k!}\langle[\eta \otimes^k \eta], \Big[\frac{\partial^k}{\partial t_{j_1}, .., \partial t_{j_k}}\ell_i(x_i, t)\Big]\rangle + ..\Big] \qquad (11)$$

We move expectation operator inside both brackets and take expectation of only the first term in the inner product. Using $\eta = \sigma_t \odot \epsilon$, we get $E_\epsilon[\eta \otimes^k \eta] = [\sigma_t \otimes^k \sigma_t] \odot E_\epsilon[\epsilon \otimes^k \epsilon]$. Using these in Eq. (11) yields the required result.

The first term of Result 1, $\ell_i(x_i, t)$ (after ignoring $\frac{1}{\sigma_{xi}^2}$), would be the only term in the cost function if the latent space were deterministic. The rest of the terms are additional in stochastic training. Each of these terms is an inner product of two tensor, the first being $[\sigma_t \otimes^k \sigma_t] \odot E_\epsilon[\epsilon \otimes^k \epsilon]$, and the second being the kth order partial derivative tensor $\Big[\frac{\partial^k}{\partial t_{j_1}, .., \partial t_{j_k}}\ell_i(x_i, t)\Big]$. We can thus consider the first tensor as providing penalizing weights to different partial derivatives in the second tensor. Since each inner product is added to the cost, we are minimizing them during optimization. This gives two important implications:

1. For sufficiently large samples, $E_\epsilon[\epsilon \otimes^k \epsilon]$ must be close to central moments of isotropic Gaussian. However, in practice, the number of samples of ϵ remains constant. As we move to the higher order moment tensors, we can expect that they do not converge to that of the standard Gaussian. This, luckily, works in our favor. Since we are minimizing $\frac{1}{k!}\langle[\sigma_t \otimes^k \sigma_t] \odot E_\epsilon[\epsilon \otimes^k \epsilon], \Big[\frac{\partial^k}{\partial t_{j_1}, .., \partial t_{j_k}}\ell_i(x_i, t)\Big]\rangle$ for each order, the inner product can be vanished for

arbitrary ϵ only by driving partial derivative tensors towards zero. Therefore, minimizing the sum of all the inner product for arbitrary ϵ would minimize most of the terms in the partial derivative tensor. From Proposition 1, this corresponds to minimizing the variation of function ℓ_i, and consequently variation of the total error function ℓ according to Eq. (10). Hence, additional terms in the stochastic latent space formulation contributes to decreasing the variation $V[f]$ and consequently the generalization gap.

2. Not all the partial derivatives are equally weighted in the cost function. Due to the presence of weighting tensor $[\boldsymbol{\sigma}_t \otimes^k \boldsymbol{\sigma}_t]$ in the first tensor of inner product, different partial derivative terms are penalized differently according to the value of $\boldsymbol{\sigma}_t$. Combination of the KL divergence term in Eq. (9) with T_1 tries to increase standard deviation, $\boldsymbol{\sigma}_t$ towards 1 whenever it does not significantly increase the cost T_1: higher value of $\boldsymbol{\sigma}_t$ penalizes the partial derivatives of a certain direction more heavily, making the cost flatter in some directions than other.

Strictly speaking, Proposition 1 requires cross partial derivatives to be small throughout the domain of latent variable, which is not included in the above analysis. It however should not significantly affect the observation that, compared to deterministic formulation, the stochastic formulation decreases the variation $V[f]$.

5   Experiments and Results

Since it is not possible to obtain real TMP data, the reconstruction network is trained on simulated data pairs of $\boldsymbol{y}$ and $\boldsymbol{x}$. We focus on evaluating three generalization tasks of the network: to learn how to reconstruct under the prior physiological knowledge given in simulation data while generalizing to (1) unseen pathological conditions in $\boldsymbol{x}$, (2) unseen geometrical variations in $\boldsymbol{y}$ that are irrelevant to $\boldsymbol{x}$, and (3) real clinical data.

5.1   Generalizing Outside the Training Distribution of TMP

Dataset and Implementation Details: We simulated training and test sets using three human-torso geometry models. Spatiotemporal TMP sequences were generated using the Aliev-Panfilov (AP) model [2], and projected to the body-surface potential data with 40 dB SNR noises. Two parameters were varied when simulating the TMP data: the origin of excitation (Exc) and abnormal tissue properties representing myocardial scar. Training data were randomly selected with regard to these two parameters. Test data were selected such that values in these two parameters differed from those used in training in four levels: (1) Scar: Low, Exc: Low, (2) Scar: Low, Exc: High, (3) Scar: High, Exc: Low, and (4) Scar: High, Exc: High, where Scar/Exc indicates the parameter being varied and High/Low denotes the level of difference (therefore difficulty) from the training data. For example, Scar: Low, Exc: High test ECG data was simulated with

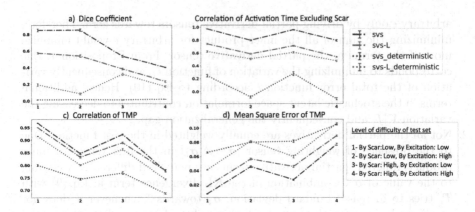

Fig. 2. Reconstruction accuracy of different architectures at the presence of test data at different levels of pathological differences from training data.

Table 1. Accuracy of different architectures at reconstructing unseen pathological conditions

Method \Metric	MSE	TMP Corr.	AT Corr.	Dice Coeff.
svs stochastic	**0.037 ± 0.021**	**0.885 ± 0.061**	**0.885 ± 0.072**	**0.645 ± 0.181**
svs deterministic	0.075 ± 0.013	0.77 ± 0.038	0.12 ± 0.13	0.01 ± 0.006
svs-L stochastic	0.068 ± 0.023	0.838 ± 0.053	0.601 ± 0.074	0.28 ± 0.154
svs-L deterministic	0.067 ± 0.02	0.84 ± 0.053	0.57 ± 0.052	0.165 ± 0.092
Greensite	–	–	0.514 ± 0.006	0.138 ± 0.005

region of scar similar to training but origin of excitation very different from that used in training.

For all four models being compared (svs stochastic/deterministic and svs-L stochastic/deterministic), we used ReLU activation functions in both the encoder and decoder, ADAM optimizer [9], and a learning rate of 10^{-3}. Each neural network was trained on approximately 2500 TMP simulations on each geometry. In addition to the four neural networks, we included a classic TMP inverse reconstruction method (Greensite) designed to incorporate temporal information [5]. On each geometry, approximately 300 cases were tested for each of the four difficulty levels. We report the average and standard deviation of the results across all three geometry models.

Results: The reconstruction accuracy was measured with four metrics: (1) mean square error (MSE) of the TMP sequence, (2) correlation of the TMP sequence, (3) correlation of TMP-derived activation time (AT), and (4) dice coefficients of the abnormal scar tissue identified from the TMP sequence. As summarized in Fig. 2 and Table 1, in all test cases with different levels of pathological differences from the training data, the stochastic version of each architecture was consistently more accurate than its deterministic counterpart. In addition, most of the networks delivered a higher accuracy than the classic Greensite method

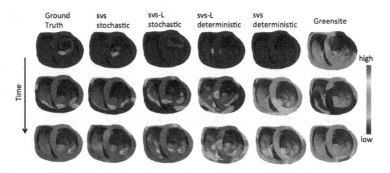

Fig. 3. Examples of TMP sequences reconstructed by different methods being compared.

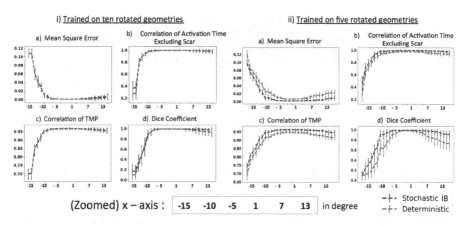

Fig. 4. Comparison of TMP reconstruction by stochastic *vs.* deterministic networks using training data with a (i) high and (ii) low amount of variations in geometrical factors irrelevant to TMP. Values along the x axis shows the degree of rotation of the heart relative to the training set, *i.e.*, cases in the center of the x-axis are the closest to the training data.

(which does not preserve TMP signal shape and thus its MSE and correlation of TMP was not reported), and the accuracy of the *svs* stochastic architecture was significantly higher than the other architectures. These observations are reflected in the examples of reconstructed TMP sequences in Fig. 3.

5.2 Generalization to Geometrical Variations Irrelevant to TMP

Dataset and Implementation Details: TMP data were simulated as described in the previous section, but on a single heart-torso geometry. ECG data were simulated from TMP with controlled geometrical variations by rotating the heart along Z-axis at different angles ($-20°$ to $+20°$ at the interval of $1°$). We trained the network to reconstruct TMP using ECG simulated by (i)

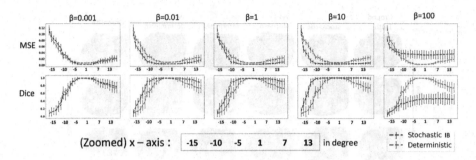

Fig. 5. Comparison of stochastic *vs.* deterministic architectures at different values of β. At $\beta = 10$, the error stays low and flat for a large range of deviation in angles in stochastic architecture.

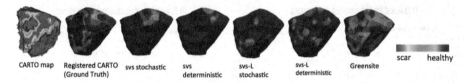

Fig. 6. Comparison of scar region identified by different architectures and the Greensite method with reference to *in vivo* voltage maps.

using five rotation angles from $-2°$ to $2°$, (ii) ten rotation angles from $-4°$ to $+5°$. We then compared the stochastic and deterministic *svs* networks on test ECG generated by the rest of the rotation angles. The network architecture and training details were the same as described in the previous section. Test ECG sets at each rotation angle were generated from 250 TMP signals with different tissue properties and origins of excitation and we report the mean and standard deviation of results for each angle.

Results: As summarized in Fig. 4(ii), when trained on a small interval of five rotation values, the stochastic information bottleneck consistently improves the ability of the network to generalize to geometrical values outside the training distribution. This margin of improvement also increases as we move further away from the training set, *i.e.* as we go left or right from the centre, and seems to be more pronounced when measuring the dice coefficient of the detected scar. When trained on a larger interval of ten rotation values, however, this performance gap diminishes as shown in Fig. 4(i). This suggests that the encoder-decoder architecture with compressed latent space can naturally learn to remove variations irrelevant to the network output, although the use of stochastic information bottleneck allows the network to generalize from a smaller number of training examples.

To understand how the parameter β in the information bottleneck loss $\mathcal{L}_{IB}$ plays a role in generalization, we repeated the above experiments with different values of β. As shown in Fig. 5, as we increase β, the generalization ability of the network first increases and then degrades reaching optimum value at $\beta = 10$.

5.3 Generalization to Real Data: A Feasibility Study

Finally, we tested the presented networks – trained on simulated data as described earlier – on clinical 120-lead ECG data obtained from a patient with scar-related ventricular tachycardia. From the reconstructed TMP sequence, the scar region was delineated based on TMP duration and compared with low-voltage regions from *in-vivo* mapping data. As shown in Fig. 6, because the network is directly transferred from the simulated data to real data, the reconstruction accuracy is in general lower than that in synthetic cases. However, similar to the observations in synthetic cases, the svs stochastic model is able to reconstruct the region of scar that is the closest to the *in-vivo* data.

6 Conclusion

To our knowledge, this is the first work that theoretically investigate the generalization of inverse reconstruction networks through the two different perspectives of stochasticity and information bottleneck, supported by carefully designed experiments in real-world applications. Note that the inequality $\mathcal{L}_{IB} \geq loss_{IB} + D_{KL}(p(\boldsymbol{w})\|r(\boldsymbol{w}))$ suggests that the minimization of $\mathcal{L}_{IB}$ puts an additional constraint (on top of $loss_{IB}$) which requires the marginal $p(\boldsymbol{w})$ to be close to a predefined $r(\boldsymbol{w})$. It is possible that the choice of $r(\boldsymbol{w})$ might also play a role in generalization and will be reserved for future investigations. Future works will also extend the presented study to a wider variety of medical image reconstruction problems.

References

1. Alemi, A., Fischer, I., Dillon, J., Murphy, K.: Deep variational information bottleneck. In: ICLR (2017). https://arxiv.org/abs/1612.00410
2. Aliev, R.R., Panfilov, A.V.: A simple two-variable model of cardiac excitation. Chaos, Solitons Fractals **7**(3), 293–301 (1996)
3. Bahdanau, D., Cho, K., Bengio, Y.: Neural machine translation by jointly learning to align and translate. arXiv preprint arXiv:1409.0473 (2014)
4. Ghimire, S., Dhamala, J., Gyawali, P.K., Sapp, J.L., Horacek, M., Wang, L.: Generative modeling and inverse imaging of cardiac transmembrane potential. In: Frangi, A.F., Schnabel, J.A., Davatzikos, C., Alberola-López, C., Fichtinger, G. (eds.) MICCAI 2018. LNCS, vol. 11071, pp. 508–516. Springer, Cham (2018). https://doi.org/10.1007/978-3-030-00934-2_57
5. Greensite, F., Huiskamp, G.: An improved method for estimating epicardial potentials from the body surface. IEEE TBME **45**(1), 98–104 (1998)
6. Han, Y.S., Yoo, J., Ye, J.C.: Deep residual learning for compressed sensing ct reconstruction via persistent homology analysis. arXiv preprint arXiv:1611.06391 (2016)

7. Hardy, G.H.: On double Fourier series and especially those which represent the double zeta-function with real and incommensurable parameters. Quart. J. Math **37**(5), 53–79 (1906)
8. Kawaguchi, K., Bengio, Y., Verma, V., Kaelbling, L.P.: Towards understanding generalization via analytical learning theory. arXiv preprint arXiv:1802.07426 (2018)
9. Kingma, D.P., Ba, J.: Adam: a method for stochastic optimization. In: ICLR (2015)
10. Kingma, D.P., Welling, M.: Auto-encoding variational bayes. In: ICLR (2013)
11. Lucas, A., Iliadis, M., Molina, R., Katsaggelos, A.K.: Using deep neural networks for inverse problems in imaging: beyond analytical methods. IEEE Sig. Process. Mag. **35**(1), 20–36 (2018)
12. Luchies, A.C., Byram, B.C.: Deep neural networks for ultrasound beamforming. IEEE Trans. Med. Imaging **37**(9), 2010–2021 (2018)
13. Mao, X., Shen, C., Yang, Y.B.: Image restoration using very deep convolutional encoder-decoder networks with symmetric skip connections. In: Advances in Neural Information Processing Systems, pp. 2802–2810 (2016)
14. Pathak, D., Krahenbuhl, P., Donahue, J., Darrell, T., Efros, A.A.: Context encoders: feature learning by inpainting. In: Proceedings of the IEEE Conference on Computer Vision and Pattern Recognition, pp. 2536–2544 (2016)
15. Plonsey, R.: Bioelectric phenomena (1969)
16. Sutskever, I., Vinyals, O., Le, Q.V.: Sequence to sequence learning with neural networks. In: Advances in Neural Information Processing Systems, pp. 3104–3112 (2014)
17. Tishby, N., Pereira, F.C., Bialek, W.: The information bottleneck method. arXiv preprint physics/0004057 (2000)
18. Wang, L., Zhang, H., Wong, K.C., Liu, H., Shi, P.: Physiological-model-constrained noninvasive reconstruction of volumetric myocardial transmembrane potentials. IEEE Trans. Biomed. Eng. **57**(2), 296–315 (2010)
19. Zhu, B., Liu, J.Z., Cauley, S.F., Rosen, B.R., Rosen, M.S.: Image reconstruction by domain-transform manifold learning. Nature **555**(7697), 487 (2018)

Disease Modeling

Event-Based Modeling with High-Dimensional Imaging Biomarkers for Estimating Spatial Progression of Dementia

Vikram Venkatraghavan[1]([✉]), Florian Dubost[1], Esther E. Bron[1],
Wiro J. Niessen[1,2], Marleen de Bruijne[1,3], Stefan Klein[1],
and for the Alzheimer's Disease Neuroimaging Initiative

[1] Biomedical Imaging Group Rotterdam, Department of Medical Informatics and
Radiology, Erasmus MC, Rotterdam, The Netherlands
v.venkatraghavan@erasmusmc.nl
[2] Faculty of Applied Sciences, Delft University of Technology,
Delft, The Netherlands
[3] Department of Computer Science, University of Copenhagen,
Copenhagen, Denmark

Abstract. Event-based models (EBM) are a class of disease progression
models that can be used to estimate temporal ordering of neuropathological changes from cross-sectional data. Current EBMs only handle scalar
biomarkers, such as regional volumes, as inputs. However, regional aggregates are a crude summary of the underlying high-resolution images,
potentially limiting the accuracy of EBM. Therefore, we propose a novel
method that exploits high-dimensional voxel-wise imaging biomarkers:
n-dimensional discriminative EBM (nDEBM). nDEBM is based on an
insight that mixture modeling, which is a key element of conventional
EBMs, can be replaced by a more scalable semi-supervised support vector machine (SVM) approach. This SVM is used to estimate the degree of
abnormality of each region which is then used to obtain subject-specific
disease progression patterns. These patterns are in turn used for estimating the mean ordering by fitting a generalized Mallows model. In order to
validate the biomarker ordering obtained using nDEBM, we also present
a framework for Simulation of Imaging Biomarkers' Temporal Evolution (SImBioTE) that mimics neurodegeneration in brain regions. SIm-
BioTE trains variational auto-encoders (VAE) in different brain regions
independently to simulate images at varying stages of disease progression. We also validate nDEBM clinically using data from the Alzheimer's
Disease Neuroimaging Initiative (ADNI). In both experiments, nDEBM
using high-dimensional features gave better performance than state-of-
the-art EBM methods using regional volume biomarkers. This suggests
that nDEBM is a promising approach for disease progression modeling.

V. Venkatraghavan and F. Dubost—Contributed equally to the study.

ⓒ Springer Nature Switzerland AG 2019
A. C. S. Chung et al. (Eds.): IPMI 2019, LNCS 11492, pp. 169–180, 2019.
https://doi.org/10.1007/978-3-030-20351-1_13

1   Introduction

In 2015, approximately 46.8 million people were estimated to be living with dementia, and by 2050 this number is expected to have increased to 131.5 million [11]. Dementia is characterized by a cascade of neuropathological changes which are quantified using several imaging and non-imaging biomarkers. Understanding how the different biomarkers progress from normal to abnormal state after disease onset enables precise estimation of disease severity in an objective and quantitative way. This can help in identifying individuals at risk of developing dementia as well as monitor the effectiveness of preventive and supportive therapies.

Event-based models (EBM) are a class of disease progression models that estimate the order in which biomarkers become abnormal during disease progression using cross-sectional data [5,6,13,14]. It was reported in a recent paper on discriminative EBM (DEBM) [13] that the EBMs are very sensitive to the quality of biomarkers used for building the model. Hence, to infer the neuropathological changes that occur during dementia accurately, good quality biomarkers are important.

An essential step in an EBM involves mixture modeling to obtain biomarker distributions in normal and abnormal classes [5,13]. This restricts the current EBMs to only handle scalar biomarkers. In case of imaging biomarkers, regional volumes from structural MRIs are often used [5,9,13–15]. However, regional volumes are a crude summary of the high-dimensional information available from structural MRI, resulting in suboptimal EBM performance, as shall be demonstrated later in this paper. Therefore, we propose a novel method that exploits voxel-wise imaging biomarkers: n-dimensional discriminative EBM (nDEBM).

Estimating the accuracy of ordering obtained by EBMs is not feasible as ground-truth ordering is not known for a disease. In order to validate the proposed method and compare its accuracy with that of existing state-of-the-art EBM methods, we also present a framework for Simulation of Imaging Biomarkers' Temporal Evolution (SImBioTE). SImBioTE uses variational auto-encoders (VAE) to simulate neurodegeneration in brain regions. These regions are represented by a vector in the latent space of the VAE. Synthetic brain regions were created by sampling latent representations corresponding to target degrees of abnormality which were determined by a ground-truth ordering of disease progression. The generated synthetic brain regions were used as inputs for nDEBM, and the regional aggregates were used as inputs for state-of-the-art EBMs to evaluate the accuracies.

2   nDEBM

In Sect. 2.1, a brief introduction to the current DEBM [13] model is given. Section 2.2, presents a novel framework to use semi-supervised SVMs in DEBM for estimating posterior probabilities of abnormality for high-dimensional biomarkers. In Sect. 2.3, we use these posterior probabilities to estimate severity of disease progression in an individual.

2.1 DEBM

In a cross-sectional dementia dataset (X) of M subjects (consisting of cognitively normal (CN) and patients with dementia (DE)), let X_j denote a measurement of biomarkers for subject $j \in [1, M]$, consisting of N scalar biomarker values $x_{j,i}$. As dementia is characterized by a cascade of neuropathological changes that occurs over several years, even CN subjects can show some abnormal biomarker values. On the other hand, in DE subjects, a proportion of biomarkers may still have normal values, especially in patients at an early disease stage. This leads to label noise in the data and hence clinical labels cannot directly be propagated to individual biomarkers. The DEBM model introduced in [13], similar to previously proposed EBMs [5,6,14], fits a Gaussian mixture model (GMM) to construct the normal and abnormal distributions. These are used to compute pre-event and post-event likelihoods $p(x_{j,i}|\neg E_i)$ and $p(x_{j,i}|E_i)$ respectively, where an event E_i is defined as the corresponding biomarker becoming abnormal. The mixing parameters are used as prior probabilities to convert these likelihoods to posterior probabilities $p(\neg E_i|x_{j,i})$ and $p(E_i|x_{j,i})$.

$p(E_i|x_{j,i})\forall i$ are used to estimate the subject-specific orderings s_j. s_j is established such that:

$$s_j \ni p(E_{s_j(1)}|x_{j,s_j(1)}) > p(E_{s_j(2)}|x_{j,s_j(2)}) > ... > p(E_{s_j(N)}|x_{j,s_j(N)}) \qquad (1)$$

Finally, DEBM computes the central event ordering S from the subject-specific estimates s_j. To describe the distribution of s_j, a generalized Mallows model is used. The central ordering is defined as the ordering that minimizes the sum of distances to all subject-specific orderings s_j, with probabilistic Kendall's Tau being the distance measure.

2.2 n-Dimensional Biomarker Progression

It was reported in [13] that the accuracy of EBMs depends on the quality of biomarkers used to build the model. Greater separability of individual biomarkers results in estimation of more accurate event ordering. We hypothesize that high-dimensional imaging biomarkers can increase the separability between the normal and abnormal groups, thus improving the accuracy when used as inputs to EBMs. The use of GMM in EBMs however restricts it to using only scalar or low-dimensional biomarkers as GMMs do not scale well to high-dimensional features. SVMs do scale well to high-dimensional features, but a supervised soft-margin SVM cannot be used because of the large amounts of label noise (upto one third of the elderly CN population could be in pre-symptomatic stages of DE [12]). In this section, we present a way in which scalable semi-supervised SVM classifiers can be used within the DEBM framework with high-dimensional inputs.

Let $X_{j,i}$ denote the high-dimensional imaging biomarker for brain region i. Since the clinical diagnosis of the subject cannot be propagated to each region, the labels cannot be trusted while training a classifier. If we were to train a classifier trusting these labels, independently on each biomarker $(X_{\forall j,i})$, we hypothesize that labels of the data close to the decision boundary or on either side of it cannot be completely trusted for that biomarker. For identifying the labels that cannot be trusted for a biomarker, we propose to train a linear classifier assuming equal class-priors. Fitting a non-linear classifier risks over-fitting to the wrongly-labeled data whereas class-priors derived from labeled data could be misleading as some of the labels might be wrong, for that biomarker.

For biomarker $X_{\forall j,i}$, subjects whose labels are preserved are considered as labeled data $(X_{L,i})$. Subjects whose labels have been rejected, along with any prodromal subjects in the dataset are considered as unlabeled data $(X_{U,i})$. Semi-supervised classifiers can be used in this context for obtaining the decision boundary for each biomarker.

To identify the subjects for whom labels can be trusted when considering $X_{\forall j,i}$, we first train a linear SVM $(f_{0;i})$ based on CN and DE subjects. After rejecting labels that cannot be trusted (with distance $d_{0;i} < |d_t|$ from the decision boundary), we use semi-supervised learning with EM [8] using linear SVM with subject-specific costs [2] $(f_{1;i}, ..., f_{k+1;i})$ to iteratively refine the decision boundary. The algorithm for this semi-supervised classification is given below:

Algorithm 1. Semi-Supervised SVM Learning with Subject-specific weights

---

1: **for** $i \in \{1...N\}$ **do**
2:     Train $f_{0;i}$ with $X_{\forall j \in \{CN,DE\},i}$ as inputs
3:     $d_{0;\forall j,i} \leftarrow$ prediction of $X_{\forall j,i}$ using $f_{0;i}$
4:     **for** $j \in \{1...M\}$ **do**
5:         **if** $d_{0;j,i} > |d_t|$ **then:** $X_{L,i} \leftarrow X_{j,i}$
6:         **else:** $X_{U,i} \leftarrow X_{j,i}$
7:     Estimate $\hat{p_0}(E_i|X_{U,i})$ from $d_{0;U,i}$ (using Platt scaling [10]).
8:     Train $f_{1;i}$ using $X_{\forall j,i}$ using $|\hat{p_0}(E_i|X_{U,i}) - \hat{p_0}(\neg E_i|X_{U,i})|$ as weights of $X_{U,i}$.
9:     Estimate $\hat{p_1}(E_i|X_{U,i})$ from $d_{1;U,i}$
10:    $k \leftarrow 1$
11:    **while** $||\hat{p}_k(E_i|X_{U,i}) - \hat{p}_{k-1}(E_i|X_{U,i})||^2 < \epsilon$ **do**
12:        Train $f_{k+1;i}$ using $X_{\forall j,i} \ni |\hat{p}_k(E_i|X_{U,i}) - \hat{p}_k(\neg E_i|X_{U,i})|$ are weights of $X_{U,i}$.
13:        Estimate $\hat{p}_{k+1}(E_i|X_{U,i})$ from $d_{k+1;U,i}$.
14:        $k \leftarrow k + 1$
15:    Estimate $\hat{p}_{k+1}(E_i|X_{\forall j,i})$ from $d_{k+1;\forall j,i}$
16:    $p(E_i|X_{j,i}) \leftarrow \hat{p}_{k+1}(E_i|X_{j,i})$

---

d_t was chosen such that such that 5% of correctly classified data closest to decision boundary are treated as unlabeled. The weights for $X_{U,i}$ in the above algorithm is motivated based on [3]. It is done because unlabeled data close to the decision boundary are not the ideal support vectors. The samples which are farther away from the decision boundary of the previous iteration can be trusted more as support vectors for the next iteration of training.

2.3 Patient Staging

Patient staging refers to the process of positioning individuals on a disease progression timeline characterized by the obtained event ordering. Patient stage (Υ_j) is computed as an expectation of event-centers (λ_n) with respect to $p(n, S, X_j)$, where n denotes the possible discrete stages in the timeline characterized by N biomarker events. Event-centers are the positions of the biomarker events on a normalized disease progression timeline $[0, 1]$, that capture relative distances between events.

$$\Upsilon_j = \frac{\sum_{n=1}^{N} \lambda_n p(n, S, X_j)}{\sum_{n=1}^{N} p(n, S, X_j)} \tag{2}$$

$p(k, S, X_j)$ can be expressed in-terms of posterior probabilities of events obtained from semi-supervised SVM as:

$$p(n, S, X_j) \propto \prod_{i=1}^{n} p\left(E_{S(i)} | X_{j,S(i)}\right) \times \prod_{i=n+1}^{N} p\left(\neg E_{S(i)} | X_{j,S(i)}\right) \tag{3}$$

3 SImBioTE: A Validation Framework

For validating classical EBMs and nDEBM in a unified framework, we extend the framework developed in [16] for simulating datasets consisting of scalar biomarkers, to be capable of generating datasets with realistic voxel-wise imaging biomarkers. It was built on the assumption that the trajectory of biomarker progression follows a sigmoid. Using a similar assumption, we consider the degree of abnormality in different regions $(a_{j,i})$ follows a sigmoidal trajectory.

$$a_{j,i}(\Psi) = \frac{1}{1 + \exp(-\rho_i(\Psi - \xi_{j,i}))} + \epsilon \tag{4}$$

Ψ denotes disease stage of a subject which we take to be a random variable distributed uniformly throughout the disease timeline. ϵ is the equivalent of measurement noise, which represents randomness in the measurement of abnormality. ρ_i signifies the rate of progression of a biomarker, which we take to be equal for all subjects for all biomarkers. It was shown in [13] that the performance of EBMs is similar for equal $\rho_i \forall i$ and unequal ρ_i. $\xi_{j,i}$ denotes the disease stage at which the biomarker becomes abnormal.

After randomly choosing degrees of abnormalities for different regions, we use a variational autoencoder (VAE) [7] for each region i, to generate 3D images of these brain regions at a target degree of abnormality $a_{j,i}(\Psi)$. VAEs are neural networks consisting of two main components: an encoder E which projects input images into a lower dimensional space $\mathbb{R}^K$ called the latent space, and a decoder D which generates images from their hidden representation in the latent space $Z \in \mathbb{R}^K$. Once the VAE has been trained using a large dementia dataset, a latent representation $Z_{j,i;t}$ corresponding to the target degree of abnormality $a_{j,i}(\Psi)$ can be sampled in the latent space. The decoder D then generates a 3D image $D(Z_{j,i;t})$ corresponding to $a_{j,i}(\Psi)$. Below we describe the VAE used in this work, and the sampling strategy in the latent space.

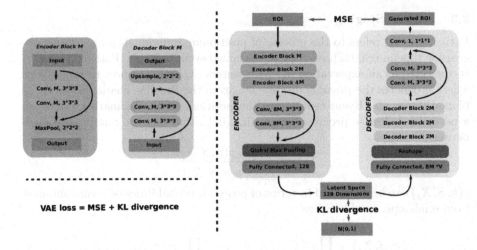

Fig. 1. Architecture of the variational autoencoder.

3.1 Implementation of the Convolutional Variational Autoencoder

Figure 1 summarizes the architecture of our VAE. We use a ReLU activation after each convolutional layer, except after the last $1*1*1$ convolutional layer. We implemented the loss function as proposed by Kingma and Welling [7], with mean-square-error (MSE) and Kullback-Leibler divergence. We optimized the network with Adadelta [17].

3.2 Sampling Strategy in the Latent Space

To navigate in the latent space $\mathbb{R}_i^K$ of region i, we use Euclidean geometry. We first build a scale vector U_i in the latent space to describe the range of the disease from CN to DE. In order to generate a point $Z_{j,i;t} \in \mathbb{R}_i^K$ at the target degree of abnormality $a_{j,i}(\Psi)$, we first randomly sample a point $Z_{j,i;s} \in \mathbb{R}_i^K$, and translate it along the direction of the scale vector U_i until we reach the target abnormality $a_{j,i}(\Psi)$.

Scale Vector from Cognitively Normal to Dementia. To build the scale vector U_i, we first compute the latent representations of all the images of region i in the training dataset by projecting these images in the latent space $\mathbb{R}_i^K$ using the encoder E. Then we use the binary labels – CN and DE – of each subject j to compute the means $\mu_{i;CN} \in \mathbb{R}_i^K$ and $\mu_{i;DE} \in \mathbb{R}_i^K$, and standard deviations $\sigma_{i;CN} \in \mathbb{R}_i^K$ and $\sigma_{i;DE} \in \mathbb{R}_i^K$ for each of the two categories respectively.

This is followed by computing the vector joining the two mean points as $u_i = \mu_{i;DE} - \mu_{i;CN}$. The idea is to create a vector U_i spanning the range of the disease progression, from CN to DE. However, u_i joins only the means, if we want to capture the whole distribution, we need to lengthen this vector by a multiple of the standard deviations, on both sides: for instance by $3\sigma_{i;CN}$ in the CN side, and $3\sigma_{i;DE}$ on the DE side. To do so, we compute the scalar projections of the standard deviations as $\sigma_{i;CNp} = |\sigma_{i;CN}.\widehat{u}_i|$ and $\sigma_{i;DEp} = |\sigma_{i;DE}.\widehat{u}_i|$, where $\widehat{u}_i = u_i/||u_i||_2$. Now we can compute the new origin point (CN) as $O = \mu_{i;CN} - 3\sigma_{i;CNp}\widehat{u}_i$, and the new end point (DE) as $M = \mu_{i;DE} + 3\sigma_{i;DEp}\widehat{u}_i$. Finally, we can compute $U_i = M - O$. Note that $\widehat{U}_i = U_i/||U_i||_2 = \widehat{u}_i$.

Navigation for Generation. We first randomly sample a point $Z_{j,i;s}$ using the mean and standard deviation of the latent representations of all subjects j for region i. The degree of abnormality $a_{j,i;s}$ of this randomly sampled point $Z_{j,i;s}$ can be computed as $a_{j,i;s} = OZ_{j,i;s}.\widehat{U}_i/||U_i||_2$. To reach the target point $Z_{j,i;t}$, we need to translate the randomly sampled point $Z_{j,i;s}$. This now can be done by computing $Z_{j,i;t} = Z_{j,i;s} + (a_{j,i;t} - a_{j,i;s})U_i$. To generate the corresponding brain region we can now use the decoder and compute $D(Z_{j,i;t})$.

4   Experiments and Results

This section describes the experiments performed to validate the proposed nDEBM algorithm and also compare it with classical EBM [5] and DEBM [13] algorithms.

4.1   ADNI Data

We considered 1737 ADNI subjects (417 CN, 106 with significant memory concern (SMC), 872 with mild cognitive impairment (MCI) and 342 AD subjects) who had a 1.5T structural MRI (T1w) scan at baseline. This was followed by multi-atlas brain extraction using the method described in [4]. Gray matter (GM) volumes of segmented regions were regressed on age, sex and intra-cranial volume (ICV) and the effects of these factors were subsequently corrected for. Student's t-test between CN and AD was performed on these confounding factor corrected GM volumes and 15 regions with smallest p-values were retained. They were subsequently used as inputs for DEBM and EBM [5] models. The optimization routine proposed in [13] was used to train the GMM in these two models.

The T1w images were registered to a common template space based on the method used in [4]. Probabilistic tissue segmentations were obtained for white matter (WM), GM, and cerebrospinal fluid on the T1w image using the unified tissue segmentation method [1]. The voxel-wise GM density maps were computed based on the Jacobian of the local deformation map and the probabilistic GM volume. The GM density maps from the corresponding 15 regions were used as inputs for nDEBM.

Model Validation. Since the groundtruth ordering is not known in a clinical setting, validation of these models was done based on the resulting patient stages for classifying AD subjects from CN as well as for classifying MCI non-converters (MCI-nc) from converters (MCI-c)[1]. We performed 10-fold cross-validation with 10 repetitions. The training set was used to train the three models. The disease timeline created during training was used to stage the patients in the test-set.

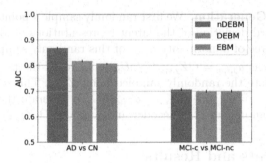

Fig. 2. AUC measures when patient stages of nDEBM, DEBM and EBM were used for classifying AD vs CN (left) and MCI-c vs MCI-nc (right). The error bar represents the standard deviation in 10 random repetitions.

Figure 2 shows the results of 10 random repetitions of 10-fold cross-validation on ADNI dataset. The error-bar shows the standard deviation of the AUCs when the patient stages obtained from nDEBM, DEBM and EBM were used to classify AD vs CN and MCI-c vs MCI-nc.

Uncertainty in Estimation. Variation of the positions of the biomarker events on a normalized disease progression timeline (event-centers) estimated by nDEBM and DEBM was studied by creating 100 bootstrapped samples of the data and applying nDEBM on those samples[2].

Figure 3 shows event-centers estimated by nDEBM and DEBM along with the uncertainty in their estimations. The biomarkers are ordered along the y-axis based on the event-ordering obtained by nDEBM.

4.2   Simulation Data

In our experiments, $\xi_{j,i}$ $\forall j$ are random variables with $\mathbb{N}(\mu_{\xi_i}, \Sigma_{\xi_i})$. μ_{ξ_i} were equally spaced for different i. The value of Σ_{ξ_i} was set to be $\Delta\xi$ where $\Delta\xi$ is the difference in μ_{ξ_i} of adjacent events. ρ_i was considered to be equal for all

---

[1] MCI converters are subjects who convert to AD within 3 years of baseline measurement.

[2] EBM was left out of this experiment as the concept of event-centers was not introduced for EBM.

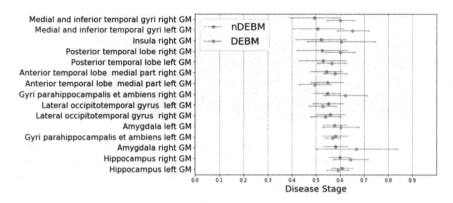

Fig. 3. Variation of event-centers estimated by nDEBM and DEBM in 100 bootstrapped samples of the ADNI data. The error bar represents the standard deviation of the respective event-centers.

biomarkers. Ψ of the simulated subjects were distributed uniformly throughout the disease timeline.

We first trained 15 VAEs (one per selected region) on the GM density maps of the ADNI dataset. Then we generated - as detailed in Sect. 3 - images for these 15 regions and for 1737 artificial subjects according to pre-computed degrees of abnormality as defined in Eq. 4. These degrees of abnormality are different for each region and each subject. We repeated this process 10 times, with different random simulations. The voxel-wise GM density maps of regions were used for obtaining the ordering using nDEBM. The GM volume of the simulated regions (computed by integrating the GM density map over the region of interest) were used as biomarkers for DEBM and EBM.

SimBioTE results depicting Lateral occipitotemporal gyrus atrophy in simulated images is shown in Fig. 4. The images thus generated were used for validating different EBM methods.

The errors made by different EBM methods on SImBioTE data are shown in Fig. 5. The estimated ordering and the ground-truth orderings were compared using Kendall's Tau distance.

5 Discussions

We proposed a novel method (nDEBM) that exploits high-dimensional voxel-wise imaging biomarkers for event-based modeling using semi-supervised SVM. This was validated based on ADNI dataset, where the spatial spread of structural abnormality was estimated based on a cross-sectional dataset. However this is an indirect validation of the orderings based on accuracy of the estimated patient stages, since the ground-truth ordering for clinical data is unknown.

To unambiguously validate the orderings obtained, we also proposed a new simulation framework (SImBioTE) to simulate voxel-wise imaging biomarkers

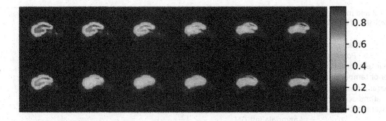

Fig. 4. An example of Lateral occipitotemporal gyrus (right) atrophy as simulated by SImBioTE. The interpolation spans the full range U_i, as described in Sect. 3. Left is normal (CN) and right is abnormal (DE). The two rows shows disease progression in two different simulated subjects.

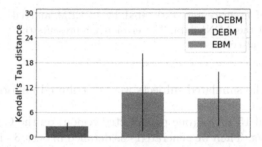

Fig. 5. Inaccuracies, as measured by Kendall's Tau distance from groundtruth, of nDEBM, DEBM and EBM. The error bar represents the standard deviation of the errors made in 10 repetitions of simulations.

based on training VAEs on different regions. It is known that GM tissue is lost in AD progression. Therefore the voxel-wise GM density maps will become darker as the disease progresses, as can be observed in Fig. 4. It was also observed in Fig. 4 that simulated regions for different subjects shows considerable variations. This shows that the simulation framework is capable of generating datasets with realistic atrophy and with good inter-subject variability. This, in combination with the scalar biomarkers' simulation framework, results in images where the disease progression in different regions can be controlled. However, a more thorough validation of the simulation framework by comparing the atrophy patterns of the simulated data with that of real-life longitudinal data is needed to understand the effect of different model parameters. Possible extensions of SImBioTE includes simulating whole brain images from these independent regions, which can be used to validate wider range of disease progression models.

The datasets simulated by SImBioTE were used for inputs for different EBMs. It was observed in Fig. 5 that the orderings obtained by nDEBM are much closer to the ground-truth as compared to DEBM and EBM. It was also observed in Fig. 2 that the patient stages obtained by nDEBM delineates AD and CN subjects much better than the ones obtained by DEBM and EBM. The AUCs of classifying MCI-c vs MCI-nc are also marginally better for nDEBM as compared to the other two methods. These experiments serve as a validation for our initial hypothesis that increasing the dimensionality of the inputs helps in better delineation of normal and abnormal regions, which increases the accuracy of the resulting ordering. It can hence be concluded that the voxelwise data helps nDEBM in estimating the disease progression more accurately than regional volumes. However, the choice of hyper-parameters in nDEBM (for e.g. d_t, SVM slack parameters) was done ad-hoc. The effect they have on the accuracy of the resulting ordering needs to be studied through more rigorous validation experiments.

The difference in event orderings obtained by nDEBM and DEBM as observed in Fig. 3 suggests that the two types of inputs can lead to very different results. Hence, computing regional aggregates, such as volumes, and using that as inputs for EBMs as done in [5,9,13–15] is not an optimal choice for estimating the spatial progression of disease.

6 Conclusion

We hypothesized that high-dimensional imaging biomarkers would result in better delineation of normal and abnormal regions thus leading to more accurate event-based models. We hence proposed a novel method (nDEBM) that exploits high-dimensional voxel-wise imaging biomarkers based on semi-supervised SVM to estimate temporal ordering of neuropathological changes in the brain structure using cross-sectional data. We also proposed a simulation framework (SImBioTE) using variational auto-encoders that mimics neurodegeneration in brain regions to validate nDEBM. Furthermore, we applied nDEBM framework to a set of 1737 subjects from ADNI dataset for clinically validating the method. In both experiments, nDEBM using high-dimensional features gave better performance than state-of-the-art EBM methods using regional volume biomarkers. This served as a validation for our initial hypothesis. nDEBM thus presents a new paradigm for estimating spatial progression of dementia.

Acknowledgement. This project has received funding from the European Union's Horizon 2020 research and innovation programme under grant agreement No. 666992. E.E. Bron is supported by the Hartstichting (PPP Allowance, 2018B011). F. Dubost is supported by The Netherlands Organisation for Health Research and Development (ZonMw) Project 104003005.

References

1. Ashburner, J., Friston, K.J.: Unified segmentation. NeuroImage **26**(3), 839–851 (2005)
2. Brefeld, U., Geibel, P., Wysotzki, F.: Support vector machines with example dependent costs. In: Lavrač, N., Gamberger, D., Blockeel, H., Todorovski, L. (eds.) ECML 2003. LNCS (LNAI), vol. 2837, pp. 23–34. Springer, Heidelberg (2003). https://doi.org/10.1007/978-3-540-39857-8_5

3. Brefeld, U., Scheffer, T.: Co-EM support vector learning. In: Proceedings of the Twenty-first International Conference on Machine Learning, ICML 2004, p. 16. ACM, New York (2004)
4. Bron, E.E., et al.: Diagnostic classification of arterial spin labeling and structural MRI in presenile early stage dementia. Hum. Brain Mapp. **35**(9), 4916–4931 (2014)
5. Fonteijn, H.M., et al.: An event-based model for disease progression and its application in familial Alzheimer's disease and Huntington's disease. NeuroImage **60**(3), 1880–1889 (2012)
6. Huang, J., Alexander, D.: Probabilistic event cascades for Alzheimer's disease. In: Advances in Neural Information Processing Systems 25, pp. 3095–3103. Curran Associates, Inc. (2012)
7. Kingma, D.P., Welling, M.: Auto-encoding variational bayes. Stat 1050, 1 (2014)
8. Nigam, K., Mccallum, A.K., Thrun, S., Mitchell, T.: Text classification from labeled and unlabeled documents using EM. Mach. Learn. **39**(2), 103–134 (2000)
9. Oxtoby, N.P., Alexander, D.C.: Imaging plus X: multimodal models of neurodegenerative disease. Curr. Opin. Neurol. **30**(4), 371–379 (2017)
10. Platt, J.: Probabilistic outputs for support vector machines and comparisons to regularized likelihood methods. Adv. Large Margin Classifiers **10**(3), 61–74 (1999)
11. Prince, M., Wimo, A., Guerchet, M., Ali, G.C., Wu, Y.T., Prina, M.: World Alzheimer's report 2015, the global impact of dementia: an analysis of prevalence, incidence, cost and trends. Alzheimer's Disease Int'l (2015)
12. Schott, J.M., Bartlett, J.W., Fox, N.C., Barnes, J., for ADNI: Increased brain atrophy rates in cognitively normal older adults with low cerebrospinal fluid $A\beta1-$ 42. Ann. Neurol. **68**(6), 825–834 (2010)
13. Venkatraghavan, V., Bron, E.E., Niessen, W.J., Klein, S.: Disease progression timeline estimation for Alzheimer's disease using discriminative event based modeling. NeuroImage **186**, 518–532 (2019)
14. Young, A.L., et al.: A data-driven model of biomarker changes in sporadic Alzheimer's disease. Brain **137**(9), 2564–2577 (2014)
15. Young, A.L., et al.: Uncovering the heterogeneity and temporal complexity of neurodegenerative diseases with subtype and stage inference. Nat. Commun. **9**, 4273 (2018)
16. Young, A.L., Oxtoby, N.P., Ourselin, S., Schott, J.M., Alexander, D.C.: A simulation system for biomarker evolution in neurodegenerative disease. Med. Image Anal. **26**(1), 47–56 (2015)
17. Zeiler, M.D.A.: An adaptive learning rate method. arxiv preprint. arXiv preprint arXiv:1212.5701 (2012)

Shape

Minimizing Non-holonomicity:
Finding Sheets in Fibrous Structures

Babak Samari, Tabish A. Syed$^{(\boxtimes)}$, and Kaleem Siddiqi

School of Computer Science and Center for Intelligent Machines,
McGill University, Montreal, Canada
{babak,tabish,siddiqi}@cim.mcgill.ca

Abstract. Oriented elements compose fibrous structures in biological tissue, and their geometry plays an important role in organ function. In the heart, for example, myocytes are stacked end on end in a particular fashion to facilitate electrical conductivity and efficient mechanical contraction. In the brain, white matter fiber tracts are neuro-anatomically partitioned into specific bundles which connect distinct brain regions. In both cases, the local geometry has been qualitatively described as being sheet-like in particular regimes. Yet, to date, few if any quantitative methods exist for finding these sheets from imaging data. We here introduce a novel computational solution to this problem, motivated by the property that a holonomic vector field is locally normal to a family of smooth surfaces. We propose an algorithm which, given an input vector field, finds a second one with which it best spans a sheet-like structure locally, by minimizing non-holonomicity. We show that our algorithm converges in theory and in practice, under reasonable assumptions about the input data, and we provide high quality sheet reconstructions from both heart wall DTI data and labeled tracts in the human brain, along with a sheet likeliness measure. Whereas sheet-like geometries have been described qualitatively in past literature, ours is the first method to provide a reconstruction of them from a single direction field. Our algorithm also admits a parallel implementation that exploits GPUs and is hence very efficient. We thus anticipate that it will find use in the community for retrieving sheets on which oriented fibrous structures lie from imaging data.

Keywords: Fibrous structures · Sheet estimation · Non-holonomicity

1 Introduction

Fibrous biological tissues are reported to be organized in sheet-like geometries in certain regimes. Examples include laminar sheets and cleavage planes in the heart wall [6,7], and sheets on which fiber tract systems in the mammalian brain are posited to lie [15]. Quantitative geometric characterizations of sheets

---

B. Samari and T. A. Syed—Equal contribution.

© Springer Nature Switzerland AG 2019
A. C. S. Chung et al. (Eds.): IPMI 2019, LNCS 11492, pp. 183–194, 2019.
https://doi.org/10.1007/978-3-030-20351-1_14

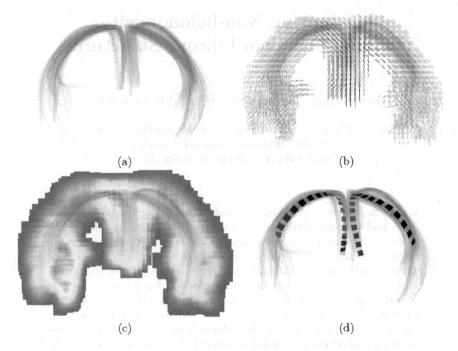

(a)   (b)

(c)   (d)

Fig. 1. (Best viewed by zooming-in on the PDF) (a) We assume as input a set of streamlines, in this example those corresponding to the left and right Fornix tracts from a Human Connectome Project (HCP) atlas. (b) We then extract a local direction field on a discrete grid, using the tangents to the streamlines. (c) The local non-holonomicity value, after convergence of our algorithm, gives a measure of the likelihood of a local sheet, with sheet probability decreasing from light blue to red using a jet colormap volumetric rendering. (d) Our estimated sheets are overlaid on the streamlines as magenta surfaces, but only in regimes found to support sheet-like geometries. (Color figure online)

in biological tissue are often based on orientation measurements from in-vivo or ex-vivo specimens, using diffusion imaging. In analyses of the heart wall, the principal and second eigenvectors of a diffusion tensor are commonly assumed to span a local sheet, with the third eigenvector giving the direction of the sheet normal [4]. This approach has shown promise in the development of models of electrical conduction in the heart wall for electrophysiology [16], and in analyses of heart wall mechanics [3]. Statistical investigations of diffusion tensor data from populations of mammalian hearts have shown, however, that the second and third eigenvalues can be very close to one another in magnitude, and thus their directions can be locally ambiguous [8,11]. As such, estimates of sheet geometries in myocardial tissue using all three eigenvectors of a diffusion tensor may not be reliable. The same is true of the mammalian brain; in regions where multiple tract systems co-exist and cross one another fiber geometry is not well characterized by a diffusion tensor.

In the human brain, the hypothesis that distinct tract systems lie on 2D sheets which intersect one another at approximately 90° angles to generate a local grid-like pattern, has been supported by qualitative considerations and visualization in [15]. Others have pointed out that distinct tract systems might span a sheet without being locally orthogonal to one another [2] and that quantitative measures of sheet geometries derived from diffusion data are desirable [1,13,14]. Yushkevich et al. have fit deformable medial models to segmented tract systems to obtain sheet-like representations of fasciculi where appropriate [18]. Motivated by the property that two vector fields span an integrable surface when the normal component of the associated Lie bracket goes to zero, Tax et al. have used this quantity to define a local sheet probability index along with robust algorithms to estimate it [13,14]. In their work the local vector field directions are chosen from the peaks of a fiber orientation distribution function. The normal component of the Lie bracket has also been shown to be effective for sheet structure visualization, via the construction of a sheet tensor in [5], while Ankele and Shultz have applied this measure directly to diffusion tensor data in [1]. Motivated by these formal approaches to sheet structure estimation based on the integrability of vector fields, we study a more general problem here, which is the reconstruction of local sheets from a *single* direction field. Such a field might arise from the principal eigenvector direction of a diffusion tensor (e.g. in the case of the heart wall) or from the tangent vectors to precomputed streamlines, e.g., in the case of labeled tract systems in the mammalian brain. Figure 1 presents an overview of our approach. We depart from past approaches by treating sheet structure estimation as an energy minimization problem, where, given the single direction field as input, we find a second vector field that is optimal with respect to spanning a local sheet with it. The optimality comes from the formal notion of holonomicity. As it turns out, this is equivalent to finding the second field as a local minimizer of the normal component of a Lie bracket. Based on these ideas, we present a gradient descent based algorithm to recover sheets, along with a proof of convergence. We also report a very efficient implementation of the algorithm using GPUs. Our application of this algorithm to mammalian heart wall orientation data from two species, rat and canine, reveals sheet geometries consistent with what has been reported only in qualitative descriptions thus far from DTI, or in observations from histological slices of heart wall tissue. Of more significance is our results on labeled tract systems from the Human Connectome Project, where we test the sheet hypothesis in a formal way. Given a tract system described as a collection of streamlines in 3D as input, we recover sheet geometries where there is support for them. As a by-product of our approach we provide high quality visualizations of the sheets in biological structures using software we have written. We anticipate that such visualizations will be useful to anatomists when examining fibrous structures in the context of their local surroundings.

2   Minimizing Non-holonomicity: Theory and Analysis

2.1   Background: Sheets and Holonomicity

Given a unit vector field $\mathbf{n}$ which is orthonormal to a family of surfaces, it can be shown that $\langle \mathbf{n}, \text{curl}\,\mathbf{n} \rangle = 0$ [17], where we use $\langle \cdot, \cdot \rangle$ to denote the inner product. Conversely, any vector field $\mathbf{n}$ such that $\langle \mathbf{n}, \text{curl}\,\mathbf{n} \rangle = 0$ is orthonormal to a family of surfaces and is said to be *holonomic*. For a general vector field $\mathbf{n}$, its degree of non-holonomicity ρ is defined as follows [17]:

$$\rho = \Big\langle \mathbf{n}, \text{curl}\,\mathbf{n} \Big\rangle.$$

Consider two orthonormal vector fields $\mathbf{u}$ and $\mathbf{v}$ such that $\mathbf{n} = \mathbf{u} \times \mathbf{v}$. It is easy to show then, that *non-holonomicity* ρ expressed in terms of $\mathbf{u}$ and $\mathbf{v}$ reduces to

$$\rho^{\mathbf{uv}} = \Big\langle \mathbf{u} \times \mathbf{v},\ [\mathbf{u}, \mathbf{v}] \Big\rangle,$$

where $[\mathbf{u}, \mathbf{v}]^i = u^j \frac{\partial v^i}{\partial x^j} - v^j \frac{\partial u^i}{\partial x^j}$ is the Lie Bracket of $\mathbf{u}$ and $\mathbf{v}$. For a pair of vector fields which span a surface, the non-holonomicity ρ vanishes identically. While this is true in the continuous case, we expect the non-holonomicity value to be small for discrete fields spanning a surface. This is the key idea behind our approach.

Given a *single* vector field $\mathbf{u}$, we consider the problem of estimating an orthonormal vector field $\mathbf{v}$, such that $\mathbf{u}$ and $\mathbf{v}$ span a sheet locally. We propose a strategy which starts with a *single* input vector field $\mathbf{u}$, and estimates an orthonormal vector field $\mathbf{v}$ by iterative minimization of an appropriate energy function.

2.2   Problem Formulation and Setup

Let $\mathbf{v}$ be the current estimate of the vector field such that $\langle \mathbf{u}, \mathbf{v} \rangle = 0$. Further, let $\rho^{\mathbf{uv}}$ be the non-holonomicity function of $\mathbf{u}$ and $\mathbf{v}$. Consider the non-holonomicity $\rho(\theta)$ corresponding to a perturbed vector field $\hat{\mathbf{v}} = \mathbf{v}(\theta)$, where θ is a scalar function which parametrizes the field $\hat{\mathbf{v}}$ with respect to field $\mathbf{v}$ in the plane perpendicular to $\mathbf{u}$. Using the definition of non-holonomicity $\rho^{\mathbf{uv}}$ given above, a straightforward computation shows that $\rho(\theta)$ is given by

$$\rho(\theta) = \rho^{\mathbf{uv}} \cos^2\theta + \rho^{\mathbf{un}} \sin^2\theta + \alpha^{\mathbf{uv}} \sin 2\theta + \nabla_{\mathbf{u}}\theta = \rho_s(\theta) + \nabla_{\mathbf{u}}\theta \qquad (1)$$

where, $\alpha^{\mathbf{uv}} = \frac{\langle \mathbf{n}, [\mathbf{u}, \mathbf{n}] \rangle - \langle \mathbf{v}, [\mathbf{u}, \mathbf{v}] \rangle}{2}$ and, $\rho^{\mathbf{uv}}$ and $\rho^{\mathbf{un}}$ are the non-holonomicity functions of the unperturbed fields $\mathbf{u}$ and $\mathbf{v}$, and $\mathbf{u}$ and $\mathbf{n}$.

Notice that for a constant perturbation function θ, $\nabla_{\mathbf{u}}\theta = 0$. Therefore $\rho(\theta) = \rho_s(\theta)$, the sinusoidal part of the $\rho(\theta)$ function which has a period of π. Further, a 180° turn of $\mathbf{v}$ leaves $\rho(\theta)$ unchanged. We know that for regions with sheet-like geometry, the spanning vector fields $\mathbf{u}$ and $\mathbf{v}$ are such that $\rho^{\mathbf{uv}} = 0$. We therefore define an energy function as follows:

$$E(\mathbf{u}, \mathbf{v}, \theta) = \rho^2(\theta). \qquad (2)$$

This energy is zero in regions where $\mathbf{u}$ and $\mathbf{v}$ span a sheet, and high in regions which are less sheet like. We can therefore pose the estimation of the vector field $\mathbf{v}$ as the following energy minimization problem:

$$\mathbf{v}^* = \arg \min_{\mathbf{v}} E(\mathbf{u}, \mathbf{v}, \theta)$$

$$\text{subject to } \langle \mathbf{u}, \mathbf{v} \rangle = 0. \tag{3}$$

2.3   Minimization Algorithm and Analysis

We solve the minimization problem (3) using an iterative gradient descent approach. We initialize with a $\mathbf{v}$, such that the orthogonality constraint $\langle \mathbf{u}, \mathbf{v} \rangle$ is satisfied. We maintain this constraint in the subsequent iterations by forcing each update to lie in the plane orthonormal to $\mathbf{u}$. At each step the varying vector field $\mathbf{v}(\theta)$ is updated using the gradient of the energy function $E(\mathbf{u}, \mathbf{v}, \theta)$. We update θ using a general discrete gradient descent update as follows:

$$\frac{\theta^{t+1} - \theta^t}{\eta} = -\frac{\partial E(\theta)}{\partial \theta}$$

$$\implies \mathbf{v}^{t+1} = \mathbf{v}(\theta^{t+1}),$$

where η is the size of the time step. The update for $\mathbf{v}$ is carried out implicitly by rotating $\mathbf{v}$ about vector $\mathbf{u}$ without explicitly using θ^{t+1}. To rotate the vector $\mathbf{v}$ by an angle β we use the rotation matrix $\mathbf{R}_\beta^{\mathbf{u}} = \cos \beta \, \mathbf{I} + \sin \beta \, [\mathbf{u}]_\times + (1 - \cos \beta)(\mathbf{u}\mathbf{u}^T)$, where $[\mathbf{u}]_\times$ is the cross-product matrix corresponding to $\mathbf{u}$. This ensures that the orthonormality constraint is satisfied at every iteration, without having to explicitly express $\mathbf{v}$ as a function of θ in the local coordinates.

One can observe that the energy E is a function not only of the values of the vector fields $\mathbf{u}$ and $\mathbf{v}$ at a point, but also of their derivatives. Therefore, the energy at a point depends on the value of the field at that point and its neighbourhood. It is quite possible, therefore, that a local point wise gradient descent update at a point, as described above, may increase the energy in the neighbourhood. In fact, a key contribution of our method is that it converges due to the following property

Proposition 1. *For an incompressible smooth vector field $\mathbf{u}$, there exists a positive η such that a gradient descent update of θ reduces the energy everywhere.*

Proof. Let $\mathbf{u}$ be the fixed input vector field and $\mathbf{v}$ be the current estimate of the second vector field. Consider the gradient of the energy function (2) at time t given by

$$\frac{\partial E(\theta)}{\partial \theta} = 2\Big(\rho_s(\theta) + \nabla_\mathbf{u}\theta\Big)\Big((\rho^{\mathbf{uu}} - \rho^{\mathbf{uv}})\sin 2\theta + 2\alpha^{\mathbf{uv}} \cos 2\theta + \operatorname{div} \mathbf{u}\Big),$$

where θ represents the perturbation with respect to the current $\mathbf{u}$ and $\mathbf{v}$.

Before the update, $\theta \equiv 0$, therefore we have

$$\frac{\partial E(\theta)}{\partial \theta}\Big|_{\theta \equiv 0} = 2\rho^{\mathbf{uv}}(2\alpha^{\mathbf{uv}} + \operatorname{div} \mathbf{u}) = \mathcal{E}_0^\rho.$$

Then, θ^{t+1} is given by

$$\theta^{t+1} = -\eta \mathcal{E}_0^\rho.$$

To prove our claim, it is sufficient to show that this update reduces the energy, so that

$$E(0) > E(-\eta \mathcal{E}_0^\rho). \tag{4}$$

For small θ we let $\sin \theta \approx \theta$, $\cos \theta \approx 1$. The condition for convergence in (4) for small positive η then reduces to

$$4\alpha^{\mathbf{uv}}(2\alpha^{\mathbf{uv}} + \operatorname{div} \mathbf{u}) + \nabla_{\mathbf{u}} \mathcal{E}_0^\rho > 0.$$

Since we have assumed that our initial fixed vector field $\mathbf{u}$ represents smoothly varying local orientation in fibrous tissue, we can assume that $\operatorname{div} \mathbf{u}$ is small, and then the convergence condition reduces to $\nabla_{\mathbf{u}} \mathcal{E}_0^\rho \gtrsim -8(\alpha^{\mathbf{uv}})^2$. For a smooth enough vector field with small divergence, we can choose a positive time step η such that the energy is reduced.

It is possible to consider a stronger smoothness condition: $|\nabla_{\mathbf{u}} \mathcal{E}_0^\rho| < 8(\alpha^{\mathbf{uv}})^2$, which helps us improve our error function and select the additional parameters, as discussed in the following section.

3   Method Evaluation and Parameter Selection

Data: In order to validate our method we carried out a few experiments with data obtained from two sources. The first is a dataset of rat and canine hearts used in [12], which is available for public download. It consists of ex-vivo diffusion tensor (DT) fits to myocardial tissue, with resolutions of $64 \times 64 \times 128$ (rat) and $300 \times 300 \times 333$ (canine) voxels, respectively. We use the principal eigenvector of the tensor, which gives an acceptable proxy for myofiber orientation [8], as our fixed vector field. The second source is a dataset of labeled fiber tract systems in the human brain, constructed from a fiber bundle atlas generated from data from the Human Connectome Project, used in the ISMRM 2015 Tractography challenge [9]. This dataset is available for public download as well. The tangents at a list of points along fiber tracts from the data were used to generate our fixed direction vector field.

Modifying the Error Function: As a corollary of our convergence analysis above, we infer from the bound on the energy gradient that a smoother energy function will have better convergence properties. This is in fact the case in practice, and we therefore used a modified error function $\hat{E}$ defined as

$$\hat{E}(\mathbf{u}, \mathbf{v}, \theta(\mathbf{x})) = \sum_{\hat{\mathbf{x}} \in Nbd(\mathbf{x})} \rho^2(\hat{\mathbf{x}}) \tag{5}$$

where $Nbd(\mathbf{x})$ is the neighbourhood of $\mathbf{x}$. We used a neighbourhood size of 3×3 in our experiments. This energy converges for a wider range of choices of the step

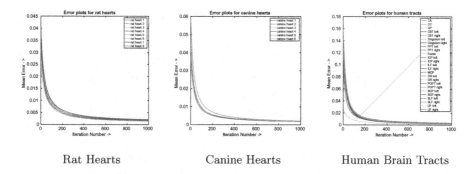

Rat Hearts   Canine Hearts   Human Brain Tracts

Fig. 2. (Best viewed by zooming-in on the PDF.) Mean error as a function of iteration number, for all examples reported in this paper.

size η. Intuitively one may understand this modification as increasing the size of the neighbourhood while calculating the deviation from sheet-like geometry at a point.

Choosing η: The convergence bound can also act as a guide to choosing the time step η, which is the only parameter other than the neighborhood size, in our approach. In accordance with the final convergence condition, we observed empirically that for brain tracts, the range of feasible η choices is smaller. This can be attributed to the more complex tract geometry in the brain compared to the heart. In fact, while larger η's worked well for simple tracts like the Inferior Longitudinal Fasciculus (ILF), more complex tract systems such as the corpus callosum (CC) required the use of a smaller η for convergence. Nonetheless, an η of 0.1, as shown in Fig. 2, resulted in smooth convergence for every tract system, as predicted by our analysis.

Convergence Rate: As shown by the plots in Fig. 2, for our 3 datasets, with $\eta = 0.1$, the mean error over all voxels in a dataset starts to flatten out after about 500 iterations. A quantitative analysis of the convergence rate is however beyond the scope of the present article, but we aim to take this up in the future.

Implementation and Runtime: We implement our algorithm in the PyTorch framework [10]. To achieve this the derivatives and the spatial average calculations for the modified energy function are formulated as convolutions. This allows for GPU-based computation which significantly reduces run-time and makes it feasible to analyze large datasets, in practical exploratory settings. We provide a comparison of run times on a CPU (Intel Core i9-7900x) and a GPU (Titan Xp), for volumes of different sizes in Table 1.

4 Sheet Reconstruction and Visualization

The output of our algorithm is a vector field **v** which is locally best in the sense of spanning a sheet with **u**, together with an energy value at each voxel

Table 1. Time taken in seconds, per iteration, for a CPU based implementation versus that taken by a GPU based implementation, for different volumes.

Sample	Size (Voxels)	CPU (s)	GPU (s)
Rat heart	$64 \times 64 \times 128$	7.9	0.1
Canine heart	$300 \times 300 \times 333$	279.3	5.6
Human brain tracts	$90 \times 108 \times 90$	11.0	0.1

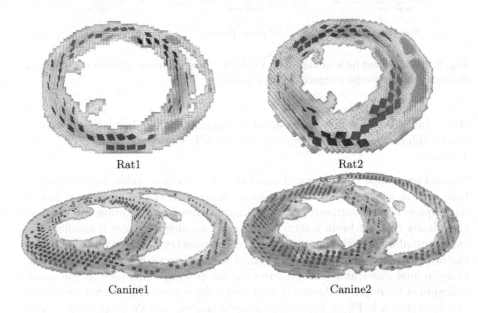

Rat1   Rat2

Canine1   Canine2

Fig. 3. (Best viewed by zooming-in on the PDF.) Sheet likelihood estimates in short axis slices of two canine and two rat hearts, illustrated with volumetric jet colormap rendering, along with our estimated sheets shown as magenta surfaces. (Color figure online)

that is proportional to non-holonomicity. We use this final energy value as a guide for exploring and reconstructing sheets in the brain and the heart, in an iterative breadth first approach. At each step we extend the sheet by a small quadrilateral sheetlet, composed of two triangular faces. The two triangular faces are generated by moving in the direction of $\mathbf{u}$ followed by $\mathbf{v}$ with a step size of around $ds = 0.2$ voxels, and then in direction $\mathbf{v}$ followed by $\mathbf{u}$. For sheet-like regions the two triangular faces are expected to share an edge. In fact, the gap between the two triangular faces is proportional to the Lie bracket $[\mathbf{u}, \mathbf{v}]$ at a point. In our visualizations we only show sheets in locations with low energy. This reconstruction process is repeated n times (with $n \approx 7$) in all four $\pm\mathbf{u}, \pm\mathbf{v}$ directions, in a breadth-first traversal manner. Since the reconstructed points are not limited to voxel locations, we use distance from already drawn vertices, r, as a criterion for adding new points. The parameter r was fixed at half the

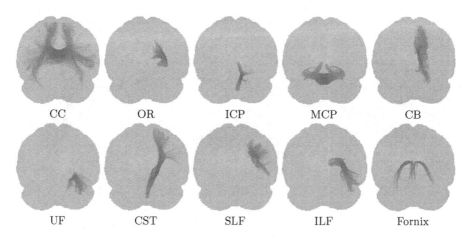

Fig. 4. The HCP tracts analysed in Fig. 5, shown in the context of their actual locations in the brain.

step size. We developed an OpenGL based visualization tool for rendering all the results presented in this paper. For the heart data, we draw sheets with uniform sampling in a given box (Fig. 3), while for the brain data, we draw sheets, when supported, at locations uniformly sampled along the tracts (Fig. 5).

5   Results

We encourage the reader to zoom-in on the electronic (PDF) version of each Figure. Figure 3 presents sheets reconstructed from diffusion tensor data for two rat hearts (top row) and two canine hearts (bottom row). In all sub-figures we show a short axis slice, with a jet colormap volume rendering of the final sheet fitting energy (energy increases from cyan to red), and with our reconstructed sheets shown as magenta surfaces. For the rat hearts we also show the direction of the principal eigenvector as an orientation field. In both species, there is clear support for both axial sheets in the wall of the left ventricle (LV), consistent with the laminar organization reported via histology in early work [7], as well as regimes of more circumferential sheets. The geometry of sheets in the septum is more complex, being predominantly circumferential, and exhibiting a degree of fanning. The right ventricle (RV) also shows sheet-like geometries for the canine hearts, while for the rats the RV is squashed due to imaging conditions. Finally, the LV papillary muscles are associated with a higher energy, and thus a lower likelihood of sheets, consistent with the property that along them muscle cells are oriented in the long axis direction. The sheet fitting energy is also high at the junctions of the LV and RV.

Moving to the human brain, Fig. 1 (bottom left) shows sheet fitting energy rendered as a jet colormap for the Fornix tract, with our recovered sheets shown as magenta surfaces (bottom right). We then consider many other tract systems,

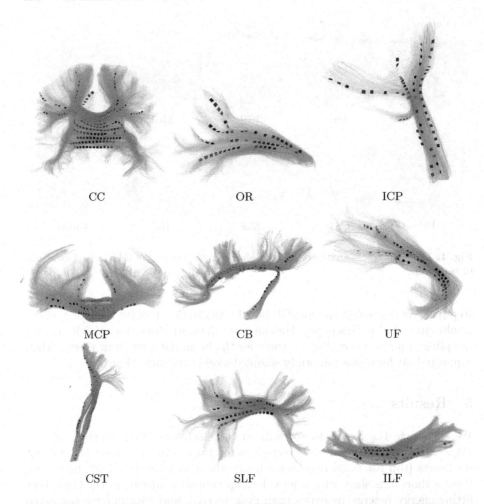

CC   OR   ICP

MCP   CB   UF

CST   SLF   ILF

Fig. 5. (Best viewed by zooming-in on the PDF.) Tract systems from an HCP atlas are shown with green streamlines, with the estimated sheets (where present) shown as magenta surfaces: corpus callosum (CC), optic radiation (OR), inferior cerebellar peduncle (ICP), middle cerebellar peduncle (MCP), cingulum bundle (CB), uncinate fasciculus (UF), corticospinal tract (CST), superior longitudinal fasciculus (SLF), and inferior longitudinal fasciculus (ILF). (Color figure online)

which are shown in the context of their actual positions in the full brain in Fig. 4. For several of these we have chosen the left hemisphere tract to analyze. A number of these tract systems (CC, CB, SLF, Fornix) have been considered in cross species qualitative investigations of sheet geometry in [15], but with no explicit sheet reconstruction. Our recovered sheets for these tracts, where we find support, are depicted as magenta surfaces in Fig. 5. The corresponding sheet fitting energies are rendered as a volumetric jet colormap in Fig. 6. It is clear from Figs. 1, 5 and 6 that whereas certain regimes of these tracts are indeed sheet-

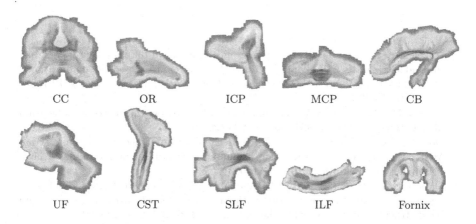

Fig. 6. (Best viewed by zooming-in on the PDF.) The HCP tracts analysed in Fig. 5, shown superimposed on the final sheet fitting energy, visualized using volume rendering with a jet colormap (energy increases from cyan to red). (Color figure online)

like (e.g. the two main arms of the Fornix, and the middle section of the CC), others, such as the fanning regions, are not. Our method allows for navigation and labeling of a tract by sheet confidence, and for the quantitative recovery of subtle shape properties that thus far have been described only qualitatively. For example, the CST is more tube like, providing little local evidence of sheet geometries in most parts, while the MCP, SLF and ILF have large sheet-like regions.

6   Conclusion

Past analyses of tract geometry in the human brain have asked the question whether *two* local directions, often taken to be the peak directions of a fiber orientation distribution function [13,14], or the first and second principal directions of a diffusion tensor [1], provide support for sheets. These attempts have had success in designing sheet probability measures by considering the normal component of the Lie bracket. The problem we have studied here is different in a subtle way, namely, we have asked whether a *single* direction field derived from fibrous tissue supports sheet-like geometries. We have designed an efficient algorithm to minimize non-holonomicity that converges, provides actual reconstructions and high quality visualizations of sheets on which myofibers in the heart are organized, or sheets on which fiber tract systems in the brain might lie, and gives a local measure of sheet likeliness. Such an algorithm could now be used to settle questions concerning the geometric organization of tract systems as suggested in [15], in a quantitative and principled way.

Acknowledgments. We are grateful to NSERC (Canada) and FRQNT (Québec) for funding that has supported this research.

References

1. Ankele, M., Schultz, T.: A sheet probability index from diffusion tensor imaging. In: Kaden, E., Grussu, F., Ning, L., Tax, C.M.W., Veraart, J. (eds.) Computational Diffusion MRI. MV, pp. 141–154. Springer, Cham (2018). https://doi.org/10.1007/978-3-319-73839-0_11

2. Catani, M., Bodi, I.: Dell'Acqua: comment on "the geometric structure of the brain fiber pathways". Science **337**(6102), 1605 (2012)

3. Dou, J., Tseng, W.Y.I., Reese, T.G., Wedeen, V.J.: Combined diffusion and strain MRI reveals structure and function of human myocardial laminar sheets in vivo. Magn. Reson. Med. **50**(1), 107–113 (2003)

4. Gilbert, S.H., Benson, A.P., Li, P., Holden, A.V.: Regional localisation of left ventricular sheet structure: integration with current models of cardiac fibre, sheet and band structure. Eur. J. Cardio-Thorac. Surg. **32**(2), 231–249 (2007)

5. Haije, T.C.J.D.: Finsler geometry and diffusion MRI. Ph.D. thesis, Eindhoven University of Technology (2017)

6. Helm, P., Beg, M.F., Miller, M.I., Winslow, R.L.: Measuring and mapping cardiac fiber and laminar architecture using diffusion tensor MR imaging. Ann. N. Y. Acad. Sci. **1047**(1), 296–307 (2005)

7. LeGrice, I.J., Smaill, B.H., Chai, L.Z., Edgar, S.G., Gavin, J.B., Hunter, P.J.: Laminar structure of the heart: ventricular myocyte arrangement and connective tissue architecture in the dog. Am. J. Physiol. **269**(2), H571–82 (1995)

8. Lombaert, H., et al.: Human atlas of the cardiac fiber architecture: study on a healthy population. IEEE T-MI **31**(7), 1436–1447 (2012)

9. Maier-Hein, K.H., et al.: The challenge of mapping the human connectome based on diffusion tractography. Nat. Commun. **8**(1), 1349 (2017)

10. Paszke, A., et al.: Automatic differentiation in pytorch (2017)

11. Peyrat, J.M., Sermesant, M., Pennec, X., Delingette, H., Xu, C., et al.: A computational framework for the statistical analysis of cardiac diffusion tensors: application to a small database of canine hearts. IEEE T-MI **26**(11), 1500–1514 (2007)

12. Savadjiev, P., Strijkers, G.J., Bakermans, A.J., Piuze, E., Zucker, S.W., Siddiqi, K.: Heart wall myofibers are arranged in minimal surfaces to optimize organ function. Proc. Natl. Acad. Sci. **109**(24), 9248–9253 (2012)

13. Tax, C.M., et al.: Sheet probability index (SPI): characterizing the geometrical organization of the white matter with diffusion MRI. NeuroImage **142**, 260–279 (2016)

14. Tax, C.M., et al.: Quantifying the brain's sheet structure with normalized convolution. Med. Image Anal. **39**, 162–177 (2017)

15. Wedeen, V.J., Rosene, D.L., Wang, R., Dai, G., et al.: The geometric structure of the brain fiber pathways. Science **335**(6076), 1628–1634 (2012)

16. Young, R.J., Panfilov, A.V.: Anisotropy of wave propagation in the heart can be modeled by a riemannian electrophysiological metric. Proc. Natl. Acad. Sci. **107**(34), 15063–15068 (2010)

17. Yu, A.: The Geometry of Vector Fields. Gordon & Breach Publ. (2000)

18. Yushkevich, P.A., Zhang, H., Simon, T.J., Gee, J.C.: Structure-specific statistical mapping of white matter tracts. NeuroImage **41**(2), 448–461 (2008)

Learning Low-Dimensional Representations of Shape Data Sets with Diffeomorphic Autoencoders

Alexandre Bône[(⊠)], Maxime Louis, Olivier Colliot, Stanley Durrleman,
and the Alzheimer's Disease Neuroimaging Initiative

ARAMIS Lab, ICM, Inserm U1127, CNRS UMR 7225,
Sorbonne University, Inria, Paris, France
{alexandre.bone,stanley.durrleman}@icm-institute.org

Abstract. Contemporary deformation-based morphometry offers parametric classes of diffeomorphisms that can be searched to compute the optimal transformation that warps a shape into another, thus defining a similarity metric for shape objects. Extending such classes to capture the geometrical variability in always more varied statistical situations represents an active research topic. This quest for genericity however leads to computationally-intensive estimation problems. Instead, we propose in this work to learn the best-adapted class of diffeomorphisms along with its parametrization, for a shape data set of interest. Optimization is carried out with an auto-encoding variational inference approach, offering in turn a coherent model-estimator pair that we name diffeomorphic auto-encoder. The main contributions are: (i) an original network-based method to construct diffeomorphisms, (ii) a current-splatting layer that allows neural network architectures to process meshes, (iii) illustrations on simulated and real data sets that show differences in the learned statistical distributions of shapes when compared to a standard approach.

1 Introduction

Medical imaging represents a unique challenge for statisticians: massive amounts of high-resolution data conceal high-stake information that, if correctly processed, could help describe and understand pathological conditions at the population level, or classify and predict clinical status at the individual level. In the case of anatomical imaging, information lies in the geometry of the imaged structures. When faced with such a data set, the most basic statistical questions are then: what is the typical geometry? How much does this specific individual deviate from this average?

Summarizing a data set of shapes in those terms consist in performing an adapted mean-variance analysis, that respects the intrinsic data structure. Pioneered two centuries ago by D'Arcy Thomson [12], deformation-based morphometry quantifies differences between shape objects – such as images or extracted

© Springer Nature Switzerland AG 2019
A. C. S. Chung et al. (Eds.): IPMI 2019, LNCS 11492, pp. 195–207, 2019.
https://doi.org/10.1007/978-3-030-20351-1_15

meshes – via ambient-space deformations that warp one into the other. Contemporary approaches construct non-linear smooth invertible deformations, diffeomorphisms, by following streamlines of "velocity" vector fields which can be either static (stationary velocity fields theory, SVF) [14] or dynamic (large deformation diffeomorphic metric mapping, LDDMM) [1,9]. In any case, those approaches define large parametric classes of diffeomorphisms, which can be searched to compute the optimal transformation that warps a shape as close as possible to some target. The intensity of this deformation can then be used as a proxy to define a similarity metric, and finally learn the induced Fréchet mean shape and the associated variance [5,11].

Recent efforts focused on proposing new parametric classes of diffeomorphisms. In [4], the authors propose a variation of the LDDMM construction where the parametrization of the diffeomorphisms is independent of the shapes on which they act, allowing unified handling of meshes – with or without point correspondence – and images. Even more recently, [6] generalizes the LDDMM framework by defining an extended class of diffeomorphisms parametrized by "modules" which encode local translations, scalings, or rotations. However, finding the structure of the deformations that will best capture shape variability is a very difficult task in practice, and learning it from the data often leads to intractable optimization problems. Coming from the deep learning research horizon, more and more contributions propose to change the optimization task into a prediction one: the optimal parameters coding for the desired diffeomorphism are directly predicted by a deep network, after its supervised or unsupervised training [2,15]. The used deformation models are either SVF or LDDMM-based i.e. well-established generic approaches, fixed throughout the learning procedure.

This work proposes to *learn* the best-adapted class of diffeomorphisms along with its parametrization for a shape data set of interest, thanks to a network-based deformation method. Optimization is carried out with a auto-encoding variational inference approach [8], offering in turn a coherent model-estimator pair that we name "diffeomorphic auto-encoder" (DAE). The main contributions of this paper are: (i) an original method to construct diffeomorphisms by integrating dynamic velocity fields which are defined as the image of segments of $\mathbb{R}^n$ by a neural network; (ii) the introduction of the current-splatting layer that allows a network architecture to process mesh objects; (iii) the provided illustrations on both simulated and real data sets that show differences in the learned statistical distributions of shapes, when compared with a more standard LDDMM approach. A special care has been given to the scalability and versatility of the proposed method, which is designed to tackle statistical inference problems on high-dimensional shape data sets, with few requirements about the data structure. Section 2 details the method for constructing diffeomorphisms; Sect. 3 introduces the statistical atlas model; Sect. 4 presents the variational inference algorithm used for estimation. Section 5 gives experimental results, Sect. 6 discusses perspectives and concludes.

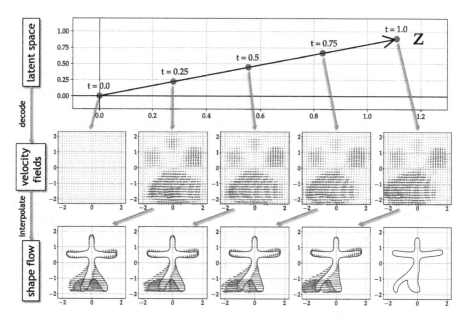

Fig. 1. Deformation mechanics: diffeomorphism are obtained by following the streamlines of dynamic velocity fields, which are themselves defined as the image of latent-space segments by a non-linear mapping represented in practice by a network. The parameters of this decoding mapping will be optimized for each new application, therefore adapting the core deformation mechanics to the considered data set.

2   Deformation Mechanics

Similarly to LDDMM, diffeomorphisms are constructed by integrating dynamic "velocity" fields over a unit interval. Those velocity fields path are taken as the image of an abstract "latent-space" segment through a neural network. Once learned, the parameters of this "decoding" neural network determine a non-linear parametrization of the obtained diffeomorphisms by the "latent" representations.

Let Ω be an open and bounded set of the ambient space $\mathbb{R}^d$ with $d \in \{2, 3\}$. Let $n, s \in \mathbb{N}^\star$ and $D_\theta : \mathbb{R}^n \to C_0^s(\Omega, \mathbb{R}^d)$ an infinitely differentiable mapping that associate to any $z \in \mathbb{R}^n$ a s-smooth vanishing vector field v on Ω. This mapping is called "decoder", and is taken under the form of a neural network with parameters θ. For the rest of this paper, the decoder D_θ is structured with three fully connected layers followed by four deconvolutional layers, with $tanh$ activation functions for all layers except the last one. For any $z \in \mathbb{R}^n$, assuming that the path $t \in [0, 1] \to v_t = D_\theta(z \cdot t)$ is s-absolutely integrable, i.e. that $\int_0^1 \|v_t\|_{s,\infty} < \infty$ with $\|v\|_{s,\infty} = \sum_{k=0}^s \|\nabla^k v\|_\infty$, implies that there exist an unique flow of diffeomorphisms $t \to \phi_t$ such that $\partial_t \phi_t = v_t \circ \phi_t$ and $\phi_0 = \mathrm{Id}_\Omega$ [16]. For such paths, we note $\Phi_\theta : z \to \phi_1$ the mapping that associates the diffeomorphism reached at unit time when integrating the "velocity" vector field path decoded from the segment $t \to z \cdot t$. The integrated vector fields are called "velocity" fields by analogy with fluid mechanics, where particles $x \in \mathbb{R}^d$ follow the streamlines of a dynamic flow $t \rightarrow v_t$. Under integrability conditions of this flow, we have defined a θ-parametric class of diffeomorphisms, indexed by the Euclidian vector space $\mathbb{R}^n$ which we call the "latent" space. In practice, the integrability condition will be explicitly enforced by adding a dedicated regularity term to the optimized loss function, with the introduction of a corresponding Lagrange multiplier λ.

Figure 1 illustrates the discrete version of those deformation mechanics: a single latent-space parameter $z \in \mathbb{R}^n$ with n typically small (here $n = 2$) encodes for a flow of diffeomorphisms of the ambient space $\mathbb{R}^d$ (here $d = 2$) that can in turn deform any shape object. A fixed number T of uniformly distributed samples of the latent-space segment $t \rightarrow z \cdot t$ are decoded by the same neural network D_θ into a set of T corresponding velocity fields discretized on a fixed and regular "deformation" grid G_d. Those velocity fields are then successively linearly interpolated on the shape to deform, and integrated according to a forward Euler scheme. We further impose that all layers of the decoder are without bias, ensuring that $\Phi_\theta(0_{\mathbb{R}^n}) = \mathrm{Id}_\Omega$. Note finally that D_θ is infinitely differentiable, enforcing some temporal smoothness of the decoded velocity fields $t \rightarrow D_\theta(z \cdot t)$.

3   Atlas Model

3.1   Generative Statistical Model

Let $y = (y_i)_i$ be a data set of N shapes. For $i = 1, ..., N$, we model the observations y_i as a random deformation of a template shape y_0:

$$y_i \overset{\text{iid}}{\sim} \mathcal{N}_\mathcal{E}\left(\Phi_\theta(z_i) \cdot y_0, \sigma_\epsilon^2\right) \quad \text{with} \quad z_i \overset{\text{iid}}{\sim} \mathcal{N}(0, I_n) \tag{1}$$

under the constraint that the $\Phi_\theta(z_i)$ are diffeomorphisms. The latent individual variables $z_i \in \mathbb{R}^n$ encode the deformations that warp the template y_0 into each observed shape y_i. Note that the template is encoded by $z_0 = 0$, by construction.

Scalability and versatility concerns are at the core of the proposed method: note that no particular assumption on the nature of shapes has been made so far. The density function of the "normal" distribution $\mathcal{N}_\mathcal{E}$ assumed on the observed y_i can be generically noted: $p(y_i|z_i; \theta, y_0) \propto \exp\left(-d_\mathcal{E}[y_i, \Phi_\theta(z_i) \cdot y_0]^2 / 2 \cdot \sigma_\epsilon^2\right)$ where $d_\mathcal{E}$ is an extrinsic distance measure on shapes. If the considered shapes are images – of fixed dimension – or meshes with point-to-point correspondence, the simple ℓ^2 metric is a natural and convenient choice: $d_\mathcal{E}(y^\alpha, y^\beta)^2 = \left\|y^\beta - y^\alpha\right\|_{\ell^2}^2$. In the case of mesh data without point correspondence, the current [13] representation can be used to construct a well-defined distance metric between shapes, at the expense of the characteristic scale hyper-parameter $\sigma_\mathcal{E}$. Noting respectively $(c_k)_{k=1,...,K}$ and $(n_k)_{k=1,...,K}$ the centers and normals of the segments or triangles forming the connectivity of the manipulated meshes, we then define:

$$d_\mathcal{E}(y^\alpha, y^\beta)^2 = \sum_{k=1}^{K^\alpha} \sum_{l=1}^{K^\beta} \exp\left[-\left\|c_l^\beta - c_k^\alpha\right\|^2 / \sigma_\mathcal{E}^2\right] \cdot (n_k^\alpha)^\top \cdot n_l^\beta. \tag{2}$$

3.2   Comparison with LDDMM-Based Approaches

From a generative point of view, the proposed model associates to any latent-space z_i a deformation and, in turn, a shape. From a learning perspective, estimating the shared parameters θ and y_0 learns a new n-dimensional representation of shapes. This global approach could straightforwardly be followed within the already-established LDDMM framework. Using intuitive notations, LDDMM diffeomorphisms could be noted $\Phi(m_i)$ where the "momentum" parameter m_i is of imposed dimensions – typically large. Note that the mapping Φ is not indexed by some θ: deformation mechanics are fixed. In order to represent the geometrical variability in a more compact way, the momenta can be constrained to span a vector space of chosen dimension by specifying $m_i = A \cdot z_i$ where $z_i \sim \mathcal{N}(0, I_n)$ is a n-dimensional vector and A is a matrix parameter to learn. This model is named "principal geodesic analysis" (PGA) in [17], in reference to the PCA-like prior on the momenta covariance. Our approach goes a step further by breaking the linear relationship between the latent-space representations and the associated velocity fields. The learned representations when introducing a non-linear network are evaluated in Sect. 5 by comparison with the PGA approach.

4   Network-Based Variational Inference

4.1   Rationale

Our goal is to estimate both the template shape y_0 and the parameters θ of the decoder which parametrize the geometry of the learned n-dimensional manifold of deformations, under the constraint of diffeomorphic $\Phi_\theta(z_i)$. In the ideal case, we would also like to determine the posterior distribution $p(z_i|y_i; \theta, y_0)$, which would give us low-dimensional latent-space representations of the individual registrations of y_i on y_0, in a probabilistic sense. Knowing this posterior would also allow to instantly register any new shape y_{N+1} to y_0. Being intractable, we approximate it by a parametric distribution $q(z_i|y_i; \vartheta)$ that we model as an uncorrelated Gaussian of $\mathbb{R}^n$. We estimate ϑ jointly with θ and y_0. We note E_ϑ the parametric "encoding" function that associates to any y_i the mean and diagonal covariance of the approximate posterior $q(z_i|y_i; \vartheta)$. This mapping is taken under the form of a neural network, composed of four convolution and one fully-connected layers, with $tanh$ activation functions for all layers except the last.

This global optimization approach is know as variational Bayes [7]. The idea of introducing a network encoding function comes from [8]. Figure 2 presents the final "diffeomorphic auto-encoder" (DAE) model-estimator pair.

4.2   Encoding Image and Mesh Shapes

In the case of images, the encoding network E_ϑ directly acts on the pixel values. In the case of meshes, a preliminary "current-splatting" [3,5] operation is performed on a regular grid G_s in order to represent this mesh as a d-channels

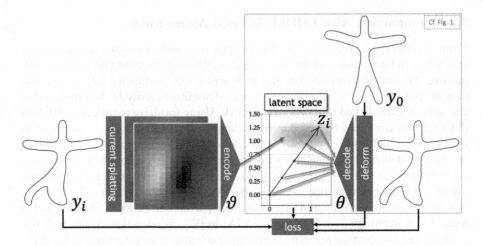

Fig. 2. Global architecture of the diffeomorphic auto-encoder (DAE). An observation y_i is encoded as a normal probability distribution, from which is sampled a latent representation $z_i \in \mathbb{R}^n$. The latent-space segment $[0, z_i]$ is then decoded into a dynamic velocity field, which is integrated into a diffeomorphism of the ambient space $\mathbb{R}^d$. This deformation is applied to a template shape y_0 to produce a reconstruction of the original shape y_i. The parameters of the encoder ϑ, of the decoder θ, and the template shape y_0 are estimated by stochastic gradient descent. To encode meshes, a preliminary current-splatting is performed before feeding y_i to the network.

image, which is then fed to the encoder network (see Fig. 2). With the notations of Eq. (2) and σ_S a characteristic length hyper-parameter, the d-channel splatting intensity $\mathcal{S}_{y_i}(x)$ at any physical location $x \in \mathbb{R}^d$ for the mesh y_i writes:

$$\mathcal{S}_{y_i}(x) = \sum_{k=1}^{K} \exp\left[-\|x - c_k\|^2 / \sigma_S^2\right] \cdot n_k. \tag{3}$$

4.3   Diffeomorphic Constraint as a Regularity Term

As discussed in Sect. 2, preventing the integral over $[0, 1]$ of the s-Sobolev norm of the decoded velocity field paths $t \to D_\theta(z_i \cdot t)$ from going to infinity is enough to ensure diffeomorphic deformations $\Phi_\theta(z_i)$. This constraint is therefore simply transformed into a regularity term. Rather than penalizing the s-Sobolev norm, we choose to penalize an equivalent norm, introduced in [18]. For any $v, w \in D_\theta(\mathbb{R}^n)$, let $\langle ., . \rangle_S$ the Sobolev metric such that $\langle v, w \rangle_S = \int_\Omega S(v)^\top \cdot w$ with $S = (\mathrm{Id} - \alpha \cdot \Delta)^s$, noting $(.)^\top$ the transposition operator and $\Delta(.)$ the Laplacian one. S is a symmetric positive-definite differential operator when the scale parameter verifies $\alpha > 0$. We note $\|.\|_S$ the induced norm. For faster computation, this norm will in practice be evaluated in the Fourier domain (see [18]).

Introducing the Lagrange multiplier λ, we define the Sobolev regularity loss:

$$\mathcal{R}_s(\theta, \vartheta; y_i) = \lambda \cdot \int_{t \in [0,1]} \int_{z_i \in \mathbb{R}^n} \left\| D_\theta(z_i \cdot t) \right\|_S^2 \cdot q(z_i | y_i; \vartheta) \cdot dz_i \cdot dt \qquad (4)$$

$$\approx \frac{\lambda}{T \cdot L} \sum_{t=1}^{T} \sum_{l=1}^{L} \left\| D_\theta\left(z_i^{(l)} \cdot \frac{t-1}{T-1}\right) \right\|_S^2 = \mathcal{R}'_s(\theta, \vartheta; y_i) \qquad (5)$$

where $z_i^{(l)} \overset{iid}{\sim} q(.|y_i; \vartheta)$ for $l = 1, ..., L$, and T is the number of Euler time-steps.

4.4   Loss Function

The loss writes $\mathcal{L}(y_i; \theta, \vartheta, y_0) = \mathcal{A}(y_i; \theta, \vartheta, y_0) + \mathcal{R}_{kl}(y_i; \theta, \vartheta) + \mathcal{R}_s(y_i; \theta, \vartheta)$, with:

$$\mathcal{A}(y_i; \theta, \vartheta, y_0) = -\int \log p(y_i | z_i; \theta, y_0) \cdot q(z_i | y_i; \vartheta) \cdot dz_i \approx -\frac{1}{L} \sum_{l=1}^{L} \log p(y_i | z_i^{(l)}; \theta, y_0)$$

$$(6)$$

where $z_i^{(l)} \overset{iid}{\sim} q(.|y_i; \vartheta)$, and $\mathcal{R}_{kl}(y_i; \theta, \vartheta) = \mathrm{KL}\big[q(z_i | y_i; \vartheta) \| p(z_i)\big]$, $\mathrm{KL}(.\|.)$ denoting the Kullback-Leibler divergence operator.

Noting $\mathcal{A}'$ the Monte-Carlo approximation of the attachment term $\mathcal{A}$ given by Eq. (6), the discrete loss function that is actually minimized writes $\mathcal{L}'(y_i; \theta, \vartheta, y_0) = \mathcal{A}'(y_i; \theta, \vartheta, y_0) + \mathcal{R}_{kl}(y_i; \theta, \vartheta) + \mathcal{R}'_s(y_i; \theta, \vartheta)$. The Kullback-Leibler regularity term $\mathcal{R}_{kl}$ can be analytically derived as a function of the mean and variance of the approximate posterior distribution $q(z_i | y_i; \vartheta)$ [8].

4.5   Optimization Details

Minimization of $\mathcal{L}'(y_i; \theta, \vartheta, y_0)$ is performed by stochastic gradient descent. Gradients with respect to the parameters θ, ϑ, y_0 are automatically computed thanks to the auto-differentiation library from the PyTorch project [10]. The numerical gradient of the loss $\mathcal{L}'$ with respect to the template shape y_0 is spatially smoothed with a Gaussian kernel of standard deviation σ_y before being applied by the gradient-based method. This operation is highly beneficial in practice when dealing with noisy data, ensuring that the original topology of the template shape is conserved [4]. The so-called reparametrization trick detailed in [8] ensures that gradients with respect to the encoder parameters ϑ are computable across the sampling procedure. In this same article, the authors report that drawing only $L = 1$ sample per data point is reasonable as long as the Adam batches are large enough; the same strategy will be adopted in this paper, with batches of size 32. Code available at: github.com/alexandrebone/deepshape/releases/tag/v0.0.1.

5   Experiments

For all subsequent experiments, the parameters of the Sobolev metric are $\alpha = 0.5$ and $s = 3$. The corresponding Lagrange multiplier is fixed to $\lambda = 1$. Finally, forward Euler integration is numerically carried out with $T = 11$ steps. Our DAE is compared to the LDDMM-based PGA model, briefly introduced in Sect. 3.2.

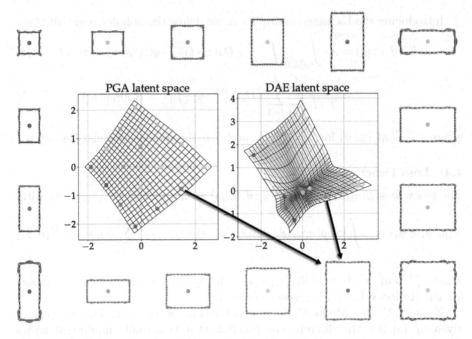

Fig. 3. [Center] Latent spaces learned by PGA and DAE. Each node of the plotted grids in solid black correspond to one of the 441 simulated rectangles. The interleaved dotted grey grid in the DAE space corresponds to the additional 400 test rectangles. [Outer] A subsample of 16 training rectangles are plotted in dotted black lines; a color code allows their identification in the latent spaces. The PGA and DAE reconstructions are plotted in red and light blue respectively. (Color figure online)

5.1   Learned Latent Space with Simulated Rectangle Meshes

A data set of $N = 441$ rectangle meshes of $\mathbb{R}^2$ is simulated: all are centered on the origin, but vary in their length and width which are independently and regularly distributed between 0.5 and 1.5. Those meshes are simulated with point correspondence: the noise model is therefore simply based on the ℓ^2 metric, with $\sigma_\epsilon = 0.01$. The remaining chosen parameters are $\sigma_S = \sigma_y = 0.2$, respectively for the splatting and template gradient smoothing operations. We first learn a PGA model with $n = 2$ components with a deformation scale fixed to 0.1, and then learn our DAE model, initialized on the PGA results.

Figure 3 represents the learned latent spaces. Both methods have correctly learned the variations in length and width of the dataset. The PGA latent space is quite regular, when the DAE one seems to feature more complex spatial relationships. DAE seems to create more curvature in the latent space. We observe also that the DAE reconstructions match more tightly the training points: the mean square errors are $1.55 \times 10^{-4} (\pm 1.22 \times 10^{-4})$ and $3.43 \times 10^{-6} (\pm 2.17 \times 10^{-6})$ in the PGA and DAE cases respectively. The ability to better match observations is certainly the consequence of allowing many more degrees of freedom in the parametrization of the diffeomorphisms. Whether the induced curvature in the latent space is a also a consequence of this construction still need to be understood. A second data set of $N = 400$ rectangles of length and width independently and regularly distributed between 0.525 and 1.475 is simulated and encoded in the DAE latent space (see Fig. 3). Note that this operation is virtually instantaneous. After subsequent decoding, the reconstruction error amounts to 3.40×10^{-6} ($\pm 1.69 \times 10^{-6}$), indicating a very good generalization performance.

5.2   Generalization to Test Data with Hippocampi Meshes

A total of 324 right hippocampi meshes are segmented from baseline T1-weighted magnetic resonance (MR) images of the ADNI database, after standard alignment preprocessing. The obtained meshes are without point correspondence: the current noise model will be used, with a kernel width $\sigma_{\mathcal{E}} = 5\,mm$ and an uncertainty parameter of $\sigma_{\epsilon} = 0.1$. Other spatial parameters are chosen equal: $\sigma_S = \sigma_y = 5\,mm$. We learn the PGA and DAE models in dimension $n = 10$, on $N = 162$ training meshes, and then personalize them to the second testing half. The deformation scale parameter for the PGA is taken equal to 10 mm, and the same current metric is used for both methods.

Table 1 gives the obtained reconstruction and generalization errors. The DAE model better fits the training data, when the PGA model better generalizes. Note however that the personalization of the PGA model to a new hippocampus requires to solve an optimization problem, which is done with a gradient method, when the learned encoder gives quasi-instantaneous results in the case of the DAE. Refining this initial guess with a gradient method, the so-called DAE+ performance improves, and gives generalization residuals smaller on average the intrinsic uncertainty on the data – which is indicated in the first column. This uncertainty has been computed by preprocessing the secondary MR images (same subject, same visit, same machine) available in the ADNI database into hippocampi meshes, and computing the current-metric residual with the primary measurements. A statistical meaning can be given to this DAE versus DAE+ distinction: recalling the encoder is probabilistic i.e. outputs the normal density distribution $q(z_i|y_i; \vartheta)$, the reported DAE generalization performance directly evaluates the decoded average $E[q(z_i|y_i; \vartheta)]$ when the DAE+ computes a MAP

Table 1. Reconstruction and generalization residuals (in mm^2), measured with the current metric (scale parameter of 5 mm). The data noise is evaluated by leveraging the secondary MR images available in the ADNI database. The DAE+ column refers to a gradient-descent-based refinement of the encoded test data points.

	Data noise	PGA	DAE	DAE+
Reconstruction	85.2 ± 40.1	66.7 ± 11.5	**32.6 ± 6.0**	-
Generalization	85.2 ± 40.1	**67.7 ± 12.6**	116.8 ± 20.0	74.7 ± 16.1

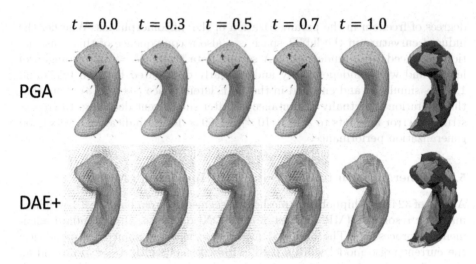

Fig. 4. Estimated diffeomorphic deformation of the PGA and DAE templates (leftmost meshes) onto a test hippocampus (rightmost red meshes). The dynamic PGA momenta and the DAE velocity fields are indicated by arrows, colored according to their magnitude. The current-metric PGA residual is $68.4 \, \text{mm}^2$, the DAE+ $75.4 \, \text{mm}^2$. (Color figure online)

estimate against the full q distribution, so the comparison with PGA which also seeks for the MAP is more fair.

Figure 4 plots the deformation of the PGA and DAE templates onto a test hippocampus. The residuals values are $68.4 \, \text{mm}^2$, $126.7 \, \text{mm}^2$ (not plotted) and $75.4 \, \text{mm}^2$ for the PGA, DAE and DAE+ methods respectively. The rightmost figures superimpose the target mesh with the fully-deformed templates. Both templates are globally similar, the PGA one being however quite smoother. The deformation fields, represented by the arrows, seem to mainly act in the same "neck" region of the hippocampi. The final registration quality is difficult to evaluate by eye, due to the noise on the original meshes.

5.3   Modes of Variability and Classification with Brain MR Images

We now consider a data set of $N = 160$ brain T1-weighted MR images from the ADNI project: 54 are from control subjects (CN), 53 from subjects presenting mild cognitive impairments (MCI), and the last 53 from patients diagnosed with Alzheimer's disease (AD). The images are aligned with an affine transformation in a preprocessing step. The simple ℓ^2 metric is used on the voxel values for the noise model, with an uncertainty parameter $\sigma_\epsilon = 1/255$. The template update smoothing is done with $\sigma_y = 1 \, \text{mm}$. The PGA and DAE representations are learned in dimension $n = 3$, the PGA scale parameter being fixed to $1 \, \text{cm}$.

Figure 5 plots the components of a PCA fitted a posteriori on the latent representations of the training images for the DAE, as well as the first axis

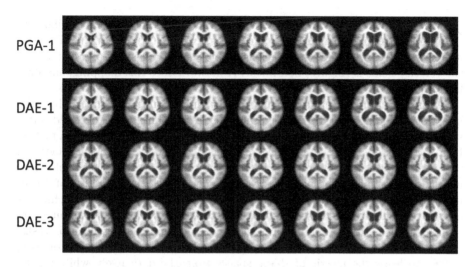

Fig. 5. First principal axis determined with the PGA approach, and all three principal axes computed with the DAE model. For each axis are plotted the shapes deviating by $-1.5, -1, -0.5, 0, 0.5, 1, 1.5$ times the standard deviation from the template y_0. Note in particular that the central column plots the learned PGA and DAE templates y_0.

of variability computed with the PGA. The first components of variability (top rows) explain respectively 59.0% and 56.7% of the captured variance by the PGA and DAE models, and clearly correspond to the ventricle size variability, which is known to be a marker of Alzheimer's disease. Table 2 gives the classification scores obtained by a 11-nearest-neighbors classifier, evaluated in a leave-one-out fashion. Note that 11 is a prime number, thus avoiding ties in the voting process. Scores are in all cases above the chance threshold, and even reach an accuracy of 85.0% in the CN versus AD classification task, based on the DAE latent representations. If both representations are pooled together, the 3-classes performance slightly increases to 62.5%, suggesting some complementarity.

Table 2. Leave-one-out classification scores obtained with a 11-nearest-neighbors classifier, taking the learned PGA or DAE latent representations as input.

	CN/MCI/AD	CN/AD	CN/MCI	MCI/AD
PGA	58.8%	84.1%	67.3%	**71.7%**
DAE	**61.3%**	**85.0%**	67.3%	68.9%

6   Discussion and Perspectives

We have presented and illustrated a method that jointly learns an atlas model and a class of diffeomorphisms from a data set of shapes. Diffeomorphisms are then parametrized by low-dimensional latent-space parameters. Similarly to LDDMM, those diffeomorphisms are constructed by integrating dynamic velocity fields. Unlike LDDMM, the relationship between latent-space parameters and the velocity fields is (highly) non-linear. A network does this mapping, and only little assumptions are made: infinite differentiability and absence of bias.

A theoretical perspective would be to determine conditions under which the image of the latent-space by this mapping defines a manifold. The decoded velocity field paths would then be geodesics for the push-forwarded Euclidian metric. In a second step, if an equivalence relationship could be established between the pushforward and the Sobolev metrics, the somewhat extrinsic Sobolev regularity term might not be needed anymore to ensure the construction of diffeomorphisms. Practical perspectives are numerous, and include speed benchmarks against contemporary statistical shape analysis softwares, network architecture refinement for better overfitting prevention, joint training on classification tasks.

The use of neural networks for generating diffeomorphisms is a promising avenue to learn the metric of shape spaces from the data itself, while raising several challenging theoretical questions.

References

1. Beg, F., Miller, M., Trouvé, A., Younes, L.: Computing large deformation metric mappings via geodesic flows of diffeomorphisms. IJCV **61**, 139–157 (2005)
2. Dalca, A.V., Balakrishnan, G., Guttag, J., Sabuncu, M.R.: Unsupervised learning for fast probabilistic diffeomorphic registration. arXiv preprint: arXiv:1805.04605 (2018)
3. Durrleman, S.: Statistical models of currents for measuring the variability of anatomical curves, surfaces and their evolution. Ph.D. thesis (2010)
4. Durrleman, S., et al.: Morphometry of anatomical shape complexes with dense deformations and sparse parameters. NeuroImage **101**, 35–49 (2014)
5. Gori, P., et al.: A Bayesian framework for joint morphometry of surface and curve meshes in multi-object complexes. Med. Image Anal. **35**, 458–474 (2017)
6. Gris, B., Durrleman, S., Trouvé, A.: A sub-riemannian modular framework for diffeomorphism-based analysis of shape ensembles. SIAM J. Imaging Sci. **11**(1), 802–833 (2018)
7. Jordan, M.I., Ghahramani, Z., Jaakkola, T.S., Saul, L.K.: An introduction to variational methods for graphical models. Mach. Learn. **37**(2), 183–233 (1999)
8. Kingma, D.P., Welling, M.: Auto-encoding variational bayes. Stat **1050**, 10 (2014)
9. Miller, M.I., Trouvé, A., Younes, L.: Geodesic shooting for computational anatomy. J. Math. Imaging Vis. **24**(2), 209–228 (2006)
10. Paszke, A., et al.: Automatic differentiation in pytorch (2017)
11. Pennec, X.: Intrinsic statistics on riemannian manifolds: basic tools for geometric measurements. J. Math. Imaging Vis. **25**(1), 127–154 (2006)
12. Thompson, D.W., et al.: On Growth and Form (1942)
13. Vaillant, M., Glaunès, J.: Surface matching via currents. In: Christensen, G.E., Sonka, M. (eds.) IPMI 2005. LNCS, vol. 3565, pp. 381–392. Springer, Heidelberg (2005). https://doi.org/10.1007/11505730_32

14. Vercauteren, T., Pennec, X., Perchant, A., Ayache, N.: Symmetric log-domain diffeomorphic registration: a demons-based approach. In: Metaxas, D., Axel, L., Fichtinger, G., Székely, G. (eds.) MICCAI 2008. LNCS, vol. 5241, pp. 754–761. Springer, Heidelberg (2008). https://doi.org/10.1007/978-3-540-85988-8_90
15. Yang, X., Kwitt, R., Styner, M., Niethammer, M.: Quicksilver: fast predictive image registration-a deep learning approach. NeuroImage **158**, 378–396 (2017)
16. Younes, L.: Shapes and Diffeomorphisms. Applied Mathematical Sciences, Springer, Heidelberg (2010). https://books.google.fr/books?id=SdTBtMGgeAUC
17. Zhang, M., Fletcher, P.T.: Bayesian principal geodesic analysis in diffeomorphic image registration. In: Golland, P., Hata, N., Barillot, C., Hornegger, J., Howe, R. (eds.) MICCAI 2014. LNCS, vol. 8675, pp. 121–128. Springer, Cham (2014). https://doi.org/10.1007/978-3-319-10443-0_16
18. Zhang, M., Fletcher, P.T.: Fast diffeomorphic image registration via Fourier-approximated lie algebras. Int. J. Comput. Vis. **127**, 1–13 (2018)

Diffeomorphic Medial Modeling

Paul A. Yushkevich[1]([⊠]), Ahmed Aly[1], Jiancong Wang[1], Long Xie[1],
Robert C. Gorman[2], Laurent Younes[3], and Alison M. Pouch[1]

[1] Department of Radiology, University of Pennsylvania Perelman School of Medicine,
Philadelphia, USA
pauly2@pennmedicine.upenn.edu
[2] Department of Surgery, University of Pennsylvania Perelman School of Medicine,
Philadelphia, USA
[3] Department of Applied Mathematics and Statistics, Johns Hopkins University,
Baltimore, USA

Abstract. Deformable shape modeling approaches that describe objects
in terms of their *medial axis* geometry (e.g., *m-reps* [10]) yield rich geometrical features that can be useful for analyzing the shape of sheet-
like biological structures, such as the myocardium. We present a novel
shape analysis approach that combines the benefits of medial shape modeling and diffeomorphometry. Our algorithm is formulated as a problem of matching shapes using diffeomorphic flows under constraints that
approximately preserve medial axis geometry during deformation. As the
result, correspondence between the medial axes of similar shapes is main-
tained. The approach is evaluated in the context of modeling the shape
of the left ventricular wall from 3D echocardiography images.

1 Introduction

In medical image analysis, *deformable medial models* (or *medial representations*)
[5,10,13] are frequently used to characterize the shape of anatomical structures
that have sheet-like geometry, such as the cerebral cortex, the myocardium, or
knee cartilage. They are deformable models that directly characterize the *medial
axes* of objects. The medial axis (or *skeleton*) of an object is a set of manifolds
formed by all points inside of the object that are equidistant to two or more
points on its boundary [3]. The distance from the medial axis to the boundary
describes the local thickness of objects. For sheet-like anatomical objects, the
shape of the medial axis can be a useful proxy for overall shape, and local
thickness is frequently an important biological measurement.

Medial axes of 3D objects can be easily derived using various skeletonization
approaches (e.g., [9]). However, even small perturbations of the boundary of an
object can result in a significant reconfiguration of the medial axis. This makes
it difficult to use medial axes derived by skeletonization in statistical shape

---

This work is supported by NIH grants AG056014, EB017255, HL103723, HL141643.

A. C. S. Chung et al. (Eds.): IPMI 2019, LNCS 11492, pp. 208–220, 2019.
https://doi.org/10.1007/978-3-030-20351-1_16

analysis. Deformable medial modeling techniques such as *m-reps* [10] overcome this challenge by explicitly controlling the configuration of the medial axis of the model during deformation (i.e., keeping the number and connectivity of the surfaces in the medial axis fixed). For many classes of anatomical objects such models can approximate the shape of individual objects with good accuracy, while allowing the features derived from the medial axis to be compared across subjects. Deformable medial models have been used to perform statistical shape analysis for various sheet-like brain structures, myocardium and heart valves, abdominal organs, etc. Medial models have also been used to impose geometrical constraints on automatic segmentation of sheet-like structures, e.g., imposing prior knowledge about heart wall thickness during myocardium segmentation [11]. Medial modeling methods include *m-reps* [10] and *s-reps* [5] (which approximate medial axis surfaces using discrete primitives), *cm-reps* [12] (which use splines and subdivision surfaces to model medial axis surfaces), and *boundary-constrained m-reps* [13] (which implicitly model medial geometry by imposing symmetry constraints on a boundary-based model).

This paper addresses a significant limitation of existing medial modeling approaches: they lack a built-in mechanism to prevent models from folding or self-intersecting during deformation; and they do not provide a natural way to extrapolate model transformations to deformations of the ambient space. In recent years, the field of statistical shape analysis has embraced an approach based on *flows of diffeomorphisms*. In this *"diffeomorphometry"* approach [8], shapes are expressed in terms of smooth invertible transformations that deform a canonical *template shape* into each shape of interest. Diffeomorphometry provides a concrete way to impose a metric on the space of shapes, based on the amount of deformation required to map one shape into another, and gives rise to rigorous algorithms for shape interpolation, computation of mean shapes, and other statistics. Diffeomorphometry also allows transformations between shapes to be extended naturally to diffeomorphic transformations of the ambient space, e.g., allowing shape correspondences to be extrapolated to image correspondences.

We propose an algorithm that combines the benefits of deformable medial models (access to intuitive geometric features like thickness) and diffeomorphometry (physically motivated transformation model, rigorous mathematical foundation, invertibility). Our algorithm is formulated as a problem of matching shapes using diffeomorphic flows under constraints that approximately preserve medial axis geometry during deformation. Our approach leverages a general framework for incorporating geometric constraints into diffeomorphic shape matching developed by Arguillère et al. [1]. To our knowledge, this is the first paper to integrate diffeomorphometry and deformable medial modeling. Our experiments focus on demonstrating the feasibility of this method in the context of matching synthetic and real-world anatomical shapes.

2   Materials and Methods

In this section, we first briefly introduce *flows of diffeomorphisms* for shape analysis. We then review the basic concepts of *medial geometry* and define a special class of *diffeomorphic flows that preserve medial geometry*. We then frame the problem of diffeomorphic medial modeling for point-set representations of 3D shapes and implement it using the general *constrained diffeomorphometry* framework developed by Arguillère et al. [1].

2.1   Flows of Diffeomorphisms for Shape Analysis

In diffeomorphometry, collections of shapes (e.g., hippocampi of different individuals) are represented as diffeomorphic transformations of some template shape $\mathcal{O}$. Following [2], diffeomorphic transformations $\{\phi : \mathbb{R}^n \to \mathbb{R}^n\}$ form a group under composition. *Flows of diffeomorphisms* are generated by the ordinary differential equation:

$$\frac{\partial \phi(x,t)}{\partial t} = v(\phi(x,t),t), \qquad \phi(x,0) = x, \qquad t \in [0,1], \qquad (1)$$

where $v : \mathbb{R}^n \times [0,1] \to \mathbb{R}^n$ is a time-varying vector field, called the *velocity field*, that satisfies certain smoothness constraints [8]. Let us write ϕ_t as shorthand for $\phi(\cdot,t)$ and v_t for $v(\cdot,t)$. Applying the diffeomorphism ϕ_t to $\mathcal{O}$ yields a new shape $\phi_t \mathcal{O} = \{x \in \mathbb{R}^n : \phi_t^{-1}(x) \in \mathcal{O}\}$. When comparing shapes, computing shape statistics, or performing shape-based segmentation, a common need is to find a deformation of $\mathcal{O}$ that matches some target shape $\mathcal{O}_{\text{trg}}$ (or some target image I_{trg}) at time $t = 1$, while applying the least total deformation to the space $\mathbb{R}^n$. This is formulated by treating vector fields v_t as elements of a reproducing kernel Hilbert space $\mathcal{H}$ with kernel K, and defining the *kinetic energy* of a diffeomorphic flow generated by v as $E_{\text{kin}}[v] = \frac{1}{2} \int_0^1 \|v_t\|_{\mathcal{H}}^2 \, dt$, where $\| \cdot \|_{\mathcal{H}}$ is the norm in $\mathcal{H}$. Since pairs of shapes might not have exact correspondence, the shape matching problem is often relaxed to that of approximate shape matching by adding a data attachment term $g(\phi_1 \mathcal{O})$ that measures goodness of fit between the deformed template $\phi_1 \mathcal{O}$ and $\mathcal{O}_{\text{trg}}$ (or I_{trg}) to the energy functional:

$$E[v] = \alpha \, g(\phi_1 \mathcal{O}) + E_{\text{kin}}[v]. \qquad (2)$$

Diffeomorphic flows that minimize $E[v]$ are geodesics in the group of diffeomorphisms. This gives rise to a powerful machinery for statistical shape analysis, in which distances between shapes $\mathcal{O}$ and $\mathcal{O}_{\text{trg}}$ are defined as the kinetic energy of the diffeomorphic flow that minimizes (2) [8]. Using this machinery, well-posed algorithms for statistical shape analysis have been developed [8].

2.2   Medial Axis Geometry

The medial axis is the locus formed by the centers of all maximal inscribed balls in an object [3]. Formally, consider a closed object $\mathcal{O} \subset \mathbb{R}^3$ with no holes and a smooth boundary $\mathcal{B_O}$. Let $B_{x,r} = \{y \in \mathbb{R}^3 : |y-x| \leq r\}$ denote a ball with center x and radius r. $B_{x,r}$ is called a *maximal inscribed ball (MIB)* in $\mathcal{O}$ if $B_{x,r} \subset \mathcal{O}$ and there exists no larger ball $B_{x',r'} \subset \mathcal{O}$ that contains $B_{x,r}$. The *medial axis* of $\mathcal{O}$ is the set of all tuples $(x,r) \in \mathbb{R}^3 \times \mathbb{R}^+$ such that $B_{x,r}$ is an MIB in $\mathcal{O}$. We will call the x-component of the medial axis (i.e., set of all MIB centers) the *medial scaffold* of $\mathcal{O}$, and denote it $\mathcal{M_O}$, and we will call the r-component the *radial scalar field*, denoted $\mathcal{R_O}$. Generically[1], $\mathcal{M_O}$ consists of a set of surfaces, called *medial surfaces*. These medial surfaces are bounded by curves that include curve segments that are shared by multiple medial surfaces, called *seam curves*, and curve segments that belong to just one medial surface, called *free edges*. As shown in [4], MIBs centered on the interior of medial surfaces are tangent to $\mathcal{B_O}$ at two points. MIBs centered on seam curves are tangent to $\mathcal{B_O}$ at three points, and MIBs centered along free edges are tangent to $\mathcal{B_O}$ at just one point. Each point in $\mathcal{B_O}$ belongs to exactly one MIB.

2.3   Medial Structure Preservation Under Diffeomorphic Flow

A flow ϕ acting on an object $\mathcal{O}$ is called *medial-preserving* if $\phi_t \mathcal{M_O} = \mathcal{M}_{\phi_t \mathcal{O}}$ for all $t \in [0,1]$, i.e., the medial scaffold of the transformed object coincides with the transformed medial scaffold of the original object. Medial preserving flows maintain point-wise correspondences on the medial scaffold as the object deforms, allowing statistical analysis of properties derived from the medial axis, such as thickness. By contrast, arbitrary diffeomorphic flows that are not medially preserving may cause the medial scaffold to change structure, e.g., by adding new surfaces or reconfiguring their geometry [4]. **The aim of this paper is to perform approximate shape matching using medial-preserving flows.**

Let the tuple of points $\{b_1, \ldots, b_n; x\}$ be called a *medial tuple* in $\mathcal{O}$ if there exists an MIB centered on x that is tangent to $\mathcal{B_O}$ at points $b_1, \ldots, b_n$. Let ϕ be a flow of diffeomorphisms that satisfies the following property: for every medial tuple $Z = \{b_1, \ldots, b_n; x\}$ in $\mathcal{O}$ and every time $t \in [0,1]$, the transformed tuple at time t, denoted $\phi_t Z = \{\phi_t(b_1), \ldots, \phi_t(b_n); \phi_t(x)\}$, is also a medial tuple in $\phi_t \mathcal{O}$. Then it can be shown (proof omitted due to limited space) that ϕ is medially preserving. Let us denote $\phi_t Z$ as $Z^t = \{b_1^t, \ldots, b_n^t; x^t\}$. To check if the tuple Z^t (with $n > 1$) is a medial tuple in $\phi_t \mathcal{O}$ it suffices to check three conditions:

$$(x^t - b_i^t) \perp T_{b_i^t} \qquad \forall i \in [1,n] \tag{3}$$

$$|x^t - b_i^t| = |x^t - b_1^t| \qquad \forall i \in [2,n] \tag{4}$$

$$|x^t - b'| \geq |x^t - b_1^t| \qquad \forall b' \in \phi_t \mathcal{B_O}, \tag{5}$$

where $T_{b_i^t}$ denotes the tangent plane to the boundary surface $\phi_t \mathcal{B_O}$ at the point b_i^t. Conditions (3) and (4) ensure that x^t is the center of a ball that is tangent to $\phi_t \mathcal{B_O}$ at points $b_1, \ldots, b_n$, and condition (5) ensures that this ball is inscribed in

---

[1] A property of $\mathcal{O}$ is considered "generic" if it is invariant to small smooth perturbations of $\mathcal{O}$. For example, the centers of the MIBs in a perfect cylinder form a line, but a small perturbation breaks this perfect symmetry.

$\phi_t \mathcal{O}$, and thus an MIB in $\phi_t \mathcal{O}$. Note that conditions (3) and (4) only involve local geometry of $\phi_t \mathcal{B}_\mathcal{O}$ around the tuple, while condition (5) requires the knowledge of the entire $\phi_t \mathcal{B}_\mathcal{O}$. In practice, it appears to be sufficient to only enforce the first two conditions, and we conjecture that diffeomorphic flows that satisfy only (3) and (4) for all Z^t with $n > 1$ are medially preserving.

2.4   Optimal Control Framework for Diffeomorphometry

Above, we defined a set of local geometric constraints that we want flows of diffeomorphisms to satisfy. We now briefly summarize a framework for constrained diffeomorphic shape matching developed by Arguillère et al. in [1]. We restrict our attention to shapes represented by point sets, which is relevant for the implementation of medial constraints in this paper.

Let $q^0 = \{q_1^0, \ldots, q_k^0\}$ be a finite set of points in $\mathbb{R}^n$, e.g., a set of landmarks sampled on the boundary (and perhaps on the interior) of the template shape $\mathcal{O}$. Let q^t denote the positions of these points at time t, i.e., $q^t = \phi_t q^0 = \{\phi_t(q_1^0), \ldots, \phi_t(q_k^0)\}$. Let us express the data attachment term $g(\phi_1 \mathcal{O})$ purely in terms of these landmarks, i.e., $g(\phi_1 \mathcal{O}) = g(q^1)$. The matching of $\mathcal{O}$ to the target shape/image then takes the form of minimizing the energy

$$E[v] = \alpha\, g(q^1) + \frac{1}{2} \int_0^1 \|v_t\|_{\mathcal{H}}^2 \, dt, \tag{6}$$

where ϕ_t is related to v via (1). This is a kind of optimal control problem, in which v is a "control", i.e., a function that affects the paths of points q^0 and guides them towards their target locations. It is a remarkable fact that this problem can be restated as a problem involving a much simpler set of controls associated with each landmark. As proven in [1], if v is a minimizer of $E[v]$ in (6), then v can be interpolated from a set of vector-valued functions $u(t) = \{u_1(t) : [0,1] \to \mathbb{R}^n, \ldots, u_k(t) : [0,1] \to \mathbb{R}^n\}$ associated with the landmarks. The interpolation is via the kernel K of the Hilbert space $\mathcal{H}$. For every t,

$$v_t(x) = \sum_{j=1}^{k} K(x, q_j^t)\, u^j(t). \tag{7}$$

The function $u_i(t)$ is called the *momentum* of the landmark q_i^0 and can be visualized as a vector placed at each point along the path traced by q_i^0. In general, the kernel $K(x,y)$ is a matrix-valued function, but in most practical applications, it is chosen to be of the form $K(x,y) = \eta(|x-y|)\mathcal{I}_{n \times n}$, where $\eta : \mathbb{R} \to \mathbb{R}$ is a radial basis kernel. As in [1], we use a Gaussian kernel $\eta(z) = e^{-0.5\, z^2/\sigma^2}$.

Given the interpolation formula (7), $\|v_t\|_{\mathcal{H}}$ and subsequently $E[v]$ can be expressed entirely in terms of the momenta $u(t)$:

$$E[u] = \alpha\, g(q^1) + \frac{1}{2} \int_0^1 \underbrace{\sum_{i=1}^{k} \sum_{j=1}^{k} u_i(t)^T K(q_i^t, q_j^t) u_j(t)}_{\|v_t\|_{\mathcal{H}}^2} \, dt, \tag{8}$$

where the landmark positions are updated according to:

$$\dot{q}_i^t = v_t(q_i^t) = \sum_{j=1}^{k} K(q_i^t, q_j^t)\, u^j(t). \tag{9}$$

Diffeomorphometry methods often take advantage of the fact that minimizers of $E[u]$ are geodesics in the group of diffeomorphisms and thus are determined by the initial momentum $u(0)$. However, here we are concerned with minimizing $E[u]$ subject to a set of constraints $C_1, \ldots, C_L$, each in the form $C_l(q^t) = 0$. Arguillère et al. [1] propose two strategies for solving such problems: as an initial momentum problem where geodesics are computed by projection of $\dot{q}_i^t$ into the null space of the constraints; and using an *Augmented Lagrangian (AL)* method in which optimization is over the complete momentum $u(t)$ and the constraints are added as penalty terms to $E[u]$. We adopt the AL-based method, which is easier to implement and is numerically more stable, but converges slowly [1].

In the AL method, minimization of $E[u]$ subject to constraints $\{C_l(q^t) = 0\}$ is achieved as a series of unconstrained problems, indexed by $m = 1, \ldots, M$. A set of L Lagrange multiplier functions $\lambda_l^m : [0,1] \to \mathbb{R}$ corresponding the constraints is introduced, initialized $\lambda_l^1(t) = 0$. At iteration m, the following energy is minimized:

$$E_{\mathrm{AL}}^m[u] = E[u] + \int_0^1 \sum_{l=1}^{L} \left[\frac{\mu^m}{2} C_l(q^t)^2 - \lambda_l^m(t) C_l(q^t) \right] \mathrm{d}t, \tag{10}$$

where μ^m is a scalar weight. The Lagrange multipliers and weights are updated at each iteration as

$$\lambda_l^{m+1}(t) = \lambda_l^m(t) - \mu^m C_l(q^t); \qquad \mu^{m+1} = \mu^m \cdot \mathring{\mu},$$

where $\mathring{\mu} = 10$ is a constant scaling factor. Minimization of (10) only requires computing the gradient of $E_{\mathrm{AL}}^m[u]$ with respect to $u(t)$, which involves solving an ODE backwards in time, as specified in [1, Remark 24].

2.5   Medial Constraints for Point Set Diffeomorphometry

In this paper, we adapt the Arguillère et al. [1] approach to the problem of matching shapes using medial-preserving flows of diffeomorphisms. To reduce the problem to point sets, we relax the constraints (3) and (4) to a finite set of medial tuples $Z_1, \ldots, Z_p$ in $\mathcal{O}$, rather than for the infinite set of all medial tuples in $\mathcal{O}$. We also discretize the time dimension. Although by enforcing constraints (3) and (4) for a discrete set of tuples and timepoints no longer guarantees the exact preservation of medial structure by the diffeomorphic flow, in practice, solving the discrete problem results in near-preservation of medial structure, i.e., $\mathcal{M}_{\phi_t \mathcal{O}} \simeq \phi_t \mathcal{M}_{\mathcal{O}}$, which is sufficient in order to perform statistical shape analysis using point correspondences between $\mathcal{M}_{\mathcal{O}}$ and $\phi_t \mathcal{M}_{\mathcal{O}}$.

Given a template object $\mathcal{O}$, the medial tuples $Z_1, \ldots, Z_p$ in $\mathcal{O}$ are sampled "regularly" from among all medial tuples in $\mathcal{O}$. Such sampling is nontrivial, because regular sampling of the x's on the medial scaffold results in irregular sampling of b's on the boundary, and vice-versa. Since constructing a template is a one-off task, we manually sample medial tuples in the template object $\mathcal{O}$ using a GUI tool. The tool computes the approximate medial scaffold $\mathcal{M}_{\mathcal{O}}$ using pruned Voronoi skeletonization [9]. Samples are taken along the seams and free edges in $\mathcal{M}_{\mathcal{O}}$ as well as on the surfaces forming $\mathcal{M}_{\mathcal{O}}$. Samples are organized into a triangle mesh, which is then inflated of both sides of each triangle to create a boundary triangle mesh. Template-building is shown in Fig. 1(a).

The Arguillère et al. approach [1] is applied as follows. We let q^0 consist of all of the points contained in the tuples $Z_1, \ldots, Z_p$. Each tuple Z_i indexes n_i boundary landmarks and one medial landmark. Let $\mathfrak{B}[i, j]$ denote the index of the j-th boundary landmarks in Z_i and let $\mathfrak{M}[i]$ denote the index of the medial point in Z_i. Then, at time t, the transformed i-th medial tuple is given by $Z_i^t = \{q_{\mathfrak{B}[i,1]}^t, \ldots, q_{\mathfrak{B}[i,n_i]}^t; q_{\mathfrak{M}[i]}^t\}$. We formulate a set of constraints that are discrete equivalents of the constraints (3) and (4).

Constraint (3) requires the vector $q_{\mathfrak{B}[i,j]}^t - q_{\mathfrak{M}[i]}^t$ to be orthogonal to $\phi_t \mathcal{B}_{\mathcal{O}}$ at the point $q_{\mathfrak{B}[i,j]}^t$. A pair of vectors spanning the tangent plane to $\phi_t \mathcal{B}_{\mathcal{O}}$ at $q_{\mathfrak{B}[i,j]}^t$ can be approximated as the weighted sum of the coordinates of adjacent boundary vertices, e.g., using the Loop tangent scheme [14, p.71]. We can write these tangent vectors as $W_{i,j}^1 q^t$ and $W_{i,j}^2 q^t$ where $W_{i,j}^1$ and $W_{i,j}^2$ are sparse $3 \times k$ matrices. The discrete equivalents of constraints (3) and (4) are then:

$$\left(q_{\mathfrak{B}[i,j]}^t - q_{\mathfrak{M}[i]}^t\right)^T W_{i,j}^\gamma q^t = 0 \quad \forall j \in [1, n_i], \gamma = 1, 2,$$
$$\left|q_{\mathfrak{B}[i,j]}^t - q_{\mathfrak{M}[i]}^t\right|^2 - \left|q_{\mathfrak{B}[i,1]}^t - q_{\mathfrak{M}[i]}^t\right|^2 = 0 \quad \forall j \in [2, n_i]. \tag{11}$$

Following Pizer et al. [10], we refer to the vectors $q_{\mathfrak{B}[i,j]}^t - q_{\mathfrak{M}[i]}^t$ as *spokes* (as in spokes on a bicycle wheel). The constraints state that spokes must be orthogonal to the boundary and that the lengths of the spokes must be equal. When monitoring AL optimization, we describe the extent to which the constraints are violated in terms of two related intuitive metrics: *spoke-normal deviation*, which measures the angle between the spoke $q_{\mathfrak{B}[i,j]}^t - q_{\mathfrak{M}[i]}^t$ and the boundary normal vector at $q_{\mathfrak{B}[i,j]}^t$; and *spoke-spoke mismatch*, which measures the maximum relative error between the lengths of two spokes in the tuple Z^t.

2.6   Data Attachment Term

Various data attachment terms can be used. When the target locations q_i^{trg} of the boundary and/or medial landmarks are given, a simple sum of square distances (SSD) attachment term is used: $g(q^1) = \sum_{i \in \Upsilon} |q_i^1 - q_i^{\text{trg}}|^2$, where Υ denotes the subset of landmarks with given target locations. When fitting a model to a target binary image $\mathcal{I}_{\text{trg}}$, we define $g(q^1)$ as an approximation of the Dice similarity coefficient (DSC) between the interior of $\phi_1 \mathcal{O}$ and the foreground region of the target binary image. The DSC attachment term leverages the triangulation of the boundary and medial surfaces created when medial tuples are sampled. Points in a 3D wedge formed by each medial triangle and the corresponding boundary triangle are sampled regularly, and the image $\mathcal{I}_{\text{trg}}$ is sampled at each sample point. Each sample point is also assigned a volume element. Integrating the sampled intensity values times the volume element yields an approximation of overlap volume, while the volume of $\phi_t \mathcal{O}$ is computed by just integrating the volume element. The volume of the foreground region in $\mathcal{I}_{\text{trg}}$ is known a priori. This allows DSC and its gradient with respect to q^1 to be computed.

2.7 Numerical Implementation

The AL minimization is implemented in C++ using CPU multi-threading. ODEs to compute $E_{\text{AL}}^m[u]$ and its gradient are solved numerically using Euler's method with 40 time steps. Unconstrained minimization (10) at each AL iteration is performed using a pseudo-Newton method (LBFGS) and is allowed to proceed until the change in $E_{\text{AL}}[u]$ (or $E_{\text{AL}}[u, \eta, \rho]$) falls below a tolerance threshold, usually for 1000–4000 iterations. Constraints, which are a mix of quadratic and linear expressions, are implemented as sparse matrix-vector multiplication. The scaling factor $\hat{\mu}$ in the AL algorithm is set to 10, while the initial value of μ is set experimentally, as is the data attachment term weight, α and the standard deviation σ of the Gaussian kernel.

3 Experiments and Results

We perform experiments on synthetic and real-world anatomical shapes, with the focus on demonstrating the feasibility of matching templates to target shapes using medial-preserving diffeomorphic flows.

3.1 Synthetic Shape Example

We use a toy example to show that our method can match shapes with branching medial axes, a problem that not all medial modeling approaches can solve (e.g., not [12]). We created two 3D shapes that have a medial axis consisting of three surfaces joining along a single seam curve, as follows. First, we manually painted a binary 3D object and smoothed it to create a surface labeled "source shape" in Fig. 1. We then flipped the binary image about the x-axis and performed diffeomorphic deformable image registration between the original image and the flipped image. The resulting warp was applied to the source shape, yielding the shape labeled as "target shape" in Fig. 1. By using deformable registration, we obtained point-wise correspondences between the two shapes.

To create the initial template medial model, we used a GUI tool as described in Sect. 2.5. The Voronoi skeleton of the "source shape" (after additional smoothing) is shown in Fig. 1(a) along with the medial points sampled from the skeleton and the triangulation of the medial points. The medial mesh shown in Fig. 1(a)

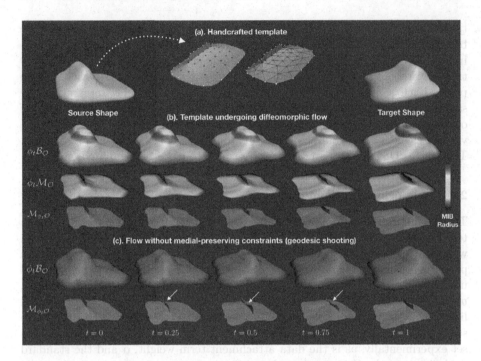

Fig. 1. Template generation and shape matching in the toy example. (a) Manual template construction by sampling tuples from the skeleton of the source shape. (b) Medial-preserving diffeomorphic flow between the template and a target shape. The deforming medial scaffold of the template ($\phi_t \mathcal{M}_\mathcal{O}$) is in close agreement with the Voronoi skeleton of the deforming template ($\mathcal{M}_{\phi_t \mathcal{O}}$), *which illustrates that medial preservation constraints are working.* (c) When analogous same shape matching (between $\mathcal{B}_\mathcal{O}$ and $\mathcal{B}_{\phi_1 \mathcal{O}}$) is performed using point set geodesic shooting *without medial preservation constraints,* the Voronoi skeleton of the deforming object changes structure and bifurcates (yellow arrows). (Color figure online)

was inflated and subdivided once using the Loop scheme [7] and then fitted to the "source shape" in Fig. 1 using the deformable medial modeling method in [13]. This yielded an initial template for which the medial constraints (11) are fully satisfied. The boundary and the medial model of this template are visualized in Fig. 1(b) under $t = 0$.

We then fitted the template to the target shape using our medially-constrained diffeomorphometry approach. We initialized the fitting using the SSD data attachment term, with target landmark locations obtained by applying the image registration warp to the template's boundary landmarks. This was done using a single AL iteration with $\mu = 1$, since the goal was only to initialize the subsequent DSC-based optimization. We then performed full AL optimization with the DSC data attachment term, and with μ increasing from 0.001 to 10 over several AL iterations. Figure 2 plots the change in the data attachment, kinetic energy, total constraint violation, spoke-normal deviation, and spoke-spoke mismatch over the course of optimization. As μ increases (>0.1), the data attachment term begins to retreat from its highest values in order to satisfy the constraints. However, the resulting practical gain at higher values of μ is very small, as the maximal normal-spoke deviation and spoke-spoke mismatch are already quite small for $\mu = 0.1$: about $1°$ and 1%, respectively, and don't decrease dramatically as μ increases. The flow visualized in Fig. 1(b) corresponds to the solution with $\mu = 0.1$, which may be considered the "sweet spot" of the optimization.

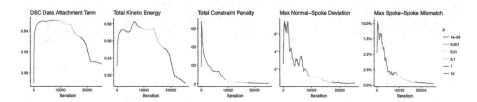

Fig. 2. Data attachment, kinetic energy, and constraints over the course of AL optimization for synthetic shape matching.

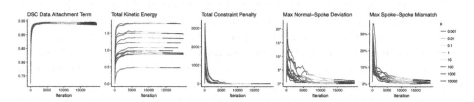

Fig. 3. Data attachment, kinetic energy, and constraints over the course of AL optimization for the 14 LV wall matching cases.

The three rows of shapes in Fig. 1(b) correspond to the evolving template boundary ($\phi_t \mathcal{B}_{\mathcal{O}}$), the evolving template medial scaffold ($\phi_t \mathcal{M}_{\mathcal{O}}$), and the Voronoi skeleton of the evolving template (an approximation of $\mathcal{M}_{\phi_t \mathcal{O}}$). Critically, $\phi_t \mathcal{M}_{\mathcal{O}}$ and $\mathcal{M}_{\phi_t \mathcal{O}}$ are highly consistent, indicating that our *medial preservation constraints are working*. By contrast, Fig. 1(c) shows that *conventional point set diffeomorphometry does not preserve medial axis structure*. We performed point set geodesic shooting between the boundary of our template ($\mathcal{B}_{\mathcal{O}}$) and the boundary of the fitted template ($\mathcal{B}_{\phi_1 \mathcal{O}}$) and extracted the Voronoi skeleton of the evolving shape. As pointed out by the yellow arrows in Fig. 1(c), the skeleton undergoes structural change during deformation.

3.2   3D Echocardiography Data

To demonstrate the feasibility of diffeomorphic medial modeling on real-world imaging datasets, we use our approach to model the shape of the left ventricle

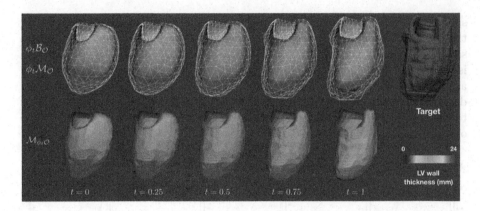

Fig. 4. Example of shape matching in the LV wall dataset. The top row shows the deforming medial scaffold (colored by thickness = 2× MIB radius) and the deforming boundary as a white wireframe. The bottom row shows the Voronoi skeleton of the deforming boundary, again emphasizing the preservation of medial scaffold structure during deformation.

(LV) wall in a dataset of 14 transesophageal 3D echocardiograms acquired prior to heart valve surgery. The dataset includes images from 8 patients who underwent surgery for ischemic mitral regurgitation (IMR) and 6 patients who did not have surgery. The LV wall was manually segmented at systole in each case by trained raters. The first IMR case was used to construct a template medial model using the same approach as in the toy example. Affine registration guided by five manually-placed landmarks was performed between the binary segmentation images of the first IMR case and all other cases. This was needed to correctly line up the LV outflow tract between cases. To initialize our medially-constrained diffeomorphometry approach with the affine registration parameters, we first performed one iteration of AL optimization with the SSD data attachment term, where the affine-transformed template landmarks were treated as target locations q^{trg}. We then performed multiple iterations of AL optimization with the DSC data attachment term. Figure 3 plots the DSC data attachment term, kinetic energy, total constraint penalty, maximum spoke-normal deviation and maximum spoke-spoke mismatch over the course of AL optimization. Fitting performance was highly consistent across the 14 cases, with final Dice coefficient ranging between 0.935 and 0.945 for all cases, and the maximum normal-spoke deviation and spoke-spoke mismatch having ranges $0.04° - 1.08°$ and $0.1\%-2.2\%$ respectively. Overall, this demonstrates excellent ability of medial-preserving diffeomorphic flows to fit real-world anatomical shapes. Figure 4 shows an example of the LV template deforming to match an individual case. As in the toy example, the preservation of the template's medial scaffold is demonstrated by excellent consistency between the deforming medial scaffold of the template ($\phi_t \mathcal{M}_{\mathcal{O}}$) and the Voronoi skeleton of the deforming template ($\mathcal{M}_{\phi_t \mathcal{O}}$).

4   Discussion and Conclusions

To our knowledge the method presented here is the first attempt to directly combine medial modeling and diffeomorphometry (an indirect approach to combining cm-reps and diffeomorphometry was recently proposed by Hong et al. [6]). The current paper demonstrates the feasibility of shape matching with this approach, but additional work is needed to extend all the tools of computational anatomy [8] (e.g., computing mean shapes or principal geodesics) to diffeomorphic medial modeling. A limitation of our approach is its high computational burden, with thousands of iterations needed for AL optimization to converge and each iteration having cost quadratic in the number of landmarks. The heart shape experiments were performed in an hour per case on a 16-core CPU. An open-source C++ implementation of our method is at https://github.com/pyushkevich/cmrep.

References

1. Arguillère, S., Trélat, E., Trouvé, A., Younes, L.: Shape deformation analysis from the optimal control viewpoint. Journal de mathématiques pures et appliquées **104**(1), 139–178 (2015)
2. Arnold, V.I.: Sur la géométrie différentielle des groupes de lie de dimension infinie et ses applicationsa l'hydrodynamique des fluides parfaits. Ann. Inst. Fourier **16**(1), 319–361 (1966)
3. Blum, H., Nagel, R.N.: Shape description using weighted symmetric axis features. Pattern Recogn. **10**(3), 167–180 (1978)
4. Giblin, P.J., Kimia, B.B.: On the local form and transitions of symmetry sets, medial axes, and shocks. Int. J. Comput. Vis. **54**(1–3), 143–157 (2003)
5. Hong, J., Vicory, J., Schulz, J., Styner, M., Marron, J.S., Pizer, S.M.: Non-euclidean classification of medically imaged objects via S-reps. Med. Image Anal. **31**, 37–45 (2016)
6. Hong, S., Fishbaugh, J., Gerig, G.: 4D continuous medial representation by geodesic shape regression. In: 2018 IEEE 15th International Symposium on Biomedical Imaging (ISBI 2018), pp. 1014–1017. IEEE (2018)
7. Loop, C., DeRose, T.: Generalized B-spline surfaces of arbitrary topology. In: Computer Graphics (ACM SIGGRAPH Proceedings), pp. 347–356 (1990)
8. Miller, M.I., Trouvé, A., Younes, L.: Geodesic shooting for computational anatomy. J. Math. Imaging Vis. **24**(2), 209–228 (2006)
9. Näf, M., Kübler, O., Kikinis, R., Shenton, M., Székely, G.: Characterization and recognition of 3D organ shape in medical image analysis using skeletonization. In: Workshop on Mathematical Methods in Biomedical Image Analysis, pp. 139–150. IEEE Computer Society (1996)
10. Pizer, S.M., et al.: Deformable m-reps for 3D medical image segmentation. Int. J. Comput. Vis. **55**(2), 85–106 (2003)
11. Sun, H., Frangi, A.F., Wang, H., Sukno, F.M., Tobon-Gomez, C., Yushkevich, P.A.: Automatic cardiac MRI segmentation using a biventricular deformable medial model. Med. Image Comput. Comput. Assist. Interv. **13**(Pt 1), 468–475 (2010)
12. Yushkevich, P.A., Zhang, H., Gee, J.: Continuous medial representation for anatomical structures. IEEE Trans. Med. Imaging **25**(2), 1547–1564 (2006)

13. Yushkevich, P.A., Zhang, H.G.: Deformable modeling using a 3D boundary representation with quadratic constraints on the branching structure of the blum skeleton. Inf. Process. Med. Imaging **23**, 280–291 (2013)
14. Zorin, D., Schröder, P., Derose, T., Kobbelt, L., Levin, A., Sweldens, W.: Subdivision for modeling and animation. In: SIGGRAPH Course Notes. ACM, New York (2000)

Controlling Meshes via Curvature: Spin Transformations for Pose-Invariant Shape Processing

Loïc Le Folgoc[1(✉)], Daniel C. Castro[1], Jeremy Tan[1], Bishesh Khanal[2], Konstantinos Kamnitsas[1], Ian Walker[1], Amir Alansary[1], and Ben Glocker[1]

[1] BioMedIA, Imperial College London, London, UK
l.le-folgoc@imperial.ac.uk
[2] King's College London, London, UK

Abstract. We investigate discrete spin transformations, a geometric framework to manipulate surface meshes by controlling mean curvature. Applications include surface fairing – flowing a mesh onto say, a reference sphere – and mesh extrusion – *e.g.*, rebuilding a complex shape from a reference sphere and curvature specification. Because they operate in curvature space, these operations can be conducted very stably across large deformations with no need for remeshing. Spin transformations add to the algorithmic toolbox for pose-invariant shape analysis. Mathematically speaking, mean curvature is a shape invariant and in general fully characterizes closed shapes (together with the metric). Computationally speaking, spin transformations make that relationship explicit. Our work expands on a *discrete* formulation of spin transformations. Like their smooth counterpart, discrete spin transformations are naturally close to conformal (angle-preserving). This quasi-conformality can nevertheless be relaxed to satisfy the desired trade-off between area distortion and angle preservation. We derive such constraints and propose a formulation in which they can be efficiently incorporated. The approach is showcased on subcortical structures.

1 Introduction

Generative shape models are tremendously useful in commputational anatomy (shape representation, population analysis), medical imaging and computer vision (segmentation, tracking), computer graphics and beyond. Most approaches to statistical shape analysis fundamentally rely on registration, from landmark based representations and active shape models [1,4,25], to medial representations [14] and Principal Geodesic Analysis [9], to deformable registration and diffeomorphometry [8,33]. Registration is known to be a source of bias in shape analysis, but is often a necessary 'evil' because input data does not come pre-aligned in a common reference frame (or *pose*). In contrast, the shape information of interest is often invariant to the object pose. Our main motivation is to investigate geometric tools that can open the way to learned, *pose-invariant*

© Springer Nature Switzerland AG 2019
A. C. S. Chung et al. (Eds.): IPMI 2019, LNCS 11492, pp. 221–234, 2019.
https://doi.org/10.1007/978-3-030-20351-1_17

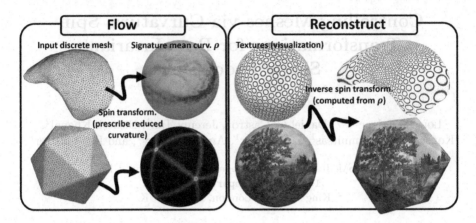

Fig. 1. Discrete spin transformations allow for controlling meshes via the mean curvature invariant. (a) Input face edge-constraint nets are flowed to a reference shape in the homotopy class (*e.g.* the unit sphere $\mathcal{S}^2$). Information required to recompute the original shape up to pose and scale is summarized within a scalar field ρ. (b) The inverse spin transformation is retrieved. Texture coordinates mapped onto the reference sphere are pushed forward with the extruded mesh. Note the preservation of texture, from which deformations are seen to be quasi-conformal. Top row: putamen. Bottom: icosahedron.

generative shape models (specifically, curves and 3D surfaces). The key insight is that mean curvature is pose-invariant and generally characterizes the shape *losslessly*. This work investigates spin transformations as the algorithmic tool to computationally implement this insight. The cornerstone of the framework lies in a gracefully simple equation that relates a spin transformation $\phi\colon \mathcal{F} \to \mathbb{H}$ (one quaternion per face in the mesh) to a change $\mu\colon \mathcal{F} \to \mathbb{R}$ in the mean curvature via a first-order differential operator D_e:

$$D_e\phi = \mu\phi. \tag{1}$$

Typically, a desired change of curvature is specified via μ, yielding a transformation ϕ from which a new shape can be constructed. The present work demonstrates this concept and shows its applicability to manipulate (flow and extrude) closed shapes in a stable manner across large deformations. Section 3 reviews the discrete geometric setting, *i.e.* (i) the geometric objects to which the framework applies, (ii) discrete mean curvature, (iii) background on quaternions as similarity transformations in $\mathbb{R}^3$. Section 4 introduces discrete spin transformations. Within the framework of spin transformations, the task of flowing a mesh onto a reference shape and that of extruding a shape back from the reference are highly symmetric: both rely on the ability to compute a transformation based on prescribed curvature and area changes. Section 5 gives an overview of the proposed procedure. Section 6 discusses applications and results.

2   Related Work

Pose-Invariant Shape Analysis. Spectral shape descriptors [28,29], built from the spectrum and eigenfunctions of the Laplace(–Beltrami) operator, have achieved popularity in this context, spanning a variety of applications *e.g.*, object retrieval [2], shape dissimilarity quantification [17], analysis of anatomical structures [10,26,31], transfer of structural and functional data [20,27]. Spectral representations pose two challenges: firstly, going back from the spectral descriptor to the corresponding shape is difficult; and secondly, they tend to discard fine-grained, local information in favor of global shape properties and symmetries. To supplement the intrinsic Laplace–Beltrami operator, the *extrinsic* Dirac operator [19], which carries more information about the shape immersion, has recently been investigated for shape analysis. Geometric deep learning [3] provides the toolset to analyze *functions* over a *fixed* graph. It remains unclear how to analyze *graphs* themselves. The present work contributes with a lossless and invertible mechanism for turning a mesh into a function (the curvature) over a reference template (say, a sphere).

Shape Flows, Large Deformations, Conformal Maps. Mean curvature flow is the archetypal algorithm for fairing, in part due to its simplicity and intuitive appeal. However mesh quality tends to degrade quickly throughout the flow, requiring tedious monitoring and remeshing to reduce artefacts and prevent singularities [16]. Furthermore it is not suitable for mesh extrusion. Conformal maps are often perceived as the gold standard in such contexts, and spin transformations originate from this perspective [5,6]. Several discretized and discrete quasi-conformal frameworks have been proposed (*e.g.*, [18,22]) on top of an incredibly rich body of theoretical work. Conformal maps have found a natural application in the context of brain mapping [11,13] by mapping the cortical surface to a reference domain. Rather than strictly on conformality, our focus here is on a parametrization of large deformations that (1) works from the shape invariant mean curvature (2) allows to efficiently flow between any shape and a reference. It is more generally related in spirit to large diffeomorphic frameworks [21,30] that can flow a shape from a template and (pose-equivariant) vector field. Our work expands on the framework of *discrete* spin transformations as introduced by Ye et al. [32]. One of the appeals of a discrete framework is to bypass *discretization* errors by design and to offer a consistent definition of discrete geometric concepts such as curvature. We introduce the framework to the community and contribute (i) with an optimization strategy that gives finer-grained control over deformations; (ii) by deriving constraints within this formulation for integrability on general topologies, and area preservation; (iii) by exploring its potency for mesh extrusion.

3   Discrete Geometric Setting

Face Edge-Constraint Nets. Our work focuses on the case of closed compact orientable surfaces in $\mathbb{R}^3$ and follows the discrete geometric setting introduced by

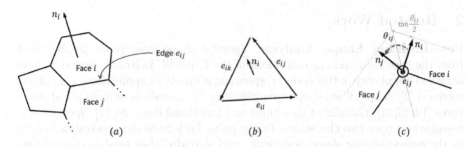

Fig. 2. Face edge-constraint nets: (a) faces are general polygons; (b) face edges are oriented (counter-clockwise); (c) θ_{ij} is the bending angle, positive if the edge is convex; the edge integrated mean curvature $H_{ij} = |e_{ij}| \tan(\theta_{ij}/2)$ is the signed created area for face i above e_{ij} when faces i and j are offset by a unit length 1 in the direction of their normals.

Ye et al. [32]. Surfaces are discretized as face edge-constraint nets, generic constructs that encompass but are not restricted to standard triangulated meshes. Let $\mathcal{G} = (\mathcal{V}, \mathcal{F}, \mathcal{E})$ denote the net combinatorics, resp. its vertices, faces and edges. Adjacent faces meet along a single edge. Edges are shared by exactly two adjacent faces. Faces can be arbitrary polygons (such as with simplex meshes [7]). In addition, let each face be assigned a unit normal n, such that for any two adjacent faces i and j joined along edge e_{ij} $((i,j) \in \mathcal{E})$, the normals satisfy the looser condition $n_i + n_j \perp e_{ij}$. $\mathcal{X} = (\mathcal{G}, n)$ is called a face edge-constraint net. For instance standard triangulations with normals orthogonal to faces are face edge-constraint nets.

Discrete Mean Curvature. Let $\mathcal{X}$ be a net. $\mathcal{X}$ is orientable and, without loss of generality, directed edges e_{ij} are traversed in the direction towards which they point when cycling over vertices of face i. This lets us orient the dihedral angle θ_{ij} between planes $P_i \triangleq \mathrm{span}\{n_i, e_{ij}\}$ and $P_j \triangleq \mathrm{span}\{n_j, e_{ij}\}$. For standard triangulations, θ_{ij} is just the bending angle between faces. The *integrated mean curvature* on edge e_{ij} (Fig. 2(c)) is defined as $H_{ij} \triangleq |e_{ij}| \tan(\theta_{ij}/2)$. The integrated mean curvature on *face* i is the sum of its integrated edge curvatures: $H_i \triangleq \sum_{j \in \mathcal{N}(i)} H_{ij}$. The discrete mean curvature $h_i \triangleq H_i / A_i$ follows by turning H_i into a density over the face. With this, the discrete mean curvature satisfies a discrete counterpart to Steiner's formula. Steiner's formula is a characterization of mean curvature that relates it to the relative change of area when offsetting the surface in the normal direction n by a distance t (replace A_i by an infinitesimal area element dA in Eq. (2) for the original formula):

$$A_i^{(t)} = A_i(1 + h_i t + \mathcal{O}(t^2)). \tag{2}$$

Geometry in the Quaternions. Quaternions $\mathbb{H}$ provide a natural algebraic language for geometry in $\mathbb{R}^3$, much like complex numbers for planar geometry. Let $\{1, \mathbf{i}, \mathbf{j}, \mathbf{k}\}$ denote a basis for $\mathbb{H}$. Elements $v \triangleq (v_x, v_y, v_z) \in \mathbb{R}^3$ are identified with pure imaginary quaternions $v_x \mathbf{i} + v_y \mathbf{j} + v_z \mathbf{k} \in \mathrm{Im}\,\mathbb{H} \triangleq \mathrm{span}\{\mathbf{i}, \mathbf{j}, \mathbf{k}\}$, so that surfaces are naturally immersed in Im $\mathbb{H}$. Denote by $\bar{q} \triangleq a - (b\mathbf{i} + c\mathbf{j} + d\mathbf{k})$ the quaternionic conjugate of $q \triangleq a + b\mathbf{i} + c\mathbf{j} + d\mathbf{k} \in \mathbb{H}$. The norm $|q|$ of q is defined as the square root of $\bar{q}q = a^2 + b^2 + c^2 + d^2$. All $q \neq 0$ admit an inverse $q^{-1} = \bar{q}/|q|^2$. Again like complex numbers, quaternions admit a polar decomposition $q = se^{\theta u} = s(\cos(\theta) + \sin(\theta)u)$ with $u \in \text{Im } \mathbb{H}$ a unit vector, which makes their geometric meaning more explicit. Indeed, $v \mapsto qvq^{-1}$, also known as conjugation by q, expresses rotation around u by an angle 2θ. In the same vein, the expression $\tilde{v} = qv\bar{q}$ conveniently expresses a similarity transformation: $\tilde{v}$ corresponds to v rotated around u by 2θ and rescaled by s^2.

Hyperedges. Every edge in the net $\mathcal{X}$ is associated with a quaternion E_{ij} dubbed *hyperedge*, with real part equal to the integrated mean curvature H_{ij} at the edge, and imaginary part equal to the embedding $e_{ij} \in \text{Im } \mathbb{H}$ of the edge:

$$E_{ij} \triangleq H_{ij} + e_{ij} \in \mathbb{H}. \tag{3}$$

Hyperedges are the fundamental structure on which discrete spin transformations act. They summarize all the geometric information that, along with the mesh combinatorics, allows to reconstruct the discrete surface immersion (See footnote 1). With that, spin transformations are introduced in a straightforward manner.

4   Discrete Spin Transformations

Discrete Spin Transformations. A discrete spin transformation ϕ associates a single quaternion ϕ_i with each face i of a face edge-constraint net. The transformation acts on hyperedges E_{ij} and face normals n_i as follows:

$$\begin{aligned} E_{ij} &\mapsto \tilde{E}_{ij} = \bar{\phi}_i E_{ij} \phi_j, \\ n_i &\mapsto \tilde{n}_i = \phi_i^{-1} n_i \phi_i. \end{aligned} \tag{4}$$

The elegance of the construct lies in the fact that Eq. (4) does transform a face edge-constraint net into another edge-constraint net. This is easily checked (cf. [32]), with the main elements of the proof stemming from the geometric interpretation of hyperedges (See footnote 1) and from the constraint on face normals. Furthermore, discrete spin transformations $E \to_\phi \tilde{E}$ are trivially invertible: $\tilde{E} \to_{\phi^{-1}} E$. The *integrability* condition that each face in the new net closes ($\sum_j \tilde{E}_{ij} \in \mathbb{R}$) is equivalent to the existence of a real valued function $\rho : i \mapsto \rho_i \in \mathbb{R}$ over faces such that:

$$D_{\mathcal{X}}\phi = \rho A \phi. \tag{5}$$

Equation (5) is the cornerstone of the framework. $D_{\mathcal{X}}$ is henceforth referred to as the *intrinsic* Dirac operator. $D_{\mathcal{X}}$ sends a quaternionic function over faces to another one such that $(D_{\mathcal{X}}\phi)_i \triangleq \sum_j E_{ij}\phi_j$. Left multiplying both sides by $\bar{\phi}_i$, the closedness constraint on faces is immediately apparent: $\bar{\phi}_i(D_{\mathcal{X}}\phi)_i = \sum_j \tilde{E}_{ij}$

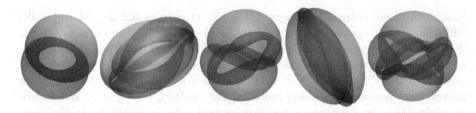

Fig. 3. A few leading eigenvectors of the intrinsic Dirac operator for the unit sphere, visualized as surface immersions (color map: eigenvector magnitude). (Color figure online)

must be real-valued. For ease of exposition, the expression in the introduction is formulated using a slightly different yet immediately related operator, the *extrinsic* Dirac operator $(D_e\phi)_i \triangleq \sum_j E_{ij}(\phi_j - \phi_i) = (D_{\mathcal{X}}\phi)_i - H_i\phi_i$. It also discards the normalization by A as in [32]. The proposed normalization however mirrors more faithfully the smooth counterpart of the present setting (see *e.g.* [15]).

The intrinsic Dirac operator $D_{\mathcal{X}}$ creates an explicit relationship between a spin transformation ϕ and the discrete (resp. integrated) mean curvature $\tilde{h}$ (resp. $\tilde{H}$) of the new net, namely $\bar{\phi}_i(D_{\mathcal{X}}\phi)_i = \tilde{H}_i \triangleq \tilde{h}_i\tilde{A}_i$ as long as the new net closes. Coupling with Eq. (5),

$$\tilde{h}_i\tilde{A}_i = \rho_i A_i|\phi_i|^2. \tag{6}$$

When $\phi := 1$ is the identity transform, $\rho_i = h_i = \tilde{h}_i$. For smooth $|\phi_i|$ and from Eq. (4), $\rho_i\sqrt{A_i} \approx \tilde{h}_i\sqrt{\tilde{A}_i}$. In other words, ρ_i jointly describes the mean curvature and length element. This quantity is precisely known as the mean curvature half-density $h|df|$ in the smooth setting, and is generally in one-to-one correspondence with a given shape. Finally, with the *extrinsic* Dirac operator, the corresponding μ describes a *change* in half-density instead: $\tilde{h}_i\tilde{A}_i = (h_i + \mu_i)A_i|\phi_i|^2$.

Dirac Operators. Dirac operators $D_{\mathcal{X}}$ and D_e have a number of properties that make them appealing for various tasks in shape analysis. $D_{\mathcal{X}}$ and D_e are self-adjoint operators. Dirac operators relate to square roots of the Laplace–Beltrami operator L. Whereas L captures the intrinsic manifold geometry and is invariant by isometry, the Dirac operators can disambiguate much more about the surface *immersion* into $\mathbb{R}^3$. We refer the reader to [19,32] for a discussion from this perspective. The eigenvectors of Dirac operators all satisfy Eq. (5) and thus provide new immersions of the abstract manifold into $\mathbb{R}^3$ (new transformed $\tilde{\mathcal{X}}$). The first (null) eigenvector of D_e is trivial. $D_{\mathcal{X}}$ cannot have a null eigenvalue for closed surfaces (*e.g.* spherical topology) of practical interest in the present work, since that would result in a minimal closed surface with everywhere zero mean curvature. The smallest eigenvector of $D_{\mathcal{X}}$ provides a generally non-trivial immersion with higher smoothness than the original shape (lower Willmore energy $\int |h|^2 dA$). Ye et al. [32] explore this mechanism for the purpose of surface fairing. The next leading eigenvectors give some geometric insight into $D_{\mathcal{X}}$ (Fig. 3). In this work however, we investigate a strategy closely related to [6] with a fine-grained control over the surface deformations.

5   Algorithms

Remark 51. *Quaternions q admit representations $M[q]$ as 4×4 real matrices (Eq. (7)), so that standard linear algebra libraries can be used to solve quaternionic linear systems. In particular, $M[\bar{q}] = M[q]^\mathsf{T}$, thus Hermitian (quaternionic) forms are represented by real symmetric matrices. We denote real vectors and matrix representations below with upright bold symbols.*

$$M[q] \triangleq \begin{bmatrix} a & -b & -c & -d \\ b & a & -d & c \\ c & d & a & -b \\ d & -c & b & a \end{bmatrix}. \tag{7}$$

Overview. The scalar function ρ introduced in Sect. 4 provides the primary degrees of freedom for mesh manipulation, and it tightly relates to mean curvature. Of course only a subset of functions ρ can be associated with some ϕ such that the integrability condition Eq. (5) is satisfied. Namely, $D_\rho \triangleq D - \rho$ should have a null eigenvalue. This leads Crane et al. [5] to solve for the smallest eigenvalue γ and eigenvector ϕ, yielding a solution of Eq. (5) up to a small constant shift: $D\phi = (\rho + \gamma)\phi$. We propose instead to formulate the objective $D_\rho\phi \simeq 0$ as a minimization problem. This gives fine-grained control to add specifications (*e.g.* smoothness, area distortion), many of which can be efficiently expressed as linear(ized) constraints or quadratic regularizers, within a unified formulation. Thus finding ϕ amounts to solving a quadratic problem:

$$\underset{\phi}{\mathrm{argmin}}\ \underbrace{\phi^\mathsf{T}(\mathbf{D}_\rho\mathbf{A}^{-1}\mathbf{D}_\rho)\phi}_{D_\rho\phi\simeq 0} + \underbrace{(\phi - 1)^\mathsf{T}\alpha\mathbf{R}(\phi - 1)}_{\text{regularization}}, \tag{8}$$

under a set of linear constraints on ϕ. $\mathbf{A}$ is a diagonal matrix of face areas. In practice we set $\mathbf{R}$ to $\mathbf{A} + \beta\mathbf{L}_f$, where $\mathbf{L}_f$ is an integrated Laplacian over faces. The eigensystem actually solved in [5] closely relates to the simplest case where there are no constraints and $\beta := 0$.

Overall, the procedure is as follows: prescribe a scalar function ρ for a target shape or curvature change (Sect. 6); then solve for the spin transformation ϕ (Eq. (8)); finally compute new hyperedges (Eq. (4)) and solve a linear system for the new vertex coordinates (Eq. (9)). The steps are typically iterated over, resulting in a flow.

Computing the New Immersion. Let transformed edges $\tilde{e}_{ij} = \mathrm{Im}\,\tilde{E}_{ij}$ be indexed by their start and end vertices $v \to v'$. Vertex coordinates $\tilde{f} \colon v \in V \mapsto \tilde{f}_v$ satisfy $\tilde{f}_{v'} - \tilde{f}_v = \tilde{e}_{v \to v'}$. In practice, we solve the mathematically equivalent (See footnote 1) linear system

$$\Delta\tilde{f} = \nabla \cdot \tilde{e}, \tag{9}$$

where Δ and $\nabla\cdot$ are the standard discrete (cotangent) mesh Laplacian and divergence operators [23]. This method of integration is robust to numerical errors. The Laplacian and divergence are computed w.r.t. either the source (e) or target ($\tilde{e}$) mesh metric (with empirically identical results). A benefit of working from a discrete setting is that no discretization error is introduced from ϕ to the corresponding $\tilde{f}$.

Geometrically Constrained Flows. The proposed formulation (Eq. (8)) enables fine-grained control over the flow by prescribing additional constraints. For instance, the method extends to topologies beyond spherical by adding an *exactness* constraint (See footnote 1). The mapping can also be encouraged to preserve angles (*i.e.* conformality) and minimize area distortion. Conformality is key in preserving mesh quality across exceptionally large deformations, which prevents considerable loss of numerical stability. It is intuitively described as circles being locally transformed into circles, or indeed texture-preserving (Fig. 1). Quasi-conformality is inherent to the present framework. From Eq. (4), the relative length of edges is preserved as soon as $|\phi_i|$ varies smoothly across faces. On the other hand large area distortion can be introduced, particularly in regions of high curvature. In some applications, we may prefer to trade off some distortion of angles for a better preservation of areas. We note again from Eq. (4) that the magnitude $|\phi_i|^4$ of the spin transformation relates to the local change of area. Thus scale changes $\log \tilde{A}_i/A_i$ (up to global rescaling) can be penalized via a linearized soft constraint over ϕ (See footnote 1).

Filtering in Curvature Space. As described in [6] in a related setting, the flow of the spin transformation can also be altered by directly manipulating ρ. The rate of change for geometric features of various scales can be tweaked by manipulating its frequency spectrum. Moreover some constraints can be efficiently enforced by orthogonal projection of ρ onto a linear subspace. In particular, we derive[1] alternative integrability conditions in the form of simple linear constraints on ρ, for the proposed discrete geometric framework.

6   Applications

This section showcases the approach on a collection of structured meshes of subcortical structures from the UK Biobank database [24]. The typical mesh size is of a few thousand nodes (up to 20k). The framework was implemented in numpy. The tool mostly relies on efficient (sparse) linear algebra. Experiments were run on a standard laptop (i7-8550U CPU @ 1.80 GHz).

Surface Fairing. Surface fairing is the process of producing successively smoother approximations of a mesh geometry f. Most algorithms proceed by

---

[1] cf. supplementary material, available at arxiv.org/abs/1903.02429.

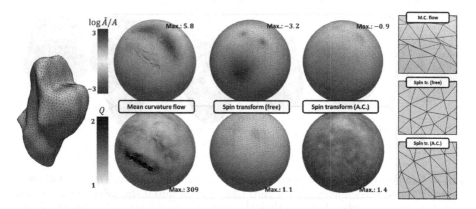

Fig. 4. Example surface flow of a subcortical structure (brain stem) to the reference sphere. Comparison of discrete spin transformations with an incompressible mean curvature (MC) flow. (Left) The brain stem. (Middle) Area distortion (top row, 0 distortion is best) and conformality error (bottom row, $Q = 1$ is best) displayed over the reference geometry. (Right) Zoom on the flowed triangulated mesh (A.C. $\equiv$ area constraint flow; free $\equiv$ unconstrained). Unlike MC flows, spin transformations naturally preserve the triangulation quality and are numerically stable. The area constrained variant yields a reasonable trade-off between preserving angles and areas without introducing unexpected artefacts.

minimizing a fairing energy, such as the membrane energy $E_M(f) \triangleq \int_S |\nabla f|^2 dA$ or the Willmore functional $E_W(f) \triangleq \int_S h^2 dA$. Recalling that $\Delta f = h\boldsymbol{n}$ and ignoring the dependence of Δ on f, gradient descent on E_M (resp. E_W) yields $\dot{f} \propto \Delta f$ ($\dot{f} \propto \Delta^2 f$). The former yields the widespread *mean curvature flow* $\dot{f} \propto -h\boldsymbol{n}$ that iteratively evolves points along the surface normal $\boldsymbol{n}$ with a magnitude proportional to the mean curvature h. Crane et al. [6] first suggested in the context of spin transformations to optimize E_W directly w.r.t. h, yielding the simple flow $\dot{h} := h$ *in curvature space*. A benefit of the approach is to decouple time and spatial integration, yielding numerically stable solutions across large time steps. We follow the same strategy. The prescribed change of curvature $\delta h := -\tau h$ is then (optionally filtered and) integrated into a new surface immersion $\tilde{f}$, by computing the corresponding spin transformation as per Sect. 5. Specifically, for a given target curvature $\bar{h}_i$ (say $h_i + \delta h_i$) and area $\bar{A}_i$, we let $\rho_i := \bar{h}_i \sqrt{\bar{A}_i / A_i}$ (Sect. 4). The standard unconstrained optimization (Eq. (8)) regularized with the face Laplacian $\mathbf{L}_f$ (or one of its powers) yields quasi-conformal transformations (Fig. 1). Large steps $\tau = 0.5\text{--}1$ typically remain stable. Whether ϕ is numerically integrable can be checked by monitoring the discrepancy between edges $\tilde{E}$ integrated as per Eq. (4), and edges recomputed from $\tilde{f}$ (*after* getting $\tilde{f}$ from Eq. (9)). The closedness generally holds within a few percent across several large steps without an explicit constraint, and within 10^{-6} with an explicit constraint (See footnote 1). A trade-off between conformality and area distortion is achieved by weighing in a soft constraint on the square norm of the logarithmic area distortion (Fig. 4).

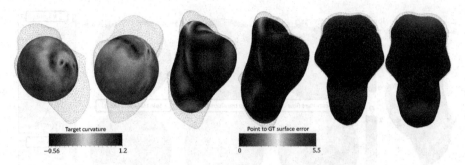

Fig. 5. Example extrusion of a brain stem from the reference sphere. The original shape is overlaid as a wireframe. (1st and 2nd) Close to the initial stage. The target mean curvature map is displayed, rather than the reconstruction error. Note that the shape flow in the next stages intuitively matches the information captured in these maps. (3rd and 4th) Intermediate stages in the flow, with overlayed reconstruction error. (5th to last) Reconstructed mesh from two views.

Comparison to Mean Curvature Flow. The procedure is compared with an incompressible mean curvature flow. Incompressibility is enforced to make the flow *less* prone to develop singularities, by adding a balloon energy $\langle h \rangle \boldsymbol{n}$, where $\langle h \rangle = \int_S h dA$ is the average mean curvature. Two metrics of interest, defined over the mesh surface, are the conformality error Q and the logarithmic area distortion $\epsilon_s = \log \tilde{A}/A$ (after normalising to the same total area). The quality factor Q measures how close-to-conformal a transformation is, as the ratio of the largest to smallest eigenvalues of the Jacobian of the mapping from f to $\tilde{f}$. For a conformal deformation, Q is identically 1 throughout the mesh. However the area distortion ϵ_s may become significant. Figure 4 exemplifies the general observation that the mean curvature flow realises a suboptimal trade-off between angle and area preservation. As expected, unconstrained discrete spin transformations are quasi-conformal. Unavoidable area distortion is introduced but mesh elements retain their original quality (right column, top and middle). To contrast, the mean curvature flow arbitrarily destroys the mesh quality, angle and area ratios in regions of high curvature. Area constrained discrete spin transformations implement a sensible compromise, whereby (i) area distortion is lessened; (ii) numerical stability is preserved; (iii) the conformal error increases rather uniformly over the entire mesh, leading to a graceful, slower loss of mesh quality. For surface fairing to a sphere, averaged over a random subset of 100 meshes in the dataset and taking the *maximum* over the mesh surface, we get the following – mean curvature flow: $Q = 97 \pm 165$, $\epsilon_s = 4.1 \pm 1.5$; unconstrained spin transformation: $Q = 1.42 \pm 0.08$, $\epsilon_s = 2.9 \pm 0.3$; area constrained: $Q = 1.7 \pm 0.2$, $\epsilon_s = 0.85 \pm 0.05$. For the area constrained spin transform, the maximum area discrepancy simply reflects a user-specified soft target.

Mesh Extrusion. The task is now to reconstruct ("extrude") a shape of interest back from a reference sphere, given its mean curvature h^* and area A^* mapped onto the sphere surface. There is to our knowledge very little done in that direction, even in related work [6,32]. To emphasize, we only wish to recover the original mesh up to *pose* and scale. Encoding scale presents little difficulty, and shape is invariant under changes of pose. To evaluate the reconstruction accuracy, we rigidly align and rescale the extruded shape to the original one, and compute the maximum distance from points on the extruded mesh to the original surface. The strategy for extrusion closely mirrors that of mesh fairing, whereby we get $\bar{h}_i$ from $\delta h_i := h_i^\star - h_i$, and set $\rho_i := \bar{h}_i \sqrt{A_i^\star / A_i}$. As a preliminary comment, note that the degree of challenge regarding mesh extrusion critically depends on the exact experimental setting and goal, as contrasted in the two following settings. The first experiment aims to estimate the accuracy that can be reached in the best scenario (somewhat upper bounded by the registration error). We take a collection of 300 subcortical meshes from the UK Biobank (incl. brain stems, caudate, putamen, accumbens, amygdala, hippocampus, thalamus, palladium) and flow them onto the unit sphere. We do not perform remeshing, only interpolating relevant maps to nodes and back to faces. We then directly reconstruct the mesh as described above. On average over the dataset, the maximum point-to-surface error is of 0.4mm. The distribution of error is widely spread over different structures, the most challenging being caudates (1.4) and hippocampi (1.2); and the least ones being the accumbens, amygdala, palladium and thalamus ($\sim$0.01–0.02). This matches our expectations, given that caudates and hippocampi are in fact highly non spherical. Thus very significant area or angle distortion is introduced when mapping onto the sphere. The second experiment investigates a more challenging setup, whereby the flowed surface is remapped onto a reference sphere with uniform meshing. Shape-specific vertex density as well as face aspect ratio, which reflect the area and angle distortion introduced during the fairing, are thus discarded. We experiment with a set of 100 brain stems (Fig. 5), which represent a happy medium between the most challenging and trivial structures, with a maximum reconstruction error of 1.4 ± 0.3 mm (2–4%). For the most challenging structures, various strategies to guide the reconstruction using either additional information obtained during the flow, or multiscale approaches with hierarchical encoding could be considered. This is left to explore in future work.

7   Conclusion

We have presented a method to manipulate surface meshes across very large deformations by prescribing mean curvature (half-density). The framework is well suited for mesh fairing and extrusion, *e.g.* to map shapes to, or back from a unit sphere. As a perspective, we believe the approach to have potential for pose-invariant shape analysis, specifically for *generative* modeling. Indeed mean curvature together with the metric generally is in one-to-one correspondence with the (closed) shape; this is in particular true for a spherical topology. We have shown how spin transformations computationally implement this insight. Therefore the shape *geometry* could be losslessly encoded as a scalar *function* on a template, making the modeling task more amenable to *learning*. In the smooth setting, spin transformations are a subgroup of conformal maps. This partly explains their numerical stability across large flow steps, a property inherited in the discrete setting. However, conformal maps can introduce significant area distortion, *e.g.* when flowing highly curved objects. An advantage of *discrete* spin transformations is to relax exact conformality, and allow the user to trade off angle for area preservation.

Acknowledgments. This work is supported by the EPSRC (grant ref no. EP/P023509/1) and the European Research Council (ERC) under the European Union's Horizon 2020 research and innovation programme (grant agreement No. 757173, project MIRA, ERC-2017-STG). DC is also supported by CAPES, Ministry of Education, Brazil (BEX 1500/15-05). KK is supported by the President's PhD Scholarship of Imperial College London. IW is supported by the Natural Environment Research Council (NERC).

References

1. Belongie, S., Malik, J., Puzicha, J.: Shape matching and object recognition using shape contexts. IEEE Trans. Pattern. Anal. Mach. Intell. **24**(4), 509–522 (2002)
2. Bronstein, A.M., Bronstein, M.M., Guibas, L.J., Ovsjanikov, M.: Shape Google: geometric words and expressions for invariant shape retrieval. ACM Trans. Graph. **30**(1), 1 (2011)
3. Bronstein, M.M., Bruna, J., LeCun, Y., Szlam, A., Vandergheynst, P.: Geometric deep learning: going beyond Euclidean data. IEEE Sig. Process. Mag. **34**(4), 18–42 (2017)
4. Cootes, T.F., Taylor, C.J., Cooper, D.H., Graham, J.: Active shape models - their training and application. Comput. Vis. Image Underst. **61**(1), 38–59 (1995)
5. Crane, K., Pinkall, U., Schröder, P.: Spin transformations of discrete surfaces. In: ACM Transactions on Graphics, vol. 30, p. 104. ACM (2011)
6. Crane, K., Pinkall, U., Schröder, P.: Robust fairing via conformal curvature flow. ACM Trans. Graph. **32**(4), 61 (2013)
7. Delingette, H.: General object reconstruction based on simplex meshes. IJCV **32**(2), 111–146 (1999)
8. Durrleman, S., et al.: Morphometry of anatomical shape complexes with dense deformations and sparse parameters. NeuroImage **101**, 35–49 (2014)
9. Fletcher, P.T., Lu, C., Pizer, S.M., Joshi, S.: Principal Geodesic Analysis for the study of nonlinear statistics of shape. IEEE TMI **23**(8), 995–1005 (2004)
10. Germanaud, D., et al.: Larger is twistier: spectral analysis of gyrification (SPANGY) applied to adult brain size polymorphism. NeuroImage **63**(3), 1257–1272 (2012)
11. Gu, X., Wang, Y., Chan, T.F., Thompson, P.M., Yau, S.T.: Genus zero surface conformal mapping and its application to brain surface mapping. IEEE TMI **23**(8), 949–958 (2004)
12. Hoffmann, T., Ye, Z.: A discrete extrinsic and intrinsic Dirac operator. arXiv (2018)
13. Hurdal, M.K., Stephenson, K.: Discrete conformal methods for cortical brain flattening. Neuroimage **45**(1), S86–S98 (2009)

14. Joshi, S., Pizer, S., Fletcher, P.T., Yushkevich, P., Thall, A., Marron, J.S.: Multi-scale deformable model segmentation and statistical shape analysis using medial descriptions. IEEE T Med. Imaging **21**(5), 538–550 (2002)
15. Kamberov, G., Pedit, F., Pinkall, U.: Bonnet pairs and isothermic surfaces. Duke Math. J. **92**(3), 637–644 (1998)
16. Kazhdan, M., Solomon, J., Ben-Chen, M.: Can mean-curvature flow be modified to be non-singular? In: Computer Graphics Forum, vol. 31, pp. 1745–1754. Wiley Online Library (2012)
17. Konukoglu, E., Glocker, B., Criminisi, A., Pohl, K.M.: WESD-weighted spectral distance for measuring shape dissimilarity. IEEE TPAMI **35**(9), 2284–2297 (2013)
18. Lam, W.Y., Pinkall, U.: Infinitesimal conformal deformations of triangulated surfaces in space. Discret. Comput. Geom. **60**(4), 831–858 (2018)
19. Liu, H.T.D., Jacobson, A., Crane, K.: A Dirac operator for extrinsic shape analysis. In: Computer Graphics Forum, vol. 36, pp. 139–149. Wiley Online Library (2017)
20. Lombaert, H., Arcaro, M., Ayache, N.: Brain transfer: spectral analysis of cortical surfaces and functional maps. In: Ourselin, S., Alexander, D.C., Westin, C.-F., Cardoso, M.J. (eds.) IPMI 2015. LNCS, vol. 9123, pp. 474–487. Springer, Cham (2015). https://doi.org/10.1007/978-3-319-19992-4_37
21. Lorenzi, M., Ayache, N., Pennec, X.: Schild's ladder for the parallel transport of deformations in time series of images. In: Székely, G., Hahn, H.K. (eds.) IPMI 2011. LNCS, vol. 6801, pp. 463–474. Springer, Heidelberg (2011). https://doi.org/10.1007/978-3-642-22092-0_38
22. Luo, F.: Combinatorial Yamabe flow on surfaces. CCM **6**(05), 765–780 (2004)
23. Meyer, M., Desbrun, M., Schröder, P., Barr, A.H.: Discrete differential geometry operators for triangulated 2-manifolds. In: Hege, H.C., Polthier, K. (eds.) Visualization and Mathematics III. MATHVISUAL, pp. 35–57. Springer, Heidelberg (2003). https://doi.org/10.1007/978-3-662-05105-4_2
24. Miller, K.L., et al.: Multimodal population brain imaging in the uk biobank prospective epidemiological study. Nat. Neurosci. **19**(11), 1523 (2016)
25. Myronenko, A., Song, X.: Point set registration: coherent point drift. IEEE Trans. Pattern Anal. Mach. Intell. **32**(12), 2262–2275 (2010)
26. Niethammer, M., et al.: Global medical shape analysis using the Laplace-Beltrami spectrum. In: Ayache, N., Ourselin, S., Maeder, A. (eds.) MICCAI 2007. LNCS, vol. 4791, pp. 850–857. Springer, Heidelberg (2007). https://doi.org/10.1007/978-3-540-75757-3_103
27. Ovsjanikov, M., Ben-Chen, M., Solomon, J., Butscher, A., Guibas, L.: Functional maps: a flexible representation of maps between shapes. ACM Trans. Graph. **31**(4), 30 (2012)
28. Raviv, D., Bronstein, M.M., Bronstein, A.M., Kimmel, R.: Volumetric heat kernel signatures. In: ACM Workshop on 3D Object Retrieval, pp. 39–44. ACM (2010)
29. Reuter, M., Wolter, F.E., Peinecke, N.: Laplace-Beltrami spectra as 'Shape-DNA' of surfaces and solids. Comput.-Aided Des. **38**(4), 342–366 (2006)
30. Vaillant, M., Glaunès, J.: Surface matching via currents. In: Christensen, G.E., Sonka, M. (eds.) IPMI 2005. LNCS, vol. 3565, pp. 381–392. Springer, Heidelberg (2005). https://doi.org/10.1007/11505730_32
31. Wachinger, C., Golland, P., Kremen, W., Fischl, B., Reuter, M., ADNI, et al.: Brainprint: a discriminative characterization of brain morphology. NeuroImage **109**, 232–248 (2015)

32. Ye, Z., Diamanti, O., Tang, C., Guibas, L., Hoffmann, T.: A unified discrete framework for intrinsic and extrinsic Dirac operators for geometry processing. In: Computer Graphics Forum, vol. 37, pp. 93–106. Wiley Online Library (2018)
33. Zhang, M., Fletcher, P.T.: Bayesian Principal Geodesic Analysis for estimating intrinsic diffeomorphic image variability. Med. Image Anal. 25(1), 37–44 (2015)

Registration

Local Optimal Transport for Functional Brain Template Estimation

T. Bazeille[1($\boxtimes$)], H. Richard[1], H. Janati[1,2], and B. Thirion[1]

[1] Inria, CEA Neurospin, Saclay, France
thomas.bazeille@inria.fr
[2] CREST ENSAE, Palaiseau, France

Abstract. An important goal of cognitive brain imaging studies is to model the functional organization of the brain; yet there exists currently no functional brain atlas built from existing data. One of the main roadblocks to the creation of such an atlas is the functional variability that is observed in subjects performing the same task; this variability goes far beyond anatomical variability in brain shape and size. Function-based alignment procedures have recently been proposed in order to improve the correspondence of activation patterns across individuals. However, the corresponding computational solutions are costly and not well-principled. Here, we propose a new framework based on optimal transport theory to create such a template. We leverage entropic smoothing as an efficient means to create brain templates without losing fine-grain structural information; it is implemented in a computationally efficient way. We evaluate our approach on rich multi-subject, multi-contrasts datasets. These experiments demonstrate that the template-based inference procedure improves the transfer of information across individuals with respect to state of the art methods.

Keywords: Brain · Atlas inference · fMRI · Functional alignment

1 Introduction

Brain Anatomical and Functional Variability. There is a very large biological variability between human brains, influenced by both genetic, developmental as well as environmental factors. It results in conspicuous anatomical differences, that have traditionally been characterized as diffeomorphic transformations and compensated by dedicated algorithms (see [1] for an application-oriented overview). Functional imaging, such as functional Magnetic Resonance Imaging (fMRI) also detects variations of activity across brain regions and thus provides a potential marker of variation in the functional organization of the brain i.e. the involvement of different neural modules when performing a given task. However, so far very little work has been dedicated to leverage fMRI contrasts to learn better correspondences between brains.

© Springer Nature Switzerland AG 2019
A. C. S. Chung et al. (Eds.): IPMI 2019, LNCS 11492, pp. 237–248, 2019.
https://doi.org/10.1007/978-3-030-20351-1_18

Capturing Functional Variability in Brain Responses. The implicit tenet of most analyses is that only anatomical information can be leveraged to estimate accurate correspondences between brains, while the unmatched functional variability is treated as a residual [2]. It might, at best, be reduced by smoothing; however, smoothing has been shown to create artificial overlaps of different functional territories, yielding biased models of functional organization (see e.g. [3]).

Meanwhile, the progressive improvement of fMRI contrast-to-noise ratio and resolution, as well as the development of *deep phenotyping* approaches, in which subjects were scanned under many conditions (e.g. [4,5]) opens a new perspective, namely that of using the acquired functional contrasts to learn interindividual correspondences. Diffeomorphic registrations were proposed to match functional variability across individuals [6] or features obtained in resting-state fMRI data [7], thus assuming a strong spatial regularity of the correspondence. This diffeomorphicity constraint was abandoned in other works, in particular in the popular *hyperalignment* framework [8,9], that attempts to identify and match activation patterns in the visual cortex without imposing strong regularity conditions. Following this line of research, direct functional correspondences obtained from resting-state fMRI data have been used to directly map functional areas across individuals [10,11]. While Hyperalignment is currently used to pool data across individuals to boost brain activity classification (see for e.g. [12]), it is not applied in more traditional group studies. Even if free correspondences potentially yield good alignment for two individuals, this framework has a hard time producing a subject independent model—a template.

Specifically, two core questions are still open: *(i)* What family of transformations should be allowed for cross-subject matching? In particular, should the transformations have some spatial regularity? *(ii)* How to estimate templates under weakly constrained deformation models?

Our Contribution. Following the intuitions that lead to the development of hyperalignment—map features across individuals under weak spatial constraints—we develop a novel framework based on optimal transport (OT), that is well suited to the estimation of explicit transformation models. In particular, we leverage the regularization procedures tied to this problem, namely entropic smoothing; we introduce spatial constraints in the matching by relying on local regions. Locality also clearly benefits to computational efficiency.

Second, we introduce an efficient template estimation procedure based on this OT deformation model. We evaluate the models by their ability to predict unseen data in new subjects, and benchmark the OT-based model against alternatives, including diffeomorphic registration, on two datasets that contain rich functional information in groups of subjects.

2   Theory

Notations. Let $p \in \mathcal{N}$, we denote $[p]$ the set of integers from 1 to p. Let $\mathbf{x} \in \mathbb{R}^d$, $\delta_{\mathbf{x}}$ will denote the Dirac mass at location $\mathbf{x}$. Given a brain region comprising

p voxels, we consider the d-dimensional signals observed in these voxels $\mathbf{x} = \{\mathbf{x}_1, ..., \mathbf{x}_p\}$. Here, these d-dimensional signals correspond to d activation maps observed in a given subject. We denote by $\mathbf{X}$ the $p \times d$ matrix obtained by concatenating the vectors in $\mathbf{x}$. $\| \|_F$ denotes Frobenius norm, and $tr(.)$ the trace operator.

Correspondences from an Optimal Transport Geometry Perspective. Let us consider the set $\mathbf{x}^s$ of functional signals in a given subject s. Following the intuitions of [10], the p vectors $\{\mathbf{x}_1^s, ..., \mathbf{x}_p^s\}$ together make up a measure μ^s lying on a latent manifold $\mathcal{F}_s$ embedded in $\mathbb{R}^d$. The discrete measure μ^s with positive weights $\mathbf{w}^s > 0$ and support $\{\mathbf{x}_1^s, ..., \mathbf{x}_p^s\} \in \mathcal{F}_s$ is defined as $\mu^s = \sum_{i=1}^{p} \mathbf{w}_i^s \delta_{\mathbf{x}_i^s}$. Note that in the present framework $\mathbf{w}^s = [\frac{1}{p}...\frac{1}{p}]$.

The difference between two measures $\mu^s = \sum_{i=1}^{p} \mathbf{w}_i^s \delta_{\mathbf{x}_i^s}$ and $\mu^t = \sum_{i=1}^{q} \mathbf{w}_i^t \delta_{\mathbf{x}_i^t}$, reflects the differences between individuals s and t. However, for $s \neq t$, the support of the $\mathcal{F}_s$ and $\mathcal{F}_t$ manifolds are distinct in general: two subjects do not exhibit the same set of responses, due to intrinsically different brain organization. Directly computing Kullback-Leibler divergence between μ^s and μ^t is useless, as non-coincident support leads to infinite values; fixing this mismatch by smoothing induces a loss of information. By contrast, the Wasserstein distance between μ^s and μ^t is well-defined [13]. In this framework, distance evaluation is tightly linked to functional alignment, as it is formulated as the task of finding an optimal coupling $\mathbf{R}^* \{\mathbf{x}_1^s, ..., \mathbf{x}_p^s\} \rightarrow \{\mathbf{x}_1^t, ..., \mathbf{x}_q^t\}, \mathbf{R} \in \mathbb{R}_+^{p \times q}$ Enforcing signal conservation and optimality of the alignment cost $\mathbf{C}(\mathbf{x}^s, \mathbf{x}^t)$ yields:

$$\mathbf{R}^* = \min_{\mathbf{R}} \sum_{i,j} \mathbf{R}_{i,j} \mathbf{C}(\mathbf{x}^s, \mathbf{x}^t)_{i,j} \tag{1}$$

$$\text{s.t. } \left(\sum_j \mathbf{R}_{i,j}\right)_i = w_i^s \text{ and } \left(\sum_i \mathbf{R}_{i,j}\right)_j = w_j^t \tag{2}$$

If both subjects functional data share a common number of voxels (i.e. $p = q$), and we search for a deterministic coupling (where each source has only one target voxel), this falls back to the optimal matching problem and makes $\mathbf{R}$ a permutation matrix minimal with respect to $\mathbf{C}(\mathbf{x^s}, \mathbf{x^t})$, that can be calculated through the Hungarian algorithm [14].

Kantorovich Relaxation. In general, admissible couplings in (1) are probabilistic, i.e. they can split the mass of a source location towards several target locations and their coefficients $\mathbf{R}_{i,j}$ encode the mass flow between points $\mathbf{x}_i^s$ and $\mathbf{x}_j^t$ [15].

One possibility, explored in [16] in the context of the MEG inverse problem, is to match the multi-dimensional signal distributions across subjects using a spatial-distance-based cost—matching preferentially voxels that are close in 3D space. The authors had to resort to unbalanced OT to deal with the variation of mass between subjects. With this formulation, μ^s and μ^t should be positive and of same norm, whereas functional signals usually have diverse amplitude across subjects and exhibit both positive and negative values, in proportions that vary across individuals. This approach requires to introduce several additional parameters to deal with unbalanced transport model. We chose another path here, closer to the hyperalignment concept [8], which is to transport voxels according to the functional information they carry. To do so, we use the discrepancy of the functional features as a cost function between voxels:

$$\forall i, j \in [p] \times [q], \, \mathbf{C}(\mathbf{x}^s, \mathbf{x}^t)_{i,j} = \|\mathbf{x}_i^s - \mathbf{x}_j^t\|_2^2$$

and couple the input measures μ^s and μ^t, where all voxels have a constant weight, respectively $1/p$ and $1/q$.

Entropic Regularization. We define the entropy of a coupling as

$$h(\mathbf{R}) = -\sum_{i,j} \mathbf{R}_{i,j}(\log(\mathbf{R}_{i,j}) - 1)$$

and use it as regularization function in Eq. 2, which becomes:

$$\mathbf{R}^{OT} = \min_{\mathbf{R}} \sum_{i,j} \mathbf{R}_{i,j} \mathbf{C}(\mathbf{X^s}, \mathbf{X^t})_{i,j} - \epsilon h(\mathbf{R}) \text{ s.t. } \left(\sum_j \mathbf{R}_{i,j}\right)_i = \frac{1}{p}, \left(\sum_i \mathbf{R}_{i,j}\right)_j = \frac{1}{q} \quad (3)$$

The entropic term makes the objective function ϵ-strongly convex, hence leading to a unique optimal solution for a given ϵ. Besides making computation of transport faster using Sinkhorn algorithm [17], this entropic regularization also acts as a smoothing of the solution.

Other Functional Alignment Methods. We may consider other transformations ϕ that map μ^s to μ^t as linear couplings $\mathbf{R}$ that predict the stacked feature values $\mathbf{X}^t$ from $\mathbf{X}^s$, under some given constraints ($\mathbf{R} \in \mathcal{R}$):

$$\mathbf{R}^* = \underset{\mathbf{R} \in \mathcal{R}}{argmin} \|\mathbf{R}(\mathbf{X^s}) - \mathbf{X^t}\|_F^2 \quad (4)$$

Hyperalignment [8], search a scaled orthogonal transformation $\mathbf{R} = \sigma\mathbf{Q}$ s.t. $\mathbf{Q}^T\mathbf{Q} = \mathbf{Id}, \sigma \in \mathbb{R}_+$. With this model, Eq. 4 is equivalent to the well-studied scaled Procrustes problem, solvable in closed form using the singular value decomposition of $\mathbf{X}^s\mathbf{X}^{t^T}$: $(\mathbf{U}, \mathbf{\Sigma}, \mathbf{V}) = \text{SVD}(\mathbf{X}^s\mathbf{X}^{t^T})$:

$$\mathbf{R}^{so} = \sigma\mathbf{Q} \text{ where } (\sigma, \mathbf{Q}) = \left(\frac{tr(\mathbf{\Sigma})}{\|\mathbf{X^s}\|_F^2}, \mathbf{UV}\right)$$

In the case where $p = q$, permutations and every coupling acceptable in strict optimal transport sense (Eq. 2) are part of this broader class of orthogonal transforms. By contrast, entropic regularization (Eq. 3) yields a non-orthogonal solution in general. It is possible to further relax the orthogonality constraint, by simply looking for a linear coupling $\mathbf{R}$ with a small norm. For computational efficiency, we consider here ℓ_2 norm penalization, yielding $\min_{\mathbf{R}}\|\mathbf{X}^t - \mathbf{R}\mathbf{X}^s\|_F^2 +$ $\frac{\lambda}{2}\|\mathbf{R}\|_2^2$. Using such a model, the alignment problem boils down to a ridge regression also solvable in closed form:

$$\mathbf{R}^{ridge} = \mathbf{X}^t\mathbf{X}^{sT}(\mathbf{X}^{sT}\mathbf{X}^\mathbf{s} + \lambda\mathbf{I_d})^{-1}$$

Full Brain Alignment. Although we aim at building a full-brain functional atlas, applying the above models to full brain suffers from two related issues: *(i)* it may create some non-local correspondences (e.g. cross-hemisphere swap) that are not neuroanatomically plausible; *(ii)* it is computationally heavy if not intractable.

In [9] functional alignment is used with a *searchlight* approach. In this popular procedure in neuroimaging an algorithm is applied on a set of 3D balls of radius r covering the brain. Regions described by multiple balls are predicted by averaging the prediction in each ball. Although this procedure does produce local correspondences, it is computationally costly. One needs approximately $\frac{p}{r^3}$ balls to ensure that all voxels are covered. Furthermore, the aggregation of several balls destroys the local structure enforced by the algorithms within each ball (sparsity, smoothness, orthogonality...).

We propose instead parcellation-based alignment. In a first step we do a functional clustering of data to find local non-overlapping clusters $c_1, \cdots, c_C$ of voxels with common activity patterns. In each of these clusters we find the optimal alignment transform and concatenate these local transforms to recover a full-brain transform with the desired regularities. Formally the optimal alignment transform to align two subjects $\mathbf{x}_{train}^s$ and subject $\mathbf{x}_{train}^t$ on the training session is obtained by solving the problem in each cluster $c \in \{c_1, \cdots, c_C\}$:

$$\mathbf{R}^*[c] = \mathbf{R}^*(\mathbf{X}_{train}^s[c], \mathbf{X}_{train}^t[c]), \text{with } * \in \{OT, so, ridge\} \tag{5}$$

On the test session $\mathbf{X}_{test}^t$ is predicted using $\mathbf{X}_{test}^s$ by:

$$\forall c \in \{c_1, \cdots, c_C\}\, \mathbf{X}_{test}^t[c] = \mathbf{R}^\star[c]\mathbf{X}_{test}^s[c] \tag{6}$$

Several algorithms perform well for functional clustering, in this study we used a computationally efficient recursive K-means method, where, for a target number of k regions, a first clustering into $\sqrt{k}$ pieces is obtained, and each of them is clustered in turn into $\sqrt{k}$ parts. Solving problem 3 or 4 within a local region constrains the solution to remain local and acts as a regularizer.

Template Inference. Pairwise correspondences do not scale well with many individuals. A template measure $\mathbf{T}$ is needed, which can be obtained by solving

$$\min_{\mathbf{T},\mathbf{R}_1...\mathbf{R}_n} \sum_{i=1}^{n}\|\mathbf{R}_s(\mathbf{T}) - \mathbf{X}^s\|_\star^2 \tag{7}$$

for the chosen loss $\|.\|_\star$ (Wasserstein or Frobenius). We solve it through alternate minimization iterating over:

- a **R**-step of independent alignment of the current template to every sample, thus estimating $\mathbf{R}_i, i = 1..n$
- a T-step where **T** is regressed to minimize jointly its distance to the samples.

$$\min_{\mathbf{R}_s} \|\mathbf{R}_s(\mathbf{T}) - \mathbf{X}^s\|_\star^2, \forall s \in [n] \qquad\qquad \mathbf{R}\text{-step}$$

$$\min_{\mathbf{T}} \sum_{s=1}^{n} \|\mathbf{R}_s(\mathbf{T}) - \mathbf{X}^s\|_\star^2 \qquad\qquad T\text{-step}$$

Note that, for all norms considered here, the T-step results in a quadratic problem solved by conjugate gradient. As initialization, we define first alignment operators list as identity, thus the first T-step is $\min_{\mathbf{T}} \sum_{s=1}^{n} \|\mathbf{T} - \mathbf{X}^s\|_2^2$ and the first template is the sample mean. In practice, we run 4 iterations of the alternate minimization, as we found that was sufficient for convergence.

Complexity Analysis. We recapitulate the algorithmic complexity of the OT algorithm for $p = q$. While the Hungarian algorithm finds an optimal (deterministic) permutation in a complexity of $O(p^3)$, Sinkhorn find a τ-approximate solution of the unregularized problem in $O(p^2\log(p)\tau^{-3})$ operations [13]. If the brain contains P voxels divided evenly into k clusters, the overall complexity of the problem is thus $O(\frac{P^2}{k}\log(\frac{P}{k})\tau^{-3})$. Increasing k thus reduces the computational burden; on the other hand, choosing k too large yields small clusters, hence reduces the benefit of OT. In the following experiments, we set $k = 200$.

3   Experiments

Datasets. To benchmark these methods and assess their prediction accuracy, we ran experiments on two datasets, where individual data were previously registered in MNI-space following standard procedure (SPM12 software called though Nipype for IBC, HCP pipeline for HCP). The "Individual Brain Charting" (IBC) [5] contains scans of the same 13 participants for a wide variety of cognitive tasks. The data were acquired using a 3 T scanner (acquisition resolution of 1.5 mm resampled at 3 mm after spatial normalization). We worked directly on activation maps: for a given functional contrast, they associate an activation statistic with each voxel.

We learn alignment between subjects between $d = 53$ contrasts derived from data acquired with antero-posterior (AP) EPI phase encoding; to assess the quality of our predictions, we also use 53 contrasts acquired in separate sessions using the same experimental paradigms with posterior-anterior (PA) EPI phase encoding. Note that the resulting AP/PA distortions were estimated and corrected with FSL's topup software prior to image pre-processing. Human Connectome Project (HCP) [18] is the collection of neuroimaging and behavioral data on 1,200 normal young adults, aged 22–35. For our experiment we focused on 20 randomly chosen subjects. For each, we used the $d = 25$ statistical maps available in both left-to-right(LR) and right-to-left(RL) phase encoding, resampled

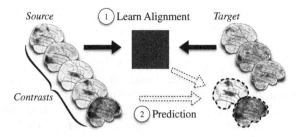

Fig. 1. Pairwise prediction of target subject from aligned source subject

at 3 mm after spatial normalization. We learn alignment between subjects using LR images and assess prediction on RL acquisitions.

Pairwise Alignment Benchmarks. In pairwise prediction, we first learn the optimal alignment operator between a source and a target subject on training data. We then use this alignment and supplementary images of the source subject to predict additional data of the target subject and score this prediction against the true target subject images using a prediction metric (see Fig. 1).

We use this straightforward set-up on IBC and HCP datasets to compare prediction performance of the alignment methods presented above, applied on a parcellation of the brain: (i) Scaled-Orthogonal Transform, (ii) Ridge Regression, (iii) Optimal Permutation, (iv) OT with entropic smoothing. We compare these to two baselines, the identity transform (that predicts the target subject as the source subject data), and a multi-purpose state-of-the-art diffeomorphic medical image registration algorithm: symmetric image normalization (SyN) [19]. SyN yields a diffeomorphic mapping maximizing Mattes mutual information between local regions. Since it works only for scalar images, it was applied only on the principal components of the training set of images. In a second experiment, we study the influence of the amount entropic regularization used in OT loss on both datasets. Obviously some pairs of subjects have more similar functional data than others. To make our evaluation process robust to this variability, we tested every method on the same set of 20 pairs of subjects chosen randomly

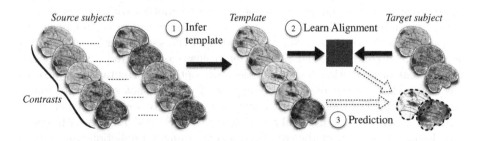

Fig. 2. Template-based prediction of left-out subject

in each dataset. Our implementation relies on Nilearn for data handling, open-source solvers (Scikit-learn, POT for Sinkhorn, antspy for SyN).

Template-Based Alignment Benchmarks. To evaluate template-based prediction accuracy, we split the IBC dataset randomly into two folds of 7 and 6 subjects. We inferred the template from the train subjects across every AP and PA contrast. We then learned an alignment operator between each of the test subject and the template using AP contrasts and try to predict their PA contrasts that we scored using predictions metrics (see Fig. 2). We compare the results of the same methods quantitatively in terms of prediction loss. In a third experiment, we infer a template on which we learn alignment for all subjects using AP data. We then apply these alignments to left out PA data to bring all our subject in a common space. In this common space, we a run a one sample-test and compare the group effects detected by each method, for specific conditions.

Prediction Metrics. To measure the quality of our prediction $\mathbf{R}_i(\mathbf{X})$, at the voxel level, against the ground truth $\mathbf{Y}$, we defined η^2, the normalized reconstruction error, as:

$$\eta^2_\star(\mathbf{Y}, \mathbf{Y}_i, \mathbf{X}) = 1 - \frac{\sum_{i=1}^n (\mathbf{Y}_i - \mathbf{R}_i \mathbf{X})^2}{\sum_{i=1}^n \mathbf{Y}_i^2},$$

where $\star$ stands for identity, ridge, scaled orthogonal, OT. An η^2 value of 0 means that the quality of the prediction is equivalent to predicting 0 along all the dimensions. A perfect prediction yields a value of 1. To focus on the prediction improvement that can be made through alignment - independently of the preexisting distance between data to align - we assess performance quantitatively using a reconstruction ratio R_{η^2}. This ratio is also defined at voxel level and is superior to 0 if the voxel is predicted better by aligned data than by raw data.

$$R_{\eta^2_\star}(\mathbf{Y}, R, \mathbf{X}) = 1 - \frac{\sum_{i=1}^n (\mathbf{Y}_i - \mathbf{R}_i \mathbf{X})^2}{\sum_{i=1}^n (\mathbf{Y}_i - \mathbf{X}_i)^2} = 1 - \frac{1 - \eta^2_\star(\mathbf{Y}, \mathbf{R}_i, \mathbf{X})}{1 - \eta^2_{id}(\mathbf{Y}, Id, \mathbf{X})}$$

4   Results

Pairwise Alignment. Figure 3 shows that functional alignment methods generally improve prediction quality from one subject to another with respect to the identity, though not uniformly over the cortex. Sensory and motor regions typically obtain high scores, showing the stability of the signals across subjects in these areas; by contrast, other regions obtain low scores overall. Syn offers no improvement of prediction scores, nor does the optimal permutation of voxels. This means that a strict one-to-one mapping of voxels is not suitable for functional alignment. For the three other methods, we clearly see different behavior between regions with high signal-to-noise ratio (SNR) and regions with lower SNR. Figure 4(a-b), report the compared distributions of predictions ratios R_{η^2} on IBC and HCP datasets and are consistent with previous observations. Ridge

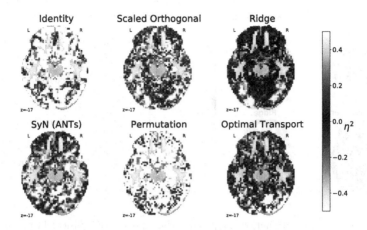

Fig. 3. Prediction score $\eta^2(\mathbf{Y}, \mathbf{R}, \mathbf{X})$ of target subject 9 using alignment with subject 15 (IBC dataset, z $= -17$ mm).

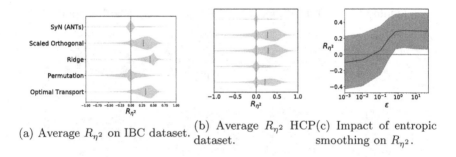

(a) Average R_{η^2} on IBC dataset.

(b) Average R_{η^2} HCP dataset.

(c) Impact of entropic smoothing on R_{η^2}.

Fig. 4. Pairwise prediction: (a), (b) alignment score of methods on 20 pairs of IBC/HCP datasets. (c) Effect of entropic regularization (OT) IBC dataset.

and OT outperform all other methods on IBC dataset whereas Scaled Orthogonal and Ridge perform slightly better on HCP dataset. Figure 4(c), shows that entropic regularization strongly improves prediction scores up to an inflexion point.

Template Alignment. In Fig. 5, we can observe that prediction accuracy is strongly improved by the use of a learned template in most brain regions, which establishes that functional alignment performs well to estimate cross-subject correspondences and identify a latent brain activity template. It also validates that our template estimation procedure manages to capture some of the inter-subject variability in its mapping process.

Figure 5 shows that Scaled orthogonal, Ridge and Optimal transport are equally accurate at predicting new subject data overall. However they do so in dissimilar ways. Ridge regression tend to predict 0 in regions with low SNR. This strong smoothing effect comes at the expense of providing predictions that are not very precise for high SNR regions. On the contrary, Optimal Transport

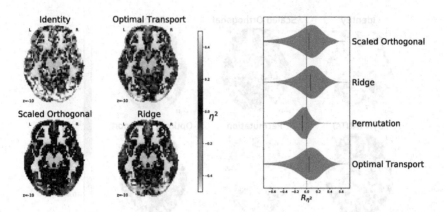

Fig. 5. Template-based prediction: map yields the score of IBC-subject 11 missing data prediction. Plot shows prediction ratio distributions across test subjects, i.e. gain from alignment over prediction from group average.

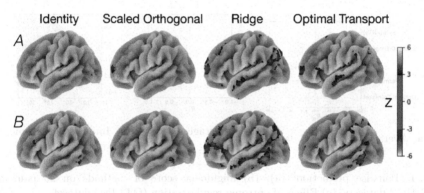

Fig. 6. 1 sample test *Zscores* after aligning IBC subjects to template. 2 conditions: (A) *Match (hcp-relational task)* (B) *0 back place (hcp-wm task)*

makes large mistakes in low SNR regions but predicts high-SNR regions more accurately. This behavior is desirable in a template-building procedure since it better preserves specificity and structure in functional signal.

We finally consider a realistic use case, where test data would be functionally aligned in view of a group study (one-sample t-test). We present the ensuing group-level brain maps, projected on the cortical surface, in Fig. 6, for 2 contrasts. The *Match* contrast (borrowed from a visual comparison task on artificial textures), shows that both ridge and optimal transport recover regions in the anterior and posterior segments of the superior temporal sulcus that would not be detected using standard approaches, or scale-orthogonal functional alignment. For the *0-back place* contrast, borrowed from a visual matching task on place images, OT- and Ridge-based alignment recover regions in the temporo occipital junction and inferior parietal sulcus that would not be detected using standard approaches, nor by scale-orthogonal functional alignment. In particular, place sensitive regions of the ventral and dorsal visual cortex seem to have been sucessfully recovered by the functional alignment approach.

5 Discussion

We demonstrated in this work that functional alignment can be used to infer a template that captures a good-enough level of detail to generalize to data from new subjects. This confirms prior results from [8,9], but we moreover introduced a principled way to build brain templates in this framework. Among the possible approaches to identify correspondences and infer a template, weakly-regularized ones proved to be particularly efficient: local ridge regression is clearly the less structured method, yet it yields high accuracy, typically higher than the more constrained local Procrustes alignment; smooth OT performed better than non-smooth OT. Eventually, the most constrained approach, Syn, did not perform well on this task. Importantly, these results do not reflect mere overfit, as the predictions are made on images not used for alignment and template inference. Additional extensions can be brought to the current framework:

- First, remove the reliance on a fixed parcellation of the brain, that is probably suboptimal to identify cross-subjects correspondences. This can be done by ensembling results obtained from multiple parcellations [20]. This should improve accuracy, albeit at a higher computation cost.
- Second, learn correspondences between subjects and toward a common template from resting-state data, following the ideas in [7,11]. This will be especially useful since resting-state data are more and more frequently used in group studies and represent the standard for brain organization studies.

Acknowledgments. This project has received funding from the European Union's Horizon 2020 Research and Innovation Programme under Grant Agreement No. 785907 (HBP SGA2).

References

1. Klein, A., et al.: Evaluation of 14 non linear deformation algorithms applied to human brain MRI registration. Neuroimage **46**(3), 786–802 (2009)
2. Thirion, B.: Functional neuroimaging group studies. In: Thompson, W., Ombao, H., Lindquist, M., Aston, J. (eds.) Handbook of Neuroimaging Data Analysis, pp. 335–354. Chapman and Hall and CRC, Boca Raton (2016). Chap 12
3. Fedorenko, E., Behr, M.K., Kanwisher, N.: Functional specificity for high-level linguistic processing in the human brain. Proc. Nat. Acad. Sci. **108**(39), 16428–16433 (2011)
4. Barch, D.M., et al.: Function in the human connectome: task-fMRI and individual differences in behavior. Neuroimage **80**, 169–189 (2013)
5. Pinho, A.L., et al.: Individual brain charting, a high-resolution fMRI dataset for cognitive mapping. Sci. Data **5**, 180105 (2018)

6. Sabuncu, M.R., Singer, B.D., Conroy, B., Bryan, R.E., Ramadge, P.J., Haxby, J.V.: Function-based intersubject alignment of human cortical anatomy. Cereb. Cortex **20**, 130 (2010)

7. Nenning, K.H., Liu, H., Ghosh, S.S., Sabuncu, M.R., Schwartz, E., Langs, G.: Diffeomorphic functional brain surface alignment: functional demons. NeuroImage **156**, 456–465 (2017)

8. Haxby, J.V., et al.: A common, high-dimensional model of the representational space in human ventral temporal cortex. Neuron **72**(2), 404–416 (2011)

9. Guntupalli, J.S., Hanke, M., Halchenko, Y.O., Connolly, A.C., Ramadge, P.J., Haxby, J.V.: A model of representational spaces in human cortex. Cereb. Cortex **26**(6), 2919–2934 (2016)

10. Langs, G., et al.: Learning an Atlas of a cognitive process in its functional geometry. In: Székely, G., Hahn, H.K. (eds.) IPMI 2011. LNCS, vol. 6801, pp. 135–146. Springer, Heidelberg (2011). https://doi.org/10.1007/978-3-642-22092-0_12

11. Langs, G., et al.: Identifying shared brain networks in individuals by decoupling functional and anatomical variability. Cereb. Cortex **26**(10), 4004–4014 (2016)

12. Güçlü, U., van Gerven, M.A.J.: Deep neural networks reveal a gradient in the complexity of neural representations across the ventral stream. J. Neurosci. **35**(27), 10005–10014 (2015)

13. Peyré, G., Cuturi, M.: Computational optimal transport. arXiv e-prints, page arXiv:1803.00567, March 2018

14. Munkres, J.: Algorithms for the assignment and transportation problems. J. Soc. Ind. Appl. Math. **5**(1), 32–38 (1957)

15. Kantorovitch, L.: On the translocation of masses. Manag. Sci. **5**(1), 1–4 (1958)

16. Gramfort, A., Peyré, G., Cuturi, M.: Fast optimal transport averaging of neuroimaging data. CoRR, abs/1503.08596 (2015)

17. Cuturi, M.: Sinkhorn distances: lightspeed computation of optimal transport. In: Advances in Neural Information Processing Systems, pp. 2292–2300 (2013)

18. Van Essen, D.C., et al.: The WU-minn human connectome project: an overview. Neuroimage **80**, 62–79 (2013)

19. Avants, B.B., Epstein, C.L., Grossman, M., Gee, J.C.: Symmetric diffeomorphic image registration with cross-correlation: evaluating automated labeling of elderly and neurodegenerative brain. Med. Image Anal. **12**(1), 26–41 (2008)

20. Hoyos-Idrobo, A., Varoquaux, G., Thirion, B.: Towards a faster randomized parcellation based inference. In: PRNI 2017–7th International Workshop on Pattern Recognition in NeuroImaging, Toronto, Canada, June 2017

Unsupervised Deformable Registration for Multi-modal Images via Disentangled Representations

Chen Qin[1,2]([⊠]), Bibo Shi[2], Rui Liao[2], Tommaso Mansi[2], Daniel Rueckert[1], and Ali Kamen[2]

[1] Department of Computing, Imperial College London, London, UK
c.qin15@imperial.ac.uk
[2] Digital Services, Digital Technology & Innovation, Siemens Healthineers, Princeton, NJ, USA

Abstract. We propose a fully unsupervised multi-modal deformable image registration method (UMDIR), which does not require any ground truth deformation fields or any aligned multi-modal image pairs during training. Multi-modal registration is a key problem in many medical image analysis applications. It is very challenging due to complicated and unknown relationships between different modalities. In this paper, we propose an unsupervised learning approach to reduce the multi-modal registration problem to a mono-modal one through image disentangling. In particular, we decompose images of both modalities into a common latent shape space and separate latent appearance spaces via an unsupervised multi-modal image-to-image translation approach. The proposed registration approach is then built on the factorized latent shape code, with the assumption that the intrinsic shape deformation existing in original image domain is preserved in this latent space. Specifically, two metrics have been proposed for training the proposed network: a latent similarity metric defined in the common shape space and a learning-based image similarity metric based on an adversarial loss. We examined different variations of our proposed approach and compared them with conventional state-of-the-art multi-modal registration methods. Results show that our proposed methods achieve competitive performance against other methods at substantially reduced computation time.

1 Introduction

Different medical image modalities, such as Magnetic Resonance Imaging (MRI), Computed Tomography (CT), and Positron Emission Tomography (PET), show unique tissue features at different spatial resolutions. In clinical practice, multiple image modalities must often be fused for diagnostic or interventional purpose, providing the combination of complementary information. However, images from different modalities are often acquired with different scanners and at different time points with some intra-patient anatomical changes. It is of great importance to register multi-modal images for an accurate analysis and interpretation.

© Springer Nature Switzerland AG 2019
A. C. S. Chung et al. (Eds.): IPMI 2019, LNCS 11492, pp. 249–261, 2019.
https://doi.org/10.1007/978-3-030-20351-1_19

Multi-modal image registration is a challenging problem, due to the unknown and complex relationship between the intensity distributions of the images to be aligned. Also, there could be presence of features in one modality but missing in another. Previous multi-modal image approaches either rely on information theoretic measures such as mutual information or on landmarks being identified in both images. However, information theoretic measures often ignores spatial information, and anatomical landmarks cannot always be localized in both images. Furthermore, landmark detection can be time-consuming or impossible in image-guided intervention.

In this paper, we propose a novel unsupervised registration method for aligning intra-subject multi-modal images, without the need of ground truth deformation fields, aligned multi-modal image pairs or any anatomical landmarks during training. To address this, our main idea is to learn a parameterized registration function via reducing the multi-modal registration problem to a mono-modal one in latent embedding space. In particular, our method decomposes images into a domain-invariant latent shape representation and a domain-specific appearance code based on the multi-modal unsupervised image-to-image translation framework (MUNIT) [9]. With the assumption that the intrinsic shape deformation between multi-modal image pairs is preserved in the domain-invariant shape space, we propose to learn an unsupervised diffeomorphic registration network directly based on the disentangled shape representations. A similarity criterion thus can be defined in the latent space, minimizing the latent shape distance between warped moving image and target one. Additionally, a complimentary learning-based similarity metric is also proposed, which is defined via an adversarial loss to distinguish whether a pair of images are sufficiently aligned or not in the image domain. Since transformation is learned from a domain-invariant space, the method is directly applicable to bi-directional multi-modal registration without extra efforts.

Our main contributions can be summarized as follows: First, we present a learning-based unsupervised multi-modal deformable image registration method that does not require any aligned image pairs or anatomical landmarks. Second, we propose to learn a *bi-directional* registration function based on disentangled shape representation by optimizing the proposed similarity criterion defined on both latent and image space. Third, we demonstrate that our proposed methods are competitive to state-of-the-art multi-modal image registration solutions in terms of accuracy, and have a much faster speed. To the best of our knowledge, this is the first work investigating a *fully unsupervised* deep learning based method for *multi-modal* deformable image registration. Though our work is currently demonstrated on 2D images, it can be readily extended for 3D volumes.

Related Work: One category of the classical and standard methods for multi-modal registration are information theory based approaches, which utilize mutual information (MI) as a similarity measure to align multi-modal images. It showed a great success in rigid registration of multi-modal medical images, and later its variations such as normalized MI and local MI etc. [16] have also been proposed to tackle deformable registration. However, such methods are often based on intensity probability distribution, and thus ignore spatial information of anatomical structures. An alternative way to address multi-modal image registration problem is to reduce the problem to a mono-modal one. They either synthesize one modality from another or map both modalities to a common domain. In order to reduce the appearance gap between different modalities, image synthesis can be achieved by taking advantage of prior knowledge on physical properties of imaging devices [19] or capturing intensity relationships using learning-based methods [3]. As to mapping both modalities to a common space, the assumption is that both modalities share the same anatomical structure or feature, and thus can be used to establish meaningful correspondences.

In recent years, many deep learning approaches have also been proposed in image registration domain. In supervised setting, these methods require ground truth deformation fields during the training process. However, as ground truth deformations are rarely available, they commonly synthetically generate geometric deformations as ground truth and then transform one of the image pairs [10,20]. Some other methods employ kind of weakly-supervised way for image registration, where they rely on the alignment of multiple labelled corresponding anatomical structures for individual image pairs during the training [8]. On the other hand, for unsupervised deformable image registration, most current approaches proposed to use convolutional neural networks [2,17] or probabilistic framework [4,12] with a spatial transformation function [11], which were trained by minimizing conventional image similarity metrics. Instead of using specific similarity metrics, Fan et al. [5] proposed a similar registration network which was trained along with learning a similarity measure by using a discriminator network to judge whether a pair of images are sufficiently aligned. However, these unsupervised methods mainly focus on mono-modal image registration.

2   Proposed Method

Our goal is to learn a multi-modal deformable registration network in a fully unsupervised manner: without ground truth deformation fields, anatomical landmarks, or aligned multi-modal image pairs for training. We achieve this by embedding images of different modalities into a domain-invariant space via image disentangling, where any meaningful geometrical deformation can be directly derived in the latent space. Our method mainly consists of three parts: image disentangling network via unpaired image-to-image translation, a deformable registration network in the disentangled latent space and an adversarial network that implicitly learns a similarity metric in image space. A schematic illustration of our method is shown in Figs. 1 and 2.

2.1   Image Disentangling via Unpaired Image-to-Image Translation

Huang et al. [9] and Lee et al. [13] have proposed to solve unpaired image-to-image translation problem through disentangled image representations, where

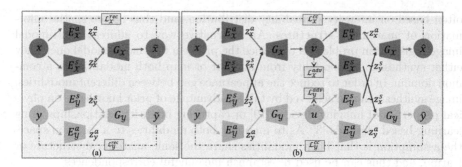

Fig. 1. Image-to-image translation framework (Sect. 2.1). x and y are sample images in $\mathcal{X}$ and $\mathcal{Y}$ domain respectively. $\{E_\mathcal{X}^s, E_\mathcal{Y}^s\}$ and $\{E_\mathcal{X}^a, E_\mathcal{Y}^a\}$ are corresponding shape encoders and appearance encoders. $\{G_\mathcal{X}, G_\mathcal{Y}\}$ are image generators. (a) Image self-reconstruction with $\{\tilde{x}, \tilde{y}\}$ reconstructed from $\{x, y\}$. (b) Image-to-image translation and cross-cycle reconstruction. $\{u, v\}$ are translated images from $\{x, y\}$ to domain $\{\mathcal{Y}, \mathcal{X}\}$ respectively. $\{\hat{x}, \hat{y}\}$ are cross-cycle reconstructed images. Black dotted lines and tilde notation indicate the consistency between variables.

images are embedded into a domain-invariant attribute space and a domain-specific attribute space, as shown in Fig. 1. As described and shown in [9], domain-invariant attribute mainly captures the underlying spatial structure, and domain-specific attribute corresponds to the rendering of structure that is determined by imaging physics in our application. This approach formed the basis of our work. We briefly describe its main concept below that is related to our following registration work.

Let $x \in \mathcal{X}$ and $y \in \mathcal{Y}$ denote unpaired images from two different domains, or in our application, two different imaging modalities. As illustrated in Fig. 1, image x is disentangled into a shape (content) code z_x^s in a domain-invariant space $\mathcal{S}$ and an appearance code z_x^a in a domain specific space $\mathcal{A}_\mathcal{X}$, where $E_\mathcal{X}^s$ and $E_\mathcal{X}^a$ encode x to z_x^s and z_x^a respectively. The generator $G_\mathcal{X}$ generates images conditioned on both shape and appearance vectors. Image-to-image translation is performed by swapping the latent codes in two domains, such as $v = G_\mathcal{X}(z_x^a, z_y^s)$ so that image y is translated to target domain $\mathcal{X}$. To train the framework for image-to-image translation and achieve representation disentanglement, a bidirectional reconstruction loss is used which comprises image self-reconstruction loss and latent reconstruction loss, i.e.,

$$\mathcal{L}_\mathcal{X}^{rec} = \mathbb{E}_x \big[\|G_\mathcal{X}(E_\mathcal{X}^s(x), E_\mathcal{X}^a(x)) - x\|_1 \big], \tag{1a}$$

$$\mathcal{L}_{\mathcal{X}^s}^{lat} = \mathbb{E}_{x,y} \big[\|E_\mathcal{Y}^s(G_\mathcal{Y}(z_x^s, z_y^a)) - z_x^s\|_1 \big], \tag{1b}$$

$$\mathcal{L}_{y^a}^{lat} = \mathbb{E}_{x,y} \big[\|E_\mathcal{Y}^a(G_\mathcal{Y}(z_x^s, z_y^a)) - z_y^a\|_1 \big]. \tag{1c}$$

In order to better preserve the shape information, we also propose to incorporate an extra loss term to ensure cross-cycle consistency [13]:

$$\mathcal{L}^{cc} = \mathcal{L}_\mathcal{X}^{cc} + \mathcal{L}_\mathcal{Y}^{cc} = \mathbb{E}_{x,y} \big[\|G_\mathcal{X}(E_\mathcal{Y}^s(u), E_\mathcal{X}^a(v)) - x\|_1 + \|G_\mathcal{Y}(E_\mathcal{X}^s(v), E_\mathcal{Y}^a(u)) - y\|_1 \big]. \tag{2}$$

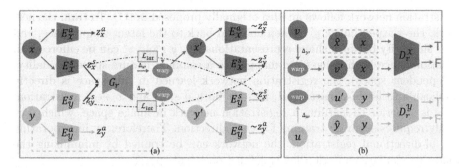

Fig. 2. Overview architecture of the proposed models. (a) Multi-modal image registration via disentangled representations (Sect. 2.2). x' and y' are warped images from x and y. (b) Learning-based similarity metric in image space. u, v and $\hat{x}$, $\hat{y}$ are translated and reconstructed images respectively adopted from Fig. 1. (a)+(b) Multi-modal image registration via combined metrics (Sect. 2.3). G_r is the registration network in latent space. $D_r^{\mathcal{X}}, D_r^{\mathcal{Y}}$ are discriminators in image space.

Besides, adversarial losses $L_{\mathcal{X}}^{adv}$ and $L_{\mathcal{Y}}^{adv}$ are employed to match the distribution of translated images to the image distribution in the target domain. Overall, our image-to-image translation network is trained by a weighted sum of image self-reconstruction loss, latent representation reconstruction loss, adversarial loss and the cross-cycle consistency loss. For more details, please refer to [9,13].

2.2 Multi-modal Image Registration via Disentangled Representations

With image-to-image translation and disentangled attributes being learned, we are able to reduce multi-modal registration problem to a mono-modal one by embedding images onto the domain-invariant latent space and learn the deformation there. A explanatory figure of our proposed network is shown in Fig. 2(a).

Specifically, images from different modalities are disentangled into a shared shape space $\mathcal{S}$ and different appearance spaces $\mathcal{A}_{\mathcal{X}}$ and $\mathcal{A}_{\mathcal{Y}}$ respectively. The latent shape representations z_x^s and z_y^s contain high-level structure information of images which is capable of restoring the original image by combining with the appearance code. Relying on this, we propose to learn a deformable registration network by aligning images via these disentangled shape representations. When registering a moving image $y \in \mathcal{Y}$ to a fixed image $x \in \mathcal{X}$, the structure of the warped moving image $y' \in \mathcal{Y}$ should be close to that of the fixed one while keeping the appearance unchanged. Therefore, a similarity criterion for training the registration network can be defined in the disentangled latent shape space. Specifically, we propose to learn a diffeomorphic registration network that receives latent shape representations as inputs and predicts a velocity field w. Deformation Δ between moving and fixed images is defined as an exponential map with respect to the velocities: $\Delta = \exp(w)$, which is implemented by an exponentiation layer as proposed in [12]. The detailed architecture of the registration network follows an idea originally proposed in [17]. To train the network, the warped image y' is then encoded back to the latent shape space, and thus similarity between shape representations $E_{\mathcal{Y}}^s(y')$ and z_x^s can be enforced. In addition, since both images are mapped to a common feature space (modality-independent space), the registration network learned in this space is directly applicable to be **bi-directional**, i.e., for both $y \rightarrow x$ and $x \rightarrow y$ registration. This is superior to learning a registration network in image space, which normally requires separate training for each direction. Therefore, by incorporating the bi-directional registration, the network can be trained by minimizing the following similarity metric that is defined on latent space:

$$\mathcal{L}_{lat} = \mathbb{E}_{x,y}\big[\|E_{\mathcal{Y}}^s(y') - z_x^s\|_1 + \|E_{\mathcal{X}}^s(x') - z_y^s\|_1\big] + \lambda_\Delta\big[\mathcal{H}(\nabla_{i,j}\Delta_{y'}) + \mathcal{H}(\nabla_{i,j}\Delta_{x'})\big], \quad (3)$$

where we penalize the gradients of the deformation fields $\Delta_{y'}$ and $\Delta_{x'}$ using an approximation of Huber loss [17] $\mathcal{H}(\nabla_{i,j}\Delta) = \sqrt{\epsilon + \sum_{m=i,j}(\nabla_i\Delta m^2 + \nabla_j\Delta m^2)}$ along both i and j directions to ensure the smoothness. λ_Δ is a regularization parameter for a balance (trade-off) between different terms, and $\epsilon = 0.01$.

2.3 Multi-modal Image Registration via Combined Metrics

While disentangled latent shape representations can effectively capture high-level structural information, training with a latent similarity criterion only could possibly ignore some detailed structure deformations. To compensate this, we propose to combine the latent similarity criterion with an additional learning-based similarity metric in image space, as shown in Fig. 2(b).

Similarly, here we define the learning-based similarity metric in image space also via image-to-image translation. However, during image-to-image translation, there could inevitably exist some mismatch of distributions between synthesized images and target images, especially when appearance distributions of real images are complex. Thus, mono-modal registration methods based on intensity similarities may not be sufficient. Therefore, instead of using a specific intensity-based similarity measure, similar to [5], we propose to learn a similarity metric function formulated by a patch GAN discriminator, which is trained to distinguish if a pair of image patches is well-aligned or not. Different from [5], to mitigate influence of distribution mismatch, we utilize the cross-cycle consistency of the translation network when designing the real pairs (well-aligned) and fake pairs (registered by network), i.e., $\{G_{\mathcal{X}}(E_{\mathcal{Y}}^s(u), E_{\mathcal{X}}^a(v)), x\}$ and $\{v', x\}$, where v' indicates the corresponding warped images of v. This is to enforce the discriminator to learn structure alignment instead of distribution differences. Architecture of discriminators follows the design of the feature encoder in registration network. Overall, we formulate the combined problem using the improved Wasserstein GAN (WGAN-GP) [6]: the image registration network G_r (generator) and two discriminators $D_r^{\mathcal{X}}$ and $D_r^{\mathcal{Y}}$ can be trained via alternatively optimizing the respective composite loss functions:

$$\mathcal{L}_{D_r^{\mathcal{X}}} = \mathbb{E}_{\tilde{q} \sim \mathbb{P}_f} \left[D_r^{\mathcal{X}}(\tilde{q}) \right] - \mathbb{E}_{q \sim \mathbb{P}_r} \left[D_r^{\mathcal{X}}(q) \right] + \lambda_{grad} \cdot \mathcal{L}_{grad}^{\mathcal{X}} \tag{4a}$$

$$\mathcal{L}_{D_r^{\mathcal{Y}}} = \mathbb{E}_{\tilde{p} \sim \mathbb{P}_f} \left[D_r^{\mathcal{Y}}(\tilde{p}) \right] - \mathbb{E}_{p \sim \mathbb{P}_r} \left[D_r^{\mathcal{Y}}(p) \right] + \lambda_{grad} \cdot \mathcal{L}_{grad}^{\mathcal{Y}} \tag{4b}$$

$$\mathcal{L}_{G_r} = -\mathbb{E}_{\tilde{q} \sim \mathbb{P}_f} \left[D_r^{\mathcal{X}}(\tilde{q}) \right] - \mathbb{E}_{\tilde{p} \sim \mathbb{P}_f} \left[D_r^{\mathcal{Y}}(\tilde{p}) \right] + \alpha \mathcal{L}_{lat}, \tag{4c}$$

where $D_r^{\mathcal{X}}$ and $D_r^{\mathcal{Y}}$ are two discriminators for the bi-directional registration to distinguish real pairs and fake pairs in $\mathcal{X}$ and $\mathcal{Y}$ domain. $\{q, \tilde{q}\}$ and $\{p, \tilde{p}\}$ are {real, fake} pairs sampled from $\mathcal{X}$ and $\mathcal{Y}$ respectively. $\mathcal{L}_{grad}^{\mathcal{X}}$ is the gradient penalty for the discriminator $D_r^{\mathcal{X}}$ which can be expressed as the form of $\mathcal{L}_{grad}^{\mathcal{X}} = \mathbb{E}_{\hat{q} \sim \mathbb{P}_{\hat{q}}} \left[\left(\| \nabla_{\hat{q}} D_r^{\mathcal{X}}(\hat{q}) \|_2 - 1 \right)^2 \right]$ with $\hat{q}$ sampled uniformly between q and $\tilde{q}$, and the same with $\mathcal{L}_{grad}^{\mathcal{Y}}$. α is a parameter to balance between the learning-based image space similarity metric and the latent space similarity measure.

3 Experiments

3.1 Datasets

We used two datasets for evaluation: one with clinical meaningful deformations in single modality (COPDGene) and one with real well-aligned multi-modality images (BraTS). In this case, we can have control over image-to-image translation quality and predicted deformation respectively.

COPDGene.[1] The COPDGene study is a multicenter observational study to analyze genetic susceptibility for the development of chronic obstructive pulmonary disease (COPD) [18]. High-quality, volumetric lung CT scans were acquired to capture full inspiration cycle of each subject using a standardized imaging protocol. CT scans were reconstructed with slice thicknesses of 0.625, 0.75, or 0.9 mm depending on the CT scanner manufacturer, with corresponding slice intervals of 0.625, 0.5, and 0.45 mm, respectively. In our experiment, 1000 subjects are randomly retrieved for evaluation, with end inspiration and expiration volumes being used to derive the underlying breathing motion. Each pair of volumes was rigidly pre-aligned, cropped, and down-sampled into a 3D volume with size of $128 \times 128 \times 128$ and resolution of 2.5 mm. We randomly split the 1000 subjects into 800/100/100 for train/test/validation, and on each subject we extract middle 10 slices. To simulate a multi-modality image registration problem, we synthesized a new modality using an intensity transformation $cos(I \cdot \pi)$ as proposed in [22] followed by Gaussian blurring and intensity normalization. Deformations were estimated between end inspiration and expiration frames of real CT and synthesized images.

BraTS'17. The Brain Tumour Segmentation (BraTS) 2017 dataset is obtained from the MICCAI BraTS 2017 challenge [1,15]. Specifically, it provides a large

[1] The COPDGene study (NCT00608764) was funded by NHLBI U01 HL089897 and U01 HL089856 and also supported by the COPD Foundation through contributions made to an Industry Advisory Committee comprised of AstraZeneca, Boehringer-Ingelheim, GlaxoSmithKline, Novartis, and Sunovion.

dataset of multi-modal MRI scans (native T1, T2, T2-FLAIR, and T1Gd) for patients with glioblastomas. Overall, the available training set consists of 285 cases, and for each case four image modalities were standardized into a 3D volume in size of 240 × 240 × 155 with 1 mm isotropic resolution. In our experiments, we utilize the T1 and T2-weighted images to define a multi-modality dataset to demonstrate the effect of our proposed approach. The set is randomly split into 225/30/30 for train/validation/test, and central 20 slices of each subject were extracted. As provided T1 and T2 images are already aligned, we generated synthetic deformation fields by spatially transforming one of the modality (T1) using elastic transformations on control points followed by Gaussian smoothing. The synthetic deformation is only used as ground truth (GT) for evaluations.

3.2   Experimental Settings

Implementation Details: For image-to-image translation, we built our network based on MUNIT implementation with changes as discussed in Sect. 2.1. The network is trained using the default settings as in [9]. Our registration network adopts the same architecture as in [17] with an additional exponentiation layer [12] as the last layer. In our implementation, we pre-train the image-to-image translation network using unpaired images, and then multi-modal registration and discriminator networks are trained. Our networks are implemented on PyTorch, using Adam optimizer for training with a learning rate of 0.0001. Hyper-parameters were chosen based on the performance on validation set, with $\lambda_{grad} = 10$ and $\lambda_{\Delta} = 1$. Run time reported for each method was tested on the same PC with 32G RAM, 3.6 GHz CPU, and Quadro P4000 GPU.

Evaluation Measures: For COPDGene dataset, we evaluate the registration accuracy indirectly via provided lung segmentation masks, as no ground truth deformation fields are available. Dice score, mean contour distance (MCD) and Hausdorff distance (HD) are computed between lung masks of fixed and warped moving images. For BraTS dataset, synthetic deformation fields are used as GT, thus pixel-wise root mean square error $(RMSE(\Delta))$ is calculated for the evaluation. Also, as pairs of aligned images are available, pixel-wise intensity error $(RMSE(I))$ can be calculated when transforming back the deformed image. Additionally, for both datasets, analysis of Jacobian matrix $J_{\Delta}(m) = \nabla\left(\Delta(m)\right)$ were conducted on the dense deformation fields Δ of each pixel m. Gradients of $J_{\Delta}(m)$ (Grad Det-Jac) are calculated as a metric to show the smoothness of Jacobian. Besides, average run time of each method is reported.

Competing Methods: We compare with two well-established multi-modal image registration methods: A mutual information based approach using the **Elastix** toolbox [14] and the **MIND** approach [7]. Also, we compare with the diffeomorphic Demons method [21] which can deal with multi-modal images using the proposed learned image-to-image translation network. Specifically, we first translate the appearance of the moving image to that of the fixed image and then run the diffeomorphic Demons algorithm on the image pair. We term this

Table 1. Evaluation of multi-modal registration on COPDGene dataset in terms of average Dice score, MCD, HD (unit: pixel), run time (GPU/CPU) and Grad Det-Jac ($\times 10^{-2}$) of each deformation field.

Method	Avg. dice	MCD	HD	Grad Det-Jac	Time(s)
MIND [7]	0.9365 (0.0822)	1.168 (0.798)	11.129 (5.736)	4.52 (0.40)	-/12.09
Elastix [14]	0.9497 (0.0822)	0.934 (0.760)	9.970 (5.772)	2.29 (0.61)	-/105.66
I2I+DiffDem	0.9347 (0.0676)	1.274 (0.923)	11.477 (5.434)	6.14 (0.39)	2.45/3.96
I2I+GAN	0.9553 (0.0444)	0.912 (0.628)	9.383 (4.977)	2.28 (0.45)	0.12/2.81
UMDIR-GAN	0.9613 (0.0357)	0.819 (0.546)	9.188 (4.981)	**2.19** (0.48)	**0.07/1.62**
UMDIR-Lat	0.9603 (0.0349)	0.823 (0.462)	8.469 (4.491)	2.73 (0.80)	**0.07/1.62**
UMDIR-LaGAN	**0.9672** (0.0280)	**0.710** (0.436)	**8.257** (4.432)	2.79 (0.60)	**0.07/1.62**

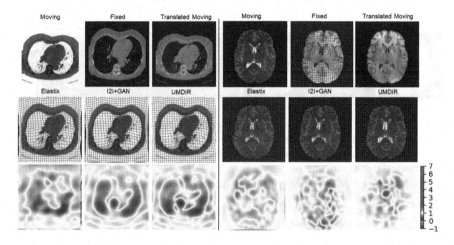

Fig. 3. Visualization results of our model against baseline methods, where warped moving images, corresponding estimated deformation fields and Jacobian determinant are shown. Left: COPDGene data; Right: BraTS data with GT overlaid on Fixed image.

method as **I2I+DiffDem**. A hierarchical multiresolution optimization scheme was used for all. Parameters were determined via searching on the validation set of each dataset separately while considering both the registration accuracy and speed. Results reported are best performance we can achieve. In addition, as no other deep learning based unsupervised multi-modal registration has been proposed yet, here we employ a diffeomorphic extension of existing monomodal registration method [5] that is enabled for multi-modal images similarly as I2I+DiffDem, termed as **I2I+GAN**. Its registration network architecture follows Sect. 2.2 where instead of estimating deformation Δ, velocity field is estimated to ensure the diffeomorphism. Its discriminator has also been adapted for multi-modality as discussed in Sect. 2.3. Finally, we term variants of our proposed method as **UMDIR-Lat**, **UMDIR-GAN** and **UMDIR-LaGAN**, corresponding to models shown in Fig. 2(a), (b) and (a)+(b).

Table 2. Evaluation of bi-directional multi-modal registration on BraTS dataset in terms of RMSE(Δ) (unit: pixel) and Grad Det-Jac ($\times 10^{-2}$) for T2 $\rightarrow$ T1 registration, and RMSE(I) for the inverse direction. Average run time (GPU/CPU) is also provided.

Method	T2 $\rightarrow$ T1		T1 $\rightarrow$ T2		Time(s)
	RMSE(Δ)	Grad Det-Jac	RMSE(I)	Grad Det-Jac	
MIND [7]	1.266 (0.253)	3.58 (0.25)	**0.045** (0.011)	3.60 (0.24)	-/18.98
Elastix [14]	1.260 (0.225)	1.23 (0.14)	0.089 (0.013)	1.22 (0.17)	-/66.97
I2I+DiffDem	1.391 (0.183)	**0.83** (0.13)	0.057 (0.015)	**0.87** (0.14)	0.81/4.44
I2I+GAN	1.250 (0.218)	1.30 (0.11)	0.074 (0.014)	2.10 (0.43)	0.20/6.44
UMDIR-GAN	1.202 (0.196)	1.35 (0.14)	0.067 (0.010)	1.88 (0.32)	**0.08/3.60**
UMDIR-Lat	1.146 (0.232)	1.04 (0.14)	0.067 (0.012)	1.37 (0.41)	**0.08/3.60**
UMDIR-LaGAN	**1.126** (0.214)	0.97 (0.11)	0.064 (0.010)	1.05 (0.20)	**0.08/3.60**

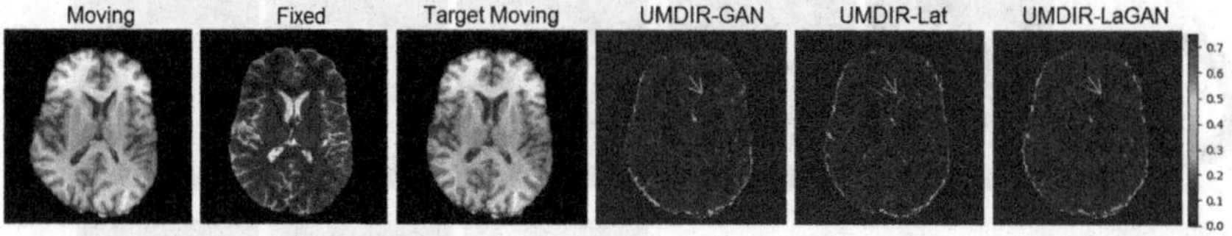

Fig. 4. Comparison between variants of proposed methods for T1 to T2 registration. Error maps are pixel-wise intensity differences between warped images and target moving images. Red arrows indicate regions where UMDIR-Lat outperforms UMDIR-GAN, and yellow arrows point out regions where UMDIR-GAN outperforms UMDIR-Lat. Combined metrics shows better performance than each of them separately. (Color figure online)

3.3   Results

First, we evaluated the performance of our methods on COPDGene data. The quantitative results for this are shown in Table 1. The registration performance is evaluated via measuring the Dice score, MCD and HD between warped lung segmentation at expiration and the GT lung segmentation at inspiration, as well as the gradient of Jacobian determinant. It can be seen that compared to the baseline methods, both traditional multi-modal registration methods and image-to-image translation plus mono-modal registration methods, our proposed UMDIR methods outperforms them in terms of Dice, MCD and HD with Grad Det-Jac smaller than or in the same range with other competing methods. In particular, success of training with latent similarity criterion implies that the learned domain-invariant attribute is capable of extracting and preserving intrinsic shape feature that is informative enough to guide the geometrical transformation for registration. In addition, Fig. 3 displays the warped moving images along with their corresponding deformation fields and Jacobian determinant, where it can be observed that our proposed model is able to achieve high accuracy with smooth and regular deformation fields. Furthermore, by combining both latent similarity and cross-cycle adversarial similarity metrics, we see a further improvement of performance on the COPDGene dataset in terms of accuracy, which indicates that these two metrics could be complementary. In terms of registration speed, our proposed methods are significantly faster than traditional baseline methods. In particular, the UMDIR methods are faster than I2I+GAN, as they learn the registration network directly from latent representations, bypassing the image-to-image translation stage. Note that the translated moving images in Fig. 3 are only used in the I2I+DiffDem and I2I+GAN.

Additionally, we also evaluated the bi-directional multi-modal registration performance on BraTS dataset, where ground truth deformation fields are available from T2 to T1, and ground truth aligned images are known for the T1 to T2 registration. Note that our proposed latent method can realize such bi-directional registration directly without any further training, while other competing methods need to be optimized or trained separately for both T1 $\rightarrow$ T2 and T2 $\rightarrow$ T1 directions. Quantitative results are shown in Table 2, with RMSE(Δ) and Grad Det-Jac calculated for T2 $\rightarrow$ T1, and RMSE(I) for T1 $\rightarrow$ T2. An example of visualization results is shown in Fig. 3. From both quantitative and qualitative results, it can be seen that the proposed UMDIR methods can achieve competitive registration performance compared with other competing methods and also with smooth and regular deformations. Though MIND achieved a lower RMSE(I) for T1 $\rightarrow$ T2 registration, this is at the cost of separate training for each direction. Our proposed methods deliver a one-shot bi-directional solution in a noticeably higher processing speed. In addition, learning registration directly from disentangled latent representations bypasses the image-to-image translation stage, which can potentially avoid problems caused by the image translation quality such as image noises or hallucinations that can lead to inaccurate registration. This possibly explains the better performance of our proposed methods against I2I with mono-modal registration methods. On the other hand, to examine the differences of latent similarity criterion and cross-cycle adversarial similarity metric as well as the benefits of combined metrics, in Fig. 4, we compared the registration performance with different metrics in the inverse direction (T1 $\rightarrow$ T2) by visualizing the pixel-wise intensity RMSE. It can be observed that by combining these two complementary metrics, UMDIR-LaGAN is able to preserve the advantages of each metric and produces more accurate registration.

4   Conclusion

In this paper, we have presented a novel deep learning based model for fully unsupervised multi-modal deformable image registration. The proposed models reduce the multi-modal registration problem to a mono-modal one via exploiting the disentangled latent embedding that is learned from an unpaired image-to-image translation framework. For training the registration network, we proposed a distance loss in latent shape space and a cross-cycle adversarial loss defined in image space as similarity metrics. Experimental results showed improvements of our proposed models against other conventional approaches in terms of both accuracy and speed.

For future work, we will further investigate the impact of joint training of MUNIT and UMDIR networks on registration accuracy. It could be helpful to refine the image-to-image translation network during the training of the registration network, so that the domain-invariant attribute can be better enforced to be equivalent to the shape that could be represented via geometrical transformations. Additionally, we will also extend the application of our model on real 3D volumes via patch-based methods for efficient training.

Disclaimer: This feature is based on research, and is not commercially available. Due to regulatory reasons its future availability cannot be guaranteed.

References

1. Bakas, S., et al.: Advancing the cancer genome atlas glioma MRI collections with expert segmentation labels and radiomic features. Sci. Data **4**, 170117 (2017)
2. Balakrishnan, G., Zhao, A., Sabuncu, M.R., Guttag, J., Dalca, A.V.: An unsupervised learning model for deformable medical image registration. In: CVPR, pp. 9252–9260 (2018)
3. Cao, X., Yang, J., Gao, Y., Guo, Y., Wu, G., Shen, D.: Dual-core steered non-rigid registration for multi-modal images via bi-directional image synthesis. MedIA **41**, 18–31 (2017)
4. Dalca, A.V., Balakrishnan, G., Guttag, J., Sabuncu, M.R.: Unsupervised learning for fast probabilistic diffeomorphic registration. In: Frangi, A.F., Schnabel, J.A., Davatzikos, C., Alberola-López, C., Fichtinger, G. (eds.) MICCAI 2018. LNCS, vol. 11070, pp. 729–738. Springer, Cham (2018). https://doi.org/10.1007/978-3-030-00928-1_82
5. Fan, J., Cao, X., Xue, Z., Yap, P.-T., Shen, D.: Adversarial similarity network for evaluating image alignment in deep learning based registration. In: Frangi, A.F., Schnabel, J.A., Davatzikos, C., Alberola-López, C., Fichtinger, G. (eds.) MICCAI 2018. LNCS, vol. 11070, pp. 739–746. Springer, Cham (2018). https://doi.org/10.1007/978-3-030-00928-1_83
6. Gulrajani, I., Ahmed, F., Arjovsky, M., Dumoulin, V., Courville, A.C.: Improved training of Wasserstein GANs. In: NIPS, pp. 5767–5777 (2017)
7. Heinrich, M.P., et al.: MIND: modality independent neighbourhood descriptor for multi-modal deformable registration. MedIA **16**(7), 1423–1435 (2012)
8. Hu, Y., et al.: Weakly-supervised convolutional neural networks for multimodal image registration. MedIA **49**, 1–13 (2018)
9. Huang, X., Liu, M.-Y., Belongie, S., Kautz, J.: Multimodal unsupervised image-to-image translation. In: Ferrari, V., Hebert, M., Sminchisescu, C., Weiss, Y. (eds.) ECCV 2018. LNCS, vol. 11207, pp. 179–196. Springer, Cham (2018). https://doi.org/10.1007/978-3-030-01219-9_11
10. Ilg, E., Mayer, N., Saikia, T., Keuper, M., Dosovitskiy, A., Brox, T.: Flownet 2.0: evolution of optical flow estimation with deep networks. In: CVPR (2017)
11. Jaderberg, M., Simonyan, K., Zisserman, A., Kavukcuoglu, K.: Spatial transformer networks. In: NIPS, pp. 2017–2025 (2015)
12. Krebs, J., Mansi, T., Mailhé, B., Ayache, N., Delingette, H.: Unsupervised probabilistic deformation modeling for robust diffeomorphic registration. In: Stoyanov, D., et al. (eds.) DLMIA/ML-CDS -2018. LNCS, vol. 11045, pp. 101–109. Springer, Cham (2018). https://doi.org/10.1007/978-3-030-00889-5_12

13. Lee, H.-Y., Tseng, H.-Y., Huang, J.-B., Singh, M., Yang, M.-H.: Diverse image-to-image translation via disentangled representations. In: Ferrari, V., Hebert, M., Sminchisescu, C., Weiss, Y. (eds.) ECCV 2018. LNCS, vol. 11205, pp. 36–52. Springer, Cham (2018). https://doi.org/10.1007/978-3-030-01246-5_3
14. Marstal, K., Berendsen, F., Staring, M., Klein, S.: SimpleElastix: a user-friendly, multi-lingual library for medical image registration. In: CVPR Workshops (2016)
15. Menze, B.H., et al.: The multimodal brain tumor image segmentation benchmark (BRATS). TMI **34**(10), 1993 (2015)
16. Pluim, J.P., Maintz, J.A., Viergever, M.A.: Mutual-information-based registration of medical images: a survey. TMI **22**(8), 986–1004 (2003)
17. Qin, C., et al.: Joint learning of motion estimation and segmentation for cardiac MR image sequences. In: Frangi, A.F., Schnabel, J.A., Davatzikos, C., Alberola-López, C., Fichtinger, G. (eds.) MICCAI 2018. LNCS, vol. 11071, pp. 472–480. Springer, Cham (2018). https://doi.org/10.1007/978-3-030-00934-2_53
18. Regan, E.A., et al.: Genetic epidemiology of COPD (COPDGene) study design. J. COPD **7**(1), 32–43 (2011)
19. Roche, A., Pennec, X., Malandain, G., Ayache, N.: Rigid registration of 3-D ultrasound with MR images: a new approach combining intensity and gradient information. TMI **20**(10), 1038–1049 (2001)
20. Uzunova, H., Wilms, M., Handels, H., Ehrhardt, J.: Training CNNs for image registration from few samples with model-based data augmentation. In: Descoteaux, M., Maier-Hein, L., Franz, A., Jannin, P., Collins, D.L., Duchesne, S. (eds.) MICCAI 2017. LNCS, vol. 10433, pp. 223–231. Springer, Cham (2017). https://doi.org/10.1007/978-3-319-66182-7_26
21. Vercauteren, T., Pennec, X., Perchant, A., Ayache, N.: Non-parametric diffeomorphic image registration with the demons algorithm. In: Ayache, N., Ourselin, S., Maeder, A. (eds.) MICCAI 2007. LNCS, vol. 4792, pp. 319–326. Springer, Heidelberg (2007). https://doi.org/10.1007/978-3-540-75759-7_39
22. Yaman, M., Kalkan, S.: An iterative adaptive multi-modal stereo-vision method using mutual information. J. Vis. Commun. Image Representation **26**, 115–131 (2015)

Learning Motion

Real-Time 2D-3D Deformable Registration with Deep Learning and Application to Lung Radiotherapy Targeting

Markus D. Foote[1]([✉]) [iD], Blake E. Zimmerman[1] [iD], Amit Sawant[2],
and Sarang C. Joshi[1]

[1] Scientific Computing and Imaging Institute, Department of Bioengineering,
University of Utah, Salt Lake City, UT, USA
foote@sci.utah.edu
[2] School of Medicine, Department of Radiation Oncology, University of Maryland,
Baltimore, MD, USA

Abstract. Radiation therapy presents a need for dynamic tracking of a target tumor volume. Fiducial markers such as implanted gold seeds have been used to gate radiation delivery but the markers are invasive and gating significantly increases treatment time. Pretreatment acquisition of a respiratory correlated 4DCT allows for determination of accurate motion tracking which is useful in treatment planning. We design a patient-specific motion subspace and a deep convolutional neural network to recover anatomical positions from a single fluoroscopic projection in real-time. We use this deep network to approximate the nonlinear inverse of a diffeomorphic deformation composed with radiographic projection. This network recovers subspace coordinates to define the patient-specific deformation of the lungs from a baseline anatomic position. The geometric accuracy of the subspace deformations on real patient data is similar to accuracy attained by original image registration between individual respiratory-phase image volumes.

Keywords: Therapy Target Tracking · Lung cancer · Real-time · Computed Tomography · Fluoroscopy · Deep learning · Convolutional neural network · Motion Analysis · Image registration · Computational Anatomy

1 Introduction

According to the United States Centers for Disease Control and Prevention, lung cancer is the leading cause of cancer death, accounting for 27% of all cancer deaths in the United States [22]. Accurate estimation of organ movement and normal tissue deformations plays a crucial role in dose calculations and treatment decisions in radiation therapy of lung cancer [3]. State-of-the-art radiation treatment planning uses 4D (3D + time) respiratory correlated computed

© Springer Nature Switzerland AG 2019
A. C. S. Chung et al. (Eds.): IPMI 2019, LNCS 11492, pp. 265–276, 2019.
https://doi.org/10.1007/978-3-030-20351-1_20

tomography (4D-RCCT) scans as a planning tool to deliver radiation dose to the tumor during treatment [6] and minimize dose to the healthy tissue and vital organs. Understanding respiratory motion allows for more accurate treatment planning and delivery, resulting in more targeted dose delivery to only the tumor.

While general motion patterns in radiotherapy patients are relatively well understood, cycle-to-cycle variations remain a significant challenge and may account for observed discrepancies between predictive treatment plan indicators and clinical patient outcomes, especially due to an increased irradiated volume which limits adequate dose to the target [18]. Gating methods have been developed but require implanted markers and lengthen treatment time. Real-time motion tracking using magnetic resonance imaging is only applied within the 2D imaging slices due to time constraints for imaging [4]. Accurate and fast noninvasive target tracking that accounts for real-time cycle-to-cycle variations in respiratory motion is a recognized need in radiotherapy [9,19].

In this paper, we propose to use 4D-RCCT acquired at treatment planning time to develop a finite low dimensional patient specific space of deformations and use treatment time single angle fluoroscopy imaging in conjunction with deep convolutional neural network to recover the full deformations of the anatomy during treatment. The constant time inference capability of convolutional neural networks allows real-time recovery of the anatomic position of the tumor target and surrounding anatomy using radiographic images of the treatment area acquired using fluoroscopy. We envision our framework to be incorporated as the target position monitoring subsystem in a conformal radiotherapy system [19]. The proposed method eliminates the need for invasive fiducial markers while still producing targeted radiation delivery during variable respiration patterns. While this framework requires training of the model on a per-patient basis, only inference is required during treatment. Inference of the deep convolutional network and subsequent linear combination of patient-specific motion components can be calculated faster than real-time and drive motion-tracking of conformal radiotherapy treatment.

The proposed framework begins by creating motion subspace from CT registration among the respiratory phase images. This motion subspace is then used to generate many respiratory phase fluoroscopic images with known subspace coordinates. These labeled fluoroscopic images serve as a training dataset for a deep convolutional neural network that recovers the motion subspace coordinates. Motion coordinates recovered by the deep neural network from unseen fluoroscopy define a linear combination of deformation components that form a full 3D deformation that is represented in the 2D fluoroscopic image.

2   Related Work

2.1   Low-Rank Respiratory Motion Models

The respiratory cycle exhibits low-rank behavior and hysteresis, leading to application of principal component analysis to study the deformation of lungs and other organs through time [8]. Sabouri *et al.* 2017 has used such a PCA approximations of the respiratory cycle to correlate the lung's principal deformations to respiratory markers directly observable during treatment such as body surface tracking during conformal radiation therapy [17]. PCA has also been applied to MR-based image guidance in radiotherapy [4].

2.2 Rank Constrained Density Motion Estimation

Our real-time tracking procedure is based on the rank-constrained diffeomorphic density matching framework, summarized here for completeness (see [1,2,14,15] for details). In general, the rank-constrained diffeomorphic density matching problem produces a registration between multiple image volumes that is explained by only a few principal components of deformation – less than the total number of volumes. The deformation set matrix rank is non-smooth and therefore unfit for optimization. Instead, the nuclear norm is used as a smooth and convex surrogate. The deformation set matrix is constructed with each vectorized deformation field as a row,

$$
X = \begin{bmatrix} \varphi_1^{-1}(x) - x \\ \varphi_2^{-1}(x) - x \\ \vdots \\ \varphi_{N-1}^{-1}(x) - x \end{bmatrix} = \{\varphi_i^{-1}(x) - x\} \tag{1}
$$

where φ_i^{-1} is the inverse of the deformation from the i-th image in the image series to a selected reference image. We thus define the nuclear norm for deformations between N images as

$$
\|X\|_* = \sum_i^{N-1} |\sigma_i(X)|, \tag{2}
$$

where σ_i are the singular values. As there are $N-1$ deformations between N images, giving only $N-1$ singular values σ.

As CT measures the linear attenuation coefficient which is proportional to the true density, 4DCT volumes are interpreted as densities, thus values change with compression or expansion. A density $I\,dx$ is acted upon by a diffeomorphism φ to compensate for changes of the density by the deformation:

$$
(\varphi, I\,dx) \mapsto \varphi_*(I\,dx) = (\varphi^{-1})^*(I\,dx) = (|D\varphi^{-1}|I \circ \varphi^{-1})\,dx \tag{3}
$$

where $|D\varphi^{-1}|$ denotes the Jacobian determinant of φ^{-1}. The Riemannian geometry of the group of diffeomorphisms with a suitable Sobolev H^1 metric is linked to the Riemannian geometry of densities with the Fisher-Rao metric [1,7,10]. The Fisher-Rao metric is used as the measure for similarity due to the property that it is invariant to the action of diffeomorphisms:

$$
d_F^2(I_0\,dx, I_1\,dx) = \int_\Omega \left(\sqrt{I_0} - \sqrt{I_1}\right)^2 dx. \tag{4}
$$

The linkage between a suitable Sobolev H^1 metric and the Fisher-Rao metric allows for evaluation of the distance in the space of diffeomorphisms in closed form. The Fisher-Rao metric, an incompressibility measure, and surrogate rank measure can then be used to match a set of densities by minimizing the energy functional:

$$E(\{\varphi_i\}) = \sum_{i}^{N-1} \left[\int_{\Omega} \left(\sqrt{|D\varphi_i^{-1}| I_i \circ \varphi_i^{-1}} - \sqrt{I_0} \right)^2 dx \right.$$
$$\left. + \int_{\Omega} \left(\sqrt{|D\varphi_i^{-1}|} - 1 \right)^2 f \, dx \right] + \alpha \sum_{i}^{N-1} |\sigma_i (\{\varphi_i^{-1}(x) - x\})| \, (5)$$

where I_0 is a chosen base or reference density and I_i are the other $N-1$ densities in the series. The first term here penalizes dissimilarity between the two densities. The second term penalizes deviations from a volume-preserving deformation. The penalty function f acts as weighting of the volume-preserving measure. The final term penalizes the surrogate rank of the subspace in which the set of deformations exist. We use a gradient flow and iterative soft thresholding for optimizing the above energy functional. This optimization produces a related set of rank-optimized deformations with improved geometric accuracy over other registration methods due to the increased physiologic relevance of the low-rank deformations which match well with the general forward-reverse process of the inhale-exhale cycle, along with hysteresis in other components [2].

2.3   Digitally Reconstructed Radiographs

For a given 4D-RCCT dataset, it is sufficient for training to simulate the 2D projection images at different respiratory states from the 3D volumes acquired at different states. These digitally reconstructed radiographs (DRR) are commonly used for radiation therapy planning. This allows for simulation of the 2D projections that would be acquired at the different phases of breathing throughout a state-of-the-art radiotherapy treatment [16,19]. A point $(u, v) \in \mathbb{R}^2$ in the DRR projection image is defined by the line integral of linear attenuation coefficients (values in the CT volume) over distance l from the x-ray source to the projection image [9,20,21]. The path can be written as $p(s) = (s(u - u_0), s(v - v_0), sl)$ where $s \in [0, 1]$ and (u_0, v_0) is the piercing point, or the unique point in the projection image that is closest to the x-ray source. The DRR operation generates a 2D projection of the 3D CT volume that can be used for training in place of actual radiography recordings. These projections closely approximate the fluoroscopic images acquired during a state-of-the-art radiotherapy treatment session.

3   Methodology

3.1   Motion Subspace Learning

A 10-phase respiratory correlated 4D-RCCT of a lung cancer patient for treatment planning from the University of Maryland was provided in anonymized form. Each 3D volume in the 4D-RCCT dataset is $512 \times 512 \times 104$ with resolution $0.976 \times 0.976 \times 3$ mm. These 10 3D CT volumes, each representing a distinct respiratory phase, are used for rank constrained density registration as described by Foote et al. [2] to produce 9 rank-optimized deformation fields that map to the full-exhale phase volume from each of the other phase volumes. The low-rank subspace of the space of diffeomorphisms in which the rank-optimized deformation components exist is determined via principal component analysis (PCA).

3.2 Training Dataset Generation

A dataset for training is generated by calculating DRR projections through a deformed reference CT volume The deformation applied to the reference volume is calculated as a linear combination of rank-optimized components. Only the first two rank-optimized components are used as they explain 99.7% of the deformation data (Table 1). The weights for this linear combination are generated as a dense grid of 300 evenly spaced points in first rank-optimized component direction and 200 evenly spaced points in the second (60000 total samples for training). The value of the maximum weight is set as 150% and 110% of the maximum magnitude of the corresponding rank-optimized component for the first and second directions, respectively. These weights serve as the target for training and are then used to calculate a linear combination of the rank-optimized component deformations. The resulting grid of deformations are calculated and applied to the full-exhale 4D-RCCT volume using PyCA [13] (Fig. 1). DRR images are calculated by ray casting and integrating along a cone-beam geometry of the fluoroscope through the deformed full-exhale 4DCT volume [16, 20, 21]. The geometry setup for the DRR generation is similar to the geometry that would be found in a current radiotherapy treatment linear accelerator's imaging accessories, such as the Varian TrueBeam. Specifically, the x-ray source was positioned laterally from the center of the CT volume. The center of the virtual detector for the projection image was then positioned 150 cm horizontally from the source, through the CT volume, with a 1024×768 pixel array with spatial resolution 0.388×0.388 mm. DRR images were preprocessed before training with variance equalization, normalizing the image intensities to $[0, 1]$, histogram equalization, and 2×2 average downsampling.

3.3 Network Architechture

The mapping from rank-optimized component weights to a projection image is highly nonlinear as it includes both a diffeomorphic deformation and radiographic projection. We aim to approximate the inverse of this mapping with a deep convolutional neural network as a multi-output continuous regression problem. A promising network architecture for this application is DenseNet [5]. DenseNet has achieved state-of-the-art performance on several datasets while using fewer parameters and decreasing over-fitting. The direct connections between constant spatial layers allow for reusing features learned from previous

Table 1. Data explanation power of cumulative rank-optimized components of deformation from rank-constrained density deformation optimization. These values are calculated from the normalized cumulative sum of eigenvalues.

Number of included components	Percentage of dataset explained
1	0.90115488
2	0.99739416
3	0.99865254
4	0.99973184
5	0.99989146
6	0.99996631
7	0.99999949
8	1.0

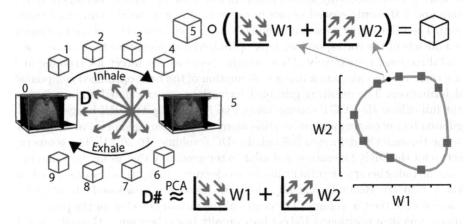

Fig. 1. Dataset generation overview. The deformations from rank constrained motion estimation are decomposed using PCA. Coordinates within the PCA space are used to generate a new deformation field, which is then applied to the reference CT volume. The resulting volume is used for DRR projection.

layers and improve the flow of gradients throughout the network. Additionally, DenseNet is ideal for real-time applications due to reduced model complexity and depth.

We use an efficient DenseNet model in PyTorch tailored to our application so that single-channel images are used as input [11,12]. The rank-optimized component weights used to produce the projection image are the regression points (Fig. 2). Summarized here for completeness, the DenseNet architecture convolves each input with a kernel size of 3 and filter number of $2 \times k$ before being input to the first dense block, where k is the growth rate. Each subsequent dense block consists of 8 convolutional layers all with filter size of 3 and a growth rate of 4.

The 4 convolutional layers within a dense block are each preceded by a batch normalization layer and a rectified linear unit (ReLU) layer. The output from a dense block enters a transition block where batch normalization and non-linear activation are followed by a convolutional feature map reduction layer (compression = 0.5) and spatial reduction factor of 2 in each dimension using max-pooling. A total of 4 dense and transition blocks are used to reduce the spatial dimensions to final feature maps. The final layer of the network was a linear layer that regresses the feature maps to the rank-optimized component weights.

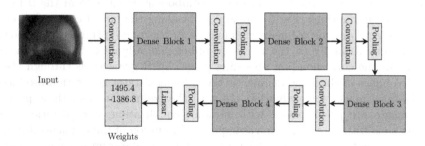

Fig. 2. DenseNet architecture used to learn the inverse deformation-projection estimate. Each dense block represents a group of 4 feature layers and growth rate 4 with an included transition layer. A final linear layer recovers the weights for deformation components.

4   Results

For our experiments, we use a 10-phase RCCT of a lung radiotherapy patient as the source data. Rank-optimized deformations were calculated as described by Foote *et al.* and summarized in Sect. 2.2 using the full-exhale (Phase 5) CT volume as a reference. Using PCA, rank-optimized components of these deformations were determined and used to generate a DRR training dataset as described in Sect. 3.2. In Sect. 4.1 we outline the specific training procedure for the neural network. Then in Sect. 4.2 we test the neural network against unseen data from a breathing model. Finally, Sect. 4.3 describes generalization of the trained model on the phases of the RCCT dataset that were not used in training dataset generation.

4.1   Training and Test Performance

The network is trained for 300 epochs using a L_1 loss function with a learning rate of 0.1 and batch size of 2048. The L_1 loss independently penalizes each deformation component which avoids preferential fitting of the larger-weighted component at any point. The learning rate is decreased by a factor of 5 when the training loss plateaus within a relative threshold of 10^{-4} for the last 20 epochs. The dataset is randomly split 80-20 between training and on-line testing to monitor for over-fitting during training. Training for 300 epochs completes in under 2 h on a single Nvidia Quadro GV100 GPU.

4.2 Spline Model Deformation Validation

A motion-subspace-based breathing model was created using a spline interpolation of the first two rank-optimized component weights from the 9 rank-optimized deformations (Fig. 3). At any point along the model curve, the coordinate weights provide a linear combination of the rank-optimized component deformations to apply to the reference full-exhale volume to obtain a model volume for the corresponding breathing phase. DRR projections through these model volumes in the same manner as the training dataset generation produced fluoroscopic images for evaluation. As with the training images, these projection images are preprocessed with variance equalization, normalization, histogram equalization, and 2× downsampling. Evaluation of these images through the trained network recovers the weights of the rank-optimized components. Inference on a single Nvidia Quadro GV100 GPU has a throughput of 1113 images/second with the same PyTorch implementation – significantly faster than real-time. The relation of these weights to the original spline model is shown in Fig. 3.

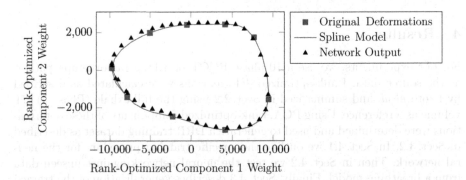

Fig. 3. Deformation component weights for each of the 9 original components (blue squares) are control points for the spline-based breathing model (red line). DRR images derived from the weights along this spline model are input to the network. Resulting inferred weights (black triangles) closely align with the model. (Color figure online)

Accuracy of the deformation recovered from the inferred weights is measured by maximum deformation distance error compared to the reconstruction of these deformations with the two rank-optimized deformation component weights directly from the model. From the 40 model points, the maximum error between the applied deformation and the recovered deformation was 1.22 mm.

4.3   RCCT Phase Patient Data and Geometric Validation

Until this point, DRR images derived from 9 of the 10 original 4DCT volumes have not been used as input for the network for either training or previous testing. Rather than a synthetic spline model of respiratory phases, we now use the original CT volumes captured at 9 stages of the respiratory cycle. These CT volumes inherently contain deformations that have not been included in any training or evaluation to this point, as the rank-constrained motion estimation produces imperfect deformations to these CT images. No deformation is applied to these CT volumes as each volume represents this intrinsic respiratory deformation relative to the full-exhale anatomical state. Evaluation of our framework on these intrinsic deformations effectively projects the true deformation into our 2-dimensional motion subspace.

Exactly as in training dataset generation, DRR images through these (undeformed) volumes are calculated and preprocessed with variance equalization, normalization, histogram equalization, and downsampling. Evaluation of the network gives rank-optimized deformation component weights describing the intrinsic deformations that can be compared in the subspace of motion component weights with the weights directly recovered from original rank-constrained density motion estimation (Fig. 4).

These weights produced by the network are used to reconstruct a deformation field as a linear combination of the rank-optimized deformation component fields. We calculate and report the error as a difference from the original rank-constrained motion estimation deformation distance that is recovered by both our deep learning framework in Fig. 5. Errors for the deformation recovered at each CT phase are also calculated against the deformations from rank-constrained motion estimation (Table 2).

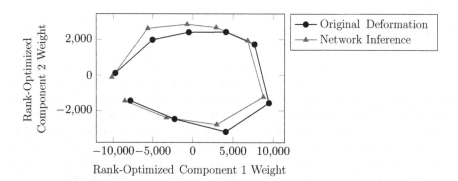

Fig. 4. Weights of rank-optimized deformation components recovered by network on real patient CT data (red triangles) align well with original deformation weights for rank-optimized components (black circles). The respiratory cycle proceeds clockwise around the loop. (Color figure online)

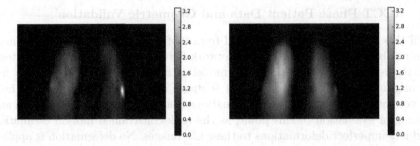

Fig. 5. Slice of error map of calculated deformation error recovered by the deep learning framework. Phase 0 (left) and 9 (right) are selected as representative examples. Both general and localized errors are similar to the axial resolution of the CT scan (3 mm).

Table 2. Deformation distance error for each phase's recovered deformation.

Phase	Average distance error (mm)	Maximum distance error (mm)
0	0.136	3.92
1	0.212	3.15
2	0.132	2.58
3	0.291	8.98
4	0.223	6.62
6	0.201	4.15
7	0.286	6.96
8	0.252	9.55
9	0.183	5.07

5   Discussion

In this paper, we have shown that estimation of anatomic position in the presence of breathing variability is possible with the combination of (1) rank-constrained density motion estimation for determination of motion components and (2) deep learning for subsequent identification of the weights of motion components in real-time. While this framework is extensible to dimensions higher than 2, the rank-constrained nature of the deformation fields produces accurate results using only two dimensions. This level of accuracy is a trade-off against the curse of dimensionality in both the dataset size and computational cost of training; however, using rank-constrained deformation components increases the accuracy of resulting deformations with the same number of dimensions.

The speed and accuracy attained by this framework is suitable for inclusion as a tumor position monitoring component of a conformal radiation therapy system. Determination of 3D tumor location from noninvasive 2D radiographic projections via deep learning instead of variational optimization approaches to the 2D-3D deformation determination problem provides real-time results for conformal radiation therapy for lung tumors.

Acknowledgements. This work was partially supported through research funding from the National Institute of Health (R01 CA169102 and R03 EB026132). Additional support was provided by internal funding from the Huntsman Cancer Institute. The authors are grateful for the support of NVIDIA Corporation by providing the GPU used for this research.

References

1. Bauer, M., Joshi, S., Modin, K.: Diffeomorphic density matching by optimal information transport. SIAM J. Imaging Sci. **8**(3), 1718–1751 (2015). https://doi.org/10.1137/151006238
2. Foote, M., Sabouri, P., Sawant, A., Joshi, S.: Rank constrained diffeomorphic density motion estimation for respiratory correlated computed tomography. In: Cardoso, M., et al. (eds.) GRAIL/MFCA/MICGen -2017. LNCS, vol. 10551, pp. 177–185. Springer, Cham (2017). https://doi.org/10.1007/978-3-319-67675-3_16
3. Geneser, S., Hinkle, J., Kirby, R., Wang, B., Salter, B., Joshi, S.: Quantifying variability in radiation dose due to respiratory-induced tumor motion. Med. Image Anal. **15**(4), 640–649 (2011). https://doi.org/10.1016/j.media.2010.07.003
4. Ha, I.Y., Wilms, M., Handels, H., Heinrich, M.P.: Model-based sparse-to-dense image registration for realtime respiratory motion estimation in image-guided interventions. IEEE Trans. Biomed. Eng. **66**(2), 302–310 (2019). https://doi.org/10.1109/TBME.2018.2837387
5. Huang, G., Liu, Z., van der Maaten, L., Weinberger, K.Q.: Densely connected convolutional networks. In: 2017 IEEE Conference on Computer Vision and Pattern Recognition (CVPR), pp. 2261–2269. IEEE, July 2017. https://doi.org/10.1109/CVPR.2017.243
6. Keall, P.J., Joshi, S., Vedam, S.S., Siebers, J.V., Kini, V.R., Mohan, R.: Four-dimensional radiotherapy planning for DMLC-based respiratory motion tracking. Med. Phys. **32**(4), 942–951 (2005). https://doi.org/10.1118/1.1879152
7. Khesin, B., Lenells, J., Misiołek, G., Preston, S.C.: Geometry of diffeomorphism groups, complete integrability and Geometric statistics. Geom. Funct. Anal. **23**(1), 334–366 (2013). https://doi.org/10.1007/s00039-013-0210-2
8. Li, R., et al.: On a PCA-based lung motion model. Phys. Med. Biol. **56**(18), 6009–6030 (2011). https://doi.org/10.1088/0031-9155/56/18/015
9. Markelj, P., Tomaževič, D., Likar, B., Pernuš, F.: A review of 3D/2D registration methods for image-guided interventions. Med. Image Anal. **16**(3), 642–661 (2012). https://doi.org/10.1016/j.media.2010.03.005. https://linkinghub.elsevier.com/retrieve/pii/S1361841510000368
10. Modin, K.: Generalized hunter-saxton equations, optimal information transport, and factorization of diffeomorphisms. J. Geom. Anal. **25**(2), 1306–1334 (2015). https://doi.org/10.1007/s12220-014-9469-2
11. Paszke, A., et al.: Automatic differentiation in PyTorch. In: NIPS-W (2017)
12. Pleiss, G., Chen, D., Huang, G., Li, T., van der Maaten, L., Weinberger, K.Q.: Memory-efficient implementation of DenseNets. arXiv preprint http://arxiv.org/abs/1707.06990, July 2017

13. Preston, J., Hinkle, J., Singh, N., Rottman, C., Joshi, S.: PyCA: python for computational anatomy. https://bitbucket.org/scicompanat/pyca
14. Rottman, C., Bauer, M., Modin, K., Joshi, S.C.: Weighted diffeomorphic density matching with applications to thoracic image registration. In: 5th MICCAI Workshop on Mathematical Foundations of Computational Anatomy (MFCA 2015), pp. 1–12 (2015)
15. Rottman, C., Larson, B., Sabouri, P., Sawant, A., Joshi, S.: Diffeomorphic density registration in thoracic computed tomography. In: Ourselin, S., Joskowicz, L., Sabuncu, M.R., Unal, G., Wells, W. (eds.) MICCAI 2016. LNCS, vol. 9902, pp. 46–53. Springer, Cham (2016). https://doi.org/10.1007/978-3-319-46726-9_6
16. Rottman, C., McBride, L., Cheryauka, A., Whitaker, R., Joshi, S.: Mobile C-arm 3D reconstruction in the presence of uncertain geometry. In: Navab, N., Hornegger, J., Wells, W.M., Frangi, A.F. (eds.) MICCAI 2015. LNCS, vol. 9350, pp. 692–699. Springer, Cham (2015). https://doi.org/10.1007/978-3-319-24571-3_83
17. Sabouri, P., et al.: A novel method using surface monitoring to capture breathing-induced cycle-to-cycle variations with 4DCT. In: 59th Annual Meeting of the American Association of Physicists in Medicine, Denver, CO (2017). http://www.aapm.org/meetings/2017AM/PRAbs.asp?mid=127&aid=37742
18. Sawant, A., et al.: Investigating the feasibility of rapid MRI for image-guided motion management in lung cancer radiotherapy. BioMed. Res. Int. **2014** (2014). https://doi.org/10.1155/2014/485067
19. Sawant, A., et al.: Management of three-dimensional intrafraction motion through real-time DMLC tracking. Med. Phys. **35**(5), 2050–2061 (2008). https://doi.org/10.1118/1.2905355
20. Sherouse, G.W., Novins, K., Chaney, E.L.: Computation of digitally reconstructed radiographs for use in radiotherapy treatment design. Int. J. Radiat. Oncol. Biol. Phys. **18**(3), 651–658 (1990). https://doi.org/10.1016/0360-3016(90)90074-T
21. Staub, D., Murphy, M.J.: A digitally reconstructed radiograph algorithm calculated from first principles. Med. Phys. **40**(1) (2013). https://doi.org/10.1118/1.4769413
22. U.S. Cancer Statistics Working Group: U.S. Cancer Statistics Working Group. United States Cancer Statistics: 1999–2014 Incidence and Mortality Web-based Report. Atlanta: U.S. Department of Health and Human Services, Centers for Disease Control and Prevention and National Cancer Institute. Technical report, Centers for Disease Control and Prevention and National Cancer Institute (2017). https://nccd.cdc.gov/uscs/

Deep Modeling of Growth Trajectories for Longitudinal Prediction of Missing Infant Cortical Surfaces

Peirong Liu[1], Zhengwang Wu[2], Gang Li[2], Pew-Thian Yap[2(✉)], and Dinggang Shen[1,2(✉)]

[1] Department of Computer Science, University of North Carolina at Chapel Hill, Chapel Hill, NC, USA
[2] Department of Radiology and BRIC, University of North Carolina at Chapel Hill, Chapel Hill, NC, USA
{ptyap,dgshen}@med.unc.edu

Abstract. Charting cortical growth trajectories is of paramount importance for understanding brain development. However, such analysis necessitates the collection of longitudinal data, which can be challenging due to subject dropouts and failed scans. In this paper, we will introduce a method for longitudinal prediction of cortical surfaces using a spatial graph convolutional neural network (GCNN), which extends conventional CNNs from Euclidean to curved manifolds. The proposed method is designed to model the cortical growth trajectories and jointly predict inner and outer cortical surfaces at multiple time points. Adopting a binary flag in loss calculation to deal with missing data, we fully utilize all available cortical surfaces for training our deep learning model, without requiring a complete collection of longitudinal data. Predicting the surfaces directly allows cortical attributes such as cortical thickness, curvature, and convexity to be computed for subsequent analysis. We will demonstrate with experimental results that our method is capable of capturing the nonlinearity of spatiotemporal cortical growth patterns and can predict cortical surfaces with improved accuracy.

Keywords: Graph Convolutional Neural Networks ·
Infant cortical surfaces · Longitudinal prediction · Shape Analysis ·
Missing data

1 Introduction

Temporal mapping of cortical changes is crucial for understanding normal and abnormal brain development. However, such analysis requires longitudinal followup scans, which can be challenging to acquire due to subject dropouts and failed scans. The easiest way to deal with missing data is by discarding the data of subjects with missing scans. Though convenient, this approach discards a huge amount of useful information and leaves a smaller subset of data for analysis with

© Springer Nature Switzerland AG 2019
A. C. S. Chung et al. (Eds.): IPMI 2019, LNCS 11492, pp. 277–288, 2019.
https://doi.org/10.1007/978-3-030-20351-1_21

reduced statistical sensitivity. To make full use of available data, we introduce in this paper a deep learning approach to predicting missing surfaces.

Meng et al. [14] recently employed random forest for longitudinal prediction of infant cortical thickness in an incomplete dataset. They first imputed the missing data and then used the imputed dataset to train their prediction model. While effective, their method is limited in the following ways: (i) Cortical surfaces need to be mapped onto a common sphere, which is a time consuming process that can lose surface topological information; (ii) Prediction is limited to cortical attributes, such as thickness; the actual surfaces are not generated, (iii) Cortical attributes are predicted at each time point independently, disregarding temporal consistency, and (iv) The imputed surfaces, when used for training, can introduce errors. Another attempt to predict cortical surfaces was carried out by Rekik et al. [19], where they proposed a learning-based framework for predicting dynamic postnatal changes in the cortical shape based on the cortical surfaces at birth using varifold metric for surface regression. Their method however requires full longitudinal scans, which are not always available.

To address the above-mentioned limitations, we propose in this paper a method for the longitudinal prediction of cortical surfaces based on a spatial graph convolutional neural network (GCNN). We first parametrize cortical surfaces spatially using intrinsic local coordinate systems. This allows us to implement an effective means of surface convolution. Such convolution mechanism is incorporated in the graph convolution layers of a dual-channel network that caters to the prediction of both inner and outer cortical surfaces, with vertex-wise cortical thickness as constraint. Longitudinal consistency is enforced by ensuring that the predicted surfaces at not only the final time point, but also the intermediate time points, match actual brain surfaces in the training set. We further adopt a binary flagging mechanism to ensure that the loss associated with a nonexistent surface is not contributing to back-propagation. Our network is hence flexible and does not require complete longitudinal data for training. Each available cortical surface can contribute to the learning of the growth trajectories for prediction purposes. Experimental results illustrate that the proposed method can accurately predict the non-linear cortical growth with longitudinal consistency. The predicted surfaces allow cortical attributes such as cortical thickness to be computed for further analysis.

2   Materials

This study is approved by the Institutional Review Board of the University of North Carolina (UNC) School of Medicine. 37 healthy infants were recruited and scanned longitudinally at 1, 3, and 6 months of age (see Table 1). The acquired T1-weighted (T1w) and T2-weighted (T2w) MR images were processed using the UNC Infant Cortical Surface Pipeline [10] to obtain the inner and outer surfaces and their vertex-to-vertex correspondences for each hemisphere. The surfaces were then align to a common space using the 4D infant cortical surface atlas described in [24] for cross-sectional and longitudinal correspondences. Each cortical surface of left and right hemisphere is represented as a mesh formed by uniform non-intersecting triangles. Mathematically, the mesh can be represented as a graph $\mathcal{G} = (\mathcal{V}, \mathcal{F})$, where $\mathcal{V}$ is the vertex set and $\mathcal{F} \subset \mathcal{V} \times \mathcal{V} \times \mathcal{V}$ is the set of triangular faces, each connecting three vertices.

Table 1. Data availability.

Availability	All $1^{st}, 3^{rd}, 6^{th}$	Only $1^{st}, 3^{rd}$	Only $1^{st}, 6^{th}$
Number of subjects	23	5	9

3   Methods

In this section, we will first introduce how spatial convolution can be defined on cortical surfaces represented as graphs. Then, we will introduce our GCNN framework for longitudinally consistent prediction of cortical surfaces.

3.1   Local Geodesic Polar Grids

Each cortical surface is represented as a triangular mesh $\mathcal{G} = (\mathcal{V}, \mathcal{F})$ associated with a vertex-wise feature map $f : \mathcal{V} \mapsto \mathcal{R}$, $f(\mathcal{V}) = \{f(v) : v \in \mathcal{V}\}$. Unlike the various global parametrizations for Euclidean domains, the lack of meaningful global parametrizations for surface meshes [3] forces us to parametrize $\mathcal{G}$ in intrinsic coordinate systems. Following [9], for every vertex $v_i \in \mathcal{V}$, we build a geodesic disc $\mathcal{D}_{v_i} = \{v'|\rho(v', v_i) \leq \rho_\mathcal{D}\} \subset \mathcal{V}$ ($\rho_\mathcal{D}$ is taken as 1% of the geodesic diameter of the entire surface mesh [13]). Then, $\mathcal{D}_{v_i}$ is partitioned into a polar grid with N_ρ geodesics bins and M_θ angular bins, via geodesic outward shooting and unfolding [8]. Therefore, within the grid $\mathcal{D}_{v_i}$, the local geodesic polar coordinate for any vertex $v_j \in \mathcal{D}_{v_i}$ is (ρ_{ij}, θ_{ij}), with ρ_{ij} and θ_{ij} denoting the geodesic distance and the angular distance between v_i and v_j, respectively. For the whole mesh $\mathcal{G}$, this local parameterization can be written as a sparse matrix $(\mathbf{P}, \mathbf{\Theta})$, with $\mathbf{P} = (\rho_{ij})_{|\mathcal{V}| \times |\mathcal{V}|}$, $\mathbf{\Theta} = (\theta_{ij})_{|\mathcal{V}| \times |\mathcal{V}|}$, and $i, j = 1, ..., |\mathcal{V}|$.

3.2   Spatial Convolution on Cortical Surfaces

Surface Patch Uniformization. With local parametrization for the whole surface mesh $\mathcal{G}$, local surface patches can be extracted within each geodesic polar grid D_v (Sect. 3.1). However, the distributions of vertices on the patches extracted at different vertices are not necessarily uniform [3]. As in [15], we map surface patches to a common template domain. Specifically, the template contains $N_\rho \times N_\theta$ virtual vertices $\{v_{kl}^{virtual} \in \mathcal{D}_v : k = 1, ..., N_\rho, l = 1, ..., N_\theta\}$ at the intersections of $N_\rho \times N_\theta$ bins (Fig. 1). Feature maps f on the virtual vertices can be obtained by weighted interpolation on $\mathcal{D}_v$ based on the actual vertices $\{v'\} \subset \mathcal{D}_v$:

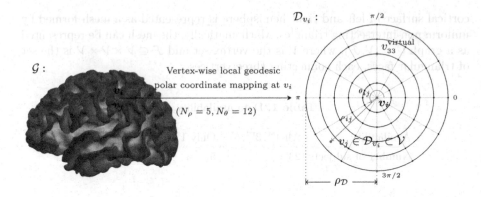

Fig. 1. A local geodesic polar grid $\mathcal{D}_{v_i}$ (5 ρ-bins, 12 θ-bins) constructed at vertex v_i on a surface mesh $\mathcal{G}$. v_j is an actual vertex, v_{33}^{virtual} is a virtual vertex located at the intersection of 3rd ρ-bin and 3rd θ-bin.

$$f(\mathcal{D}_v) = \{f(v_{kl}^{\text{virtual}}) : k = 1, ..., N_\rho, l = 1, ..., N_\theta\}, \quad v \in V \tag{1}$$

$$f(v_{kl}^{\text{virtual}}) = \sum_{v' \in \mathcal{D}_v} w_{kl}(\boldsymbol{u}_v(v'))f(v'), \quad (k,l) \in \{1,...,N_\rho\} \times \{1,...,N_\theta\} \tag{2}$$

where $\boldsymbol{u}_v(v') = (\rho(v,v'), \theta(v,v'))$ denotes the local geodesic polar coordinate of v' in relation to v, $\{w_{kl}(\cdot)\}$ are the parametric Gaussian kernels adopted from [15]:

$$w_{kl}(\boldsymbol{u}) = \exp\left\{-\frac{1}{2}(\boldsymbol{u} - \boldsymbol{u}_{kl})^T \sum_{kl}^{-1}(\boldsymbol{u} - \boldsymbol{u}_{kl})\right\} \tag{3}$$

where the mean vectors $\{\boldsymbol{u}_{kl} \in \mathcal{R}^{2 \times 1}\}$ and the diagonal covariance matrices $\{\sum_{kl} \in \mathcal{R}^{2 \times 2}\}$ are learnable. The parametric kernels with extra degrees of freedom generalize the fixed local Gaussian kernels in [13], and naturally solve the origin ambiguity of angular coordinates caused by geodesic polar grids construction in Sect. 3.1.

Spatial Convolution. With the uniform surface patches, we can define the convolution filter γ as a real function field on $\mathcal{D}_v$:

$$\gamma(\mathcal{D}_v) = \{\gamma(v_{kl}^{\text{virtual}}) : k = 1, ..., N_\rho, l = 1, ..., N_\theta\}, \quad v \in V. \tag{4}$$

We define the spatial convolution on cortical surface meshes as

$$(f * \gamma)(v) = \sum_{k=1}^{N_\rho}\sum_{l=1}^{N_\theta}(f \cdot \gamma)(v_{kl}^{\text{virtual}}), \quad v_{kl}^{\text{virtual}} \in \mathcal{D}_v, \quad v \in V \tag{5}$$

where $\{\gamma(v_{kl}^{\text{virtual}})\}$ are learnable filter coefficients. A spatial graph convolutional layer (Fig. 2) consists of two sub-layers that perform (a) Local surface patch uniformization via Eq. (1); and (b) Spatial convolution via Eq. (5).

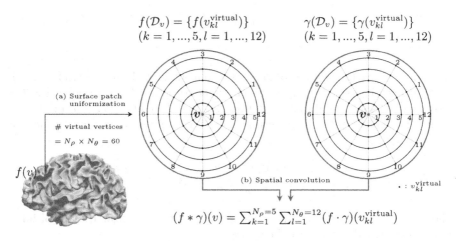

Fig. 2. Spatial graph convolutional layer. Each surface patch extracted by grid $\mathcal{D}_v$ has 5 ρ-bins and 12 θ-bins, resulting in 60 learnable Gaussian kernels (Eq. (3)) for surface patch uniformization. The uniformization step makes it possible to implement the convolution as a scalar product between the patch feature maps and the filter coefficients $\gamma(\mathcal{D}_v)$. Spatial convolution across the entire triangular mesh $\mathcal{G}$ is similar to Cartesian convolution.

3.3   Longitudinal Surface Prediction

Given the baseline (1st month) inner ('in') and outer ('out') cortical surfaces of an infant subject, i.e., $\{\mathcal{G}_1^{\text{in}} = (\mathcal{V}_1^{\text{in}}, \mathcal{F}_1^{\text{in}}), \mathcal{G}_1^{\text{out}} = (\mathcal{V}_1^{\text{out}}, \mathcal{F}_1^{\text{out}})\}$, we train a spatial GCNN to predict the inner and outer cortical surfaces at later time points (3rd month and 6th month).

Input - Local Parameterization Matrices. Locally parametrized baseline inner and outer cortical surface pair: $I_{\text{G}} = \{\mathcal{G}_1^{\text{in}} = (\mathbf{P}_1^{\text{in}}, \boldsymbol{\Theta}_1^{\text{in}}), \mathcal{G}_1^{\text{out}} = (\mathbf{P}_1^{\text{out}}, \boldsymbol{\Theta}_1^{\text{out}})\}$.

Input - Local Shape Descriptors. Local shape information is captured by computing the geometric relationship between a vertex and its neighbors. Specifically, we define the vertex-wise neighborhood difference map $I_{\text{ND}}^{\text{in}}(\mathcal{V})$ associated with baseline inner cortical surface $\mathcal{G}_1^{\text{in}}$ as

$$I_{\text{ND}}^{\text{in}}(v) = \{(x_1^{\text{in}}(v) - x_1^{\text{in}}(w), y_1^{\text{in}}(v) - y_1^{\text{in}}(w), z_1^{\text{in}}(v) - z_1^{\text{in}}(w)) : w \in \mathcal{N}(v)\}, \quad (6)$$

where $(x_1^{\text{in}}(v), y_1^{\text{in}}(v), z_1^{\text{in}}(v))$ refers to the xyz-coordinates of vertex v on $\mathcal{G}_1^{\text{in}}$ at the 1st month, $\mathcal{N}^{(1)}(v)$ is a set of vertices adjacent to v determined by triangular faces. Likewise, the neighborhood difference map of the baseline outer cortical surface $\mathcal{G}_1^{\text{out}}$ is

$$I_{\text{ND}}^{\text{out}}(v) = \{(x_1^{\text{out}}(v) - x_1^{\text{out}}(w), y_1^{\text{out}}(v) - y_1^{\text{out}}(w), z_1^{\text{out}}(v) - z_1^{\text{out}}(w)) : w \in \mathcal{N}(v)\}. \quad (7)$$

where $(x_1^{\text{out}}(v), y_1^{\text{out}}(v), z_1^{\text{out}}(v))$ refers to the xyz-coordinates of vertex v on $\mathcal{G}_1^{\text{out}}$ at the 1st month.

Output - Growth Deformations. The output growth maps $O_M(\mathcal{V})$ associated with cortical surface $\mathcal{G}_M$ at the M-th month ($M = 3, 6$) are defined as the vertex-wise displacements of the surface to the M-month from the prior time point. More specifically, the growth maps of inner and outer cortical surfaces at the 3rd month are

$$\begin{cases} O_3^{\text{in}}(v) = (x_3^{\text{in}}(v) - x_1^{\text{in}}(v), y_3^{\text{in}}(v) - y_1^{\text{in}}(v), z_3^{\text{in}}(v) - z_1^{\text{in}}(v)), \\ O_3^{\text{out}}(v) = (x_3^{\text{out}}(v) - x_1^{\text{out}}(v), y_3^{\text{out}}(v) - y_1^{\text{out}}(v), z_3^{\text{out}}(v) - z_1^{\text{out}}(v)), \end{cases} \quad (8)$$

where subscript '3' denotes the 3rd month. Similarly, the growth maps of inner and outer cortical surfaces at the 6th month are

$$\begin{cases} O_6^{\text{in}}(v) = (x_6^{\text{in}}(v) - x_3^{\text{in}}(v), y_6^{\text{in}}(v) - y_3^{\text{in}}(v), z_6^{\text{in}}(v) - z_3^{\text{in}}(v)), \\ O_6^{\text{out}}(v) = (x_6^{\text{out}}(v) - x_3^{\text{out}}(v), y_6^{\text{out}}(v) - y_3^{\text{out}}(v), z_6^{\text{out}}(v) - z_3^{\text{out}}(v)). \end{cases} \quad (9)$$

The cortical thickness at vertex $v \in \mathcal{V}$ is computed based on the inner and outer cortical surface pair $(\mathcal{G}_M^{\text{in}}, \mathcal{G}_M^{\text{out}})$ at the M-th month as

$$\text{thickness}_M(v) = \|(x_M^{\text{out}}(v) - x_M^{\text{in}}(v), y_M^{\text{out}}(v) - y_M^{\text{in}}(v), z_M^{\text{out}}(v) - z_M^{\text{in}}(v))\|. \quad (10)$$

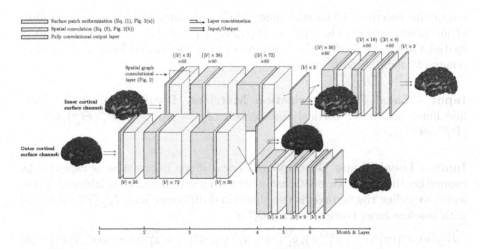

Fig. 3. GCNN longitudinal prediction network. Each graph convolutional layer consists of a surface patch uniformization sub-layer (blue blocks) with 60 learnable Gaussian kernels, followed by a spatial convolution sub-layer (gray blocks) with feature map sizes of 36, 72, 36, 18, 9, 3. Note that the surface uniformization sub-layers do not change feature map size. (Color figure online)

Network Architecture. The proposed longitudinal prediction network has two independent prediction channels with the same architecture to cater to the inner and outer cortical surfaces (see Fig. 3). The depth of the network increases with time, allowing more complex mappings to be learned as prediction further in time needs to be carried out. At each target time point M (i.e., 3rd, 6th month), the network outputs the predicted cortical surface displacements (i.e., $O_M^{\text{in}}, O_M^{\text{out}}$ in Eqs. (8) and (9)). Additionally, at the 3rd month, the hidden feature maps from the 3rd spatial graph convolution sub-layer will be concatenated with the predicted surface displacements at 3rd month to be fed together into the next (4th) surface patch uniformization sub-layer for prediction at the 6th month. Layer concatenation as described above can be interpreted as gathering of dynamic growth momentum (hidden features at the 3rd month) and static status (cortical geometry at the 3rd month). During training, the cortical growth across all time points are learned as a whole, promoting the temporal consistency of longitudinal predictions. The network architecture is generic and can be modified to take into consideration more time points by increasing network depth and adding more output and concatenation layers.

Loss Functions. We employ L^2-norm, denoted as $\text{Loss}_{\text{displacement}}^M$, to measure the errors in the predicted vertex displacements O_M^{in} and O_M^{out} of the inner and outer cortical surfaces at the M-th month ($M = 3, 6$). We also include a cortical thickness loss term to constrain the spatial consistency between the predicted $\mathcal{G}_M^{\text{in}}$ and $\mathcal{G}_M^{\text{out}}$:

$$\text{Loss}_{\text{thickness}}^M = \sum_{v \in \mathcal{V}} |\text{thickness}^{\text{p}}(v) - \text{thickness}^{\text{g}}(v)|, \tag{11}$$

where $\text{thickness}^{\text{p}}(\cdot)$ and $\text{thickness}^{\text{g}}(\cdot)$ are the predicted and ground-truth thickness, respectively.

To fully utilize the incomplete data (see Table 1), we use a binary flag to indicate the nonexistence (flag '0') or existence (flag '1') of a ground-truth surface. The flag is used to ensure that the loss associated with a nonexistent surface is not contributing to back-propagation. More specifically, this is achieved by defining the total loss of the network as

$$\text{Loss} = \sum_{M=3,6} \text{flag}^M \cdot (\alpha \cdot \text{Loss}_{\text{displacement}}^M + (1 - \alpha) \cdot \text{Loss}_{\text{thickness}}^M). \tag{12}$$

where α $(0 < \alpha < 1)$ controls the relative contributions of $\text{Loss}_{\text{displacement}}^M$ and $\text{Loss}_{\text{thickness}}^M$. As a consequence, our network is flexible and does not require longitudinal data that are complete at all $1^{\text{st}}, 3^{\text{rd}}$ and 6th months for training. Each available ground-truth cortical surface can contribute to the learning of the growth trajectories.

4 Experiments

We compared the proposed longitudinal prediction network (GCNN-LP) with two methods: (1) Affine transformation (AF) [7]; (2) Independent prediction networks (GCNN-IPs). Specifically, the GCNN-IP for surface prediction at the 3rd month is implemented by removing all layers after the output layer for the 3rd month in GCNN-LP. GCNN-IP for the 6th month is implemented by removing the output and concatenation layers of GCNN-LP at the 3rd month. All inputs and outputs of GCNN-IPs are the same as those defined in GCNN-LP.

We chose 3 infant subjects (see Table 1) with data available at 1st, 3rd and 6th months for testing. Other subjects were used for training. For each surface mesh $\mathcal{G}$, in total the number of vertices $|\mathcal{V}| = 10242$ and the number of triangular faces $|\mathcal{F}| = 20480$. Local geodesic polar grids with radius $\rho_D = 2\,\text{mm}$ were constructed on the baseline inner and outer cortical surfaces. Each grid was partitioned into 60 bins ($N_\rho = 5, N_\theta = 12$), as shown in Fig. 1. The corresponding 60 learnable Gaussian kernels (Eq. (3)) were initialized with random means and variances. Training for each model was performed with 25k maximum updates using Adam, 10^{-4} learning rate for the first 5k iterations, and 10^{-5} for the remaining iterations.

To quantitatively evaluate the prediction results, we computed the median absolute error (MAE) for both cortical surface (cs) and cortical thickness (ct) predictions:

$$\text{MAE}_{cs} = \text{median}_{v\in\mathcal{V}}\{\|(x^p(v) - x^g(v), y^p(v) - y^g(v), z^p(v) - z^g(v))\|\}, \quad (13)$$

$$\text{MAE}_{ct} = \text{median}_{v\in\mathcal{V}}\{|\text{thickness}^p(v) - \text{thickness}^g(v)|\} \quad (14)$$

where 'p' and 'g' denote the prediction and ground-truth, respectively.

Table 2 summarizes the prediction performance of the different methods. Compared with AF, the better performance of all GCNN models in predicting cortical surfaces indicates that GCNNs are capable of learning the non-linearity in cortical growth, which cannot be captured by AF. The smaller errors achieved

Table 2. Quantitative comparison of AF, GCNN-IP, and GCNN-LP at the 3rd and 6th months using median absolute errors (MAE) averaged across testing subjects.

Month	Method	Cortical thickness	Inner surface	Outer surface
		MAE$_{ct}$ (mm)	MAE$_{cs}$ (mm)	
3	AF	1.2029	4.2784	4.1332
	GCNN-IP	0.3656	2.4702	2.5020
	GCNN-LP	**0.3166**	**2.4436**	**2.4755**
6	AF	1.6035	4.5378	5.4352
	GCNN-IP	0.3857	2.3764	2.5386
	GCNN-LP	**0.3277**	**2.0932**	**2.2568**

by GCNNs over AF in cortical thickness prediction validate the spatial consistency between the inner and outer cortical surfaces predicted by GCNNs. GCNN-LP yields greater accuracy than GCNN-IP in all prediction tasks.

Figure 4 shows the vertex-wise surface prediction errors in terms of L^2 Euclidean distances of corresponding vertices on the inner and outer surfacess. The corresponding error maps for cortical thickness computed from the predicted cortical surfaces are shown in Fig. 5. Clearly, GCNN-LP and GCNN-IP yield much smaller prediction errors than AF across different cortical regions.

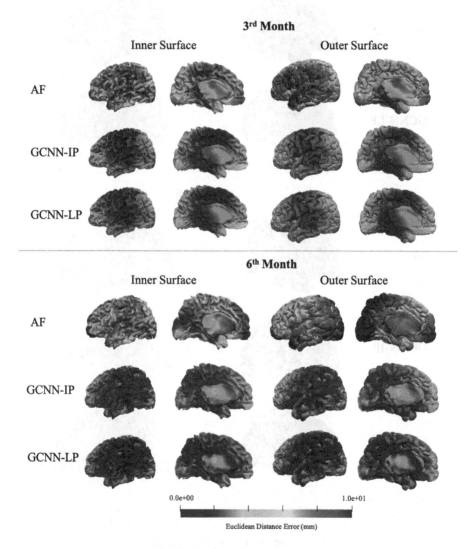

Fig. 4. Surface prediction errors.

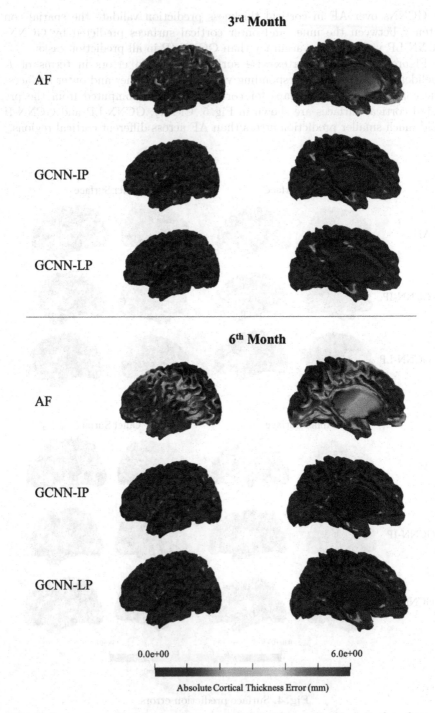

Fig. 5. Errors in cortical thickness computed from the predicted cortical surfaces.

5   Conclusion

We propose a novel longitudinally consistent prediction method, based on spatial graph convolutional neural network, for the prediction of infant cortical surfaces. Our method is able to learn intrinsic, non-linear growth features via spatial convolution directly applied on the cortical surfaces. Predicting the cortical growth across all target time points within a single network, the proposed method models the growth trajectories with temporal consistency. Experimental results demonstrated that our method is capable of capturing the growth trajectories for accurate longitudinal surface prediction.

Acknowledgment. This work was supported in part by NIH grants (MH117943, EB006733, AG041721, and MH100217).

References

1. Boscaini, D., Masci, J., Melzi, S., Bronstein, M.M., Castellani, U., Vandergheynst, P.: Learning class-specific descriptors for deformable shapes using localized spectral convolutional networks. Comput. Graph. Forum (2015)
2. Boscaini, D., Masci, J., Rodolà, E., Bronstein, M.M.: Learning shape correspondence with anisotropic convolutional neural networks. In: Neural Information Processing Systems (NeurIPS) (2016)
3. Bronstein, M.M., Bruna, J., LeCun, Y., Szlam, A., Vandergheynst, P.: Geometric deep learning: going beyond euclidean data. IEEE Signal Process. Mag. **34**, 18–42 (2017)
4. Bruna, J., Zaremba, W., Szlam, A., LeCun, Y.: Spectral networks and deep locally connected networks on graphs. In: International Conference on Learning Representations (ICLR) (2014)
5. Defferrard, M., Bresson, X., Vandergheynst, P.: Convolutional neural networks on graphs with fast localized spectral filtering. In: Neural Information Processing Systems (NeurIPS) (2016)
6. Fischl, B.: Freesurfer. NeuroImage **62**, 774–781 (2012)
7. Kanatani, K.: Statistical Optimization for Geometric Computation: Theory and Practice. Elsevier Science Inc., New York (1996)
8. Kimmel, R., Sethian, J.A.: Computing geodesic paths on manifolds. Proc. National Acad. Sci. (PNAS) **95**, 8431–8435 (1998)
9. Kokkinos, I., Bronstein, M.M., Litman, R., Bronstein, A.M.: Intrinsic shape context descriptors for deformable shapes. In: Computer Vision and Pattern Recognition (CVPR) (2012)
10. Li, G., Nie, J., Wu, G., Wang, Y., Shen, D.: Consistent reconstruction of cortical surfaces from longitudinal brain MR images. NeuroImage **59**, 3805–3820 (2011)
11. Liu, G., Lin, Z., Yan, S., Sun, J., Yu, Y., Ma, Y.: Robust recovery of subspace structures by low-rank representation. IEEE Trans. Pattern Anal. Mach. Intell. **35**, 171–184 (2013)
12. Long, J., Shelhamer, E., Darrell, T.: Fully convolutional networks for semantic segmentation. In: Computer Vision and Pattern Recognition (CVPR) (2015)
13. Masci, J., Boscaini, D., Bronstein, M.M., Vandergheynst, P.: Geodesic convolutional neural networks on Riemannian manifolds. In: International IEEE Workshop on 3D Representation and Recognition (3DRR) (2015)

14. Meng, Y., Li, G., Gao, Y., Lin, W., Shen, D.: Learning-based subject-specific estimation of dynamic maps of cortical morphology at missing time points in longitudinal infant studies. Hum. Brain Mapp. **37**, 4129–41417 (2016)
15. Monti, F., Boscaini, D., Masci, J., Rodolà, E., Svoboda, J., Bronstein, M.M.: Geometric deep learning on graphs and manifolds using mixture model CNNs. In: Computer Vision and Pattern Recognition (CVPR) (2017)
16. Niepert, M., Ahmed, M., Kutzkov, K.: Learning convolutional neural networks for graphs. In: International Conference on Machine Learning (ICML) (2016)
17. Niethammer, M., Huang, Y., Vialard, F.-X.: Geodesic regression for image timeseries. In: Fichtinger, G., Martel, A., Peters, T. (eds.) MICCAI 2011. LNCS, vol. 6892, pp. 655–662. Springer, Heidelberg (2011). https://doi.org/10.1007/978-3-642-23629-7_80
18. Pathan, S., Hong, Y.: Predictive image regression for longitudinal studies with missing data. In: Medical Imaging with Deep Learning (MIDL) (2018)
19. Rekik, I., Li, G., Lin, W., Shen, D.: Predicting infant cortical surface development using a 4D varifold-based learning framework and local topography-based shape morphing. Med. Image Anal. **28**, 1–12 (2015)
20. Rekik, I., Li, G., Yap, P.T., Chen, G., Lin, W., Shen, D.: Joint prediction of longitudinal development of cortical surfaces and white matter fibers from neonatal MRI. Neuroimage **152**, 411–424 (2017)
21. Scarselli, F., Gori, M., Tsoi, A.C., Hagenbuchner, M., Monfardini, G.: The graph neural network model. IEEE Trans. Neural Netw. **20**(1), 61–80 (2009)
22. Wardetzky, M., Mathur, S., Kälberer, F., Grinspun, E.: Discrete Laplace operators: no free lunch. In: Eurographics Symposium on Geometry Processing (2007)
23. Wee, C.Y., Yap, P.T., Shen, D.: Prediction of Alzheimer's disease and mild cognitive impairment using cortical morphological patterns. Hum. Brain Mapp. **34**, 3411–3425 (2013)
24. Wu, Z., Li, G., Meng, Y., Wang, L., Lin, W., Shen, D.: 4D infant cortical surface atlas construction using spherical patch-based sparse representation. In: Descoteaux, M., Maier-Hein, L., Franz, A., Jannin, P., Collins, D.L., Duchesne, S. (eds.) MICCAI 2017. LNCS, vol. 10433, pp. 57–65. Springer, Cham (2017). https://doi.org/10.1007/978-3-319-66182-7_7

Functional Imaging

Integrating Convolutional Neural Networks and Probabilistic Graphical Modeling for Epileptic Seizure Detection in Multichannel EEG

Jeff Craley[1]([⊠]), Emily Johnson[2], and Archana Venkataraman[1]

[1] Department of Electrical and Computer Engineering,
Johns Hopkins University, Baltimore, USA
jcraley2@jhu.edu
[2] Department of Neurology,
Johns Hopkins Medical Institute, Baltimore, USA

Abstract. Manual seizure detection in clinical electroencephalography (EEG) is time consuming and requires extensive training. In addition, the seizure origin and spreading pattern is valuable for therapeutic planning but cannot always be manually disambiguated. Prior work in automated seizure detection has focused on engineering new features that better capture the seizure activity. However, these methods ignore crucial information in the data and are not sensitive enough to track the seizure propagation. In this work we introduce a hybrid Probabilistic Graphical Model-Convolutional Neural Network (PGM-CNN) for seizure tracking in multichannel EEG. Our model leverages the power of deep learning for data driven analysis of the raw EEG time series while retaining clinically relevant information through the latent PGM prior. We validate our hybrid model on clinical EEG data from two hospitals with distinct patient populations. Our system achieves better detection performance than baseline methods, which exclusively use PGMs or neural networks.

1 Introduction

Epilepsy affects nearly 3.5 million people in the United States and is associated with a fivefold increase in mortality rate [1]. It has been estimated that 20–40% of epilepsy patients are medically refractory and do not respond to anti-epileptic drugs [2]. Subsequent treatments for these patients rely on clinicians being able to detect, and if appropriate, localize seizure activity in the brain. Due to the heterogeny of epilepsy disorders, scalp electroencephalography (EEG) recordings are critical for diagnosis and treatment planning. Typical in-patient evaluations for epilepsy involve continuous EEG recordings, sometimes for days. These recordings are manually inspected for seizure activity, a process which is time consuming, requires years of training, and is prone to human error.

Feature Engineering for EEG Analysis: Automated seizure detection has been an active field of research for the past three decades. Most algorithms

© Springer Nature Switzerland AG 2019
A. C. S. Chung et al. (Eds.): IPMI 2019, LNCS 11492, pp. 291–303, 2019.
https://doi.org/10.1007/978-3-030-20351-1_22

follow a two-stage machine learning pipeline consisting of (1) feature extraction from the EEG signal over short time windows, followed by (2) a binary classifier to identify seizure versus non-seizure intervals [3]. This end-to-end pipeline was exemplified by Shoeb et al. [4] where power features in different frequency bands were used in conjunction with a support vector machine classifier.

Prior work in the seizure detection community has focused largely on the feature extraction step. For example, Andrzejak et al. [5] noted that EEG during seizures exhibited a different degree of non-linearity than EEG recorded during baseline, inspiring the application of non-linear signal processing and chaos theory to EEG analysis. Similarly, Güler et al. [6] used Lyapunov exponents to discriminate between seizure and non-seizure EEG. While the above methods are promising, the generalization power is fundamentally limited by the chosen features. In addition, they perform classification independently for each time window and do not capture the seizure origin or manifestation.

Craley et al. [7] introduced a novel approach for seizure detection that used a Coupled Hidden Markov Model (CHMM) to track the propagation of a seizure across the scalp. However, this method relied on carefully selected features in order to learn a highly structured likelihood function. Despite leading to good performance, feature extraction focused specifically on a small number of spectral features. These features, combined with likelihood scoring using a restricted set of functions, likely missed relevant seizure information. In contrast, here we rely on data-driven strategies using deep architectures to directly learn more effective representations and analysis functions.

Data-Driven Representation Learning: Traditional representation learning techniques solve auxiliary problems in the pursuit of representations with desirable properties. While these properties are often useful, there are no guarantees that they are most appropriate for a given task. Alternatively, deep networks learn representations that capture facets of the data directly applicable to the task at hand [8]. This improved analytical power can come at the cost of interpretability, as these features may lack inuitive explanation.

This paper presents an integrated framework for epileptic seizure detection that blends the interpretability of Probabilistic Graphical Models (PGMs) with advancements in deep learning. Our PGM leverages the CHMM [7] for automated seizure tracking. We augment this PGM with a Convolutional Neural Network (CNN) likelihood model. Our PGM-CNN strategy can automatically learn the EEG features relevant for detection from limited amounts of training data. We demonstrate our PGM-CNN framework on multichannel EEG data acquired from two hospitals with distinct patient populations. Our PGM-CNN framework correctly identifies more of the annotated seizure activity in both datasets than comparable baseline methods. This performance suggests a new direction for automated seizure tracking in clinical EEG.

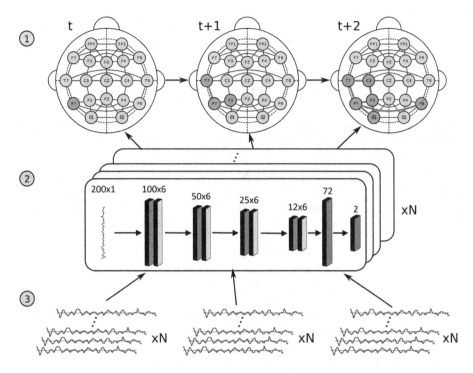

Fig. 1. Detail of the inference procedure. Time flows to the right while information flows upwards. In the third row, we depict the raw EEG signal. The signal from each channel is fed into a dedicated CNN for scoring in the second row. The first row depicts a hypothetical seizure spreading through the propagation network of the CHMM.

2   Integrating PGMs and Deep Learning

Figure 1 outlines our modeling strategy. Raw EEG signal from each channel in row three is fed directly into the CNNs in row two, where one CNN is trained for each channel. The CNNs score the signal for seizure activity and feed this information into the CHMM prior shown in row 1. The CHMM fuses these scores across the scalp and through time to perform posterior inference for seizure activity. Below, we formalize the mathematical relationships and inference procedure.

2.1   PGM Prior Based on the Coupled Hidden Markov Model

The PGM prior couples the hidden states of each EEG channel according to the previous states of the neighboring and contralateral channels [7]. For each channel i, we let the underlying seizure state at time t be represented by the variable $X_i^t \in \{0, 1, 2\}$ corresponding to pre-seizure baseline, seizure activity, and post-seizure baseline, respectively. The corresponding EEG data is represented by Y_i^t. We define the aunts of channel i, $au(i)$, as the neighbors in the graphs shown in Fig. 1 and indicate the states of the ensemble of aunts of channel i at time t with $\mathbf{X}_{au(i)}^{t}$. The joint probability distribution can be written

$$P(\mathbf{X}, \mathbf{Y}) = \prod_{i=1}^{N} P(Y_i^0 \mid X_i^0) \prod_{t=1}^{T} P(Y_i^t \mid X_i^t) P(X_i^t \mid \mathbf{X}_{au(i)}^{t-1}, X_i^{t-1}), \qquad (1)$$

where N indicates the number of channels and T is the length of the recording. Notice that we assume all channels are initially in baseline (i.e. $X_i^0 = 0$, $\forall i$) and have thus omitted the distribution over the initial state.

The transition probability $P(X_i^t \mid \mathbf{X}_{au(i)}^{t-1}, X_i^{t-1})$ for each chain depends only on the aunt states and the state of the chain in the previous timestep. These probabilities are encoded in a left-to-right time-inhomogenous transition matrix $\mathbf{A}_i^t$ where $P(X_i^t = k \mid X_i^{t-1} = j, X_{au(i)}^{t-1}) = A_{i,jk}^t$ as follows:

$$\mathbf{A}_i^t = \begin{bmatrix} 1 - g_i^t & g_i^t & 0 \\ 0 & 1 - h_i^t & h_i^t \\ 0 & 0 & 1 \end{bmatrix}. \qquad (2)$$

Here g_i^t and h_i^t correspond to the probability that a channel enters or exits the seizure state, respectively. We model these probabilities as logistic regressions

$$\log\left(\frac{g_i^t}{1 - g_i^t}\right) = \rho_0 + \rho_1 \eta_i^t, \qquad \log\left(\frac{h_i^t}{1 - h_i^t}\right) = \phi_0 + \phi_1 \eta_i^t \qquad (3)$$

such that ρ_0 corresponds to the base rate of seizure onset for each individual channel while ρ_1 corresponds to the influence of the aunt channels on the seizure onset. Likewise, the parameters ϕ_0 and ϕ_1 govern offset in an identical way.

2.2   Nonparameteric Likelihood via Convolutional Neural Networks

CNNs have become standard in computer vision due to their ability to learn spatially invariant features across multiple scales [8]. At a high level, the early layers learn simple features, such as edge detectors, while subsequent layers learn more and more complicated features. CNNs are also becoming popular for one-dimensional and time series data, where they provide a valuable alternative to the standard Recurrent Neural Network (RNN). While RNNs have been particularly effective in analyzing short sequences, CNNs with large receptive fields can be trained much faster than RNNs for long sequences. In addition, CNNs are restricted to learning highly structured functions composed of convolutions, which reduces their ability to overfit when training data is limited [8]. While CNNs are powerful tools for data analysis, they suffer from a lack of interpretability. However, from a clinical standpoint, we are primarily concerned with the seizure propagation patterns, as opposed to the underlying feature representation. Our hybrid approach captures the clinically relevant information by using a directly interpretable PGM prior while giving the CNN free rein over the data likelihood to improve EEG signal analysis, resulting in gains in detection performance.

One important caveat to integrating a CNN data likelihood is that, by default, a CNN is trained for posterior inference. Namely, given the input data Y_i^t, the CNN will output a soft class assignment of seizure versus baseline, i.e. $P(X_i^t \mid Y_i^t)$. In contrast, the joint distribution in Eq. (1) relies on the data likelihood, $P(Y_i^t \mid X_i^t)$. We can obtain this factor by applying Bayes' rule:

$$P(Y_i^t \mid X_i^t) = \frac{P(X_i^t \mid Y_i^t)P(Y_i^t)}{P(X_i^t)} \propto \frac{P(X_i^t \mid Y_i^t)}{P(X_i^t)}. \tag{4}$$

Notice that we ignore the marginal probability $P(Y_i^t)$, as this term is the same regardless of the class label, and we only require data likelihoods up to a constant factor for posterior inference. Hence, we can rescale the CNN output by $P(X_i^t)$ to arrive at a surrogate likelihood term [9]. We approximate $P(X_i^t)$ by the proportion of seizure versus baseline in the dataset, i.e.

$$\hat{P}(X = 1) = \frac{\#\,\text{seizure windows}}{\#\,\text{windows}}, \qquad \hat{P}(X = 0) = 1 - \hat{P}(X = 1). \tag{5}$$

The rescaling of the discriminative posterior in Eq. (4) using the approximate prior over states in Eq. (5) will serve as the likelihood in our PGM-CNN model.

2.3   Fitting the PGM-CNN Model

We fit the PGN-CNN using a variational algorithm, similar to the one in [7]. We approximate the latent posterior as the product of independent HMM chains.

$$P(\mathbf{X} \mid \mathbf{Y}) \approx Q(\mathbf{X}) = \prod_{i=1}^{N} \frac{1}{Z_{Q_i}} Q_i(\mathbf{X}_i) = \prod_{i=1}^{N} \frac{1}{Z_{Q_i}} \prod_{t=1}^{T} T_i^t(X_i^t \mid X_i^{t-1}) E_i^t(X_i^t). \tag{6}$$

The factors $E_i^t(X_i^t)$ and $T_i^t(X_i^t \mid X_i^{t-1})$ encode the emission and transition terms of the approximating HMMs, respectively.

Posterior Inference: We infer the latent posterior distribution by iteratively running the forward-backward algorithm [10] over each of the individual chains, while holding the remaining chains constant. The forward-backward algorithm calculates the following posterior statistics under the distribution Q:

$$\tilde{\gamma}_i^t(j) := E_{Q_i}\left[\mathbb{1}(X_i^t = j)\right] \qquad \tilde{\xi}_i^t(j, k) := E_{Q_i}\left[\mathbb{1}(X_i^t = j, X_i^{t+1} = k)\right].$$

The variational form of $T_i^t(X_i^t \mid X_i^{t-1})$ closely resembles the original transition distribution but is now based on the statistics $\{\tilde{\gamma}_i^t(j), \tilde{\xi}_i^t(j, k)\}$. The emission parameters are the original likelihood multiplied by a correction factor $\alpha_i^t(\cdot)$.

$$E_i^t(0, 2) = p(Y_i^t \mid X_i^t = 0, 2)\alpha_i^t(0), \qquad E_i^t(1) = p(Y_i^t \mid X_i^t = 1)\alpha_i^t(1)$$

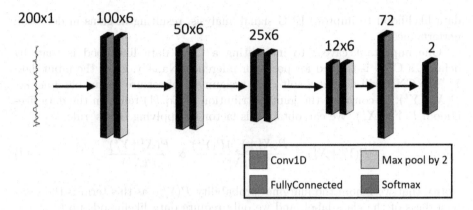

Fig. 2. Convolutional neural network architecture used in this work

$$\alpha_i^t(z) \approx \sum_{j \in au(i)} \left[\tilde{\xi}_j^t(0,0) \left(-\rho_0 - \rho_1 \left(\nu_j^{t+1} + z \right) \right) \right.$$

$$- \tilde{\gamma}_j^t(0) \log \left(1 + e^{-\rho_0 - \rho_1 \left(\nu_j^{t+1} + z \right)} \right) + \tilde{\xi}_j^t(1,1) \left(-\phi_0 - \phi_1 \left(\nu_j^{t+1} + z \right) \right)$$

$$\left. - \tilde{\gamma}_j^t(1) \log \left(1 + e^{-\phi_0 - \phi_1 \left(\nu_j^{t+1} + z \right)} \right) \right] \quad (7)$$

The factor shown in Eq. (7) encodes the influence of the aunts in the following timestep. In this term we define $\nu_i^t = \sum_{j \in au(i)} X_j^t$. We use Newton's method to learn the transition parameters $\{\rho_0, \rho_1, \phi_0, \phi_1\}$ based on the inferred $Q(\mathbf{X})$.

Neural Network Implementation: We implemented the CNN in PyTorch. The CNN consists of 4 convolution and pool layers as shown in Fig. 2. Each layer uses 6 channels with a kernel size of 5 samples and 2 sample zero padding to maintain a constant size. A LeakyReLU activation, where LeakyReLU$(x) = \max(0, x) + 0.01 \cdot \min(0, x)$, is applied at each layer. A max pooling operation with a kernel size of 2 and a stride of 2 is applied, halving the size of the representation at each layer. After the final convolution, the hidden units are concatenated and passed to a single linear layer for classification using a softmax activation.

During experimentation in the design of this network, we investigated similar architectures of varying depths, numbers of channels, and activation functions. Networks with saturating activations failed to train in some cases, perhaps due to the presence of artifact with extreme amplitudes. We found the LeakyReLU to be the most robust, likely due to the fact that it does not saturate.

The CNNs were trained discriminatively with a cross entropy loss function prior to posterior inference. We trained separate CNN classifiers for each EEG channel to capture behavior specific to different parts of the scalp. Stochastic gradient descent was performed using the Adam optimizer with a batch size of 32 samples and a learning rate of 0.5. We trained each CNN for 60 epochs, which was sufficient to achieve reliable performance without overfitting.

3 Evaluation

3.1 Baseline Comparisons

We compare our PGM-CNN detection performance to baseline methods ranging from simple classifiers on hand selected features to a fully CNN strategy. The features used in [7] (sum of spectral components and line-length) were used for all non-CNN baselines. Recordings were randomly assigned to 5-folds for cross validation. Training was performed on 4 folds while the remaining fold was used for testing. The baseline methods are summarized below.

CNN: We implement an end-to-end deep learning pipeline based on the CNN classification architecture described in Sect. 2.3. This comparison evaluates the predictive value of the CNN without the smoothing in the PGM prior.

CHMM: We implement the original CHMM model proposed in [7] which assumes a Gaussian Mixture Model (GMM) likelihood using the suggested parameter settings. This comparison will evaluate the performance gain in using a non-parametric likelihood with data driven learning from the raw EEG signal.

ANN: Similar to the CNN baseline, we evaluate the performance of the predefined features as inputs for an Artificial Neural Network (ANN) classifier. Due to the relatively small feature space we opted for a small ANN shown in Fig. 3 to avoid overfitting. Our networks are composed of two hidden layers with 10 units each. Each layer is fully connected with Rectified Linear Unit (ReLU) activations. The final output layer contains two nodes with a softmax activation applied. Thus the final layer represents the posterior probability of a hidden state given the associated feature vector.

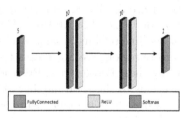

Fig. 3. Artificial neural network used for seizure detection in this work.

GMM: Finally, we implement a simple GMM classifier based on the precomputed EEG features. The inclusion of this baseline allows us to evaluate the relative performance of the CNN, ANN, and parametric GMM likelihoods directly without the inclusion of the latent seizure spreading prior.

3.2 Performance Metrics

Our performance metrics are based on the maximum a posterior (MAP) estimate of baseline versus seizure for each method and are presented as averages across test folds. Since the clinical seizure annotations tend to be overly generous and do not contain spatial information about onset, we aggregate the True Positives (TP), True Negatives (TN), False Positives (FP), and False Negatives (FN) across all windows, channels, and all seizure recordings. In general, the recordings contain muscle artifact directly following the seizure which confounds

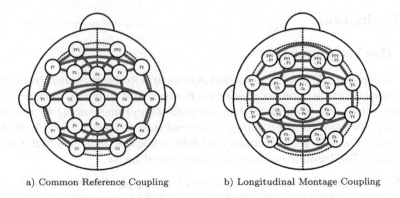

a) Common Reference Coupling   b) Longitudinal Montage Coupling

Fig. 4. Propagation paths for the (a) common reference and (b) longitudinal montage.

the offset for all methods. Therefore, we count any seizure classification occuring within the annotated seizure region as TP. However any contiguous classifications continuing past the annotated offset is not counted in our evaluation statistics.

Below we detail the summary statistics computed for each model. True Positive Rate (TPR), also known as recall, represents the total rate of correct classification. False Positive Rate (FPR) represents the rate of incorrect classification of baseline regions as seizure after excluding classifications beginning within the seizure region. We calculate a lower bound on the Area Under the Curve (AUC) using these two metrics. Precision (P) details the ratio of correct seizure classifications to the total number of seizure classifications. In addition to AUC, the F1 score offers a similar summary by computing the harmonic mean of P and TPR. Mathematically, these statistics are given by:

$$TPR = \frac{\sum_{i=1}^{N} TP_i}{\sum_{i=1}^{N} (TP_i + FN_i)} \qquad FPR = \frac{\sum_{i=1}^{N} FP_i}{\sum_{i=1}^{N} (TN_i + FP_i)}$$

$$P = \frac{\sum_{i=1}^{N} TP_i}{\sum_{i=1}^{N} (TP_i + FP_i)} \qquad F1 = 2\frac{P \cdot R}{P + TPR}$$

$$AUC = FPR \cdot TPR/2 + (1 - FPR)(1 + TPR)/2.$$

4   Experimental Results

Data and Preprocessing: Epileptic seizures are extremely heterogeneous. For example, generalized seizures manifest across the entire cortex at once, whereas focal seizures originate from a single area and may spread to other regions of the cortex. Given this heterogeneity, we evaluate our algorithm on two datasets. The first is taken from the Johns Hopkins Hospital (JHH) and contains 90 seizures from 15 adult patients with focal epilepsy. The second is a publicly available

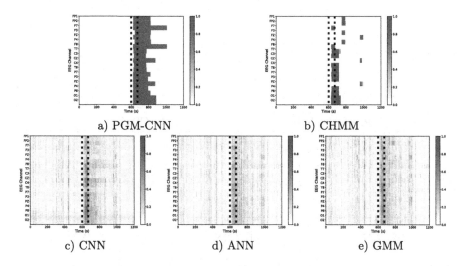

a) PGM-CNN   b) CHMM

c) CNN   d) ANN   e) GMM

Fig. 5. Estimated posteriors for a single seizure from the JHH dataset. EEG channels are shown on the y-axis and time proceeds in the x-direction. The first row shows models with a CHMM prior. The second row shows channel-wise classifications.

Table 1. Results for the both datasets

	JHH dataset					CHB dataset				
Trial	TPR	FPR	AUC	P	F1	TPR	FPR	AUC	P	F1
PGM-CNN	**0.45**	0.010	**0.72**	<u>0.79</u>	**0.57**	**0.61**	0.013	**0.80**	<u>0.74</u>	**0.67**
CHMM	0.37	0.0083	0.68	**0.80**	0.50	0.571	**0.0067**	0.78	**0.83**	**0.67**
CNN	0.19	0.010	0.59	0.62	0.28	0.27	0.0071	0.63	0.70	0.39
DNN	0.11	**0.0070**	0.55	0.58	0.18	0.23	0.0071	0.61	0.66	0.34
GMM	0.18	0.015	0.58	0.52	0.27	0.26	0.010	0.62	0.61	0.37

dataset from Children's Hospital Boston (CHB) of unspecified epilepsy types [4]. We used 185 recordings from this dataset from 24 pediatric patients.

Besides the patient populations, another difference between the two datasets is the acquisition protocol. The JHH dataset contains the original recordings of the 10/20 international system in common reference. In contrast, the CHB dataset uses the longitudinal montage, which forms difference channels by subtracting the signals in neighboring electrodes. We specify a propagation network appropriate for this montage as shown in Fig. 4b. This coupling preserves neighboring and contralateral relationships on the scalp from the original prior.

Our recordings contain one seizure and up to ten minutes of pre- and post-seizure baseline. For the CHB data, these segments were clipped from the original release. EEG channels were low and highpass filtered at 50 and 1.6 Hz, respectively. A notch filter at 60 Hz was applied to remove any remaining power supply artifact. As in [7], 4 spectral features and one line-length feature were extracted

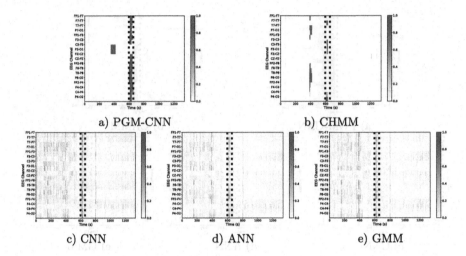

a) PGM-CNN   b) CHMM

c) CNN   d) ANN   e) GMM

Fig. 6. Example posteriors from the CHB dataset. CHMM and likelihood models are shown in the first and second rows, respectively.

from 1 s windows with a 250 ms overlap. The CNN model was trained directly on the raw EEG signal from the 1 s windows.

Detection Performance. Table 1 reports the seizure detection performance averaged across the testing folds for both the JHH and CHB datasets. We have reported True Positive Rate (TPR), False Positive Rate (FPR), Area Under the Curve (AUC), Precision (P), and F1, as described in Sect. 3.2.

Our PGM-CNN dramatically outperforms all of the baseline methods on the JHH dataset. The only drawback is a slightly higher FPR, since our CNN shows more sensitivity to seizure activity, and classifies slightly more baseline as seizure. Despite the numerical increase in FPR, the increased sensitivity is valuable in the clinic, particularly when augmenting the expert manual inspections. Moreover, these spurious detections are compensated by more accurate true detections, which are reflected in the AUC, precision, and F1 measures. We emphasize that our evaluation metrics are much more conservative than in prior studies, which is why the TPR seems uniformly low. Instead of measuring singular detections within the annotated seizure period, we aggregate over channels and windows. This allows us to evaluate not only correct detections of seizures but *how much seizure activity* our algorithms are capable of discerning.

Interestingly, the same detection trends are seen in the CHB data, despite our PGM spreading prior being designed for focal and not generalized seizures. The PGM-CNN achieves the best TPR and AUC as well as a comparable F1 score. In short our flexible data likelihood based on the CNN allows us to learn complex data representations that better separate seizure from baseline. This leads to better detection rates, which is valuable for clinical planning.

Finally, we note that the channel-wise baselines are uniformly bad. Detecting seizure activity is, in general, a relatively difficult problem. Both seizure and

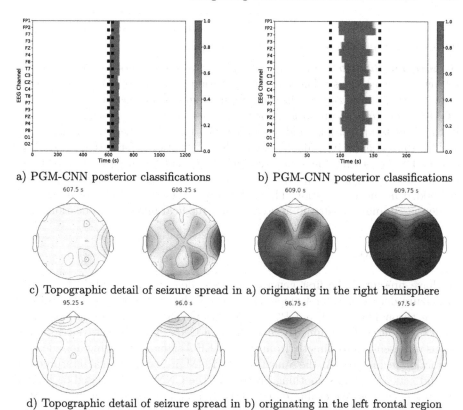

a) PGM-CNN posterior classifications

b) PGM-CNN posterior classifications

c) Topographic detail of seizure spread in a) originating in the right hemisphere

d) Topographic detail of seizure spread in b) originating in the left frontal region

Fig. 7. Example seizure tracking from the JHH dataset. (a, b) Posteriors for all channels. (c, d) Topographic detail showing posterior onsets in clinically annotated regions.

baseline contain high amplitude muscle artifact, which confound the detection over short time windows. In addition, the data distributions are highly overlapping, with seizure activity often resembling normal behavior. The effect of the prior in the PGM-CNN and CHMM for data fusion across channels is apparent.

Figures 5 and 6 show the classification posteriors of each model for an example seizure in the JHH and CHB datasets, respectively. EEG channels are presented on the y-axis while the x-axis shows time. The dashed black lines correspond to annotations for seizure onset and offset. Red indicates the posterior probabilities of the seizure state. The PGM-CNN correctly classifies more of the annotated seizure in Fig. 5 than any of the other models. Each model incorrectly activates during the period immediately following the seizure, responding to the presence of artifact. However, the CNN likelihood model places more confidence in the seizure region, allowing for more correct classification. In contrast, the ANN and GMM identify strong seizure-like activity in the artifact following the actual seizure, causing an incorrect classification by the CHMM [7]. In Fig. 6 the PGM-CNN correctly classifies more of the annotated seizure than the CHMM but makes a false positive, while the CHMM classifies only a small portion of the seizure and responds strongly to the artifact prior to the seizure.

Seizure Localization: Surgical resection is the standard-of-care for medically refractory focal epilepsy. The latent propagation prior of our PGM-CNN has the potential to aid in seizure localization. Figure 7 shows two classifications from the PGM-CNN. Clinical annotations for the seizure in (a) and (c) suggest an origin in the right temporal lobe and spreading left. Likewise, the annotations in (b) and (d) suggest a left frontal lobe onset. The localization information provided by our model agrees with the annotated foci. Remarkably, this spreading behavior is *learned in a completely unsupervised manner* based on the clinical hypotheses embedded in the PGM prior. This result highlights the promise of integrating model-based and data-driven approaches for medical imaging applications.

5   Conclusion

We have presented the first generative model-deep learning hybrid for epileptic seizure detection. Our framework captures the spatio-temporal spread of a seizure through a structured PGM prior, while allowing for a complex likelihood function that is implicitly learned via a CNN. This data driven approach learns representations directly from the raw EEG signal, improving upon feature extraction techniques. At the same time the PGM preserves clinical interpretability and acts as a local smoothing process for the CNN outputs based on limited training examples. We evaluate our method on clinical data from two hospitals with distinct patient populations. In both cases, our PGM-CNN achieved higher true positive detection and AUC than any of the baseline methods.

Future work will explore alternate deep learning architectures with larger receptive fields and evaluate the effectiveness of training multichannel CNNs for fusing information across the scalp. In addition, modeling improvements such as restrictions on allowed onsets and enforcement of concurrent offsets across channels would likely reduce false positives and is an ongoing direction of work.

Acknowledgments. This work was supported by a JHMI Synergy Award (Venkataraman/Johnson) and NSF CAREER 1845430 (Venkataraman).

References

1. Zach, M., et al.: National and state estimates of the numbers of adults and children with active epilepsy - United States, 2015. CDC MMWR **66**, 821–825 (2017)
2. French, J.A.: Refractory epilepsy: clinical overview. Epilepsia **48**, 3–7 (2007)
3. Osorio, I., Zaveri, H.P., Frei, M.G., Arthurs, S.: Epilepsy: the Intersection of Neurosciences, Biology, Mathematics, Engineering, and Physics. CRC Press, Boca Raton (2016)
4. Shoeb, A.H., Guttag, J.V.: Application of machine learning to epileptic seizure detection. In: International Conference on Machine Learning, pp. 975–982 (2010)

5. Andrzejak, R.G., et al.: Indications of nonlinear deterministic and finite-dimensional structures in time series of brain electrical activity: dependence on recording region and brain state. Phys. Rev. E **64**(6), 061907 (2001)
6. Güler, N.F., et al.: Recurrent neural networks employing Lyapunov exponents for EEG signals classification. Expert Syst. Appl. **29**(3), 506–514 (2005)
7. Craley, J., Johnson, E., Venkataraman, A.: A novel method for epileptic seizure detection using coupled hidden markov models. In: Frangi, A.F., Schnabel, J.A., Davatzikos, C., Alberola-López, C., Fichtinger, G. (eds.) MICCAI 2018. LNCS, vol. 11072, pp. 482–489. Springer, Cham (2018). https://doi.org/10.1007/978-3-030-00931-1_55
8. Goodfellow, I., Bengio, Y., Courville, A.: Deep Learning. MIT Press, Cambridge (2016). http://www.deeplearningbook.org
9. Hinton, G., et al.: Deep neural networks for acoustic modeling in speech recognition: the shared views of four research groups. IEEE Signal Process. Mag. **29**(6), 82–97 (2012)
10. Murphy, K.P.: Machine Learning: A Probabilistic Perspective. MIT Press, Cambridge (2012)

A Novel Sparse Overlapping Modularized Gaussian Graphical Model for Functional Connectivity Estimation

Zhiyuan Zhu[1], Zonglei Zhen[2], and Xia Wu[1(✉)]

[1] College of Information Science and Technology, Beijing Normal University,
Beijing, China
wuxia@bnu.edu.cn
[2] Faculty of Psychology, Beijing Normal University, Beijing, China

Abstract. Neural mechanisms underlying brain functional systems remain poorly understood, the problem of estimating statistically robust and biologically meaningful functional connectivity by limited functional magnetic resonance imaging (fMRI) time series containing complex noises remains an open field. Addressing this issue, motivated by recent studies, which have highlighted that brain existing functional overlapping modularized patterns, we propose a novel sparse overlapping modularized Gaussian graphical model (SOMGGM) that estimates functional connectivity by modularizing the connection patterns and allowing each brain region belonging to multiple modules. Extensive experimental results demonstrate that the proposed SOMGGM not only has more power to accurately estimate functional connectivity network structure, but also improves feature extraction and enhances the performance in the brain neurological disease diagnosis task. Additionally, SOMGGM can help to find the brain regions assigned to multiple network modules which are likely important hub nodes. In general, the proposed SOMGGM offers a new computational methodology for brain functional connectivity estimation.

Keywords: Functional connectivity · fMRI ·
Sparse inverse covariance estimation · Overlapping modules ·
Gaussian graphical model

1 Introduction

Brain functional connectivity (FC) has held great promise in diagnosis of neurological diseases because of which can be seen as reflecting brain's functional organization [1]. The progression of many brain neurological diseases are closely associated with the dysfunction of multiple specific FCs [2]. In recent years, in order to better understanding the construction of human brain connectomes, FC has been widely used in predicting human behaviors or diagnosing brain neurological disease [3, 4]. In particular, FC has proven to be effectively in delineating biomarkers for many neuropsychiatric conditions.

Because of low signal-noise rate character of fMRI and big cost of imaging, statistical power comes to be a major concern to improve the performance of FC

© Springer Nature Switzerland AG 2019
A. C. S. Chung et al. (Eds.): IPMI 2019, LNCS 11492, pp. 304–315, 2019.
https://doi.org/10.1007/978-3-030-20351-1_23

estimation. Previous studies have shown that sparse Gaussian graphical model (SGGM) with computing the inverse covariance (IC, also called precision matrix) has been used as a more promising statistical method than conventional Pearson's correlation to estimate FC in eliminating the common signals and reducing noise effects, mainly because the off-diagonals of computed IC matrix have one-to-one correspondence with partial correlations, hence avoiding spurious effects in network modeling [5]. The ℓ_1-norm regularization to the IC matrix resulted in the estimated results sparse, which could force spurious and noisy connections to zero, thus all other connections can be better estimated.

However, previous methods of using SGMM only focus on each brain region existing as an individual or just belonging to one network for FC estimation, these pure data-driven SGGM approaches do not take the advantage of modular spatial overlapped prior knowledge, which would be short comprehensive to learn the intrinsic FC. In the neuroscience field, recent researches widely suggest that there exist multiple concurrent brain functional patterns, which are functional modular spatial overlapped and interacts with each other to jointly realize the total brain function during specific task performance [6, 7]. This important property of many real-world networks has never been considered in graph learning model, which would bring about a consequence that overlapping modules of neurons subserving different functions are likely to go unnoticed owing to the spatial averaging. Intuitively, we hypothesize that the property of incorporating modular spatial overlapped prior in SGGM may capture additional dimension information of brain connectivity and thus enhance neurological clinical diagnosis.

In this paper, we propose a novel method called SOMGGM (sparse overlapping modularized Gaussian graphical model) to estimate FC by incorporating spatial overlapping modularized characteristics. To verify the effectiveness of the proposed method, this work aims to answer three key open questions: (1) whether SOMGGM can precisely extract the intrinsic association in brain functional systems; (2) whether the incorporating spatial overlapping modularized approach can gain more statistical power of representing individual characteristics for improving prediction result of the severity of depression symptoms, the improved result can better help to explore what FC features that contributed to the prediction; (3) what are the spatial overlapping mechanisms of FC discovered by SOMGGM.

We address the first question by two simulated fMRI data which have the ground truth that can be used to verify estimated accuracy. For the second one, we use SOMGGM to identify the severity of depression symptoms in a prediction task and compare the performance of SOMGGM with other state-of-the-art methods. The edges (FCs) with high contributing weights for the prediction can be seen as important factor in determining the deterioration of depression. To answer the third one, the key innovation of SOMGGM is to allow for overlap between brain modules, which can be used for exploring modular spatial overlapped condition of each brain region.

2 Method

The framework of the proposed estimating method is illustrated in Fig. 1. Firstly, the preprocessed fMRI images from individuals are first registered into a standard space and aligned with the automated anatomical labeling (AAL) atlas. After extracting fMRI signals from the whole regions of interest (ROIs), the proposed method is used to jointly learn the structure of FC network and the assignment of ROIs into modules. As results, the estimated precision matrix and modules assignment matrix are obtained which can respectively represent brain function connectivity and modules overlapped conditions.

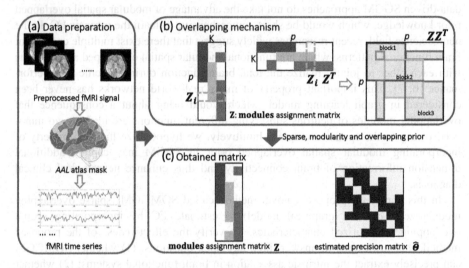

Fig. 1. The framework of SOMGGM to estimate brain functional connectivity from fMRI signals. (a) The signal to be used for estimating FC. (b) The overlapping mechanism in SOMGGM framework. (c) Learning Z and $\widehat{\Theta}$ iteratively.

Following we will give a brief description of the sparse Gaussian graphical model (SGGM) which is a state-of-the-art method for estimating a well-conditioned sparse IC matrix, then introduce our proposed SOMGGM that modularizes the connection patterns and allows free overlap between brain modules.

2.1 Sparse Gaussian Graphical Model

We suppose that the brain has been parceled into p ROIs, $\{x^{(1)}, x^{(2)}, \ldots, x^{(p)}\} \in X_{t,}$, where $X_t \in R^m$, $t = 1, 2, \ldots, n$ time points. We aim to learn a well-conditioned sparse IC matrix $\sum^{-1} \in p \times p$ on the basis of n observations. It can be formulated as the following optimization problem [8]:

$$\hat{\Theta} = argmax_{\Theta \geq 0} \ log \ det \ \Theta - tr(S\Theta) - \lambda \|\Theta\|_1 \tag{1}$$

Where the solution $\hat{\Theta}$ is an estimate of $\sum^{-1}$, S denotes the empirical covariance matrix, λ is set to a non-negative value to control the strength of the ℓ_1 penalty that applied to the elements of Θ. It is clear that the ℓ_1 penalty will force the matrix structure become sparse, which can effectively remove redundant or spurious connections in FC. Note that the solution amounts to maximizing a penalized log-likelihood of a multivariate Gaussian distribution. Some optimization algorithms such as quadratic inverse covariance [9] or proximal method [10] can be used to efficiently solve Eq. (1) problem.

Discussion. It is well known that $\hat{\Theta}$ determines the conditional independence structure of the p variables that can represent the FC between brain ROIs, there is an edge between the ith and jth brain region if the (i, j) element of $\hat{\Theta}$ is non-zero. As the toy examples shown in Fig. 2(a), the FC built by conventional method may have a large number of spurious connections (gray scatters). After applying the sparse constraint at each brain region independently, as shown in Fig. 2(b), sparse constraint results in retaining smaller number of connections, which can make the estimation of FC more robust by limited samples.

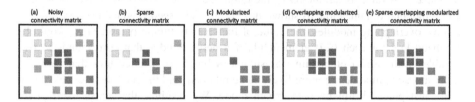

Fig. 2. The intuition behind incorporating modular spatial overlapped prior in the estimation of optimized functional connectivity.

2.2 Sparse Overlapping Modularized Gaussian Graphical Model

Since fMRI is an indirect reflection of brain activity and it is widely reported the fact that brain functional activity is organized with modular spatial overlapped structure, addressing this issue, we propose to establish a Gaussian graphical model that can exhibits the specific structure. The proposed SOMGGM incorporating modular spatial overlapped as a structural prior into Eq. (1) can be summarized as:

$$\hat{\Theta} = argmax_{\Theta \geq 0, Z \in \mathcal{D}} \ log \ det \ \Theta - tr(S\Theta) - \lambda_1 \|\Theta\|_* - \lambda_2 (\|\Theta\|_1 - tr(ZZ^T|\Theta|)), \tag{2}$$

$$\text{subject to } \|Z\|_2 \leq \tau, \|Z_i\|_2 \leq 1, \|Z\|_F \leq \beta, \ (i \in \{1, \ldots p\}),$$

The Eq. (2) can be also re-written as:

$$\hat{\Theta} = argmax_{\Theta \geq 0, Z \in \mathcal{D}} \ log \ det \ \Theta - tr(S\Theta) - \lambda_1 \|\Theta\|_* - \sum_{i,j} \lambda_2 \left(1 - \left(ZZ^T\right)_{ij}\right) |\Theta_{i,j}|, \quad (3)$$

$$\text{subject to } \|Z\|_2 \leq \tau, \|Z_i\|_2 \leq 1, \|Z\|_F \leq \beta, \ (i \in \{1, \ldots p\}),$$

Where λ_1 and λ_2 are non-negative tuning parameter. Notably, different from SGGM, SOMGGM combines a formulated as $\|\Theta\|_*$ and $tr(ZZ^T|\Theta|)$, which encourages Θ to be modularized and have overlapping characteristics. As shown in Fig. 1(b), Z is a real matrix of size $p \times K$, where K is the total number of modules. The ith row of Z, denoted by Z_i, can be interpreted for the variable $x^{(i)}$ as a low-rank embedding, which showing its modularized assignment scores, the pattern of weakened sparsity of ZZ^T would index the regions covered by all K modules. The similar embedding between $x^{(i)}$ and $x^{(j)}$ would encourage $|\Theta_{ij}|$ to be non-zero.

Discussion. However, just having sparse constraints is not enough, because sometimes the real connections are also eliminated. A prior information that is more in line with the true state of the brain can help to estimate brain functional connectivity network more accurately from fMRI signals with low signal-to-noise ratio. Specifically, comparing with SGGM, the proposed method adds other two terms. The first added term introduces low rank constraint $\|\Theta\|_*$, the tuning parameter λ_1 would prompt to achieve strong modular organization, as shown in Fig. 2(c). The second added term encourages to have overlapping modules, the value of the sparsity tuning parameter λ_2 would be penalized less for each (i,j) element Θ_{ij} if a network edge that corresponds to two variables with similar embedding, as shown in Fig. 2(d). This ensures that variables under the same module are more likely to be retained, and the modules can be overlap freely just purely learnt by data driven mode. We combine the sparse overlapping modules to estimate FC patterns, as shown in Fig. 2(e).

Parameter Selection. Matrix Z is constrained by the set $\mathcal{D} \subset [-1,1]^{p \times K}$, which also satisfied the following constraints: (1) $\|Z_i\|_2 \leq 1$. This constraint ensures each (i,j) element's regularization parameter is non-negative. (2) $\|Z\|_F \leq \beta$. This global constraint on Z that prevents all regularization parameters from becoming zero $(\forall i,j : (ZZ^T)_{ij} = 1)$. (3) $\|Z\|_2 \leq \tau$. This constraint guards against the case that all variables are assigned to one module. (4) $\tau = \frac{\beta}{\sqrt{K}}$. This guarantees that there are K non-empty modules at least. In our experiments, the hyper-parameter $\beta = \sqrt{\frac{p}{2}}$, which means that each variable is allowed to get on average half of its largest possible squared norm.

Update Θ with Z Fixed. The block coordinate descent method was adopted to learn Z and Θ iteratively. When fixing Z, we can deduce the following formula

$$\hat{\Theta} = argmax_{\Theta \geq 0, Z \in \mathcal{D}} \ log \ det \ \Theta - tr(S\Theta) - \lambda_1 \|\Theta\|_* - \sum_{(i,j)} \Lambda_{i,j} |\Theta_{ij}|, \quad (4)$$

Where $\Lambda_{i,j} = \lambda_2(1 - (ZZ^T)_{ij})$, the last term can be seen as the SGGM with edge-specific sparse regularization parameters $\Lambda_{i,j}$. Equation (4) is a convex problem and we solve it by adopting an existing mature solution by SGGM with incorporating a modularity prior algorithm [11].

Update Z with Θ Fixed. When Θ is fixed, the problem (2) becomes

$$maximize_{Z \geq 0} \ tr(ZZ^T|\Theta|), \tag{5}$$

$$\text{subject to } \|Z\|_2 \leq \tau, \|Z_i\|_2 \leq 1, \|Z\|_F \leq \beta, \ (i \in \{1, \dots p\}),$$

This special penalty formula used in network models was first proposed by [12]. Equation (5) is equivalent to the following:

$$maximize_{W \geq 0} \ tr(W|\Theta|), \tag{6}$$

$$\text{subject to } rank(W) \leq K, W \leq \tau^2 I, diag(W) \leq 1, tr(W) \leq \beta^2,$$

Where W is a $p \times p$ matrix, K is the number of modules, I is the identity matrix of p. The problem (5) is a semi-defined problem, a method recently proposed by Hosseini et al. can be used to solve the convex optimization problem respect to W [12].

2.3   Obtaining Overlapping Modules from Dependent Matrix Z

After the SOMGGM algorithm converges, an estimated precision matrix $\hat{\Theta}$ and a modules assignment matrix Z can be obtained. For the matrix Z, it provides the variables contained information in each K modules. Each variable is allowed to be assigned to multiple modules which prompts the result of overlapping mechanism.

3   Materials

3.1   Synthetic Data

Self-constructed Simulated Data. In this experiment, we set up three overlapping modules without scattered points intuitively. Similar to Kudela et al. [13], we used the function mvrnorm() from the library "MASS" of the statistical computing and graphics software R (http://www.r-project.org) to generate random time series data. The generated data subject to multivariate normal distribution by the user-specified mean vector and covariance matrix. Here, the mean vectors were determined by real human data time-series based on the AAL atlas, the covariance matrix was computed from the ground truth correlation matrix. As a result, a ninety-dimensional time series of 300 points with adding thermal white noise of standard deviation 1% (of mean signal level) were obtained. The designed binarized ground truth correlation matrix with overlapped modularity was shown in Fig. 3(a).

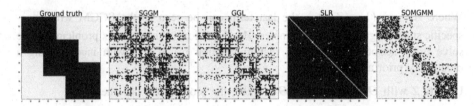

Fig. 3. The estimated functional connectivity matrices in self-constructed simulated data.

Open Simulated Data. NetSim [14], which is widely used as a standard simulated data, was generated using dynamic causal modeling - a generative network model aimed to quantify the interaction and dynamics between neurons. NetSim is comprised of 28 different brain networks with different levels of complexity to simulate rich and realistic fMRI time series, such as these conditions: high and low dimensionality, stronger connections, more connections, etc. For each simulated FC ground truth, the data is available for 50 "subjects" are generated which contains 200 time-series sampled with TR of 3 s Thus, a total of 1400 synthetic dataset that can be used for testing.

3.2 Real Data and Preprocessing

75 adult patients with major depressive disorder (MDD) (42 females, mean age 34.84) were recruited. HAMA was recorded for representing individual severity of depression symptoms. All of the resting state functional imaging scans were acquired on a 3.0-Tesla scanner with the following parameters: TR = 2000 ms, TE = 30 ms, FA = 90°, matrix size = 64 × 64, FOV = 220 mm × 220 mm, total 240 volumes, slice thickness = 3.5 mm, skip = 0.6 mm, and slice number = 33. The data preprocessing was performed using SPM8 (http://www.fil.ion.ucl.ac.uk/spm) software. Each fMRI scan contained a total of 240 time points; the first 10 volumes were discarded due to signal stabilization and the adaptation of subjects to the noise of the scanner. Subsequently, slicing time correction and realignment, spatial normalization into the standard stereotaxic space, and smoothing of image volumes with an 8 × 8 × 8 FWHM Gaussian kernel were performed. The network regions were defined by the AAL template which parcels the whole brain without cerebellum into 90 non-overlapped ROIs. For each of the 90 ROIs, the mean resting-state fMRI time series were calculated by averaging the GM-masked BOLD signals among all voxels within the particular ROI.

4   Experiment and Results

To verify the effectiveness of our proposed FC estimation method, we used simulated data sets which had the ground truth to assess the accuracy of the estimation result. Furthermore, to verify if the method can learn more precise functional connectivity network structure which improves feature extraction, we utilized the intrinsic FC represented by the proposed method based on a real fMRI data set, and then used the estimated FC to predict the severity of depression symptoms at the individual level. A better description of the relationship between FC and the severity of depression symptoms is of great significance for the treatment of depression in understanding brain function mechanisms.

Several previous studies have used the designed GGM to estimate brain functional connectivity. For instance, Huang, et al. firstly used the classic SGGM model which had been introduced in the front to explore the sparse brain networks in Alzheimer's patients [15]. Varoquaux et al. developed a group-graphical lasso (GGL) modeling approach to improve the estimation of a subject's network based on group time series data to constraint the intrinsic randomness from sample's short time series [16]. Qiao et al. proposed a sparse low-rank (SLR) graph learning method which could get a sparse modularized FC network structure [11]. In this experiment, we used the three state-of-the-art methods as competitors.

Estimating FC on Simulated Data. Since all the GGM methods have the regularized parameters to control sparse degree and other peculiar properties, the regularized parameters involved in estimating FC may significantly affect the FC structures, thus all the four methods were under a grid search method to conduct their regularized parameters. For each regularized parameter, we used candidate values in [0.1, 0.2, 0.3, 0.4, 0.5, 0.6, 0.7, 0.8, 0.9, 1, 2, 4, 8, 16, 32]. The parameter with the best performance was reserved as the final result. Notably, as the ground truth in the two simulated data is sparse, however, Pearson correlation (PC) method doesn't have the characteristics of obtaining sparse result, we didn't conduct PC for comparison.

For illustrating the estimation results on simulated data, we used the same method with Ryali et al. [17]. For each estimation result, the binary views were used for presentation and statistics. As our ground truth and results were all sparse, we regarded the result applied to the estimated connection strengths as a binary classification problem, the valued edges were seen as one class and the null ones as the other. Since it is not enough to get only high precision or recall, accuracy and F1-score were compared.

$$\text{Accuracy} = \frac{TP + TN}{TP + FN + FP + TN} \tag{7}$$

$$\text{F1-score} = \frac{2 \cdot precision * recall}{precision + recall} \tag{8}$$

Figure 3 shows each estimated sparse graph matrix, it's easy to notice that only the proposed method keeps the original outline best. Table 1 shows the estimated accuracy and F1-score results in self-constructed simulated data. The best performance on the self-constructed simulated data demonstrates that the proposed model has a better ability to estimate overlapping modularized characteristics of fMRI data.

Table 2 shows the results on NetSim. Our model has no significant performance improvements, the main reason maybe that NetSim does not take adding the simulation of overlapping modularized features into account. Although NetSim simulates many other complex conditions, our model can still keep high-level performance as better as other state-of-the-art methods. This demonstrates that our model not only has better ability to estimate overlapping modularized relationships, but also maintains excellent performance on general tasks.

Table 1. Accuracy and F1-score results on the self-constructed simulated data.

Methods	SGGM	GGL	SLR	SOMGGM
Accuracy	0.5914	0.5691	0.5365	**0.64**
F1-score	0.5749	0.5262	0.4989	**0.6061**

Table 2. The mean Accuracy and F1-score results for all simulated data on NetSim

Methods	SGGM	GGL	SLR	SOMGGM
Mean Accuracy	0.8881	**0.8975**	0.7322	0.8959
Mean F1-score	0.8839	0.8927	0.7154	**0.8935**

Prediction Framework and Feature Selection/Extraction. Once we obtained the FCs for all subjects, the next task is using the estimated FCs as features to predict the severity of depression symptoms. In this study, all edges in the FC matrix were selected as features, the severity of depression symptoms could be expressed by HAMA scores. As we had 90 ROIs, thus the feature dimensionality was 4005, the features greatly exceeded the number of observable subject information. At the same time, we expected to retain more predictive contribution features as possible, one widely used method is ridge regression, which employs a spherical Gaussian prior that assumes equal and independent variance for all parameters. We applied ridge regression model to predict depression symptoms. An introduction to the object function of ridge algorithm and prediction framework is detailed as follows.

$$\min_\beta \sum_{i=1}^{N} \left(f(x_i) - y_i \right)^2 + \lambda \sum_{j=1}^{P} \left\| \beta_j \right\|^2, \tag{9}$$

Where β_j is the regression coefficient for the jth feature and λ is used to control the trade-off between the prediction error of the training data and L2-norm regularization.

A nested leave-one-out cross validation (LOOCV) method was used for the prediction framework, where the outer loop to estimate prediction accuracy and the inner loop to determine the optimal parameter selection. Regarding the λ choices, a grid search was employed, the λ was set with $[e^{-5}, e^{-4}, \ldots, e^3, e^4, e^5]$. Each edge of the estimated FC was extracted to construct the feature vector. After the training procedure was accomplished, the features (i.e., connectivity edges) with a nonzero regression coefficient/weight in the models of all outer LOOCV loops can be deemed as contributing edges for the prediction of depression symptoms.

Prediction of the Severity of Depression Symptoms from FC. Similar to the procedure above in FC estimated, the grid search method was also used in ridge regression model to selected regularized parameters for all the FCs estimated by the four sparse GMM method. As Pearson correlation is the most widely used method, the FC obtained by Pearson correlation was also used for the prediction task. Figure 4(a) shows the prediction results, it illustrated that the proposed measure had the best performance in predicting the severity of depression symptoms ($r = 0.3158$, $p < 0.001$, permutation test), which demonstrated that the modular spatial overlapped prior helped to improve FCs' ability to diagnose brain neurological diseases.

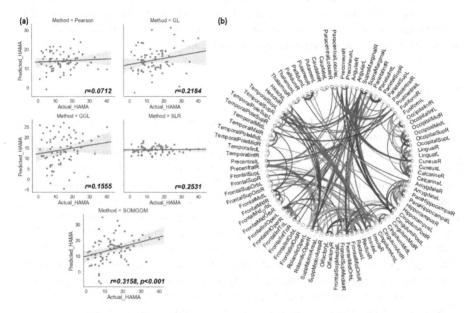

Fig. 4. (a) Prediction results: correlation between actual and predicted HAMA. (b) The most contributing edges. The thickness of each arc denotes the contributing power of the corresponding connection. The color of each arc is randomly assigned just for better visualization. (Color figure online)

Contributing Edges (of FCs). When the training procedure was accomplished, the reserved edges of the optimal prediction results were considered as important edges/features that relate to the predicted performance. A better predictive model means that its features are more effective. As SOMGGM got the best predictive performance, the top 15% contributed edges by SOMGGM are shown in Fig. 4(b). The contribution weights of the left hemisphere connections are significantly higher than that of the right hemisphere, which is consistent with the previous neuroimaging reports that left hemisphere showed significantly changes in connectivity strengths of patients with depression [18].

The Overlapping Probability of Each Brain Region (Node). The key innovation of SOMGGM is to allow for overlap between modules, each brain region may exist in multiple modules, we can obtain the conditions of the brain regions belonging to each module from the learnt estimated parameters **Z**. The assignment results of each region were calculated. In order to find the difference from the health, the overlapping probability for another 70 healthy controls were also computed, there was no significant age or gender difference (39 females, mean age 35.2, $p = 0.87$, t-test). The healthy controls used the same conditions as the depression processing flow in the scanning process and regularization parameters selection. A more overlapping situation means more likely to be a hub node that plays a central role in the brain's functional mechanisms. Intuitively, we found that the Caudate with left hemisphere in MDDs are weaker overlapped than healthy controls. This is consistent with a large number of previous studies, that is, the symptomatic manifestations of MDD are closely related to the decreased function and volume reduction of Caudate [19].

5   Conclusion

In this paper, inspired by the fact that brain functional connectivity networks are spatial overlapped by multiple concurrent functional patterns, we proposed a novel sparse graphical model with incorporating modular spatial overlapped prior to estimate FC. We showed on synthetic data that SOMGGM has excellent performance as well as other state-of-the-art methods. In addition, the SOMGGM can better estimate network structure in modular spatial overlapped conditions, which is considered to be an important feature of brain function activity. We further applied the estimated FC patterns by SOMGGM to predict the severity of depression symptoms, more significantly better improving the prediction results demonstrated that SOMGGM has high discrimination power and great potentials in computer-aided diagnosis of brain neurological diseases. Additionally, the brain regions of overlapping mechanism can be mined via the proposed innovative data-driven method. This work points that the modular spatial overlapped prior may provide insights for better estimating FC and exploring the brain functional mechanisms.

Acknowledgment. This work was supported by the General Program of National Natural Science Foundation of China (Grant No. 61876021) and Fundamental Research Funds for the Central Universities (Grant No. 2017EYT36).

References

1. Greicius, M.D., Krasnow, B., Reiss, A.L., Menon, V.: Functional connectivity in the resting brain: a network analysis of the default mode hypothesis. Proc. Natl. Acad. Sci. **100**(1), 253–258 (2003)
2. Menon, V.: Large-scale brain networks and psychopathology: a unifying triple network model. Trends cogn. Sci. **15**(10), 483–506 (2011)
3. Huang, H., Liu, X., Jin, Y., Lee, S.W., Wee, C.Y., Shen, D.: Enhancing the representation of functional connectivity networks by fusing multi-view information for autism spectrum disorder diagnosis. Hum. Brain Mapp. **40**, 833–854 (2018)
4. Shen, X., et al.: Using connectome-based predictive modeling to predict individual behavior from brain connectivity. Nat. Protocols. **12**(3), 506 (2017)

5. Ng, B., Varoquaux, G., Poline, J.B., Thirion, B.: A Novel sparse group Gaussian graphical model for functional connectivity estimation. Inf. Process. Med. Imaging **23**, 256–267 (2013)
6. Yuan, J., et al.: Spatio-temporal modeling of connectome-scale brain network interactions via time-evolving graphs. Neuroimage **180**, 350–369 (2017)
7. Gorka, A.X., Torrisi, S., Shackman, A.J., Grillon, C., Ernst, M.: Intrinsic functional connectivity of the central nucleus of the amygdala and bed nucleus of the stria terminalis. Neuroimage **168**, 392–402 (2018)
8. Friedman, J., Hastie, T., Tibshirani, R.: Sparse inverse covariance estimation with the graphical lasso. Biostatistics **9**(3), 432–441 (2008)
9. Hsieh, C.-J., Dhillon, I.S., Ravikumar, P.K., Sustik, M.A.: Sparse inverse covariance matrix estimation using quadratic approximation. In: Advances in Neural Information Processing Systems, pp. 2330–2338 (2011)
10. Combettes, P.L., Pesquet, J.-C.: Proximal splitting methods in signal processing. In: Bauschke, H., Burachik, R., Combettes, P., Elser, V., Luke, D., Wolkowicz, H. (eds.) Fixed-Point Algorithms for Inverse Problems in Science and Engineering, vol. 49, pp. 185–212. Springer, New York (2011). https://doi.org/10.1007/978-1-4419-9569-8_10
11. Qiao, L., Zhang, H., Kim, M., Teng, S., Zhang, L., Shen, D.: Estimating functional brain networks by incorporating a modularity prior. NeuroImage **141**, 399–407 (2016)
12. Hosseini, M.J., and Lee, S.-I.: Learning sparse gaussian graphical models with overlapping blocks. In: Advances in Neural Information Processing Systems, pp. 3808–3816 (2016)
13. Kudela, M., Harezlak, J., Lindquist, M.A.: Assessing uncertainty in dynamic functional connectivity. NeuroImage **149**, 165–177 (2017)
14. Smith, S.M., et al.: Network modelling methods for FMRI. Neuroimage **54**(2), 875–891 (2011)
15. Huang, S., et al.: Learning brain connectivity of Alzheimer's disease by sparse inverse covariance estimation. Neuroimage **50**(3), 935–949 (2010)
16. Varoquaux, G., Gramfort, A., Poline, J.-B., Thirion, B.: Brain covariance selection: better individual functional connectivity models using population prior. In: Advances in Neural Information Processing Systems, pp. 2334–2342 (2010)
17. Ryali, S., Chen, T., Supekar, K., Menon, V.: Estimation of functional connectivity in fMRI data using stability selection-based sparse partial correlation with elastic net penalty. NeuroImage **59**(4), 3852–3861 (2012)
18. Carballedo, A., et al.: Functional connectivity of emotional processing in depression. J. Affect. Disord. **134**(1–3), 272–279 (2011)
19. Pizzagalli, D.A., et al.: Reduced caudate and nucleus accumbens response to rewards in unmedicated individuals with major depressive disorder. Am. J. Psychiatry **166**(6), 702–710 (2009)

White Matter Imaging

Asymmetry Spectrum Imaging for Baby Diffusion Tractography

Ye Wu, Weili Lin, Dinggang Shen, Pew-Thian Yap$^{(\boxtimes)}$,
and the UNC/UMN Baby Connectome Project Consortium

Department of Radiology and BRIC, University of North Carolina, Chapel Hill, USA
ptyap@med.unc.edu

Abstract. Fiber tractography in baby diffusion MRI is challenging due
to the low and spatially-varying diffusion anisotropy, causing most tractography algorithms to yield streamlines that fall short of reaching the
cortex. In this paper, we introduce a method called asymmetry spectrum
imaging (ASI) to improve the estimation of white matter pathways in the
baby brain by (i) incorporating an asymmetric fiber orientation model
to resolve subvoxel fiber configurations such as fanning and bending, and
(ii) explicitly modeling the range (or *spectrum*) of typical diffusion length
scales in the developing brain. We validated ASI using in-vivo baby diffusion MRI data from the Baby Connectome Project (BCP), demonstrating that ASI can characterize complex subvoxel fiber configurations and
accurately estimate the fiber orientation distribution function in spite of
changes in diffusion patterns. This, in turn, results in significantly better
diffusion tractography in the baby brain.

1 Introduction

In diffusion magnetic resonance imaging (DMRI) [1], the local directional information is a direct consequence of the directional preference, i.e., anisotropy, of
water diffusion, shaped by microstructural barriers such as cell membranes and
myelin. Tractography algorithms are significantly affected by changes in diffusion
anisotropy and are typically designed to traverse areas of high anisotropy while
avoiding areas of low anisotropy. In the developing brain where the anisotropy is
typically low owing to on-going myelination, far fewer voxels are included in the
pathway at birth than later time points. As the axonal membranes are more per-
meable to water than myelin sheets, the degree of anisotropy is less pronounced
in the absence of myelin [2]. Structural connectivity analysis relies on tractography and therefore tractograms of insufficient quality will result in inaccurate
connectomes.

Local fiber orientation at each voxel is typically encoded in a fiber orientation distribution function (FODF), which is typically determined based on

This work was supported in part by NIH grants (NS093842, EB022880, MH104324 and
1U01MH110274), a research grant from Nestec Ltd., and the efforts of the UNC/UMN
Baby Connectome Project Consortium.

© Springer Nature Switzerland AG 2019
A. C. S. Chung et al. (Eds.): IPMI 2019, LNCS 11492, pp. 319–331, 2019.
https://doi.org/10.1007/978-3-030-20351-1_24

techniques such as multi-tissue constrained spherical deconvolution (MTCSD) [3], taking into account response functions (RFs) specific to white matter (WM), gray matter (GM), and cerebrospinal fluid (CSF). However, MTCSD is limited in that it uses a fixed set of RFs throughout the whole brain, ignoring the spatial changes in hindered and restricted diffusion, which is typical in the developing brain due to ongoing myelination. Moreover, MTCSD lacks the capability to deal with complex axonal trajectory configurations such as fanning and bending due to its inherent assumption that the FODF is antipodal symmetric.

In this paper, we introduce a method called asymmetry spectrum imaging (ASI) to allow subvoxel orientation asymmetry and to take into account a spectrum of hindered/restricted diffusion. To capture white matter configurations such as bending and fanning to mitigate gyral bias, we will incorporate information from neighboring voxels to estimate *asymmetric* FODFs (AFODFs). We will extend the MTCSD model to account for positive orientations and negative orientations separately in order to capture the asymmetry of the underlying fiber geometry in a local neighborhood. We will estimate the AFODF at each voxel by enforcing orientation continuity across voxels. Unlike [4–6], our approach is formulated as a convex problem and does not require initialization with precomputed symmetric FODFs. Moreover, our algorithm provides the global solution for multiple voxels simultaneously instead of solving for each voxel individually. To account for the effects of changes in microstructural properties (e.g., anisotropy) on infant tractography, we will further extend our AFODF model described above to account for the whole diffusion spectrum ranging from intra-axonal restriction diffusion to extra-axonal hindrance diffusion. This will address the limitations of MTCSD, where only one response function is used to represent each tissue type (i.e., WM, GM, and CSF). Such fixed response functions do not account for the changes in diffusion properties and will cause false-positive orientations [7]. Accounting for the whole spectrum of diffusion characteristics will allow the FODFs to be estimated accurately despite changes in microstructural properties.

2   Method

2.1   Multi-tissue Spherical Deconvolution

MTCSD [3] voxel-wisely decomposes the diffusion signal profile $S_{\mathbf{p}}(\mathbf{g})$ for diffusion gradient $\mathbf{g} \in \mathbb{S}^2$ and voxel location $\mathbf{p} \in \mathbb{R}^3$ based on three tissue types (anisotropic: WM, isotropic: GM and CSF) in the form of spherical convolution of an antipodal and axially symmetric response function (RF) [8] $R(\mathbf{g}, \mathbf{u})$ and an antipodal symmetric FODF $F_{\mathbf{p}}(\mathbf{u})$:

$$S_{\mathbf{p}}(\mathbf{g})/S_{\mathbf{p}}(0) = \int_{\mathbf{u} \in \mathbb{S}^2} R^{\mathrm{WM}}(\mathbf{g}, \mathbf{u}) F_{\mathbf{p}}(\mathbf{u}) d\mathbf{u} + h_{\mathbf{p}}^{\mathrm{GM}} R^{\mathrm{GM}}(\mathbf{g}) + h_{\mathbf{p}}^{\mathrm{CSF}} R^{\mathrm{CSF}}(\mathbf{g}), \quad (1)$$

where $h_{\mathbf{p}}^{\mathrm{GM}}$ and $h_{\mathbf{p}}^{\mathrm{CSF}}$ are the volume fractions indicating the contributions of GM and CSF, respectively. $S_{\mathbf{p}}(0)$ is the baseline signal without diffusion sensitization. The antipodal symmetry limits the FODF in representing complex configurations such as fanning and bending. To circumvent this limitation, we extend the MTCSD framework by incorporating information from voxel neighborhoods to allow FODF asymmetry.

2.2 Asymmetric Fiber Orientation Distribution Functions (AFODFs)

FODFs are often estimated with some form of regularization [8,9]. In ASI, we employ the fiber continuity constraint. A fiber streamline leaving a voxel $\mathbf{p}$ along direction $\mathbf{u}$ should enter the next voxel $\mathbf{q} \in \mathcal{N}_\mathbf{p}$ along direction $-\mathbf{u}$, where $\mathcal{N}_\mathbf{p}$ is a neighborhood of $\mathbf{p}$. We minimize the discontinuity of $F_\mathbf{p}(\cdot)$ along direction $\mathbf{u}$ by

$$\min \Phi(\mathbb{F}) = \min \sum_\mathbf{p} \int_{\mathbf{u} \in \mathbb{S}^2} \left| F_\mathbf{p}(\mathbf{u}) - \frac{1}{K_{\mathbf{p},\mathbf{u}}} \sum_{\mathbf{q} \in \mathcal{N}_\mathbf{p}} W(\langle \hat{\mathbf{v}}_{\mathbf{p},\mathbf{q}}, \mathbf{u} \rangle) F_\mathbf{q}(\mathbf{u}) \right| d\mathbf{u}, \quad (2)$$

where $\mathbb{F} = \{F_\mathbf{p}\}$, $W(\langle \hat{\mathbf{v}}_{\mathbf{p},\mathbf{q}}, \mathbf{u} \rangle)$ is a directional probability distribution function (PDF) dependent on the angular difference between $\mathbf{u}$ and $\hat{\mathbf{v}}_{\mathbf{p},\mathbf{q}} = (\mathbf{q} - \mathbf{p})/\|\mathbf{q} - \mathbf{p}\|$, and $K_{\mathbf{p},\mathbf{u}} = \sum_{\mathbf{q} \in \mathcal{N}_\mathbf{p}} W(\langle \hat{\mathbf{v}}_{\mathbf{p},\mathbf{q}}, \mathbf{u} \rangle)$ is a normalization factor. We choose $W(\cdot)$ to be the von Mises-Fisher distribution with reference direction $\hat{\mathbf{v}}_{\mathbf{p},\mathbf{q}}$ [10].

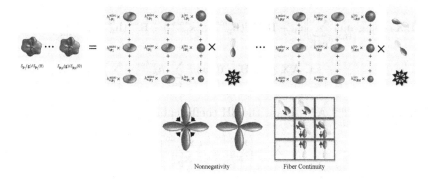

Fig. 1. ASI problem formulation with non-negativity and fiber continuity constraints.

2.3 Asymmetry Spectrum Imaging (ASI)

To capture changes in hindered/restricted diffusion across voxels, ASI employs a spectrum of RFs. Unlike the fixed set of RFs used in MTCSD, the spectrum of RFs in ASI allows the AFODF to be estimated correctly in spite of the changes in diffusion patterns. In ASI, the signal is represented by

$$S_\mathbf{p}(\mathbf{g})/S_\mathbf{p}(0) = \int_{\mathbf{u} \in \mathbb{S}^2} \sum_{i=1}^n h_{i,\mathbf{p}}^{\text{aniso}} R_i^{\text{aniso}}(\mathbf{g}, \mathbf{u}) F_\mathbf{p}(\mathbf{u}) d\mathbf{u} + \sum_{j=1}^m h_{j,\mathbf{p}}^{\text{iso}} R_j^{\text{iso}}(\mathbf{g}), \quad (3)$$

where n and m are the respective lengths of the anisotropic and isotropic spectra, which consist of a series of response functions with volume fractions $\{h_{i,\mathbf{p}}^{aniso}\}$ and $\{h_{j,\mathbf{p}}^{iso}\}$.

We denote the spherical harmonic (SH) coefficients of the signal $S_\mathbf{p}(\mathbf{g})/S_\mathbf{p}(0)$ and the AFODF $F_\mathbf{p}(\mathbf{u})$ as vectors $\mathbf{s}_\mathbf{p}$ and $\mathbf{x}_\mathbf{p}^{aniso}$, whereas the rotational harmonic coefficients of the response functions $R_1^{aniso}(\mathbf{g}, \mathbf{u}), \ldots, R_n^{aniso}(\mathbf{g}, \mathbf{u})$ as matrix $\mathbf{R}^{aniso} = [\mathbf{R}_1^{aniso}, \cdots, \mathbf{R}_n^{aniso}]$. By letting $\mathbf{h}_\mathbf{p}^{aniso} = [h_{1,\mathbf{p}}^{aniso}, \cdots, h_{n,\mathbf{p}}^{aniso}]^\top$ and $\mathbf{h}_\mathbf{p}^{iso} = [h_{1,\mathbf{p}}^{iso}, \cdots, h_{m,\mathbf{p}}^{iso}]^\top$, Eq. (3) can be written as

$$\mathbf{s}_\mathbf{p} = \mathbf{R}^{aniso}(\mathbf{h}_\mathbf{p}^{aniso} \otimes \mathbf{x}_\mathbf{p}^{aniso}) + \mathbf{R}^{iso}(\mathbf{h}_\mathbf{p}^{iso} \cdot \mathbf{x}_\mathbf{p}^{iso}), \qquad (4)$$

where $\otimes$ denotes the Kronecker tensor product and $\cdot$ denotes the dot product. $\mathbf{R}^{iso}$ and $\mathbf{x}_\mathbf{p}^{iso}$ are the rotational harmonic coefficients and the *zero*-th SH coefficient for the isotropic component, respectively. We require the volume fractions to sum to unity, i.e., $\sum_{i=1}^n h_{i,\mathbf{p}}^{aniso} + \sum_{j=1}^m h_{j,\mathbf{p}}^{iso} = 1$.

2.4   Problem Formulation

We group the signal vectors of N voxels at locations $\mathbb{P} = \{\mathbf{p}_1, \mathbf{p}_2, \ldots, \mathbf{p}_N\}$ as columns of matrix $\mathbf{S}$ and the SH coefficients of the corresponding AFODF given by ASI as columns in matrix $\mathbf{X}$. With a set of directions $\mathbb{U} = \{\mathbf{u}_1, \mathbf{u}_2, \ldots, \mathbf{u}_K\}$, we aim to solve the SH coefficients of the N voxels simultaneously as follows (Fig. 1):

$$(\hat{\mathbf{H}}, \hat{\mathbf{X}}) = \arg \min_{(\mathbf{H}, \mathbf{X})} \sum_{\mathbf{p} \in \mathbb{P}} \left\| \mathbf{s}_\mathbf{p} - \mathbf{R}^{aniso}(\mathbf{h}_\mathbf{p}^{aniso} \otimes \mathbf{x}_\mathbf{p}^{aniso}) - \mathbf{R}^{iso}(\mathbf{h}_\mathbf{p}^{iso} \cdot \mathbf{x}^{iso}) \right\|_2^2 + \lambda \Phi(\mathbb{F})$$

$$\text{s.t. } \mathbf{AX} \succeq 0, \ \mathbf{H} \succeq 0, \text{ and } \sum_{i=1}^n h_{i,\mathbf{p}}^{aniso} + \sum_{j=1}^m h_{j,\mathbf{p}}^{iso} = 1, \ \forall \mathbf{p} \in \mathbb{P}.$$

$$(5)$$

Matrix $\mathbf{A} = [\mathbf{A}^{aniso} \ \mathbf{A}^{iso}]$ maps the SH coefficients

$$\mathbf{X} = \begin{bmatrix} \mathbf{x}_{\mathbf{p}_1}^{ansio} & \cdots & \mathbf{x}_{\mathbf{p}_N}^{ansio} \\ \mathbf{x}_{\mathbf{p}_1}^{iso} & \cdots & \mathbf{x}_{\mathbf{p}_N}^{iso} \end{bmatrix} \qquad (6)$$

to the AFODF amplitudes at directions specified by $\mathbb{U}$ for imposing AFODF nonnegativity, i.e., $\mathbf{AX} \succeq 0$. The volume fractions, represented by

$$\mathbf{H} = \begin{bmatrix} \mathbf{h}_{\mathbf{p}_1}^{ansio} & \cdots & \mathbf{h}_{\mathbf{p}_N}^{ansio} \\ \mathbf{h}_{\mathbf{p}_1}^{iso} & \cdots & \mathbf{h}_{\mathbf{p}_N}^{iso} \end{bmatrix}, \qquad (7)$$

are also required to be non-negative. $\Phi(\mathbb{F})$ defined in (2) is computed only for the anisotropic portion of the AFODF. If we let

$$\widehat{\mathbf{W}}(\mathbf{u}) = \begin{bmatrix} \widehat{W}(\mathbf{p}_1, \mathbf{p}_1, \mathbf{u}) & \cdots & \widehat{W}(\mathbf{p}_N, \mathbf{p}_1, \mathbf{u}) \\ \vdots & \ddots & \vdots \\ \widehat{W}(\mathbf{p}_1, \mathbf{p}_N, \mathbf{u}) & \cdots & \widehat{W}(\mathbf{p}_N, \mathbf{p}_N, \mathbf{u}) \end{bmatrix}, \qquad (8)$$

with

$$\widehat{W}(\mathbf{p},\mathbf{q},\mathbf{u}) = \begin{cases} \frac{W(\langle \hat{\mathbf{v}}_{\mathbf{p},\mathbf{q}},\mathbf{u} \rangle)}{K_{\mathbf{p},\mathbf{u}}}, & \mathbf{q} \in \mathcal{N}_{\mathbf{p}}, \\ 0, & \text{otherwise,} \end{cases} \tag{9}$$

and define the operator $\circ$ as

$$\mathbf{A}^{\text{aniso}}\mathbf{X}^{\text{aniso}} \circ \widehat{\mathbf{W}} = \left[(\mathbf{A}^{\text{aniso}}\mathbf{X}^{\text{aniso}})_1 \widehat{\mathbf{W}}(\mathbf{u}_1), \dots, (\mathbf{A}^{\text{aniso}}\mathbf{X}^{\text{aniso}})_K \widehat{\mathbf{W}}(\mathbf{u}_K) \right]^{\top}, \tag{10}$$

where $(\mathbf{A}^{\text{aniso}}\mathbf{X}^{\text{aniso}})_i$ is the i-th row of $\mathbf{A}^{\text{aniso}}\mathbf{X}^{\text{aniso}}$ and corresponds to direction $\mathbf{u}_i$, problem (5) can be rewritten as

$$(\hat{\mathbf{H}}, \hat{\mathbf{X}}) = \arg \min_{(\mathbf{H},\mathbf{X})} \sum_{\mathbf{p} \in \mathbb{P}} \left\| \mathbf{s}_{\mathbf{p}} - \mathbf{R}^{\text{aniso}}(\mathbf{h}_{\mathbf{p}}^{\text{aniso}} \otimes \mathbf{x}_{\mathbf{p}}^{\text{aniso}}) - \mathbf{R}^{\text{iso}}(\mathbf{h}_{\mathbf{p}}^{\text{iso}} \cdot \mathbf{x}_{\mathbf{p}}^{\text{iso}}) \right\|_2^2 +$$

$$\lambda \left\| \mathbf{A}^{\text{aniso}}\mathbf{X}^{\text{aniso}} \circ \widehat{\mathbf{W}} - \mathbf{A}^{\text{aniso}}\mathbf{X}^{\text{aniso}} \right\|_F^2$$

$$\text{s.t. } \mathbf{AX} \succeq 0, \ \mathbf{H} \succeq 0, \text{ and } \sum_{i=1}^{n} h_{i,\mathbf{p}}^{\text{aniso}} + \sum_{j=1}^{m} h_{j,\mathbf{p}}^{\text{iso}} = 1, \ \forall \mathbf{p} \in \mathbb{P},$$

$$\tag{11}$$

where λ is a user-defined regularization parameter. We solve for $\hat{\mathbf{H}}$ and $\hat{\mathbf{X}}$ of all voxels concurrently using the alternating direction method of multipliers (ADMM) [11].

3 Experimental Results

3.1 Numerical Simulation

We evaluated ASI using numerical simulations for a range of diffusion anisotropy. A single fiber population at various diffusion anisotropy was simulated with a gradient table identical to the in-vivo dataset (see Sect. 3.3). Figure 2 indicates that the FODFs given by MTCSD are gradually dispersed as the signal anisotropy decreases. The FODFs given by ASI remain consistent despite changes in anisotropy.

3.2 Phantom Data

We used Phantomas [12] to generate *in silico* data (SNR = 30) with different configurations: branching, bending, and fanning. The gradient table of the in-vivo data was used. We used a fixed axial diffusivity (D_{L}) of $2 \times 10^{-3}\,\text{mm}^2/\text{s}$ and a range of radial diffusivity (D_{T}) from $0.1 \times 10^{-3}\,\text{mm}^2/\text{s}$ to $1.1 \times 10^{-3}\,\text{mm}^2/\text{s}$ with step size $0.2 \times 10^{-3}\,\text{mm}^2/\text{s}$. Figures 3 (branching), 4 (bending), and 5 (fanning) indicate that the FODFs given by ASI remain consistent despite changes in anisotropy. To evaluate which signal model better explains the data, we computed the normalized mean-squared error (NMSE) between the simulated signal and the predicted signal. Figure 6 confirms that the ASI signal model matches the diffusion signal better, compared with MTCSD and the AFODF model described in [10].

Signal profiles

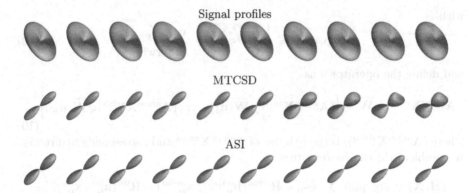

MTCSD

ASI

Fig. 2. FODFs estimated for signal profiles with decreasing anisotropy (from left to right).

$D_T/D_L = 0.05$ $D_T/D_L = 0.25$ $D_T/D_L = 0.35$ $D_T/D_L = 0.45$

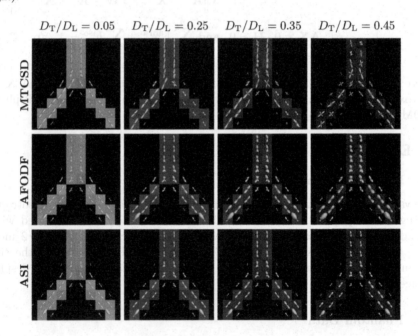

Fig. 3. Min-max normalized FODFs given by MTCSD, AFODF, and ASI.

3.3   In-Vivo Data

DMRI data of two infant subjects (19 days and 54 days of age), acquired via the Baby Connectome Project (BCP), were used for evaluation. The data were collected with 1.5 mm isotropic resolution with $b = 500, 1000, 1500, 2000, 2500, 3000\,s/mm^2$, using a total of 144 gradient directions, and 6 non-diffusion-weighted images, multi-band with a factor of 5, and positive and negative phase

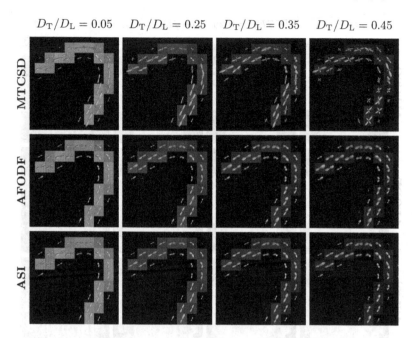

Fig. 4. Min-max normalized FODFs given by MTCSD, AFODF, and ASI.

encoding in the anterior-posterior direction. The total scan time was approximately 13 min per subject.

We examined the brain region where fibers from the corpus callosum (CC), the corona radiata (CR), and the superior longitudinal fasciculus (SLF) cross. Figure 7 shows that the AFODFs given by ASI correctly reflect the complex WM fiber configurations, such as branching in the red box and crossing in the blue box. Figure 8 shows that the FODFs estimated via ASI are more anisotropic and reflect well the WM structure. The tissue-specific fiber response functions for MTCSD and AFODF were estimated for each b-shell based on [13]. We also varied the anisotropy of the response function [14] in MTCSD and AFODF and evaluated the NMSE of the predicted signal. Figure 9 shows that the signal predicted by the ASI signal model best matches the data.

We extended the direction getter mechanism described in [15], which originally caters to symmetric FODFs, to work with asymmetric FODFs and extracted five tracts-of-interest using RecoBundles [15] (see Figs. 10 and 11). Note that the same seeds (brain mask) were used for tractography and streamlines less than 20 mm were removed. Figures 10 and 11 indicate that the tracts-of-interest can be recovered well in the 19-day-old and 54-day-old infant subjects using ASI but not MTCSD and AFODF.

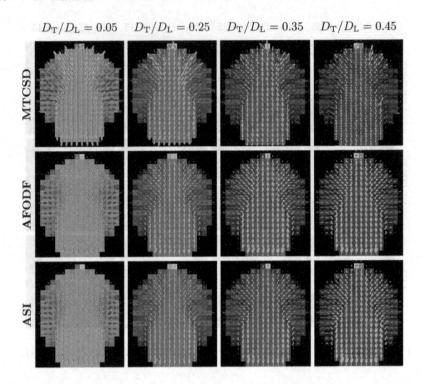

Fig. 5. Min-max normalized FODFs given by MTCSD, AFODF, and ASI.

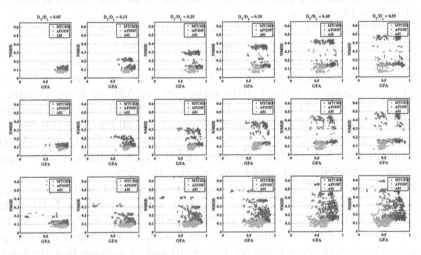

Fig. 6. NMSE of predicted signal as a function of GFA (Top: branching; Middle: bending; Bottom: fanning).

MTCSD   AFODF   ASI

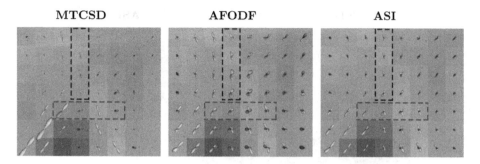

Fig. 7. Close-up views of FODFs given by MTCSD, AFODF, and ASI. (Color figure online)

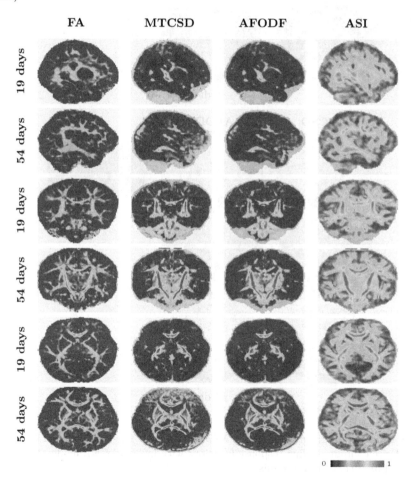

Fig. 8. FA and GFA maps of FODFs estimated by the different methods.

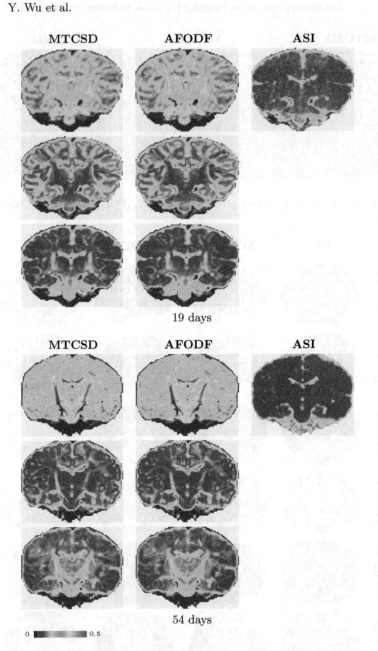

Fig. 9. NMSE maps given by MTCSD, AFODF and ASI. The FODFs for MTCSD and AFODF are computed using response functions with low (top row), moderate (middle row), and high (bottom row) anisotropy.

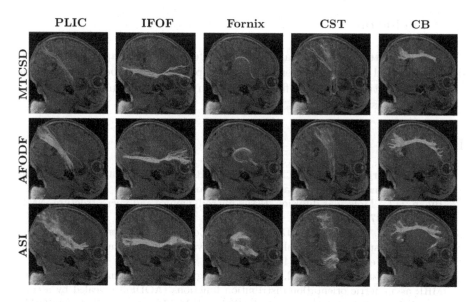

Fig. 10. Five tracts-of-interest given by MTCSD, AFODF, and ASI for the 19-day-old infant subject.

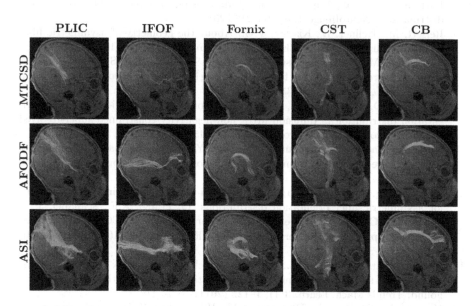

Fig. 11. Five tracts-of-interest given by MTCSD, AFODF, and ASI for the 54-day-old infant subject.

4 Conclusion

We have presented a method, called ASI, for effective tractography in the developing brain. ASI allows characterization of complex subvoxel fiber configurations and accurate estimation of the fiber orientation distribution function in spite of changes in diffusion patterns.

References

1. Johansen-Berg, H., Behrens, T.E.: Diffusion MRI: From Quantitative Measurement to in Vivo Neuroanatomy. Academic Press, Cambridge (2013)
2. Bihan, D.L.: Molecular diffusion, tissue microdynamics and microstructure. NMR Biomed. **8**, 375–386 (1995)
3. Jeurissen, B., Tournier, J.D., Dhollander, T., Connelly, A., Sijbers, J.: Multi-tissue constrained spherical deconvolution for improved analysis of multi-shell diffusion MRI data. NeuroImage **103**, 411–426 (2014)
4. Cetin, S., Ozarslan, E., Unal, G.: Elucidating intravoxel geometry in diffusion-MRI: asymmetric orientation distribution functions (AODFs) revealed by a cone model. In: Navab, N., Hornegger, J., Wells, W.M., Frangi, A.F. (eds.) MICCAI 2015. LNCS, vol. 9349, pp. 231–238. Springer, Cham (2015). https://doi.org/10.1007/978-3-319-24553-9_29
5. Bastiani, M., et al.: Improved tractography using asymmetric fibre orientation distributions. NeuroImage **158**, 205–218 (2017)
6. Reisert, M., Kellner, E., Kiselev, V.G.: About the geometry of asymmetric fiber orientation distributions. IEEE Trans. Med. Imaging **31**(6), 1240–1249 (2012)
7. Parker, G., Marshall, D., Rosin, P.L., Drage, N., Richmond, S., Jones, D.K.: A pitfall in the reconstruction of fibre ODFs using spherical deconvolution of diffusion MRI data. Neuroimage **65**, 433–448 (2013)
8. Tournier, J.D., Calamante, F., Connelly, A.: Robust determination of the fibre orientation distribution in diffusion MRI: non-negativity constrained super-resolved spherical deconvolution. NeuroImage **35**(4), 1459–1472 (2007)
9. Auría, A., Daducci, A., Thiran, J.P., Wiaux, Y.: Structured sparsity for spatially coherent fibre orientation estimation in diffusion MRI. NeuroImage **115**, 245–255 (2015)
10. Wu, Y., Feng, Y., Shen, D., Yap, P.-T.: A multi-tissue global estimation framework for asymmetric fiber orientation distributions. In: Frangi, A.F., Schnabel, J.A., Davatzikos, C., Alberola-López, C., Fichtinger, G. (eds.) MICCAI 2018. LNCS, vol. 11072, pp. 45–52. Springer, Cham (2018). https://doi.org/10.1007/978-3-030-00931-1_6
11. Boyd, S., Parikh, N., Chu, E., Peleato, B., Eckstein, J., et al.: Distributed optimization and statistical learning via the alternating direction method of multipliers. Found. Trends Mach. Learn. **3**(1), 1–122 (2011)
12. Caruyer, E., Daducci, A., Descoteaux, M., Houde, J.C., Thiran, J.P., Verma, R.: Phantomas: a flexible software library to simulate diffusion MR phantoms. In: ISMRM (2014)
13. Dhollander, T., Raffelt, D., Connelly, A.: Unsupervised 3-tissue response function estimation from single-shell or multi-shell diffusion MR data without a co-registered T1 image. In: ISMRM Workshop on Breaking the Barriers of Diffusion MRI, vol. 5 (2016)

14. Bastiani, M., et al.: Automated processing pipeline for neonatal diffusion MRI in the developing Human Connectome Project. NeuroImage **185**, 750–763 (2018)
15. Garyfallidis, E., et al.: Dipy, a library for the analysis of diffusion MRI data. Front. Neuroinf. **8**, 8 (2014)

A Fast Fiber k-Nearest-Neighbor Algorithm with Application to Group-Wise White Matter Topography Analysis

Junyan Wang[✉] and Yonggang Shi

Laboratory of Neuro Imaging (LONI),
USC Stevens Neuroimaging and Informatics Institute,
Keck School of Medicine of USC, Los Angeles, CA 90033, USA
junyan.wang@loni.usc.edu

Abstract. Finding the fiber k-nearest-neighbors (k-NN) is often essential to brain white matter analysis yet it is computationally prohibitive, and no efficient approximation to it is known to the best of our knowledge. We observe a strong relationship between the point-wise distances and tract-wise distances. Based on this observation, we propose a fast algorithm for approximating the k-NN distances of large fiber bundles with point-wise K-NN algorithm, and we call it the *fast fiber k-NN algorithm*. Furthermore, we apply our fast fiber k-NN algorithm to white matter topography analysis, which is an emerging problem in brain connectomics reasearch. For the latter task, we first propose to quantify the white matter topography by metric embedding, which gives rise to the first anatomically meaningful fiber-wise measure of white matter topography to the best of our knowledge. In addition, we extend the individual white matter topography analysis to group-wise analysis using the k-NN fiber distances computed with our fast algorithm. In our experiments, (a) we find that our fast fiber k-NN algorithm reasonably approximates the ground-truth distance at 1–2 percent of its computational cost, (b) we also verify the anatomical validity of our proposed topographic measure, and (c) we find that our fast fiber k-NN algorithm performs identically well compared with the exhaustive fiber distance computation, for the group-wise white matter topography analysis for 792 subjects from the Human Connectome Project.

This work was in part supported by the National Institute of Health (NIH) under Grant RF1AG056573, R01EB022744, U01EY025864, U01AG051218, P41 EB015922, P50AG05142. Data used in this paper were provided by the Human Connectome Project, WU-Minn Consortium (Principal Investigators: David Van Essen and Kamil Ugurbil; 1U54MH091657) funded by the 16 NIH Institutes and Centers that support the NIH Blueprint for Neuroscience Research; and by the McDonnell Center for Systems Neuroscience at Washington University.

A. C. S. Chung et al. (Eds.): IPMI 2019, LNCS 11492, pp. 332–344, 2019.
https://doi.org/10.1007/978-3-030-20351-1_25

1   Introduction

Tractography based on diffusion magnetic resonance imaging (dMRI) is currently the only method for in vivo and non-invasive measurement of structural connectivity of the brain. In recent years, tremendous progress has been made to improve the quality of tractography [12,14]. In our work, we are focused on analyzing the fiber tracts generated by tractography.

1.1   Fiber Distance Computation

Large-scale white matter fiber analysis has become an emerging technique for brain research [9,11,13], in which the k-nearest-neighbor (k-NN) fiber distance computation is usually an essential step. However, it is often intractable to compute the k-NN fiber distances for massive fiber set from a population of subjects, and the existing powerful fiber analysis methods are not applicable to those large-scale studies. As the first contribution of this work, we propose a fast algorithm for approximating the k-NN fiber distance, which is the first of this type to the best of our knowledge, and we call it the *fast fiber k-NN algorithm*. Our idea is motivated by the observation that the fiber-wise k-NN distance is strongly related to point-wise K-NN distance. In the remainder of this paper, we use K-NN to denote point-wise K-nearest-neighbor and k-NN to denote fiber-wise k-nearest-neighbor. Since the K-NN pointwise distance can be computed efficiently with well-established fast algorithms, e.g. the celebrated k-d tree algorithm [2], the computational cost for the k-NN fiber distance can also be greatly reduced. The experimental results show that our fast fiber k-NN reasonably approximates the ground-truth fiber k-NN distance at significantly smaller computational cost.

1.2   Characterizing Whole Brain White Matter Topography

Recently, the study of brain topography has been gaining renewed interest [7]. However, the study of white matter topography is often based on qualitative methods [17], and mathematical modeling of the whole brain white matter topography of fiber tracts has not been properly explored until very recently. In [10], Lambert et al. proposed a model of tractography topographic gradient defined on white matter voxels based on the voxel-wise structural connectivity computed from the fiber tracts. However, the brain white matter is formed by nerve fibers and the topography for the fiber tracts has not been defined. The most related work is [15,16], in which a local measure of the topographic regularity of fiber tracts is proposed. However, this model does not characterize how each fiber is organized with respect to other fibers in the rest of the whole brain.

1.3   Method Overview

Our model is based on the notion of metric embedding of fiber curves, and it maps each curve to a vector in a finite dimensional vector space. Since the mapping is isomorphic and nearly-isometric, we consider that the resultant finite dimensional embedding space and the fiber curve space are equivalent in their geometrical construct, and the topography of the fibers is characterized by the statistical and geometrical analysis of the embedding vectors. Although fiber embedding has been proposed for fiber analysis [8,11], this is the first time that it is used to represent white matter topography and it is also the first anatomically meaningful model of fiber-wise white matter topography to the best of our knowledge. Furthermore, we propose to extend the fiber embedding of individual subjects to group-wise embedding with the k-NN tract distance computed with our fast algorithm, and this leads up to a novel method for aligning the embedding vectors across different individual subjects based on an orthognality-constrained least square formulation. The experimental results show that the topographic vectors well characterize the white matter organization, and the approximate distance computed from our fast fiber k-NN algorithm is almost identical to the ground-truth distance for group-wise white matter topography analysis.

2 Fast Approximation of k-Nearest-Neighbor Fiber Distance

2.1 Theoretical Relationship Between the K-NN Point Distance and the k-NN Fiber Distance

Without loss of generality, in the theoretical discussions presented here we treat a fiber as a point set, and we consider a fiber bundle as a collection of point sets. Our main idea of the fast approximation of the k-NN fiber distance lies in the following theorem.

Theorem 1. *Suppose we are given a collection of point sets, denoted as Γ, and two point sets X, Y belonging to Γ, i.e. $X, Y \in \Gamma$, and suppose $N_\Gamma^K(y)$ is the set of the K-NN points of a point $y \in Y$ within Γ and the point-wise K-NN is defined by point-wise distance $d(\cdot, \cdot)$, additionally if $N_\Gamma^K(y) \cap X \neq \emptyset$, then*

$$d_X(y) = \min_{x \in X} d(x, y) = \min_{x \in N_\Gamma^K(y) \cap X} d(x, y) \qquad (1)$$

This theorem shows that we do not require the entire set, or fiber, X to compute $d_X(y)$, but we would only require the pointwise K-NN computed beforehand, which lays the theoretical basis of our method. The proof is omitted due to page length limit.

According to Theorem 1, if $\forall y \in Y$, $N_\Gamma^K(y) \cap X \neq \emptyset$, we can rewrite a common fiber distance as follows:

$$d_H(X, Y) = \max_{y \in Y} \min_{x \in X} d(x, y) = \max_{y \in Y} \min_{x \in N_\Gamma^K(y) \cap X} d(x, y) \qquad (2)$$

which is also known as the one-sided Hausdorff distance.

In addition, we observe that $\forall y \in Y$, $N_\Gamma^K(y) \cap X \neq \emptyset$ actually implies that X and Y are really *close-by*. This can be described formally as

Proposition 1. *Suppose* $\forall y \in Y,\ N_\Gamma^K(y) \cap X \neq \varnothing$

$$d_H(X, Y) \leq \max_{y \in Y} R(N_\Gamma^K(y)) \tag{3}$$

where $R(N_\Gamma^K(y)) = \max_{z \in N_\Gamma^K(y)} d(z, y)$ *may be called the radius of* $N_\Gamma^K(y)$.

Proposition 1 can be proven by upper-bounding Eq. (2).

2.2   Fast Fiber k-NN Approximation

Our idea for fast fiber k-NN is to approximate the fiber k-NN, and the corresponding distances can be computed using Eq. (1). The previous observations motivate us to relate the size of $N_\Gamma^K(y) \cap X$ with the closeness of fibers, and we propose a fiber k-NN-likeness measure based on the size of $N_\Gamma^K(y) \cap X$ as follows:

$$\delta^K(X|Y) = \frac{1}{|Y|} \sum_{y \in Y} |N_\Gamma^K(y) \cap X| \tag{4}$$

where $|\cdot|$ is the cardinality, or size, of a set. X with larger $\delta^K(X|Y)$ is considered closer to Y, which gives rise to our definition of the key notion of this work:

Definition 1 (Approximate fiber k-NN). *We define the approximate fiber k-NN in* Γ *for fiber* Y *as the set* $\mathfrak{N}_\Gamma^k(Y) = \{X^1, X^2, \cdots, X^k\}$, *if* $\exists K$ *such that* $\delta^K(X|Y) \geq \delta^K(X'|Y)$ *for* $\forall X \in \mathfrak{N}_\Gamma^k(Y)$ *and* $\forall X' \notin \mathfrak{N}_\Gamma^K(Y)$.

where the k is usually much smaller than the K value in the point-wise K-NN.

At this point, we show the main point of this work that Eq. (4) can be *computed efficiently* without resorting to all pairwise fiber distances based on the following observations.

Definition 2 (Point-to-tract mapping). *For fiber bundle* $T = \{t^1, t^2, \cdots, t^N\}$, *where each fiber is defined by a point set as* $t^i = \{\mathbf{x}_1^i, \mathbf{x}_2^i, \cdots, \mathbf{x}_{m_i}^i\}$, *if we denote the set of all points on all fibers as* $P = \{\mathbf{x}_1, \mathbf{x}_2, \cdots, \mathbf{x}_M\}$, *the injection mapping* $PT : i \in \{\forall i' | \mathbf{x}_{i'} \in P\} \mapsto j \in \{\forall j' | t_{j'} \in T\}$ *is called a* **point-to-tract mapping.**

The fiber bundles are stored as a point set in benchmark file formats of fiber bundles, such as the `trk` and `tck` files, and this mapping is inherently provided with the tract files.

Proposition 2 (Indicator of tract neighbors). *Suppose* $N_\Gamma^K(y)$ *is a set of point indices and* $N_\Gamma^K(Y)$ *denotes the union of the indices of tracts containing points belonging to the K-NN of certain* $y \in Y$, *i.e.* $N_\Gamma^K(Y) = \bigcup_{y \in Y} PT(N_\Gamma^K(y))$. *We have*

$$\delta^K(X|Y) > 0 \text{ iff } X \in N_\Gamma^K(Y) \tag{5}$$

This proposition is proven by definition of PT, i.e. Definition 2, definition of $N_\Gamma^K(y)$ and definition of $\delta^K(X|Y)$. It shows us that we can easily identify the union set $N_\Gamma^K(Y)$ and compute Eq. (4) for this set only.

In addition, we can see that it is also straightforward to compute $|N_\Gamma^K(y) \cap X|$ for Eq. (4), since

$$|N_\Gamma^K(y) \cap X| = m_{PT(N_F^K(y))}(i(X)) \tag{6}$$

where $i(X)$ is the index of X and $m_A(x)$ is the multiplicity of x in the multiset A. In addition, it is also straightforward to identify every fiber X with $\delta^k(X|Y) > 0$ for fixed Y based on the following theorem.

Combining Eqs. (1) and (4), we obtain our fast fiber k-NN algorithm summarized in Algorithm 1.

Algorithm 1. Fast fiber k-NN algorithm

Input : **Tractogram 1** $T_1 = \{t_1^1, t_1^2, t_1^3 ..., t_1^{N_1}\}$, **Tractogram 2**
$T_2 = \{t_2^1, t_2^2, t_2^3 ..., t_2^{N_2}\}$, **Point Neighborhood size** K, **Fiber Neighborhood Size** k $(k \ll K)$

Output: k-NN fiber distance $d^k(T_1, T_2)$

1 $PT_2 \leftarrow$ point_id_to_tract_id (T_2);
2 **for** $i = 1$ **to** N_1 **by** 1 **do**
3     $t_1 \leftarrow T_1(i)$;
4     $D_i^{|t_1| \times K}, ID_i^{|t_1| \times K} \leftarrow$ pt_knnsearch (T_2, t_1, K) % point-wise K-NN producing K-NN distances D_i and the neighbor set ID_i;
5     $N_{T_2}^K(t_1) \leftarrow PT_2(ID_i)$;
6   **for** j in $\mathcal{N}_{T_2}^K(t_1)$ **do**
7 | $\delta^K(j|t_1) \leftarrow$ Eq. (4);
8   **end**
9     $\mathfrak{N}_{T_2}^k(t_1) \leftarrow$ sort$(\delta^K(j|t_1),$ top $k)$;
10   **for** t_2 in $\mathfrak{N}_{T_2}^k(t_1)$ **do**
11   **for** $j = 1$ **to** $|t_1|$ **by** 1 **do**
12 | $\{N_{T_2}^K(t_1) \cap t_2\} \leftarrow$ find$(PT_2(ID_i(j,:)) == t_2)$;
13 | $\hat{d}(j) \leftarrow \min(D_i(j, \{N_{T_2}^K(t_1) \cap t_2\})$ % by Eq. (1);
14   **end**
15         $d^k(i, t_2) \leftarrow \max\limits_{1 \leq j \leq |t_1|} \hat{d}(j)$ % max is used as a matter of choice;
16   **end**
17 **end**

---

3 Group-Wise White Matter Topography Analysis

Our idea for fiber-wise white matter topography measure is based on the notion called metric embedding [1], and specifically we adopt the Euclidean embedding, a.k.a. the classical Multidimensional Scaling (cMDS) [3], which tries to represent the data in complex form as low-dimensional vectors in Euclidean space while preserving the distances in the original space of the data, The embedding space will then faithfully represent the geometry of the orginal data.

3.1   White Matter Topography Characterized by Isometric Euclidean Embedding

Basic Formulations of MDS. The cMDS embedding can be obtained by using the following steps [3]:

$$(a)\ \mathbf{B} = P\left[-\frac{1}{2}\mathbf{D}^{(2)}\right]P,\ (b)\ \mathbf{E}\mathbf{\Lambda}\mathbf{E}^T = \texttt{svd}(\mathbf{B}),\ (c)\ \mathbf{Z}_p = \mathbf{E}_p\mathbf{\Lambda}_p^{\frac{1}{2}} \tag{7}$$

where P is known as the centering matrix defined as $P_{ij} = 1 - \frac{1}{n}, \forall i = j$ and $P_{ij} = -\frac{1}{n}, \forall i \neq j$ where n is the number of samples, $\mathbf{D}^{(2)}$ is the input squared distance matrix, $\mathbf{Z}_p$ and $\mathbf{E}_p$ are the first p columns of $\mathbf{Z}$ and $\mathbf{E}$, and $\mathbf{\Lambda}_p$ is the top-left $p{\times}p$ block matrix of $\mathbf{\Lambda}$ where p is the embedding dimension. In this work, we adopt all the eigenvectors associated with positive eigenvalues for embedding.

The Geometry of Fibers in the Embedding Space. Based on the MDS formulation, we can infer that more contrast on the values of embedding vectors can be seen for geometrically more distant fibers. In addition, the significance of each dimension of the embedding vectors in terms of its contribution in forming the target distance is naturally characterized by the corresponding eigenvalues:

Theorem 2.

$$\|\mathbf{B} - \mathbf{z}_i\mathbf{z}_i^T\|_F = \sqrt{\sum_{j \neq i}\lambda_j^2} \tag{8}$$

where $\Lambda = \mathrm{diag}(\lambda_1, \lambda_2, ...)$ *are the eigenvalues associated with the eigenvectors* $\mathbf{E} = [\mathbf{e}_1, \mathbf{e}_2, ...]$.

The proof is omitted due to page length limit.

In conclusion, the embedding space coincide with the metric-distance geometry of the original fibers, and each dimension characterizes the geometrical organization of the fibers. Furthermore, they resemble the classic yet vague notion of topographic gradients in the neuroscience literature, and, here, we call them the *topographic vectors*.

3.2   Group-Wise White Matter Topography Analysis

To extend the individual white matter topography analysis to group-wise analysis, we will need to characterize the embedding vectors in a group of subjects. Our idea is based on the conventional group-wise analysis of volumetric data in which the brain voxels are registered and then analyzed across the group.

A technical problem in the group-wise analysis is that the topographic vectors computed on parallel for each individual may be misaligned, largely due to the fact that $\mathbf{B} = \mathbf{ZZ}^T = \mathbf{ZRR}^T\mathbf{Z}^T$, where $\mathbf{R}^{p \times p}$ is an arbitrary orthogonal matrix. Therefore, we propose to additionally align the topographic vectors by finding the optimal orthogonal transformation $\mathbf{R}$. Without loss of generality, here we consider the case for two subjects. Let the two fiber bundles be denoted as T_1 and T_2. Their topographic vectors are denoted as $\mathbf{Z}_1^{N^1 \times p}$ and $\mathbf{Z}_2^{N^2 \times p}$. Similar to the volumetric studies, we propose to establish the fiber correspondences first based on the k-NN fiber distance. Suppose we consider T_1 as a fixed reference, we can find the subset of $\mathbf{Z}_2$ corresponding to $\mathbf{Z}_1$, which is denoted as $\mathbf{Z}_{21}^{N^1 \times p}$. Then, our formulation for cross-subject embedding alignment reads:

$$\mathbf{Z}_{21}^* = \mathbf{Z}_{21}\mathbf{R}^*, \quad \mathbf{R}^* = \underset{\mathbf{RR}^T = \mathbf{I}}{\arg\min} \|\mathbf{Z}_{21}\mathbf{R} - \mathbf{Z}_1\|_F^2 \tag{9}$$

To solve this problem we first rewrite the objective function as

$$\|\mathbf{Z}_{21}\mathbf{R} - \mathbf{Z}_1\|_F^2 = \|\mathbf{U}_{21}\mathbf{\Lambda}_{21}\mathbf{V}_{21}^T\mathbf{R} - \mathbf{Z}_1\|_F^2 = \|\mathbf{R} - \mathbf{V}_{21}\mathbf{\Lambda}_{21}^{-1}\mathbf{U}_{21}\mathbf{Z}_1\|_F^2 \tag{10}$$

which is in the typical form of orthogonality-constrained least-square problem and it admits a closed-form solution [5]:

$$\mathbf{Z}_{21}^* = \mathbf{Z}_{21}\mathbf{R}^*, \quad \mathbf{R}^* = \mathbf{U}^*\mathbf{V}^{*T} \tag{11}$$

where $[\mathbf{U}^*, \mathbf{D}^*, \mathbf{V}^*] = \mathrm{svd}(\mathbf{V}_{21}\mathbf{\Lambda}_{21}^{-1}\mathbf{U}_{21}\mathbf{Z}_1)$.

After the alignment, we recompute the aligned topographic vectors with local smoothing: $\widetilde{\mathbf{z}}_{21}^i = \sum_{\mathbf{z}_{21}^j \in N_{\mathbf{z}_{21}^i}^k} W_{ij}\mathbf{z}_{21}^j{}^*$, where $W_{ij} = \frac{\exp(-\|\mathbf{z}_{21}^i - \mathbf{z}_{21}^j\|^2/\sigma^2)}{\sum_{\mathbf{z}_{21}^j \in N_{\mathbf{z}_{21}^i}^k} \exp(-\|\mathbf{z}_{21}^i - \mathbf{z}_{21}^j\|/\sigma^2)}$ and we used $k = 10$ and $\sigma^2 = 10$ in this definition. Note that we adopt the pointwise distances between $\mathbf{Z}_{21}^*$ and $\mathbf{Z}_1$ to alleviate the errors in the fiber distance caused by registration error and distance approximation error. Upon completing the topographic vector alignment, we can perform statistical analysis for all topographic vectors.

4   Results

4.1   Materials

In our experiment, we use the minimally preprocessed dMRI data of 792 subjects from the Human Connectome Project (HCP) dataset [6]. A whole brain tractogram of 10,000 fibers is generated for each subject by using MRtrix3 [14], resulting in a massive fiber set to pairwise distance computation. Afterwards, a tract-density image (TDI) is generated for each tractogram and then a nonrigid warp field is generated by registering 791 TDI images to a reference TDI image using ANTs. All tractograms are subsequently warped by using the warp field, such that all tractograms are aligned to the same image space.

Note that the tract "distance" $d_X()$ defined by Eq. (2) is asymmetric and it is not a metric distance. In this work, we adopt the symmetric fiber distance measure in the following form: $d_{min}(X,Y) = \min(d_H(X,Y), d_H(Y,X))$, by which short fibers are considered to be part of close-by long fibers. Our method is readily applicable to distance measures based on the one-sided Hausdorff distance and it can be generalized to many other measures based on the form of $d_X(y)$ defined in Eq. (1).

4.2 Efficient Distance Approximation

We evaluate our fast fiber k-NN distance computation against exhaustive pairwise computation, since the latter produces the ground-truth distances. The point-wise neighborhood sizes in our method are $K = 100, 200, ..., 1000$. The tract-wise neighborhood size for our method is always set to $k_1 = 10$ and the neighborhood sizes for the exhaustive fiber distance computation are $k_2 = 10, 20, \cdots, 100$. We first evaluate our method in terms of: (a) the number of overlapped fiber sets in the tract neighborhood from both methods, and (b) the linear correlation of the distances. The results are shown in Fig. 1. We only show the overlap histograms for a small number of combinations of parameters due to paper length limit. From the histograms, we observe that our method gives high neighborhood overlap rate with the exhaustive distance computation when $k_2 = 10$. Particularly, our method with $k_1 = 10$ gives almost perfect overlap with the exhaustive distance computation when $k_2 = 20$, meaning that our fast fiber 10-NN almost surely lies in the ground-truth fiber 20-NNs. In addition to the neighborhood construction, we also observe that the fast fiber k-NN distances for $k_1 = 10$ computed by our method is also accurate for $K \geq 500$.

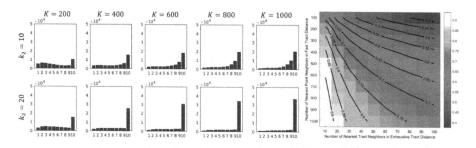

Fig. 1. Comparison of our method with exhaustive fiber distance computation. The bar plots on the left are the histograms of size of overlapped neighbor set. The image on the right shows the linear correlation of the two distances.

Furthermore, we calculate the mean neighborhood size overlap, mean(k^*), for different K values, and we also calculate the speed-up ratio of our method, denoted by r, which is defined as the computation time of exhaustive fiber distance computation divided by that of our method. The results are shown in Fig. 2. The baseline computational cost for the exhaustive fiber distance computation is 15826.47 s in MATLAB on a normal PC with Intel i7-6820HQ CPU and 32 GB ram. On the contrary, our method requires only couples of minutes to achieve 7 or 8 neighborhood overlap. To further quantify the performance, we fit the scatter points of the mean neighborhood size overlap $m = \text{mean}(k^*)$ and speed-up ratio r to two curves against K, as shown in Fig. 2. The results are summarized in Table 1, where we show the parameters of the fitting curves and the fitting scores. We also present the projected values of m and r for $K = 2000$ and 6000. From the predictions we can observe that we could increase K to achieve almost perfect distance approximation, but at the computational cost almost identical to that of the exhaustive method.

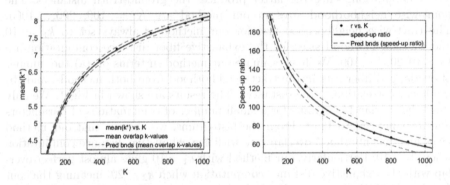

Fig. 2. Effectiveness and efficiency of our method. The solid curves are least-squared curve fitting of the points. The dashed lines are 95% confidence bounds of the prediction curves.

Table 1. Performance curve parameters and predictions

Curves	a	b	c	RMSE	R-square	$K = 2000$	$K = 6000$
$m(K) = aK^b + c$	−27.77	−0.2561	12.79	0.03581	0.9993	8.82	9.79
$r(K) = aK^b + c$	1130	−0.3145	−72.2	2.985	0.9962	31.26	1.04

4.3 Individual White Matter Topography Analysis

Quality of Individual Embedding. For the individual analysis, we require the whole pairwise distance matrix for each tractogram. After the MDS for all aligned 792 whole brain tractograms, we obtain the topographic vectors. The maximum embedding dimensions associated with positive eigenvalues are 16 or 17. The dimensions of the topographic vectors are arranged in descending order by the magnitude of the eigenvalues. The linear correlation between the ground-truth distance and the embedding distance is 0.98 ± 0.0032, meaning that the embedding is nearly isometric and stable.

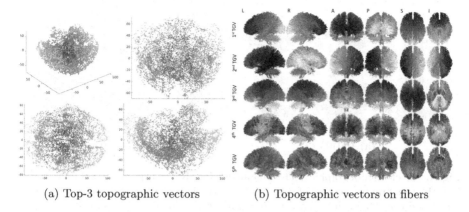

(a) Top-3 topographic vectors   (b) Topographic vectors on fibers

Fig. 3. Individual white matter topography. The colors of the points correspond to the norm of the vectors.

Anatomical Interpretations of the Topographic Vectors. The top-3 topographic vectors (TGV) associated with the largest-3 eigenvalues are shown in Fig. 3(a). Interestingly, the point cloud of the top-3 topographic vectors resembles the shape of a brain and we observe at least two layers of structures. To further investigate this unanticipated finding, we plot the fibers using the [0,1]-normalized topographic values as the lightness in gray colormap with QIT [4], and the results are shown in Fig. 3(b). We find that the top-3 topographic values on the fibers, somehow, show clear gradients in the three principal anatomical directions, namely anterior-posterior, left-right and superior-inferior. In addition, the fourth dimension separates the motor fibers passing through brainstem and cerebellum from all other fibers, and the fifth dimension gives some contrast for the association fibers near the frontal cortex and visual cortex. In addition, by combining the point cloud and fiber visualizations, we deduce that the outer layer of the point cloud is largely formed by associative fibers and the inner layer corresponds to the long fibers.

4.4 Group-Wise White Matter Topography Analysis

We used $k_1 = 10$ and $K = 500$ for the fast fiber k-NN distances for this experiment, and we compare our fast k-NN fiber distance computation with the exhaustive fiber distance computation for this task.

The topographic vectors from different subjects can be largely misaligned, as shown in the top rows of Fig. 4. After our alignment proposed in Sect. 3.2, the topographic vectors are visually well aligned to the reference topographic vectors.

The performance of our fast k-NN fiber distance computation for group-wise white matter topography anlaysis is quantitatively assessed by comparing the aligned topographic vectors computed via our fast fiber k-NN algorithm with the ones computed with exhaustive fiber distance computation. We used two measures to quantify the performance: (a) element-wise Pearson linear correlation of

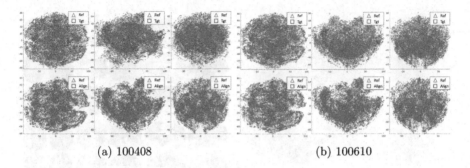

(a) 100408   (b) 100610

Fig. 4. Effect of topographic vector alignment for HCP subjects 100408 and 100610. Ref: the topographic vectors of reference subject. Tgt: the topographic vectors of the target subject. Align: the aligned topographic vectors of the target subject.

all topographic vectors denoted as `corr`, (b) average RMSE of the topographic vectors for single dimension. The statistics are summarized in Table 2, according to which our method produces topographic vectors almost identical to the ones given by exhaustive fiber distance computation in terms of linear correlation. Note that the range of each dimension of the topographic vectors is around ±100. The absolute difference between the results from the two distance computation methods is also negligible. Furthermore, alignments with both of the two distances achieve high fidelity, in terms of mean of RMSE, and reproducibility, in terms of standard deviation of RMSE, when comparing the alignment results with the reference data.

Finally, we present the top-3 group-wise topographic vectors computed using our fast fiber k-NN method for the 792 subjects in Fig. 5. Comparing with the individual top-3 topographic vectors, the group-wise topographic vectors form a more smooth boundary and more regular internal organization.

Remark on Computational Cost. The most time-consuming part of the group-wise white matter topography analysis is the MDS for individual subjects, which requires the full pairwise distance computation, and it usually takes hours for a single subject to complete. Hence, we distributed this task on our server and the entire analysis with our fast method is completed within couples of hours.

Table 2. Performance of group-wise white matter topography analysis

Measures	FFD vs. GTD	Original vs. GTD	Fidelity and reproducibility	
			FFD vs. Ref	GTD vs. Ref
`corr`	0.989 ± 0.0027	0.0002 ± 0.004	0.968 ± 0.0034	0.972 ± 0.0028
RMSE	2.43 ± 0.24	24.71 ± 0.23	4.39 ± 0.25	4.14 ± 0.20

FFD: Fast Fiber Distance (Our method); GTD: Ground-Truth Distance (Exhaustive fiber distance computation); Original: Target topographic vectors without alignment

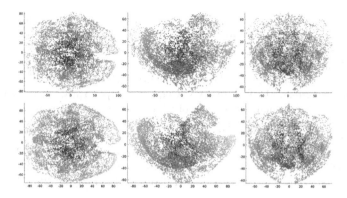

Fig. 5. Top-3 group-average topographic vectors (2nd row) comparing with the individual top-3 topographic vectors (1st row). The colors of the points correspond to the norm of the vectors.

5 Conclusion

In this work, we proposed a novel fast fiber k-NN algorithm that reasonably approximates the ground-truth k-NN distances of large fiber set at significantly reduced computational cost. We also proposed a novel mathematical model of fiber-wise white matter topography, and the results are anatomically meaningful. In addition, we proposed a novel workflow for group-wise white matter topography analysis, and we found that our fast fiber k-NN algorithm achieves the results almost identical to those computed with the ground-truth distances. For future work, we would apply the fast fiber k-NN distance algorithm to other fiber analysis problems, e.g. fiber clustering and registration, and we would apply the group-wise white matter topography analysis to identify subtle white matter damages for, such as, early diagnosis of Alzheimer's disease.

References

1. Abraham, I., Bartal, Y., Neiman, O.: Advances in metric embedding theory. Adv. Math. **228**(6), 3026–3126 (2011)
2. Bentley, J.L.: Multidimensional binary search trees used for associative searching. Commun. ACM **18**(9), 509–517 (1975)
3. Borg, I., Groenen, P.J.: Modern Multidimensional Scaling: Theory and Applications. Springer, Heidelberg (2005). https://doi.org/10.1007/0-387-28981-X
4. Cabeen, R.P., Laidlaw, D.H., Toga, A.W.: Quantitative imaging toolkit: software for interactive 3D visualization, processing, and analysis of neuroimaging datasets. In: Proceedings of the International Society for Magnetic Resonance in Medicine (2018)
5. Gibson, W.: On the least-squares orthogonalization of an oblique transformation. Psychometrika **27**(2), 193–195 (1962)

6. Glasser, M.F., et al.: The minimal preprocessing pipelines for the human connectome project. Neuroimage **80**, 105–124 (2013)
7. Jbabdi, S., Sotiropoulos, S.N., Behrens, T.E.: The topographic connectome. Curr. Opin. Neurobiol. **23**(2), 207–215 (2013)
8. Jianu, R., Demiralp, C., Laidlaw, D.: Exploring 3D DTI fiber tracts with linked 2D representations. IEEE Trans. Vis. Comput. Graph. **15**(6), 1449–1456 (2009)
9. Jin, Y., et al.: Automatic clustering of white matter fibers in brain diffusion MRI with an application to genetics. Neuroimage **100**, 75–90 (2014)
10. Lambert, C., Simon, H., Colman, J., Barrick, T.R.: Defining thalamic nuclei and topographic connectivity gradients in vivo. Neuroimage **158**, 466–479 (2017)
11. O'Donnell, L.J., Westin, C.F.: Automatic tractography segmentation using a high-dimensional white matter atlas. IEEE Trans. Med. Imaging **26**(11), 1562–1575 (2007)
12. Poulin, P., et al.: Learn to track: deep learning for tractography. In: Descoteaux, M., Maier-Hein, L., Franz, A., Jannin, P., Collins, D.L., Duchesne, S. (eds.) MICCAI 2017. LNCS, vol. 10433, pp. 540–547. Springer, Cham (2017). https://doi.org/10.1007/978-3-319-66182-7_62
13. Siless, V., Chang, K., Fischl, B., Yendiki, A.: Anatomicuts: hierarchical clustering of tractography streamlines based on anatomical similarity. Neuroimage **166**, 32–45 (2018)
14. Tournier, J., Calamante, F., Connelly, A., et al.: MRtrix: diffusion tractography in crossing fiber regions. Int. J. Imaging Syst. Technol. **22**(1), 53–66 (2012)
15. Wang, J., Aydogan, D.B., Varma, R., Toga, A.W., Shi, Y.: Topographic regularity for tract filtering in brain connectivity. In: Niethammer, M., et al. (eds.) IPMI 2017. LNCS, vol. 10265, pp. 263–274. Springer, Cham (2017). https://doi.org/10.1007/978-3-319-59050-9_21
16. Wang, J., Aydogan, D.B., Varma, R., Toga, A.W., Shi, Y.: Modeling topographic regularity in structural brain connectivity with application to tractogram filtering. NeuroImage **183**, 87–98 (2018)
17. Wedeen, V.J., et al.: The geometric structure of the brain fiber pathways. Science **335**(6076), 1628–1634 (2012)

Posters

Posters

3D Organ Shape Reconstruction from Topogram Images

Elena Balashova[1,2(✉)], Jiangping Wang[2], Vivek Singh[2], Bogdan Georgescu[2],
Brian Teixeira[2], and Ankur Kapoor[2]

[1] Department of Computer Science, Princeton University, Princeton, NJ, USA
sizikova@cs.princeton.edu
[2] Siemens Healthineers, Digital Services, Digital Technology and Innovation,
Princeton, NJ, USA

Abstract. Automatic delineation and measurement of main organs such as liver is one of the critical steps for assessment of hepatic diseases, planning and postoperative or treatment follow-up. However, addressing this problem typically requires performing computed tomography (CT) scanning and complicated post-processing of the resulting scans using slice-by-slice techniques. In this paper, we show that 3D organ shape can be automatically predicted directly from topogram images, which are easier to acquire and have limited exposure to radiation during acquisition, compared to CT scans. We evaluate our approach on the challenging task of predicting liver shape using a generative model. We also demonstrate that our method can be combined with user annotations, such as a 2D mask, for improved prediction accuracy. We show compelling results on 3D liver shape reconstruction and volume estimation on 2129 CT scans (This feature is based on research, and is not commercially available. Due to regulatory reasons its future availability cannot be guaranteed).

Keywords: Organ shape reconstruction · Organ delineation ·
Generative modelling · Data-driven modelling · Deep learning

1 Introduction

In medical imaging, observing realistic organ shape is a critical step in enabling health care professionals gain a better insight into patients' body. Accurate depiction of internal organs, such as liver, often allows for more accurate health screening and early diagnosis, as well as planning of procedures such as radiation therapy to target specific locations in the human body. Delineating 3D organ shape from 2D X-ray images is an extremely difficult and unsolved problem in bio-medical engineering today due to visual ambiguities and information loss as a result of projection. The goal of this problem is to accurately predict the shape of the observed 3D organ given a single image.

Existing liver delineation techniques typically produce organ shape from computed tomography (CT) scans. The procedures to obtain these scans involve

© Springer Nature Switzerland AG 2019
A. C. S. Chung et al. (Eds.): IPMI 2019, LNCS 11492, pp. 347–359, 2019.
https://doi.org/10.1007/978-3-030-20351-1_26

long patient-doctor interaction time, costly machinery, and exposure to a high dose of radiation. The practical challenges in obtaining these scans may preclude obtaining accurate organ depictions. In addition, existing delineation tools [30] would delineate (either automatically or semi-automatically) the two-dimensional shape in each slice of the three-dimensional CT volume and combine the set of predictions into a three-dimensional shape. The intermediate processing may introduce an additional source of error to the overall shape prediction quality due to the lack of spatial context.

The key idea of this paper is to reconstruct 3D organ shape from topograms, which are projected 2D images from tomographic devices, such as X-ray [26]. These types of images can be much more easily obtained and are often used by medical professionals for planning purposes [18,24]. Motivated by the significant advances in deep learning techniques for organ segmentation [31] and representation learning on 3D data [8,21,25], we pose the problem of organ reconstruction as the task of predicting 3D shape from a single image. Further, we describe an automatic delineation procedure that outputs the shape from the topogram image only, as well as a semi-automatic extension, where we allow the user to outline the approximate two-dimensional mask and use it (in conjunction with the topogram) to obtain a more accurate 3D shape prediction.

Our system has two components: a generative shape model, composed of a shape encoder and decoder, and an encoder from 2D observations (topogram only or topogram and mask). The shape encoder and decoder form a variational auto-encoder (VAE) [14] generative model in order to represent each shape observation using a compact low-dimensional representation. The topogram and optional mask encoders (whose architectures are similar to [29]) map the partial observations from images (and masks when provided) to the coordinates of the corresponding shape observations. The entire system is optimized end-to-end in order to simultaneously infer shapes from topogram image observations and to learn the underlying shape space. This allows us to simultaneously learn a generative shape space covering complex shape variations from the 3D supervisions and infer the shapes from input 2D observations. To validate our approach, we collected a new medical dataset of 2129 abdominal CT scans and topogram images, and evaluated the proposed approach on the challenging tasks of 3D liver reconstruction and volume prediction. The contributions of our work are:

- An automatic and a semi-automatic approach to perform 3D organ reconstruction from 2D topograms, allowing automatic 3D shape prediction from the topogram only and a more refined prediction where 2D mask annotation is available.
- An evaluation of our method on accurate 3D organ volume estimation and reconstruction applications.

2   Related Work

In the medical imaging domain, extraction and visualization of 3D organs is a key step in clinical applications such as surgical planning and post-surgical assessment, as well as pathology detection and disease diagnosis. Of particular interest is the liver, which can exhibit highly heterogeneous shape variation that makes it even more difficult to segment. Previously, liver volume was segmented semi-automatically [9] or automatically using statistical shape models [10], sigmoid-edge modelling [6], graph-cut [15] and others (see [19] for an overview). Recently, automatic deep learning based methods [4,5,17] have been shown to provide impressive results on this task. However, these methods need a CT scan procedure, which is costly and requires a high radiation exposure. On the other hand, X-ray and topogram images are easier to obtain, require less radiation, and are often used by medical professionals for planning purposes [18,24].

Shape extraction from X-ray is particularly complex as its projective nature can contain complex or fuzzy textures, boundaries and anatomical part overlap [31]. To mitigate these challenges, traditional methods use prior knowledge, such as motion patterns [32] or intensity and background analysis [22], in order to perform X-ray segmentation. More recent methods [23] focus on learning to segment using deep neural networks. For example, [1] decomposes X-ray into non-overlapping components, [30] uses a generative adversarial network (GAN) [29] to improve segmentation quality, and [31] applies unpaired image-image translation techniques to learn to segment X-ray by observing CT scan segmentation. These methods achieve remarkable results on 2D shape delineation and segmentation tasks.

In parallel, in the computer vision domain, deep generative 3D shape models based on variational auto-encoder networks (VAE) [8,25] and generative adversarial networks (GAN) [29] have shown superior performance in learning to generate complex topologies of shapes. Combined with a mapping from image space, these methods are able to infer 3D shape predictions from 2D observations. To obtain more detailed and accurate predictions, input annotations, such as landmarks or masks, are often used to guide the synthesis process. [3] incorporates 2D landmarks for alignment optimization of a skinned vertex-based human shape model to image observations. [12] and [27] applies landmark annotations to guide synthesis of observed 3D shape in input images. [2] uses landmarks and [7] incorporates silhouettes to formulate additional objective terms to improve performance in 3D shape reconstruction and synthesis problems.

To the best of our knowledge, we are the first to propose both automatic and semi-automatic approaches to 3D organ shape reconstruction from topograms.

3 Overview

An overview of our training pipeline can be seen in Fig. 1. Our system consists of several key components: a generative shape model and a set of encoders from 2D observations. The generative model is composed of an encoder and a decoder, where the encoder maps the 3D shapes of organs to their coordinates in the latent space and the decoder reconstructs the shapes back from their coordinates. The first observation encoder is the topogram encoder that maps two-dimensional observations to the coordinates of the corresponding shapes. The second observation encoder is the joint topogram and mask encoder that predicts the latent

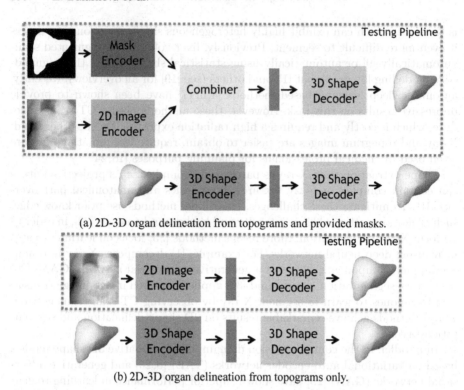

(a) 2D-3D organ delineation from topograms and provided masks.

(b) 2D-3D organ delineation from topograms only.

Fig. 1. Overview of our system. We train a generative model from a collection of 3D shapes, and learn to map from topograms (see Fig. 1(b)) or topograms and user-provided 2D masks (see Fig. 1(a)) to reconstructed 3D shapes of the observed organ. For both methods, the training phase involves training the generative model (3D shape encoder and decoder) jointly with the 2D observation encoders (topogram (blue), or topogram (blue), mask (green) and their combiner (brown)) in an end-to-end procedure described in Sect. 3. During testing, only the 2D observations are necessary for 3D shape prediction. (Color figure online)

coordinate of the organ shape given the 2D mask and topogram. The mask information, when provided, helps generate a more accurate prediction.

The organ shape prediction approach is very general, and can be used for organs other than human liver. The technique requires access to a database of shape and X-ray (two-dimensional observation) pairs. We demonstrate an accuracy improvement using user input in the form of 2D masks. Other types of input that can be encoded using a neural network can also be applied in place of masks to improve prediction accuracy.

Generative Model. As input, our system receives a set of examples $E = \{(s,i)\}$ where $s \in S$ is the example shape and $i \in I$ is the corresponding topogram image observation. The generative model $G = (Q, P)$ consists of an encoding component Q and a decoding component P. Here $Q(z|s)$ maps shape s to its latent coordinate z in the stochastic low dimensional space distributed according to prior distribution $p(z)$ and $P(s|z)$ maps the latent coordinate z back to the shape space S. The loss function of the generative model is composed of a reconstruction loss L_{rec} and a distribution loss L_{dist}, as is typical for variational auto-encoder training. L_{rec} is the binary cross entropy (BCE) error that measures the difference between the ground truth shape $s \in S$ and the predicted shape $s' \in S$:

$$L_{rec}(s, s') = -\frac{1}{N} \sum_{n=1}^{N} s_n \log s'_n + (1 - s_n) \log (1 - s'_n) \tag{1}$$

where $N = 64^3$. L_{dist} is the distribution loss that enforces the latent distribution of z_1 to match its prior distribution $L_{dist}(z_1) = \mathrm{KL}(Q(z|s)\|p(z))$, where $p(z) = \mathcal{N}(\mu, \sigma^2)$ and α_1, α_2 are the weights applied to each type of loss.

The 3D shape encoder maps an observation, represented with a 64 by 64 by 64 voxel grid, to its 200-dimensional latent vector z. The normal distribution parameters are defined $\mu = 0$ and $\sigma = 1$, as is customary for variational auto-encoder models. The architecture of the encoder consists of five convolutional layers with output sizes $64, 128, 256, 512, 200$, kernel size 4 for each layer, and padding sizes 1,1,1,1 and 0. The convolutional layers are separated by batch-normalization [11] and ReLU layers [20]. The 3D shape decoder takes as input a single 200-dimensional latent vector z, and predicts a 64 by 64 by 64 voxelized representation of shape. The decoder architecture mirrors that of the encoder.

Topogram Encoder. Given a generative model G, we can learn a topogram image encoder I_1, so that for each observation $(s, i) \in E$, the image i is mapped to the coordinate location $\hat{z} = I_1(i)$ such that the reconstructed shape $G(\hat{z})$ and the ground truth shape s are as close as possible. The image encoder loss is the binary cross entropy (BCE) loss $L_{rec}(s, G(\hat{z}))$ as defined in Eq. 1.

The topogram encoder I_1 takes a 1 by 256 by 256 topogram image, and outputs a 200-dimensional latent shape vector $\hat{z}$. It consists of five convolutional layers with the number of outputs $64, 128, 256, 512, 200$, kernel sizes $11, 5, 5, 5, 8$ and strides $4, 2, 2, 2, 1$, separated by batch-normalization [11] and rectified linear units (ReLU) [20].

Topogram and Mask Encoder. For each observation $(s, i) \in E$, given a topogram i and a mask $k = Pr(s) \in K$, where $Pr(\cdot)$ is defined to be an orthographic projection operator, we train the joint topogram and mask encoder I_2 that outputs $\tilde{z} = I_2(i, k)$ so that $G(\tilde{z})$ and s are as close as possible. The loss of I_2 is defined to be the binary cross entropy (BCE) error $L_{rec}(s, G(\tilde{z}))$, as defined Eq. 1. We also enforce an additional mask loss:

$$L_{mask}(k, \tilde{k}) = -\sum_{n=1}^{N} k_n \log \tilde{k}_n + (1 - k_n) \log (1 - \tilde{k}_n).$$

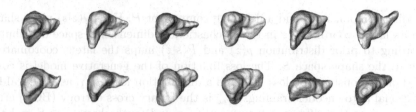

Fig. 2. Visualization of example 3D shape variations of the liver in the collected medical dataset of abdominal CT scans. The shapes represent a complex assortment typical of this organ.

that ensures that the input mask k and the projected mask $\tilde{k}$ of the predicted shape (i.e. $\tilde{k} = Pr(G(\tilde{z}))$) match.

The topogram and mask encoder I_2 consists of a topogram encoder branch, a mask encoder branch, and a common combiner network (see Fig. 1), so that the observations are mapped to a common latent coordinate $\tilde{z}$. The topogram encoder branch has the same architecture as the topogram encoder in Sect. 3 and maps the topogram to an intermediate 200-dimensional feature v_1. The mask encoder branch receives a 1 by 64 by 64 binary mask image which it maps to a 200-dimensional vector v_2 using five convolutional layers with kernel sizes of $3, 3, 3, 3, 3$ and strides $4, 2, 2, 2, 2$, separated by batch-normalizations [11] and rectified linear units (ReLU) [20]. v_1 and v_2 are then concatenated and run through the the combiner network consisting of a single fully connected layer to predict a joint 200-dimensional latent coordinate $\tilde{z}$.

Combined Training. To train the models, we optimize the all the components of the system together in an end-to-end training process using the combined objective:

$$L = \alpha_1 L_{rec}(s, s') + \alpha_2 L_{KL} + \alpha_3 L_{rec}(s, G(\bar{z})) + \alpha_4 L_{mask}(k, \tilde{k}),$$

where $\bar{z} = \tilde{z}$ if training the topogram-mask encoder, and $\bar{z} = \hat{z}$ when training the topogram-only encoder. Note that $\alpha_1 L_{rec}(s, s')$ is the reconstruction loss of the VAE and $\alpha_3 L_{rec}(s, G(\bar{z}))$ is the 2D-3D reconstruction loss. It is also possible to train the above model without the shape encoder, i.e. $\alpha_1 = 0$ and $\alpha_2 = 0$.

In all experiments, we use $\alpha_1 = 50.0$, $\alpha_2 = 0.1$, $\alpha_3 = 50.0$ and $\alpha_4 = 0.0001$ if the mask is provided as input (see Sect. 3) or $\alpha_4 = 0$ otherwise (for topogram only approach). All models are trained using Adam optimizer [13] with learning rate 0.0001 for 250 epochs and batch size of 32.

4   Experimental Results and Discussion

We perform extensive quantitative and qualitative experiments of our method on the difficult tasks of estimating 3D shape of the human liver and predicting its volume. Due to their heterogeneous and diffusive shape, automatic liver segmentation is a very complex problem. Using our method we can accurately estimate the 3D shape of the liver from a 2D topogram image and optionally a 2D mask. We use voxel grids as our base representation, and visualize results using 2D projections or 3D meshes obtained using marching cubes [16].

We investigate the effect of shape context provided by the mask observations by evaluating a baseline where 3D shape is predicted directly from the mask. We also quantitatively compare our method to an adversarial baseline [28] approach.

4.1 Dataset

To conduct an experimental evaluation, we collected 2129 abdominal CT scans (3D volumetric images of the abdomen covering the liver organ) from several different hospital sites. The liver shapes were segmented using volumetric segmentation approach [30] and topograms and masks are extracted via 2D projection. Examples from the dataset as well as the provided annotations are shown in Fig. 2. We use 1554 scans for training, and 575 for testing.

We demonstrate several direct applications of our method: three-dimensional shape reconstruction with corresponding two-dimensional liver delineation through projection and organ volume prediction.

4.2 Organ Shape Reconstruction from Topograms

Given a learned generative model of liver shapes and an image encoder which estimates a latent space vector given a topogram image (and mask, if given), we predict the 3D liver shape, and project it back onto the topogram image plane to perform two-dimensional delineation. Visually delineating accurate shape from topograms is particularly difficult due to visual ambiguities, such as color contrast and fuzzy boundaries. Our method can predict the three-dimensional shapes automatically from the topogram, and refine the prediction, given a two-dimensional mask annotation.

Qualitative Evaluation. In Fig. 3, we visualize the 3D reconstruction results. The first column is a visualization of the input topogram, the second column is the visualization of the ground truth 3D shape, the third column is the visualization of the result of the topogram-only approach, the fourth column is the visualization of the result of the topogram+mask approach, and the fifth and sixth columns are visualizations of projected masks of the corresponding two approaches, overlaid with the ground truth masks. Each row corresponds to a different example.

Both proposed methods are able to capture significant variation in the observed shapes, such as a prominent dome on the right lobe in Example 1 and shape of the left lobe in Example 5. The topogram+mask method is able to convey more topological details compared to the topogram-only method: an elongated interior tip in Examples 1 and 4, protrusion off left lobe in Examples

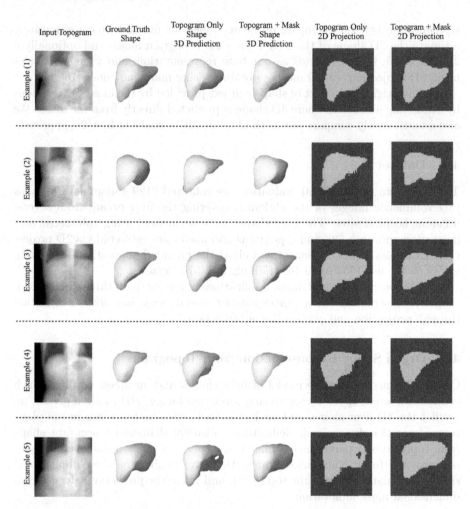

Fig. 3. Sample examples of 3D reconstruction. The input topograms are shown in first column, the ground truth shapes are shown in second column, and the predicted shapes are shown in purple (third column - topogram only approach, fourth column - topogram + mask approach). The projected masks of the corresponding approaches, overlaid with the ground truth masks, are shown in the fifth and sixth columns, respectively. The ground truth mask is shown in pink, and the predicted mask is shown in light purple (the predicted background segmentation is dark purple) (Color figure online).

2 and 3, and overall topology in Example 5, where the mask-based method corrects the hole artifact introduced by the topogram-only method. Overall, the surfaces in predictions from the mask-based method are visually closer to the ground truth.

We also project the 3D predictions directly on the input topograms (see Fig. 4). This allows us to visualize the corresponding inferred 2D segmentation.

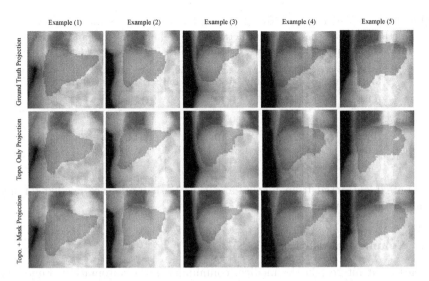

Fig. 4. Sample 2D projections of the predicted organ shapes. The ground truth projections are shown in first row, the topogram only prediction projections are shown in second row, and the topogram+mask projections are shown in third row. By predicting the 3D shape of the organ, we are also able to generate an accurate 2D segmentation of the input topograms via projection.

The shape reconstruction network (in both topogram only and topogram+mask methods) learns to emphasize on characteristic parts of the organ shape, such as the curves in the right lobe and interior tip.

Quantitative Evaluation. Several metrics can be used to quantitatively compare 3D shape reconstructions (see [4] for details). We provide a quantitative evaluation using two popular volume-based metrics (Intersection over Union (IoU) and Dice coefficients) and a surface-based metric (Hausdorff distance) in Table 1. The topogram+mask approach outperforms the topogram only approach according to all of the metrics, but especially according to Hausdorff distance, which is very sensitive to shape variations such as critical cases of incorrect tip or bulge presence prediction.

Shape Context. It is important to investigate whether the provided mask provides too much context, rendering the problem of 3D shape prediction a much easier task. We thus train a mask-only baseline that learns to reconstruct 3D shape directly from mask (no topogram image provided). In Table 1, we compare the performance of this baseline and the two methods that receive the topogram as input. The mask only method is unable to achieve the same quality of results as the topogram-based methods, generating significantly lower mean IoU and Dice errors, and a much larger Hausdorff error. The topogram images contain important information, such as shape layout, that is complementary to

Table 1. Quantitative comparison of the mask only, topogram only and topogram+ mask methods on 3D shape reconstruction using volumetric (IoU and Dice metrics) and surface-based metrics (Hausdorff distance).

Metric (mean)	Mask only	Topogram only	Topogram + mask
IOU	0.58	0.78	**0.82**
Dice	0.73	0.87	**0.90**
Hausdorff	28.28	7.10	**5.00**

the context extracted from masks, and thus both inputs are needed for high quality reconstruction.

4.3 Volume Calculation

Of particular interest in the medical community is the automatic volume measurement of main organs. Our method predicts the 3D shape, which we can directly use to measure organ volume. In Table 2, we evaluate our proposed approaches on the task of volume prediction. We use the volume of the voxelized 3D segmentation of the liver, obtained from segmentation of the 3D CT, as the ground truth. Given the 3D shape prediction, we measure the predicted volume as the number of voxels in the generated shape (which can be converted to milliliters (mL) using scanning configuration parameters). We report the volume error prediction $V_f = \|V_{pred} - V_{gt}\|/V_{gt}$ where V_{pred} and V_{gt} are the volumes of the predicted and ground truth organs, respectively.

On average, we are able to predict liver volume to 6% error with the topogram+mask method and to 10% error with the topogram only method. The mask-only based method is unable to predict volume accurately, since it cannot predict the correct 3D topology (see Sect. 4.2).

Table 2. Mean volume error (V_f) evaluation and comparison.

Metric	Mask only	Topogram only	Topogram + mask
Volume error (V_f)	0.34	0.10	**0.06**

4.4 Comparison to Adversarial Approaches

We also compare our method to an adversarial baseline (3D VAE-GAN [29]) which is another commonly used generative modelling approach. We train this baseline with the same architecture and hyperparameters described in [29]. We observe that the discriminator in this baseline would typically encourage more uniform predictions compared to our VAE-based method, thus discouraging generation of more diverse shape topologies. Quantitatively, this method achieves

Table 3. Comparison of the variational autoencoder (VAE) based approaches to a generative adversarial network (GAN) based approach on volume prediction and shape reconstruction tasks.

	Volume prediction	Shape reconstruction		
	Volume error (V_f)	IoU	Dice	Hausdorff
Variational autoencoder (VAE) (without/with mask)	0.10/**0.06**	0.78/**0.82**	0.87/**0.90**	7.10/**5.00**
Adversarial (3D-GAN) [29]	0.21	0.61	0.75	10.50
Performance difference	109%/250%	22%/26%	14%/17%	48%/110%

lower quality results than the both VAE-based methods (see Table 3), especially in surface-based error and volume error due to its tendency to predict an average shape irrespective of the input.

4.5 Conclusion and Future Work

3D organ shape reconstruction from topograms is an extremely challenging problem in medical imaging. Among other challenges, it is a difficult problem because the input X-ray images can contain projection artifacts that reconstruction methods need to handle, in addition to predicting the topology of occluded and unseen parts the three-dimensional organ. The core insight of this work is that, despite the visual ambiguities present in this type of imagery, it is possible to predict 3D organ shape directly from topograms. It is also possible to improve the quality of the prediction by providing supplementary two-dimensional shape information in the form of masks.

This work is only a first step towards performing more accurate and reliable 3D organ shape reconstruction. It would be interesting to investigate the performance of our approach on organs other than liver, such as lung or heart, and explore other types of user inputs and annotations that can improve the reconstruction quality. Also, it would be critical to study why 2D to 3D mapping is possible, and what types of neural networks (in this work we focused on the VAE) are best suited for modelling the shape space and achieving high reconstruction accuracy. Further, categorizing the dataset according to data perturbations, such as fatty liver, tumors, liver disease, age or gender, one should study how these factors affect the performance accuracy. Finally, it would be important to analyze how X-ray can help improve reconstruction accuracy when 3D scans are available and extracting liver shape can be posed as a 3D shape segmentation problem. We hope this work will inspire other approaches that apply generative 3D modelling techniques to reconstructing and predicting organ shapes.

Acknowledgements. We thank Daguang Xu for help with anatomical part labelling and discussions; Thomas Funkhouser, Terrence Chen, Kai Ma, and members of the Princeton Graphics and Vision Group for helpful suggestions; Sungheon Gene Kim,

Linda Moy, Krzysztof Geras, and Kyunghyun Cho for discussions on medical applications of the proposed method. This work was supported by Siemens Healthcare and NSF-GRFP.

References

1. Albarqouni, S., Fotouhi, J., Navab, N.: X-ray in-depth decomposition: revealing the latent structures. In: Descoteaux, M., Maier-Hein, L., Franz, A., Jannin, P., Collins, D.L., Duchesne, S. (eds.) MICCAI 2017. LNCS, vol. 10435, pp. 444–452. Springer, Cham (2017). https://doi.org/10.1007/978-3-319-66179-7_51
2. Balashova, E., Singh, V., Wang, J., Teixeira, B., Chen, T., Funkhouser, T.: Structure-aware shape synthesis. In: 3DV, pp. 140–149. IEEE (2018)
3. Bogo, F., Kanazawa, A., Lassner, C., Gehler, P., Romero, J., Black, M.J.: Keep it SMPL: automatic estimation of 3D human pose and shape from a single image. In: Leibe, B., Matas, J., Sebe, N., Welling, M. (eds.) ECCV 2016. LNCS, vol. 9909, pp. 561–578. Springer, Cham (2016). https://doi.org/10.1007/978-3-319-46454-1_34
4. Christ, P.F., et al.: Automatic liver and tumor segmentation of CT and MRI volumes using cascaded fully convolutional neural networks. arXiv preprint arXiv:1702.05970 (2017)
5. Dou, Q., Chen, H., Jin, Y., Yu, L., Qin, J., Heng, P.-A.: 3D deeply supervised network for automatic liver segmentation from CT volumes. In: Ourselin, S., Joskowicz, L., Sabuncu, M.R., Unal, G., Wells, W. (eds.) MICCAI 2016. LNCS, vol. 9901, pp. 149–157. Springer, Cham (2016). https://doi.org/10.1007/978-3-319-46723-8_18
6. Foruzan, A.H., Chen, Y.W.: Improved segmentation of low-contrast lesions using sigmoid edge model. Int. J. Comput. Assist. Radiol. Surg. 11(7), 1267–1283 (2016)
7. Gadelha, M., Maji, S., Wang, R.: 3D shape induction from 2D views of multiple objects. In: 3DV, pp. 402–411. IEEE (2017)
8. Girdhar, R., Fouhey, D.F., Rodriguez, M., Gupta, A.: Learning a predictable and generative vector representation for objects. In: Leibe, B., Matas, J., Sebe, N., Welling, M. (eds.) ECCV 2016. LNCS, vol. 9910, pp. 484–499. Springer, Cham (2016). https://doi.org/10.1007/978-3-319-46466-4_29
9. Häme, Y., Pollari, M.: Semi-automatic liver tumor segmentation with hidden Markov measure field model and non-parametric distribution estimation. Med. image Anal. 16(1), 140–149 (2012)
10. Heimann, T., et al.: Comparison and evaluation of methods for liver segmentation from CT datasets. IEEE Trans. Med. Imaging 28(8), 1251–1265 (2009)
11. Ioffe, S., Szegedy, C.: Batch normalization: accelerating deep network training by reducing internal covariate shift. arXiv preprint arXiv:1502.03167 (2015)
12. Kar, A., Tulsiani, S., Carreira, J., Malik, J.: Category-specific object reconstruction from a single image. In: CVPR, pp. 1966–1974 (2015)
13. Kingma, D.P., Ba, J.: Adam: a method for stochastic optimization. arXiv preprint arXiv:1412.6980 (2014)
14. Kingma, D.P., Welling, M.: Auto-encoding variational Bayes (2014)
15. Li, G., Chen, X., Shi, F., Zhu, W., Tian, J., Xiang, D.: Automatic liver segmentation based on shape constraints and deformable graph cut in CT images. IEEE Trans. Image Process. 24(12), 5315–5329 (2015)
16. Lorensen, W.E., Cline, H.E.: Marching cubes: a high resolution 3D surface construction algorithm. In: ACM Siggraph Computer Graphics, vol. 21, pp. 163–169. ACM (1987)

17. Lu, F., Wu, F., Hu, P., Peng, Z., Kong, D.: Automatic 3D liver location and segmentation via convolutional neural network and graph cut. Int. J. Comput. Assist. Radiol. Surg. **12**(2), 171–182 (2017)
18. Mayo-Smith, W.W., Hara, A.K., Mahesh, M., Sahani, D.V., Pavlicek, W.: How I do it: managing radiation dose in CT. Radiology **273**(3), 657–672 (2014)
19. Mharib, A.M., Ramli, A.R., Mashohor, S., Mahmood, R.B.: Survey on liver CT image segmentation methods. Artif. Intell. Rev. **37**(2), 83 (2012)
20. Nair, V., Hinton, G.E.: Rectified linear units improve restricted boltzmann machines. In: ICML, pp. 807–814 (2010)
21. Qi, C.R., Su, H., Nießner, M., Dai, A., Yan, M., Guibas, L.J.: Volumetric and multi-view CNNs for object classification on 3D data. In: CVPR, pp. 5648–5656 (2016)
22. Qin, B., et al.: Accurate vessel extraction via tensor completion of background layer in X-ray coronary angiograms. Pattern Recogn. **87**, 38–54 (2019)
23. Ronneberger, O., Fischer, P., Brox, T.: U-net: convolutional networks for biomedical image segmentation. In: Navab, N., Hornegger, J., Wells, W.M., Frangi, A.F. (eds.) MICCAI 2015. LNCS, vol. 9351, pp. 234–241. Springer, Cham (2015). https://doi.org/10.1007/978-3-319-24574-4_28
24. Schertler, T., et al.: Dual-source computed tomography in patients with acute chest pain: feasibility and image quality. Eur. Radiol. **17**(12), 3179–3188 (2007)
25. Sharma, A., Grau, O., Fritz, M.: VConv-DAE: deep volumetric shape learning without object labels. In: Hua, G., Jégou, H. (eds.) ECCV 2016. LNCS, vol. 9915, pp. 236–250. Springer, Cham (2016). https://doi.org/10.1007/978-3-319-49409-8_20
26. Sioutos, N., de Coronado, S., Haber, M.W., Hartel, F.W., Shaiu, W.L., Wright, L.W.: NCI thesaurus: a semantic model integrating cancer-related clinical and molecular information. J. Biomed. Inf. **40**(1), 30–43 (2007)
27. Vicente, S., Carreira, J., Agapito, L., Batista, J.: Reconstructing PASCAL VOC. In: CVPR, pp. 41–48 (2014)
28. Wu, J., et al.: Single image 3D interpreter network. In: Leibe, B., Matas, J., Sebe, N., Welling, M. (eds.) ECCV 2016. LNCS, vol. 9910, pp. 365–382. Springer, Cham (2016). https://doi.org/10.1007/978-3-319-46466-4_22
29. Wu, J., Zhang, C., Xue, T., Freeman, B., Tenenbaum, J.: Learning a probabilistic latent space of object shapes via 3D generative-adversarial modeling. In: Advances in Neural Information Processing Systems, pp. 82–90 (2016)
30. Yang, D., et al.: Automatic liver segmentation using an adversarial image-to-image network. In: Descoteaux, M., Maier-Hein, L., Franz, A., Jannin, P., Collins, D.L., Duchesne, S. (eds.) MICCAI 2017. LNCS, vol. 10435, pp. 507–515. Springer, Cham (2017). https://doi.org/10.1007/978-3-319-66179-7_58
31. Zhang, Y., Miao, S., Mansi, T., Liao, R.: Task driven generative modeling for unsupervised domain adaptation: application to X-ray image segmentation. In: Frangi, A.F., Schnabel, J.A., Davatzikos, C., Alberola-López, C., Fichtinger, G. (eds.) MICCAI 2018. LNCS, vol. 11071, pp. 599–607. Springer, Cham (2018). https://doi.org/10.1007/978-3-030-00934-2_67
32. Zhu, Y., Prummer, S., Wang, P., Chen, T., Comaniciu, D., Ostermeier, M.: Dynamic layer separation for coronary DSA and enhancement in fluoroscopic sequences. In: Yang, G.-Z., Hawkes, D., Rueckert, D., Noble, A., Taylor, C. (eds.) MICCAI 2009. LNCS, vol. 5762, pp. 877–884. Springer, Heidelberg (2009). https://doi.org/10.1007/978-3-642-04271-3_106

A Cross-Center Smoothness Prior for Variational Bayesian Brain Tissue Segmentation

Wouter M. Kouw[1](✉), Silas N. Ørting[1], Jens Petersen[1], Kim S. Pedersen[1], and Marleen de Bruijne[1,2]

[1] University of Copenhagen, Universitetsparken 1, DK-2100 Copenhagen Ø, Denmark
wmkouw@gmail.com
[2] Erasmus Medical Center Rotterdam, Dr. Molewaterplein 50, 3015 GE Rotterdam, The Netherlands

Abstract. Suppose one is faced with the challenge of tissue segmentation in MR images, without annotators at their center to provide labeled training data. One option is to go to another medical center for a trained classifier. Sadly, tissue classifiers do not generalize well across centers due to voxel intensity shifts caused by center-specific acquisition protocols. However, certain aspects of segmentations, such as spatial smoothness, remain relatively consistent and can be learned separately. Here we present a smoothness prior that is fit to segmentations produced at another medical center. This informative prior is presented to an unsupervised Bayesian model. The model clusters the voxel intensities, such that it produces segmentations that are similarly smooth to those of the other medical center. In addition, the unsupervised Bayesian model is extended to a semi-supervised variant, which needs no visual interpretation of clusters into tissues.

Keywords: Variational inference · Bayesian transfer learning · Image segmentation

1 Introduction

Many modern automatic brain tissue segmentation methods are based on machine learning models. One of the limitations of these models is that they generalize poorly beyond the domain of the data they are trained on. In medical imaging, an example of a domain is the medical center itself. Data collected at different centers varies due to experimental, acquisition and annotation protocols. Most notably, the voxel intensity distributions of MR images are different, which means the mapping from scans to segmentations differs between centers. As a result, tissue classification models trained on examples from one center tend to perform poorly on data from another center [21].

W. M. Kouw—Supported by a contribution from the Niels Stensen Fellowship.

A. C. S. Chung et al. (Eds.): IPMI 2019, LNCS 11492, pp. 360–371, 2019.
https://doi.org/10.1007/978-3-030-20351-1_27

But not all factors of variation are inconsistent across centers. Although the segmentations are different for each patient, certain aspects remain consistent. One such aspect is the spatial *smoothness* of each tissue. Radiologists and MR imaging experts know how smooth a segmentation is supposed to look like, and use this knowledge when segmenting a new scan. Essentially, we would like to give the tissue classifier that information as well. Our goal is to learn from segmentations at other medical centers and incorporate that knowledge into a Bayesian model for tissue segmentation.

1.1 Related Work

In transfer learning and domain adaptation, a model learns from a *source* domain and aims to generalize to a differently distributed *target* domain [10,16]. In Bayesian transfer learning, the source domain can be interpreted as prior knowledge for the target task [8,17]. For instance, in natural language processing, a document classification task can be performed using a Bayesian linear classifier trained on a bag-of-word encoding of the document [17]. Instead of imposing a weakly informative prior on how important each word of the dictionary is for the document classification task, one could fit the prior on data from Wikipedia. That produces a stronger, more informative prior over how important each word is. To our knowledge, no Bayesian transfer learning models have been proposed for medical imaging tasks. Our interest is to study what forms of prior knowledge can be obtained from large open access labeled data sets, and how that knowledge can be exploited for a specific task.

Hidden Markov Random Field (MRF) models are a form of Bayesian models for image segmentation. They pose a hidden state for each voxel that accounts for some intrinsic latent structure of the image [22]. For tissue segmentation, the latent state is assumed to be the tissue of the voxel, while the observed voxel intensity value is a sample from a probabilistic observation model. The observation model specifies the causal relations between the latent image and the observed image [1,24]. Such assumptions are not unreasonable for the case of MR imaging, where T1 relaxation times depend on the tissue of the voxel.

Inference in hidden MRF's is often done through Monte Carlo sampling [23]. However, sampling remains a computationally expensive procedure. An alternative is to use variational inference, where the joint distribution of an intractable Bayesian model is approximated [4,7]. Variational inference is often much faster than sampling, depending on the form of the approximating distribution. We will employ variational Bayes to infer the underlying tissues of an observed MRI scan.

1.2 Outline

In Sect. 2, we will discuss a Bayesian model for tissue segmentation along with a hidden Markov Random Field prior. The variational approximation and the general inference procedure is presented in Sect. 2.1. Section 3 covers how to fit the MRF prior to segmentations produced at other medical centers. We perform a series of experiments in Sect. 4 where we pair up data sets from different medical centers. Model extensions and limitations are discussed in Sect. 5 and we draw conclusions in Sect. 6.

2   Method

Let $X \in [0,1]^{H \times W \times D}$ be an MR image and $Y \in \{0,1\}^{H \times W \times K}$ be its segmentation. H and W are the height of the width of the image, respectively, with $N = H \cdot W$ as the total number of voxels. D refers to the number of channels of the image, which could be stacked filter response maps or additional modalities. In this paper, we consider only the MR image (i.e. $D = 1$), but the update equations in Sect. 2.3 are general. K corresponds to the number of tissues in the segmentation, also referred to as classes. Observed voxels are marked as x. Voxel labels are marked as y and consist of $\{0,1\}$-valued vectors with 1 on the k-th index if that voxel belongs to class k (a.k.a. *one-hot* vectors).

2.1   Bayesian Model

We assume a causal model $Y \to X$, such that the tissue causes the voxel intensity value. The measurement instrument, i.e. the MRI scanner, maps tissues to voxel intensities f, but imposes noise on the observation: $x = f(y) + \epsilon$. The mapping f between Y and X is assumed to vary across experimental and acquisition protocols. We model the likelihood function of observing X from Y with a Gaussian mixture model, with one component for each tissue:

$$p(X \mid Y; \pi, \mu, \Lambda) = \prod_{i=1}^{N} \prod_{k=1}^{K} \left[\pi_k \, \mathcal{N}(x_i \mid \mu_k, \Lambda_k^{-1}) \right]^{y_{ik}}. \tag{1}$$

The parameter π_k is the proportion coefficient, μ_k is the mean intensity and Λ_k is the precision of the k-th tissue. Note that this likelihood assumes that voxels are independent of each other, which is not valid in MR images. We model spatial relationships in Sect. 2.2 which introduces dependencies between pixels.

We select a Dirichlet distribution as the prior for the tissue proportions and a Normal-Wishart as the prior for the mean and precision parameters:

$$\pi_k \sim \mathcal{D}(\alpha_{0k}), \qquad \mu_k \sim \mathcal{N}(\upsilon_{0k}, (\gamma_{0k} \Lambda_k)^{-1}), \qquad \Lambda_k \sim \mathcal{W}(\nu_{0k}, \Delta_{0k}).$$

The α_0 are called the Dirichlet distribution's concentration parameters, υ_0 the hypermeans, γ_0 are precision-scaling hyperparameters, ν_0 are the degrees of freedom of the Wishart distribution and Δ_0 are the hyperprecisions. These priors are conjugate to the Gaussian likelihood.

2.2   Hidden Potts - Markov Random Field

Spatial properties of images can be described using Markov Random Fields. In general, MRF's describe interactions between nodes in a graph by defining a probability distribution – to be precise, a Gibbs distribution – over configurations of states at the nodes [22]. The Markov property allows us to model this distribution in terms of local interactions. The Ising model is a classical MRF model, which describes the pairwise interactions between a binary-valued image pixel and its direct neighbours (i.e. up, down, left, right). The Potts model is its multivariate extension, using K states.

We use the Potts model to capture how often a voxel's label is equal to the labels of its neighbours. In other words, how *smooth* the segmentation is. The model incorporates a set of parameters, $\beta = (\beta_1, \dots, \beta_K)$, that explicitly describes each tissue's smoothness. By fitting a hidden Potts model to a series of segmentations, it can act as an informative prior in the Bayesian model – a point we discuss in more detail in Sect. 3.

Hidden Potts models are usually defined for whole images. However, that induces a partition function with a discrete sum over K^N states, which is computationally intractable. Instead, we consider a local variant, where voxels depend only on their direct neighbours δ_i [12,13]:

$$p(Y \mid \beta) = \prod_{i=1}^{N} p(y_i \mid y_{\delta_i}, \beta).$$

Voxels in the center of the image have four neighbours (i.e. up, down, left, right), while edge and corner voxels have three and two neighbours, respectively. Taking its logarithm, the Potts model has the following form:

$$\log p(y_i \mid y_{\delta_i}, \beta) = \sum_{k=1}^{K} \beta_k y_{ik} \sum_{j \in \delta_i} y_{jk} - \log \sum_{\{y'\}} \exp \left(\sum_{k=1}^{K} \beta_k \, y'_k \sum_{j \in \delta_i} y_{jk} \right) \quad (2)$$

$$= \sum_{k=1}^{K} \beta_k y_{ik} \sum_{j \in \delta_i} y_{jk} - \log \sum_{k=1}^{K} \exp \left(\beta_k \sum_{j \in \delta_i} y_{jk} \right). \quad (3)$$

The sum with the subscript $\{y'\}$ in (2) denotes summing over all possible states of y (i.e. $[1,0,\dots 0]$, $[0,1,\dots,0]$, $\dots$, $[0,0,\dots,1]$). Since y is a one-hot vector, it multiplies the terms in the sum that involve the k-th tissue with 1 and multiplies the other terms with 0. All but one term drop out, which means the sum over $\{y'\}$ can be simplified to a sum over classes, as in (3).

2.3 Variational Approximation

The hidden Potts-MRF describes spatial relationships in the segmentation and acts as a prior on the Gaussian mixture model. Including the hidden Potts model, the joint distribution of the full model becomes:

$$p(X, Y, \pi, \mu, \Lambda \mid \beta)$$
$$= p(X \mid Y, \pi, \mu, \Lambda) \, p(Y \mid \beta) \, p(\pi \mid \alpha) \, p(\mu \mid v, (\gamma\Lambda)^{-1}) \, p(\Lambda \mid v, \Delta). \quad (4)$$

In the following, the likelihood parameters are summarized as $\theta = (\pi, \mu, \Lambda)$. With the inclusion of the hidden Potts-MRF, the posteriors cannot be derived analytically. We perform a variational approximation of the joint distribution using a distribution over the segmentation and the likelihood parameters, $q(Y, \theta \mid \beta)$ [4]. This approximation relates to the marginal log-likelihood as follows:

$$
\begin{aligned}
\log p(X \mid \beta) &= \log \int \int p(X, Y, \theta \mid \beta) \; d\theta \; dY \\
&= \log \int \int q(Y, \theta \mid \beta) \frac{p(X, Y, \theta \mid \beta)}{q(Y, \theta \mid \beta)} \; d\theta \; dY \\
&\geq \int \int q(Y, \theta \mid \beta) \log \frac{p(X, Y, \theta \mid \beta)}{q(Y, \theta \mid \beta)} \; d\theta \; dY \; = \; \mathcal{L}(q). \quad (5)
\end{aligned}
$$

$\mathcal{L}(q)$ is a function of the approximating distribution q and is called the evidence lower bound. Here, the dependence on the hyperparameters is left out for notational convenience. We only maintain the dependence on β, as it is of importance in Sect. 3. In this framework, the objective is to find a parametric form for the variational approximation distribution $q(Y, \theta \mid \beta)$ such that it matches the true distribution as well as possible [4].

For computational reasons, we make the mean-field assumption that the segmentation and the likelihood parameters are independent of each other: $q(Y, \theta \mid \beta) = q(Y \mid \beta) \, q(\theta)$ [4]. The optimal form of each factor can be found by dropping terms in the lower bound that do not depend on the factor in question (as they are constants in the optimization procedure), and deriving the analytical solutions to the remaining expectations. For latent factor $q(Y \mid \beta)$, terms in the numerator and denominator of (5) not involving Y and β are ignored, producing:

$$
\begin{aligned}
\mathcal{L}(q) &\propto \int \int q(Y \mid \beta) \, q(\theta) \log \frac{p(X \mid Y, \theta) \, p(Y \mid \beta)}{q(Y \mid \beta)} \; d\theta \; dY \\
&= \int q(Y \mid \beta) \log \frac{\exp \left(\int q(\theta) \, \log p(X \mid Y, \theta) \, + \log p(Y \mid \beta) \, d\theta \right)}{q(Y \mid \beta)} \; dY. \quad (6)
\end{aligned}
$$

Note that in (6), the expectation with respect to the other factor, $q(\theta)$, is moved to the numerator. It can now be seen that the latent factor is optimal when: $\log q^*(Y \mid \beta) \propto \mathbb{E}_\theta \big[\log p(X \mid Y, \theta) \big] + \log p(Y \mid \beta)$. Using the full Bayesian model specified in (4) and the hidden Potts from (3), the i-th voxel of the segmentation factor can be written as [4]:

$$
\begin{aligned}
&\log q^*(y_i \mid \beta) \\
&\propto \mathbb{E}_{\pi, \mu, \Lambda} \Big[\sum_{k=1}^{K} y_{ik} \log \pi_k \mathcal{N}(x_i \mid \mu_k, \Lambda_k^{-1}) \Big] + \log p(y_i \mid y_{\delta_i}, \beta) \\
&\propto \sum_{k=1}^{K} y_{ik} \Big(\mathbb{E}_{\pi_k} \big[\log \pi_k \big] + \mathbb{E}_{\mu_k, \Lambda_k} \big[\log \mathcal{N}(x_i \mid \mu_k, \Lambda_k^{-1}) \big] + \beta_k \sum_{j \in \delta_{ik}} y_{jk} \Big), \quad (7)
\end{aligned}
$$

where

$$\mathbb{E}_{\pi_k}\big[\log \pi_k\big] = \psi(\alpha_k) - \psi\Big(\sum_{k=1}^{K}\alpha_k\Big),$$

$$\mathbb{E}_{\mu_k, \Lambda_k}\big[\log \mathcal{N}(x_i \mid \mu_k, \Lambda_k^{-1})\big] = -\frac{D}{2}\log 2\pi + \frac{1}{2}\mathbb{E}_{\Lambda_k}\big[\log|\Lambda_k|\big] - \frac{1}{2}\mathbb{E}_{\mu_k, \Lambda_k}\big[\tilde{x}_{ik}\big],$$

$$\mathbb{E}_{\Lambda_k}\big[\log|\Lambda_k|\big] = \sum_{d=1}^{D}\psi\big[(\nu_k + 1 - d)/2\big] + D\log 2 + \log|\Delta_k|,$$

$$\mathbb{E}_{\mu_k, \Lambda_k}\big[\tilde{x}_{ik}\big] = \frac{D}{\gamma_k} + \nu_k(x_i - \upsilon_k)\Delta_k(x_i - \upsilon_k)^\top,$$

and $\tilde{x}_{ik} = (x_i - \mu_k)\Lambda_k(x_i - \mu_k)^\top$. ψ refers to the digamma function.

In Eq. 7, we recognize a multinomial distribution: $\log q^*(y_i \mid \beta) \propto \sum_{k}^{K} y_{ik}\log r_{ik}$. The proportionality is due to the ignored terms. As these terms only serve to normalize the probabilities to the $[0, 1]$ interval, we can replace their computation by the following normalization: $\rho_i = r_{ik}/\sum_{k=1}^{K} r_{ik}$ [4]. The ρ_{ik} are called the responsibilities, referring to the probability for the i-th voxel to belong to the k-th class. Note that β has not been integrated out. It will be estimated in a cross-medical center fashion (see Sect. 3).

Similar steps are taken to compute an optimal form for $q(\theta)$. This time, we ignore all terms in the ratio in (5) that do not depend on θ:

$$\mathcal{L}(q) \propto \int\int q(Y \mid \beta)\, q(\theta)\log\frac{p(X \mid Y, \theta)\, p(\theta)}{q(\theta)}\, d\theta\, dY$$

$$= \int q(\theta)\log\frac{\exp\big(\int q(Y \mid \beta)\,\log p(X \mid Y, \theta) + \log p(\theta)\, dY\big)}{q(\theta)}\, d\theta. \qquad (8)$$

The factor $q(\theta)$ is optimal when: $\log q^*(\theta) \propto \mathbb{E}_Y\big[\log p(X \mid Y, \theta)\big] + \log p(\theta)$. This is a well-known result (the choice of a Gaussian likelihood with conjugate priors is made often) and extensive derivations are widely available [4]. It produces the following update equations:

$$\alpha_k = \alpha_{0k} + S_k^0, \qquad \gamma_k = \gamma_{0k} + S_k^0, \qquad \nu_k = \nu_{0k} + S_k^0,$$

$$\upsilon_k = (\gamma_{0k}\upsilon_{0k} + S_k^1) / (\gamma_{0k} + S_k^0),$$

$$\Delta_k^{-1} = \Delta_{0k}^{-1} + S_k^2 + \frac{\gamma_{0k}S_k^0}{\gamma_{0k} + S_k^0}(S_k^1 - \upsilon_k)(S_k^1 - \upsilon_k)^\top, \qquad (9)$$

where parameters with the subscript 0 belong to the priors and

$$S_k^0 = \sum_{i=1}^{N}\rho_{ik}, \qquad S_k^1 = \sum_{i=1}^{N}\rho_{ik}x_i, \qquad S_k^2 = \sum_{i=1}^{N}\rho_{ik}(x_i - S_k^1)(x_i - S_k^1)^\top.$$

Note that the smoothness parameters β affect these hyperparameter estimates through the estimates of the responsibilities ρ_{ik}.

Inference consists of iteratively computing the responsibilities based on the current posterior hyperparameters followed by updating the posterior hyperparameters given the new responsibilities. This procedure, known as variational Bayes, is halted when the change in values between iterations is smaller than a set threshold [4,5,13].

2.4   Semi-supervised Model

Unsupervised models are limited by the fact that cluster assignments are not tied to tissue labels. Manually labeling one voxel per tissue overcomes this limitation. In order to incorporate the given voxel labels, a split in the likelihood function between labeled samples and unlabeled samples needs to be introduced [11]:

$$p(X, \tilde{Y} \mid Y;\; \theta) = \prod_{j \in O} \prod_{i \notin O} \prod_{k=1}^{K} \left[\pi_k \mathcal{N}(x_j \mid \mu_k, \Lambda_k^{-1}) \right]^{\tilde{y}_{jk}} \left[\pi_k \mathcal{N}(x_i \mid \mu_k, \Lambda_k^{-1}) \right]^{y_{ik}},$$

where $\tilde{Y}$ are the observed labels, Y are the unobserved labels and $O \subset [1, \ldots N]$ is the subset of indices that are observed.

To derive a semi-supervised hidden Potts Gaussian mixture requires substituting the unsupervised likelihood from (1) in the Bayesian model in (4) with the above semi-supervised likelihood. Using the same derivations as throughout Sect. 2, this results in equivalent update equations for both the $q(Y \mid \beta)$ and $q(\theta)$ with the following exception: the responsibilities of the observed voxels are fixed to $\rho_{ik} = 1.0$ if class k was observed, and to $\rho_{im} = 0.0$ for $m \neq k$. These responsibilities remain fixed throughout the variational optimization procedure.

2.5   Initialization of Posterior Hyperparameters

Variational inference is a form of non-convex optimization, which means that different initializations lead to different local optima. Several initializations for variational mixture models have been proposed, most notably k-means for unsupervised Gaussian mixtures [15]. In that case, the responsibilities ρ of a point are set by the negative exponential of the distance to each cluster center.

For the semi-supervised model, the responsibilities can be initialized based on the distance to the given labeled voxels. This corresponds to k-nearest-neighbour classifier. As long as the number of labeled pixels is small, this remains computationally efficient.

3   Cross-Center Empirical Bayes

The Potts model can be fit to other segmentations using a maximum likelihood approach. First, it is treated as a likelihood function in its own right, with Y

as the observed variable dependent on the smoothing parameters β. Using the log-likelihood, the estimator becomes:

$$\hat{\beta} = \underset{\beta \in \mathbb{R}^+}{\arg\max} \sum_{i=1}^{N} \log p(y_i \mid y_{\delta_i}, \beta).$$

This log-likelihood function is convex in β, which means the optimal smoothing parameters can be obtained using gradient descent. Its partial derivative with respect to β is:

$$\frac{\partial}{\partial \beta} \log p(y_i \mid y_{\delta_i}, \beta) = \sum_{k=1}^{K} y_{ik} \bar{y}_{ik} - \sum_{l=1}^{K} \bar{y}_{il} \exp\left(\beta_l \bar{y}_{il}\right) / \left[\sum_{m=1}^{K} \exp\left(\beta_m \bar{y}_{im}\right) \right].$$

where $\bar{y}_{ik} = \sum_{j \in \delta_i} y_{jk}$. Using a constrained optimization procedure, where all β's are lower bounded by 0, we can obtain a point estimate for each β_k.

4   Experiments

We perform a series of cross-center brain tissue segmentation experiments. The goal is to assign each pixel in the MR image the label "background", "cerebro-spinal fluid", "gray matter", or "white matter". One data set will act as the source and another as the target. For the sake of comparison, we include single-center experiments, where β cannot be learned and is subsequently set to 0.1. All classification errors are computed using the brain mask. In other words, we ignore all mistakes in the skull and outlying regions. With the unsupervised models, each cluster is interpreted as one of the tissues, so that classification errors can be computed. To test the performance gain that can be achieved with a small amount of supervision, we provide the semi-supervised models with 1 voxel label per tissue from the target image, sampled at random. The experiments are repeated 10 times.

4.1   Data Sets

We will make use of 3 publicly available data sets: Brainweb1.5T, MRBrainS13, and IBSR. Each data set originates from one medical center. Brainweb1.5T is based on 20 realistic phantoms from Brainweb [2] and an MRI simulator (SIMRI; [3]). The simulator was set to use TE, TR and flip angle parameters of the 1.5T scanner in the Rotterdam Scan Study [9]. MRBrainS13 is a grand challenge for medical image tissue segmentation methods containing 5 scans for training [14]. The scans are 3T and have been fully manually annotated. IBSR is a classical data set of 18 patients and is automatically segmented but manually corrected [18]. Skulls are stripped off in all scans. Figure 1 visualizes examples from these sets.

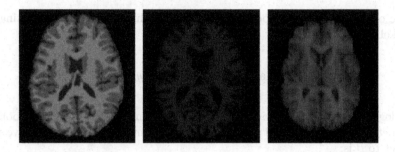

Fig. 1. Example scans. (Left) Brainweb1.5T, (middle) MRBrainS13 and (right) IBSR.

4.2   Segmentation Methods

We will compare the following methods: firstly, a U-net consisting of a mirrored VGG16 architecture pre-trained on ImageNet and fine-tuned on labeled data from the source medical center [19,20]. This method represents the performance of a state-of-the-art tissue segmentation model without taking center-based variation into account. Secondly, we take both an unsupervised and a semi-supervised variational Gaussian mixture model (UGM, SGM), initialized using k-means and 1-nearest-neighbours respectively. Thirdly, an unsupervised and a semi-supervised hidden Potts Gaussian mixture (UHP, SHP) are taken, also initialized using k-means and 1-nearest-neighbours. Comparing these with the previous two models shows the influence of smoothing the segmentations. Lastly, we train a 1-nearest-neighbours (1NN) based on the labeled voxels (1 per tissue) in the target image, as a baseline supervised tissue classifier. The maximum number of training iterations is set to 30 for all methods.

4.3   Results

We present mean classification errors (with standard errors of the means over 10 repetitions) of each method in Table 1. Firstly, comparing the performances of UHP and SHP in the experiments off the diagonal (multi-center) with their performances on the diagonal (single-center) shows that the learned smoothness parameters are more effective than the chosen ones. Secondly, the errors of the hidden Potts models versus the standard Gaussian mixtures tend to be lower or similar (UHP $<=$ UGM and SHP $<=$ SGM). Thirdly, the semi-supervised models tend to outperform the unsupervised ones (SGM $<$ UGM and SHP $<$ UHP). Taken the performance of 1NN into account, it shows that even 1 label per tissue is very informative. U-net performs poorly as it is not aware of the intensity and contrast shifts between data sets.

Figure 2 shows examples of each segmentation method on the MRBrainS13 data set, with Brainweb1.5T as the source center. For the unsupervised models we only show boundaries between clusters, to indicate that interpretation remains a necessary step. A couple of observations can be made: firstly, the hidden Potts models produce smoother segmentations. Secondly, the U-net

Table 1. Mean classification error and standard errors of the means (in brackets) of each of the segmentation models on all pairwise combinations of one data set as the source (rows) and another as the target (columns).

	Methods	Brainweb1.5T	MRBrainS13	IBSR
Brainweb1.5T	U-net	-	0.448 (.008)	0.384 (.019)
	1NN	0.117 (.027)	0.288 (.019)	0.518 (.075)
	UGM	0.142 (.044)	0.339 (.023)	0.525 (.088)
	SGM	0.116 (.031)	0.268 (.017)	0.527 (.089)
	UHP	0.147 (.053)	0.337 (.023)	0.511 (.087)
	SHP	0.117 (.032)	0.253 (.017)	0.519 (.078)
MRBrainS13	U-net	0.257 (.003)	-	0.589 (.022)
	1NN	0.103 (.010)	0.282 (.018)	0.513 (.075)
	UGM	0.112 (.024)	0.345 (.022)	0.521 (.090)
	SGM	0.102 (.011)	0.282 (.021)	0.502 (.093)
	UHP	0.119 (.030)	0.344 (.018)	0.507 (.091)
	SHP	0.102 (.008)	0.277 (.020)	0.503 (.076)
IBSR	U-net	0.334 (.007)	0.425 (.015)	-
	1NN	0.102 (.005)	0.282 (.064)	0.492 (.034)
	UGM	0.125 (.037)	0.369 (.071)	0.508 (.039)
	SGM	0.103 (.015)	0.260 (.043)	0.502 (.039)
	UHP	0.123 (.023)	0.350 (.068)	0.509 (.041)
	SHP	0.103 (.008)	0.255 (.049)	0.496 (.041)

over-predicts white matter in the whole image. Thirdly, the 1-nearest-neighbours classifier over-predicts background voxels in fluid regions. Lastly, all methods favour white matter over gray matter in ambiguous regions.

5 Discussion

Although segmentations remain relatively consistent across medical centers compared to the scans, annotator variation can be quite large. This is especially true if medical centers teach different annotation protocols. To account for this type of variation, it would be more appropriate to capture the uncertainty in smoothness and infer the posterior over β [13].

In our formulation, the hidden Potts-MRF acts as a spatial regularizer on the responsibilities estimated by the variational mixture model. Spatial regularizers are not uncommon, but are often employed on the observed data: most models incorporate information on the smoothness in X to estimate Y. Here, we explicitly look at smoothness in Y.

A limitation of the current model is that it is not appropriate for abnormality or pathology detection. That would require a different number of components for

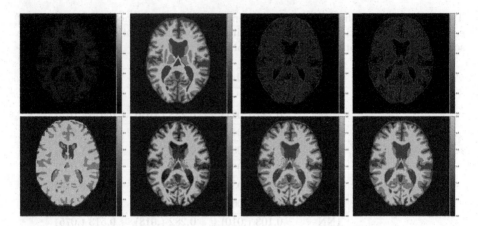

Fig. 2. Segmentations with Brainweb1.5T as source and MRBrainS13 as target data. Top row, from left to right: original scan, true segmentation, unsupervised Gaussian mixture (UGM), unsupervised hidden Potts (UHP). Bottom row: U-net, 1-nearest-neighbour, semi-supervised Gaussian mixture (SGM), semi-supervised hidden Potts (SHP). Purple = background, blue = cerebro-spinal fluid, green = gray matter and yellow = white matter. (Color figure online)

images *with* pathologies versus images *without* pathologies. However, it should be possible to extend variational Gaussian mixture models to incorporate a variable amount of components. In that case, the component weights are not modeled using a Dirichlet distribution, but a Dirichlet process [6].

6 Conclusion

We proposed to tackle center-specific variation in medical imaging data sets with Bayesian transfer learning. We fitted a spatial smoothness prior on the segmentations produced in one medical center and used this informative prior to perform brain tissue segmentation at the target center. Our results show improvements over non-spatially smoothed segmentations, and improvements with learned smoothness parameters over chosen ones.

References

1. Ashburner, J., Friston, K.J.: Unified segmentation. NeuroImage **26**(3), 839–851 (2005)
2. Aubert-Broche, B., Griffin, M., Pike, G.B., Evans, A.C., Collins, D.L.: Twenty new digital brain phantoms for creation of validation image data bases. IEEE Trans. Med. Imaging **25**(11), 1410–1416 (2006)
3. Benoit-Cattin, H., Collewet, G., Belaroussi, B., Saint-Jalmes, H., Odet, C.: The SIMRI project: a versatile and interactive MRI simulator. J. Magn. Reson. **173**(1), 97–115 (2005)

4. Bishop, C.M.: Pattern Recognition and Machine Learning. Springer, Heidelberg (2006)
5. Blaiotta, C., Cardoso, M.J., Ashburner, J.: Variational inference for medical image segmentation. Comput. Vis. Image Underst. **151**, 14–28 (2016)
6. Blei, D.M., Jordan, M.I., et al.: Variational inference for dirichlet process mixtures. Bayesian Anal. **1**(1), 121–143 (2006)
7. Blei, D.M., Kucukelbir, A., McAuliffe, J.D.: Variational inference: a review for statisticians. J. Am. Stat. Assoc. **112**(518), 859–877 (2017)
8. Finkel, J.R., Manning, C.D.: Hierarchical bayesian domain adaptation. In: Conference of the North American Chapter of the Association for Computational Linguistics, pp. 602–610 (2009)
9. Ikram, M.A., et al.: The Rotterdam scan study: design update 2016 and main findings. Eur. J. Epidemiol. **30**(12), 1299–1315 (2015)
10. Kouw, W.M., Loog, M.: A review of single-source unsupervised domain adaptation. arXiv:1901.05335 (2019)
11. Krijthe, J.H., Loog, M.: Implicitly constrained semi-supervised linear discriminant analysis. In: International Conference on Pattern Recognition, pp. 3762–3767 (2014)
12. Liu, J., Zhang, H.: Image segmentation using a local GMM in a variational framework. J. Math. Imaging Vis. **46**(2), 161–176 (2013)
13. McGrory, C.A., Titterington, D.M., Reeves, R., Pettitt, A.N.: Variational Bayes for estimating the parameters of a hidden Potts model. Stat. Comput. **19**(3), 329 (2009)
14. Mendrik, A.M., et al.: MRBrainS challenge: online evaluation framework for brain image segmentation in 3T MRI scans. Comput. Intell. Neurosci. **2015**, 1 (2015)
15. Nasios, N., Bors, A.G.: Variational learning for Gaussian mixture models. IEEE Trans. Syst. Man Cybern. **36**(4), 849–862 (2006)
16. Pan, S.J., Yang, Q., et al.: A survey on transfer learning. IEEE Trans. Knowl. Data Eng. **22**(10), 1345–1359 (2010)
17. Raina, R., Ng, A.Y., Koller, D.: Constructing informative priors using transfer learning. In: International Conference on Machine Learning, pp. 713–720 (2006)
18. Rohlfing, T.: Image similarity and tissue overlaps as surrogates for image registration accuracy: widely used but unreliable. IEEE Trans. Med. Imaging **31**(2), 153–163 (2012)
19. Ronneberger, O., Fischer, P., Brox, T.: U-net: convolutional networks for biomedical image segmentation. In: Navab, N., Hornegger, J., Wells, W.M., Frangi, A.F. (eds.) MICCAI 2015. LNCS, vol. 9351, pp. 234–241. Springer, Cham (2015). https://doi.org/10.1007/978-3-319-24574-4_28
20. Simonyan, K., Zisserman, A.: Very deep convolutional networks for large-scale image recognition. arXiv:1409.1556 (2014)
21. Van Opbroek, A., Ikram, M.A., Vernooij, M.W., De Bruijne, M.: Transfer learning improves supervised image segmentation across imaging protocols. IEEE Trans. Med. Imaging **34**(5), 1018–1030 (2015)
22. Wang, C., Komodakis, N., Paragios, N.: Markov random field modeling, inference & learning in computer vision & image understanding: a survey. Comput. Vis. Image Underst. **117**(11), 1610–1627 (2013)
23. Winkler, G.: Image Analysis, Random Fields and Markov Chain Monte Carlo methods: A Mathematical Introduction, vol. 27. Springer, Heidelberg (2012)
24. Zhang, Y., Brady, M., Smith, S.: Segmentation of brain MR images through a hidden Markov random field model and the expectation-maximization algorithm. IEEE Trans. Med. Imaging **20**(1), 45–57 (2001)

A Graph Model of the Lungs with Morphology-Based Structure for Tuberculosis Type Classification

Yashin Dicente Cid[1]([✉]) [iD], Oscar Jimenez-del-Toro[1,2,3] [iD],
Pierre-Alexandre Poletti[3] [iD], and Henning Müller[1,2] [iD]

[1] University of Applied Sciences Western Switzerland (HES-SO),
Sierre, Switzerland
yashin.dicente@hevs.ch
[2] University of Geneva, Geneva, Switzerland
[3] University Hospitals of Geneva (HUG), Geneva, Switzerland

Abstract. Pulmonary tuberculosis (TB) is still an important cause of death worldwide, even after being almost eradicated 40 years ago. Early identification of TB in computed tomography (CT) scans can influence therapeutical decisions, thus improving patient outcome. In this paper, a graph model of the lungs is proposed for the classification of TB types using local texture features in thorax CT scans of TB patients. Based on lung morphology, an automatic patient-specific lung field parcellation was initially computed. Local visual features were then extracted from each region and were used to build a personalized lung graph model. A new graph-based patient descriptor enables comparisons between lung graphs with a different number of nodes and edges, encoding the distribution of several node measures from graph theory. The proposed model was trained and tested on a public dataset of 1,513 CT scans of 994 TB patients. The evaluation was performed on data from a scientific challenge together with 39 participant algorithms, obtaining the best unweighted Cohen kappa coefficient of 0.24 in a 5-class setup with 505 test CTs. Even though each lung graph has a unique structure, the proposed method was able to identify key texture changes associated with the different manifestations of TB.

Keywords: Lung graph model · Texture analysis ·
Tuberculosis type classification

1 Introduction

Tuberculosis (TB) is a bacterial infection that remains a persistent threat and an important cause of death worldwide even after being almost eradicated around 40 years ago [21]. TB is usually clinically confined to the respiratory system, although it can spread to any organ in immunocompromised patients [4]. Medical imaging, *i.e.* computed tomography (CT), has a major role in TB detection and

© Springer Nature Switzerland AG 2019
A. C. S. Chung et al. (Eds.): IPMI 2019, LNCS 11492, pp. 372–383, 2019.
https://doi.org/10.1007/978-3-030-20351-1_28

associated treatment decisions, including the length of a therapy course [3]. For pulmonary TB, diagnostic imaging is particularly challenging, as the radiological signs can mimic those of other diseases, sometimes causing a delay in the start of a proper treatment strategy [15]. Moreover, early treatment can slow disease progression and reduce mortality associated with TB [2].

Since 2017, the ImageCLEF Tuberculosis challenge has been organized, promoting the development of automatic algorithms for TB type classification using a large dataset of CT scans[1]. The method proposed by Sun *et al.* trained a recurrent neural network with 2D patches and obtained the top scores in the 2017 edition of this task [19]. In 2018, Liauchuk *et al.* obtained the best scores both in unweighted Cohen kappa coefficient and overall classification accuracy [13]. They developed a lesion-based TB descriptor and trained a random forest classifier for this task. The results from both challenges show that for some TB types other algorithms obtained a higher classification accuracy, which supports the notion that there is still room for improvement [9].

Graph modeling is a complete framework that was previously proposed for brain connectivity analysis [16,20] but has rarely been applied to other organs. Graph methods divide the brain into fixed anatomical regions and compare neural activations between regions [17]. Following a similar approach, Dicente *et al.* participated in the ImageCLEF 2017 Tuberculosis challenge [8] with a graph model of the lungs with fixed structure [5]. The approach consisted of first dividing the lung into a fixed number of regions and then creating a graph where each node represented a lung region and the edges encoded (dis)similarities between regional texture features inside the regions. During the 2017 challenge multiple combinations of pruning levels of the complete graph were tested and different similarity measures between the regional texture features [5]. In the ImageCLEF 2018 Tuberculosis challenge [9] the best model of 2017 [10] ranked second in terms of accuracy in the TB type classification task. Moreover, with the same graph model patients with pulmonary hypertension were identified, which is a very challenging task if only visual inspection of CT scans is performed [7]. Nevertheless, this graph model and all its variations were always built on a fixed initial parcellation of the lungs, *i.e.* a geometrical atlas with 36 regions.

In this work we present a new graph model of the lungs with an underlying structure derived from the morphology of the lung and not based on a geometric division. We first divide the lung volume into homogeneous regions using a generalization for 3D volumes of the SLIC (Simple Linear Iterative Clustering) algorithm [1,18]. This technique generates a varying number of regions for each patient and therefore the graph structure differs in each patient. The graph-based descriptor of the lungs is then defined using measures from graph theory. To be able to compare the benefits of using this new lung division instead of a fixed structure to construct a graph model, we used the same regional descriptors and the same similarity measure between regions as Dicente *et al.* in [10]. We also used the same training and test dataset of the ImageCLEF 2018 TB type classification task to evaluate the outcomes.

---

[1] https://www.imageclef.org/2017/tuberculosis, as of 1 March 2019.

2   Methods

This section first describes the dataset used in our experiments and then details the steps involved in the creation of this novel graph model: (1) division of the lung fields into regions; (2) extraction of local texture features in each region; and (3) construction of a lung graph encoding the comparison between the regional features of adjacent regions. Finally, the definition of a new graph-based patient descriptor is detailed.

2.1   Dataset

We used the publicly available dataset of the TB type classification task of ImageCLEF tuberculosis 2018 [9]. This dataset consists of 1,513 CT scans of 994 TB patients along with the TB type and patient age at the moment of the scan, split into 1,008 scans for training and 550 for testing. The dataset contains automatically generated masks of the lungs obtained with the method described in [6]. For each patient there are between 1 and 9 CT scans acquired at different time points. All scans of the same patient were diagnosed with the same TB type by expert radiologists. Figure 1 shows one example for each of the five TB types. Figure 2 shows examples of two patients with three CT scans each. The numbers of CT scans and patients for each TB type are shown in Table 1. Only the CT images and lung masks provided were used without using any additional meta-data *i.e.* age.

Table 1. Dataset distribution of the ImageCLEF 2018 TB type classification task. Data taken from [9].

Patient set	Num. Pats. (CT series)			
	Train		Test	
Type 1 (T1) – Infiltrative	228	(376)	89	(176)
Type 2 (T2) – Focal	210	(273)	80	(115)
Type 3 (T3) – Tuberculoma	100	(154)	60	(86)
Type 4 (T4) – Miliary	79	(106)	50	(71)
Type 5 (T5) – Fibro–cavernous	60	(99)	38	(57)
Total patients (CTs)	**677**	**(1,008)**	**317**	**(505)**

Data Preprocessing: Our approach uses rotation-invariant 3D texture descriptors that require having isometric voxels. We first made the 3D images and the lung masks isometric. After analyzing the multiple resolutions and the inter-slice distances in the dataset, we opted for a voxel size of 1 mm in all three dimension to capture a maximum of the available information.

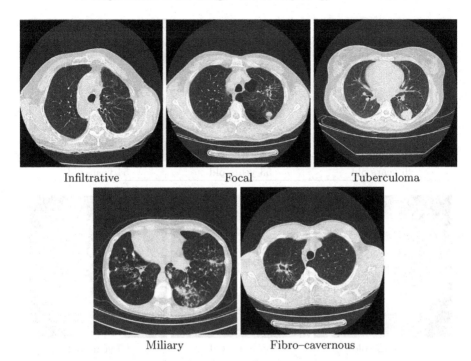

Infiltrative   Focal   Tuberculoma

Miliary   Fibro–cavernous

Fig. 1. CT slices of five patients from the ImageCLEF 2018 TB dataset, each one presenting a different TB type.

2.2 Lung Parcellation

Once we obtain the isometric volumes, we divide the lung area into homogeneous regions based on the HU information using a generalization for 3D volumes of the SLIC algorithm [1]. We used an initial step size s of 30 voxels (equivalent to 30 mm) followed by a refinement step where any supervoxel containing fewer than $\frac{s^3}{2}$ voxels (13,500) was merged with the most similar adjacent supervoxel. The initial step size and the refinement procedure were empirically established to obtain a reasonable number of regions with a minimum volume that can contain meaningful texture information. Figure 3 shows the supervoxelization result for one image in the dataset. The resulting lung parcellations contained between 43 and 325 regions, with an average of 170 regions per patient.

2.3 Regional 3D Texture Features

For each region r of a given lung parcellation, two texture feature descriptors were extracted: the Fourier-based histogram of oriented gradients (FHOG) [14] and the locally-oriented 3D Riesz-wavelet transform (3DRiesz) [11]. These descriptors were extracted using the same configuration as in [10] to compare to a strong baseline. FHOG was computed using 28 3D directions for the histogram,

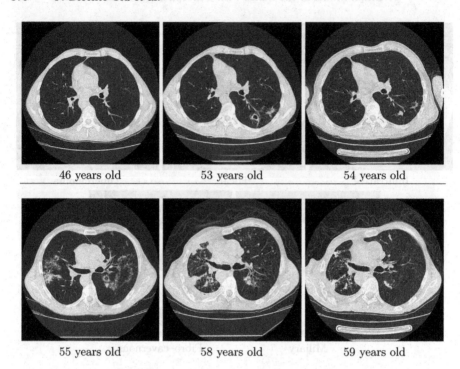

|46 years old | 53 years old | 54 years old|

|55 years old | 58 years old | 59 years old|

Fig. 2. Examples of two patients in the ImageCLEF 2018 TB dataset, each one with three CT scans acquired at different time points. Each row contains a slice of the three scans of a patient ordered by the patient age at the moment they were taken. The three CT images of the first row were labeled as having TB type 1 (infiltrative) while the three series in the second row are of type 4 (miliary).

obtaining a 28-dimensional feature vector per image voxel v ($\mathbf{f}_H(v) \in \mathbb{R}^{28}$). For 3DRiesz we used the 3rd-order Riesz-wavelet transform, with 4 scales and 1st-order alignment (see [11]). The feature vector for a single voxel was defined as the absolute Riesz response along the 4 scales, obtaining a 40-dimensional feature vector ($\mathbf{f}_{\mathcal{R}}(v) \in \mathbb{R}^{40}$). Finally, the average and standard deviation of these two descriptors were obtained for each region r: $\boldsymbol{\mu}_H(r)$, $\boldsymbol{\sigma}_H(r)$, $\boldsymbol{\mu}_{\mathcal{R}}(r)$, and $\boldsymbol{\sigma}_{\mathcal{R}}(r)$.

2.4   Graph Model of the Lungs

Using the patient-specific lung parcellation defined in Sect. 2.2 and the regional texture descriptors detailed in Sect. 2.3, we create an undirected edge-weighted graph model as defined in [10]. This means: given a division of the lungs with n regions $\{r_1, \ldots, r_n\}$, we define a *graph model of the lungs* $\mathcal{G} = (\mathcal{N}, \mathcal{E})$ as a set of n nodes $\mathcal{N} = \{N_1, \ldots, N_n\}$ connected by a set of m edges $\mathcal{E}$. An undirected edge $E_{i,j}$ with associated weight $w_{i,j}$ exists between nodes N_i and N_j if regions r_i and r_j are 3D adjacent in the lung parcellation. The weight $w_{i,j}$ is defined as the correlation distance between the regional feature vectors. Figure 4 contains a 3D visualization of the graph using the patient-specific lung parcellation.

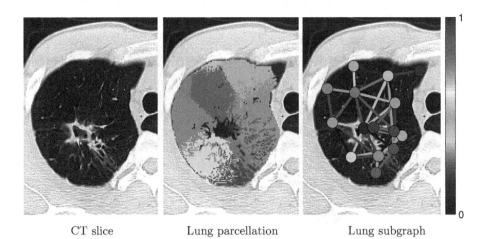

CT slice   Lung parcellation   Lung subgraph

Fig. 3. From left to right: Cropped CT slice of a patient with fibro-cavernous TB shown in Fig. 1, the automatically generated supervoxelization (or lung parcellation) and the subgraph containing the nodes that correspond to the regions present in the cropped CT slice. This subgraph contains 25 nodes and 42 edges, whereas the full graph of this patient contained 233 nodes and 2,035 edges (see Fig. 4). The color of the nodes matches the color of the region that they represent. The edges are colored according to their weight and are normalized between 0 and 1. For this example we used as weight the correlation distance between the average absolute Riesz response in each region $\mu_H(r)$ (see Sect. 2.3). (Color figure online)

2.5   Graph-Based Patient Descriptor

Dicente *et al.* defined in [10] a graph model of the lungs containing the same number of nodes and the same edges for all patients. Therefore, a graph-based patient descriptor w_p was defined as the collection of weights in the graph, sorted with respect to their position in the adjacency matrix. Our graph model of the lungs on the other hand contains a varying number of nodes (and edges) for each patient and the above mentioned approach can not be used. We described each graph with a fixed number of graph measures in order to compare graphs of different patients.

For each node N in the graph $\mathcal{G}$ we computed five graph centrality measures: the weighted degree $d^w(N)$, the relative weighted degree $d^r(N) = \frac{d^w(N)}{d(N)}$ (the weighted degree divided by the degree), the weighted closeness $c^w(N)$, the relative weighted closeness $c^r(N) = \frac{c^w(N)}{d(N)}$ (the weighted closeness divided by the degree) and the weighted betweenness $b^w(N)$. Each of these measures provided different information about the importance of each node inside the graph (see Fig. 5). Considering the entire set of nodes $\mathcal{N}$ in $\mathcal{G}$, each of these five measures results in a distribution: $D_{\mathcal{G}}^w = \{d^w(N)\}$, $D_{\mathcal{G}}^r = \{d^r(N)\}$, $C_{\mathcal{G}}^w = \{c^w(N)\}$, $C_{\mathcal{G}}^r = \{c^r(N)\}$ and $B_{\mathcal{G}}^w = \{b^w(N)\}$, where $N \in \mathcal{N}$. Then, we described each of these distributions using 10 equidistant percentiles from 0 to 100 (step size of

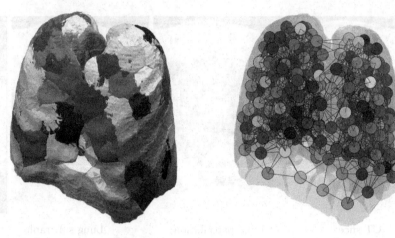

Lung parcellation   Lung graph

Fig. 4. Morphology-based lung parcellation and graph derived from it. Each region is identified by a node and the edges are defined between nodes of 3D-adjacent regions in the lung parcellation. The color of the nodes corresponds to the color of the lung region that they represent. (Color figure online)

11.$\overline{1}$), with percentiles 0 ($\pi_1(X)$) and 100 ($\pi_{10}(X)$) being the minimum and maximum values in the distribution, respectively. Let $\boldsymbol{\pi}(X) = (\pi_1(X), \ldots, \pi_{10}(X))$ be the vector composed of the 10 percentiles $\pi_k(X)$ of a distribution X. Our graph-based patient descriptor is then defined as:

$$\boldsymbol{\omega}(\mathcal{G}) = (\mu_w, \boldsymbol{\pi}(D_\mathcal{G}^w), \boldsymbol{\pi}(D_\mathcal{G}^r), \boldsymbol{\pi}(C_\mathcal{G}^w), \boldsymbol{\pi}(C_\mathcal{G}^r), \boldsymbol{\pi}(B_\mathcal{G}^w))$$

where μ_w is the mean of the weights in the graph.

For each patient p with graph model $\mathcal{G}_p$, its graph-based patient descriptor $\boldsymbol{\omega}(\mathcal{G}_p)$ belongs to $\mathbb{R}^{51}$. From now on, $\boldsymbol{\omega}(\mathcal{G}_p)$ is referred to as $\boldsymbol{\omega}_{\mathbf{f},p}$, where $\mathbf{f}$ corresponds to the regional feature used to build the graph $\mathcal{G}_p$.

Concatenation of Patient Descriptors: As mentioned in Sect. 2.3, four regional features were computed in each region of the lung parcellation ($\mu_H(r)$, $\sigma_H(r)$, $\mu_\mathcal{R}(r)$, and $\sigma_\mathcal{R}(r)$) providing complementary information about the texture and its variability. Given a patient p, a different weighted graph (same nodes and edges but different weights) was obtained from each of these textural features. The final patient descriptor $\hat{\boldsymbol{\omega}}_p$ used in our experiments was defined as the concatenation of the four graph-based patient descriptors:

$$\hat{\boldsymbol{\omega}}_p = (\boldsymbol{\omega}_{\mu_H,p}, \boldsymbol{\omega}_{\sigma_H,p}, \boldsymbol{\omega}_{\mu_\mathcal{R},p}, \boldsymbol{\omega}_{\sigma_\mathcal{R},p}) \in \mathbb{R}^{204}.$$

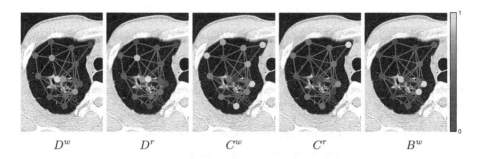

Fig. 5. Visualization of the distribution along the graph shown in Fig. 3 of the five graph measures extracted in each node of the graph. From left to right: Weighted degree D^w, relative weighted degree D^r, weighted closeness C^w, relative weighted closeness C^r and weighted betweenness B^w. For better visualization, the values of each measure are normalized between 0 and 1 considering only the values in the nodes present in the depicted slice.

3   Experimental Setup

We applied Z-score normalization to each dimension of the descriptor vectors $\hat{\omega}_p$ using the mean and standard deviation computed on the training set vectors. Then, we used linear discriminant analysis (LDA) as a dimensionality reduction technique and as a classifier algorithm in a 5-class setup. The optimization of the LDA classifier was done using 10-fold cross-validation with random sampling without repetition and grid search over the parameter space.

The ImageCLEF TB dataset contained more than one CT scan for several patients (see Sect. 2.1). In our experiments we treated each CT scan as a different instance. However, since the evaluation by the ImageCLEF organizers was done at a patient level, we combined the predictions of the CT images of each patient to obtain a final predicted class per patient. This combination was obtained by averaging the probabilities of the LDA classifier. The final evaluation on the test set was done by the ImageCLEF organizers using the same measures as the ones reported during the challenge: the unweighted Cohen kappa coefficient and the accuracy. Moreover, the true positive rate (TPR) of each class was provided.

4   Results

Table 2 shows the results obtained by our approach and by the top three groups that participated in the ImageCLEF 2018 TB type classification task: the *UIIP_BioMed* [13], the *fau_ml4cv* [12] and the *MedGIFT* [10] groups. All results were provided by the ImageCLEF 2018 TB organizers. The approach of Dicente *et al.* participated as the MedGIFT group. The results obtained by our new graph model are much higher than the ones obtained by the MedGIFT group using a related approach and slightly higher than the winner of the challenge in terms of Cohen's kappa. Figure 6 contains the confusion matrix of our approach and Fig. 7 shows the true positive rate (TPR) of our approach and the 3 best participants.

Table 2. Results obtained by our approach and by the 3 best participants in the ImageCLEF 2018 TB type classification task.

Group name	Kappa	Accuracy
Our approach	**0.2385**	0.4196
UIIP_BioMed [13]	0.2312	**0.4227**
fau_ml4cv [12]	0.1736	0.3533
MedGIFT [10]	0.1706	0.3849

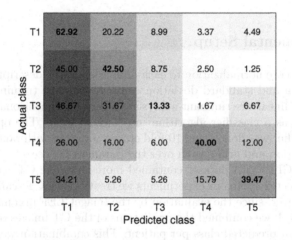

Fig. 6. Confusion matrix of our approach in %.

5   Discussion

In this work we used a graph model with an underlying structure that it is based on the morphology of the lungs. The comparison between graphs of different patients was then translated to the comparison of the distributions along each graph for five graph measures, extracted in each node. The selected node measures are both local (considering only the weights of incident edges to a given node) and global (considering the whole structure of the graph). In Fig. 5, it can be seen how the selected node measures are complementary and each of them highlights different but relevant nodes. The manual analysis of several graphs revealed that the distributions of these measures usually did not follow a normal distribution and therefore the use of central moment statistics was not

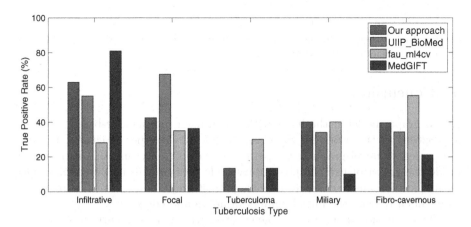

Fig. 7. True positive rate (%) for each TB type obtained by our approach and the top 3 groups participating in the ImageCLEF 2018 TB task.

appropriate. The use of percentiles as distribution descriptors allowed to encode the proportion of important nodes (for a given node measure) and their level of importance inside the graph. Since the number of nodes per graph was 170 on average (see Sect. 2.2) the use of 10 percentiles, including the percentiles 0 and 100, allowed us to describe each distribution in a summarized form that still kept the shape of the distribution.

In order to see the effect of using this new morphology-based structure instead of a fixed structure, we used the same regional texture features and the same weight definition as Dicente *et al.* in [10]. The results, both in terms of accuracy and kappa value, clearly show the benefits of using our new graph structure (see Sect. 4) instead of the one used by the MedGIFT group, indicating that the global structure of the same texture information is as important as the local information.

The analysis of the confusion matrix shown in Fig. 6 shows the strong effect produced by the unbalanced dataset. Patients with TB type 1 and 2 (T1 and T2) were much more frequent in the dataset than the other three TB types. This generated a bias in the classification of the test set towards these two classes since the optimization of our classifier was done using the overall cross-validation accuracy. Moreover, in the training phase we considered each CT scan as a different patient (see Sect. 3), therefore creating an even stronger effect towards classes T1 and T2 due to their higher proportion of scans (see Table 1). Analyzing the TPR for each TB type in Fig. 7, the MedGIFT and UIIP_BioMed groups seem to have had a similar bias towards classes T1 and T2, but it is not the case for the fau_m4cv group that obtained a similar TPR for all the classes. In this task, the unweighted Cohen kappa coefficient is a better measure of the performance of the algorithms due to its invariance to unbalanced datasets. It indicates the level of agreement between the predicted labels and the ground truth labels considering their prior probability in the dataset, and therefore giving more importance to matches in rare classes than in frequent classes. All the results provided by the ImageCLEF organizers are reported in this work. Paired statistics between the algorithms could not be computed since individual results per patient were not available.

6 Conclusions

A new graph model of the lungs with a non-fixed morphology-based structure is proposed in this work for the classification of TB types in chest CT scans. We present a novel graph-based patient descriptor encoding the distributions inside the graph of five complementary node measures using percentiles. This technique allows us to characterize each patient graph in the same feature space, independently from the initial number of nodes and edges.

The evaluation in a public challenge strengthens the comparison of this new graph model against the other 39 participating algorithms, obtaining the top unweighted Cohen kappa coefficient and the second best overall classification accuracy. Although the obtained results are promising, better scores would be required to apply this model in medical practice. Nevertheless, the use of the same regional texture features and weight definition than in the graph model from the MedGIFT group shows the benefits of our new morphology-based structure. This confirms the importance of encoding the overall structure along the lung using similar tissue patterns.

Acknowledgments. This work was partly supported by the Swiss National Science Foundation in the PH4D project (grant agreement 320030-146804).

References

1. Achanta, R., Shaji, A., Smith, K., Lucchi, A., Fua, P., Süsstrunk, S.: SLIC superpixels compared to state-of-the-art superpixel methods. IEEE Trans. Pattern Anal. Mach. Intell. **34**(11), 2274–2282 (2012)
2. Andreu, J., Caceres, J., Pallisa, E., Martinez-Rodriguez, M.: Radiological manifestations of pulmonary tuberculosis. Eur. J. Radiol. **51**(2), 139–149 (2004)
3. Blumberg, H.M., Burman, W.J., Chaisson, R.E., Daley, C.L., et al.: American thoracic society/centers for disease control and prevention/infectious diseases society of America: treatment of tuberculosis. Am. J. Respir. Crit. Care Med. **167**(4), 603 (2003)
4. Burrill, J., Williams, C.J., Bain, G., Conder, G., Hine, A.L., Misra, R.R.: Tuberculosis: a radiologic review. Radiographics **27**(5), 1255–1273 (2007)
5. Dicente Cid, Y., Batmanghelich, K., Müller, H.: Textured graph-based model of the lungs: application on tuberculosis type classification and multi-drug resistance detection. In: Bellot, P., et al. (eds.) CLEF 2018. LNCS, vol. 11018, pp. 157–168. Springer, Cham (2018). https://doi.org/10.1007/978-3-319-98932-7_15
6. Dicente Cid, Y., Jimenez-del-Toro, O., Depeursinge, A., Müller, H.: Efficient and fully automatic segmentation of the lungs in CT volumes. In: Goksel, O., Jimenez-del-Toro, O., Foncubierta-Rodriguez, A., Müller, H. (eds.) Proceedings of the VISCERAL Challenge at ISBI, pp. 31–35. No. 1390 in CEUR Workshop Proceedings, April 2015

7. Dicente Cid, Y., Jiménez-del-Toro, O., Platon, A., Müller, H., Poletti, P.-A.: From local to global: a holistic lung graph model. In: Frangi, A.F., Schnabel, J.A., Davatzikos, C., Alberola-López, C., Fichtinger, G. (eds.) MICCAI 2018. LNCS, vol. 11071, pp. 786–793. Springer, Cham (2018). https://doi.org/10.1007/978-3-030-00934-2_87
8. Dicente Cid, Y., Kalinovsky, A., Liauchuk, V., Kovalev, V., Müller, H.: Overview of ImageCLEFtuberculosis 2017 - predicting tuberculosis type and drug resistances. In: CLEF 2017 Labs Working Notes. CEUR Workshop Proceedings, 11–14 September 2017, Dublin, Ireland. CEUR-WS.org (2017). http://ceur-ws.org
9. Dicente Cid, Y., Liauchuk, V., Kovalev, V., Müller, H.: Overview of image CLEF tuberculosis 2018 - detecting multi-drug resistance, classifying tuberculosis type, and assessing severity score. In: CLEF 2018 Working Notes. CEUR Workshop Proceedings, 10–14 September 2018, Avignon, France. CEUR-WS.org (2018). http://ceur-ws.org
10. Dicente Cid, Y., Müller, H.: Texture-based graph model of the lungs for drug resistance detection, tuberculosis type classification, and severity scoring: Participation in Image CLEF 2018 tuberculosis task. In: CLEF 2018 Working Notes. CEUR Workshop Proceedings, 10–14 September 2018, Avignon, France. CEUR-WS.org (2018). http://ceur-ws.org
11. Dicente Cid, Y., Müller, H., Platon, A., Poletti, P.A., Depeursinge, A.: 3-D solid texture classification using locally-oriented wavelet transforms. IEEE Trans. Image Process. **26**(4), 1899–1910 (2017)
12. Ishay, A., Marques, O.: Ensemble of 3D CNNs with multiple inputs for tuberculosis type classification. In: CLEF 2018 Working Notes. CEUR Workshop Proceedings, 10–14 September 2018, Avignon, France. CEUR-WS.org (2018). http://ceur-ws.org
13. Liauchuk, V., Tarasau, A., Snezhko, E., Kovalev, V., Gabrielian, A., Rosenthal, A.: ImageCLEF 2018: Lesion-based TB-descriptor for CT image analysis. In: CLEF2018 Working Notes. CEUR Workshop Proceedings, 10–14 September 2018, Avignon, France. CEUR-WS.org (2018). http://ceur-ws.org
14. Liu, K., Skibbe, H., Schmidt, T., Blein, T., Palme, K., Brox, T., Ronneberger, O.: Rotation-invariant hog descriptors using fourier analysis in polar and spherical coordinates. Int. J. Comput. Vis. **106**(3), 342–364 (2014)
15. Parra, J.A.C., Zúñiga, N.M., Lara, C.S.: Tuberculosis "the great imitator": false healing and subclinical activity. Indian J. Tuberc. **64**(4), 345–348 (2017)
16. Richiardi, J., Bunke, H., Van De Ville, D., Achard, S.: Machine learning with brain graphs. IEEE Sig. Process. Mag. **30**, 58 (2013)
17. Richiardi, J., Eryilmaz, H., Schwartz, S., Vuilleumier, P., Van De Ville, D.: Decoding brain states from fMRI connectivity graphs. NeuroImage **56**(2), 616–626 (2011). https://doi.org/10.1016/j.neuroimage.2010.05.081
18. Schabdach, J., Wells, W.M., Cho, M., Batmanghelich, K.N.: A likelihood-free approach for characterizing heterogeneous diseases in large-scale studies. In: Niethammer, M., et al. (eds.) IPMI 2017. LNCS, vol. 10265, pp. 170–183. Springer, Cham (2017). https://doi.org/10.1007/978-3-319-59050-9_14
19. Sun, J., Chong, P., Tan, Y.X.M., Binder, A.: ImageCLEF 2017: ImageCLEF tuberculosis task - the SGEast submission. In: CLEF 2017 Working Notes. CEUR Workshop Proceedings, 11–14 September 2017, Dublin, Ireland. CEUR-WS.org (2017). http://ceur-ws.org
20. Varoquaux, G., Gramfort, A., Poline, J., Thirion, B.: Brain covariance selection: better individual functional connectivity models using population prior. In: NIPS, vol. 10, pp. 2334–2342 (2010)
21. World Health Organization, et al.: Global tuberculosis report 2016 (2016)

A Longitudinal Model for Tau Aggregation in Alzheimer's Disease Based on Structural Connectivity

Fan Yang[1,2], Samadrita Roy Chowdhury[1,2], Heidi I. L. Jacobs[2],
Keith A. Johnson[2], and Joyita Dutta[1,2(✉)]

[1] Department of Electrical and Computer Engineering,
University of Massachusetts Lowell, Lowell, MA, USA
[2] Massachusetts General Hospital and Harvard Medical School,
Boston, MA, USA
dutta.joyita@mgh.harvard.edu

Abstract. Tau tangles are a pathological hallmark of Alzheimer's disease (AD) with strong correlations existing between tau aggregation and cognitive decline. Studies in mouse models have shown that the characteristic patterns of tau spatial spread associated with AD progression are determined by neural connectivity rather than physical proximity between different brain regions. We present here a network diffusion model for tau aggregation based on longitudinal tau measures from positron emission tomography (PET) and structural connectivity graphs from diffusion tensor imaging (DTI). White matter fiber bundles reconstructed via tractography from the DTI data were used to compute normalized graph Laplacians which served as graph diffusion kernels for tau spread. By linearizing this model and using sparse source localization, we were able to identify distinct patterns of propagative and generative buildup of tau at a population level. A gradient descent approach was used to solve the sparsity-constrained optimization problem. Model fitting was performed on subjects from the Harvard Aging Brain Study cohort. The fitted model parameters include a scalar factor controlling the network-based tau spread and a network-independent seed vector representing seeding in different regions-of-interest. This parametric model was validated on an independent group of subjects from the same cohort. We were able to predict with reasonably high accuracy the tau buildup at a future time-point. The network diffusion model, therefore, successfully identifies two distinct mechanisms for tau buildup in the aging brain and offers a macroscopic perspective on tau spread.

Keywords: Alzheimer's disease · Network diffusion · Tau ·
Structural connectivity · PET · DTI

Supported by the National Institute on Aging grant K01AG050711.

A. C. S. Chung et al. (Eds.): IPMI 2019, LNCS 11492, pp. 384–393, 2019.
https://doi.org/10.1007/978-3-030-20351-1_29

1   Introduction

Alzheimer's disease (AD) is a progressive neurodegenerative disorder which is the leading cause of dementia in the elderly. Extracellular amyloid-β (Aβ) plaques and intracellular tau neurofibrillary tangles, the two hallmark pathologies of this disease, are believed to play a key mechanistic role in AD [8]. Studies show that misfolded tau pathology in the medial temporal lobe is an important biomarker for neurodegeneration in preclinical AD [3]. Unlike Aβ, tau exhibits an anatomically stereotypical propagation pattern in the brain. A growing body of evidence indicates that tau spreads through the brain from neurons to nearby neurons in a prion-like fashion [5,11–14]. Studies in mouse models have shown that the characteristic patterns of tau spatial spread associated with AD progression are determined by neural connectivity rather than physical proximity between different brain regions [1]. Comprehension of neurodegenerative pathogenesis requires the understanding of proliferation and accumulation mechanisms of tau [10]. Network diffusion models [7,17,18] have had reasonable success predicting dementia patterns and as well as modeling the relationship between structural and functional connectivity in the human brain. In this paper, we present a network diffusion model for tau propagation that seeks to characterize – at a macroscopic level – its relationship with the axonal pathway distributions captured by the brain's structural connectivity network.

In recent years, a number of novel positron emission tomography (PET) radiotracers have enabled *in vivo* visualization of tau burden. Recent studies report that ^{18}F-flortaucipir PET imaging of tau [20] allows *in vivo* Braak staging based on tracer uptake measures and that the spatial distribution patterns of the tracer mirror clinical and neuroanatomical variability in AD [9,15,19]. Here we use longitudinal ^{18}F-flortaucipir tau PET data collected at two time-points for obtaining regional tau measures. White matter fiber bundles generated via diffusion tensor imaging (DTI) are used to compute the structural connectivity network graphs for each subject.

In Sect. 2, we present the derivation and implementation of the network diffusion model. The data processing and analysis details are provided in Sect. 3, while our main findings are reported in Sect. 4. In Sect. 5, we summarize this work, discuss its strengths and limitations, and present our envisioned future directions.

2   Theory

2.1   Network Diffusion Model

We model the accumulation of tau as a diffusion process on a brain network graph defined as $\mathcal{G} = (\mathcal{V}, \mathcal{E})$ where the ith node, $\nu_i \in \mathcal{V}$, represents the ith gray matter parcellation or region-of-interest (ROI), $|\mathcal{V}| = N$ is the number of ROIs, and $\epsilon_{ij} \in \mathcal{E}$ represents fiber connectivity between node ν_i and node ν_j. The regional tau burden is a time-varying signal defined on the graph $\mathcal{G}$ and can be represented as a vector $\boldsymbol{x}(t) = \{x(\nu_i, t), \nu_i \in \mathcal{V}\}$, $\boldsymbol{x}(t) \in \mathbb{R}^N$. $\boldsymbol{x}(t)$ is the solution to a first order partial differential equation, usually referred to as the *network diffusion equation*:

$$\frac{\partial \boldsymbol{x}(t)}{\partial t} = -\beta \boldsymbol{L} \boldsymbol{x}(t), \tag{1}$$

where $\boldsymbol{L} \in \mathbb{R}^{N \times N}$ is the static graph Laplacian matrix based on DTI, which captures the structural connectivity of an individual subject's brain. Solutions to (1) are of the form:

$$\boldsymbol{x}(t) = e^{-\beta L(t-t_0)} \boldsymbol{x}(t_0), \tag{2}$$

where $\boldsymbol{x}(t_0)$ is the initial tau burden at time t_0. To model proteopathic tau seeding [6] in addition to network-dependent spread, we add a source term $\boldsymbol{s}(t)$ to (1) as follows:

$$\frac{\partial \boldsymbol{x}(t)}{\partial t} = -\beta \boldsymbol{L} \boldsymbol{x}(t) + \boldsymbol{s}(t). \tag{3}$$

For $\boldsymbol{s}(t) = \boldsymbol{\alpha} \delta(t - t_0^+)$, an impulsive source at $t = t_0^+$, the solution to this equation is:

$$\boldsymbol{x}(t) = e^{-\beta L(t-t_0)} \boldsymbol{x}_0 + e^{-\beta L(t-t_0^+)} \boldsymbol{\alpha} u(t - t_0^+), \tag{4}$$

where $u(t - t_0^+)$ is the unit step function at t_0^+. In subsequent analyses, we replace t_0^+ with t_0 in the second term.

2.2 Longitudinal Two Time-Point Model

For longitudinal two time-point tau PET datasets, t_0 represents the time-point at which a baseline tau PET scan is performed and t represents a second time-point at which either a follow-up tau PET scan is performed or at which the tau burden is to be predicted using the network diffusion model. For simplicity, we denote the tau buildup at t_0 and t by $\boldsymbol{x}_0$ and $\boldsymbol{x}_t$ respectively and the time gap as $\Delta t = t - t_0$. For preclinical AD, tau accumulation occurs at a slow rate. Using this rationale, we linearize (4) via the relationship:

$$e^{-\beta L(t-t_0)} \simeq \boldsymbol{I} - \beta \boldsymbol{L}(t - t_0). \tag{5}$$

Accordingly, the solution can be approximated as:

$$\boldsymbol{x}_t = [\boldsymbol{I} - \beta \boldsymbol{L} \Delta t] (\boldsymbol{x}_0 + \boldsymbol{\alpha}). \tag{6}$$

For ease of notation, we denote:

$$\boldsymbol{H}(\beta) = \boldsymbol{I} - \beta \boldsymbol{L} \Delta t. \tag{7}$$

We can estimate the parameters $\boldsymbol{\alpha}$ and β by minimizing the data fidelity cost function:

$$\min_{\beta, \boldsymbol{\alpha}} \frac{1}{2} \| \boldsymbol{H}(\beta)(\boldsymbol{x}_0 + \boldsymbol{\alpha}) - \boldsymbol{x}_t \|_2^2. \tag{8}$$

The unknowns in this model are $\boldsymbol{\alpha}$ and β. For group-level prediction, we extend (8), which is an individual model, to a jointly fitted model for the entire cohort where, $k = 1, 2, \ldots M$, M being the number of subjects. We modify (7) to incorporate the index k as follows:

$$H^{(k)}(\beta) = I - \beta L^{(k)} \Delta t^{(k)}. \tag{9}$$

The new group-level data fidelity cost function is as follows:

$$\Phi_{DF}(\boldsymbol{\alpha}, \beta) = \sum_k \frac{1}{2} \|H^{(k)}(\beta)(\boldsymbol{x}_0^{(k)} + \boldsymbol{\alpha}) - \boldsymbol{x}_t^{(k)}\|_2^2. \tag{10}$$

To ensure a spatially sparse distribution of tau seeds, we introduce an L^1 penalty on $\boldsymbol{\alpha}$. To ensure small values of β, which is the basis of linearization, we introduce an L^2 penalty on β. The penalty terms are grouped together as a combined regularization function given by:

$$\Phi_R(\boldsymbol{\alpha}, \beta) = \lambda_1 |\boldsymbol{\alpha}| + \frac{1}{2} \lambda_2 \beta^2, \tag{11}$$

where λ_1 and λ_2 are regularization parameters.

2.3 Implementation

We use an alternating gradient descent strategy to solve the associated constrained optimization problem:

$$(\hat{\boldsymbol{\alpha}}, \hat{\beta}) = \arg \min_{\boldsymbol{\alpha} \geq 0, \beta \geq 0} \Phi(\boldsymbol{\alpha}, \beta), \tag{12}$$

$$\Phi(\boldsymbol{\alpha}, \beta) = \Phi_{DF}(\boldsymbol{\alpha}, \beta) + \Phi_R(\boldsymbol{\alpha}, \beta). \tag{13}$$

The partial derivatives with respect to β are computed as follows:

$$\frac{\partial \Phi_{DF}}{\partial \beta} = \sum_k \left[-\Delta t^{(k)} L^{(k)} (\boldsymbol{x}_0^{(k)} + \boldsymbol{\alpha}) \right]^T \left[H^{(k)}(\beta)(\boldsymbol{x}_0^{(k)} + \boldsymbol{\alpha}) - \boldsymbol{x}_t^{(k)} \right], \tag{14}$$

$$\frac{\partial \Phi_R}{\partial \beta} = \lambda_2 \beta. \tag{15}$$

The partial gradients with respect to $\boldsymbol{\alpha}$ are computed as follows:

$$\nabla_{\boldsymbol{\alpha}} \Phi_{DF} = \sum_k \left[H^{(k)} \right]^T \left[H^{(k)}(\beta)(\boldsymbol{x}_0^{(k)} + \boldsymbol{\alpha}) - \boldsymbol{x}_t^{(k)} \right], \tag{16}$$

$$\nabla_{\boldsymbol{\alpha}} \Phi_R = \lambda_1 \mathbf{1}, \tag{17}$$

where $\mathbf{1}$ represents a vector with all entries equal to the number 1. In deriving (17), we rely on the fact that our constrained optimization algorithm restricts the solution for $\boldsymbol{\alpha}$ to the non-negative orthant where the L^1 norm is differentiable.

3   Experiments

3.1   Data Description

All experiments relied on data from the Harvard Aging Brain Study (HABS) [4], which is an ongoing longitudinal study aimed at revealing the differences between normal aging and preclinical AD. Datasets available from this study include longitudinal data of neuropsychological scores as well as multimodality neuroimaging data.

3.2   Subject Information

We applied the model to 62 subjects (75.85 ± 6.18 years, 37 females) from HABS with T1-weighted high-resolution anatomical MR images, diffusion MR images, and two time-point ^{18}F-flortaucipir PET scans for tau.

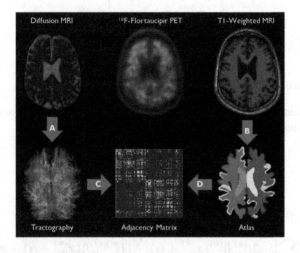

Fig. 1. Sample ^{18}F-flortaucipir PET, diffusion MR, and T1-weighted MR images, the FreeSurfer atlas, and a sample weighted adjacency matrix. White matter fiber tracts were reconstructed from the diffusion MR images via tractography (step A) using the software MedINRIA. The T1-weighted anatomical reference images were segmented by means of deformable registration to match the FreeSurfer atlas (step B). Fiber counting was performed on the segmented diffusion image volumes to derive pairwise inter-region connection strengths thereby yielding an adjacency matrix (steps C and D). The mean ^{18}F-flortaucipir specific binding was computed for the FreeSurfer ROIs.

3.3   Data Acquisition and Processing

The overall data preprocessing workflow is depicted in Fig. 1. All MR imaging was performed on a Siemens Tim Trio 3T MR scanner with a 12-channel phased-array head coil. High-resolution, T1-weighted MR images were obtained using an MPRAGE pulse sequence.

DTI Processing. Diffusion MRI data preprocessing comprised correction of subject motion, eddy current distortion correction, and tensor model estimation. The first two steps were performed using FSL [2] while the last step was processed in MedINRIA [21]. We also enabled the embedded feature of automatic brain extraction during tensor model estimation. Diffusion tensor maps of fractional anisotropy (FA), mean diffusivity, axial diffusivity, and radial diffusivity were computed. After DTI data preprocessing, deterministic tractography was performed using MedINRIA. Tractography comprises seeding, propagation, and termination of streamlines indicative of fiber pathways. The seeding and termination of these pathways is determined by the starting and stopping FA threshold values, which were set at 0.07 and 0.1 respectively in accordance with literature-suggested numbers for the adult brain. The minimum length for a streamline to be considered a valid representation of a fiber pathway was set to 10 mm.

To adjust for linear shifts in head position and scale within the same subject, each T1-weighted scan was registered to the corresponding diffusion MR scans using FSL with 9-parameter registration based on a mutual information cost function. We retained only the tracts starting and ending at the 112 FreeSurfer-defined cortical and subcortical ROIs. The reconstructed streamlines or tracts were counted for each pair of ROIs leading to pairwise connection strengths used to construct a 112×112 adjacency matrix.

PET Acquisition and Processing. PET images were acquired on a Siemens (Knoxville, TN) ECAT HR+ scanner (3D mode, 63 image planes, 15.2-cm axial field of view, 5.6-mm transaxial resolution, and 2.4-mm slice interval). ^{18}F-flortaucipir scans were performed 80–100 min after a 9.0–11.0 mCi bolus injection in four 5-minute frames.

Each attenuation-corrected PET image frame was verified for adequacy of counts and absence of head motion during imaging. For anatomical reference, the ^{18}F-flortaucipir PET image from each subject was rigidly co-registered with the corresponding T1-weighted MR image using SPM8 [16]. FreeSurfer ROIs were mapped into the PET native space. We calculate the standardized uptake value ratio (SUVR) for each of the 112 ROIs using FreeSurfer's cerebellar gray ROI mean as the reference.

4   Results

4.1   Parameter Estimation

The model parameters α and β were computed from two time-point data for the 62-subject cohort described in Sect. 3.2. Figure 2 shows the differential aggregation of tau across the two time-points averaged over the cohort and split into propagative and generative components. Tau aggregation in disparate regions of the brain is differently impacted by the diffusive spread vs. generative buildup.

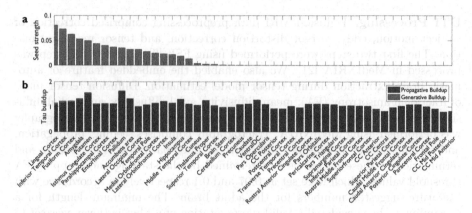

Fig. 2. Tau seeding and spread at different ROIs. (a) Spatially sparse sources (localized seeds) identified by the network diffusion model sorted in descending order of strength. (b) The corresponding relative extents of tau buildup in different anatomical ROIs via spread alone (propagative buildup) and seeding-induced spread (generative buildup).

Consistent with our understanding of early AD, some of the strongest seeding effects were observed in several medial temporal areas such as the inferior temporal lobe, fusiform gyrus, entorhinal cortex, and the parahippocampal gyrus. Several limbic and subcortical regions also exhibited prominent roles in tau seeding.

4.2   Model Validation

Model parameters estimated for the 62-subject-group were validated using an independent group of 10 subjects. This validation dataset contained ^{18}F-flortaucipir PET scans at three distinct time-points (t_1, t_2, t_3). α and β computed from the 62-subject dataset were used to predict tau at t_2 from tau at t_1 and tau at t_3 from tau at t_2 for the 10-subject dataset. Figure 3 shows predicted vs. observed scatter plots for time-point combinations (t_1, t_2) and (t_2, t_3). Table 1 shows goodness-of-fit measures for the predicted vs. observed data, including the sum of squares due to error (SSE), R^2, adjusted R^2, and root-mean-square error (RMSE). Our results indicate high prediction accuracy for (t_1, t_2) and diminished accuracy for (t_2, t_3).

Table 1. Model validation: goodness-of-fit between predicted and observed tau

Time-points	SSE	R^2	Adjusted R^2	RMSE
(t_1, t_2)	5.449	0.8803	0.8802	0.0698
(t_2, t_3)	19.24	0.6207	0.6204	0.1312

a

b

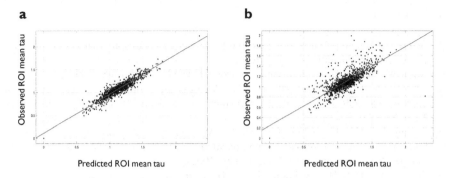

Fig. 3. Scatter plots showing predicted vs. observed ROI mean tau values. (a) Tau at time-point t_2 predicted from tau at time-point t_1. (b) Tau at time-point t_3 predicted from tau at time-point t_2. Linear regression lines are shown in blue. (Color figure online)

5 Conclusion

We presented here a macroscopic model of tau spread and seeding based on structural networks derived from DTI and longitudinal tau measures based on ^{18}F-flortaucipir PET. The model relies on a linearized solution to the network diffusion equation and incorporates a spatially sparse source term capturing network-independent seeding. The model parameters were computed using data from 62 HABS subjects with diffusion MR data and two time-point ^{18}F-flortaucipir PET data. The fitted model parameters were validated on an independent group of 10 subjects with longitudinal ^{18}F-flortaucipir PET available at three time-points. The parametric model identified strong network-independent seeding in several anatomical areas believed to play prominent roles in preclinical AD.

One key limitation of the existing implementation is that it is based on a linear approximation motivated by the availability of only two temporal samples in the longitudinal tau PET study. Since the model parameters were estimated for an early cross-section of the preclinical AD population, the model's accuracy is expected to diminish for later disease stages. The model exhibited higher accuracy when applied to data from the first two time-points of the validation dataset. As expected, the accuracy was lower for data from the second and third time-points. It is understandable that, for these cases, the approximate linear model exhibits a greater divergence relative to the original exponential model.

We have demonstrated the effectiveness of a network diffusion approach to model and predict tau aggregation based on structural connectivity. Our model identified distinct patterns of network-based propagative and network-independent generative buildup of tau in an elderly cohort. Our future work would involve extending this implementation to fit a piecewise linear model to three time-point datasets as they gradually become available in greater numbers for the HABS cohort.

References

1. Ahmed, Z., et al.: A novel in vivo model of tau propagation with rapid and progressive neurofibrillary tangle pathology: the pattern of spread is determined by connectivity, not proximity. Acta Neuropathol. **127**(5), 667–683 (2014)
2. Andersson, J.L.R., Sotiropoulos, S.N.: An integrated approach to correction for off-resonance effects and subject movement in diffusion MR imaging. Neuroimage **125**, 1063–1078 (2016)
3. Arriagada, P.V., Growdon, J.H., Hedley-Whyte, E.T., Hyman, B.T.: Neurofibrillary tangles but not senile plaques parallel duration and severity of Alzheimer's disease. Neurology **42**(3 Pt 1), 631–639 (1992)
4. Dagley, A., et al.: Harvard aging brain study: dataset and accessibility. Neuroimage **144**(Pt B), 255–258 (2017)
5. Frost, B., Diamond, M.I.: Prion-like mechanisms in neurodegenerative diseases. Nat. Rev. Neurosci. **11**(3), 155–159 (2010)
6. Holmes, B.B., et al.: Proteopathic tau seeding predicts tauopathy in vivo. Proc. Natl. Acad. Sci. USA **111**(41), E4376–4385 (2014)
7. Hu, C., Hua, X., Ying, J., Thompson, P.M., Fakhri, G.E., Li, Q.: Localizing sources of brain disease progression with network diffusion model. IEEE J. Sel. Top. Sig. Process. **10**(7), 1214–1225 (2016)
8. Hyman, B.T., et al.: National Institute on Aging-Alzheimer's Association guidelines for the neuropathologic assessment of Alzheimer's disease. Alzheimers Dement. **8**(1), 1–13 (2012)
9. Johnson, K.A., et al.: Tau positron emission tomographic imaging in aging and early Alzheimer disease. Ann. Neurol. **79**(1), 110–119 (2016)
10. Kaufman, S.K., Del Tredici, K., Thomas, T.L., Braak, H., Diamond, M.I.: Tau seeding activity begins in the transentorhinal/entorhinal regions and anticipates phospho-tau pathology in Alzheimer's disease and PART. Acta Neuropathol. **136**(1), 57–67 (2018)
11. Lace, G., et al.: Hippocampal tau pathology is related to neuroanatomical connections: an ageing population-based study. Brain **132**(Pt 5), 1324–1334 (2009)
12. Lee, S.J., Desplats, P., Sigurdson, C., Tsigelny, I., Masliah, E.: Cell-to-cell transmission of non-prion protein aggregates. Nat. Rev. Neurol. **6**(12), 702–706 (2010)
13. Nussbaum, J.M., et al.: Prion-like behaviour and tau-dependent cytotoxicity of pyroglutamylated amyloid-β. Nature **485**(7400), 651–655 (2012)
14. Nussbaum, J.M., Seward, M.E., Bloom, G.S.: Alzheimer disease: a tale of two prions. Prion **7**(1), 14–19 (2013)
15. Ossenkoppele, R., et al.: Tau PET patterns mirror clinical and neuroanatomical variability in Alzheimer's disease. Brain **139**(Pt 5), 1551–1567 (2016)
16. Penny, W.D., Friston, K.J., Ashburner, J.T., Kiebel, S.J., Nichols, T.E.: Statistical Parametric Mapping: The Analysis of Functional Brain Images. Elsevier, Amsterdam (2011)
17. Raj, A., Kuceyeski, A., Weiner, M.: A network diffusion model of disease progression in dementia. Neuron **73**(6), 1204–1215 (2012)
18. Raj, A., LoCastro, E., Kuceyeski, A., Tosun, D., Relkin, N., Weiner, M.: Network diffusion model of progression predicts longitudinal patterns of atrophy and Metabolism in Alzheimer's disease. Cell Rep. **10**, 359–369 (2015)
19. Schwarz, A.J., et al.: Regional profiles of the candidate tau PET ligand 18F-AV-1451 recapitulate key features of Braak histopathological stages. Brain **139**(5), 1539–1550 (2016)

20. Shoup, T.M., et al.: A concise radiosynthesis of the tau radiopharmaceutical, [(18) F]T807. J. Labelled Comp. Radiopharm. **56**(14), 736–740 (2013)
21. Toussaint, N., Souplet, J.C., Fillard, P.: MedINRIA: medical image navigation and research tool by INRIA. In: Medical Image Computing and Computer Assisted Intervention, vol. 7 (2007)

Accurate Nuclear Segmentation with Center Vector Encoding

Jiahui Li, Zhiqiang Hu$^{(\boxtimes)}$, and Shuang Yang

SenseTime Research, Beijing, China
{lijiahui,huzhiqiang,yangshuang1}@sensetime.com

Abstract. Nuclear segmentation is important and frequently demanded for pathology image analysis, yet is also challenging due to nuclear crowdedness and possible occlusion. In this paper, we present a novel bottom-up method for nuclear segmentation. The concepts of Center Mask and Center Vector are introduced to better depict the relationship between pixels and nuclear instances. The instance differentiation process are thus largely simplified and easier to understand. Experiments demonstrate the effectiveness of Center Vector Encoding, where our method outperforms state-of-the-arts by a clear margin.

1 Introduction

Pathology has long been regarded as the gold standard for medical diagnosis, especially cancer-related diagnosis. Nuclear segmentation is one of the most important and frequently demanded tasks of pathology image analysis, acting as the building block for nuclear statistical analysis such as size, density, counts, etc., which in turn contribute to cancer grading, therapy planning and outcome prediction. On the other hand, nuclear segmentation is laborious, tedious, and prone to errors for manual processing, and challenging for automatic methods due to nuclear crowdedness and possible occlusion.

Nuclear segmentation aims to segment out the nuclear areas from the backgrounds, as well as differentiate nuclear instances. The task can be well formulated as an instance segmentation problem. For the instance segmentation problem, there are two main frameworks, namely top-down and bottom-up. The top-down framework begins by localizing object instances, commonly in the form of bounding boxes, and then performs the segmentation within the bounding box. Mask R-CNN and its variants [4,9,13] are of the state-of-the-art top-down models. The bottom-up framework, on the contrary, performs the semantic segmentation on the whole image firstly, and differentiate instances with post-processing based on prior knowledge about the objects [3,5,8,19]. With the incorporation of prior knowledge, the bottom-up methods are challenging to design, but may perform better than general-purpose top-down counterparts.

In this work we focus on bottom-up methods. Among the previous works [1,2, 6,10–12,16–18,20–22,24–26], Xing et al. [21] proposed a two-class Convolutional Neural Network (CNN) based method for the first-step semantic segmentation

© Springer Nature Switzerland AG 2019
A. C. S. Chung et al. (Eds.): IPMI 2019, LNCS 11492, pp. 394–404, 2019.
https://doi.org/10.1007/978-3-030-20351-1_30

that predicts inside and outside mask, and differentiate nuclear instances by carefully-designed distance transform and region growth. However, the method suffers from under-segmentation, especially for crowded nuclei. As a follow-up, Kumar et al. [11] extended the model to a three-class CNN, which predicts boundary mask in addition to inside and outside mask. They also proposed an anisotropic region growth method for instance differentiation, based on estimated probabilities in the three masks. Despite the decent improvement compared with Xing et al. [21], the Kumar et al. [11] method has at least three limitations:

1. A simple boundary mask takes limited advantage of overall information. For example, distance information is not explicitly modeled.
2. The boundary targets during training are sensitive to the nuclear annotations. Different annotators may deliver slightly different annotations even for the same nucleus, but in this case the boundaries will become totally different. Since the annotations can never be perfect, the sensitivity will make the model harder to learn.
3. The instance differentiation process is complex. Multiple thresholds are applied to control the region growth algorithm. The process behaves more like ad-hoc rules and is hard to tune and understand.

In this paper, we propose a novel method for nuclear segmentation that overcomes the aformentioned shortcomings. As shown in Fig. 1, our method begins by Fully Convolutional Neural Network (FCN) [14,15] for semantic segmentation. Instead of predicting boundaries, our method estimates the Center Mask, Center Vector, as well as the common Inside Mask. The Center Mask encodes the center regions of nuclei, the target of which during training is generated by morphological operations and distance thresholding. The Center Vector, on the other hand, encodes for each inside-nucleus pixel the relative displacement with respect to the centers. It contains two channels, for horizontal and vertical directions respectively. During inference, the center region of each nuclear instance is firstly derived by applying connected component analysis to the predicted Center Mask, and then each inside-nucleus pixel (predicted by Inside Mask after some processing) is assigned to a center region according to the predicted Center Vector. Pixels with Center Vector not pointing to any center region are assigned to the nearest center region. Finally we refine the Instance Mask, for example filling the holes, to remove the artifacts.

Compared with Kumar et al. [11], the concept of Center Vector in our method takes into consideration the distance with respect to the centers, instead of the dichotomous boundary labels, so we utilize more information for the model to separate touching nuclei. Also, our method is less sensitive to the annotations. For slighted perturbed annotations, only a tiny fraction of Center Vector targets will be affected, and the model can still learn well based on the majority of correct supervisions. Lastly, the Center Vector guides the pixels to find its center. The relationship between pixels and nuclear instances is clear with the concept of Center Vector. The process is straightforward, easier to understand and implement.

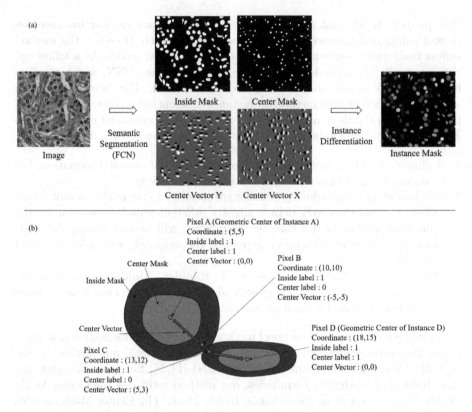

Fig. 1. (a) Overview of our framework: We apply Fully Convolutional Neural Network (FCN) for semantic segmentation and predicts Inside Mask, Center Mask and Center Vector, which are then utilized in instance differentiation to generate Instance Mask. (b) Illustration of Center Mask and Center Vector. Center Mask encodes the center region of nuclei, while Center Vector encodes the relative displacement of each inside-nucleus pixel with respect to the corresponding center.

We perform extensive experiments on the dataset released by Kumar et al. [11]. The quantitative results demonstrate the superiority of our method in performance. Our method outperforms state-of-the-arts by a clear margin. We also conduct ablation studies to investigate the benefits gained by introducing Center Vector, both in training phase and in inference phase. Finally, we show qualitative results to give an insight why the proposed pipeline is better than a boundary-prediction method.

Our contributions are summarized as follows:

1. We introduce the concepts of Center Mask and Center Vector to better depict the relationship between pixels and nuclear instances.
2. Based on the Center Vector Encoding, we present a pipeline for nuclear segmentation, easy to understand and implement.

3. Our model achieves state-of-the-art performance in the challenging dataset released by Kumar et al. [11]. Besides, experiments demonstrate the benefits of Center Vector for better instance differentiation.

2   Center Vector Encoding

As shown in Fig. 1(a), the entire pipeline consists of two parts: semantic segmentation and instance differentiation. We apply Fully Convolutional Neural Network (FCN) [14] for semantic segmentation and predicts Inside Mask, Center Mask and Center Vector, which are then utilized in instance differentiation to generate Instance Mask.

2.1   Center Mask and Center Vector in Semantic Segmentation

Center Mask and Center Vector are the core concepts of our work. The Center Mask encodes the center regions of nuclei. The target center region of a nuclear instance during training is calculated as follows: The instance mask for the nuclear instance is firstly processed with morphological erosion, and then we calculate the distance from each pixel to the boundary in the eroded mask, and take as the center region those pixels with distance larger than a threshold. The operations mainly aim to ensure center regions of touching nuclei to separate.

The Center Vector, on the other hand, encodes the relative displacement of each inside-nucleus pixel with respect to the corresponding center. The center C_i for a nuclear instance i is defined as the geometric center of the instance mask, and is denoted as $C_i = \left(\tilde{X}_i, \tilde{Y}_i\right)$. For each pixel $P_{ij} = (X_{ij}, Y_{ij})$ within the instance i, the Center Vector ΔP_{ij} of the pixel is defined as

$$\Delta P_{ij} = P_{ij} - C_i = \left(X_{ij} - \tilde{X}_i, Y_{ij} - \tilde{Y}_i\right) \tag{1}$$

For pixels not belonging to any nuclear instance, i.e. the backgrounds, the Center Vector is not defined, and the corresponding loss is ignored during training. See Fig. 1(b) for an illustration of the concepts of Center Mask and Center Vector.

Compared with boundary encoding [11], the Center Vector encodes the distance between pixels and centers instead of the dichotomous boundary labels, and thus contains richer information. The Center Vector is smooth inside a nuclear instance, making it easier for the model to learn, but changes sharply in the boundary areas, especially in the boundary of touching nuclei, forcing the model to pay more attention to the boundaries. Moreover, Center Vector is less sensitive to the annotation perturbation. Even if annotation areas are slightly enlarged or reduced, for example due to different annotation styles by different annotators, only a tiny fraction of Center Vector targets will be affected, and the model can still learn well based on the majority of correct supervision.

Finally, the Inside Mask simply contains all the foreground pixels – pixels within the overall region of some nuclear instance. For an input image, the Inside Mask and Center Mask are of the same shape as the image, with 1 channel each in the semantic segmentation output; Center Vector contains 2 channels for horizontal and vertical directions respectively, and is also of the same shape as the input image.

2.2   Instance Differentiation

During inference, the semantic segmentation model outputs three kind of prediction: Inside Mask, Center Mask and Center Vector, from which we will derive the final Instance Mask. To this end, we firstly perform the connected component analysis to the Inside Mask, and remove regions which have no intersection with Center Mask. This serves as a kind of false positive suppression. On the other hand, we also perform the connected component analysis to the Center Mask, and takes each resulting region as the center region of one nuclear instance. Finally we will assign pixels in the false-positive-suppressed Inside Mask to the center regions: Pixels in the Center Mask are directly assigned to the corresponding center region without considering the Center Vector; For pixels not in the Center Mask but in the Inside Mask, we assign them to the center region their Center Vector points to, or the nearest center region in case that their Center Vector does not point to any valid center region. Minor refinement are applied afterwards, for example filling the holes, to remove the artifacts.

With the concepts of Center Mask and Center Vector, the instance differentiation process is straightforward and easy to understand. To summarize, the Center Mask represents the center region of each nuclear instance, while the Center Vector links the pixels to the corresponding center regions.

3   Experiments

3.1   Implementations

It is worthy noting that our method does not rely on any particular network architecture for the semantic segmentation model. For implementation we use Deep Layer Aggregation (DLA) [23] for the network architecture in this paper. DLA extends common network structures with deep aggregations. The term deep aggregation refers to aggregations that are nonlinear, compositional and going through multiple stages. DLA introduces two types of deep aggregations: Iterative Deep Aggregation and Hierarchical Deep Aggregation. Iterative Deep Aggregation merges layers iteratively, while Hierarchical Deep Aggregation aggregates layers in a tree-like hierarchical manner. With these two types of deep aggregations, the network can better fuse information from multiple layers and scales, and thus achieves better performance in various classification and segmentation problems. Figure 2 illustrates the Iterative Deep Aggregation and Hierarchical Deep Aggregation introduced by DLA.

For the loss function, we utilize a combination of pixel-wise cross entropy (CE) loss and Intersection-Over-Union (IOU) loss for the optimization of Inside Mask (IM) and Center Mask (CM) estimation. For Center Vector (CV, with

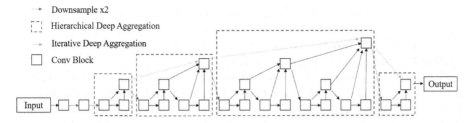

Fig. 2. Illustration of the Iterative Deep Aggregation and Hierarchical Deep Aggregation introduced by Deep Layer Aggregation. Iterative Deep Aggregation merges layers iteratively, while Hierarchical Deep Aggregation aggregates layers in a tree-like hierarchical manner.

CV_X and CV_Y for two directions) with continuous target values, we apply pixelwise mean square (MS) loss. Please see (2), (3), and (4) for detailed formulations, where y_i and p_i are targets and predictions for pixel i respectively, i.e., class labels/probabilities for CE and IOU loss but distance targets/estimations for MS loss. Finally, the total loss is a weighted summation of all the aforementioned losses, as shown in (5), where α, β, γ are the balancing parameters.

$$l_{CE} = \sum_{S\in\{IM,CM\}} \sum_{i\in S} y_i \log(p_i) + (1 - y_i)\log(1 - p_i) \tag{2}$$

$$l_{IOU} = \sum_{S\in\{IM,CM\}} 1 - \frac{\sum_{i\in S} y_i p_i}{\sum_{i\in S} y_i + \sum_{i\in S} p_i - \sum_{i\in S} y_i p_i} \tag{3}$$

$$l_{MS} = \sum_{S\in\{CV_X,CV_Y\}} \sum_{i\in S} (p_i - y_i)^2 \tag{4}$$

$$l = \alpha l_{CE} + \beta l_{IOU} + \gamma l_{MS} \tag{5}$$

We use DLA-34 for the model. The model is implemented in Pytorch 0.4. We train the model for 2000 epochs. Using SGD as the optimizer, learning rate is initially set as 0.01 and decayed polynomially. Batchsize is 4 and weight decay is 0.0001. In loss function we set $\alpha = 10$, $\beta = 10$, $\gamma = 1$ to balance different losses.

3.2   Dataset and Evaluation Metric

We perform extensive experiments on the dataset released by Kumar et al. [11] to evaluate the proposed method. The dataset consists of 30 Hematoxylin and Eosin (H&E) stained images, all of which are of the size 1000×1000 pixels. Nuclear instances are carefully annotated so as to generate the instance mask for each image. The images come from multiple organs: 4 organs (breast, kidney, liver and prostate) have 6 images each, while another 3 organs (bladder, colon and stomach) have 2 images each. Following the same principle as Kumar et al. [11], that is test data must contain images from organs never seen in train data, we sample 4 images from each of 4 majority-class organs (breast, kidney, liver and prostate), a set of 16 images in total for training and put the rest for test. The multi-organ diversity and zero-shot setting make the problem even more challenging, but closer to clinical practice.

The performance of nuclear segmentation solutions is evaluated based on the metric Aggregated Jaccard Index (AJI) [11]. AJI penalizes both segmentation errors and instance differentiation errors, and is a balancing metric for a comprehensive evaluation. We summarize the AJI calculation steps listed in [11] as the Eq. (6), where $\{G_i\}_{i=1}^M$ and $\{P_j\}_{j=1}^N$ denote the set of annotated nuclei and predicted nuclei, respectively; $f(i) = \mathrm{argmax}_j |G_i \bigcap P_j| / |G_i \bigcup P_j|$ assigns best-match prediction to each annotated nuclear instance; $[N] = \{1, 2, ..., N\}$ and $f([N]) = \{f(1), f(2), ..., f(N)\}$ are convenient notations.

$$\text{AJI} = \frac{\sum_{i=1}^M |G_i \bigcap P_{f(i)}|}{\sum_{i=1}^M |G_i \bigcup P_{f(i)}| + \sum_{j \in [N] \setminus f([M])} |P_j|} \tag{6}$$

$$\text{IOU} = \frac{|G \bigcap P|}{|G \bigcup P|} \tag{7}$$

$$\text{Dice} = \frac{2|G \bigcap P|}{|G| + |P|} \tag{8}$$

To investigate the error modes, we also apply two metrics originally designed for the semantic segmentation task: Intersection-Over-Union (IOU) and Dice. Please refer to (7) and (8) for detailed formulations, where $G = \bigcup_{i=1}^M G_i$ and $P = \bigcup_{j=1}^N P_j$ are the global annotations and predictions, respectively. Note that IOU is the upper bound of AJI: We have

$$\sum_{i=1}^M |G_i \bigcap P_{f(i)}| \leq |G \bigcap P| \tag{9}$$

and

$$\sum_{i=1}^M |G_i \bigcup P_{f(i)}| + \sum_{j \in [N] \setminus f([M])} |P_j| \geq |G \bigcup P| \tag{10}$$

leading to

$$\text{AJI} = \frac{\sum_{i=1}^M |G_i \bigcap P_{f(i)}|}{\sum_{i=1}^M |G_i \bigcup P_{f(i)}| + \sum_{j \in [N] \setminus f([M])} |P_j|} \leq \frac{|G \bigcap P|}{|G \bigcup P|} = \text{IOU} \tag{11}$$

Dice is yet the upper bound of IOU. As a result, the metrics IOU and Dice can be used for distinguishing instance differentiation errors from segmentation errors.

3.3   Results

In Table 1 we show the performance comparison of our method against state-of-the-art methods: CNN2 [21] for two-class CNN (Inside, Outside) and CNN3 [11] for three-class CNN (Inside, Outside, Boundary). We omit IOU scores since they are not reported in the literature. From the comparison it is clear to see that our method outperforms the state-of-the-arts by a large margin, both with respect to the instance-level AJI metric and with respect to the segmentation-level Dice metric.

We also perform ablation studies to investigate the benefits gained from the design. We train the semantic segmentation model to predict Inside Mask and Center Mask only, and differentiate instances by Random Walker [7] seeded with center regions derived from Center Mask predictions. We term this setting as V1. Further for the setting V2, we add Center Vector supervisions during training,

Table 1. Performance comparison of our method against state-of-the-art methods: CNN2 [21] for two-class CNN (Inside, Outside) and CNN3 [11] for three-class CNN (Inside, Outside, Boundary).

Organs	AJI			Dice		
	CNN2	CNN3	Ours	CNN2	CNN3	Ours
Breast	0.425	0.538	0.601	0.646	0.718	0.819
Liver	0.371	0.516	0.601	0.610	0.688	0.797
Kidney	0.407	0.508	0.487	0.656	0.722	0.737
Prostate	0.228	0.573	0.615	0.704	0.792	0.792
Bladder	0.319	0.437	0.557	0.715	0.781	0.815
Colon	0.308	0.521	0.452	0.664	0.739	0.745
Stomach	0.379	0.446	0.612	0.855	0.895	0.848
Overall	0.348	0.508	**0.561**	0.693	0.762	**0.793**

Table 2. Results of ablation studies. Center Vector is not utilized in V1, only during training in V2, and both during training and inference in V3. We add results from CNN3 [11] for comparison.

Organs	AJI				IOU				Dice			
	CNN3	V1	V2	V3	CNN3	V1	V2	V3	CNN3	V1	V2	V3
Breast	0.538	0.597	0.595	0.601	None	0.699	0.677	0.694	0.718	0.822	0.807	0.819
Liver	0.516	0.598	0.573	0.601	None	0.672	0.646	0.663	0.688	0.803	0.784	0.797
Kidney	0.508	0.496	0.483	0.487	None	0.606	0.574	0.585	0.722	0.754	0.727	0.737
Prostate	0.573	0.600	0.626	0.615	None	0.645	0.648	0.655	0.792	0.784	0.786	0.792
Bladder	0.437	0.504	0.544	0.557	None	0.673	0.677	0.693	0.781	0.799	0.803	0.815
Colon	0.521	0.441	0.437	0.452	None	0.614	0.560	0.594	0.739	0.763	0.717	0.745
Stomach	0.446	0.558	0.593	0.612	None	0.734	0.717	0.736	0.895	0.846	0.835	0.848
Overall	0.508	0.542	0.550	**0.561**	None	**0.664**	0.663	0.663	0.762	**0.794**	0.791	0.793

but we ignore the Center Vector output during inference and also apply Random Walker [7]. In this case, Center Vector serves as a way to facilitate training. Finally the setting V3 is the entire method we describe above, where Center Vector is utilized both in training and during inference.

Table 2 shows the results of ablation studies. We add results from CNN3 [11] for comparison. The performance gain of V1 from CNN3 [11] mainly attributes to the better Deep Layer Aggregation (DLA) [23] architecture. Comparing V1, V2 and V3, the AJI score is increasing, which demonstrates the effectiveness of Center Vector, both in training and during inference. However, the IOU and Dice scores are largely comparable for V1, V2 and V3, showing that Center Vector works mainly from suppressing errors in the instance differentiation step.

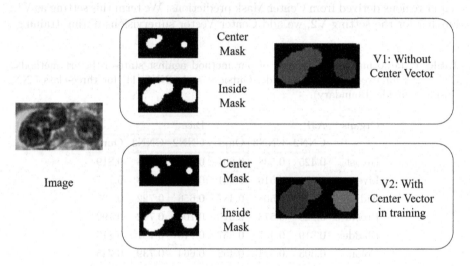

Fig. 3. Qualitative results from V1 and V2: The V2 model, with Center Vector during training, learns to better separate touching nuclei in the Center Mask.

We also display some qualitative results to give an insight why Center Vector is effective, as shown in Figs. 3 and 4. Figure 3 compares qualitative results from V1 and V2. The V2 model, with Center Vector during training, learns to better separate touching nuclei in the Center Mask, showing that Center Vector supervision guides the model to concentrate more in the center regions and learn better Center Mask estimation. On the other hand, Fig. 4 compares V2 with V3, where the models differ only in the instance differentiation step. It can be seen that Random Walker method in V2 tends to separate touching nuclei with a "straight cut" while Center Vector generates more natural and realistic boundaries.

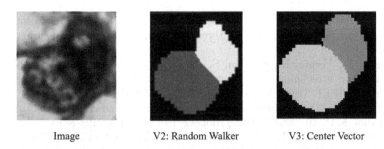

Image   V2: Random Walker   V3: Center Vector

Fig. 4. Qualitative results from V2 and V3: Random Walker method in V2 tends to separate touching nuclei with a "straight cut" while Center Vector generates more natural and realistic boundaries.

4 Conclusion

We present a novel bottom-up method for nuclear segmentation. The concepts of Center Mask and Center Vector are introduced to better depict the relationship between pixels and nuclear instances. Based on the Center Vector Encoding, we develop a pipeline for nuclear segmentation, easy to understand and implement. Experiments demonstrate the effectiveness of Center Vector Encoding, where our method outperforms state-of-the-arts by a clear margin.

References

1. Arbelle, A., Raviv, T.R.: Microscopy cell segmentation via adversarial neural networks. In: 2018 IEEE 15th International Symposium on Biomedical Imaging, ISBI 2018, pp. 645–648. IEEE (2018)
2. Bamford, P.: Automating cell segmentation evaluation with annotated examples. In: APRS Workshop on Digital Image Computing, pp. 21–25 (2003)
3. Belsare, A., Mushrif, M., Pangarkar, M.: Breast epithelial duct region segmentation using intuitionistic fuzzy based multi-texture image map. In: 2017 14th IEEE India Council International Conference (INDICON), pp. 1–6. IEEE (2017)
4. Chen, L.C., Hermans, A., Papandreou, G., Schroff, F., Wang, P., Adam, H.: MaskLab: instance segmentation by refining object detection with semantic and direction features. arXiv preprint arXiv:1712.04837 2 (2018)
5. Cui, Y., Zhang, G., Liu, Z., Xiong, Z., Hu, J.: A deep learning algorithm for one-step contour aware nuclei segmentation of histopathological images. CoRR abs/1803.02786. http://arxiv.org/abs/1803.02786 (2018)
6. Fu, D., Xie, X.S.: Reliable cell segmentation based on spectral phasor analysis of hyperspectral stimulated raman scattering imaging data. Anal. Chem. **86**(9), 4115–4119 (2014)
7. Grady, L.: Random walks for image segmentation. IEEE Trans. Pattern Anal. Mach. Intell. **28**(11), 1768–1783 (2006)
8. Gurcan, M.N., Boucheron, L., Can, A., Madabhushi, A., Rajpoot, N., Yener, B.: Histopathological image analysis: a review. IEEE Rev. Biomed. Eng. **2**, 147 (2009)
9. He, K., Gkioxari, G., Dollár, P., Girshick, R.: Mask R-CNN. In: 2017 IEEE International Conference on Computer Vision (ICCV), pp. 2980–2988. IEEE (2017)

10. Ho, D.J., Fu, C., Salama, P., Dunn, K.W., Delp, E.J.: Nuclei segmentation of fluorescence microscopy images using three dimensional convolutional neural networks (2017)
11. Kumar, N., Verma, R., Sharma, S., Bhargava, S., Vahadane, A., Sethi, A.: A dataset and a technique for generalized nuclear segmentation for computational pathology. IEEE Trans. Med. Imaging **36**(7), 1550–1560 (2017)
12. Li, G., et al.: 3D cell nuclei segmentation based on gradient flow tracking. BMC Cell Biol. **8**(1), 40 (2007). https://doi.org/10.1186/1471-2121-8-40
13. Liu, S., Qi, L., Qin, H., Shi, J., Jia, J.: Path aggregation network for instance segmentation. CoRR abs/1803.01534. http://arxiv.org/abs/1803.01534 (2018)
14. Long, J., Shelhamer, E., Darrell, T.: Fully convolutional networks for semantic segmentation. In: Proceedings of the IEEE Conference on Computer Vision and Pattern Recognition, pp. 3431–3440 (2015)
15. Ronneberger, O., Fischer, P., Brox, T.: U-Net: convolutional networks for biomedical image segmentation. CoRR abs/1505.04597. http://arxiv.org/abs/1505.04597 (2015)
16. Sadanandan, S.K., Ranefall, P., Le Guyader, S., Wählby, C.: Automated training of deep convolutional neural networks for cell segmentation. Sci. Rep. **7**(1), 7860 (2017)
17. Stegmaier, J., et al.: Cell segmentation in 3D confocal images using supervoxel merge-forests with CNN-based hypothesis selection. In: 2018 IEEE 15th International Symposium on Biomedical Imaging, ISBI 2018, pp. 382–386. IEEE (2018)
18. Su, H., Yin, Z., Huh, S., Kanade, T.: Cell segmentation in phase contrast microscopy images via semi-supervised classification over optics-related features. Med. Image Anal. **17**(7), 746–765 (2013)
19. Wang, P., Hu, X., Li, Y., Liu, Q., Zhu, X.: Automatic cell nuclei segmentation and classification of breast cancer histopathology images. Sig. Process. **122**, 1–13 (2016)
20. Wang, Z., Li, H.: Generalizing cell segmentation and quantification. BMC Bioinform. **18**(1), 189 (2017)
21. Xing, F., Xie, Y., Yang, L.: An automatic learning-based framework for robust nucleus segmentation. IEEE Trans. Med. Imaging **35**(2), 550–566 (2016)
22. Yin, Z., Bise, R., Chen, M., Kanade, T.: Cell segmentation in microscopy imagery using a bag of local Bayesian classifiers. In: 2010 IEEE International Symposium on Biomedical Imaging: From Nano to Macro, pp. 125–128. IEEE (2010)
23. Yu, F., Wang, D., Shelhamer, E., Darrell, T.: Deep layer aggregation. arXiv preprint arXiv:1707.06484 (2017)
24. Zhang, X., Liu, W., Dundar, M., Badve, S., Zhang, S.: Towards large-scale histopathological image analysis: Hashing-based image retrieval. IEEE Trans. Med. Imaging **34**(2), 496–506 (2015)
25. Zhang, X., Xing, F., Su, H., Yang, L., Zhang, S.: High-throughput histopathological image analysis via robust cell segmentation and hashing. Med. Image Anal. **26**(1), 306–315 (2015)
26. Zhou, Y., Kuijper, A., Heise, B., He, L.: Cell segmentation using level set method. NA (2007)

Bayesian Longitudinal Modeling of Early Stage Parkinson's Disease Using DaTscan Images

Yuan Zhou[1]([✉]) and Hemant D. Tagare[1,2]

[1] Department of Radiology and Biomedical Imaging, Yale University,
New Haven, CT 06510, USA
zhouyuanzxcv@gmail.com
[2] Department of Biomedical Engineering, Yale University,
New Haven, CT 06520, USA

Abstract. This paper proposes a disease progression model for early stage Parkinson's Disease (PD) based on DaTscan images. The model has two novel aspects: first, the model is fully coupled across the two caudates and putamina. Second, the model uses a new constraint called *model mirror symmetry* (MMS). A full Bayesian analysis, with collapsed Gibbs sampling using conjugate priors, is used to obtain posterior samples of the model parameters. The model identifies PD progression subtypes and reveals novel fast modes of PD progression.

Keywords: Parkinson's Disease · Disease progression model · Bayesian analysis

1 Introduction

Parkinson's Disease (PD) is a common neurodegenerative disease characterized by loss of dopaminergic neurons, and accompanied by progressively worsening clinical motor and non-motor symptoms. PD is also a heterogeneous disease; it exhibits vastly different rates of progression in different subjects.

DaTscan imaging is the commercial name for SPECT imaging with 123 I-FP-CIT. DaTscans measure the local density of presynaptic dopamine transporters (DaT). Dopaminergic neural loss decreases DaT density and is visible as signal loss in DaTscan images. Our goal is to model the progression of PD as it manifests in DaTscans. We use the Parkinson's Progression Marker Initiative (PPMI) dataset, described in more details in Sect. 2.

For quantitative analysis, intensity values in every voxel of a DaTscan are converted to Striatal Binding Ratios (SBR). The SBR at voxel v is defined as $SBR_v = (I_v - \mu)/\mu$, where I_v is the intensity in voxel v and μ is the mean (or median) intensity in the occipital lobe [8]. SBR is a measure of DaT density in the voxel. The sum or the mean of the SBR in a brain region is taken as a measure of DaT density in the region.

A. C. S. Chung et al. (Eds.): IPMI 2019, LNCS 11492, pp. 405–416, 2019.
https://doi.org/10.1007/978-3-030-20351-1_31

DaTscan and PD characteristics that are important in modeling early stage PD are listed below. Our model takes these characteristics into account:

1. *Disease Stages*: PD progresses along stages called Braak Stages [3]. Early stage PD affects the striatum, with the putamen affected more than the caudate.
2. *Coupled Progress*: Early stage PD is also asymmetric; one brain hemisphere is affected more than the other hemisphere [7]. As the disease progresses, the disease becomes symmetric, demonstrating a coupling between ROIs.
3. *Exponential Loss*: SBR loss in the striatum due to PD progression is approximately exponential [1,6].
4. *Heterogeneity*: PD is a heterogeneous disease, with patients progressing at different rates and exhibiting variable clinical symptoms. Different PD subtypes have been proposed using clinical symptoms (MDS-UPDRS ratings), e.g. rigidity-dominant vs. tremor-dominant [4], or early-onset vs. late-onset [13]. To the best of our knowledge, the existence of image-based progression subtypes has not yet been reported in the literature. One of our goals is to investigate such subtypes.

Besides these previously known properties, we identify a new property called *model mirror symmetry* (MMS) which is critical in reducing the dimension of the model:

1. *Model Mirror Symmetry*: Progression from the asymmetric state to the symmetric state does not depend on the hemisphere that the disease originally affected. This implies that the progression model should remain invariant if left hemisphere voxels (or regions) are swapped with right hemisphere voxels (or regions). We call this *model mirror symmetry*.

The above properties suggest that PD progression in DaTscan images can be modeled as a mixture of linear dynamical systems (LDS), where the transition matrices of the dynamical systems are constrained to be centrosymmetric. This is explained further in Sect. 3.1. We fit the model using a Bayesian methodology: collapsed Gibbs sampling (Sect. 4.1) and Bayesian model selection for the optimal number of mixture components (Sect. 4.2). Sampling avoids entrapment in spurious local maxima, a common problem in maximum-likelihood methods and the EM algorithm.

Modeling brain disease progression is a relatively new problem. Using prior knowledge (about toxic protein aggregation followed by transmission along neuronal pathways) graph theoretic approaches have been proposed for Alzheimer's disease progression, e.g. [14]. Other approaches use discrete event models or generalized linear time models for disease progression [5,9]. Regression of image features with longitudinal clinical scores are also used for disease progression modeling [17]. Most of these methods are applied to MRI images of Alzheimer's disease. DaTscans have a lower resolution than MRI images and contain very different kind of information (DaT density rather than structural information). MRI-based models are not directly applicable to DaTscans.

2   Data

The PPMI dataset has 449 early stage PD subjects. The subjects are imaged at baseline and approximately at 1, 2, 4, and 5 years out. Not all subjects have a complete time series. And the time series for different subjects has slightly different timings. The PPMI DaTscan images are registered to the MNI space; but, we did find some misregistered images in the data. We preprocessed PPMI data to eliminate subjects with only a single scan, and subjects with misregistered images (using a simple non-parametric correlation test). In the end, data from 365 subjects survived, and entered the analysis. Of these subjects, 320 subjects had 3 or more scans, 130 subjects had 4 or more scans, and 3 subjects had 5 scans.

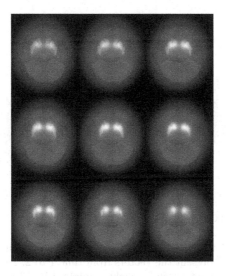

Fig. 1. Caudates (red), putamina (green), and occipital lobe (blue) ROIs superimposed on the mean baseline DaTscan image (36th - 44th slices shown). (Color figure online)

Since early stage PD mostly affects the caudate and putamen, we modeled the mean SBR in the two caudates and putamina. The MNI atlas was used to identify caudates and putamina, and manual ROI (similar to the one in [18]) was created for the occipital lobe (Fig. 1 shows these regions on 9 slices). Figure 2 shows mean SBR time series for the 365 surviving subjects. The time series for left and right caudates and the left and right putamina are shown in different plots. For each subject, the sequence of the mean SBRs are shown as blue, orange, yellow, and purple arrows which correspond to data from time 1 to 2, 2 to 3, 3 to 4, and 4 to 5 respectively. Note that, modulo noise, the data are symmetric around the 45° line. The figure shows that any model that fits well to this data should remain invariant if the "left" and "right" labels are swapped. This is model mirror symmetry.

3   Disease Progression Model

3.1   Time Series Model

The four mean SBRs are arranged in a 4 by 1 vector $\mathbf{x}$ in the order: left caudate (LC), left putamen (LP), right putamen (RP), and right caudate (RC). Note that $\mathbf{x} \in \mathbb{R}^D$ with $D = 4$. This vector is the feature we extract from every image, and our goal is to model the time series of this feature for all subjects.

Keeping in mind that SBR is known to decay exponentially in PD, a continuous time evolution model for $\mathbf{x}$ is the linear differential equation: $\frac{d\mathbf{x}}{dt} = \mathbf{A}\mathbf{x}$ where $\mathbf{A} \in \mathbb{R}^{D \times D}$. Since $\mathbf{A}$ is not required to be diagonal, this model captures coupled progression between the caudates and putamina.

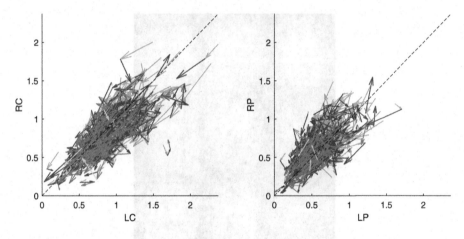

Fig. 2. Time series of the mean SBR in the caudates and putamina. Blue, orange, yellow, purple arrows represent the vectors from time 1 to 2, 2 to 3, 3 to 4, and 4 to 5 respectively. LC = left caudate, RC = right caudate, LP = left putamen, RP = right putamen. (Color figure online)

Next, we account for the fact that the longitudinal time series for each subject is discrete and not necessarily uniformly sampled in time. Letting $\mathbf{x}_{i1}, \ldots, \mathbf{x}_{iT_i}$ denote the discrete time series for the ith subject, and letting Δt_{ij} denote the difference in time between the jth and the $(j+1)$th imaging times, the differential equation can be discretized as $\frac{\mathbf{x}_{i,j+1} - \mathbf{x}_{ij}}{\Delta t_{ij}} = \mathbf{A}\mathbf{x}_{ij} + \boldsymbol{\epsilon}_{ij}$, where we assume that the noise $\boldsymbol{\epsilon}_{ij}$ has a Gaussian distribution, $\boldsymbol{\epsilon}_{ij} \sim \mathcal{N}\left(0, \sigma^2 \mathbf{I}_D\right)$. Denoting the entire time series for the subject as $\mathbf{x}_i = \{\mathbf{x}_{i1}, \mathbf{x}_{i2}, \ldots, \mathbf{x}_{iT_i}\}$, we have

$$p\left(\mathbf{x}_i | \mathbf{A}, \sigma^2\right) = p\left(\mathbf{x}_{i1}\right) \prod_{j=1}^{T_i-1} p\left(\mathbf{x}_{i,j+1} | \mathbf{x}_{i,j}, \mathbf{A}, \sigma^2\right) = \frac{p\left(\mathbf{x}_{i1}\right) e^{-\frac{1}{2\sigma^2} \sum_j \|\mathbf{v}_{ij} - \mathbf{A}\mathbf{x}_{ij}\|^2}}{(2\pi\sigma^2)^{(T_i-1)D/2} \prod_j \Delta t_{ij}^D},$$

$$(1)$$

where $\mathbf{v}_{ij} = \frac{\mathbf{x}_{i,j+1} - \mathbf{x}_{ij}}{\Delta t_{ij}}$ and $p(\mathbf{x}_{i1}) = \mathcal{N}(\mathbf{x}_{i1}|\mathbf{0}, \Sigma)$ with Σ estimated from all the $\mathbf{x}_{i1}$.

Next, we impose MMS:

Definition 1. $\pi : \mathbb{R}^D \to \mathbb{R}^D$ *is a symmetric permutation if* $(\pi(\mathbf{x}))_i = (\mathbf{x})_{D-i+1}$ *for* $i = 1, \cdots, D$, *and* $(\mathbf{x})_k$ *refers to the kth component of vector* $\mathbf{x}$. *A* $D \times D$ *matrix* $\mathbf{A}$ *is centrosymmetric if* $\pi(\mathbf{Ax}) = \mathbf{A}\pi(\mathbf{x})$ *for all* $\mathbf{x}$, *where* π *is a symmetric permutation.*

Because of how LC, LP, RP, and RC are arranged in $\mathbf{x}$, swapping right and left hemisphere ROIs corresponds to applying a symmetric permutation to $\mathbf{x}$. Thus, MMS implies that $\mathbf{A}$ should be a centrosymmetric matrix. The set of all $D \times D$ centrosymmetric matrices forms a subspace of all $D \times D$ matrices. This subspace has dimension $\lceil D^2/2 \rceil$, hence the number of parameters for fitting the data is reduced by approximately half. Also, if a centrosymmetric matrix has distinct eigenvalues, its eigenvectors are either symmetric or skew-symmetric [16]. We will see the importance of this property when interpreting results.

Let $\mathbf{e}_j$ be a vector of the form $[\ldots, 1, \ldots, 1, \ldots]^T$ where 1 only appears at the jth position and the $(D^2 - j + 1)$th position and the other components are zero. Then, any centrosymmetric matrix $\mathbf{A}$ can be represented as $\mathrm{vec}(\mathbf{A}) = \mathbf{Ea}$ where $\mathbf{E} = [\mathbf{e}_1, \ldots, \mathbf{e}_{\lceil D^2/2 \rceil}]$ is the basis and $\mathbf{a}$ contains the coordinates for expressing $\mathrm{vec}(\mathbf{A})$ in this basis. Hence, the density $p(\mathbf{x}_i|\mathbf{A}, \sigma^2)$ in (1) can be reorganized as $p(\mathbf{x}_i|\mathbf{a}, \sigma^2)$:

$$p(\mathbf{x}_i|\mathbf{a}, \sigma^2) = \frac{h_i}{\sigma^{d_i}} e^{-\frac{1}{2\sigma^2}[\mathbf{a}^T \Lambda_i \mathbf{a} - 2\mu_i^T \mathbf{a} + \epsilon_i]} \tag{2}$$

where

$$h_i = \frac{\mathcal{N}(\mathbf{x}_{i1}|\mathbf{0}, \Sigma)}{(2\pi)^{(T_i-1)D/2} \prod_{j=1}^{T_i-1} \Delta t_{ij}^D}, \quad \epsilon_i = \sum_{j=1}^{T_i-1} \mathbf{v}_{ij}^T \mathbf{v}_{ij}, \quad d_i = (T_i - 1)D,$$

$$\Lambda_i = \mathbf{E}^T \left(\sum_{j=1}^{T_i-1} \mathbf{x}_{ij}\mathbf{x}_{ij}^T \otimes \mathbf{I}_D \right) \mathbf{E}, \quad \mu_i = \mathbf{E}^T \sum_{j=1}^{T_i-1} \mathrm{vec}\left(\mathbf{v}_{ij}\mathbf{x}_{ij}^T \right). \tag{3}$$

Note that $h_i, \Lambda_i, \mu_i, \epsilon_i$ are functions of $\mathbf{x}_i$, but the dependence is not explicitly shown to simplify notation. For Bayesian analysis we will need conjugate priors for $\mathbf{a}, \sigma^2$ and a posterior predictive probability density for $\mathbf{x}$. The quadratic form for $\mathbf{a}$ in Eq. (2) is either strictly positive definite or positive semi-definite depending on the length of the time series. In either case, the density belongs to the exponential family and a conjugate prior is available [2]. For completeness, we state the conjugate prior and the posterior for the specific form in (2):

Theorem 1. *Suppose* $\mathbf{x}_i$, $i = 1, \ldots, N$ *are conditionally independent random variables, with densities given by Eq. (2) where* Λ_i *is symmetric. Then,* $\mathbf{X} = \{\mathbf{x}_1, \ldots, \mathbf{x}_N\}$ *has a conjugate prior in the form of normal-inverse-gamma (NIG)*

$$p(\mathbf{a}, \sigma^2|\mu_0, \Lambda_0, \nu_0, \kappa_0) = NIG(\mathbf{a}, \sigma^2|\mu_0, \Lambda_0, \nu_0, \kappa_0)$$
$$= \mathcal{N}(\mathbf{a}|\mu_0, \sigma^2\Lambda_0^{-1}) IG(\sigma^2|\nu_0, \kappa_0) \tag{4}$$

where Λ_0 is positive definite, and $IG(x|a,b) = \frac{b^a}{\Gamma(a)}x^{-(a+1)}e^{-\frac{b}{x}}$. Because the prior is conjugate, the posterior is also NIG

$$p\left(\mathbf{a},\sigma^2|\mathbf{X},\boldsymbol{\mu}_0,\Lambda_0,\nu_0,\kappa_0\right) = NIG\left(\mathbf{a},\sigma^2|\boldsymbol{\mu}_p,\Lambda_p,\nu_p,\kappa_p\right) \tag{5}$$

with

$$\nu_p = \nu_0 + \frac{\sum_i d_i}{2}, \; \Lambda_p = \Lambda_0 + \sum_i \Lambda_i, \; \boldsymbol{\mu}_p = \Lambda_p^{-1}\left(\Lambda_0\boldsymbol{\mu}_0 + \sum_i \boldsymbol{\mu}_i\right),$$

$$\kappa_p = \kappa_0 + \frac{1}{2}\left(\boldsymbol{\mu}_0^T\Lambda_0\boldsymbol{\mu}_0 + \sum_i \epsilon_i - \boldsymbol{\mu}_p^T\Lambda_p\boldsymbol{\mu}_p\right).$$

In Eq. (4), $\boldsymbol{\mu}_0,\Lambda_0,\nu_0,\kappa_0$ are parameters of the prior (hyperparameters). We jointly refer to them as $\boldsymbol{\beta} = \{\boldsymbol{\mu}_0,\Lambda_0,\nu_0,\kappa_0\}$. A direct consequence of Theorem 1 is that the posterior predictive distribution has a closed form:

Corollary 1. *Suppose* $\mathbf{x}_{N+1}$ *has density given by Eq. (2) where* Λ_{N+1} *is symmetric. Then, the posterior predictive density of* $\mathbf{x}_{N+1}$ *given* $\mathbf{X} = \{\mathbf{x}_1,\ldots,\mathbf{x}_N\}$ *is*

$$p\left(\mathbf{x}_{N+1}|\mathbf{X},\boldsymbol{\beta}\right) = \int\int p\left(\mathbf{x}_{N+1}|\mathbf{a},\sigma^2\right)p\left(\mathbf{a},\sigma^2|\mathbf{X},\boldsymbol{\mu}_0,\Lambda_0,\nu_0,\kappa_0\right)d\mathbf{a}d\sigma^2$$

$$= \frac{|\Lambda_p|^{\frac{1}{2}}}{|\Lambda_p + \Lambda_{N+1}|^{\frac{1}{2}}}\frac{\Gamma\left(\nu_p + \frac{d_{N+1}}{2}\right)}{\Gamma(\nu_p)}\frac{h_{N+1}}{\kappa_p^{\frac{d_{N+1}}{2}}}\left[1 + \frac{Q}{2\kappa_p}\right]^{-\left(\nu_p + \frac{d_{N+1}}{2}\right)} \tag{6}$$

where
$$Q = \boldsymbol{\mu}_p^T\Lambda_p\boldsymbol{\mu}_p + \epsilon_{N+1} - \left(\Lambda_p\boldsymbol{\mu}_p + \boldsymbol{\mu}_{N+1}\right)^T\left(\Lambda_p + \Lambda_{N+1}\right)^{-1}\left(\Lambda_p\boldsymbol{\mu}_p + \boldsymbol{\mu}_{N+1}\right).$$

3.2   Heterogeneity and Mixture Models

The above model holds for all the subjects satisfying a single differential equation. It does not account for heterogeneity. Heterogeneity implies that different subjects may be modeled by different transition matrices $\mathbf{A}$ (as represented by their coordinates $\mathbf{a}$) and corresponding noise variances σ^2. Assuming that there are K distinct $\mathbf{a}_k$ and σ_k^2, $k = 1,\ldots,K$, then the time series for each subject can be modeled as generated by first picking a latent variable $z_i \in \{1,2,\ldots,K\}$, $i = 1,\ldots,N$, and then sampling from the distribution $p\left(\mathbf{x}_i|\mathbf{a}_{z_i},\sigma_{z_i}^2\right)$. The density of $\mathbf{x}_i$ given all $\mathbf{a}_k$ and σ_k^2 is, of course, a mixture model

$$p\left(\mathbf{x}_i|\boldsymbol{\pi},\{\mathbf{a}_l,\sigma_l^2\}\right) = \sum_{k=1}^{K} p\left(z_i = k|\boldsymbol{\pi}\right)p\left(\mathbf{x}_i|z_i = k,\{\mathbf{a}_l,\sigma_l^2\}\right) = \sum_{k=1}^{K} \pi_k p\left(\mathbf{x}_i|\mathbf{a}_k,\sigma_k^2\right),$$

where $z_i|\boldsymbol{\pi} \sim \mathrm{Cat}(\boldsymbol{\pi})$ with $\boldsymbol{\pi} = (\pi_1, \pi_2, \ldots, \pi_K)$. We call this a *mixture of linear dynamical systems* model, or *mixture LDS* for short. We are interested in estimating $\boldsymbol{\theta} = \{\boldsymbol{\pi}, \mathbf{a}_k, \sigma_k^2 : k = 1, \ldots, K\}$ for this model.

Since $\boldsymbol{\pi}$ has a categorical distribution, for Bayesian analysis we use its conjugate prior, a Dirichlet distribution $\boldsymbol{\pi}|\boldsymbol{\alpha} \sim \mathrm{Dir}(\boldsymbol{\alpha})$. For $\mathbf{a}_k, \sigma_k^2$, we use NIG as its conjugate prior, i.e. $\mathbf{a}_k, \sigma_k^2 \sim \mathrm{NIG}(\boldsymbol{\beta})$, from Theorem 1. $\boldsymbol{\alpha}$ and $\boldsymbol{\beta}$ are hyperparameters. The mixture LDS model captures all of the characteristics of PD progression listed in Sect. 1.

4 Bayesian Analysis

Bayesian analysis of the above model consists of generating samples from the posterior $p(\mathbf{z}, \boldsymbol{\theta}|\mathbf{X}, \boldsymbol{\alpha}, \boldsymbol{\beta})$ using MCMC methods, where $\mathbf{z} = (z_1, \ldots, z_N)$ is the vector of latent variables. The overall strategy is to sample from $\mathbf{z}, \boldsymbol{\pi}, \mathbf{a}_k, \sigma_k^2$ sequentially (a.k.a. Gibbs sampling). We use a collapsed Gibbs sampler for sampling $\mathbf{z}$ from $p(\mathbf{z}|\mathbf{X}, \boldsymbol{\alpha}, \boldsymbol{\beta})$, and then sample the rest from $p(\boldsymbol{\theta}|\mathbf{z}, \mathbf{X}, \boldsymbol{\alpha}, \boldsymbol{\beta})$.

4.1 Collapsed Gibbs Sampling

To sample $\mathbf{z}$, we integrate out $\boldsymbol{\theta}$ and sample from $p(\mathbf{z}|\mathbf{X}, \boldsymbol{\alpha}, \boldsymbol{\beta})$. This is collapsed Gibbs sampling and it is well known that it leads to faster convergence [12,15]. The samples of $\mathbf{z}$ are generated one component at a time based on

$$p(z_i = k|\mathbf{z}_{-i}, \mathbf{X}, \boldsymbol{\alpha}, \boldsymbol{\beta}) \propto p(z_i = k|\mathbf{X}_{-i}, \mathbf{z}_{-i}, \boldsymbol{\alpha}, \boldsymbol{\beta}) p(\mathbf{x}_i|z_i = k, \mathbf{X}_{-i}, \mathbf{z}_{-i}, \boldsymbol{\alpha}, \boldsymbol{\beta})$$
$$= p(z_i = k|\mathbf{z}_{-i}, \boldsymbol{\alpha}) p(\mathbf{x}_i|z_i = k, \mathbf{X}_{-i,k}, \boldsymbol{\beta})$$

where $\mathbf{z}_{-i} = \{z_j : j \neq i, j = 1, \ldots, N\}$ (the same for $\mathbf{X}_{-i}$), and $\mathbf{X}_{-i,k} = \{\mathbf{x}_j : j \neq i, z_j = k, j = 1, \ldots, N\}$. Assuming that $\boldsymbol{\alpha} = (\alpha/K, \ldots, \alpha/K)$, the first term in the product is easily shown to be $p(z_i = k|\mathbf{z}_{-i}, \boldsymbol{\alpha}) = \frac{N_{-i,k} + \alpha/K}{N + \alpha - 1}$, where $N_{-i,k} = \sum_{j \neq i} \mathbb{I}(z_j = k)$ and $\mathbb{I}(\cdot) = 1$ if its argument is true and zero otherwise. The second term is calculated from (6) according to Corollary 1.

To sample $\boldsymbol{\theta}$ from $p(\boldsymbol{\theta}|\mathbf{z}, \mathbf{X}, \boldsymbol{\alpha}, \boldsymbol{\beta})$, we sample $\boldsymbol{\pi}$ and then $\mathbf{a}_k, \sigma_k^2$. Sampling $\boldsymbol{\pi}$ is straightforward since $p(\boldsymbol{\pi}|\mathbf{z}, \mathbf{X}, \boldsymbol{\alpha}, \boldsymbol{\beta}) = p(\boldsymbol{\pi}|\mathbf{z}, \boldsymbol{\alpha})$ and $\boldsymbol{\pi}|\mathbf{z}, \boldsymbol{\alpha} \sim \mathrm{Dir}(\alpha/K + N_1, \ldots, \alpha/K + N_K)$. Sampling $\mathbf{a}_k, \sigma_k^2$ is done by sampling from NIG in (5) following Theorem 1 since $p(\mathbf{a}_k, \sigma_k^2|\mathbf{z}, \mathbf{X}, \boldsymbol{\alpha}, \boldsymbol{\beta}) = p(\mathbf{a}_k, \sigma_k^2|\mathbf{X}_k, \boldsymbol{\beta})$ where $\mathbf{X}_k = \{\mathbf{x}_i : z_i = k, i = 1, \ldots, N\}$.

We use weak priors by setting the hyperparameters to $\alpha = 1$ and $\boldsymbol{\beta} = (\mathbf{0}, 10^{-8}\mathbf{I}_{\lceil D^2/2 \rceil}, 10^{-3}, 10^{-3})$. For the results reported below, we use 3000 MCMC iterations with initial 40% samples discarded.

4.2 Choosing the Number of Clusters

Our model requires K, the number of clusters to be chosen a priori. We choose the number of clusters using Bayesian model selection as well as cross validation [10,11]. For cross validation, we divide the dataset into 10 subsets (10-fold cross validation). Taking each subset as test set, we use the remaining data as training set to infer the parameters $\boldsymbol{\theta}$ and then evaluate the log-likelihood of the test set.

For Bayesian model selection, we denote $\mathbf{M}_K$ for the model with K components, and $\mathcal{M} = \{\mathbf{M}_1, \ldots, \mathbf{M}_{K_{\max}}\}$. Assuming $p(K) \propto$ constant on $K = 1, \ldots, K_{\max}$, we have $p(K|\mathbf{X}, \mathcal{M}) \propto p(K) p(\mathbf{X}|\mathcal{M}, K) \propto p(\mathbf{X}|\mathcal{M}, K) = p(\mathbf{X}|\mathbf{M}_K)$. Then, finding the optimal $\hat{K} = \arg\max_K p(K|\mathbf{X}, \mathcal{M})$ is equivalent to finding the maximum of $p(\mathbf{X}|\mathbf{M}_K)$ with respect to K. The density $p(\mathbf{X}|\mathbf{M}_K)$ is evaluated by the integral

$$p(\mathbf{X}|\mathbf{M}_K) = \int p(\mathbf{X}|\boldsymbol{\theta}) \, p(\boldsymbol{\theta}|\mathbf{M}_K) \, d\boldsymbol{\theta}. \tag{7}$$

The Gibbs sampler discussed above generates samples from $p(\mathbf{z}, \boldsymbol{\theta}|\mathbf{X}, \boldsymbol{\alpha}, \boldsymbol{\beta})$. Using $p(\boldsymbol{\theta}|\mathbf{X}, \mathbf{M}_K)$ as a proposal distribution and the generated samples of $\boldsymbol{\theta}$, we evaluate the integral in (7) by importance sampling.

5   Results

Recall from Sect. 2 that time series data from 365 subjects survived preprocessing. This is the dataset that we analyze. First we determine the number of clusters, then we use the determined number of clusters to sample from the posterior of the model parameters. Finally, we interpret the mean of the posterior.

5.1   Determine the Number of Clusters

Figure 3 shows plots for Bayesian model selection (with $K_{\max} = 10$) as well as 10-fold cross validation as a function of number of clusters. In each plot, the blue curve shows the value of the log-likelihood vs. the number of clusters. The log-likelihood behavior is similar in both plots, consistent with the common understanding that empirical Bayesian and cross validation have similar results. We observed that as the number of clusters increased, empty clusters were created. In both plots, the orange curve shows the number of clusters that were not empty. Note that the log-likelihood increases with number of clusters and approximately plateaus from 4 clusters onwards. The one exception is when we initialize with 9 clusters, where Bayesian model selection gives 5 non-empty clusters with a slightly higher log-likelihood value. For cross validation, the average number of final number of clusters (over the 10 folds) remains around 4. Considering these results, we use 4 clusters for the dataset.

5.2   Interpreting the Model

Having chosen the number of clusters, Table 1 shows the mean of the posterior distribution for $\boldsymbol{\theta}$, which we take as the "fit" of the model to the data. The table does not directly show matrices $\mathbf{A}_k$, instead it shows the eigenvalues and eigenvectors of the matrices. These are easier to interpret, as we discuss below. Figure 4 shows the raw SBR time series for subjects for each cluster.

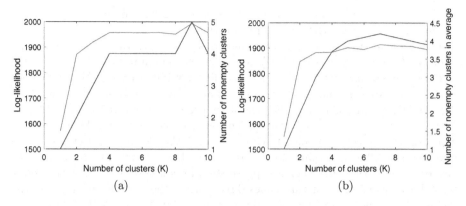

Fig. 3. Model selection using Bayesian (a) and cross validation (b). The y-axis has two scales corresponding to log-likelihood value (blue curve) and number of nonempty clusters (orange curve) separately. (Color figure online)

Table 1. $\mathbb{E}(\theta)$ from averaging the generated samples.

Class	$k = 1$				$k = 2$				$k = 3$				$k = 4$			
π_k	0.382				0.072				0.397				0.148			
σ_k	0.069				0.268				0.128				0.087			
λ^a	-0.3	-0.2	-0.2	-0.1	-0.7	-0.4	-0.4	-0.1	-0.4	-0.3	-0.1	-0.1	-0.6	-0.4	-0.2	-0.2
u	0.4	-0.3	-0.6	-0.6	0.5	0.7	-0.7	-0.6	-0.4	0.5	-0.6	0.6	0.5	-0.2	-0.6	0.6
	-0.6	0.7	-0.3	-0.4	-0.5	-0.1	-0.2	-0.4	0.6	-0.5	-0.4	0.4	-0.5	0.7	-0.4	0.4
	0.6	0.7	0.3	-0.4	0.5	-0.1	0.2	-0.4	-0.6	-0.5	0.4	0.4	0.5	0.7	0.4	0.4
	-0.4	-0.3	0.6	-0.6	-0.5	0.7	0.7	-0.6	0.4	0.5	0.6	0.6	-0.5	-0.2	0.6	0.6

[a] **A** is represented by its eigenvalues λ and eigenvectors **u**. Eigenvectors are shown to first significant digit to conserve horizontal space.

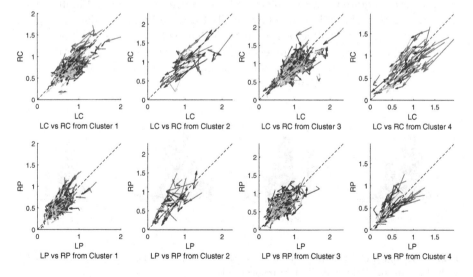

Fig. 4. Four clusters from Gibbs sampling on the whole data.

To interpret the model, first note that cluster 2 has the largest σ and the smallest π_k. Also, the SBR trajectories for this cluster (Fig. 4) are more disorganized than SBR trajectories for other clusters. Quite likely, this cluster represents additional outliers in the data. We focus on the remaining clusters. For these clusters, the eigenstructure of $\mathbf{A}_k$'s is particularly illuminating: All eigenvalues of $\mathbf{A}_k$'s are real and negative, showing that all linear combinations of SBRs decrease with time. Cluster 1 has the least negative eigenvalues, while cluster 4 has the most negative eigenvalues. Cluster 3 is intermediate. Thus cluster 4 captures the fastest evolving subjects, cluster 1 the slowest, and cluster 3 the intermediate. The eigenvalues for cluster 4 are almost twice the eigenvalues for cluster 1, suggesting that DaT loss proceeds approximately twice as fast in cluster 4. Further evidence for this comes directly from the data. Figure 5 shows the histograms of the magnitude of initial velocities ($\|\mathbf{v}_{i1}\|$) as calculated from the raw SBRs for each cluster. The medians of the histograms are 0.17, 0.61, 0.27, 0.36 respectively, which verifies our speed analysis.

The solution to a LDS $\frac{d\mathbf{x}}{dt} = \mathbf{A}\mathbf{x}$ is determined by the eigenvalues $\{\lambda_i\}$ and eigenvectors $\{\mathbf{u}_i\}$ of $\mathbf{A}$. The eigenvector determines the subspace in which the time series proceeds with the eigenvalue as the time constant. Recall from Sect. 3.1 that the eigenvectors of centrosymmetric matrices are either symmetric or skew-symmetric. This symmetry or antisymmetry represents symmetry or asymmetry of disease progression. To see this, suppose $\mathbf{u}$ is a skew-symmetric eigenvector, say $\mathbf{u} = (a, b, -b, -a)$. Because of how we have arranged the caudates and putamina in $\mathbf{x}$, this suggests that $a \times \mathrm{LC} + b \times \mathrm{LP} - (b \times \mathrm{RP} + a \times \mathrm{RC})$ goes to zero with speed λ. In other words, a skew-symmetric eigenvector and its eigenvalue capture how the asymmetry (of the linear combination $a \times \mathrm{Caudate} + b \times \mathrm{Putamen}$) between the two hemispheres decreases to zero. Similarly, a symmetric eigenvector and its eigenvalue capture how the symmetry (i.e. the weighted "mean" of the SBRs) decreases to zero. Finally, recall from Sect. 1 that the difference between SBR uptake in the caudate and putamen reflects the extent of PD in each brain hemisphere. Thus if a and b have opposite signs, then a skew-symmetric eigenvector represents asymmetry in the disease across the hemispheres, while a symmetric eigenvector represents the mean disease in both hemispheres.

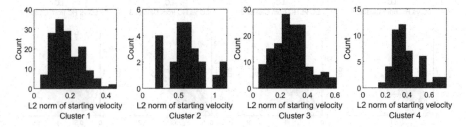

Fig. 5. Histogram of starting velocity magnitude for each cluster. The medians for the 4 clusters are 0.17, 0.61, 0.27, 0.36 respectively.

Applying this interpretation to each cluster of Table 1 gives the following: The most negative eigenvalue in each cluster has a skew-symmetric eigenvector. This implies that the loss of asymmetry of disease across hemispheres has the fastest speed of *all possible linear combinations of SBRs*. Also note that the first eigenvector in clusters 1, 3 and 4 is numerically quite similar. The next significant eigenvalue in each cluster has a symmetric eigenvector. The last eigenvector in all clusters represents the "mean" of all four regions and has the slowest eigenvalue, hence the mean (or net) SBR in the four regions is the slowest indicator of early stage PD.

6   Discussion and Conclusion

The results presented above show that PD progression as manifest in DaTscans is heterogeneous, with one subtype (cluster 4) progressing almost twice as fast as the slowest subtype (cluster 1). This is the first significant finding of this paper. The second, and potentially more interesting, finding is that within each subtype (cluster) the change in SBR asymmetry across hemispheres has a faster time constant than the change in mean SBR across hemispheres. Moreover, the change in asymmetry is the fastest change among all linear combinations of SBRs. Whether this finding can be utilized to create a sensitive disease progression index is an open question. We plan to investigate this in the future. Such a disease progression index is likely to have significant implications for clinical trials that use DaTscans.

Model mirror symmetry is also a novel idea with broader implications. Extending the MMS idea to high dimensional data (more structures, voxel level rather than ROI modeling) could be challenging as the dimension increases. One possible route to higher dimensions is to require $\mathbf{A}$ to be sparse or low rank. This will be the focus of forthcoming research.

In conclusion, this paper proposes a mixture LDS model for PD progression in DaTscans. The model reveals that progression in DaTsans is heterogeneous, with a significant range of progression time constants. The model also suggests that the change in asymmetry may be a more sensitive index of PD disease progression.

Acknowledgements. This research is supported by the NIH grant R01NS107328. We gratefully acknowledge discussions with Prof. Sule Tinaz of the Dept. of Neurology Yale University.

The data used in the preparation of this article was obtained from the Parkinson's Progression Markers Initiative (PPMI) database (up-to-date information is available at http://www.ppmi-info.org). PPMI – a public-private partnership – is funded by the Michael J. Fox Foundation for Parkinson's Research and multiple funding partners. The full list of PPMI funding partners can be found at ppmi- info.org/fundingpartners.

References

1. Au, W.L., Adams, J.R., Troiano, A., Stoessel, A.J.: Parkinson's disease: in vivo assessment of disease progression using positron emission tomography. Mol. Brain Res. **134**, 24–33 (2005)
2. Bernardo, J.M., Smith, A.F.: Bayesian Theory. Wiley, Hoboken (2009)
3. Braak, H., Tredici, K.D., Rub, U., de Vos, R.A., Steur, E.N.J., Braak, E.: Staging of brain pathology related to sporadic Parkinson's disease. Neurobiol. Aging **24**(2), 197–211 (2003)
4. Eggers, C., Kahraman, D., Fink, G.R., Schmidt, M., Timmermann, L.: Akinetic-rigid and tremor-dominant Parkinson's disease patients show different patterns of FP-CIT single photon emission computer tomography. Mov. Disord. **26**(3), 416–423 (2011)
5. Fonteijn, H.M., et al.: An event-based model for disease progression and its application in familial Alzheimer's disease and Huntington's disease. NeuroImage **60**(3), 1880–1889 (2012)
6. Hilker, R., et al.: Nonlinear progression of Parkinson disease as determined by serial positron emission tomographic imaging of striatal fluorodopa F 18 activity. Archiv. Neurol. **62**(3), 378–382 (2005)
7. Hoehn, M.M., Yahr, M.D.: Parkinsonism: onset, progression and mortality. Neurology **17**, 427–442 (1967)
8. Innis, R.B., et al.: Consensus nomenclature for in vivo imaging of reversibly binding radioligands. J. Cereb. Blood Flow Metab. **27**(9), 1533–1539 (2007)
9. Jedynak, B.M., et al.: A computational neurodegenerative disease progression score: method and results with the Alzheimer's disease Neuroimaging Initiative cohort. Neuroimage **63**(3), 1478–1486 (2012)
10. Kass, R.E., Raftery, A.E.: Bayes factors. J. Am. Stat. Assoc. **90**(430), 773–795 (1995)
11. McLachlan, G.J., Rathnayake, S.: On the number of components in a Gaussian mixture model. Wiley Interdisc. Rev.: Data Min. Knowl. Discov. **4**(5), 341–355 (2014)
12. Murphy, K.P.: Machine Learning: A Probabilistic Perspective. MIT Press, Cambridge (2012)
13. Quinn, N., Critchley, P., Marsden, C.D.: Young onset Parkinson's disease. Mov. Disord. **2**, 73–91 (1987)
14. Raj, A., Powell, F.: Models of network spread and network degeneration in brain disorders. Biol. Psychiatry: Cogn. Neurosci. Neuroimaging **3**, 788–797 (2018)
15. Sudderth, E.B.: Graphical models for visual object recognition and tracking. Ph.D. thesis, Massachusetts Institute of Technology (2006)
16. Weaver, J.R.: Centrosymmetric (cross-symmetric) matrices, their basic properties, eigenvalues, and eigenvectors. Am. Math. Mon. **92**(10), 711–717 (1985)
17. Zhou, J., Liu, J., Narayan, V.A., Ye, J.: Modeling disease progression via fused sparse group lasso. In: Proceedings of the 18th ACM SIGKDD International Conference on Knowledge Discovery and Data Mining, pp. 1095–1103. ACM (2012)
18. Zubal, I.G., Early, M., Yuan, O., Jennings, D., Marek, K., Seibyl, J.P.: Optimized, automated striatal uptake analysis applied to SPECT brain scans of Parkinson's disease patients. J. Nucl. Med. **48**(6), 857–864 (2007)

Brain Tumor Segmentation on MRI with Missing Modalities

Yan Shen and Mingchen Gao$^{(\boxtimes)}$

Department of Computer Science and Engineering,
University at Buffalo, The State University of New York, Buffalo, USA
{yshen22,mgao8}@buffalo.edu

Abstract. Brain Tumor Segmentation from magnetic resonance imaging (MRI) is a critical technique for early diagnosis. However, rather than having complete four modalities as in BraTS dataset, it is common to have missing modalities in clinical scenarios. We design a brain tumor segmentation algorithm that is robust to the absence of any modality. Our network includes a channel-independent encoding path and a feature-fusion decoding path. We use self-supervised training through channel dropout and also propose a novel domain adaptation method on feature maps to recover the information from the missing channel. Our results demonstrate that the quality of the segmentation depends on which modality is missing. Furthermore, we also discuss and visualize the contribution of each modality to the segmentation results. Their contributions are along well with the expert screening routine.

Keywords: Brain tumor segmentation · Multi-modality ·
Domain adaptation · Self-supervised learning

1 Introduction

In the United States, it is estimated that 25,000 new patients are diagnosed with brain cancer every year. While average five-year survival rate is just above one in three, early diagnosis is important to increase life quality of patients. MR imaging are the most common kinds of screening methods on brain pathology. MR images provide some primary indicators on unhealthy tissue matters, and have great impact on improved diagnosis, tumor classification and treatment planning.

While brain tumor segmentation requires professional knowledge to distinguish unhealthy tissues from healthy ones. Those tasks are expensive and limited. Computer-aided automatic segmentation tools provide an important reference for diagnosis. The automatic input-output pipeline can provide patients instant diagnosis that gives them the opportunity to have first-aid on what suspects to be a pathology.

The success of deep learning has made computer program an indispensable aid to physicians for analyzing on brain tumor development [6]. Such automatic detection methods based on multi-layer neural networks have been widely

© Springer Nature Switzerland AG 2019
A. C. S. Chung et al. (Eds.): IPMI 2019, LNCS 11492, pp. 417–428, 2019.
https://doi.org/10.1007/978-3-030-20351-1_32

applied to segmentation on brain tumors. MICCAI Brain Tumor Segmentation (BraTS) challenge collected so far the largest collection of brain tumor segmentation dataset that is publicly available. They use well-defined training and testing splits, thereby allowing us fair comparison among different approaches. Mohammad *et al.* are the first to apply deep neural network methods to segment brain tumors on BraTS dataset [4]. They use Fully Convolutional Networks (FCN) to perform pixel level classification by taking local patches as input. Their method becomes the baseline for deep learning based approach on BrainTumor Segmentation. In our knowledge, the best result on Brain Tumor Segmentation is produced by RA-UNet [8] which proposes a 3D hybrid residual attention-aware segmentation method. They achieve Dice score of 0.8863 on whole tumor segmentation. Currently, state-of-art result on BraTS dataset can even produce comparable results with human experts.

However current state-of-art brain tumor segmentation benchmark requires complete MR images in all T1, T2, T1c and Flair modalities, as provided in the dataset. Multi-modality images provide complementary information to distinguish tissues and anatomies. Segmenting brain tumors from MR images learns a complicated function on all four modalities parameterized both by anatomical morphology and local pixels values. However, in practical situations, different hospitals may follow different protocols and procedures when performing MR images. Missing one of the four modalities is common. This may pose some challenges on simultaneous available requirements of four complete modalities on MR images.

Related Work. Image segmentation a task of clustering pixels into salient image regions corresponding to their characteristics. They typical generate labels on the pixel level. Earlier time image segmentation uses handcrafted filter banks like Gaussian Kernels, Fourier Transformations, Wavelets to pre-process the image and later trains a SVM for classification. Succeeding work [16] uses statistical approach like CRF to infer a fine boundary. CRF approaches incorporates local evidence in unary assignments and models interactions between label assignment in a probabilistic graphical model. In the era of deep learning, convolutional neural networks (CNNs) are considered as the state-of-the-art in biomedical image segmentation. Deep approaches include a forward pipeline to inference target from inputs and a backward pipeline to learn network parameters. Early deep learning method on image segmentation uses FCN classification networks that perform pixels level classifications by taking local region inputs. Later approaches turn to U-Net [14] structure that include a down-sampling path to encode input images and an up-sampling path to decode feature maps to segmentation map. Further work [18] adds a RNN layer like a CRF to further refine the boundary of segmentation maps produced by U-Nets.

Deep Learning approaches for brain tumor segmentation include end-to-end U-Net [7,9], regional proposals [15], hierarchy classification [2] and level set [10]. Hierarchical models have been proposed to firstly classify pixels into background and whole tumor using T2 and Flair channels, the whole tumor is then further classified into four classes based on all four modalities [2].

There are also a number of methods proposed on dealing with missing data in medical imaging. Primitive methods include building separate models for each condition. However each model could only fit a specific combination of input modalities. Domain adaptation methods are widely used to learn a unified model that could apply for a wide spectrum of channel modes. Ganin *et al.* [3] use adversarial loss on intermediate feature maps of two domains and thus transfer the network learnt in one domain to the other. Manders *et al.* [11] use a class specific adversarial loss on feature maps to transfer the learnt network from source domain to target domain. Generative model is also proposed by Zhang *et al.* [17] to synthesize missing channel from available channels. Havaei *et al.* [5] builds a unified model from purely self-supervised training pipeline for each individual channel. And they made combined prediction on multi-channels by merging the feature maps from each channels and computing the mean and variance.

Contributions. In our paper, we use self-supervised learning by randomly removing one modality during training to enhance the model to handle the instances with a missing modality. While trained with a missing modality, we use an extra adversarial loss to ensure the modal generate similar features as in full modality situation. Rather than directly adapting one domain to another in previous methods, we consider domain diversities from different channels. We take the combined features from all the domains and adapt it to encode distribution on any of remaining channels after dropping one.

Our contributions in this paper are three folds:

- Firstly, we learn a network that can be broadly applied to tolerate on missing any modality without the need of fitting to specific combinations of remaining modalities.
- Secondly, we put forward a novel domain adaptation model. Our adaptation model uses adversarial loss to adapt feature maps from missing modalities to the one from full modalities.
- Finally, we decouple the segmentation contribution to each individual modality and thus generate on interpretations of our segmentation on four modalities of MR images.

2   Training Modality Missing Tolerant Network: A Joint Objective of Missing Modality Reconstruction and Domain Adaptation

2.1   U-Net Structure: Modality-Separate Encoding Path and Feature Fusion at Various Resolutions on Decoding Path

Our basic model architecture follows U-net, as shown in Fig. 1. Each modality is fed into the model as one channel. Blue box indicates separated encoding path of the multi-channel MR image input. Red box indicates decoding path following the encoding of multi-channel input on various levels of feature maps. Green box indicates multi-stage segmentation outputs. Encoding path includes multiple feed-forward down-sampling convolutional layers after each channel input. And it ends up with 64 features map of resolution 24 × 25 from each input channel. Individual encoding path of each channel have independent sets of parameters and have no connection with each other before decoding. Though cross-channel filter banks could be used to extract features by contrasting different input channels at early stage in a more straight-forward way, our separated feature maps on four different channels can be used to encode abstractions of segmentation information that is tolerant on channel loss. Our separately encoded feature maps are fused and decoded in our following decoding path.

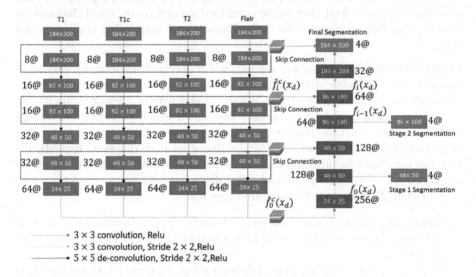

Fig. 1. The architecture of our 4 channel input segmentation network (Color figure online)

In our network's decoding path, higher resolutions of segmentation outputs are created by successively up-sampling in a bottom-up approach and mixing channel-separate feature maps at various levels. Up-sampling operations use deconvolution operators. Channel-separate feature maps created at encoding path are fused by convolution operators. The features maps at the end of encoding path from each input channel are fused to create bottle-neck feature maps at the same resolution. Two levels of inter-mediate feature maps from each input channel are fused with the feature maps created along the decoding path. We fuse intermediate feature maps from encoding path with the ones from decoding to create skip connections. Our decoding path includes a total of three stages of successive mixing and up-sampling. After each stage, we also generate a segmentation at the same level of the same resolution by convolutions. The final segmentation outputs with the same resolutions as input MR images are generated after the final stage.

We train on the lower resolution segmentation outputs at the intermediate feature maps to force our network learn a hierarchical representation of segmentation related information from coarse to fine, where the structural information is encoded at the lower resolution feature maps and the boundary level information is encoded at the higher resolution feature maps. In this way, we generate our segmentation outputs by sequentially inferring area of pathology structures and exact boundaries.

2.2   Segmentation on Missing Modality Inputs

We first define how our network infers segmentation outputs from missing channel inputs. Formally, let's denote x_d as a sample taken from the training set $\mathcal{D}$, $\mathcal{C}$ as the set of all channels in MR images. And we suppose only channels in set $\mathcal{C}_d^- \in \mathcal{C}$ are available. As we mentioned previously, our U-Net's decoding path mixes the channel-specific feature maps with the feature maps created along the decoding path and then use convolution operations to predict the probability of segmentation at various resolutions. In the condition of missing channel inputs, we set the encoding path of missing channel to zero, and keep the rest the same. For the decoding path, the feature maps are calculated as :

$$f_i(x_d) = \sum_{c \in C_d^-} \hat{W}_i^c(\hat{f}_i^c(x_d)) + W_i(f_{i-1}(x_d)), \tag{1}$$

where $\hat{W}_i^c(\cdot)$ denotes the skip convolution kernel on the same level encoding feature map $\hat{f}_i^c(x_d)$ from channel c at layer i, $W^i(\cdot)$ denotes the feed-forward convolution kernel on feature map $f_{i-1}(x_d)$ produced at the layer $(i-1)$ before along decoding path. The skip convolution feature maps $\hat{f}_i^c(x_d)$ comes from the encoding path after a 3×3 stride 1 convolution on feature map of the same size as $f_{i-1}(x_d)$. At the bottleneck layer 0, their feature maps only come from convolutions on channel-separated feature maps from encoding layers. For missing channel inputs, we only convolute on those feature maps from available channels and zero out the rest.

$$f_0^-(x_d) = \sum_{c \in C_d^-} W_0^c(\hat{f}_0^c(x_d)) \tag{2}$$

where $W_0^c(\cdot)$ denotes the convolution kernel on the feature map $\hat{f}_0^c(x_d)$ from channel c. The rest available channels for encoding path keep the same as in the architecture of full channels in described in Sect. 2.1.

2.3   Training Missing Modality Tolerant Model by Random Modality-Drop

The model proposed in Sect. 2.2 is able to train and test images with missing channels. However, the missing channels will certainly jeopardize the segmentation performance. To make our model robust to channel losses, we initiate a

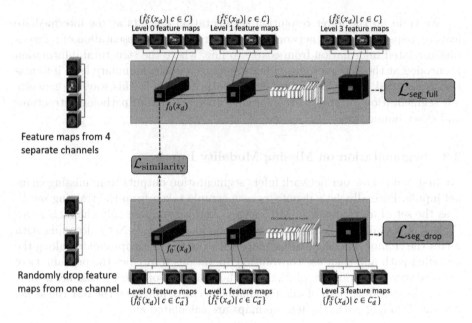

Fig. 2. Training of our brain separation networks on missing channel. Encoded feature maps from 4 separate channels are connected to decoding path in full channel input. Encoded feature maps from residue channels are connected on decoding path in missing channel input. We randomly drop one channel in a training step. Our training objective function include the reconstruction loss on full channel input and missing channel input. We also add the similarity loss on decoded feature maps from full channel input and the one from missing channel input.

process to compensate the missed modalities. We train the model by randomly dropping out an input channel. The model has independent encoding path has two benefits: (i) to learn a unique feature maps for each input channel (ii) to avoid the false co-adaptations between modalities. Our key idea is to train a model capable of producing meaningful segmentations from any arbitrary combination of available channels.

The objective function is as follows:

$$\mathcal{L}_{seg\_drop} = \sum_{k=1}^{3} \sum_{d \in \mathcal{D}} {}^{k}\mathbf{y}_d \log p_Y({}^{k}\hat{\mathbf{y}}_d | x_d^{(\mathcal{C}_d^-)}), \tag{3}$$

where $x_d^{(\mathcal{C}_d^-)}$ is the $|\mathcal{C}| - 1$ available channel inputs from x_d after we randomly drop one, ${}^{k}\mathbf{y}_d$ is the k's stage resolution of one-hot encoding of segmentation labels, $p_Y({}^{k}\hat{\mathbf{y}}_d | x_d^{(\mathcal{C}_d^-)})$ is the softmax segmentation prediction. We use a uniform distribution to seed the index of the channel to be dropped at each training step.

2.4 Domain Adversarial Similarity Loss on Bottleneck Feature Maps

The domain adversarial similarity loss [3] is used with a discriminator to adapt representations from different domains to a similar distribution. Our whole training diagram is shown in Fig. 2. We further introduce a domain adversarial similarity loss term on bottleneck feature maps for co-adaptations among abstract representations from different channels. We choose bottleneck feature maps for adaptation because it is where individually predicted abstract features are fused to produce a joint inference on high level representations for segmentations (mostly at structural level).

The outputs at bottleneck layer are the sum of convolutions from all contributing channels as shown in Eq. 3 . In the case of modality-drop, the outputs at bottleneck layer are the sum of convolutions from available channels.

The expectation of $f_0^-(x_d)$ could be written as:

$$
\begin{aligned}
\mathbb{E}[f_0^-(x_d)] &= \mathbb{E}_{\delta, x_d}[\sum_{c \in C_d^-} W_0^c(\hat{f}_0^c(x_d))] \\
&= \mathbb{E}_{\delta, x_d}[\sum_{c \in C} \delta^{(c)} W_0^c(\hat{f}_0^c(x_d))] \\
&= \mathbb{E}_{\delta|x_d}[\sum_{c \in C} \delta^{(c)} \mathbb{E}_{x_d}[W_0^c(\hat{f}_0^c(x_d))]] \\
&= \sum_{c \in \mathcal{C}} p(\delta^{(c)} \neq 0) \mathbb{E}[W_0^c(\hat{f}_0^c(x_d))]]
\end{aligned}
$$

As we use uniform distribution to choose the dropout channel on C channels input, each individual channel c is kept with probability $p(\delta^{(c)} \neq 0) = \frac{C-1}{C}$. So we have

$$
\begin{aligned}
\mathbb{E}[f_0^-(x_d)] &= \frac{C-1}{C} \mathbb{E}[\sum_{c \in \mathcal{C}} W_0^c(\hat{f}_0^c(x_d))]] \\
&= \frac{C-1}{C} \mathbb{E}[f_0(x_d)]
\end{aligned}
$$

To co-adapt the $W_0^c(\hat{f}_0^c(x_d))$ from different channels, we use adversarial loss on $f_0(x_d)$ and $\hat{f}_0(x_d)$ after compensation for the coefficient on their expectation's ratio, we use the following minimax adversarial loss to regularize the two distributions.

$$
\mathcal{L}_{similarity} = \min_\theta \max_\phi \mathbb{E}_{x_d^{(C_d^-)}}[\log D_\theta(\hat{f}_0(x_d, \phi))] + \mathbb{E}_{x_d^{(C_d)}}[\log(1 - D_\theta(\frac{C-1}{C} f_0(x_d, \phi))], \quad (4)
$$

where $D_\theta(\cdot)$ is an auxiliary discriminative network that are co-trained with our segmentation network. The total loss function of our training is

$$
\mathcal{L} = \mathcal{L}_{seg\_full} + \alpha \mathcal{L}_{seg\_drop} + \beta \mathcal{L}_{similarity} \quad (5)
$$

2.5   Prediction Relevance Analysis

Robnik-Sikonja *et al.* [13] proposed a technique for assigning relevance value to each input feature with respect to a class label. Inspired by their idea, we assign a relevance value to each input channel c with respect to segmentation label j for every pixel. The basic idea is that the relevance of a segmentation label of a channel j can be estimated by measuring how the prediction changes if we remove channel c.

We first estimate probability for class j in pixel $\hat{y}_d$ produced from full channels inputs, denoted as $\log p_Y(\hat{y}_d = j|x_d^{(\mathcal{C})})$. Then we re-estimate the class probability from missing channel c, denoted as $\log p_Y(\hat{y}_d = j|x_d^{(\mathcal{C}_c^-)})$. Once these class probabilities are estimated, we follow the definition proposed by Robnik-Sikonja *et al.* [13] to calculate the weight of evidence on class j from channel c, given as

$$\text{WE}_c(y_d^j = c|x_d^c) = \log_2(\text{odds}(p_Y(\hat{y}_d = j|x_d^{(\mathcal{C})}))) - \log_2(\text{odds}(p_Y(\hat{y}_d = j|x_d^{(\mathcal{C}_c^-)}))),$$
(6)

where $\text{odds}(a) = a/(1-a)$.

3   Experiments

Data, Data Selection and Preprocessing. We evaluate our method on BraTS17. BraTS17 contains 262 scans of glioblastoma and 199 scans of lower grade glioma. Our U-Net is trained on extracted 2D image patches which are extracted from all the 3D scans that have more than 200 non-zeros pixels (excluding the wasteful empty scans). We randomly split the extracted 3D volume data to 80% training and 20% testing. We normalize the gray value to a range of -1 to 1 for each input channel and crop the MR image on the center window of size 200×186. We follow the protocol in BraTS17 to label the four types of intra-tumoral structures, namely GD-enhancing tumor (ET-label 4), the peritumoral edema (ED-label 2), the necrotic and non-enhancing tumor (NCR/NET label 1) and the background (label 0). For MR image scans, all the ground truth labels have been manually labeled and certified by expert board-certified neuroradi-ologists. The manual labeling process is followed by a hierarchical annotation protocol. Experts firstly segment whole tumor regions by contrasting on T2 and Flair channel and separate tumor core and enhancing core from T1 and T1c channel. Experts decision are agreed by majority vote.

Evaluation. All our experiments were performed using Python 3.6 with Ten-sorFlow library [1] and run on a GTX 1080 Ti graphics processing unit using CUDA 8.0. Our models are tested on both full channel input and missing channel input. In the case of missing channel input, each time we remove one channel from full channel input. Specifically, we ran the following experiments.

Firstly, we evaluated our segmentation result quantitatively by measuring Dice score with ground-truth. We report three types of Dice scores including whole tumor, tumor core and enhancing core on 2D slice level. Our three types of Dice score were evaluated on both full channel inputs and missing channel inputs.

Secondly, we explored our segmentation results qualitatively by visualizing our results with ground truth segmentation. Our quality assessments include the segmentation region, boundary qualities and specificity/sensitivity. We evaluated our trained network's segmentation qualities on both full channel inputs and missing channel inputs.

Finally, to provide interpretations on which our prediction is based, we generated relevance map by the method we described in Sect. 2.5. This helps us to understand the role of each individual channel on the estimation of whole tumor, tumor core and enhanced core. Our model has a surplus benefit of generating meaningful interpretations as our network broadly adapts to full channel and missing channel input.

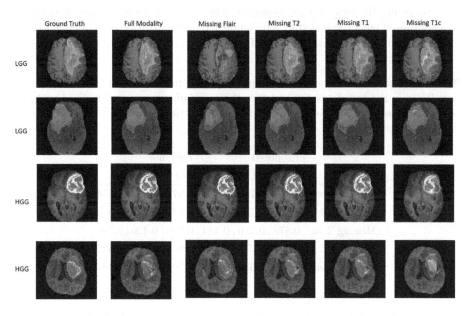

Fig. 3. Examples of the segmentation masks with missing modality compared to the ground truth. The edema area is labeled in green color. The non-enhancing core area is labeled in red color. The enhancing core area is labeled in yellow color. (Color figure online)

Quantitative Result of our Model. The segmentation result with our proposed method is shown in Table 1. In the presence of four channels, our model can be comparable with the state-of-art result in [8]. The down-grading on Dice score for three types of tumor regions from missing channel inputs complies with the result in [5]. We also have the following findings:

– Missing T1 and T2 channel would have a minor decreasing in Dice score of all three categories. This observation consists with the manual protocol of BraTs dataset. T1 verifies the tumor core segmentation from T1c channel and T2 verifies whole tumor segmentation from Flair.

- Missing T1c channel would have a substantial decreasing in Dice score for both tumor core and enhancing core, for T1c is the chief indicating channel for segmenting tumor core and enhancing core region. Missing Flair channel would have a sharp decreasing on Dice score for all three categories, for Flair is the chief indicating channel for segmenting the whole tumor.
- As shown in Fig. 3, missing Flair channel would result in a coarse locating on the whole tumor region. And missing T1c channel would result in mistaking tumor core and enhanced core region as non-core region.

To provide justification of domain adaptation loss term we introduce, we also provide an ablation experiment by training only on reconstruction loss in training process. Our baseline result is shown in Table 1. Distinct increases of Dice score in all categories are observed when trained with domain adaptation loss compared with the baseline. The qualitative visualization are consistent with the quantitative results as shown in Fig. 3.

Table 1. The dice scores for whole tumor (WT), tumor core (TC) and enhanced core (EC) on the test dataset. The left is the result of our proposed method with our adversarial loss. The right is result of our baseline method trained without our domain adaptation loss.

	Proposed			Baseline		
	WT	TC	EC	WT	TC	EC
Full channel	0.894	0.790	0.653	0.875	0.693	0.554
Missing T1	0.890	0.778	0.642	0.871	0.672	0.532
Missing T1c	0.879	0.570	0.484	0.856	0.426	0.380
Missing T2	0.893	0.775	0.643	0.865	0.660	0.521
Missing Flair	0.616	0.680	0.552	0.508	0.570	0.464

Contribution of Every Channel to Segmentation Labels. In contrast to most segmentation algorithms performed as black-boxes and evaluated purely on accuracy, we provide some insights of the decisions of segmentation networks to physicians. The physicians could weigh this information and incorporate it in the overall diagnosis process.

Figure 4 shows the contribution of each channel while predicting three types of tumors at pixel level. By weighting the prediction differences between inputting full channels and removing a specific channel, we visualize the influence of each channel to an individual segmentation label. Red color represents positive evidence, and blue color represents negative evidence from that channel to the segmentation label. We observed that, different channels contribute distinctly to different tumor types.

For example, Flair channel provides a strong positive evidence on the whole tumor regions and a negative evidence of the non-tumor regions. T2 channel refines the evidence across the boundary area. T1c channel provides supporting

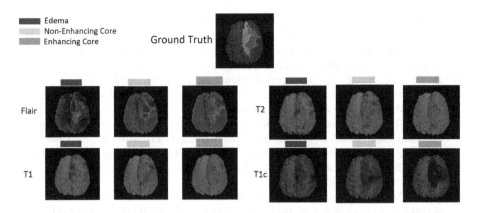

Fig. 4. Visualization of segmentation decision on different channels, using prediction relevance analysis. Red color represents positive evidence, and blue color represents negative evidence of that region. (Color figure online)

evidence both on tumor core and enhanced core area against the rest in the whole tumor area. T1 channel refines the evidence across the boundaries of tumor core area. In general, we trust the segmentation classifiers that could not only produce exact and distinct labels for each tumor type, but also provide reasonable explanations for its decisions.

4 Conclusion

We propose a brain tumor segmentation algorithm that is robust to missing modality. Our model is designed to recover the information from missing modality and is able to visualize the contribution of each channel. The comparisons between full and missing modality show the important roles of Flair and T1c on discrimination of whole tumor and tumor core, respectively. These findings are along well with the expert labeling routine [12].

References

1. Abadi, M., et al.: Tensorflow: a system for large-scale machine learning. OSDI **16**, 265–283 (2016)
2. Chen, L., Wu, Y., DSouza, A.M., Abidin, A.Z., Wismüller, A., Xu, C.: MRI tumor segmentation with densely connected 3D CNN. In: Medical Imaging 2018: Image Processing, vol. 10574, p. 105741F. International Society for Optics and Photonics (2018)
3. Ganin, Y., Lempitsky, V.: Unsupervised domain adaptation by backpropagation. In: International Conference on Machine Learning, pp. 1180–1189 (2015)
4. Havaei, M., et al.: Brain tumor segmentation with deep neural networks. Med. Image Anal. **35**, 18–31 (2017)

5. Havaei, M., Guizard, N., Chapados, N., Bengio, Y.: HeMIS: hetero-modal image segmentation. In: Ourselin, S., Joskowicz, L., Sabuncu, M.R., Unal, G., Wells, W. (eds.) MICCAI 2016. LNCS, vol. 9901, pp. 469–477. Springer, Cham (2016). https://doi.org/10.1007/978-3-319-46723-8_54
6. Hoo-Chang, S., et al.: Deep convolutional neural networks for computer-aided detection: CNN architectures, dataset characteristics and transfer learning. IEEE Trans. Med. Imaging **35**(5), 1285 (2016)
7. Isensee, F., et al.: Brain Tumor Segmentation Using Large Receptive Field Deep Convolutional Neural Networks. In: Maier-Hein, geb. Fritzsche, K., Deserno, geb. Lehmann, T., Handels, H., Tolxdorff, T. (eds.) Bildverarbeitung für die Medizin 2017. Informatik aktuell, pp. 86–91. Springer, Heidelberg (2017). https://doi.org/10.1007/978-3-662-54345-0_24
8. Jin, Q., Meng, Z., Sun, C., Wei, L., Su, R.: RA-UNet: a hybrid deep attention-aware network to extract liver and tumor in CT scans. arXiv preprint arXiv:1811.01328 (2018)
9. Kao, P.-Y., Ngo, T., Zhang, A., Chen, J., Manjunath, B.: Brain tumor segmentation and tractographic feature extraction from structural MR images for overall survival prediction. arXiv preprint arXiv:1807.07716 (2018)
10. Le, T.H.N., Gummadi, R., Savvides, M.: Deep recurrent level set for segmenting brain tumors. In: Frangi, A.F., Schnabel, J.A., Davatzikos, C., Alberola-López, C., Fichtinger, G. (eds.) MICCAI 2018. LNCS, vol. 11072, pp. 646–653. Springer, Cham (2018). https://doi.org/10.1007/978-3-030-00931-1_74
11. Manders, J., Marchiori, E., van Laarhoven, T.: Simple domain adaptation with class prediction uncertainty alignment. arXiv preprint arXiv:1804.04448 (2018)
12. Menze, B.H., et al.: The multimodal brain tumor image segmentation benchmark (BRATS). IEEE Trans. Med. Imaging **34**(10), 1993–2024 (2015)
13. Robnik-Šikonja, M., Kononenko, I.: Explaining classifications for individual instances. IEEE Trans. Knowl. Data Eng. **20**(5), 589–600 (2008)
14. Ronneberger, O., Fischer, P., Brox, T.: U-Net: convolutional networks for biomedical image segmentation. In: Navab, N., Hornegger, J., Wells, W.M., Frangi, A.F. (eds.) MICCAI 2015. LNCS, vol. 9351, pp. 234–241. Springer, Cham (2015). https://doi.org/10.1007/978-3-319-24574-4_28
15. Wang, G., Li, W., Ourselin, S., Vercauteren, T.: Automatic brain tumor segmentation using cascaded anisotropic convolutional neural networks. In: Crimi, A., Bakas, S., Kuijf, H., Menze, B., Reyes, M. (eds.) BrainLes 2017. LNCS, vol. 10670, pp. 178–190. Springer, Cham (2018). https://doi.org/10.1007/978-3-319-75238-9_16
16. Zhang, Y., Brady, M., Smith, S.: Segmentation of brain MR images through a hidden markov random field model and the expectation-maximization algorithm. IEEE Trans. Med. Imaging **20**(1), 45–57 (2001)
17. Zhang, Y., Funkhouser, T.: Deep depth completion of a single RGB-D image. In: Proceedings of the IEEE Conference on Computer Vision and Pattern Recognition, pp. 175–185 (2018)
18. Zheng, S., et al.: Conditional random fields as recurrent neural networks. In: Proceedings of the IEEE International Conference on Computer Vision, pp. 1529–1537 (2015)

Contextual Fibre Growth to Generate Realistic Axonal Packing for Diffusion MRI Simulation

Ross Callaghan$^{(\boxtimes)}$, Daniel C. Alexander, Hui Zhang, and Marco Palombo

Centre for Medical Image Computing, Department of Computer Science,
University College London, London, UK
ross.callaghan.16@ucl.ac.uk

Abstract. This paper presents ConFiG, a method for generating white matter (WM) numerical phantoms with more realistic orientation dispersion and packing density. Numerical phantoms are commonly used in the validation of diffusion MRI (dMRI) techniques so it is important that they are as realistic as possible. Current numerical phantoms either oversimplify the complex morphology of WM or are unable to produce realistic orientation dispersion at high packing density. The highest packing density and orientation dispersion achieved so far is only 20% at 10°. ConFiG takes advantage of a shift of paradigm: rather than 'packing fibres', our algorithm 'grows fibres' contextually and efficiently, attempting to produce a substrate with desired morphological priors (orientation dispersion, packing density and diameter distribution), whilst avoiding intersection between fibres. The potential of ConFiG is demonstrated by reaching the highest packing density and orientation dispersion ever, to our knowledge (25% at 35°). The algorithm is compared with a 'brute force' growth approach showing that it is much more efficient, being $\mathcal{O}(n)$ compared to the $\mathcal{O}(n^2)$ brute-force method. The application of the method to dMRI is demonstrated with simulations of diffusion-weighted MR signal in three example substrates with differing orientation-dispersions, packing-densities and permeabilities.

1 Introduction

Numerical phantoms have found much use for validating many magnetic resonance imaging (MRI) experiments. In particular, many studies employing diffusion MRI (dMRI) to study microstructural features of white matter (WM) use numerical phantoms as part of the validation process [9,10,16].

Typically, the models used in these studies represent axons in WM using simplistic geometrical representations such as parallel cylinders with uniform [9] or polydisperse [5] radii. Other studies introduce more complexity into the numerical phantoms with, for example, harmonic beading [1], spines [13] and undulation of individual fibres [11]. These studies typically only consider one

---

H. Zhang and M. Palombo—Joint senior author.

© Springer Nature Switzerland AG 2019
A. C. S. Chung et al. (Eds.): IPMI 2019, LNCS 11492, pp. 429–440, 2019.
https://doi.org/10.1007/978-3-030-20351-1_33

mode of morphological variation at a time and all of these representations over-simplify the true complexity of axonal morphology that has been investigated through ex-vivo studies using electron microscopy [7].

Another emerging application of dMRI simulations is in the direct estimation of microstructural features from a measured dMRI signal. Some recent works use fingerprinting-style techniques and machine learning to match simulated signals and the corresponding ground truth microstructure of the numerical phantom to the measured signal [6,8,12,14].

For all of these applications, synthetic models of WM that accurately represent real tissue are highly important.

Generating realistic WM numerical phantoms which accurately capture realistic microstructural features (such as dispersion, undulation, beading, etc.) at high packing densities is a major open challenge for the dMRI community. While densely packing straight, parallel, fibres is relatively easy, only a few groups have attempted to densely pack irregular, non-parallel, fibres. The highest packing density achieved so far under modest dispersion (up to $10°$) reaches only 20% [4]. These approaches typically involve the packing of fibres. That is, trying to pack a set of existing fibres together as densely as possible.

Here, we propose a completely different strategy: rather than densely 'packing' irregular fibres, we 'grow' fibres contextually, mimicking natural fibre genesis. The algorithm presented proposes a method called ConFiG (Contextual Fibre Growth) for the generation of WM numerical phantoms with more realistic orientation dispersion and packing density. Fibres are grown one-by-one following a cost function which attempts to impose the morphological priors that are input to the algorithm.

The rest of the paper is organized as follows: Sect. 2 describes ConFiG, Sect. 3 details some experiments showing the potential of the algorithm and comparing it to a brute-force approach to fibre growth and Sect. 4 summarises the contributions and discusses future work.

2   ConFiG: Contextual Fibre Growth

In this section we describe ConFiG which grows fibres one-by-one avoiding intersection between fibres whilst attempting to ensure that the resulting substrate has desired morphological properties such as orientation dispersion, diameter distribution and packing density. The algorithm is broken into a few stages:

- the definition of inputs to the algorithm
- the generation of the network on which fibres grow
- the method by which each fibre grows
- the meshing procedure to create 3D meshes

Pseudocode for the first three of these points is shown in Algorithm 1. The rest of this section details each of the above stages.

Algorithm 1. ConFiG algorithm pseudocode. Takes desired morphological priors (OD, ρ and d_0) as well as desired number of nodes in the growth network. From these initial fibre positions, targets and the growth network are generated before the main loop of the algorithm in which each fibre grows one-by-one.

procedure FIBREGROWTH(OD, ρ, d_0, numNodes)
    [startPoints, targets] ← GETINITIALPOINTS(OD, ρ, d_0)   ▷ Section 2.1
    [DT, D] ← INTIALISENETWORK(numNodes, startPoints, targets)   ▷ Section 2.2
    numFibre ← number of entries in startPoints
    for i in 1:numFibre **do**   ▷ Initialise the fibre structures
        fibres(i).node(0) = startPoints(i)
    end for
    for i in 1:numFibre **do**   ▷ Main growth loop (Section 2.3)
        terminated ← false
        j ← 0
        while not terminated **do**
            GETCANDIDATENODES(fibres(i).node(j), DT)   ▷ Figure 1a
            • candidates ← DT.nodes sharing edge with fibres(i).node(j)
            GETBESTSTEP(candidates, D, targets)   ▷ Figure 1b
            • costs ← costs for candidates from Eq. (1) given targets, D
            • bestStep ← candidate with minimum cost
            TAKESTEP(fibres(i), bestStep)   ▷ Figure 1c
            • fibres(i).node(j+1) ← bestStep
            UPDATETRIANGULATION(fibres(i), DT, D)   ▷ Figure 1d
            • segment ← vector from fibre(i).node(j) to fibre(i).node(j+1)
            • D_{new} ← distance from DT.nodes to segment
            • D ← min(D, D_{new})
            ISTERMINATED(fibres(i), targets)
            • **if** fibre(i) has reached target:
                terminated ← true
            • **elseif** fibre(i) has no possible node to move to:
                terminated ← true
            • **else**:
                terminated ← false
                j ← j + 1
        end while
    end for
end procedure

2.1 Input to the Algorithm

The morphology of the final substrate will depend on the inputs to the algorithm which can be split into two general categories: parameters defining the fibre population(s), and parameters defining the space in which fibres grow.

Fibre parameters include the desired orientation dispersion (OD), packing density (ρ) and diameter distribution ($P(d_0)$). These three parameters determine the initial settings for each individual fibre. Each fibre is defined by a starting point and a target point towards which it will grow as well as an initial fibre diameter, d_0. These parameters for each fibre are determined from OD, ρ and $P(d_0)$ by packing circles with the diameters drawn from $P(d_0)$ up to a density of ρ in 2 dimensions. Orientation dispersion is introduced by moving the target points of fibres relative to the starting points.

Alternatively, if the user wishes, the starting point, target point and diameter for each fibre can be directly input, rather than allowing ConFiG to generate them, in order to specify particular fibre configurations such as crossing fibre bundles or fanning fibres.

Each fibre is allowed to shrink its diameter if it is necessary to fit into spaces close to other fibres. The maximum amount of shrinkage permitted is a controllable parameter, specified as a percentage of the initial fibre diameter.

Due to the stochastic nature of the algorithm, the final substrate is not guaranteed to have the exact morphological properties as input in the priors, however these inputs give the target morphology that ConFiG will attempt to produce.

Parameters defining the space in which the fibres grow are used to define a discretisation of the space into a set of node points that the fibres can occupy. Ideally, the space in which the fibres can grow is a continuous space, so there are an infinite number of positions a fibre can occupy, however this is impractical, so in this algorithm the space is discretised into a finite set of nodes.

Naturally, the choice of the density and arrangement of node points will impact the substrate that is produced. Too few nodes will result in fibres that have very long, straight segments and may introduce intersections between fibres. Using more nodes will reduce overlap between fibres at the cost of more memory usage and slower growth of the fibres. The arrangement of the nodes will also affect the morphology of the final substrate. For instance, placing nodes on a uniform grid may produce fibres with unnaturally angular paths. If the density of nodes on a uniform grid becomes sufficiently high, these angular bends are insignificant compared to the diameter and the fibres will have more natural shapes. For large substrates, the number of nodes required to satisfy this condition becomes intractably large. For this reason, the nodes used are typically pseudo-randomly distributed to ensure broadly uniform coverage of the space, whilst keeping the number of nodes required lower.

2.2   Creation of the Growth Network

In order to embed information about the local environment at each node, the first step of the algorithm is generating the paths that fibres can take between the nodes as well as defining a maximum diameter that can be sustained at each node to avoid intersection which will be denoted by d_i, for a node, i. These paths define a network along which the fibres may grow.

The paths between nodes are defined by the Delaunay triangulation [3] of the nodes which creates a sparse network in which any node can be reached from any other node. This triangulation creates edges between nearby nodes, encoding information about the local connectivity at each node. Nodes that become occupied by a fibre will be inaccessible to any future fibres, which is one way in which intersection is minimised between fibres.

The maximum diameter, d_i, at each node encodes information on the amount of space available at each node. Where d_i is small, that node is close to an existing fibre, so any subsequent fibre passing through that node will have to shrink its diameter to d_i in order to prevent intersections. Allowing fibres to contextually shrink their diameter allows fibres to occupy spaces which would otherwise be unavailable.

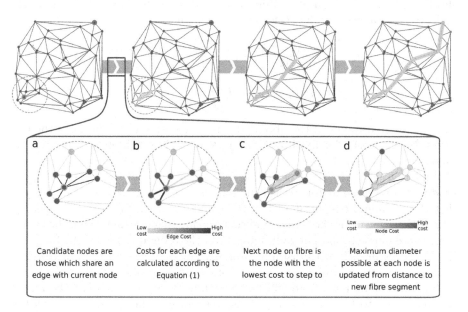

Fig. 1. Schematic overview of the fibre growth algorithm. A fibre grows sequentially, moving from one node to the next, starting from the start point (top left, green node) toward the target (top left, blue node) along the edges defined by the Delaunay triangulation. Inset: The algorithm determining which node a fibre steps to at any given iteration. (a) The possible nodes to step to are those which share an edge with the current node. (b) From the edges available costs are calculated using Eqs. (1) and (2). (c) The fibre will grow along the edge with the lowest cost. (d) From this new segment, the maximum diameter sustainable at a given node is calculated, giving each node a cost based on the maximum sustainable diameter. This cost will then be used in the calculation of edge weights (b) for future fibres. Note that although this figure illustrates the algorithm in 2D, in practice the algorithm grows fibres in 3D. (Color figure online)

2.3   Growth of a Fibre

Each individual fibre grows by moving the head of the fibre from node to node according to a cost function which attempts to ensure that the fibre moves towards its target whilst avoiding intersection. The main steps in the growth of a single fibre are shown in Fig. 1.

The first step in the growth of a fibre is determining which nodes are the possible next nodes the fibre can step to, referred to as candidate nodes. From a given starting node, s, the candidate nodes are any of the nodes which share an edge with s.

The choice of which candidate node a fibre steps to from the current node is determined by a cost function. The cost function consists of two terms, one which penalises moving away from the target point, t, and one which penalises moving to a position where d_i is low, meaning the fibre diameter would have to shrink. The cost function for a fibre at a position, s, to move to an candidate node, c, given a target point, t, is $l = l_t + f l_d$, where

$$l_t = \frac{1}{2} \cdot \frac{\|s - c\|}{1 + \|s - c\|} \cdot \left(1 - \frac{(c - s) \cdot (t - s)}{\|c - s\| \|t - s\|}\right), \tag{1}$$

$$l_d = \max\left(0, \frac{1}{d_0}(d_0 - d_i)\right), \tag{2}$$

d_0 is the desired radius of the fibre and f is a weighting factor between the two terms. In this work, f is fixed to 0.2 to more strongly weight growth toward the target.

Equation (1) is the term penalising moving away from the target. The dot product between the vector to the candidate and the vector to the target ensures that the minimum cost occurs when the candidate is directly aligned with the target. Equation (2) is the term penalising moving to a position where the radius of the fibre must shrink. For radii lower than the desired radius of the fibre, d_0, Eq. (2) grows linearly with distance from d_0. For radii greater than or equal to d_0, Eq. (2) is zero, meaning that regions of empty space are equally weighted.

The next node for a fibre will be the candidate node which has the lowest cost according to Eqs. (1) and (2). This method of finding a path through the triangulation by choosing the lowest cost node at each position amounts to a greedy best-first pathfinding approach with a heuristic given by Eqs. (1) and (2).

With the next node chosen, the value of d_i needs to be updated for other nearby nodes. All nodes have d_i set to the Euclidean distance between the node and the surface of the new section of fibre if that distance is less than the current value of d_i. This is illustrated in Fig. 1d.

Any nodes which now lie within the fibre have d_i set to zero. Nodes with $d_i = 0$ are disallowed from future steps, meaning that once a fibre has grown, no future fibres can connect to any nodes within the fibre. This, in addition to shrinking the radius of future fibres according to d_i at each node means that the fibres grow in an almost completely non-intersecting manner. Since the value of d_i is set based on fibre-to-point distances, there can be cases in which the fibres would intersect when the closest point between two fibre sections is not at one of the fibre nodes. In order to account for this, a meshing process developed which can deform fibres around one another. This is described in Sect. 2.4.

The fibre growth algorithm will output a set of fibres which are defined by a series of nodes and the diameter of the fibre at each node. These are written into the Stockley-Wheal-Cole (SWC) format [15], a format commonly used to store cellular morphology information.

2.4   Creation of Fibre Meshes

In order to create 3D meshes to be used in dMRI simulations, a meshing process was developed using 3D modelling software Blender (https://blender.org). Fibres are meshed one-by-one using the Blender "SWC Mesher" add-on (https://github.com/mcellteam/swc_mesher) which uses Blender metaballs to make a mesh.

In Blender, a metaball is an implicit surface defined as the isosurface of a so-called directing structure. This directing structure can be seen the source of a static field. For instance a spherical isosurface can be formed with a directing structure which mimics the electric field a point charge. When multiple metaballs come close to one another, the fields will combine to form a surface that merges the two spheres together. An example of metaball interactions is shown in Fig. 2.

By placing metaballs along the skeleton of each fibre, with the path and diameters given from the fibre growth algorithm, a smooth surface is formed for each fibre. It is this implicit surface, created using metaballs that the SWC mesher add-on creates. This implicit surface can be turned into an explicit surface (i.e. a mesh of vertices and faces) in Blender, which can then be refined by progressively smoothing and reducing the number of faces in the mesh to create a mesh which can be used in dMRI simulations.

This process can be used to mesh each fibre individually, however issues can arise with intersection of fibres, as mentioned in Sect. 2.3. In order to account for this, a contextual meshing algorithm was developed. The metaball surface for one fibre is created using the SWC Mesher. This surface is then turned into a mesh as described above, however the metaballs are retained. The metaball potential is then turned negative, meaning that rather than attracting any future nearby metaball surfaces, it will repel them, as shown in Fig. 2b. This means that subsequent fibres which are meshed very close to, or overlapping with existing fibres will deform organically to resolve the intersection, thus creating a series of completely non-intersecting fibre meshes which can be used by the dMRI simulator.

The deformation introduced by the contextual meshing process has two effects. As well as helping to prevent intersection between fibres, the deformation produces fibres with more organic non-circular cross sections, better mimicking realistic mythologies. This is vastly different to the majority of previous WM numerical phantoms which model fibres as circular or elliptic cylinders.

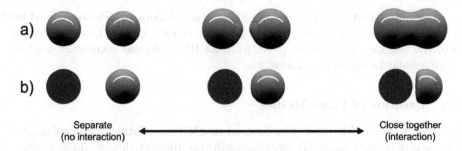

Fig. 2. Simple example of metaball interactions. (a) With two positive metaballs, the fields combine to attract the surfaces together. This is used to join individual segments into a continuous fibre. (b) With one negative metaball (indicated by the flat grey circle) the surface of the metaball is repelled from the negative metaball. This is used to deform nearby fibres around one another.

3 Experiments and Results

3.1 Demonstration of ConFiG

To demonstrate the potential of ConFiG, three substrates at different (dispersion, packing density) conditions were generated: (0°, 60%), (15°, 30%) and (35°, 25%), shown in Fig. 3a. Each substrate is grown using 5×10^6 pseudo-randomly placed source nodes for the growth network, giving a network with 3.88×10^7 edges and a mean distance between any given node and its neighbours of $0.29\,\mu$m. The packing densities chosen represent the highest densities achievable using ConFiG for each dispersion condition.

For the 0° dispersed substrate, initial diameters were drawn from a gamma distribution with mean $d_0 = 2\,\mu$m and standard deviation $\sigma_d = 0.2\,\mu$m. The 15° and 35° substrates were generated with $d_0 = 1.2\,\mu$m and $\sigma_d = 0.2\,\mu$m in order to show the flexibility of ConFiG to generate substrates with different diameter distributions as well as orientation dispersion and packing density. Diameters were limited to be permitted to shrink to 25% of the original fibre diameter in order to fit into space.

For each substrate, the Pulsed-Gradient-Spin-Echo (PGSE) signal was simulated in Camino [2] using 5×10^5 diffusing spins and 5×10^3 discrete time steps, uniformly distributed with bulk-diffusivity $D_0 = 2\,\mu$m²/ms. To show the range of simulation possibilities available, three different membrane permeabilities ($\kappa = 0, 0.0025, 0.0050\,\mu$m/ms) were also imposed. The simulated PGSE measurement parameters were: $\delta/\Delta = 1/40$ ms and 50 b-values from 0 to $9\,$ms/μm² along x-, y- and z-directions.

The corresponding direction-averaged simulated PGSE signals at different permeabilities are shown with SNR $= \infty$ in Fig. 3b and SNR $= 20$ in Fig. 3c. The signal decays to a lower value as the dispersion increases and density decreases, as expected.

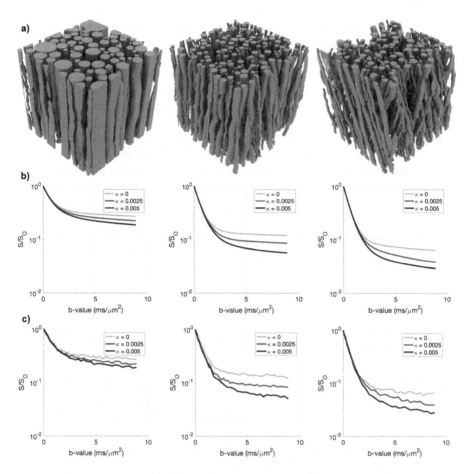

Fig. 3. (a) Example substrates (cut into $30 \times 30 \times 30\,\mu\mathrm{m}^3$ cube) from the fibre growth algorithm, left to right: Zero macroscopic dispersion (60% density), 15° of macroscopic dispersion (30% density), 35° dispersed (25% density). (b) Simulations for each substrate for varying permeabilities with SNR $= \infty$ and (c) SNR $= 20$. Units of κ are $\mu\mathrm{m}/\mathrm{ms}$.

3.2   Comparison with Brute-Force Approach

ConFiG was compared against the naïve brute-force approach to fibre growth. The brute-force approach grows fibres one segment at a time and checks for collisions between the new segment and all existing fibres. Each new segment is chosen from one of 128 candidate directions on a cone aligned with the previous segment, with each direction being weighted according to Eq. (1).

Substrates were grown with both the brute-force approach and ConFiG using the same starting and target points and initial diameters. These initial parameters were determined by packing circles with gamma distributed radii (mean $d_0 = 2\,\mu\mathrm{m}$, standard deviation $\sigma = 0.6\,\mu\mathrm{m}$) into a $40\,\mu\mathrm{m} \times 40\,\mu\mathrm{m}$ square up to a packing density of 60%. Target points were set as $40\,\mu$m directly above the starting points to define a substrate with $0°$ macroscopic orientation dispersion. This resulted in a substrate with a total of 54 initial fibres.

The fibre growth algorithm used 1×10^6 randomly distributed points for the Delaunaty triangulation giving a mean distance between points of $0.5\,\mu$m, matching the brute force approach which used a segment length of $0.5\,\mu$m for each new fibre segment.

From these initial parameters, fibres were grown using a subset of $n = 1, 5, 10, 15, 20, 25, 30, 40$ fibres and the growth was timed. Each value of n was timed 5 times with and the mean taken to reduce single-run timing fluctuations.

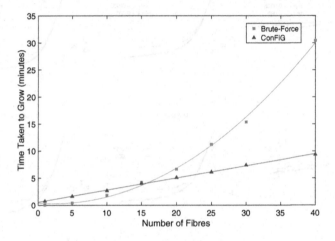

Fig. 4. Timing of brute force growth vs. the fibre growth algorithm along with a quadratic fit (brute-force) and linear fit (fibre growth algorithm). The fibre growth algorithm is clearly linear in the number of fibres, while brute force growth fits an order n^2 well.

Figure 4 shows the timing results of the brute-force approach versus the fibre growth algorithm. The fibre growth algorithm has approximately $\mathcal{O}(n)$ complexity with n being the number of fibres. Conversely, the brute-force algorithm shows $\mathcal{O}(n^2)$ complexity owing to the fact that every new segment has to check for collisions with all existing fibres.

The fibre growth algorithm has a higher $n = 0$ offset which is caused by the overhead in calculating the Delaunay triangulation for the growth network. This causes the brute-force approach to have better performance at low n, while at higher n (approaching the > 100 fibres needed for a realistic dMRI voxel) the linearity of the fibre growth algorithm gives it much faster performance.

4   Discussion and Conclusion

ConFiG shifts perspective from previous works attempting to pack together fibres, by trying to mimic natural fibre genesis. This approach represents a major step towards very high fibre packing, enabling us to reach the highest dispersion at the highest packing density reached so far, to our knowledge. Our (15°, 30%) and (35°, 25%) represent an average ~50% and ~200% improvement, respectively, over the best previously reported results of (10°, 20%) [4].

The substrates presented in Fig. 3 are just a few examples of the kinds of substrates that can be produced using our ConFiG method. By varying the setup of the morphological controls and start and target points, many different fibre configurations can be produced. Currently, fibres will attempt to grow in a straight line between the start and target points, meaning that certain configurations such as kissing bundles cannot be represented. However, the algorithm can in principle be extended to allow for series of target points, allowing the definition of a desired 'path' of a fibre.

Additionally, some input parameter settings cannot be achieved. For instance, trying to grow a substrate with both very high density and very high dispersion will result in a final substrate that does not reach the density required. The reason for this could be a combination of limitations of the algorithm in restricting growth to a discrete network and also the fact that some morphological settings are practically infeasible. This limitation, however, also applies to the fibre packing and brute force growth approaches.

One weakness of the fibre-growth algorithm is that since the fibre diameters are calculated from a fibre-to-point distance, there can still be some small amount of overlap between fibres. This is solved using the meshing process in Blender to deform the regions of slight overlap between neighbouring fibres.

To conclude, the proposed ConFiG approach, using the fully connected growth network, is shown to be more efficient than a 'brute-force' growth approach. The fact that ConFiG is linear with the number of fibres makes it far more efficient for high numbers of fibres. For instance, a realistic voxel will need hundreds or thousands of fibres which will become impractically slow for the 'brute-force' approach, whilst remaining manageable for our algorithm. This efficiency, along with the high density and orientation dispersion achieved means that ConFiG represents a promising step forward in the construction of ultra-realistic numerical phantoms of WM.

Acknowledgements. This work is supported by the EPSRC-funded UCL Centre for Doctoral Training in Medical Imaging (EP/L016478/1) and the Department of Health's NIHR-funded Biomedical Research Centre at University College London Hospitals. This work was supported by EPSRC grants EP/M020533/1 and EP/N018702/1.

References

1. Budde, M.D., Frank, J.A.: Neurite beading is sufficient to decrease the apparent diffusion coefficient after ischemic stroke. PNAS **107**(32), 14472–14477 (2010). https://doi.org/10.1073/pnas.1004841107/

2. Cook, P., Bai, Y., Seunarine, K.K., Hall, M.G., Parker, G.J., Alexander, D.C.: Camino: open-source diffusion-mri reconstruction and processing. In: 14th Scientific Meeting of the International Society for Magnetic Resonance in Medicine, vol. 14, p. 2759 (2006)
3. Delaunay, P.B.: Sur la sphere vide. Bulletin of Academy of Sciences of the USSR (1934). https://doi.org/10.1051/jphysrad:01951001207073500
4. Ginsburger, K., et al.: Improving the realism of white matter numerical phantoms: a step toward a better understanding of the influence of structural disorders in diffusion MRI. Front. Phys. 5(FEB), 1–18 (2018). https://doi.org/10.3389/fphy.2018.00012
5. Hall, M.G., Alexander, D.C.: Convergence and parameter choice for Monte-Carlo simulations of diffusion MRI. IEEE Trans. Med. Imaging 28(9), 1354–1364 (2009). https://doi.org/10.1109/TMI.2009.2015756
6. Hill, I., et al.: Deep neural network based framework for in-vivo axonal permeability estimation. In: 26th Annual Meeting of the International Society for Magnetic Resonance in Medicine (ISMRM) (2018)
7. Lee, H.H., et al.: Electron microscopy 3-dimensional segmentation and quantification of axonal dispersion and diameter distribution in mouse brain corpus callosum. bioRxiv 357491 (2018)
8. Nedjati-Gilani, G.L., et al.: Machine learning based compartment models with permeability for white matter microstructure imaging. NeuroImage (2017). https://doi.org/10.1016/j.neuroimage.2017.02.013
9. Nilsson, M., Alerstam, E., Wirestam, R., Ståhlberg, F., Brockstedt, S., Lätt, J.: Evaluating the accuracy and precision of a two-compartment Karger model using Monte Carlo simulations. J. Magn. Reson. 206(1), 59–67 (2010). https://doi.org/10.1016/j.jmr.2010.06.002
10. Nilsson, M., Lasič, S., Drobnjak, I., Topgaard, D., Westin, C.F.: Resolution limit of cylinder diameter estimation by diffusion MRI: the impact of gradient waveform and orientation dispersion. NMR Biomed. 30(7), 1–13 (2017). https://doi.org/10.1002/nbm.3711
11. Nilsson, M., Lätt, J., Ståhlberg, F., van Westen, D., Hagslätt, H.: The importance of axonal undulation in diffusion MR measurements: a Monte Carlo simulation study. NMR in Biomed. 25(5), 795–805 (2012). https://doi.org/10.1002/nbm.1795
12. Palombo, M., et al.: Machine learning based estimation of axonal permeability: validation on cuprizone treated in-vivo mouse model of axonal demyelination. In: Proceedings of the Joint Annual Meeting ISMRM-ESMRMB, Paris, France (2018)
13. Palombo, M., Ligneul, C., Hernandez-Garzon, E., Valette, J.: Can we detect the effect of spines and leaflets on the diffusion of brain intracellular metabolites? NeuroImage (2018). https://doi.org/10.1016/j.neuroimage.2017.05.003
14. Rensonnet, G., et al.: Towards microstructure fingerprinting: estimation of tissue properties from a dictionary of Monte Carlo diffusion MRI simulations. NeuroImage 184(May 2018), 964–980 (2018). https://doi.org/10.1016/J.NEUROIMAGE.2018.09.076
15. Stockley, E., Cole, H., Brown, A., Wheal, H.: A system for quantitative morphological measurement and electronic modelling of neurons: three-dimensional reconstruction. J. Neurosci. Methods 47(1–2), 39–51 (1993)
16. Zhang, H., Schneider, T., Wheeler-Kingshott, C.A., Alexander, D.C.: NODDI: practical in vivo neurite orientation dispersion and density imaging of the human brain. NeuroImage 61(4), 1000–1016 (2012). https://doi.org/10.1016/j.neuroimage.2012.03.072

DeepCenterline: A Multi-task Fully Convolutional Network for Centerline Extraction

Zhihui Guo[1], Junjie Bai[2(✉)], Yi Lu[2], Xin Wang[2], Kunlin Cao[2], Qi Song[2],
Milan Sonka[1], and Youbing Yin[2]

[1] University of Iowa, Iowa City, IA 52242, USA
[2] CuraCloud Corporation, Seattle, WA 98104, USA
junjieb@curacloudcorp.com

Abstract. A novel centerline extraction framework is reported which combines an end-to-end trainable multi-task fully convolutional network (FCN) with a minimal path extractor. The FCN simultaneously computes centerline distance maps and detects branch endpoints. The method generates single-pixel-wide centerlines with no spurious branches. It handles arbitrary tree-structured object with no prior assumption regarding depth of the tree or its bifurcation pattern. It is also robust to substantial scale changes across different parts of the target object and minor imperfections of the object's segmentation mask. To the best of our knowledge, this is the first deep-learning based centerline extraction method that guarantees single-pixel-wide centerline for a complex tree-structured object.

The proposed method is validated in coronary artery centerline extraction on a dataset of 620 patients (400 of which used as test set). This application is challenging due to the large number of coronary branches, branch tortuosity, and large variations in length, thickness, shape, etc. The proposed method generates well-positioned centerlines, exhibiting lower number of missing branches and is more robust in the presence of minor imperfections of the object segmentation mask. Compared to a state-of-the-art traditional minimal path approach, our method improves patient-level success rate of centerline extraction from 54.3% to 88.8% according to independent human expert review.

Keywords: Centerline · Deep learning · Multi-task · Attention

1 Introduction

Centerline, or skeleton, provides a concise representation of the object topology. An ideal centerline extraction algorithm generates centerline points close enough to "centers" of the object cross-sectionally, captures all "branches", and has no false positive spurious branches.

Z. Guo and J. Bai—Equal contribution.

© Springer Nature Switzerland AG 2019
A. C. S. Chung et al. (Eds.): IPMI 2019, LNCS 11492, pp. 441–453, 2019.
https://doi.org/10.1007/978-3-030-20351-1_34

Many semi-automated and automated approaches exist for centerline extraction. Morphological thinning and erosion based methods are popular in road centerline extraction [2]. However, centerlines extracted by these methods often come along with spurious branches and usually need ad-hoc post pruning.

In contrast, minimal path based centerline extraction methods guarantee a more structured centerline output by requiring explicitly specified endpoints. A *centerline distance map* (also called cost image) is generated from an object segmentation mask by methods such as Euclidean distance transform, which assigns smaller values to voxels closer to centerline and larger values to voxels farther away. A minimal path between the endpoints in the centerline distance map thus corresponds to the object centerline.

Minimal path algorithms are widely used in blood vessel centerline extraction [1,2,4,5,9]. In [4], Metz et al. adopted vesselness and region statistics as cost metrics and manually specified each branch endpoint. Gülsün et al. [1] used human selected features to compute flow field as cost image. Mirikharaji et al. [5] integrated a predefined tree topology and tubularity scores to get minimal paths. Zheng et al. [9] used a machine learning based vesselness algorithm to generate the cost image. These methods require either human crafted features/priors or manual specification of branch endpoints.

Convolutional neural networks (CNN) have been prevalent in medical image analysis recently and achieved great success. There are three advantages of CNN-based methods over traditional methods. First, multi-layer CNNs have enough capacity to learn complex functions that cannot be described by simple models. Second, CNNs do not require humans to select features and support end-to-end training. Third, a single CNN model has the ability to handle multiple tasks.

Coronary computed tomography angiography (CCTA) is a noninvasive technique widely used in clinical practice for coronary artery disease detection. Given a coronary artery segmentation mask, extracting its centerline is a prerequisite step for automatic stenosis grading, calcium evaluation, plaque evaluation and visualization [3,7]. Extracting coronary artery centerline from a segmentation mask faces multiple notable challenges. First, multiple branches, usually more than a dozen, with large intra-subject and inter-subject variations of length, thickness, and shape are presented, forming a complex tree structure. Detecting all branches without false positive is quite challenging. Second, branch diameter changes significantly from proximal to distal portion of coronary artery. The proximal end can be several times wider than the distal end. Third, tortuous course of vessel branches hinders the performance of a minimal path based algorithm, by which straight paths are inherently preferred. Fourth, imperfections of segmentation masks such as brief touching of two nearby branches could lead to incorrect bifurcation in centerline.

To address these challenges, we propose a two-head multi-task FCN which simultaneously generates a locally normalized distance map and a list of branch endpoints (Fig. 1). One head of the multi-task FCN outputs a normalized centerline distance map that is scale-invariant and robust to image segmentation imperfections. Log-transform and attention mechanism are also incorporated to increase model sensitivity. The other head of the FCN automatically detects the

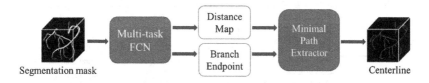

Fig. 1. Schematic workflow of DeepCenterline

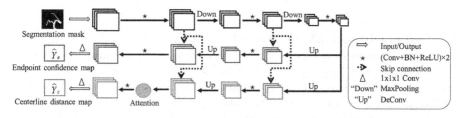

Fig. 2. The proposed multi-task FCN architecture. The input is 3D segmentation mask volume. The two tasks, centerline distance map and endpoint confidence map computation, share the same encoder path and have separate decoder paths. Skip-connections are added among features of same scale to facilitate good use of information. An attention module is added for the centerline distance map task to further boost accuracy.

sparsely distributed endpoints of the object skeleton with high accuracy. The resulting distance map and endpoint list are fed into a minimal path extractor which gives the final centerline extraction results.

2 Method

The proposed method consists of two main steps (Fig. 1): a multi-task FCN computing a locally normalized centerline distance map and a list of endpoints simultaneously, and a minimal cost path extractor taking the output of the FCN to generate a set of paths as centerline.

2.1 Multi-task FCN Architecture

The multi-task FCN accomplishes two tasks: computing a normalized centerline distance map and detecting branch endpoints. As shown in Fig. 2, the two tasks share the same encoder layers consisting of convolution (Conv), batch normalization (BN), ReLU activation function and max pooling (shown as 'Down' in Fig. 2) operations. The two tasks then have different decoder layers tailored for each task, consisting of conv, BN, ReLU, and upsampling operations. Skip connections are applied at the same scale between encoder and decoder layers to make effective use of both high-level and low-level features similar to [6]. Suppose a volumetric segmentation mask is $I^{X \times Y \times Z}$, and $\mathcal{I} = \{(x,y,z)|x \in \{1,\ldots,X\}, y \in \{1,\ldots,Y\}, z \in \{1,\ldots,Z\}\}$ denotes the set of all voxel locations in the image.

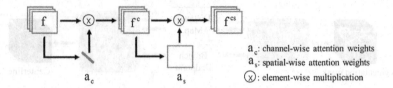

Fig. 3. Spatial-wise and channel-wise attention

Centerline Distance Map. A centerline distance map is defined as an image whose voxel intensity shows how close each voxel is to the nearest centerline point. Due to the large variations in branch radius (coronary artery proximal radius can be five times bigger than the distal radius), a straightforward Euclidean distance transform computation generates centerline distance map with largely variable range of values at different sections of the branch. To obtain a centerline consistently well-positioned in the "center" from beginning to end requires tricky balancing of cost image contrast between thick and thin sections.

To achieve the desired scale-invariance property, we propose to use FCN to generate a *locally normalized* centerline distance map. More specifically, during training, a local cross-sectional view of the segmentation mask perpendicular to the centerline tangent direction at each centerline point is obtained. Suppose the set of all foreground voxels in the cross-sectional view is $\mathcal{S}$. Then the locally normalized distance map value for voxel index $i = (x, y, z) \in \mathcal{S}$ is computed as

$$d_i = \frac{d_i^{Euc}}{\max_{i \in \mathcal{S}} d_i^{Euc}} \tag{1}$$

where d_i^{Euc} is the Euclidean distance of voxel i to the centerline point on the view. To further highlight contrast at portions closer to centerline, log-transform is applied to generate the reference centerline distance map

$$\mathbf{Y_c} = \log(\mathbf{D_c} + \delta) \tag{2}$$

where $\mathbf{D_c} = \{d_i | i \in \mathcal{I}\}$ is the locally normalized centerline distance map throughout the whole segmentation mask image I and δ is a small positive constant to avoid numerical issues. Note that the distance computation in Eqs. (1) and (2) is only carried out when generating training reference standards. During testing phase, the FCN will directly predict centerline distance map $\widehat{\mathbf{Y}}_c$.

Spatial-Wise and Channel-Wise Attention for Centerline Distance Map. Traditionally the convolutional features at different spatial locations and channels are treated equally by the following layers. However, centerline extraction is inherently a localized task. Specifically, the narrow region surrounding the underlying centerline requires most attention for best discriminating contrast. Thus, a spatial-wise attention module is proposed to weight feature maps at different spatial locations. Similarly, different channels of the feature maps can highlight different regions (some channels may focus more around centerline, while other channels may focus more on object mask boundary, etc). It also makes sense to add a channel-wise attention to weight different channels accordingly. Figure 3 shows the proposed spatial-wise and channel-wise attention module, inspired by [8]. The feature map $\mathbf{f}$ is first weighted by channel-wise attention, generating $\mathbf{f^c}$, and then weighted by the spatial attention, generating $\mathbf{f^{cs}}$.

Channel-wise attention weights different channels by vector $\mathbf{a_c} \in \mathbb{R}^C$, where $\sum_{i=1}^{C} \mathbf{a_c}(i) = 1$. To obtain this weighting vector, average pooling is first applied on each channel of the feature map to obtain a summarized channel feature vector $\mathbf{v} \in \mathbb{R}^C$. Then a convolutional layer and a ReLU nonlinearity $\sigma(\cdot)$ are added to obtain the raw attention weights $\mathbf{u} \in \mathbb{R}^C$. In Eq. (3), $*$ is the convolution operator. $\mathbf{W_c}$ is the convolutional kernel and $\mathbf{b_c}$ is the bias vector. A softmax function is applied on the raw attention weights $\mathbf{u}$ to obtain the final channel-wise attention vector $\mathbf{a_c}$, as shown in Eq. (4).

$$\mathbf{u} = \sigma(\mathbf{W_c} * \mathbf{v} + \mathbf{b_c}) \tag{3}$$

$$\mathbf{a_c}(i) = \frac{e^{\mathbf{u}(i)}}{\sum_{c=1}^{C} e^{\mathbf{u}(c)}}, \quad i \in \{1, \cdots, C\} \tag{4}$$

To apply the channel-wise attention weights, the input feature map at channel i is multiplied by attention weight $\mathbf{a_c}(i)$ to obtain channel-weighted feature map

$$\mathbf{f}_i^{\mathbf{c}} = \mathbf{a_c}(i) \cdot \mathbf{f}_i, \quad i \in \{1, \cdots, C\} \tag{5}$$

Spatial-wise attention weight matrix $\mathbf{a}_s \in \mathbb{R}^I$ is obtained similar to the channel-wise attention. The raw spatial attention map $\mathbf{q}$ is computed by applying a $1 \times 1 \times 1$ convolutional layer $\mathbf{W_s}$ with bias $\mathbf{b_s}$ and a ReLU nonlinearity $\sigma(\cdot)$ to $\mathbf{f^c}$ (Eq. (6)). Then a softmax function is used to obtain the final spatial attention weights $\mathbf{a_s}$, where $\sum_{i \in \mathcal{I}} \mathbf{a_s}(i) = 1$. The spatial attention weight is applied by multiplying $\mathbf{a_s}(i)$ with features $\mathbf{f}_i^{\mathbf{c}}$ at location i (Eq. (8)).

$$\mathbf{q} = \sigma(\mathbf{W_s} * \mathbf{f_c} + \mathbf{b_s}) \tag{6}$$

$$\mathbf{a_s}(i) = \frac{e^{\mathbf{q}(i)}}{\sum_{j \in \mathcal{I}} e^{\mathbf{q}(j)}}, \quad i \in \mathcal{I} \tag{7}$$

$$\mathbf{f}_i^{\mathbf{cs}} = \mathbf{a_s}(i) \cdot \mathbf{f}_i^{\mathbf{c}}, \quad i \in \mathcal{I} \tag{8}$$

Branch Endpoint Detection. Different from centerline distance map which consists of continuous values inside the whole segmentation mask, branch endpoints are just a few isolated points. Directly predicting these points using a voxel-wise classification or segmentation framework is not feasible due to the extreme class imbalance. To tackle the class imbalance problem, a voxel-wise endpoint confidence map is generated by constructing a Gaussian distribution around each endpoint to occupy a certain area spatially. The FCN is then trained to predict the endpoint confidence map, which has a more balanced ratio between nonzero and zero voxels.

Specifically, a spatial Gaussian field is generated around each endpoint

$$\mathbf{Y_e}(i) = \frac{1}{\sqrt{2\pi\Delta}} e^{-\frac{\mathbf{D_e}(i)^2}{\Delta^2}}, \quad i \in \mathcal{I} \tag{9}$$

where $\mathbf{D_e}(i)$ is the geodesic distance from voxel i to the nearest branch endpoint inside the segmentation mask. Δ controls the scale of the Gaussian field.

In testing phase, the predicted endpoint confidence map is thresholded by half of the maximum possible value, i.e., $0.5/\sqrt{2\pi\Delta}$. The centroid of each connected component is then returned as branch endpoints.

Loss Function. The loss function shown in Eq. (10) consists of two terms, one for the centerline distance map prediction and the other for the branch endpoint detection. We enforce the loss function to only account for regions inside the segmentation mask. Suppose the segmentation mask is $\Lambda \in \{0,1\}^{X \times Y \times Z}$. $\Lambda(x, y, z)$ is 1 for every voxel (x, y, z) inside the segmentation mask, and 0 otherwise.

$$L = \gamma \|\Lambda \odot (\mathbf{Y_c} - \widehat{\mathbf{Y}}_c)\|^2 + (1 - \gamma)\|\Lambda \odot (\mathbf{Y_e} - \widehat{\mathbf{Y}}_e)\|^2 \tag{10}$$

In Eq. (10), $\mathbf{Y_c}$ and $\widehat{\mathbf{Y}}_c$ are the reference standard and the predicted centerline distance map. $\mathbf{Y_e}$ and $\widehat{\mathbf{Y}}_e$ are the reference standard and the predicted endpoint confidence map. $\odot$ denotes the Hadamard matrix product operation, which is element-wise multiplication of two matrices. γ is a weighting factor that balances losses of centerline distance map and branch endpoint confidence map.

2.2   Minimal Path Extraction

Given a root point, a list of branch endpoints, and the underlying centerline distance map, a minimal path algorithm is used to extract the centerline of a tree-structured object.

We construct an undirected graph $G = (\mathcal{V}, \mathcal{E})$, where set $\mathcal{V}$ contains all vertices corresponding to voxels in the segmentation mask and set $\mathcal{E}$ includes all edges connecting two neighboring vertices in set $\mathcal{V}$ under a 26-neighborhood setting. On each vertex v_i, weight $w_{v_i} = \exp(\widehat{\mathbf{Y}}_c(i))$ is set according to the centerline distance map. Note that each vertex carries a weight that is smaller when the corresponding voxel is closer to the centerline location, and larger when it is farther away from centerline. Given a starting vertex $s \in \mathcal{V}$ and an ending vertex $t \in \mathcal{V}$, a minimal path between the two is defined as $\mathbf{p} = (p_1, p_2, \ldots, p_K), p_k \in \mathcal{V}, k = \{1, 2, \ldots, K\}$ such that (1). $p_1 = s$, $p_K = t$; (2). every two neighboring vertices in the path is connected by an edge; (3). the sum of vertex weights along this path is minimized (Eq. (11)).

$$\mathbf{p} = \operatorname*{argmin}_{(p_k, p_{k+1}) \in \mathcal{E}} \sum_{k=1}^{K} w_{p_k} \tag{11}$$

Such a minimal path from s to t corresponds to the desired centerline between the two points. To extract the centerline of a tree-structured object such as a coronary artery tree, one root point usually correspond to multiple branch endpoints $t_1, t_2, \ldots, t_T$. In this case, the minimal path between root point s and each endpoint $t_i, i \in \{1, 2, \ldots, T\}$ is computed respectively. Then we trace each path from the end to the start point sequentially. Once the current path intersects with some previously traced paths, it is merged into the previously traced paths. The centerline points are finally smoothed by an iterative mean filtering in a small window for smoother appearance.

3   Experiments and Results

3.1   Experimental Design

To evaluate the proposed method, 620 volumetric coronary CTA scans of 620 patients are used. The image spacing is first normalized to $0.4 \times 0.4 \times 0.4 \, \mathrm{mm}^3$. Coronary arteries and ascending aorta are segmented by a semi-automatic software with manual review and editing. The segmentation masks of coronary arteries and ascending aorta serve as input to the experiment. Since coronary artery originates from ascending aorta, the root points of each coronary vessel tree are readily available as the artery voxels connected to aorta. To simplify notation, we use *CL* as a shorthand for 'centerline'.

Manual annotations of centerline are hard to obtain due to the complex 3D structure of vessels and the single-pixel-wide requirement. Thus, during training, centerlines extracted by a state-of-the-art traditional method (called *baseline*) serve as the training reference truth for DeepCL. During testing, the degree of matching between DeepCL and baseline is first studied as a sanity check. Then various metrics requiring no "truth" centerline such as centerline to segmentation mask Hausdorff distance, and independent human expert review, are utilized to evaluate DeepCL and baseline method.

Baseline. The baseline method is also a minimal path approach. However, both branch endpoints and centerline distance map are computed by traditional methods. The centerline distance map $\mathbf{D^{Sig}}$ is derived from the Euclidean distance map $\mathbf{D^{Euc}}$ of the segmentation mask by summing three sigmoid functions to highlight the contrast in regions close to the centerline area.

$$\mathbf{D^{Sig}} = \sum_{i=1}^{3} \frac{1}{1 + \exp(-\frac{\mathbf{D^{Euc}} - \beta_i}{\alpha_i})} \tag{12}$$

Three pairs of parameters (α_i, β_i), each controlling the width and level of a contrast window, are tuned to enhance central contrast for vessel segments with large, medium, and small diameters respectively. Summing of these three sigmoid functions results in a relatively good contrast around centerline area throughout the whole vessel tree. The branch endpoints are detected as local maxima of the arrival time by a breadth first search, starting from the root point at the junction of aorta and artery to each voxel throughout the artery segmentation mask. All related parameters are tuned on a different dataset.

DeepCenterline. We randomly divided 620 scans into three dataset: 200 scans for training, 20 scans for validation and 400 scans for testing. On the training set, centerlines extracted by the baseline method are used as the reference truth. Although generated by a strong baseline method, the reference truth still contains errors such as missing branches, wrong bifurcations in case of imperfect segmentation mask, etc. The locally normalized centerline distance map and the branch endpoint confidence map are generated based on the reference truth. The parameters of the proposed method are tuned based on the validation set. The tuned model is applied to the 400 testing scans to evaluate the performance.

The input patch size is $64 \times 64 \times 64$ voxels. The standard deviation of Gaussian field Δ in Eq. (9) is set to $3\,\mathrm{mm}$. The loss weighting coefficient γ in Eq. (10) is 0.5. Our multi-task FCN network is optimized by stochastic gradient descent, with batch size of 3. Total number of epochs is 20. The initial learning rate is 10^{-2}, which is divided by a factor of 2 every 5 epochs.

Evaluation Metrics. Several evaluation metrics based on either objective metrics or independent human expert review are used for a thorough comparison of the performance of baseline method and DeepCL on the test set.

i Mean centerline to centerline distance. The mean absolute distance from centerline A to centerline B is defined as the mean of the absolute distance to the nearest point on B for every point on A.

ii Coverage percentage. A point on centerline A is covered by centerline B if the closest point on B is within half a voxel $(0.2\,\mathrm{mm})$.

iii Number of missing endpoints. The number of endpoints not found by automated algorithm is counted manually in patient-level as well as branch-level.

iv Number of scans with wrong bifurcations. This usually happens when two branches are spatially close or even briefly joined at a certain section. The centerline could wrongly consider this brief joining as a bifurcation.

v Average patient-level centerline length. The patient-level centerline length is computed as the sum of lengths of each centerline segment. In general, the less straight "shortcut" centerline takes, and/or the more branch endpoints are detected, the longer centerline will be.

vi Hausdorff distance. Hausdorff distance is defined as the maximum of distances from every artery segmentation mask voxel to the closest centerline point. Hausdorff distance shows how close each segmentation voxel is being covered by the extracted centerline.

vii Overall success rate. A centerline extraction is called fully successful when an expert reviews the centerline and determines that the centerline covers all branches sufficiently, has no spurious false positive branch, no wrong bifurcation, and no obvious deviation from the center throughout all sections.

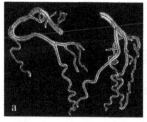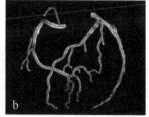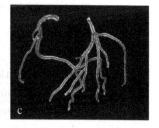

Fig. 4. Example coronary artery with: (a) very tortuous course; (b) small branches; (c) two spatially close branches. Red lines are centerlines generated by DeepCL. (Color figure online)

3.2 Results

Figure 4 displays three examples of coronary artery segmentation masks overlaid with centerlines extracted by DeepCL. For each coronary artery, radius changes substantially from the proximal to the distal side. Different coronary arteries have large variations of vessel curvature, shape and branch topology. Despite all these difficulties, our method is able to extract well-positioned centerline for all branches without false positive branches.

Table 1. Degree of matching between DeepCL and baseline method. A→B measures the distance from one point on centerline A to nearest point on centerline B.

	Baseline → DeepCL	DeepCL → baseline
Mean distance (mm)	0.066 ± 0.053	0.068 ± 0.014
Being covered by (%)	99.7 ± 0.7	99.5 ± 0.6

Matching to Baseline. Table 1 shows the degree of matching between DeepCL and baseline method. The mean centerline distance and "being covered by" percentage both shows how close/well one centerline is being covered by the other centerline. The low mean distance value and the very high coverage percentage on both direction (baseline to DeepCL and DeepCL to baseline) show that the two methods are in good alignment in general. However, a larger portion of baseline centerline points are being covered by DeepCL centerline (99.7%) by a smaller distance (0.066 mm) than the other way around (99.5%, 0.068 mm). This implies DeepCL provides slightly better coverage than baseline, which will be assessed in detail in the following analysis.

Notably, both DeepCL and baseline generate no spurious false positive branches in the extracted centerline according to visual inspection.

Performance Difference. Table 2 shows a detailed analysis regarding the difference between results generated by DeepCL and baseline. Bold items show the

Table 2. Difference in performance of DeepCL and baseline.

Metrics		Raw number #/#		Ratio %	
		Baseline	DeepCL	Baseline	DeepCL
Missing endpoint	Patient-level	170/400	**34/400**	42.5%	**8.5%**
	Branch-level	233/6048	**35/6048**	3.9%	**0.6%**
Scans with wrong bifurcation		28/400	**11/400**	7.0%	**2.8%**
CL length (mm)		308.9	**314.3**	-	-
Overall success rate		217/400	**355/400**	54.3%	**88.8%**

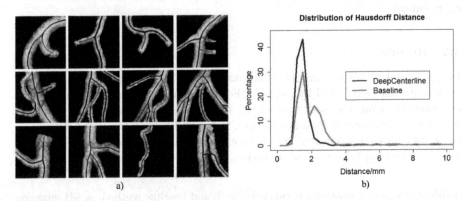

Fig. 5. Visual comparison of two methods and Hausdorff distance distributions. (a) Red is centerlines from DeepCL. Cyan is centerlines from baseline method. Green shows the overlap of both centerlines. First row: DeepCL finds branches missed by baseline method. Second row: DeepCL avoids wrong bifurcations generated by baseline. Third row: DeepCL generates centerlines well-positioned at central location, avoiding taking straight shortcuts at complex bifurcation regions or tortuous segments. The last figure with red border shows a failure case for both DeepCL and baseline. (b) Hausdorff distance distribution from voxels to the nearest centerline points for both methods. (Color figure online)

method with better performance on each metric. DeepCL finds more branch endpoints on both branch-level and patient-level. The number of wrong bifurcations shown in DeepCL is also less than that in baseline. Besides, DeepCL increased the average patient-level centerline length, due to finding of more endpoints and staying to the center instead of taking straight shortcuts at tortuous regions. Overall, the percentage of scans with successful centerline extraction without any type of error on any branch is substantially increased from 54.3% to 88.8%.

Figure 5(a) shows qualitative comparison of both methods. Compared to baseline, DeepCL shows significant improvement in finding more endpoints, reducing number of wrong centerline bifurcations at region with vessels close together, and staying at center instead of taking straight shortcut at regions with high curvature.

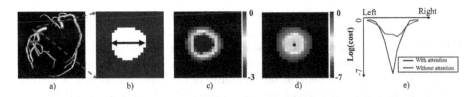

Fig. 6. Comparison of centerline distance map prediction with and without attention. (a) Coronary artery segmentation mask. (b) A cross-sectional view of segmentation mask. (c) Centerline distance map without attention module. (d) Centerline distance map with attention module. (e) Centerline distance map values at the profile line shown as double-arrowed line in (b). With attention, the centerline distance map shows a high peak around centerline instead of a plateau by the model without attention.

Figure 5(b) shows the distribution of patient-level Hausdorff distance from any segmentation mask voxel to centerline. A smaller Hausdorff distance means that *all* voxels in the segmentation mask are "covered" by a closer nearby centerline point. The majority of Hausdorff distances for DeepCL centerlines form a peak around 1.7 mm. In contrast, the baseline method has a longer tail towards higher Hausdorff distance values, with a significant percentage of scans having Hausdorff distance above 2 mm. This shows that DeepCL covers all segmentation mask voxels more closely.

Importance of Attention. Figure 6 compares the centerline distance maps generated with and without the attention module. As shown in Fig. 6(e), the centerline distance map has a clear peak around the central location by using attention. In contrast, the CL distance map generated by model without attention results in a "plateau" for a large area. If this situation occurred at regions with high curvature, then the minimal path extractor can easily pick a straight shortcut passing through non-center plateau points as the resulting centerline. This problem is greatly alleviated by utilizing the attention module to improve the centerline distance map contrast around real centerline point.

4 Discussion

The proposed method tackles multiple long-existing challenges of centerline extraction. A novel branch endpoint detection algorithm using Gaussian-field based endpoint confidence map is developed to detect the extremely sparse branch endpoints. The centerline distance map is made scale-invariant to the substantial diameter change of vessel branches from proximal to distal sections through local normalization within each cross-sectional view. The scale-invariant centerline distance map helps generate well-positioned centerline throughout all sections. Log-transform and attention module are utilized to further highlight the central locations, aiding accurate localization of the single-pixel-wide centerline. The large model capacity of FCN provides robustness to minor imperfections of segmentation masks.

Note that the reference "true" centerlines used in the training phase are results generated by the baseline method *without* manual correction, due to the difficulty of manual correction of a single-pixel-wide centerline. Despite of this disadvantage, our method achieves better performance than baseline on the test set. This shows the good generalization ability of the proposed model. A further study topic is to use our current method's output as reference standard to train another FCN model. It would be interesting to see whether this second model would further improve upon the first-generation model.

5   Conclusion

We propose a novel centerline extraction framework which combines a multi-task FCN computing a locally normalized centerline distance map and detecting branch endpoints, with a minimal path extractor. The proposed method is the first deep-learning based centerline extraction method that guarantees single-pixel-wide centerline for a complex tree-structured object. Designed to be robust to substantial scale changes at different locations and minor imperfections of segmentation mask, the proposed method generates centerlines with more complete and closer coverage of segmentation masks without false positive branches.

Acknowledgement. The authors would like to thank Xiaoyang Xu and Bin Ouyang for organizing the dataset. This study has received funding by Shenzhen Municipal Government (KQTD2016112809330877).

References

1. Gülsün, M.A., Funka-Lea, G., Sharma, P., Rapaka, S., Zheng, Y.: Coronary centerline extraction via optimal flow paths and CNN path pruning. In: Ourselin, S., Joskowicz, L., Sabuncu, M.R., Unal, G., Wells, W. (eds.) MICCAI 2016. LNCS, vol. 9902, pp. 317–325. Springer, Cham (2016). https://doi.org/10.1007/978-3-319-46726-9_37
2. Jin, D., Iyer, K.S., Chen, C., Hoffman, E.A., Saha, P.K.: A robust and efficient curve skeletonization algorithm for tree-like objects using minimum cost paths. Pattern Recogn. Lett. **76**, 32–40 (2016)
3. Kirişli, H., et al.: Standardized evaluation framework for evaluating coronary artery stenosis detection, stenosis quantification and lumen segmentation algorithms in computed tomography angiography. Med. Image Anal. **17**(8), 859–876 (2013)
4. Metz, C., Schaap, M., Weustink, A., Mollet, N., van Walsum, T., Niessen, W.: Coronary centerline extraction from CT coronary angiography images using a minimum cost path approach. Med. Phys. **36**(12), 5568–5579 (2009)
5. Mirikharaji, Z., Zhao, M., Hamarneh, G.: Globally-optimal anatomical tree extraction from 3D medical images using pictorial structures and minimal paths. In: Descoteaux, M., Maier-Hein, L., Franz, A., Jannin, P., Collins, D.L., Duchesne, S. (eds.) MICCAI 2017. LNCS, vol. 10434, pp. 242–250. Springer, Cham (2017). https://doi.org/10.1007/978-3-319-66185-8_28

6. Ronneberger, O., Fischer, P., Brox, T.: U-net: convolutional networks for biomedical image segmentation. In: Navab, N., Hornegger, J., Wells, W.M., Frangi, A.F. (eds.) MICCAI 2015. LNCS, vol. 9351, pp. 234–241. Springer, Cham (2015). https://doi.org/10.1007/978-3-319-24574-4_28
7. Xiong, G., et al.: Comprehensive modeling and visualization of cardiac anatomy and physiology from CT imaging and computer simulations. IEEE Trans. Vis. Comput. Graph. **23**(2), 1014–1028 (2017)
8. Zhang, X., Wang, T., Qi, J., Lu, H., Wang, G.: Progressive attention guided recurrent network for salient object detection. In: CVPR, pp. 714–722 (2018)
9. Zheng, Y., Tek, H., Funka-Lea, G.: Robust and accurate coronary artery centerline extraction in CTA by combining model-driven and data-driven approaches. In: Mori, K., Sakuma, I., Sato, Y., Barillot, C., Navab, N. (eds.) MICCAI 2013. LNCS, vol. 8151, pp. 74–81. Springer, Heidelberg (2013). https://doi.org/10.1007/978-3-642-40760-4_10

ECKO: Ensemble of Clustered Knockoffs
for Robust Multivariate Inference
on fMRI Data

Tuan-Binh Nguyen[1,2,4(✉)], Jérôme-Alexis Chevalier[1,2,3],
and Bertrand Thirion[1,2]

[1] Parietal Team, Inria Saclay, Saclay, France
tuan-binh.nguyen@inria.fr
[2] CEA/Neurospin, Gif-Sur-Yvette, France
[3] Telecom Paristech, Paris, France
[4] Laboratoire de Mathématiques d'Orsay, Paris, France

Abstract. Continuous improvement in medical imaging techniques allows the acquisition of higher-resolution images. When these are used in a predictive setting, a greater number of explanatory variables are potentially related to the dependent variable (the response). Meanwhile, the number of acquisitions per experiment remains limited. In such high dimension/small sample size setting, it is desirable to find the explanatory variables that are truly related to the response while controlling the rate of false discoveries. To achieve this goal, novel multivariate inference procedures, such as knockoff inference, have been proposed recently. However, they require the feature covariance to be well-defined, which is impossible in high-dimensional settings. In this paper, we propose a new algorithm, called Ensemble of Clustered Knockoffs, that allows to select explanatory variables while controlling the false discovery rate (FDR), up to a prescribed spatial tolerance. The core idea is that knockoff-based inference can be applied on groups (clusters) of voxels, which drastically reduces the problem's dimension; an ensembling step then removes the dependence on a fixed clustering and stabilizes the results. We benchmark this algorithm and other FDR-controlling methods on brain imaging datasets and observe empirical gains in sensitivity, while the false discovery rate is controlled at the nominal level.

1 Introduction

Medical images are increasingly used in predictive settings, in which one wants to classify patients into disease categories or predict some outcomes of interest. Besides predictive accuracy, a fundamental question is that of *opening the black box*, *i.e.* understanding the combinations of observations that explains the outcome. A particular relevant question is that of the importance of image features in the prediction of an outcome of interest, conditioned on other features. Such

---

T.-B. Nguyen and J.-A. Chevalier—Equal contribution.

A. C. S. Chung et al. (Eds.): IPMI 2019, LNCS 11492, pp. 454–466, 2019.
https://doi.org/10.1007/978-3-030-20351-1_35

conditional analysis is a fundamental step to allow causal inference on the implications of the signals from image regions in this outcome; see e.g. [12] for the case of brain imaging. However, the typical setting in medical imaging is that of high-dimensional small-sample problems, in which the number of samples n is much smaller than the number of covariates p. This is further aggravated by the steady improvements in data resolution. In such cases, classical inference tools fail, both theoretically and practically. One solution to this problem is to reduce the massive number of covariates by utilizing dimension reduction, such as clustering-based image compression, to reduce the number of features to a value close to n; see e.g. [4]. This approach can be viewed as the bias/variance trade-off: some loss in the localization of the predictive features—bias—is tolerated as it comes with less variance—hence higher power—in the statistical model. This is particularly relevant in medical imaging, where localizing predictive features at the voxel level is rarely important: one is typically more interested in the enclosing region.

However, such a method suffers from the arbitrariness of the clustering step and the ensuing high-variance in inference results with different clustering runs, as shown empirically in [6]. [6] also introduced an algorithm called Ensemble of Clustered Desparsified Lasso (ECDL), based on the inference technique developed in [13], that provides p-values for each feature, and controls the Family Wise Error Rate (FWER), i.e. the probability of making one or more false discoveries. In applications, it is however more relevant to control the False Discovery Rate (FDR) [3], which indicates the expected fraction of false discoveries among all discoveries, since it allows to detect a greater number of variables. In univariate settings, the FDR is easily controlled by the Benjamini-Hochberg procedure [3], valid under independence or positive correlation between features. It is unclear whether this can be applied to multivariate statistical settings. A promising method which controls the FDR in multivariate settings is the so-called knock-off inference [2,5], which has been successfully applied in settings where $n \approx p$. However, the method relies on randomly constructed knockoff variables, therefore it also suffers from instability. Our contribution is a new algorithm, called Ensemble of Clustered Knockoffs (ECKO), that *(i)* stabilizes knockoff inference through an aggregation approach; *(ii)* adapts knockoffs to $n \ll p$ settings. This is achieved by running the knockoff inference on the reduced data and ensembling the ensuing results.

The remainder of our paper is organized as follows: Sect. 2 establishes a rigorous theoretical framework for the ECKO algorithm; Sect. 3 describes the setup of our experiments with both synthetic and brain imaging data predictive problems, to illustrate the performance of ECKO, followed by details of the experimental results in Sect. 4; specifically, we benchmark this approach against the procedure proposed in [7], that does not require the clustering step, yet only provides asymptotic ($n \to \infty$) guarantees. We show the benefit of the ECKO approach in terms of both statistical control and statistical power.

2   Theory

2.1   Generalized Linear Models and High Dimensional Setting

Given a design matrix $\mathbf{X} \in \mathbb{R}^{n \times p}$ and a response vector $\mathbf{y} \in \mathbb{R}^n$, we consider that the true underlying model is of the following form:

$$\mathbf{y} = f(\mathbf{X}\mathbf{w}^*) + \sigma\epsilon, \tag{1}$$

where $\mathbf{w}^* \in \mathbb{R}^p$ is the true parameter vector, $\sigma \in \mathbb{R}^+$ the (unknown) noise magnitude, $\epsilon \sim \mathcal{N}(\mathbf{0}, \mathbf{I}_n)$ the noise vector and f is a function that depends on the experimental setting (e.g. $f = Id$ for the regression problem or e.g. $f = sign$ for the classification problem). The columns of $\mathbf{X}$ refer to the explanatory variables also called features, while the rows of $\mathbf{X}$ represent the coordinates of different samples in the feature space. We focus on experimental settings in which the number of features p is much greater than the number of samples n *i.e.* $p \gg n$. Additionally, the (true) support denoted by S is given by $S = \{k \in [p] : \mathbf{w}_k^* \neq 0\}$. Let $\hat{S}$ denotes an estimate of the support given a particular inference procedure. We also define the signal-to-noise ratio (SNR) which allows to assess the noise regime of a given experiment:

$$\mathrm{SNR} = \frac{\|\mathbf{X}\mathbf{w}^*\|_2^2}{\sigma^2 \|\epsilon\|_2^2}. \tag{2}$$

A high SNR means the signal magnitude is strong compared to the noise, hence it refers to an easier inference problem.

2.2   Structured Data

In medical imaging and many other experimental settings, the data stored in the design matrix $\mathbf{X}$ relate to *structured* signals. More precisely, the features have a peculiar dependence structure that is related to an underlying spatial organization, for instance the spatial neighborhood in 3D images. Then, the features are generated from a random process acting on this underlying metric space. In our paper, the distance between the j-th and the k-th features is denoted by $d(j, k)$.

2.3   FDR Control

In this section, we introduce the false discovery rate (FDR) and a spatial generalization of the FDR that we called δ-FDR. This quantity is important since a desirable property of an inference procedure is to control the FDR or the δ-FDR. In the following, we assume that the true model is the one defined in Sect. 2.1.

Definition 1. False discovery proportion (FDP). *Given an estimate of the support $\hat{S}$ obtained from a particular inference procedure, the false discovery proportion is the ratio of the number selected features that do not belong to the support (false discoveries) divided by the number of selected features (discoveries):*

$$FDP = \frac{\#\{k \in \hat{S} : k \notin S\}}{\#\{k \in \hat{S}\}} \tag{3}$$

Definition 2. δ-FDP. *Given an estimate of the support $\hat{S}$ obtained from a particular inference procedure, the false discovery proportion with parameter $\delta > 0$, denoted δ-FDP is the ratio of the number selected features that are at a distance more than δ from any feature of the support, divided by the number of selected features:*

$$\delta\text{-}FDP = \frac{\#\{k \in \hat{S} : \forall j \in S, \; d(j, k) > \delta\}}{\#\{k \in \hat{S}\}} \tag{4}$$

One can notice that for $\delta = 0$, the FDP and the δ-FDP refer to same quantity *i.e.* $0\text{-}FDP = FDP$.

Definition 3. False Discovery Rate (FDR) and δ-FDR. *The false discovery rate and the false discovery rate with parameter $\delta > 0$ which is denoted by δ-FDR are respectively the expectations of the FDP and the δ-FDP:*

$$FDR = \mathbb{E}[FDP],$$
$$\delta\text{-}FDR = \mathbb{E}[\delta\text{-}FDP]. \tag{5}$$

2.4 Knockoff Inference

Initially introduced by [2] to identify variables in genomics, the knockoff filter is an FDP control approach for multivariate models. This method has been improved to work with mildly high-dimensional settings in [5], leading to the so-called model-X knockoffs:

Definition 4. Model-X knockoffs [5]. *The model-X knockoffs for the family of random variables $\mathbf{X} = (X_1, \ldots X_p)$ are a new family of random variables $\tilde{\mathbf{X}} = (\tilde{X}_1, \ldots, \tilde{X}_p)$ constructed to satisfy the two properties:*

1. For any subset $\mathcal{K} \subset \{1, \ldots, p\}$: $(\mathbf{X}, \tilde{\mathbf{X}})_{swap(\mathcal{K})} \overset{d}{=} (\mathbf{X}, \tilde{\mathbf{X}})$,

  where the vector $(\mathbf{X}, \tilde{\mathbf{X}})_{swap(\mathcal{K})}$ denotes the swap of entries X_j and $\tilde{X}_j$, $\forall j \in \mathcal{K}$

2. $\tilde{\mathbf{X}} \perp\!\!\!\perp \mathbf{y} \mid \mathbf{X}$ where $\mathbf{y}$ is the response vector.

In a nutshell, knockoff procedure first creates extra null variables that have a correlation structure similar to that of the original variables. A test statistic vector is then calculated to measure the strength of the original versus its knockoff counterpart. An example of such statistic is the lasso-coefficient difference (LCD) that we use in this paper:

Definition 5. Knockoff procedure with intermediate p-values [2,5].

1. *Construct knockoff variables, produce matrix concatenation:* $[\mathbf{X}, \tilde{\mathbf{X}}] \in \mathbb{R}^{n \times 2p}$.
2. *Calculate LCD by solving*

$$\min_{\mathbf{w} \in \mathbb{R}^{2p}} \frac{1}{2} \|\mathbf{y} - [\mathbf{X}, \tilde{\mathbf{X}}]\mathbf{w}\|_2^2 + \lambda \|\mathbf{w}\|_1,$$

and then, for all $j \in [p]$, take the difference $z_j = |\hat{\mathbf{w}}_j(\lambda)| - |\hat{\mathbf{w}}_{j+p}(\lambda)|$.
3. *Compute the p-values p_j, for $j \in [p]$:*

$$p_j = \frac{\#\{k : z_k \leq -z_j\}}{p}. \tag{6}$$

4. *Derive q-values by Benjamini-Hochberg procedure:* $(q_j)_{j \in [p]} = BHq\left((p_j)_{j \in [p]}\right)$
5. *Given a desired FDR level $\alpha \in (0,1)$: $\hat{S} = \{j : q_j \leq \alpha\}$.*

Remark 1. *The above formulation is distinct from that of [2,5], but it is equivalent. We use it to introduce the intermediate variables p_j for all $j \in [p]$.*

Our first contribution is to extend this procedure computing q_j by aggregating different draws of knockoffs before applying the Benjamini-Hochberg (BHq) procedure. More precisely, we first compute B draws of knockoff variables and, using (6), we derive the corresponding p-values $p_j^{(b)}$, for all $j \in [p]$ and $b \in [B]$. Then, we aggregate them for each j in parallel, using the quantile aggregation procedure introduced in [11]:

$$\forall j \in [p], \; p_j = \text{quantile-aggregation}(\{p_j^{(b)} : b \in [B]\}) \tag{7}$$

We then proceed with the fourth and fifth steps of the knockoff procedure described in Definition 5.

2.5 Dimension Reduction

Knockoff (KO) inference is intractable in high-dimensional settings, as knockoff generation requires the estimation and inversion of covariance matrices of size $(2p \times 2p)$. Hence we leverage data structure by introducing a clustering step that reduces data dimension before applying KO inference. As in [6], assuming the features' signals are spatially smooth, it is relevant to consider a spatially-constrained clustering algorithm. By averaging the features with each clustering, we reduce the number of parameters from p to q, the number of clusters, where $q \ll p$. KO inference on cluster-based signal averages will be referred to as Clustered Knockoffs (CKO). However, it is preferable not to fully rely on a particular clustering, as a small perturbation on the input data has a dramatic impact on the clustering solution. We followed the approach used in [9] that aggregates solutions across random clusterings. More precisely, they build C different clusterings from C different random subsamples of size $\lfloor 0.7n \rfloor$ from the full sample $\mathbf{X}$, but always using the same clustering algorithm.

2.6   The Ensemble of Clustered Knockoff Algorithm

The problem is to aggregate the q-values obtained across CKO runs on different clustering solutions. To do so, we transfer the q-values from clusters (group of voxels) to features (voxels): given a clustering solution $c \in [C]$, we assign to each voxel the q-value of its corresponding cluster. More formally, if, considering the c-th clustering solution, the k-th voxel belongs to the j-th cluster denoted by $G_j^{(c)}$ then the q-value $\tilde{q}_k^{(c)}$ assigned to this voxel is: $\tilde{q}_k^{(c)} = q_j^{(c)}$ if $k \in G_j^{(c)}$. This procedure hinges on the observation that the FDR is a resolution-invariant concept—it controls the *proportion* of false discoveries. In the worst case, this results in a spatial inaccuracy of δ in the location of significant activity, δ being the diameter of the clusters. Finally, the aggregated q-value $\tilde{q}_k$ of the k-th voxel is the average of the q-values $\tilde{q}_k^{(c)}$, $c \in [C]$, received across C different clusterings: given the FDR Definition (5), FDPs can naturally be averaged. The algorithm is summarized in Algorithm 1 and represented graphically in Fig. 1.

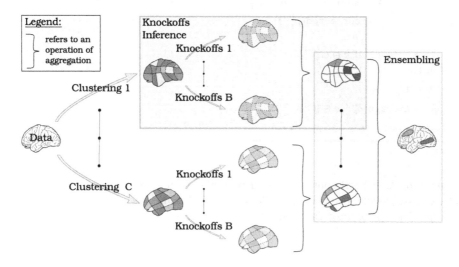

Fig. 1. Representation of the ECKO algorithm. To create a stable inference result, we introduce ensembling steps both within each cluster level and at the voxel-level, across clusterings.

2.7   Theoretical Results

Ensemble of Clustered Knockoffs (ECKO).

Algorithm 1. Full ECKO algorithm

---

input : Data matrix $\mathbf{X}_{\text{init}} \in \mathbb{R}^{n \times p}$, response vector $\mathbf{y}_{\text{init}} \in \mathbb{R}^n$;
         Clustering object Ward($\cdot$);
param: $q = 500, B = 25, C = 25$, fdr - Nominal FDR threshold;

for $c = 1, \ldots, C$ **do**

    $X_{\text{init}}^{(c)} = \texttt{resample}(X_{\text{init}})$

    $X_{\text{clustered}}^{(c)} = \texttt{Ward}(q, X_{\text{init}}^{(c)})$

    for $b = 1, \ldots, B$ **do**

       $\forall j = 1, \ldots, q :$

       $z_j^{(b,c)} \leftarrow \texttt{Knockoffs}(X_{\text{clustered}}^{(c)}, \mathbf{y}_{\text{init}}, \texttt{fdr})$

       $p_j^{(b,c)} \leftarrow \dfrac{\#\{k \in [q] : z_k^{(b,c)} \leq -z_j^{(b,c)}\}}{p}$

    end

    $\forall j = 1, \ldots, q :$

    $p_j^{(c)} \leftarrow \texttt{Aggregated}(p_j^{(b,c)}, b \in [B])$

    $q_j^{(c)} \leftarrow \texttt{BHq\_corrected}(p_j^{(c)})$

    $\forall k = 1, \ldots, p :$

    $\tilde{q}_k^{(c)} \leftarrow q_j^{(c)}$ if $k \in G_j^{(c)}$

end

$\forall k = 1, \ldots, p :$

$\tilde{q}_k \leftarrow \texttt{Average}(\tilde{q}_k^{(c)}, c \in [C])$

return $\hat{S} \leftarrow \{k \in [p] : \tilde{q}_k \leq \texttt{fdr}\}$

Theorem 1. δ-FDR control by the Ensemble of Clustered Knockoffs procedure at the voxel level. *Assuming that the true model is the one defined in* (1), *using the q-values* $\tilde{q}_k$ *defined in Sect. 2.6, the estimated support* $\hat{S} = \{k : \tilde{q}_k \leq \alpha\}$ *ensure that the δ-FDR is lower than* α.

Sketch of the proof (details are omitted for the sake of space). We first establish that the aggregation procedure yields q-values q_j^c that control the FDR. This follows simply from the argument given in the proof of Theorem 3.1 in [11]. Second, we show that broadcasting the values from clusters (q) to voxels ($\tilde{q}$) still controls the FDR, yet with a possible inaccuracy of δ, where δ is the supremum of clusters diameters: the δ-FDR is controlled. This comes from the resolution invariance of FDR and the definition of δ-FDR. Third, averaging-based aggregation of the q-values at the voxel level, controls the δ-FDR. This stems from the definition of the FDR as an expected value.

2.8   Alternative Approaches

In the present work, we use two alternatives to the proposed CKO/ECKO approach: the ensemble of clustered desparsified lasso (ECDL) [6] and the APT framework from [7]. As we already noted, ECDL is structured as ECKO. The main differences are that it relies on desparsified lasso rather than knockoff inference and returns p-values instead of q-values. The APT approach was proposed to return feature-level p-values for binary classification problems (though the generalization to regression is straightforward). It directly works at the voxel level, yet with two caveats:

- Statistical control is granted only in the $n \to \infty$ limit
- Unlike ECDL and ECKO, it is unclear whether the returned score represents marginal or conditional association of the input features with the output.

For both ECDL and APT, the returned p-values are converted to q-values using the standard BHq procedure. The resulting q-values are questionable, given that BHq is not valid under negative dependence between the input q-values [3]; on the other hand, practitioners rarely check the hypothesis underlying statistical models. We thus use the procedure in a black-box mode and check its validity a posteriori.

3   Experiments

Synthetic Data. To demonstrate the improvement of the proposed algorithm, we first benchmark the method on 3D synthetic data set that resembles a medical image with compact regions of interest that display some predictive information. The size of the weight vector $\mathbf{w}$ is $50 \times 50 \times 50$, with 5 regions of interest (ROIs) of size $6 \times 6 \times 6$. A design matrix $\mathbf{X}$ that represents random brain signal is then sampled according to a multivariate Gaussian distribution. Finally, the response vector $\mathbf{y}$ is calculated following linear model assumption with Gaussian noise, which is configured to have $SNR \approx 3.6$, similar to real data settings. An average precision-recall curve of 30 simulations is calculated to show the relative merits of single cluster Knockoffs inference versus ECKO and ECDL and APT. Furthermore, we also vary the Signal-to-Noise Ratio (SNR) of the simulation to investigate the accuracy of FDR control of ECKO with different levels of difficulty in detecting the signal.

Real MRI Dataset. We compare single-clustered Knockoffs (CKO), ECKO and ECDL on different MRI datasets downloaded from the Nilearn library [1]. In particular, the following datasets are used:

- **Haxby** [8]. In this functional-MRI (fMRI) dataset, subjects are presented with images of different objects. For the benchmark in our study, we only use the brain signal and responses for images related to faces and houses of subject 2 ($n = 216, p = 24083$).
- **Oasis** [10]. The original collection include data of gray and white matter density probability maps for 416 subjects aged 18 to 96, 100 of which have been clinically diagnosed with very mild to moderate Alzheimers disease. The purpose for our inference task is to find regions that predict the age of a subject ($n = 400, p = 153809$).

We chose $q = 500$ in all experiments for the algorithms that require clustering step (KO, ECKO and ECDL). In the two cases, we start with a qualitative comparison of the returned results. The brain maps are ternary: all regions outside $\hat{S}$ are zeroed, while regions in $\hat{S}$ get a value of $+1$ or -1, depending on whether the contribution to the prediction is positive or negative. For ECKO, a vote is performed to decide whether a voxel is more frequently in a cluster with positive or negative weight.

4   Results

Synthetic Data. A strong demonstration of how ECKO makes an improvement in stabilizing the single-clustering Knockoffs (CKO) is shown in Fig. 2. There is a clear distinction between selection of the orange area at lower right and the blue area at upper right in the CKO result, compared to the ground truth. Moreover, CKO falsely discovers some regions in the middle of the cube. By Contrast, ECKO's selection is more similar to the true 3D weight cube. While it returns a wider selection than ECKO, ECDL also claims more false discoveries, most visibly in the blue area on upper-left corner. At the same time, APT returns adequate results, but is more conservative than ECKO. Figure 3a is the result of averaging 30 simulations for the 3D brain synthetic data. ECKO and ECDL obtain almost identical precision-recall curve: for a precision of at least 90%, both methods have recall rate of around 50%. Meanwhile, CKO falls behind, and in fact it cannot reach a precision of over 40% across all recall rates. APT yields the best precision-recall compromise, slightly above ECKO and ECDL. When varying SNR (from 2^{-1} to 2^5) and investigating the average proportion of false discoveries (δ-FDR) made over the average of 30 simulations (Fig. 3b), we observe that CKO fails to control δ-FDR at nominal level 10% in general. Note that accurate δ-FDR control would be obtained with larger δ values, but this makes the whole procedure less useful. The ECDL controls δ-FDR at low SNR level. However, when the signal is strong, ECDL might select more false positives. ECKO, on the other hand, is always reliable—albeit conservative—keeping FDR below the nominal level even when SNR increases to larger magnitude.

Oasis and Haxby Dataset. When decoding the brain signal on subject 2 of the Haxby dataset using response vector label for watching 'Face vs. House', there is a clear resemblance of selection results between ECKO and ECDL. Using an

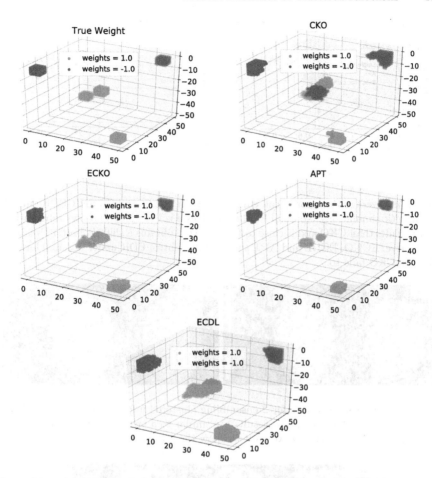

Fig. 2. Experiments on simulated data: Original 3D weight vector (top left) and inference results from CKO vs. ECKO. The single CKO run has markedly different solutions to the ground truth. Meanwhile, ECKO's solution is closer to the ground truth in the sense that altogether, it is more powerful than APT and also more precise than ECDL.

FDR threshold of 10%, both algorithms select the same area (with a difference in size), namely a face responsive region in the ventral visual cortex, and agree on the sign of the effect. However, on Oasis dataset, thresholding to control the FDR at 0.1 yields empty selection with ECDL and APT, while ECKO still selects some voxels. This potentially means that ECKO is statistically more powerful than ECDL and APT (Figs. 4 and 5).

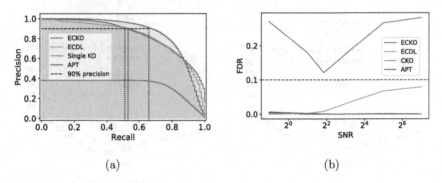

(a)   (b)

Fig. 3. (a) Average Precision-recall curve (for $SNR \approx 3.6$) and (b) SNR-FDR curve of 30 synthetic simulations. Nominal FDR control level is 10%. ECKO shows substantially better results than CKO and is close to ECDL. APT obtains a slightly better Precision-recall curve. ECKO, ECDL and APT successfully control FDR under nominal level 0.1 where as CKO fails to.

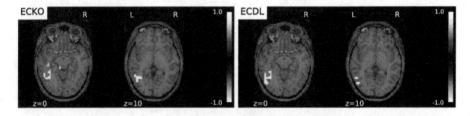

Fig. 4. Comparison of results for 2 ensembling clustered inference methods on Haxby dataset, nominal FDR = 0.1. The results are similar to a large extent. No voxel region is detected by APT, therefore we omit to show the selection outcome of the method.

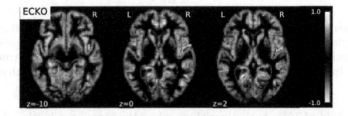

Fig. 5. Results of ECKO inference on Oasis dataset, nominal FDR = 0.1. ECKO is the only method to detect significant regions. The temporal region detected by ECKO would be detected by other approaches using a less conservative threshold.

5   Conclusion

In this work, we proposed an algorithm that makes False Discovery Rate (FDR) control possible in high-dimensional statistical inference. The algorithm is an integration of clustering algorithm for dimension reduction and aggregation technique to tackle the instability of the original knockoff procedure. Evaluating the algorithm on both synthetic and brain imaging datasets shows a consistent gain of ECKO with respect to CKO in both FDR control and sensitivity. Furthermore, empirical results also suggest that the procedure achieves non-asymptotic statistical guarantees, yet requires the δ-relaxation for FDR.

The number of clusters represents a bias-variance trade-off: increasing it can reduce the bias (in fact, the value of δ), while reducing it improves the conditioning for statistical inference, hence the sensitivity of the knockoff control. We set it to 500 in our experiments. Learning it from the data is an interesting research direction.

We note that an assumption of independence between hypothesis tests is required for the algorithm to work, which is often not the case in realistic scenarios. Note that this is actually the case for all FDR-controlling procedures that rely on the BHq algorithm. As a result, making the algorithm work with relaxed assumption is a potential direction for our future study. Furthermore, the double-aggregation procedure makes the algorithm more expensive, although it results in embarrassingly parallel loops. An interesting challenge is to reduce the computation cost of this procedure. Another avenue to explore for the future is novel generative schemes for knockoff, based e.g. on deep adversarial approaches.

Acknowledgement. This research is supported by French ANR (project FAST-BIG ANR-17-CE23-0011) and Labex DigiCosme (project ANR-11-LABEX-0045-DIGICOSME). The authors would like to thank Sylvain Arlot and Matthieu Lerasle for fruitful discussions and helpful comments.

References

1. Abraham, A., et al.: Machine learning for neuroimaging with scikit-learn. Front. Neuroinform. **8**, 14 (2014)
2. Barber, R.F., Candès, E.J.: Controlling the false discovery rate via knockoffs. Ann. Stat. **43**(5), 2055–2085 (2015). http://arxiv.org/abs/1404.5609
3. Benjamini, Y., Hochberg, Y.: Controlling the false discovery rate: a practical and powerful approach to multiple testing. J. R. Stat. Soc. Ser. B (Methodol.) **57**(1), 289–300 (1995). https://www.jstor.org/stable/2346101
4. Bühlmann, P., Rütimann, P., van de Geer, S., Zhang, C.H.: Correlated variables in regression: clustering and sparse estimation. J. Stat. Plan. Inference **143**(11), 1835–1858 (2013)
5. Candès, E., Fan, Y., Janson, L., Lv, J.: Panning for gold: model-x knockoffs for high dimensional controlled variable selection. J. R. Stat. Soc.: Ser. B (Stat. Methodol.) **80**(3), 551–577
6. Chevalier, J.-A., Salmon, J., Thirion, B.: Statistical inference with ensemble of clustered desparsified lasso. In: Frangi, A.F., Schnabel, J.A., Davatzikos, C., Alberola-López, C., Fichtinger, G. (eds.) MICCAI 2018. LNCS, vol. 11070, pp. 638–646. Springer, Cham (2018). https://doi.org/10.1007/978-3-030-00928-1_72
7. Gaonkar, B., Shinohara, R.T., Davatzikos, C.: Interpreting support vector machine models for multivariate group wise analysis in neuroimaging. Med. Image Anal. **24**(1), 190–204 (2015)

8. Haxby, J.V., Gobbini, M.I., Furey, M.L., Ishai, A., Schouten, J.L., Pietrini, P.: Distributed and overlapping representations of faces and objects in ventral temporal cortex. Science **293**(5539), 2425–2430 (2001)
9. Hoyos-Idrobo, A., Varoquaux, G., Schwartz, Y., Thirion, B.: Frem scalable and stable decoding with fast regularized ensemble of models. NeuroImage **180**, 160–172 (2018). http://www.sciencedirect.com/science/article/pii/S1053811917308182, New advances in encoding and decoding of brain signals
10. Marcus, D.S., Wang, T.H., Parker, J., Csernansky, J.G., Morris, J.C., Buckner, R.L.: Open access series of imaging studies (OASIS): cross-sectional MRI data in young, middle aged, nondemented, and demented older adults. J. Cogn. Neurosci. **19**(9), 1498–1507 (2007)
11. Meinshausen, N., Meier, L., Bhlmann, P.: P-values for high-dimensional regression. J. Am. Stat. Assoc. **104**(488), 1671–1681 (2009)
12. Weichwald, S., Meyer, T., zdenizci, O., Schlkopf, B., Ball, T., Grosse-Wentrup, M.: Causal interpretation rules for encoding and decoding models in neuroimaging. NeuroImage **110**, 48–59 (2015). http://www.sciencedirect.com/science/article/pii/S105381191500052X
13. Zhang, C.H., Zhang, S.S.: Confidence intervals for low dimensional parameters in high dimensional linear models. J. R. Stat. Soc.: Ser. B (Stat. Methodol.) **76**(1), 217–242 (2014)

Graph Convolutional Nets for Tool Presence Detection in Surgical Videos

Sheng Wang, Zheng Xu, Chaochao Yan, and Junzhou Huang$^{(\boxtimes)}$

University of Texas at Arlington, Arlington, TX 76019, USA
jzhuang@uta.edu

Abstract. Surgical tool presence detection is one of the key problems in automatic surgical video content analysis. Solving this problem benefits many applications such as the evaluation of surgical instrument usage and automatic surgical report generation. Given the fact that each video is only sparsely labeled at the frame level, meaning that only a small portion of video frames will be properly labeled, existing approaches only model this problem as an image (frame) classification problem without considering temporal information in surgical videos. In this paper, we propose a deep neural network model utilizing both spatial and temporal information from surgical videos for surgical tool presence detection. The proposed model uses Graph Convolutional Networks (GCNs) along the temporal dimension to learn better features by considering the relationship between continuous video frames. To the best of our knowledge, this is the first work taking videos as input to solve the surgical tool presence detection problem. Our experiments demonstrate the employment of temporal information offers a significant improvement to this problem, and the proposed approach achieves better performance than all state-of-the-art methods.

Keywords: Surgical video analysis · Graph convolution networks · Surgical tool detection

1 Introduction

Automatic content analysis of surgical videos recorded by an endoscopic camera in minimally invasive surgery is significant for many functions in the operating room of the future [3], such as analysis of the operation steps, review of the techniques employed, evaluation of instrument usage, and automatic surgical report generation [14]. Among all the tasks of surgical video content analysis, one crucial problem is surgical tool presence detection, to detect which surgical tools are being used at a certain time during surgery. The problem is different from surgical tool detection [16] or object detection [15,19] since it does not require the awareness of the location of surgical tools or general objects. However, the

This work was partially supported by US National Science Foundation IIS-1718853 and the NSF CAREER grant IIS-1553687.

problem is challenging due to several reasons: First, multiple surgical tools could be used at the same time. Second, different tools could have partial presence and occlusion which makes it even harder to detect. Third, since the frequencies of different surgical tools being used vary a lot, the data could be very imbalanced among certain surgical tools [17].

Existing approaches and models solve this problem by engaging multi-label image classification: sampling every frame with ground truth as an image dataset, learning features from each still image and then perform classification [2,8,10,16–18]. There are two ways of feature extraction. One is to use manually hand-crafted features or pre-designed features, e.g., SIFT features. The other is to use deep neural networks such as convolution neural networks (CNNs) to extract high-level features. After applying deep neural networks, the classification accuracy generally improves. However, one key piece that is still missing from the current methods is the information along the temporal dimension, which is the nature of videos. As shown in Fig. 1, almost all surgical tool detection datasets are labeled sparsely, i.e. the tools being used are not labeled for every frame. Only a very **tiny portion** (usually only a few percentages) of video frames are manually labeled. The insufficient label information leads to a huge challenge for the research of machine learning based surgical tool presence detection. To address this problem intuitively, the temporal information from neighbor frames could help the presence detection and should provide better performance than utilizing only the labeled image. For instance, one tool might be occluded at a certain frame and it can be very difficult to recognize it from the complex background by one single image. However, when using a continuous sequence of frames, even slight movement of the surgical tool could be noticed and help the tool get detected correctly.

To utilize the temporal information of the surgical videos for detection, it is not easy to apply current methods straightforwardly. Since almost all current surgical tool detection datasets are sparsely labeled at the frame level, using fixed length frames around the labeled image as a video could either introduce noise or lack enough temporal information. It might not offer enough temporal information when the video length is too small, while it might introduce noise when the video length is too large. Besides, if we use continuous frames around the labeled image as a video, the length of videos in this problem will not be long enough or the variation of the frame contents will not be large enough to learn long-range temporal dependency with Recurrent Neural Networks (RNNs) such as Long Short-Term Memory (LSTM) [7,21,23] for general video understanding.

In this paper, we propose a novel deep neural network model named Surgical Tool Graph Convolutional Networks (STGCN) combining the power of both Convolutional Neural Networks (CNNs) and Graph Convolutional Networks (GCNs) [12]. We model the problem as a video classification problem by using the sparsely labeled frame and the neighbor frames around it. STGCN uses DenseNet [9] as our backbone to learn the spatial features from the input images and extracts the features directly from the videos with inflated 3D DenseNet. Then it applies GCNs along the temporal dimension to learn better feature with consideration of the relationships among continuous frames. In our experiments, we demonstrate temporal information can always improve the performance by a significant amount in the detection task.

To fully demonstrate the superiority of our model, we evaluate our model on two most recently developed datasets: M2cai-tool and Cholec80 [17]. On M2cai-tool, STGCN beats the first place method of the data challenge[1] by more than 28% in mean average precision (mAP) and surpasses the previous best performance in literature as we know of. On Cholec80 dataset, the proposed STGCN improves the best performance by 10% in terms of mAP.

The contributions of this paper are summarized below:

- To the best of our knowledge, this is the first work to utilize the temporal information for surgical tool presence detection problem.
- We propose to apply GCNs to better model the temporal information from surgical videos.
- The proposed STGCN achieves state-of-the-art results with a significant gain on both M2cai-tool and Cholec80 datasets.

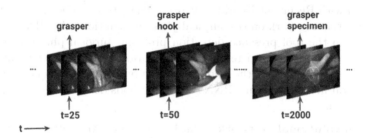

Fig. 1. Sparsely labeled surgical tool detection dataset. In this dataset, the tools being used in one image is labeled every 25 frames. Existing methods only use the labeled images for model training. In this paper, we propose to use both the labeled frame and the unlabeled frames around it as a video for model training.

2 Related Work

Surgical Tool Detection. By introducing deep neural networks to extract high-level image feature for surgical tool detection, many approaches have been developed on larger-scale datasets [2,8,10,17,18] and the overall accuracies have been improved. EndoNet [17] first proposed to use CNNs to train a tool detection model on labeled images. Since the M2cai-tool challenge, an increasing number of methods have been developed to solve this problem with M2cai-tool dataset. The winner of M2cai-tool challenge [18] modeled the problem as

---

[1] M2CAI Surgical Tool Presence Detection Challenge 2016: http://camma.u-strasbg.fr/m2cai2016/.

a multi-label image classification problem and used VGGNet and InceptionNet. The authors ensembled the results of these two deep models as the final result. After that, two methods have been proposed to further improve the detection performance by labeling extra localization information of surgical tools to the original dataset [2,10]. AGNet [8] proposed a model with two parts: one attention model as a global network to detect the areas with high possibilities to contain the surgical tools, and one local model to detect the tools from selected areas. AGNet has achieved the best performance. However, given the fact that each video is only sparsely labeled at the frame level, all these existing methods modeled surgical tool presence detection problem as an image classification problem without taking the advantage of the temporal information from unlabeled neighboring frames around the labeled frame.

Video Understanding and Surgical Video Understanding. Meanwhile, many researchers focus on video inference for the better ability of computer video understanding. A great number of cutting edge approaches have been proposed to improve the video understanding performance, and several complex datasets have been built to promote related research [1,6].

Recent video understanding work focuses on modeling long term temporal information with Recurrent Neural Networks. There has also been some surgical video understanding work on the surgical phase recognition using RNNs [11,22]. Different from the tool presence detection problem, surgical phase recognition demands to model long term temporal information on a whole surgical video, while the short video among the single labeled surgical frame does not need long term temporal modeling. Thus, RNNs based methods do not serve as a good fit in our problem.

Graph Convolutional Networks. Until recent years, very little attention has been devoted to the generalization of neural network models to more general structure such as graphs or networks [4,13]. The deep models handling the graph-like structure are named Graph Convolutional Networks (GCNs).

Our work is motivated by recent work on human recognition [20] using GCN as one crucial part of their proposed deep neural network model. In this work, the authors built a graph containing nodes corresponding to different object proposals aggregated over video frames. Different from this work, we model the feature extracted from each frame as a node and build the graph as the relationship within the continuous frames of a video segment to learn better feature with temporal information.

3   Methodology

3.1   Problem Definition

Image Classification. Existing methods for surgical tool detection models the problem as an multi-label image classification problem. Given the image x_t at frame t, models are trained to get the prediction for the input image $F(x_t)$ close to its groundtruth y_t.

Video Classification. In this paper, we propose to use not only the labeled image but also the neighbor images as a video segment for model training and evaluation. Thus, the problem becomes that given a video segment corresponding to the t frame $[x_{t-l}, ..., x_t, ..., x_{t+l}]$, where l is the number of frames before and after the labeled frame image we take into consideration, models are trained to get the prediction for the input video $F(x_{t-l}, ..., x_t, ..., x_{t+l})$ close to its groundtruth y_t.

3.2 Model Overview

As shown in Fig. 2, the proposed STGCN contains several components. To get the features from the input video, we use an inflated 3D DenseNet-121 [1,9] to get the representation of each frame in the video. We take the representation of each frame as a node and build a similarity graph on these nodes. By applying GCNs on the constructed graph, the GCNs will adaptively generate the features considering the relationships among the nodes in the graph, i.e., the temporal relationship in continuous frames. After that, we use pooling over all the nodes corresponding to continuous frames. We note the pooling layer as temporal pooling since what it does is applying the pooling on the temporal dimension. The details of each component will be discussed in the following sections.

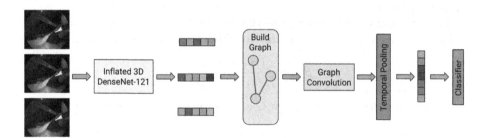

Fig. 2. The overview of the proposed STGCN.

3.3 Inflated 3D DenseNet

Different from most deep convolutional neural networks, DenseNet [9] connects all the convolutional layers in pairs when their spatial output sizes are the same. The output of each feature maps also serves as the input of all following convolutional layers. The idea is similar to Residual Networks. However, it can reuse all the features in the network. This sort of network almost exhaustively maximizes the network capacity to squeeze its spatial feature extraction and prediction power. Also, the network can alleviate the vanishing-gradient problem, strengthen feature propagation and substantially reduce the number of the parameters in the network.

In our proposed model, we use DenseNet to learn and extract spatial features for each frame in the input video. To adapt DenseNet for video input, the original DenseNet needs to be inflated to 3D ConvNet (I3D) [1,9]. That is, to support the input video of length t, a 3D kernel with $t \times k \times k$ dimensions can be inflated from a 2D $k \times k$ kernel by copying the weight t times and rescaling by $1/t$. In our implementation, we use 11 as the number of frames. The growth rate is 32 as the default number for DenseNet-121.

3.4   Graph Convolutional Networks

We apply GCNs [4] in the proposed framework to better capture the temporal relationship along the continuous frames.

Similarity Graph Building. For a video input $X = [x_{t-l}, ..., x_t, ..., x_{t+l}]$ with length N, where x_t is with the dimension of d, containing the labeled surgical tools while others not. We use the output of the fully-connected layer right after the fourth dense block from our inflated DenseNet-121 model to get the feature representations noted as $[f(x_{t-l}), ..., f(x_{t-1}), f(x_t), f(x_{t+1}), ..., f(x_{t+l})]$. We regard the representation for each frame as one vertex (node) v_k of a graph, and use the similarity S_{ij} between each pair of nodes (v_i, v_j) as the corresponding edge of the graph. Thus, the graph could reflect the temporal relationship of the continuous frames.

There are quite a few different methods to build the similarity graph. In the proposed STGCN, we use the **cosine similarity** to build the graph as

$$S_{ij} = \frac{f(x_i) \cdot f(x_j)}{\|f(x_i)\| \, \|f(x_j)\|}, \tag{1}$$

and we can get the similarity graph G after normalizing each row of S as

$$G_{ij} = \frac{e^{S_{ij}}}{\sum_{j=1}^{N} e^{S_{ij}}}. \tag{2}$$

Graph Convolutional Layer. After building the similarity graph, the graph convolutional layer could be represented as

$$Z = GXW, \tag{3}$$

where W is the weight mapping feature of each node to another dimension. The graph convolutional layer could not only map the feature as a general convolutional layer, but also take the graph information (temporal relationship among the frames in the input video) into consideration. In the surgical tool detection problem, graph convolutional layer could learn features while adaptively reference the relationship among the frames to generate the correct prediction.

The graph convolutional layers could be stacked as a deep GCNs or in general CNNs by

$$X^{(l)} = GX^{(l-1)}W^{(l-1)}, \tag{4}$$

where $X^{(l-1)}$ is the feature map as the input to current graph convolutional layer, $W^{(l-1)}$ is the weight. $X^{(l)}$ is the output of current layer as well as the input of next layer.

In our proposed model, we use a residual variation of the graph convolutional layer as

$$X^{(l)} = \sigma\left(GX^{(l-1)}W^{(l-1)}\right) + X^{(l-1)}, \tag{5}$$

where $\sigma(\cdot)$ is the activation function after the graph convolutional layer and we add $X^{(l-1)}$ to the output of the layer as a residual component.

3.5 Temporal Pooling

The feature after the last graph convolutional layer contains N features for the N frames. Then we add a temporal pooling layer to combine all the N features from N frames in the video. Temporal pooling layer has no difference than general pooling layer that it aggregates the features along the temporal dimension. It should not be a crucial factor in the performance of the proposed model since the features for the pooling layer has utilized the temporal information with GCNs. However, we still try different pooling strategies in STGCN to seek potential improvement. There are a lot of methods for pooling such as l_p pooling, average pooling, max pooling, and max-min pooling [5]. In later ablation experiments, we will show the performance of different pooling methods on Cholec80 dataset.

Given a sequence of N d-dimensional dense features after GCNs as $x^{(i)}$, where i is from 1 to N, temporal pooling pools the features along the time dimension. Assume the N-dimensional feature after temporal pooling as $\tilde{x}$, for **max temporal pooling**, $\tilde{x}_k = max(x_k^{(i)})$ where i from 1 to N, for **average temporal pooling**, $\tilde{x}_k = \frac{1}{N}\sum_{i=1}^{N} x_k^{(i)}$ and for l_p **temporal pooling**, $\tilde{x}_k = \sqrt[p]{\sum_{i=1}^{N}\left(x_k^{(i)}\right)^p}$ where k is from i to d for all temporal pooling methods. For **max-min pooling**, we apply a simple version of max-min pooling, which could be computed as:

$$\tilde{x}_k = max(x_k^{(i)}) + \alpha min(x_k^{(i)}), \tag{6}$$

where α is a hyperparameter balancing the weights of max pooling and min pooling.

4   Experiments

4.1   Implementation Details

DenseNet. We use DenseNet-121 pretrained from ImageNet to continue training on surgical tool detection datasets for a multi-label image classification. Then we inflate the trained DenseNet to 3D DenseNet. To avoid using temporal information in the inflated DenseNet, we keep all the dimension of kernels in either dense blocks or other convolutional/pooling layers as 1. Thus, all the temporal information is used in the GCNs part of the proposed model. We fix the length of the video segment around each labeled image to 11 to train the GCNs and following classifier. The DenseNet is trained with Adam optimizer with learning rate 0.0001 for 200 epochs. The learning rate will be decayed if the training loss does not decrease after three continuous training epochs.

GCNs. After extracting the feature presentation for each frame from Inflated DenseNet-121, we input the features along with the similarity graph into the GCNs. The feature we get from the inflated DenseNet-121 has the dimension of 1024. In our GCNs, we use one graph convolutional layer which maps the input feature from 1024 dimensions to 1024 dimensions. Then the temporal pooling layer is added to pool the features along the temporal dimension. After that is followed by a layer maps 1024 dimensions feature to the number of surgical tools for classification. In GCNs, both batch normalization and dropout are added after the graph convolutional layer. Batch normalization is also added before the graph convolutional layer. We train the GCNs with Adam optimizer with learning rate 0.0001 for 300 epochs. The dropout rate is set as 0.75 in our training. The same learning rate decay strategy is used as the one in training DenseNet. For max-min pooling, we fix the hyperparameter α to 0.75.

4.2   Data Description

M2cai-Tool Dataset [17]. This dataset from M2CAI surgical tool presence detection challenge contains 15 videos of laparoscopic cholecystectomy procedures from the University Hospital of Strasbourg/IRCAD (Strasbourg, France). The dataset is split into two parts: the training subset (containing 10 videos) and the testing subset (5 videos) by the challenge organizers. The videos are recorded at 25 fps and labeled at 1 fps (one labeled frame in every 25 frames). There are 23287 training samples and 12541 testing samples. The evaluation process only considers the labeled frames in testing dataset.

In this dataset, there are seven kinds of surgical tools in total as shown in Fig. 3: grasper, hook, clipper, bipolar, irrigator, scissors, and specimen bag.

Cholec80 Dataset. The Cholec80 dataset is larger than M2cai-tool dataset. It contains 40 videos (86304 labeled frames) for training and 40 videos (98194 labeled frames) for testing. The Cholec80 is also from the University Hospital of Strasbourg/IRCAD and has the same recording rate, labeling rate, and tool set as M2cai-tool dataset.

Validation Sets. For both M2cai-tool and Cholec80 datasets, we split 10% samples from training sets as validation sets. We tune our hyperparameters on the validation sets.

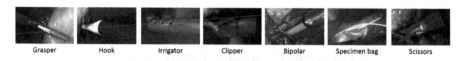

| Grasper | Hook | Irrigator | Clipper | Bipolar | Specimen bag | Scissors |

Fig. 3. The surgical tools used in M2cai-tool and Cholec80 datasets. Both of the datasets have the same seven surgical tools.

4.3 Evaluation Metric

We use the mean average precision (mAP) among the average precision (AP) on each of the seven surgical tools, which is the same as the challenge evaluation metric. To ensure a fair comparison with all the methods during and after the challenge, we exactly follow every detail of data usage and evaluation protocol used in M2CAI challenge.

4.4 Experimental Results

M2cai-Tool Dataset. In this experiment, we choose the winner's and the 3rd place's methods from the challenge, as well as three approaches after the challenge as comparison methods. Among the challenge methods, EndoNet [17] first proposed using CNN as a baseline model. The winner of the challenge [18] introduced an ensemble model of VGGNet and Inception Net. However, the highest mAP is a little above 60%. For the methods after the challenge, both Jin *et al.* [10] and Choi *et al.* [2] added location information of the tools by adding surgical tools bounding box to the dataset. These two approaches improved the mAP by 10%. AGNet [8] proposed to use an attention model to increase the detection performance. AGNet trained two cascaded deep convolutional neural networks: the first one as a global model to locate the area which has higher responses by the attention based classification network, and then the second one as a local model to classify the cropped areas with higher attention. Before our method, AGNet has the best mAP among all the approaches. We compare all these methods with our results of STGCN results. We include three variations of the proposed STGCN as side ablation experiments. STGCN (DenseNet) is the model we train and test on the labeled images without using any temporal information. STGCN (3D DenseNet + LSTM) contains the inflated 3D DenseNet as the backbone, and add an LSTM layer after it to extract the temporal information from continuous frames in the video. The difference between STGCN (3D DenseNet + GCNs) and STGCN (3D DenseNet + LSTM) is that STGCN (3D DenseNet + GCNs) uses GCNs to exploit the temporal information.

As shown in Table 1, the STGCN (DenseNet) model has achieved better performance than all existing methods. Compared to AGNet, STGCN (DenseNet) has not used any attention strategy to boost the performance to have around 2% better mAP than AGNet. By adding temporal information, the STGCN (3D DenseNet + LSTM) and the proposed STGCN (3D DenseNet) both improves our image classification model STGCN (DenseNet). With GCNs, it

Table 1. The results on M2cai-tool dataset.

Methods	Mean AP
STGCN (3D DenseNet + GCNs)	**90.24**
STGCN (3D DenseNet + LSTM)	89.03
STGCN (DenseNet)	88.27
AGNet [8]	86.8
Choi et al. [2]	72.3
Jin et al. [10]	71.8
Sheng et al. [18]	63.8
Twinanda et al. [17]	52.5

could have 1% better mAP than LSTM. Our results demonstrate that temporal information is effectively helpful for surgical tool presence detection, and GCNs is better than LSTM in this problem.

Cholec80 Dataset. We compare the proposed STGCN result with the two baseline methods ToolNet and EndoNet on this dataset in [17]. We also try the four different temporal pooling methods: l_2 pooling (STGCN(l_2)), average pooling (STGCN(avg)), max pooling (STGCN(max)), and max-min pooling (STGCN) on this dataset. Results are shown in Table 2. On this larger dataset, the proposed STGCN has better performance than the baseline methods ToolNet and EndoNet modeling the problem as a multi-label image classification problem. By utilizing the temporal information, the proposed STGCN has improved the performance around 10% in mAP.

Among all the results with different temporal pooling strategies, max-min pooling has better performance. However, the improvement is so small that it could be caused by randomness during model training. The slight difference among the four pooling methods offers support to our analysis that the graph convolutional layer has utilized the temporal information so how to aggregate the information along the temporal dimension is not sensitive, which could be convenient for model designing.

Table 2. The results on Cholec80 dataset.

	ToolNet [17]	EndoNet [17]	STGCN (l_2)	STGCN (avg)	STGCN (max)	STGCN
mAP	80.9	81.0	90.05	90.11	90.08	**90.13**

By comparing the results of the proposed STGCN with the existing methods on both M2cai-tool and Cholec80 datasets, it demonstrates that there is always significant improvement by utilizing the extra temporal information by modeling the surgical tool presence detection as a video classification problem.

Besides, with the power of GCNs, STGCN has better accuracy even compared with existing leading methods using multiple CNNs [8] or labeling additional localization ground truth [10].

5   Conclusion

Surgical tool presence detection is an essential problem for automatic surgical video analysis. To use the temporal information from the video data, we propose a novel model named STGCN which applies graph convolutional learning on continuous video frames to better use the temporal information. STGCN can directly take a video (a sequence of image frames) as input, extract both spatial and temporal features of the input and get excellent surgical tool detection precision. To the best of our knowledge, this is the first model which can take video sequences as inputs for surgical tool presence detection. On both of the two datasets to evaluate our model, STGCN has the best mean average precision. Comparing with the models that only use spatial features, we demonstrate that with GCNs, the temporal information is effective to improve surgical tool presence detection performance.

References

1. Carreira, J., Zisserman, A.: Quo vadis, action recognition? A new model and the kinetics dataset. In: 2017 IEEE Conference on Computer Vision and Pattern Recognition (CVPR), pp. 4724–4733. IEEE (2017)
2. Choi, B., Jo, K., Choi, S., Choi, J.: Surgical-tools detection based on convolutional neural network in laparoscopic robot-assisted surgery. In: 2017 39th Annual International Conference of the IEEE Engineering in Medicine and Biology Society (EMBC), pp. 1756–1759. IEEE (2017)
3. Cleary, K., Chung, H.Y., Mun, S.K.: OR 2020 workshop overview: operating room of the future. In: International Congress Series, vol. 1268, pp. 847–852. Elsevier (2004)
4. Defferrard, M., Bresson, X., Vandergheynst, P.: Convolutional neural networks on graphs with fast localized spectral filtering. In: Advances in Neural Information Processing Systems, pp. 3844–3852 (2016)
5. Durand, T., Mordan, T., Thome, N., Cord, M.: Wildcat: weakly supervised learning of deep convnets for image classification, pointwise localization and segmentation. In: IEEE Conference on Computer Vision and Pattern Recognition (CVPR 2017), vol. 2 (2017)
6. Gu, C., et al.: Ava: a video dataset of spatio-temporally localized atomic visual actions. arXiv preprint arXiv:1705.08421 (2017)
7. Hochreiter, S., Schmidhuber, J.: Long short-term memory. Neural Comput. 9(8), 1735–1780 (1997)
8. Hu, X., Yu, L., Chen, H., Qin, J., Heng, P.-A.: AGNet: attention-guided network for surgical tool presence detection. In: Cardoso, M.J., et al. (eds.) DLMIA/ML-CDS -2017. LNCS, vol. 10553, pp. 186–194. Springer, Cham (2017). https://doi.org/10.1007/978-3-319-67558-9_22

9. Huang, G., Liu, Z., Van Der Maaten, L., Weinberger, K.Q.: Densely connected convolutional networks. In: CVPR, vol. 1, p. 3 (2017)
10. Jin, A., et al.: Tool detection and operative skill assessment in surgical videos using region-based convolutional neural networks. In: 2018 IEEE Winter Conference on Applications of Computer Vision (WACV), pp. 691–699. IEEE (2018)
11. Jin, Y., et al.: SV-RCNet: workflow recognition from surgical videos using recurrent convolutional network. IEEE Trans. Med. Imaging 37(5), 1114–1126 (2018)
12. Kipf, T.N., Welling, M.: Semi-supervised classification with graph convolutional networks. arXiv preprint arXiv:1609.02907 (2016)
13. Li, R., Wang, S., Zhu, F., Huang, J.: Adaptive graph convolutional neural networks. In: Thirty-Second AAAI Conference on Artificial Intelligence (2018)
14. Loukas, C.: Video content analysis of surgical procedures. Surg. Endosc. 32(2), 553–568 (2018)
15. Ren, S., He, K., Girshick, R., Sun, J.: Faster R-CNN: towards real-time object detection with region proposal networks. In: Advances in Neural Information Processing Systems, pp. 91–99 (2015)
16. Sznitman, R., Becker, C., Fua, P.: Fast part-based classification for instrument detection in minimally invasive surgery. In: Golland, P., Hata, N., Barillot, C., Hornegger, J., Howe, R. (eds.) MICCAI 2014. LNCS, vol. 8674, pp. 692–699. Springer, Cham (2014). https://doi.org/10.1007/978-3-319-10470-6_86
17. Twinanda, A.P., Shehata, S., Mutter, D., Marescaux, J., De Mathelin, M., Padoy, N.: EndoNet: a deep architecture for recognition tasks on laparoscopic videos. IEEE Trans. Med. Imaging 36(1), 86–97 (2017)
18. Wang, S., Raju, A., Huang, J.: Deep learning based multi-label classification for surgical tool presence detection in laparoscopic videos. In: 2017 IEEE 14th International Symposium on Biomedical Imaging (ISBI 2017), pp. 620–623. IEEE (2017)
19. Wang, S., Yao, J., Xu, Z., Huang, J.: Subtype cell detection with an accelerated deep convolution neural network. In: Ourselin, S., Joskowicz, L., Sabuncu, M.R., Unal, G., Wells, W. (eds.) MICCAI 2016. LNCS, vol. 9901, pp. 640–648. Springer, Cham (2016). https://doi.org/10.1007/978-3-319-46723-8_74
20. Wang, X., Gupta, A.: Videos as space-time region graphs. In: Ferrari, V., Hebert, M., Sminchisescu, C., Weiss, Y. (eds.) ECCV 2018. LNCS, vol. 11209, pp. 413–431. Springer, Cham (2018). https://doi.org/10.1007/978-3-030-01228-1_25
21. Xu, Z., Wang, S., Zhu, F., Huang, J.: Seq2seq fingerprint: an unsupervised deep molecular embedding for drug discovery. In: Proceedings of the 8th ACM International Conference on Bioinformatics, Computational Biology, and Health Informatics, pp. 285–294. ACM (2017)
22. Yengera, G., Mutter, D., Marescaux, J., Padoy, N.: Less is more: surgical phase recognition with less annotations through self-supervised pre-training of CNN-LSTM networks. arXiv preprint arXiv:1805.08569 (2018)
23. Zhang, X., Wang, S., Zhu, F., Xu, Z., Wang, Y., Huang, J.: Seq3seq fingerprint: towards end-to-end semi-supervised deep drug discovery. In: Proceedings of the 2018 ACM International Conference on Bioinformatics, Computational Biology, and Health Informatics, pp. 404–413. ACM (2018)

High-Order Oriented Cylindrical Flux for Curvilinear Structure Detection and Vessel Segmentation

Jierong Wang[✉] and Albert C. S. Chung

Lo Kwee-Seong Medical Image Analysis Laboratory,
Department of Computer Science and Engineering,
The Hong Kong University of Science and Technology,
Kowloon, Hong Kong
{jwangdh,achung}@cse.ust.hk

Abstract. In this paper, we present a novel blood vessel structure detector, namely Oriented Cylinder Flux (*OCF*). Our method formulates blood vessels as curvilinear cylinders with circular cross-sections, incorporating two-step computations. First, *OCF* computes cross-section responses based on the normal spaces generated by two eigenvectors in the Optimally Oriented Flux (*OOF*). Second, *OCF* accumulates the cross-section responses along the curvilinear structures. We then modify *OCF* to fit into a high-order tensor framework on a unit sphere $\mathbf{S}^3$, which is able to encode multi-orientation information within a single voxel. A random walker based graphical framework is employed to measure the angular coherence among the decomposed rank-1 tensors. In the synthetic and clinical image experiments, the proposed method achieves high segmentation performance under various radii of the curvilinear structures and different levels of random noise, demonstrating that it has a strong noise-resistant ability and can be used to deal with the shrinking problem, which is one of the main problems in blood vessel segmentation.

Keywords: Oriented cylindrical flux · High-order tensor ·
Random walks

1 Introduction

Blood vessel disease is one of the most critical health problems around the world. For diagnosis purposes, vessel segmentation has been playing an important role and attracting enormous amount of attention over the past decades. Nowadays, precise vascular segmentation still remains challenging especially in small vessel structure detection and medical image segmentation with the high noise level.

In the literature, one of the major curvilinear structure tractography or segmentation methods is derived based on the order-2 tensor, which is modeled as an elliptical structure with the eigenvectors acted as the main axes of the ellipsoid.

© Springer Nature Switzerland AG 2019
A. C. S. Chung et al. (Eds.): IPMI 2019, LNCS 11492, pp. 479–491, 2019.
https://doi.org/10.1007/978-3-030-20351-1_37

The most well-known vesselness filters are derived based on the Hessian matrix [3], observing that a second order derivative can have a peak response at vessel cross-section and have an almost null response along the vessel structures. Based on the Hessian analysis, a steerable curvilinear filterbank [7] was recently proposed, computing the directional derivative of a curvilinear Gaussian trivariate function. Considering Hessian-based methods are sensitive to intensity inhomogeneity and neighboring objects, a gradient-flux based method has been proposed [11]. This method exploits the first order derivative of images and measures vessel responses in the local enclosed regions. Taking account of structure orientation, Optimally Oriented Flux (OOF) [5] is regarded as an anisotropic vessel filter, which focuses on directions that maximize the projected flux. Experiments presented in [5] have shown that OOF outperforms the Hessian-based methods and the gradient flux. However, OOF may fail in bifurcations and ends of vessels where the radii are extremely small. To enforce orientation coherence, an OOF based graphical framework combining with angular coherence measurement was formulated in [12].

However, the order-2 tensor may fail at the branches or structures with highly irregular cross-section due to pathologies. In the domain of medical imaging, Diffusion-Weighted MRI faces the similar challenges for tracking white matter tracts. To tackle the limitations raising in the DW-MRI, High Angular Resolution Diffusion Imaging (HARDI) was proposed, considering multiple diffusion gradients sampled in a unit sphere. In the context of vascular segmentation, a high-order tensor framework was presented in [2] for n-furcation modeling.

In this paper, we design an adaptive local cylindrical model and perform oriented cylinder flux to enhance vascular structures. The local region can be curvilinear when a detected point x is located inside vessels with high curvature, while cross sections of the local cylinder can have varying radii. We then apply high-order tensor analysis to enforce angular coherence between neighborhood voxels, combining with the random walker framework.

2   Methods

2.1   Oriented Cylindrical Flux

Comparing to spherical models, cylinder flux considers adjacent voxels and thus it is more robust than the spherical models. In this subsection, we will first introduce the cylinder flux model and then define the oriented cylinder flux.

Cylinder Flux Model. The cylinder flux can be expressed as follows [13],

$$f(x; r) = \frac{1}{4\pi r} \int_{-L}^{L} \int_{0}^{2\pi} v(x + h) \cdot \hat{n} d\theta dl = \frac{1}{4\pi r} \int_{-L}^{L} \int_{0}^{2\pi} v(x(l, \theta)) \cdot N(\theta) d\theta dl,$$
(1)

where $\hat{n}$ is the outward normal, $N(\theta)$ is a unit vector on the vessel cross-section centered at x perpendicular to the structure orientation n_x at x, r is the radius of the cross-section and $(2L + 1)$ is the length of the local cylinder model.

In [13], $x(l, \theta)$ was the coordinate function represented by the median position of two adjacent nodes and the local structure orientation n_x was the corresponding unit vector between them. Then, the continuous form was relaxed into a discrete formulation. The discrete cylinder flux was embedded into a graph-based framework. The main limitations of this cylinder model are that the local region cannot expand along curvilinear structures and the flux responses are computed at links rather than nodes of the graph, meaning that it cannot generate an individual feature map out of a graph-based framework. Besides, sampling in the cross-section will weaken the effects since in practice the whole circular plane cannot be fully visited.

Oriented Cylinder Flux Model. In this part, we will define an oriented local cylindrical model on each voxel in an image, whose centerline can be curvilinear and orientation is homogeneous with the object structure. To compute pixel-based cylinder responses, we modify the coordinate function in Eq. (1),

$$f(x_t; r) = \int_{-L}^{L} \int_{0}^{2\pi} v(x_{t+l} + n_{x_{t+l}} + N(\theta)) \cdot N(\theta) d\theta dl, \qquad (2)$$

where $n_{x_{t+l}}$ is the local structure orientation at x_{t+l}.

Consider the cross-section C_r centered at x with radius r. Instead of calculating the gradient flux discretely by sampling C_r, we exploit OOF responses to approximate it. Denote the resulting pairs of eigenvalues and eigenvectors in OOF as $\lambda_k(x; r)$ and $\omega_k(x; r)$, where $k \in \{1, 2, 3\}$. The approximated gradient flux at C_r is acquired based on two of the three eigenvalues,

$$\Lambda(x; r) = \pi \sqrt{(\lambda_2)^2 + (\lambda_3)^2}, \qquad (3)$$

where λ_2 and λ_3 are the median eigenvalue and the minimal eigenvalue respectively. We give a brief proof that we can use eigenvalues in OOF at x to approximate gradient flux of the cross-section centered at x. For implementation, we exploit the square form of $\Lambda(\cdot)$ to enhance the responses and normalize $\Lambda(\cdot)$ by r. The final normalized approximated gradient flux is given as,

$$\Lambda^2(x; r) = \frac{\pi \sqrt{(\lambda_2)^2 + (\lambda_3)^2}}{r}. \qquad (4)$$

Proof. From [5], we have,

$$\lambda_k(x; r) = \frac{1}{4\pi r^2} \int_{\partial S_r} ((v(x + h) \cdot \omega_k(x; r)) \omega_k(x; r)) \cdot \hat{n} dA. \qquad (5)$$

The eigenvalues solved in OOF are the amount of projected gradient flux flows out of the local sphere S_r under direction $\omega_k(\cdot)$, when S_r precisely touches the boundary of a curvilinear structure. Consider any point $y \in S_r \backslash C_r$, where C_r is the surface of the local sphere, $v(y)$ can be sufficiently small since inner intensities of curvilinear structures are ideally uniform. Thus,

$$\lambda_k(\boldsymbol{x};r) = \frac{1}{4\pi r^2}\left(\int_{\partial C_r}(\cdot)\mathrm{d}A + \int_{\partial(S_r\setminus C_r)}(\cdot)\mathrm{d}A\right) \approx \frac{1}{4\pi r^2}\int_{\partial C_r}(\cdot)\mathrm{d}A. \quad (6)$$

Then, we apply multi-scale detection scheme to the cross-section flux computation,

$$\tilde{r}(\boldsymbol{x}) = arg\max_{r_i}\Lambda^2(\boldsymbol{x};r_i), \quad \Lambda_{\tilde{r}}^2(\boldsymbol{x}) = \Lambda^2(\boldsymbol{x};\tilde{r}(\boldsymbol{x})). \quad (7)$$

With the help of $\Lambda_{\tilde{r}}^2(\boldsymbol{x})$, our cylindrical model can have cross-sections with varying radii. It is noted that the radii of cross-sections shrink at the end of vessel structures, showing that the length of a vessel segment is related to its radius. We measure their relationship on a logarithmic scale and define the lengths of the local cylinder model by using the detected scales extracted from the multi-scale scheme in cross-section flux computation,

$$L(\boldsymbol{x}) = \log(\tilde{r}(\boldsymbol{x}) + 1). \quad (8)$$

by which smaller vessels can have a relative larger cylindrical length and thus a more precise responses can be caught.

The last unknown variable is $\boldsymbol{n}_{\boldsymbol{x}}$, which is used to explore the next position in the local cylindrical region. Denote $\lambda_1(\boldsymbol{x};r)$ as the largest eigenvalue and $\boldsymbol{\omega}_1(\boldsymbol{x};r)$ as the corresponding eigenvector. We make use of $\boldsymbol{\omega}_1(\boldsymbol{x};r)$ to provide orientation information to our local model. The Oriented Cylinder Flux model can be then reformulated as,

$$f(\boldsymbol{x}_t) = \int_{-L}^{L}\Lambda_{\tilde{r}}^2(\boldsymbol{x}_{t+l} + \boldsymbol{n}_{\boldsymbol{x}_{t+l}})\mathrm{d}l = \int_{-\log(\tilde{r}(\boldsymbol{x}_t)+1)}^{\log(\tilde{r}(\boldsymbol{x}_t)+1)}\Lambda_{\tilde{r}}^2(\boldsymbol{x}_{t+l} + \boldsymbol{\omega}_1(\boldsymbol{x}_{t+l};\tilde{r}(\boldsymbol{x}_{t+l})))\mathrm{d}l. \quad (9)$$

We give a discrete version of OCF by replacing integral with summation,

$$DOCF(\boldsymbol{x}_n) = \sum_{l=-L'}^{L'}\Lambda_{\tilde{r}}^2(\boldsymbol{x}_{n+l} + \tilde{\boldsymbol{\omega}}_1(\boldsymbol{x}_{n+l};\tilde{r}(\boldsymbol{x}_{n+l}))), \quad (10)$$

where $L' = [\log(\tilde{r}(\boldsymbol{x}_t)+1)]$ and $\tilde{\boldsymbol{\omega}}_1(\boldsymbol{x}_{n+l};\tilde{r}(\boldsymbol{x}_{n+l})) = \boldsymbol{\omega}_1(\boldsymbol{x}_{n+l};\tilde{r}(\boldsymbol{x}_{n+l}))$ if $\boldsymbol{\omega}_1(\cdot)*\boldsymbol{\omega}_1(\boldsymbol{x}_n;\tilde{r}(\boldsymbol{x}_n)) \geq 0$ and $-\boldsymbol{\omega}_1(\boldsymbol{x}_{n+l};\tilde{r}(\boldsymbol{x}_{n+l}))$ otherwise.

The new metric is derived based on the concepts of OOF. Different from [13], whose local cylinder is elongated along a straight centerline between two adjacent points, our local cylindrical region has not only a curvilinear centerline but also cross-sections with varying radii. In [12], the authors also exploited the local structure orientations calculated from OOF. However, they only used the orientation between two adjoining points and encoded it into a graph-based framework. An illustration of our designed cylinder model is shown in Fig. 1.

To use oriented cylindrical flux in the computation of high-order tensor, we then modify the formula of $DOCF$ to collect the responses measurements under different projected directions as follows,

$$D(\boldsymbol{g}) = \sum_{l=-L'}^{L'}\Lambda_{\tilde{r}}^2(\boldsymbol{x}_{n+l} + \boldsymbol{g}*\Delta x)\frac{\max\{\boldsymbol{\omega}_1(\boldsymbol{x}_{n+l};\tilde{r}(\boldsymbol{x}_{n+l}))^T\boldsymbol{g}, -\boldsymbol{\omega}_1(\boldsymbol{x}_{n+l};\tilde{r}(\boldsymbol{x}_{n+l}))^T\boldsymbol{g}\}}{\|\boldsymbol{\omega}_1(\boldsymbol{x}_{n+l};\tilde{r}(\boldsymbol{x}_{n+l}))\|\|\boldsymbol{g}\|}, \quad (11)$$

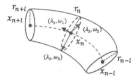

Fig. 1. An illustration for the designed model. Our model is adaptive: (a) the centerline can be curvilinear (gray dash line), stretching along ω_1; (b) cross-sections can have varying radii (e.g., $r_{n+l} \neq r_{n-l}$) and (c) length of the cylinder is a function of r_n.

which considers the angular coherence between the measured direction and the orientation estimated by the oriented cylindrical flux as the weights in the cylindrical accumulation.

2.2   High-Order Tensor Construction

In the High Angular Resolution Diffusion Imaging (HARDI), the apparent local diffusion can be estimated [8] by,

$$D(\boldsymbol{g}) = \sum_{i_1=1}^{n} \sum_{i_2=1}^{n} \cdots \sum_{i_l=1}^{n} \mathcal{D}_{i_1 i_2 \ldots i_l} g_{i_1} \cdots g_{i_l}, \tag{12}$$

where l is the order of the tensor and n is the dimension of the data. Observed from Eq. (12), it is clear that $D(\boldsymbol{g})$ is symmetric when l is even.

We adopt a 4D construction of high-order tensor proposed in [2] where the 4th dimension is determined by $D(\boldsymbol{g})$ with the purpose of suppression of the responses along some unwanted directions in the bifurcations. Equation (12) now becomes,

$$D(\boldsymbol{g}) = \sum_{i_1=1}^{4} \sum_{i_2=1}^{4} \cdots \sum_{i_l=1}^{4} \mathcal{D}_{i_1 i_2 \ldots i_l} g_{i_1} \cdots g_{i_l}. \tag{13}$$

On the left-hand size, the HARDI measurement $D(\boldsymbol{g})$ is computed in the 3D space with $\boldsymbol{g} \in \mathbb{R}^3$, while on the right-hand size $\boldsymbol{g} = (g_1, g_2, g_3, g_4)^T$, where $g_4(\boldsymbol{g}) = \frac{1}{1+\exp^{-a(D(\boldsymbol{g})-c)}}$ $(a, c > 0)$, acting as a high-pass filter that enhances the measurement responses along the direction of curvilinear structures and the bifurcations. The high-order tensor $\mathcal{D}_{i_1 i_2 \ldots i_l}$ is computed by repeated outer products with a vector **v** theoretically and thus it is totally symmetric. For an order-l tensor in n dimensions, the number of distinguished channels equals to $N = \binom{n+l-1}{l}$ [10]. Denote $[\mathcal{D}]_i$ as the i-th non-redundant element of $\mathcal{D}_{i_1 i_2 \ldots i_l}$ and $\mathbf{d} = ([\mathcal{D}]_1, [\mathcal{D}]_2, \ldots, [\mathcal{D}]_N)^T$. Let $g_{i(p)}$ denote the component of $\boldsymbol{g}$ specified by the p-th index of the i-th element in $\mathbf{d}$ and μ_i denote the number of times element i is repeated as a channel in the tensor, which equals to $\mu_i = \frac{l!}{n_1! n_2! \ldots n_l!}$, where n_j $(j = 1, \ldots, l)$ denotes the number of times index j appeared in the subscripts of element i. Then, Eq. (13) can be rewritten as,

$$D(\boldsymbol{g}) = \sum_{i=1}^{N} [\mathcal{D}]_i \mu_i \prod_{p=1}^{l} g_{i(p)}. \tag{14}$$

Let M be the number of sampled directions over the unit sphere $\mathbb{S}^2$. Given $D(\boldsymbol{g})$ and $\boldsymbol{g}$, the order-l tensor can be obtained by,

$$D(\boldsymbol{g}_m) = \tilde{\boldsymbol{g}}_m^T \mathbf{d}, \quad m = 1, \ldots, M, \tag{15}$$

where $\tilde{\boldsymbol{g}} = (\mu_1 \prod_{p=1}^{l} g_{1(p)}, \ldots, \mu_N \prod_{p=1}^{l} g_{N(p)})^T$. Let $\mathbf{D} = (D(\boldsymbol{g}_1), \ldots, D(\boldsymbol{g}_M))^T$, the high-order tensor components can be estimated via least-squares estimation,

$$\mathbf{d} = (\mathbf{G}^T \mathbf{G})^{-1} \mathbf{G}^T \mathbf{D}, \tag{16}$$

where $\mathbf{G} = (\tilde{\boldsymbol{g}}_1, \ldots, \tilde{\boldsymbol{g}}_M)^T$.

Tensor Decomposition. We apply the Tucker decomposition, which is a form of higher-order PCA, to obtain dominant orientations of the computed tensor. The Tucker format of a given tensor $\mathcal{R}$ is a decomposition as the product of a core tensor $\mathcal{G}$ and multiple matrices which relate to different core singular values along each mode. Assume a order-L tensor $\mathcal{R} \in \mathbb{R}^{I_1 \times I_2 \times \cdots \times I_L}$, the Tucker decomposition is given as follows,

$$\min_{\tilde{\mathcal{D}}} \quad \|\mathcal{D} - \tilde{\mathcal{D}}\|,$$
$$\text{subject to} \quad \tilde{\mathcal{D}} = \sum_{p_1=1}^{P_1} \sum_{p_2=1}^{P_2} \cdots \sum_{p_N=1}^{P_N} g_{p_1 p_2 \ldots p_N} u_{p_1}^{(1)} \circ u_{p_2}^{(2)} \circ \ldots \circ u_{p_N}^{(N)}, \tag{17}$$
$$= \mathcal{G} \times_1 U^{(1)} \times_2 U^{(2)} \times_3 \ldots \times_N U^{(N)},$$

where $u_{p_j}^{(i)}$ is the p_j-th column vector of $U_{p_j}^{(i)} \in \mathbb{R}^{I_i \times P_j}$, $\times_n$ represents the tensor-matrix product in mode-n, and $\circ$ represents the outer product.

In the construction of the above high order tensor, $\mathcal{D}_{i_1 i_2 \ldots i_l}$ is supersymmetric and therefore in the Tucker decomposition,

$$\tilde{\mathcal{D}} = \mathcal{G} \times_1 U \times_2 U \times_3 \ldots \times_N U. \tag{18}$$

Finally, we collect column vectors in U as the dominant orientations of the computed tensor. The number of vectors equal to the rank R defined by the user in the Tucker decomposition.

Spherical Deconvolution. The Spherical deconvolution is used to eliminate the effects of the average of multi-orientations on the detected structures. Such technique used in the HARDI is expressed by the spherical harmonic functions, assuming that the measure responses $S(\theta, \phi)$ can be regarded as the convolution of a fiber orientation density function $F(\theta, \phi)$ with an axially symmetric kernel $R(\theta)$ [9]. However, since our high-order tensor is defined in the 4D space and the computation of the spherical harmonic functions in 4D is complex, we introduce the similar technique during the tensor decomposition. The averaging effect can be regarded as an isotropic component in the measure tensor [9] and therefore before the decomposition, we let

$$\mathcal{D} := \mathcal{D} - \text{mean}(\mathcal{D}) \times e^{ol}, \tag{19}$$

where e denotes a 4D column vector with all elements one and e^{ol} represents $e \circ e \circ \ldots \circ e$ for l times.

Angular Coherence. Denote U as the result matrix decomposed from $\mathcal{D}_{i_1 i_2 \ldots i_l}$, which is computed from oriented cylindrical flux among multiple projected directions. We employ the direction information extracted from high-order tensor analysis to enhance the angular coherence between voxels. Define

$$A(v_i, v_j) = e^{\frac{\gamma |U(v_i)^T U(v_j)|}{Z}}, \tag{20}$$

where Z is the normalization factor and γ is a user-defined parameter for the sensitivity of the coherence. Note that the decomposed dominant vectors are column vectors in 4D, we can firstly normalize the vectors by the 4th dimension, treating as homogeneous vectors and then extract the components in the first 3 dimensions to map the vectors into 3D space. Consider a voxel at the bifurcation, we want such voxel to have high angular coherence with its neighborhood pixels at other branches. To achieve that, we collect the maximum value of the matrix $A(v_i, v_j)$ as the coherence response among v_i and v_j, which will be used in the random walk framework later.

2.3 High-Order OCF Connectivity Enhanced Random Walks

Random walks is an interactive, graph-based framework [4]. Given a weighted graph $G = (V, E)$, w_{ij} is the weight appointed to edge e_{ij}, which spans two vertices v_i and v_j. We assume the graph is undirected, then we have $w_{ij} = w_{ji}$. The segmentation task is done by solving the combinatorial Dirichlet problem. A combinatorial formulation of the Dirichlet integral $D[u] = \frac{1}{2} \int_\Omega |\nabla u|^2 d\Omega$ is,

$$D[x] = \frac{1}{2}(Ax)^T C(Ax) = \frac{1}{2} x^T L x = \frac{1}{2} \sum_{e_{ij} \in E} w_{ij}(x_i - x_j)^2, \tag{21}$$

where $x = (x_1, x_2, \ldots, x_n)^T$ is the probability that a walker will first reach a foreground seed starting from v_i. L is a combinatorial Laplacian matrix and A is an edge-node incidence matrix, and C is the constitutive matrix such that $L = A^T C A$. Suppose v_s are foreground seeds and v_b are background seeds, a object function is then given by minimizing $D[x]$,

$$x = arg \min_x(x^T L x) = arg \min_x \left(\sum_{e_{ij} \in E} (x_i - x_j)^2 \right), \text{s.t. } x(v_s) = 1, x(v_b) = 0. \tag{22}$$

Similar to [12], we embed the new vessel descriptor into the objective function as follows,

$$x = arg\min_{x} \sum_{e_{ij} \in E} w_{ij} c_{ij} (x_i - x_j)^2$$

$$+ \sum_{v_i \in V \setminus \{v_s, v_b\}} (DOCF(x_i) \times (x_i - 1)^2 + (1 - DOCF(x_i)) \times (x_i - 0)^2), \quad (23)$$

subject to $x(v_s) = 1, x(v_b) = 0$.

Followed by [4], we exploit the Gaussian weighting function to assign edge weights $w_{ij} = \exp(-\beta(g_i - g_j)^2)$, where β is the only parameter in random walks and g_i represents the image intensity at voxel i. c_{ij} is the coherence response between voxel i and j, which equals to $\max\{A(v_i, v_j)\}$.

3 Experiments and Results

Dataset. Experiments have been conducted on both synthetic and real clinical data. For synthetic data, we carried out two groups of experiments. The first group was a set of helix-like tubes with radii from 1 to 4 voxels and intensities from 0.5 to 1. The second group was a set of tree-like tubes with radii from 2 to 4 voxels and intensities all equal to 1. The purpose of the helix-like tube experiments is to simulate the shrinking problem in clinical data, and for tree-like tubes, we investigate the effects on vessel junctions. For the clinical experiments, we evaluated our methods on a set of healthy normal MRA images from *TubeTK* [1]. Figures 2 and 3 give the illustration for the synthetic data.

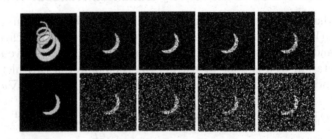

Fig. 2. First column: the original helix-like tube without noise in 3D view and in 2D view respectively. $2^{nd} - 4^{th}$ columns (from left to right and from up to bottom): helix-like tube with noise levels $\mathcal{N} \in \{0.02, 0.04, 0.06, 0.1, 0.2, 0.3, 0.4, 0.5\}$ respectively.

Experiment Setting. The proposed method has been compared with classical random walks (*RW*), Optimally Oriented Flux with direction coherence (*OOF_2016*) [12], the well-known Hessian method [3] with the same graph-based framework in [12] and the Ranking Orientation Responses of Path Operators

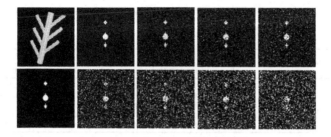

Fig. 3. First column: the original tree-like tube without noise in 3D view and in 2D view respectively. 2nd–4th columns (from left to right and from up to bottom): tree-like tube with noise levels $\mathcal{N} \in \{0.02, 0.04, 0.06, 0.1, 0.2, 0.3, 0.4, 0.5\}$ respectively.

($RORPO$) [6]. We also extracted the outcome in the first step of $DOCF$ namely cross-section flux, which is exactly $\Lambda_{\hat{r}}^2$, and $DOCF$ for evaluation. In the synthetic experiments, radii for proposed method, OOF_2016 and Hessian methods were set from 1 to 10, with steps equal to 0.5. As for $RORPO$, the minimum path length was set to 2, with factor and number of scales equal to 1.5 and 10 respectively. In the clinical tests, the range of radii for the methods mentioned was from 1 to 20, with step equal to 0.5. The minimum path length was 2, with factor and number of scales equal to 1.5 and 20 respectively. To obtain binary segmentation results, the thresholding values were optimized to the maximum accuracy by selecting the values from 0.02 to 0.8 with step equal to 0.02. In all experiments, β related to random walks and random walker based framework was set to 100. As for other parameters in the proposed method, we fixed $R = 4$, $a = 1$, $c = 0.5$ and $M = 64$. The numerical results are listed in Tables 1, 2 and 3. We employ Dice Coefficient for statistic measurements,

$$DICE = \frac{2 * |X \cap Y|}{|X| + |Y|} = \frac{2TP}{FN + FP + 2TP}, \tag{24}$$

where $|X|$, $|Y|$ are the cardinalities of set X and set Y, FN, FP and TP represent false negative, false positive and true positive respectively.

As listed in Table 1, both $\Lambda_{\hat{r}}^2$ and $DOCF$ can give good performance on tubular images in the low-noise environment. When noise level raises, traveling along local cylindrical models intensifies the ability of distinction between noise and vascular parts and thus $DOCF$ has a relative stable pattern on Dice coefficient. The high-order $DOCF$ combines the advantages of $\Lambda_{\hat{r}}^2$ and $DOCF$, expressing better performance and more stable on Dice scores among all noise levels. It is shown that the Dice scores under different orders of the computed tensor are slightly different. In our experiments, order-3 tensor fitted both helix-like tubes and tree-like tubes the best with the largest number of maximum Dice scores. From Tables 2 and 3, the high-order $DOCF$ outperforms among other methods. Both $RORPO$ and RW can achieve a high score on input images without noise. However, RW only considers intensity homogeneity of images and thus when noise appears it suffers from intensity fluctuation as well as seed

Table 1. Dice on helix-like tubes and tree-like tubes (intra-comparison on the proposed method)

Synthetic Data	Methods	Noise Level								
		0	0.02	0.04	0.06	0.1	0.2	0.3	0.4	0.5
Helix-liked Tubes	Λ_F^2	100.00%	97.12%	**96.32%**	94.66%	87.05%	88.38%	77.70%	61.08%	58.95%
	DOCF	94.52%	81.96%	80.90%	80.60%	81.10%	78.77%	75.38%	72.20%	68.99%
	Order-4 OCF	91.50%	96.46%	95.41%	**94.71%**	92.85%	88.38%	84.80%	81.44%	**78.04%**
	Order-3 OCF	100.00%	96.62%	95.37%	94.19%	93.29%	**89.82%**	**86.26%**	**82.38%**	76.58%
	Order-2 OCF	100.00%	96.39%	95.60%	94.48%	**93.66%**	89.62%	86.16%	81.27%	75.37%
Tree-liked Tubes	Λ_F^2	100.00%	92.87%	89.87%	82.86%	80.37%	78.58%	68.27%	60.05%	39.80%
	DOCF	98.50%	86.20%	85.10%	84.92%	82.98%	81.16%	77.60%	73.32%	70.00%
	Order-4 OCF	85.66%	**95.99%**	94.10%	92.92%	**92.21%**	90.01%	87.93%	85.00%	81.33%
	Order-3 OCF	100.00%	95.63%	**94.13%**	93.28%	92.20%	90.18%	**88.29%**	84.05%	**84.04%**
	Order-2 OCF	100.00%	95.79%	93.99%	**93.72%**	92.10%	**90.46%**	87.04%	**85.36%**	82.82%

sensitivity problem, leading segmentation results unpredictable. *RORPO* gives relatively good results with low noise levels, despite a sudden drop when noise becomes large. Although *OOF_2016* also leverages vascular orientation obtained from *OOF*, this method considers the dominant orientations estimated from an elliptical tensor within an ideal spherical local region, resulting in relative poor performance since the idea spherical assumption cannot actually be achieved under the noise environment.

Given the above two groups of synthetic experiments and the corresponding statistics results, we only compared high-order *OCF* with *RORPO* and *OOF_2016* qualitatively in this part. Figure 4 shows the segmentation results obtained from high-order *OCF*. As shown in Fig. 4, with the help of our local cylindrical model, high-order *OCF* can achieve promising segmentation results under high noise level and intensity fluctuation in clinical images. Comparisons with respective to vascular responses among the proposed method, *RORPO* and *OOF_2016* are shown in Fig. 5 in the first, second and third rows respectively. The responses of the proposed method and *OOF_2016* are the probability maps generated in the similar random walks frameworks. But *OOF_2016* can only obtain relatively favorable results around the Circle of Willis and fail in other regions. The region marked by the red rectangle demonstrated the ability of angular coherence derived by the high-order tensor to enhance the performance of vascular detection, with the effects of smoothing the voxels within vessel lumen. The maps shown in the second row for *RORPO* exhibited good responses for vessels. But the responses were influenced by noise, resulting in some unwanted segments in the results (see the blue rectangle region, where we changed the color of background for better visualization on noise and the unwanted segments.).

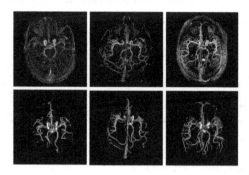

Fig. 4. First row: sample MRA images in *TubeTK*, which are Normal001, Normal002 and Normal003 respectively. Second row: the segmentation results of high-order *DOCF*.

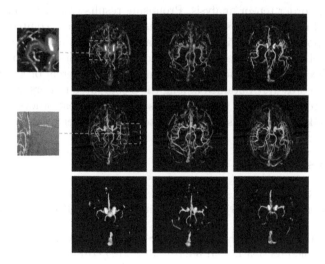

Fig. 5. Vascular responses of high-order *OCF*, *RORPO* and *OOF_2016*.

Table 2. Dice on helix-like tubes (comparison with other methods)

Synthetic Data	Methods	Noise Level								
		0	0.02	0.04	0.06	0.1	0.2	0.3	0.4	0.5
Helix-liked Tubes	*Order-4 OCF*(ours)	91.50%	96.46%	95.41%	**94.71%**	92.85%	88.38%	84.80%	81.44%	**78.04%**
	Order-3 OCF(ours)	**100.00%**	96.62%	95.37%	94.19%	93.29%	**89.82%**	**86.26%**	**82.38%**	76.58%
	Order-2 OCF(ours)	**100.00%**	96.39%	**95.60%**	94.48%	**93.66%**	89.62%	86.16%	81.27%	75.37%
	RORPO	**100.00%**	**97.80%**	88.17%	76.75%	57.44%	0.33%	0.00%	0.00%	0.00%
	OOF_2016	98.78%	92.23%	90.08%	90.50%	91.47%	89.68%	86.09%	80.79%	75.10%
	Hessian with RW	98.84%	95.94%	95.26%	94.35%	92.13%	82.92%	73.49%	62.79%	53.29%
	Random Walks	**100.00%**	51.70%	51.10%	36.72%	48.26%	49.07%	30.23%	53.92%	36.44%

Table 3. Dice on tree-like tubes (comparison with other methods)

Synthetic Data	Methods	Noise Level								
		0	0.02	0.04	0.06	0.1	0.2	0.3	0.4	0.5
Tree-liked Tubes	*Order-4 OCF*(ours)	85.66%	95.99%	94.10%	92.92%	**92.21%**	90.01%	87.93%	85.00%	81.33%
	Order-3 OCF(ours)	**100.00%**	95.63%	94.13%	93.28%	92.20%	90.18%	**88.29%**	84.05%	**84.04%**
	Order-2 OCF(ours)	**100.00%**	95.79%	93.99%	**93.72%**	92.10%	**90.46%**	87.04%	**85.36%**	82.82%
	RORPO	99.97%	**99.83%**	**95.80%**	86.18%	67.16%	0.74%	0.00%	0.00%	0.00%
	OOF_2016	99.77%	94.79%	93.74%	92.76%	90.42%	89.55%	86.54%	85.18%	81.27%
	Hessian with RW	98.73%	94.51%	93.39%	92.22%	90.45%	85.14%	75.09%	59.89%	47.01%
	Random Walks	**100.00%**	77.80%	46.93%	56.01%	26.12%	58.11%	41.76%	40.00%	54.50%

4   Conclusions

We have presented a novel 3D vascular pixel-based detector and fitted it into a high-order framework to perform vessel segmentation. We then apply the random walker framework to combine *DOCF* responses and angular coherence computed from the high-order tensor analysis. Promising results can be obtained on both synthetic and real MRA data under different levels of noise, compared with two recently proposed 3D curvilinear segmentation methods and two classical segmentation methods. Note that in the synthetic experiments and clinical tests, we separately discussed the performance of tensors with different order and most of highest Dice scores were obtained among the 3 computed tensors. Further efforts can be done to combine the tensor responses with different orders, constructing a Adaboost-liked strong tensor responses to obtain higher performance.

References

1. Aylward, S.R., Bullitt, E.: Initialization, noise, singularities, and scale in height ridge traversal for tubular object centerline extraction. IEEE TMI **21**(2), 61–75 (2002)
2. Cetin, S., Unal, G.: A higher-order tensor vessel tractography for segmentation of vascular structures. IEEE TMI **34**(10), 2172–2185 (2015)
3. Frangi, A.F., Niessen, W.J., Vincken, K.L., Viergever, M.A.: Multiscale vessel enhancement filtering. In: Wells, W.M., Colchester, A., Delp, S. (eds.) MICCAI 1998. LNCS, vol. 1496, pp. 130–137. Springer, Heidelberg (1998). https://doi.org/10.1007/BFb0056195
4. Grady, L.: Random walks for image segmentation. IEEE TPAMI **28**(11), 1768–1783 (2006)
5. Law, M.W.K., Chung, A.C.S.: An oriented flux symmetry based active contour model for three dimensional vessel segmentation. In: Daniilidis, K., Maragos, P., Paragios, N. (eds.) ECCV 2010. LNCS, vol. 6313, pp. 720–734. Springer, Heidelberg (2010). https://doi.org/10.1007/978-3-642-15558-1_52
6. Merveille, O., Talbot, H., Najman, L., Passat, N.: Curvilinear structure analysis by ranking the orientation responses of path operators. IEEE TPAMI **40**(2), 304–317 (2018)

7. Moriconi, S., Zuluaga, M.A., Jäger, H.R., Nachev, P., Ourselin, S., Cardoso, M.J.: VTrails: inferring vessels with geodesic connectivity trees. In: Niethammer, M., Styner, M., Aylward, S., Zhu, H., Oguz, I., Yap, P.-T., Shen, D. (eds.) IPMI 2017. LNCS, vol. 10265, pp. 672–684. Springer, Cham (2017). https://doi.org/10.1007/978-3-319-59050-9_53

8. Özarslan, E., Mareci, T.H.: Generalized diffusion tensor imaging and analytical relationships between diffusion tensor imaging and high angular resolution diffusion imaging. Magn. Reson. Med. **50**(5), 955–965 (2003)

9. Schultz, T., Seidel, H.P.: Estimating crossing fibers: a tensor decomposition approach. IEEE Trans. Vis. Comput. Graph. **14**(6), 1635–1642 (2008)

10. Schultz, T., Weickert, J., Seidel, H.P.: A higher-order structure tensor. In: Laidlaw, D., Weickert, J. (eds.) Visualization and Processing of Tensor Fields. MATHVISUAL, pp. 263–279. Springer, Heidelberg (2009). https://doi.org/10.1007/978-3-540-88378-4_13

11. Vasilevskiy, A., Siddiqi, K.: Flux maximizing geometric flows. IEEE TPAMI **24**(12), 1565–1578 (2002)

12. Zhang, Q., Chung, A.C.S.: 3D vessel segmentation using random walker with oriented flux analysis and direction coherence. In: Zheng, G., Liao, H., Jannin, P., Cattin, P., Lee, S.-L. (eds.) MIAR 2016. LNCS, vol. 9805, pp. 281–291. Springer, Cham (2016). https://doi.org/10.1007/978-3-319-43775-0_25

13. Zhu, N., Chung, A.C.S.: Random walks with adaptive cylinder flux based connectivity for vessel segmentation. In: Mori, K., Sakuma, I., Sato, Y., Barillot, C., Navab, N. (eds.) MICCAI 2013. LNCS, vol. 8150, pp. 550–558. Springer, Heidelberg (2013). https://doi.org/10.1007/978-3-642-40763-5_68

Joint CS-MRI Reconstruction and Segmentation with a Unified Deep Network

Liyan Sun[1], Zhiwen Fan[1], Xinghao Ding[1(✉)], Yue Huang[1], and John Paisley[2]

[1] Fujian Key Laboratory of Sensing and Computing for Smart City,
Xiamen University, Fujian, China
dxh@xmu.edu.cn
[2] Department of Electrical Engineering, Columbia University,
New York, NY, USA

Abstract. The need for fast acquisition and automatic analysis of MRI data is growing. Although compressed sensing magnetic resonance imaging (CS-MRI) has been studied to accelerate MRI by reducing k-space measurements, current techniques overlook downstream applications such as segmentation when doing image reconstruction. In this paper, we test the utility of CS-MRI when performing automatic segmentation and propose a unified deep neural network architecture called SegNetMRI for simultaneous CS-MRI reconstruction and segmentation. SegNetMRI uses an MRI reconstruction network with multiple cascaded blocks, each containing an encoder-decoder unit and a data fidelity unit, and a parallel MRI segmentation network having the same encoder-decoder structure. The two subnetworks are pre-trained and fine-tuned with shared reconstruction encoders. The outputs are merged into the final segmentation. Our experiments show that SegNetMRI can improve both the reconstruction and segmentation performance when using compressed measurements.

Keywords: Compressed sensing · Magnetic resonance imaging · Medical image segmentation

1 Introduction

Magnetic resonance imaging (MRI) is a fundamental technique for visualizing human tissue. In MRI, raw measurements come in the form of Fourier transform coefficients in "k-space" and the MRI can be viewed after an inverse 2D Fourier transform of the fully sampled k-space. Conventionally, radiologists view MRI for diagnosis. However, in areas where medical expertise may be lacking or not sufficient to meet demand, automated methods may also be useful. To this end, automatic MR image segmentation is essential because it allows for finer localization of focus. To take brain segmentation for example, usually four structures

L. Sun and Z. Fan—The co-first authors contributed equally.

© Springer Nature Switzerland AG 2019
A. C. S. Chung et al. (Eds.): IPMI 2019, LNCS 11492, pp. 492–504, 2019.
https://doi.org/10.1007/978-3-030-20351-1_38

emerge including background, gray matter (GM), white matter (WM) and cerebrospinal fluid (CSF). Lesions appearing in white matter are closely associated with various issues such as strokes and Alzheimer's disease [25].

Although rich anatomical information can be provided by MRI, it is limited by a long imaging period. This can introduce motion artifacts caused by movement of the patient [3] or induce psychological pressures brought by claustrophobia [11]. Thus accelerating imaging speed while maintaining high imaging quality is key for MRI. Compressed sensing (CS) theory [5,9], which shows the possibility of recovering signals with sub-Nyquist sampling rates, has been introduced to the field of MRI to accelerate imaging. In 2017, the US Food and Drug Administration (FDA) approved CS-MRI techniques for use by two major MRI vendors: Siemens and GE [10]. Thus, one can expect increasing deployment of CS-MRI technique in the future for real-world applications.

Current segmentation algorithms for MRI assume a "clean" (i.e., fully-sampled) image as input and, to our knowledge, do not take CS-MRI scenarios into consideration. Likewise, CS-MRI reconstruction methods do not consider their output's potential downstream use for segmentation. Although experienced human experts can make relatively robust decisions with CS-reconstructed images, the anticipated increase in the number of CS-reconstructed MRI for clinical application will call for automatic segmentation algorithms optimized for this type of data. Therefore, a joint approach to MRI reconstruction/segmentation under the compressed sensing framework is worth exploring.

In this paper, we develop a unified deep neural network called SegNetMRI for joint MRI reconstruction and segmentation with compressive measurements. The model is unified in that parameters are ultimately tuned taking both segmentation and reconstruction tasks into consideration. We build SegNetMRI on two joined networks: an MRI reconstruction network (MRN) and MRI segmentation network (MSN). The MSN is an encoder-decoder structure network and for SegNetMRI this is made up of basic blocks which each consist of an encoder-decoder and data fidelity unit. The MRN is pre-trained with pairs of artificially under-sampled MRI and their corresponding fully-sampled MRI, and the MSN is pre-trained with fully-sampled MRI and their corresponding segmentation labels. We then fine-tune the resulting unified network with MSN and MRN both sharing the same encoder component. In this way, the MRI reconstruction and segmentation models can each aid the learning of the other through shared regularization.

2   Background and Related Work

MRI Segmentation. Broadly speaking, the research in MRI segmentation can be categorized into three classes: (1) atlas-based segmentation with registration; (2) machine learning models with hand-crafted features; (3) deep learning models. Atlas-based segmentation [1,2] requires accurate registration and is time-consuming, so it is impractical for applications that require fast speed. In the second class, manually designed features are used for classification, for example

3D Haar/spatial features classified with random forests [27]. Similar to many image processing problems, these hand-crafted features are not very flexible for encoding diverse patterns within the MRI data. Recently deep learning based models have been proposed, such as a 2D convolutional neural network [19,20], a 3D convolutional neural network [6,7], and parallelized long short-term memory (LSTM) [26]. These models can learn semantic image features from data, typically leading to the state-of-the-art performance in MRI segmentation. However, these MRI segmentation models do not take the input quality into consideration, such as degradations from a sub-sampled k-space, but assume a fully-sampled MRI.

Compressed Sensing MRI. We briefly review the work in CS-MRI reconstruction. Denote the underlying vectorized MRI $x \in \mathbb{C}^{P \times 1}$, which we seek to reconstruct from the sub-sampled vectorized k-space data $y \in \mathbb{C}^{Q \times 1}$ ($Q \ll P$). CS-MRI inversion is then typically formulated as the optimization

$$x = \arg\min \|F_u x - y\|_2^2 + f_\theta(x), \tag{1}$$

where the $F_u \in \mathbb{C}^{Q \times P}$ denotes the under-sampled Fourier matrix. The ℓ_2 term is the data fidelity and $f_\theta(\cdot)$ represents a regularization with parameter θ to constrain the solution space.

The main research focus of CS-MRI is proposing better f_θ and efficient optimization techniques. In the first CS-MRI work called SparseMRI [17], wavelet domain ℓ_1 sparsity plus image total variation were imposed as regularizations. More complex wavelet variants were designed for CS-MRI in PANO [21] and GBRWT [13]. Dictionary learning techniques have also been introduced to CS-MRI, such as DLMRI [22] and BPTV [12]. These works can all be categorized as sparsity-based CS-MRI methods since they model the MRI with a "one-level" sparse prior. This prior often tends to over-smooth the resulting image.

Recently, deep neural networks have been introduced to CS-MRI. Researchers have directly applied the convolutional neural network (CNN) to learn a direct mapping from the zero-filled MRI $F_u^H y$ (obtained by zero-padding the unsampled positions in k-space) to the true MRI [28]. A deep residual architecture was also proposed for this same mapping [14]. Data fidelity terms have been incorporated into the deep neural network by [24] to add more guidance. These deep learning based CS-MRI models have achieved higher reconstruction quality and faster reconstruction speed.

Combining Visual Tasks. The combination of different visual tasks into a unified model is frequently considered in the field of computer vision. For example, a joint blind image restoration and recognition model based on sparse coding has been proposed for face recognition with low-quality images [29]. The image dehazing model AOD-Net performs detection in the presence of haze by performing dehazing during detection [15]. In the MRI field, models for 3T-obtained images have been proposed to jointly perform segmentation and super-resolution (7T) image generation [4].

3   Methodology

In this section, we give a detailed description of the proposed SegNetMRI model. First, we propose a segmentation network as baseline and test popular CS-MRI methods with this model. Next we propose an MRI reconstruction network formed by cascading basic network blocks. We show that the proposed MRI reconstruction network achieves better performance on segmentation compared with conventional sparsity-based CS-MRI models, but is still inferior to using the fully-sampled MRI. We finally propose the SegNetMRI model to merge these MRI reconstruction and segmentation approaches into an single model.

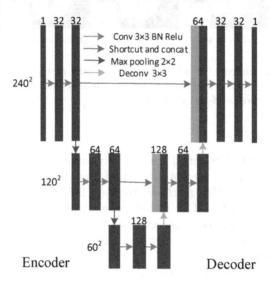

Fig. 1. The MSN architecture composed of an encoder and decoder. We use this segmentation network to compare performance using different CS-MRI reconstruction approaches as input.

3.1   Illustration: Segmentation After CS-MRI

We first test several popular CS-MRI model outputs on an automatic MRI segmentation model to assess the impact of compressed sensing for the segmentation task. As a basic segmentation model, we use the MRI segmentation network (MSN) shown in Fig. 1, which is the state-of-the-art medical image segmentation model called U-Net [23]. The segmentation encoder (SE) component uses convolution and pooling to extract features from the input image at different scales, and the segmentation decoder (SD) component uses a deconvolution operation to predict the the pixel-level segmentation class using these features. Shortcut connections are used by the model to directly send lower-layer feature information to high-layer features by concatenation.

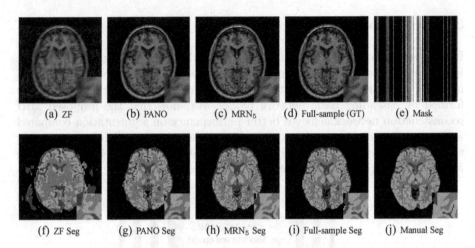

(a) ZF   (b) PANO   (c) MRN₅   (d) Full-sample (GT)   (e) Mask

(f) ZF Seg   (g) PANO Seg   (h) MRN₅ Seg   (i) Full-sample Seg   (j) Manual Seg

Fig. 2. Top: reconstructed MRI using different CS-MRI methods and a 20% sampling mask. Bottom: these MRI are segmented using an independently-trained segmentation model based on the state-of-the-art U-Net (referred to as MSN in this paper for its MRI application).

After training this MSN model using fully-sampled MRI and their ground truth segmentation labels, we test model performance using reconstructed MRI produced by various CS-MRI methods. We use a 20% Cartesian under-sampling mask as shown in Fig. 2(e). Our tested methods including the degraded zero-filled (ZF) reconstruction as baseline, PANO [21] and the proposed MRN model which will be discussed in the following section. We tuned the parameters of PANO for this problem.

We observe that the zero-filled (ZF) reconstruction in Fig. 2(a) produces a low-quality MRI, which leads to the poor segmentation performance shown in Fig. 2(f). The PANO reconstructed MRI in Fig. 2(b) is segmented better in Fig. 2(g), but is still far from satisfactory because of the loss of structural details in the reconstruction. Segmentation using the fully-sampled (FS) MRI in Fig. 2(d) is shown in Fig. 2(i). Though this isn't the ground truth segmentation, it is the segmentation performed on the ground truth MRI, and so represents an upper bound for CS-MRI on this segmentation task. The manually label segmentation is shown in Fig. 2(j). This experiment shows that while CS-MRI can substantially improve the reconstruction quality visually, the fine structural details which are important for segmentation can still be missing, leaving space for improvement.

3.2   An MRI Reconstruction Network

Deep learning for CS-MRI has the advantage of large modeling capacity, fast running speed, and high-level semantic modeling ability, which eases the integration of high-level task information compared with traditional sparsity-based CS-MRI models. Therefore, we adopt the same encoder-decoder architecture in Fig. 1 as a basic encoder-decoder unit with a global residual shortcut to reconstruction the sub-sampled MRI. Since information loss can become severe as neural network depth increases, we introduce a data fidelity (DF) unit to help correct the Fourier coefficients of the reconstructed MRI produced by the encoder-decoder architecture on the sampled positions in k-space. This takes advantage of the fact that we have accurate measurements at the under-sampled k-space locations, and so the layers of the network should not override this information. The details of the data fidelity unit can be found in [24].

The encoder-decoder architecture and data fidelity unit make up a basic block. As more blocks are stacked, the quality of the reconstructed MRI at each block gradually improves [24]. We therefore cascade N such basic units to form the MRI reconstruction network (MRN$_N$) in Fig. 3. The reconstruction encoder in different blocks extract features at different depths. Previously in Fig. 1, we observed that MRN$_5$ achieves better reconstruction performance in Fig. 2(c) than the non-deep PANO method, but the segmentation output in Fig. 2(h) (MRN→MSN) is still inferior to the fully-sampled segmentation. This motivates the following joint learning framework.

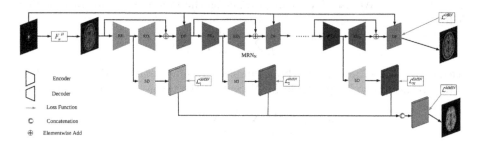

Fig. 3. The SegNetMRI structure, formed by connecting the previously discussed MRN for reconstruction (top) with MSN for segmentation (bottom).

3.3 SegNetMRI: A Unified Deep Neural Network

Using the previously discussed networks as starting points, we design a joint framework for CS-MRI reconstruction/segmentation based on deep learning. We call this joint network SegNetMRI and show its structure in Fig. 3. At a high level, the two problems are connected by a shared encoder, while having separate decoders.

To learn this model, we first pre-train two separate models. We pre-train the MRN$_N$ with under-sampled and fully-sampled MRI training pairs. Similarly, we pre-train the MSN with fully-sampled MRI and their corresponding segmentation labels. After training MSN, we discard the encoder component (SE) and keep the decoder component (SD). We then connect the single decoder component of the MSN (SD) to each of the encoder components of each MRN (called

RE_n) within each block. The resulting N outputs of the MSN decoder for each block are concatenated and merged to give the final segmentation via a 1×1 convolution. After pre-training separately and initializing the remaining parts, the parameters of SegNetMRI$_N$ (with N blocks in the MRN portion, but a single segmentation decoder duplicated N times) are then fine-tuned. Therefore, both the reconstruction and segmentation tasks share the *same* encoders, but have *separate* decoders for their respective tasks.

The rationale for using this architecture is as follows:

1. With the pre-training of MRN$_N$, the reconstruction encoder extracts basic features in different blocks. In SegNetMRI, the sharing of the reconstruction encoders between MRN and MSN means that these same features are used for both reconstruction and segmentation. This can help the two problems regularize each other.
2. The segmentation component uses information at various depths in the cascaded MRN and combines this information in the decoder. The 1×1 convolution used to merge the outputs of the segmentation decoder at each layer can be viewed as ensemble learning.

Loss Function. We use Euclidean distance as the loss function for pre-training MRN,

$$\mathcal{L}^{\mathrm{MRN}} = \frac{1}{L} \sum\nolimits_{i=1}^{L} \left\| x_i^{fs} - x_i \right\|_2^2, \tag{2}$$

where x_i^{fs} and x_i are the ith fully-sampled training image and the output of MRN, respectively. To pre-train MSN, we use the pixel-wise cross-entropy loss function

$$\mathcal{L}^{\mathrm{MSN}} = -\sum\nolimits_{i=1}^{L} \sum\nolimits_{j=1}^{N} \sum\nolimits_{c=1}^{C} t_{ijc}^{gt} \ln t_{ijc}, \tag{3}$$

where C tissue classes are to be classified. t^{gt} and t is the pixel-wise ground-truth label and the MSN-predicted label, respectively.

After pre-training MRN and MSN, we then construct and fine-tune SegNetMRI using the following loss function

$$\mathcal{L}^{\mathrm{SegNetMRI}} = \mathcal{L}^{\mathrm{MRN}} + \lambda \mathcal{L}^{\mathrm{OMSN}}. \tag{4}$$

We set $\lambda = 0.01$ in our experiments. The overall MSN (OMSN) loss, consisting of $N + 1$ loss function terms if SegNetMRI contains N blocks, is

$$\mathcal{L}^{\mathrm{OMSN}} = \frac{1}{N+1} \left(\mathcal{L}^{\mathrm{MMSN}} + \sum\nolimits_{i=1}^{N} \mathcal{L}_i^{\mathrm{SMSN}} \right), \tag{5}$$

where the $\mathcal{L}^{\mathrm{MMSN}}$ is the loss for the merged prediction and $\mathcal{L}^{\mathrm{SMSN}}$ is the loss for each sub-MSN decoder prediction.

4   Experiments and Discussions

4.1   Implementation Details

Setup. We implement all deep models on TensorFlow for the Python environment using a NVIDIA Geforce GTX 1080Ti with 11 GB GPU memory and Intel Xeon CPU E5-2683 at 2.00 GHz. We show the hyperparameter settings of encoder-decoder architecture used for both MRN and MSN in Fig. 1. We use batch normalization to stabilize training. ReLU is used as the activation function, except for the last convolutional layer of the encoder-decoder unit within each MRN block, where the identity map is applied for residual learning. We apply Xavier initialization for pre-training MRN and MSN. MSN is pre-trained for 60,000 iterations using 64×64 fully-sampled MRI patches randomly cropped (16 patches in a batch) and MRN is pre-trained for 30,000 iterations using the entire training image (4 images in a batch). We then fine-tune the SegNetMRI model for 8,000 further iterations using entire images (4 images in a batch). ADAM is chosen as optimizer. We select the initial learning rate to be 0.0005, the first-order momentum to be 0.9 and the second momentum to be 0.999.

Data. We test SegNetMRI on the MRBrainS datasets from the Grand Challenge on MR Brain Image Segmentation (MRBrainS) Workshop [18]. These datasets are acquired using 3T MRI scans. Five datasets are provided containing T1-1mm, T1, T1-IR and T2-FLAIR imaging modalities already registered and with manual segmentations. Here we use the T1 MRI data of the size 240×240 throughout the paper. We use four datasets for training (total 192 slices) and one dataset for testing (total 48 slices). We adopt the same data augmentation technique discussed in [8].

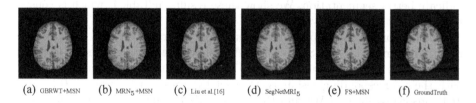

(a) GBRWT+MSN (b) MRN_5+MSN (c) Liu et al.[16] (d) $SegNetMRI_5$ (e) FS+MSN (f) GroundTruth

Fig. 4. The segmentations of the compared methods. (Color figure online)

4.2   Experimental Results

To evaluate the segmentation performance, we compare the proposed $SegNetMRI_5$ (5 blocks) with the following: (1) inputting a fully-sampled MRI into MSN (FS+MSN), which we take as ground truth performance; (2) inputting the MRN_5 reconstruction into MSN (MRN_5+MSN), i.e., no joint learning; (3) inputting the GBRWT model reconstruction into MSN (GBRWT+MSN),

Table 1. The segmentation performance of different models using DC (%), HD and AVD (%) as metrics. FS+MSN is the segmentation performance when the ground truth MRI is known. We consider FS+MSN the upper bound on performance given our chosen MSN approach.

Methods	GM			WM			CSF		
	DC	HD	AVD	DC	HD	AVD	DC	HD	AVD
GBRWT+MSN	75.55	2.24	4.21	65.56	1.90	3.10	76.50	1.77	2.69
MRN$_5$+MSN	79.36	2.06	3.57	65.76	1.88	2.96	78.43	1.64	2.33
Liu et al. [16]	83.41	1.81	2.96	78.05	1.24	1.61	77.81	1.76	2.58
SegNetMRI$_5$	**86.38**	**1.66**	**2.52**	**81.49**	**1.08**	**1.34**	**79.23**	**1.61**	**2.23**
FS+MSN	87.36	1.60	2.33	85.94	1.00	1.14	81.01	1.61	2.18

since GBRWT [13] represents the state-of-the-art performance among non-deep sparsity-based CS-MRI methods; (4) finally, we also compare with the joint framework proposed by [16], where only the reconstruction network is fine-tuned in MRN$_5$+MSN using the loss function $\mathcal{L}^{MRN} + \lambda \mathcal{L}^{MSN}$. The same under-sampling mask shown in Fig. 2(e) is again used.

We show a qualitative performance comparison in Fig. 4. We color the segmentation corresponding to white matter (yellow), gray matter (green) and cerebrospinal fluid (yellow). We observe that the proposed SegNetMRI$_5$ model provides better segmentation and approximates the ideal FS+MSN most closely, both of which are not perfect compared with the human labeling. For quantitative evaluation, we use the Dice Coefficient (DC), the 95th-percentile of the Hausdoff distance (HD) and the absolute volume difference (AVD), which are also used in the MRBrainS challenge [18]. Larger DC and smaller HD and AVD indicate better segmentation. We show these results in Table 1, which is consistent with our subjective evaluation.

In addition to the improved segmentation accuracy, we also evaluate the reconstruction quality of SegNetMRI. We show the reconstructed MRI from SegNetMRI$_5$, the joint framework from [16], MRN$_5$ and GBRWT in Fig. 5, along with their corresponding residuals. (We set the error ranges from [0 0.1] on a [0 1] pre-scaled image.) We find that SegNetMRI achieves the minimal reconstruction error, especially in the meaningful tissue regions. We also give averaged reconstruction performance measures in Table 2 using peak signal-to-noise ratio (PSNR) and the corresponding normalized mean squared error (NMSE) on all 37 test MRI. We see that the segmentation information is able to aid learning the reconstruction network as well.

Discussion. It is worth noting that the the model in [16] achieves better segmentation performance than an independently learned MRN$_5$ model (i.e., no joint learning), but that reconstruction quality is worse than MRN$_5$ both qualitatively and quantitatively. The original work in [16] is devoted to joint natural image denoising and segmentation, with segmentation taking priority. However, for the

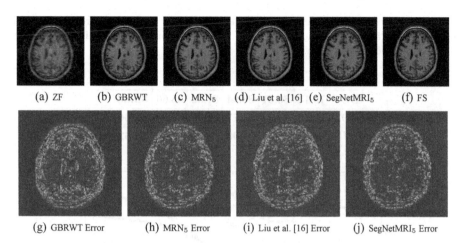

(a) ZF　　(b) GBRWT　　(c) MRN₅　　(d) Liu et al. [16] (e) SegNetMRI₅　　(f) FS

(g) GBRWT Error　　(h) MRN₅ Error　　(i) Liu et al. [16] Error　　(j) SegNetMRI₅ Error

Fig. 5. (Top) reconstructed MRI using various methods (top). (Bottom) approximation residuals.

Table 2. The averaged PSNR (dB) and NMSE on 37 test MRI.

	GBRWT	MRN₅	Liu et al. [16]	SegNetMRI₅
PSNR	31.80	33.94	33.47	**34.27**
NMSE	0.0584	0.0361	0.0388	**0.0333**

medical image analysis problem the reconstruction and segmentation performance are both important; often a radiologists will hand-segment for diagnosis, which is made more difficult by poor reconstruction. Therefore, SegNetMRI has been designed to equally weight the performance on both reconstruction and segmentation in model learning.

In $SegNetMRI_N$, the output of N MSN decoders are concatenated and merged into the final segmentation using a 1×1 convolution. This ensemble learning can make full use of the information from different depths of SegNetMRI and so produce better segmentation accuracy. To illustrate, we consider the SegNetMRI₅ result on the gray matter tissue of all test MRI. In Table 3, we show the segmentation performance of the outputs from each block in SegNetMRI₅ model without the 1×1 convolution, and we compare them with the segmentation output produced after merging the SegNetMRI₅ outputs using 1×1 convolution. It is clear that the output of SegNetMRI₅ can achieve better segmentation performance by fusing the outputs from all layers, even though individual performance is worse at shallower layers.

In Fig. 6, we show the segmentation accuracy as a function of number of blocks N using the Dice Coefficient metric. The reconstruction quality (in PSNR) improves as the number of the blocks increases in SegNetMRI, but at the expense of longer training time.

Table 3. We compare the segmentation performance of the outputs from each block in SegNetMRI5 model without using 1×1 convolution to fuse their information. SegNetMRI5 does this fusion.

GM	B_1	B_2	B_3	B_4	B_5	Merged
DC	75.15	80.31	83.64	81.02	85.66	**86.38**
HD	2.15	1.95	1.77	1.90	1.68	**1.66**
AVD	4.35	3.58	2.90	3.43	2.60	**2.52**

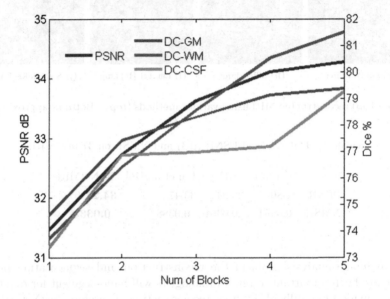

Fig. 6. The model performance of SegNetMRI$_N$ as a function of the number of blocks.

5 Conclusion

Automatic segmentation of MRI is an important problem in medical imaging, and with the recent adoption of CS-MRI by industry, segmentation techniques that take CS-MRI reconstruction into account are needed. After verifying that the two tasks suffer when done independently, we proposed a deep neural network architecture called SegNetMRI to merge the MRI reconstruction and segmentation problems into a joint framework. Our experiments show that doing simultaneous reconstruction and segmentation can positively reinforce each other, improving both tasks significantly.

Acknowledgements. This work was supported in part by the National Natural Science Foundation of China under Grants 61571382, 81671766, 61571005, 81671674, 61671309 and U1605252, in part by the Fundamental Research Funds for the Central Universities under Grant 20720160075, 20720180059, in part by the CCF-Tencent open fund and, the Natural Science Foundation of Fujian Province of China (No.

2017J01126). L. Sun conducted portions of this work at Columbia University under China Scholarship Council grant No. 201806310090.

References

1. Aljabar, P., Heckemann, R.A., Hammers, A., Hajnal, J.V., Rueckert, D.: Multi-atlas based segmentation of brain images: atlas selection and its effect on accuracy. Neuroimage **46**(3), 726–738 (2009)
2. Artaechevarria, X., Munoz-Barrutia, A., Ortiz-de Solórzano, C.: Combination strategies in multi-atlas image segmentation: application to brain MR data. IEEE Trans. Med. Imaging **28**(8), 1266–1277 (2009)
3. Atkinson, D., et al.: Automatic compensation of motion artifacts in MRI. Magn. Reson. Med. **41**(1), 163–170 (1999)
4. Bahrami, K., Rekik, I., Shi, F., Shen, D.: Joint reconstruction and segmentation of 7T-like MR images from 3T MRI based on cascaded convolutional neural networks. In: Descoteaux, M., Maier-Hein, L., Franz, A., Jannin, P., Collins, D.L., Duchesne, S. (eds.) MICCAI 2017. LNCS, vol. 10433, pp. 764–772. Springer, Cham (2017). https://doi.org/10.1007/978-3-319-66182-7_87
5. Candès, E.J., Romberg, J., Tao, T.: Robust uncertainty principles: exact signal reconstruction from highly incomplete frequency information. IEEE Trans. Inf. Theory **52**(2), 489–509 (2006)
6. Chen, H., Dou, Q., Yu, L., Qin, J., Heng, P.A.: VoxResNet: deep voxelwise residual networks for brain segmentation from 3D MR images. NeuroImage **170**, 446–455 (2017)
7. Çiçek, Ö., Abdulkadir, A., Lienkamp, S.S., Brox, T., Ronneberger, O.: 3D U-Net: learning dense volumetric segmentation from sparse annotation. In: Ourselin, S., Joskowicz, L., Sabuncu, M.R., Unal, G., Wells, W. (eds.) MICCAI 2016. LNCS, vol. 9901, pp. 424–432. Springer, Cham (2016). https://doi.org/10.1007/978-3-319-46723-8_49
8. Dong, H., Yang, G., Liu, F., Mo, Y., Guo, Y.: Automatic brain tumor detection and segmentation using U-net based fully convolutional networks. In: Valdés Hernández, M., González-Castro, V. (eds.) MIUA 2017. CCIS, vol. 723, pp. 506–517. Springer, Cham (2017). https://doi.org/10.1007/978-3-319-60964-5_44
9. Donoho, D.L.: Compressed sensing. IEEE Trans. Inf. Theory **52**(4), 1289–1306 (2006)
10. Fessler, J.A.: Medical image reconstruction: a brief overview of past milestones and future directions. arXiv preprint arXiv:1707.05927 (2017)
11. Hricak, H., Amparo, E.: Body MRI: alleviation of claustrophobia by prone positioning. Radiology **152**(3), 819–819 (1984)
12. Huang, Y., Paisley, J., Lin, Q., Ding, X., Fu, X., Zhang, X.P.: Bayesian non-parametric dictionary learning for compressed sensing MRI. IEEE Trans. Image Process. **23**(12), 5007–5019 (2014)
13. Lai, Z., et al.: Image reconstruction of compressed sensing MRI using graph-based redundant wavelet transform. Med. Image Anal. **27**, 93–104 (2016)
14. Lee, D., Yoo, J., Ye, J.C.: Deep residual learning for compressed sensing MRI. In: ISBI, pp. 15–18. IEEE (2017)
15. Li, B., Peng, X., Wang, Z., Xu, J., Feng, D.: AOD-Net: all-in-one dehazing network. In: ICCV, October 2017
16. Liu, D., Wen, B., Liu, X., Wang, Z., Huang, T.S.: When image denoising meets high-level vision tasks: a deep learning approach. In: IJCAI (2018)

17. Lustig, M., Donoho, D., Pauly, J.M.: Sparse MRI: the application of compressed sensing for rapid MR imaging. Magn. Reson. Med. **58**(6), 1182–1195 (2007)
18. Mendrik, A.M., et al.: MRBrainS challenge: online evaluation framework for brain image segmentation in 3T MRI scans. Comput. Intell. Neurosci. **2015**, 1 (2015)
19. Moeskops, P., Viergever, M.A., Mendrik, A.M., de Vries, L.S., Benders, M.J., Išgum, I.: Automatic segmentation of MR brain images with a convolutional neural network. IEEE Trans. Med. Imaging **35**(5), 1252–1261 (2016)
20. Nie, D., Wang, L., Gao, Y., Sken, D.: Fully convolutional networks for multi-modality isointense infant brain image segmentation. In: ISBI, pp. 1342–1345. IEEE (2016)
21. Qu, X., Hou, Y., Lam, F., Guo, D., Zhong, J., Chen, Z.: Magnetic resonance image reconstruction from undersampled measurements using a patch-based non-local operator. Med. Image Anal. **18**(6), 843–856 (2014)
22. Ravishankar, S., Bresler, Y.: MR image reconstruction from highly undersampled k-space data by dictionary learning. IEEE Trans. Med. Imaging **30**(5), 1028–1041 (2011)
23. Ronneberger, O., Fischer, P., Brox, T.: U-Net: convolutional networks for biomedical image segmentation. In: Navab, N., Hornegger, J., Wells, W.M., Frangi, A.F. (eds.) MICCAI 2015. LNCS, vol. 9351, pp. 234–241. Springer, Cham (2015). https://doi.org/10.1007/978-3-319-24574-4_28
24. Schlemper, J., Caballero, J., Hajnal, J.V., Price, A., Rueckert, D.: A deep cascade of convolutional neural networks for MR image reconstruction. In: Niethammer, M., Styner, M., Aylward, S., Zhu, H., Oguz, I., Yap, P.-T., Shen, D. (eds.) IPMI 2017. LNCS, vol. 10265, pp. 647–658. Springer, Cham (2017). https://doi.org/10.1007/978-3-319-59050-9_51
25. Steenwijk, M.D., et al.: Accurate white matter lesion segmentation by k nearest neighbor classification with tissue type priors (kNN-TTPs). NeuroImage Clin. **3**, 462–469 (2013)
26. Stollenga, M.F., Byeon, W., Liwicki, M., Schmidhuber, J.: Parallel multi-dimensional LSTM, with application to fast biomedical volumetric image segmentation. In: NIPS, pp. 2998–3006 (2015)
27. Wang, L., et al.: Links: learning-based multi-source integration framework for segmentation of infant brain images. NeuroImage **108**, 160–172 (2015)
28. Wang, S., et al.: Accelerating magnetic resonance imaging via deep learning. In: ISBI, pp. 514–517. IEEE (2016)
29. Zhang, H., Yang, J., Zhang, Y., Nasrabadi, N.M., Huang, T.S.: Close the loop: joint blind image restoration and recognition with sparse representation prior. In: ICCV, pp. 770–777. IEEE (2011)

Learning a Conditional Generative Model for Anatomical Shape Analysis

Benjamín Gutiérrez-Becker[(✉)] and Christian Wachinger

Artificial Intelligence in Medical Imaging (AI-Med),
Department of Child and Adolescent Psychiatry,
University Hospital, LMU Munich, Munich, Germany
benjamin.gutierrez_becker@med.uni-muenchen.de

Abstract. We introduce a novel conditional generative model for unsupervised learning of anatomical shapes based on a conditional variational autoencoder (CVAE). Our model is specifically designed to learn latent, low-dimensional shape embeddings from point clouds of large datasets. By using a conditional framework, we are able to introduce side information to the model, leading to accurate reconstructions and providing a mechanism to control the generative process. Our network design provides invariance to similarity transformations and avoids the need to identify point correspondences between shapes. Contrary to previous discriminative approaches based on deep learning, our generative method does not only allow to produce shape descriptors from a point cloud, but also to reconstruct shapes from the embedding. We demonstrate the advantages of this approach by: (i) learning low-dimensional representations of the hippocampus and showing low reconstruction errors when projecting them back to the shape space, and (ii) demonstrating that synthetic point clouds generated by our model capture morphological differences associated to Alzheimer's disease, to the point that they can be used to train a discriminative model for disease classification.

1 Introduction

Over the last decades, a variety of approaches for shape analysis have been developed for modeling the human anatomy from medical images [17]. These approaches have become a mainstay in medical image analysis, not only because of their utility in providing priors for segmentation, but also because of their value in quantifying shape changes between subjects and populations. Shape analysis helps in localizing anatomical changes, which can yield a better understanding of morphological changes due to aging and disease [7,24]. Given that the morphology of organs across a population is highly heterogeneous, modeling and quantifying these shape variations is a challenging task. Thanks to the growing availability of large-scale medical imaging datasets, we have now the possibility to model these underlying shape variations in the population more accurately. Unfortunately, working on large sample sizes comes with computational challenges, which can limit the practical application of traditional methods

© Springer Nature Switzerland AG 2019
A. C. S. Chung et al. (Eds.): IPMI 2019, LNCS 11492, pp. 505–516, 2019.
https://doi.org/10.1007/978-3-030-20351-1_39

for shape analysis [17]. In addition, imaging datasets usually come with valuable phenotypic information of the patient. This large amount of available data, paired with recent advances in machine learning, calls for the development of a data-driven and learning-based shape analysis framework that can benefit from the large amount of image data and provides a mechanism to include prior information in the analysis.

Many fields in medical image analysis have recently been revolutionized by the introduction of deep neural networks [15]. These approaches have the ability to learn complex, hierarchical feature representations that have proven to outperform hand-crafted features in a variety of applications. One of the reasons for the superior performance is their ability to model complex non-linear relationships between variables. Medical shape analysis has not been untouched by this wave and deep neural networks for disease prediction have been proposed [10,21]. Although these approaches have demonstrated the benefit of learning shape representations optimal for a given task with deep neural networks, the generation of new shapes based on low-dimensional representations has not yet been explored.

In this paper, we propose a conditional generative model for learning shape representations, which is based on a conditional variational autoencoder operating directly on unordered point clouds. Our model offers the following advantages:

(1) our framework is invariant to similarity transformations, avoiding the need to pre-align the shapes to be analyzed; (2) our network operates on point clouds, which present a raw, simple and lightweight representation that is trivial to obtain from a segmented surface; (3) our method is invariant to the ordering of the elements in the point cloud, meaning that computing correspondences between points across shapes is not necessary; (4) our method does not impose any constraints on the topology of the shapes, providing high flexibility; (5) the conditional nature of our network gives us the possibility to introduce prior knowledge in a simple manner; (6) the model scales to analyzing large shape datasets; (7) the neural network learns modes of variation that capture complex shape changes, yielding a compact representation and the generation of realistic samples.

1.1   Related Work

A large volume of work in medical shape analysis is based on point distribution models (PDMs) [3], which represent surfaces of objects as point clouds. A statistical model is built by finding correspondences between points of different shapes and by obtaining the principal modes of variation via principal component analysis. PDMs have been widely been used due to their simplicity and due to their application to segmentation through active shape models. One common drawback of PDMs is, however, that point correspondences have to be found between all shapes in a dataset. This usually involves a registration step, which is not only challenging but also computationally expensive for large databases. Moreover, homologous features may not exist when comparing shapes that are subject to strong variations, e.g., over the course of brain development. While our method is also based on point clouds, we do not require correspondences between shapes. Next to point clouds, other popular representations for shape analysis are skeletal models [18], spectral signatures [23], spherical harmonics [7], and deformations [4,16].

Conditional variational autoencoders [14,22] are an extension of the generative model in variational autoencoders by introducing a condition vector, which allows to include prior information in the autoencoder. A CVAE has recently been used in medical imaging for 3D fetal skull reconstruction from 2D ultrasound [2]. Conditional generative models have also recently become popular in the context of generative adversarial networks [8]. A conditional adversarial networks was proposed as a general-purpose solution to image-to-image translation problems [11]. In contrast to those previous work, we are proposing a conditional generative model for shape analysis on point cloud representations.

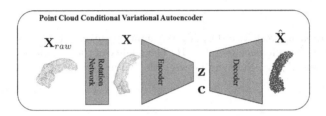

Fig. 1. Overview of our network architecture. Our framework is based on three main components: (1) a rotation network bringing the input point cloud to a canonical space, (2) an encoder approximating the posterior distribution $P_E(\mathbf{z}|\mathbf{X})$, and (3) a decoder reconstructing the point cloud by approximating the mapping $[\mathbf{z}, \mathbf{c}] \mapsto \mathbf{X}$.

2 Method

An overview of our generative model is shown in Fig. 1. Our approach is based on a CVAE that encodes a point cloud $\mathbf{X} = \{\mathbf{p}_0, \mathbf{p}_1, \ldots, \mathbf{p}_n\}$ with $\mathbf{p}_i = [x_i, y_i, z_i]$ into a set of k-dimensional latent variables $\mathbf{z} \in \Omega_z \subset \mathbb{R}^k$ and then decodes this embedding to reconstruct a point cloud $\hat{\mathbf{X}}$. Our network architecture consists of three main elements: (1) the rotation network aligning input point clouds to a canonical space, (2) the encoder aiming at finding the posterior distribution $P_E(\mathbf{z}|\mathbf{X})$, and (3) the decoder approximating the mapping $[\mathbf{z}, \mathbf{c}] \mapsto \mathbf{X}$, where $\mathbf{c} \in \mathbb{R}^m$ is a condition vector of dimension m. Our network is trained in an end-to-end fashion using a loss function, which jointly minimizes the alignment error with respect to a reference shape, the reconstruction error and the latent loss of the variational autoencoder.

Our generative model can be employed in two different ways: First, to obtain a low-dimensional embedding $\mathbf{z}$ given an input $\mathbf{X}$, which in turn can be used to perform basic operations between shapes and to compute shape statistics. Second, to generate synthetic point clouds $\hat{\mathbf{X}}$ from the learned embedding space by sampling $\mathbf{z}$ from a multivariate Gaussian and setting a condition vector $\mathbf{c}$.

2.1   Rotation Network

According to one of its most popular definitions, shape is all the geometrical information that remains when location, scale and rotational effects are filtered out from an object [13]. Thus when our network receives as input a raw point cloud $\mathbf{X}_{raw}$, we must first ensure that its output is invariant to similarity transformations (scaling, translation, and rotations).

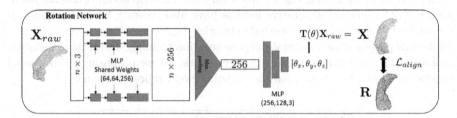

Fig. 2. Rotation network transforming the input point cloud $\mathbf{X}_{raw}$ to bring it into alignment with the reference template $\mathbf{R}$. The quality of the alignment is measured by the loss function $\mathcal{L}_{align}$. Numbers between the parenthesis are the dimensions of the layers.

Invariance to scaling and translation can be enforced by first centering an input shape $\mathbf{X}_{raw}$ around its center of mass and normalizing the point coordinates in the $[0,1]$ range. To guarantee invariance to rotation, we introduce a rotation network (Fig. 2) that learns the mapping $f(\mathbf{X_{raw}}) \mapsto \theta$, such that $\mathbf{X} = \mathbf{T}(\theta)\mathbf{X}_{raw}$ is in spatial alignment with a reference point cloud $\mathbf{R}$. The rotation matrix $\mathbf{T}(\theta)$ is parameterized by the rotation vector $\theta = [\theta_x, \theta_y, \theta_z]^T$. An important challenge when working with point cloud representations is that point clouds are in mathematical terms an order-less set. Traditional statistical shape models solve this challenge by first finding point correspondences between point clouds, therefore inducing an order to the set. Instead, we propose to use a network architecture, which is invariant to point ordering. The architecture of the rotation network and the encoder are based on PointNet [19], which operates directly on orderless point clouds. The basic operation of the rotation network is to first pass each individual point of the network through a multilayer perceptron (MLP), with shared weights among all points, projecting each 3D point to a higher dimensional representation. These representations are aggregated using the max pooling operator across all points. Max pooling is a symmetric operation, and therefore invariant to point ordering. Third, the output of the max pooling layer is fed into a MLP, which predicts the rotation parameters θ. Our transformation network therefore has the form:

$$f(\mathbf{X_{raw}}) = [\theta_x, \theta_y, \theta_z] = \text{MLP}\Big(\max_{\mathbf{p} \in \mathbf{X_{raw}}} h(\mathbf{p})\Big), \qquad (1)$$

where h corresponds to the operations of the MLP with shared weights. Note that the separate convolution of each point and the following aggregation guarantee the invariance to point ordering. Our mechanism to measure the quality of our alignment to the reference template is to measure a distance between $\mathbf{R}$ and $\mathbf{X}$. Since our framework operates on unordered point clouds, we require a metric which is permutation invariant. We use the 1-Wasserstein distance, also known as earth mover's distance (EMD) [20], defined as:

$$\mathcal{L}_{align}(\mathbf{X}, \mathbf{R}) = EMD(\mathbf{X}, \mathbf{R}) = \min_{\phi: \mathbf{X} \to \hat{\mathbf{R}}} \sum_{\mathbf{p} \in \mathbf{X}} \|\mathbf{p} - \phi(\mathbf{p})\|_1, \qquad (2)$$

where $\phi(\mathbf{p})$ is a bijection, which maps a point $\mathbf{p} \in \mathbf{X}$ to its closest point $\mathbf{r} \in \mathbf{R}$.

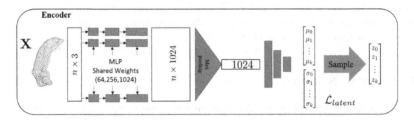

Fig. 3. Encoder network approximates the distribution $P_E(\mathbf{z}|\mathbf{X})$. The input of the network is the aligned point cloud $\mathbf{X}$ and the output is the embedding $\mathbf{z}$ generated by the normal distribution $\mathcal{N}_z(\mu, \Sigma)$. Numbers inside the parenthesis are layer sizes.

2.2   Encoder Network

The encoder seeks an approximation to the posterior distribution $P_E(\mathbf{z}|\mathbf{X})$. The architecture of the encoder is illustrated in Fig. 3. The encoder and the rotation network have a very similar architecture, since both take unordered point clouds as input and predict a vector of parameters. Two main differences exist between the rotation network and the encoder: first, the dimensions of the MLP layers of the encoder are larger, to give additional descriptive power to the encoding task; second, while the rotation network estimates rotation parameters, the encoder estimates vectors $\mu = [\mu_0, \mu_1, \dots, \mu_k]$ and $\Sigma = \text{diag}[\sigma_0, \sigma_1, \dots \sigma_k]$. These vectors are the parameters of a normal distribution $\mathcal{N}_z(\mu, \Sigma)$, which approximates the posterior $P_E(\mathbf{z}|X)$. This means that during training, given an input $\mathbf{X}$, the low-dimensional embedding $\mathbf{z}$ is obtained by drawing a sample at random from $\mathcal{N}_z$. At this stage, we introduce a latent loss for the variational autoencoder $\mathcal{L}_{latent}$ given by the Kullback-Leibler divergence between $\mathcal{N}_z$ and a Gaussian prior $\mathcal{N}(0, \mathbf{I})$. Since Σ is a diagonal matrix, the Kullback-Leibler divergence between these distributions is:

$$\mathcal{L}_{latent} = \sum_{i=1}^{k} \sigma_i + \mu_i - \log(\sigma_i) - 1. \qquad (3)$$

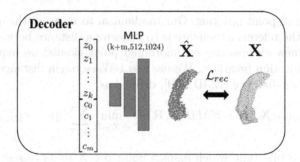

Fig. 4. Decoder network approximates the mapping $[\mathbf{z}, \mathbf{c}] \mapsto \mathbf{X}$. The input of the decoder are the embedding $\mathbf{z}$ and the condition vector $\mathbf{c}$. The output is the reconstructed point cloud $\hat{\mathbf{X}}$. The accuracy of the reconstruction is measured using the reconstruction loss $\mathcal{L}_{rec}$. Numbers inside the parenthesis are layer sizes.

2.3   Decoder Network

The last part of our framework is the decoder network (Fig. 4). The decoder maps the embedding to a reconstructed point cloud by approximating the mapping $[\mathbf{z}, \mathbf{c}] \mapsto \hat{\mathbf{X}}$. Similar to previous approaches based on CVAEs, the decoder is a fully connected MLP with 3 layers, which maps the low-dimensional representation back to a reconstruction $\hat{\mathbf{X}}$. The decoder also takes as input the vector $\mathbf{c} \in \mathbb{R}^m$, which allows our network to include conditions to the reconstruction of $\hat{\mathbf{X}}$. The quality of the reconstruction is evaluated by a reconstruction loss $L_{rec} = EMD(\mathbf{X}, \hat{\mathbf{X}})$, which measures the EMD between the input shape and its reconstruction.

The full network is trained in an end-to-end fashion using stochastic gradient descent by optimizing the loss function:

$$\mathcal{L} = \mathcal{L}_{rec} + \mathcal{L}_{align} + \mathcal{L}_{latent}. \tag{4}$$

3   Experiments

3.1   Conditional Shape Model of 3D Digits

As a first experiment, we train a generative shape model using a 3D point cloud version of the MNIST database[1] and successively sample point clouds from the low-dimensional embedding. This dataset consists of 5000 3D point clouds of handwritten digits from 0 to 9. For this experiment, we trained two separate generative models. For the first one, we set the dimension of the embedding $\mathbf{z}$ to $k = 2$, and we use a 10-dimensional one hot encoding of the class of each digit as the condition vector $\mathbf{c}$. The second model is trained under the same settings but with the condition vector $\mathbf{c}$ set to all zeros. This means that both models are essentially identical, with the important difference that the first one

---

[1] https://github.com/Harry-Zhi/3DMNIST.

is equipped with a condition vector, which allows us to give information to the network about the digit to be encoded and reconstructed. In Fig. 5, we present artificial point clouds generated by these two models. At the bottom right of Fig. 5, we show point clouds generated without the use of the condition vector **c**. Although the model is able to generate some realistically looking digits (like the 1s in the center column), the reconstructed point clouds are generally not as sharp as those generated by the conditional model. In contrast, by setting the condition vector to generate a specific digit, we are able to obtain sharp point clouds while at the same time capturing complex non-linear deformations for each digit. The digits in Fig. 5 present a very similar orientation (tilted to the right and aligned with respect to the x, y plane). This is the result of aligning the point clouds to a reference template using the rotation network. An important observation is that all digits are sampled from the same shape space Ω_z, and only the condition vector **c** changes. This means that the encoding **z** is able to encode common shape characteristics between all digits. For example, the 1st embedding dimension in Fig. 5 captures the width of the digits. It is also worth mentioning that for many typical statistical shape models, training a shape model consisting of 5000 point clouds would be impractical due to memory limitations and to the computationally expensive task of finding corresponding points between all these shapes.

3.2 Conditional Shape Model of the Hippocampus

In our second experiment, we build a shape model of the left hippocampus. Our goal is to assess shape differences between healthy controls (HC) and subjects diagnosed with Alzheimer's disease (AD). Several previous studies have established strong morphological changes in the hippocampus associated to the progression of dementia [6,7]. Magnetic resonance images of 200 subjects were randomly selected from the Alzheimer's Disease Neuroimaging Initiative (ADNI) [12] and processed with Freesurfer [5] to obtain segmentations.

For comparison, we build a statistical shape model of the hippocampus using the ShapeWorks framework [1]. ShapeWorks is a statistical shape model tool, which achieved the best performance in several shape analysis tasks in a recent comparison [9]. For our evaluation, we split the images into a training and testing set (100/100 split) and we build a statistical shape model of the left hippocampus using the training set (50 HC and 50 AD). Segmentations are pre-processed using the grooming operations included in ShapeWorks to obtain smooth hippocampi surfaces, and models of 1024 points are trained. As a condition vector **c**, we use a one hot encoding of the diagnosis of the patient ([0, 1] for HC, [1, 0] for AD). We limit our analysis to this relatively small number of samples to be able to perform a fair comparison with ShapeWorks, which is limited in the number of samples to be analyzed due to memory constraints. It is also worth mentioning that training the ShapeWorks model for 100 images took 5 h, compared to the 2 h training time for our model.

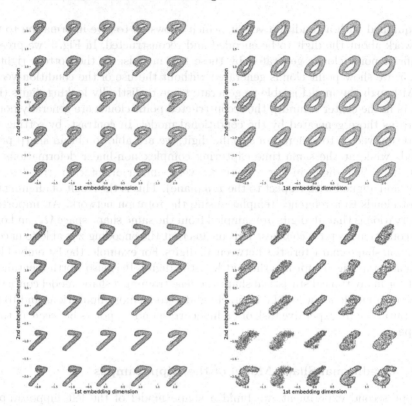

Fig. 5. Point clouds sampled from the 2D embedding space generated by training our model using the 3D MNIST dataset. On the bottom right we show 3D point clouds generated by setting the conditional vector **c** to zero. For the other figures, **c** is set to generate point clouds of the digits $9, 0$ and 7.

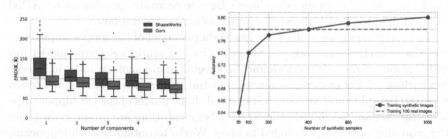

Fig. 6. Left: reconstruction error of shapes generated using either ShapeWorks or our CVAE framework with respect to the input point cloud. Right: HC vs AD Classification accuracy for a PointNet model trained either using point clouds obtained from real segmentations obtained from the ADNI database or synthetic hippocampus point clouds generated by our model.

Reconstruction Error. We first evaluate the ability of our model to obtain an accurate and compact representation of the hippocampus shape. To this end, we measure the reconstruction error between the reconstructed shapes $\hat{\mathbf{X}}$ and the input shapes $\mathbf{X}$ by evaluating $EMD(\mathbf{X}, \hat{\mathbf{X}})$. We train 5 different models with embedding dimensions ranging from $k = 1$ to $k = 5$. As a comparison, we quantify the reconstruction error of synthetic hippocampus shapes generated by ShapeWorks. The lower reconstruction errors of our method in Fig. 6 indicate that it captures the complex deformations of the hippocampi and therefore allows for a compact shape representation with few modes.

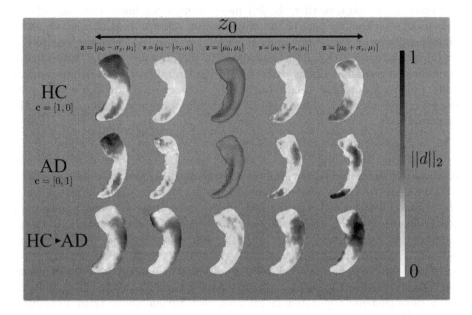

Fig. 7. Hippocampus surfaces generated using point clouds sampled from our model trained on segmented images obtained from the ADNI database. The top row corresponds to point clouds generated by setting the condition vector to generate HC shapes, and the middle row corresponds to AD. Point clouds are generated by moving along the first embedding dimension. For the top two rows, the color coding shows the deformation (measured as the absolute distance between corresponding points) between the mean and the generated point cloud. In the bottom row, the deformation between HC and AD shapes generated using the same shape embedding $\mathbf{z}$ are shown.

Effect of Conditioning the Shape Model Using a Diagnostic Label. One of the main contributions that separates our framework from previous approaches for shape analysis is the introduction of the conditional vector $\mathbf{c}$. We have observed in our experiment on the MNIST dataset that our method is able to generate realistic shapes of digits given different condition vectors $\mathbf{c}$.

To evaluate the effects of the condition vector in the model of the hippocampus shapes, we use the model trained on the previous experiment (for embedding dimension $k = 2$) and generate a set of synthetic point clouds by sampling values of z and assigning either $c = [1, 0]$ or $c = [0, 1]$ to generate synthetic hippocampus shapes corresponding to morphological characteristics associated to either HC or AD. In Fig. 7 we can observe some of the synthetic shapes generated by our model, corresponding to the mean shape (center) and shapes generated by moving across the first embedding dimension z_0. Notice that shapes in the same column correspond were generated using the same embedding z, with different condition vector c. In Fig. 7 we can observe that by moving across z_0 our model captures shape differences which are common between the HC and AD cases. For example, we observe that the left most example for both cases has a large deformation on the top part of the hippocampus. On the bottom row, we show differences between the point clouds of the top two rows, which correspond to the shape variations that our model associates to the presence of AD. These shape variations correspond to large variations in the lateral part of the hippocampus body, roughly around the CA1 subfield. These observations are in line with previous findings on shape differences of the left hippocampus associated to AD diagnosis [6, 7].

Synthesizing Training Data. A critical question to answer is whether our synthetically generated point clouds capture shape differences that are specific to AD. We assess this by generating synthetic point clouds associated to HC or AD, and training a PointNet classifier [10, 19] to discriminate between hippocampi belonging either to HC or AD subjects. We experiment with synthetic datasets generated by our model of sizes: 50, 100, 200, 400, 600, and 1000. For each dataset, a separate PointNet classifier is trained. We compare the classification accuracy of our model with a PointNet classifier trained using the 100 samples of the training set directly, without the use of the generative model. The results in Fig. 6 show that our generated samples are realistic enough to train a classifier relying solely on the synthetic images. Interestingly, our generator allow us to sample an arbitrary number of samples, giving us the possibility to boost the accuracy of the classifier by increasing artificially the size of the dataset.

4   Conclusions

In this work, we have presented a conditional generative model to model anatomical shapes. This model is able to generate low-dimensional shape representations taking as input unordered point clouds, without the need of finding point correspondences between them. We have demonstrated that our model can be used to encode complex shape variations using a low-dimensional embedding and we have shown that by introducing a conditional vector, we are able to obtain more accurate reconstructions. We have demonstrated the properties of our generative model by creating realistically looking synthetic shapes, which can even be used to train deep learning based models. This has the potential to enable the use of powerful models in scenarios where the amount of annotated data is limited. On the hippocampus experiments, we operated on relatively small sample sizes to ensure a fair comparison to previous approaches, but on the MNIST data we demonstrated that our network scales to datasets with thousands of shapes. Our network facilitates processing of large datasets, since we do not require expensive operations for finding point correspondences between samples. We believe that our framework can be used to analyze other anatomical structures and more importantly the use of different condition vectors, which include diverse phenotypic information.

Acknowledgments. This work was supported in part by DFG and the Bavarian State Ministry of Education, Science and the Arts in the framework of the Centre Digitalisation. Bavaria (ZD.B).

References

1. Cates, J., Fletcher, P.T., Styner, M., Hazlett, H.C., Whitaker, R.: Particle-based shape analysis of multi-object complexes. In: Metaxas, D., Axel, L., Fichtinger, G., Székely, G. (eds.) MICCAI 2008. LNCS, vol. 5241, pp. 477–485. Springer, Heidelberg (2008). https://doi.org/10.1007/978-3-540-85988-8_57
2. Cerrolaza, J.J., et al.: 3D fetal skull reconstruction from 2DUS via deep conditional generative networks. In: Frangi, A.F., Schnabel, J.A., Davatzikos, C., Alberola-López, C., Fichtinger, G. (eds.) MICCAI 2018. LNCS, vol. 11070, pp. 383–391. Springer, Cham (2018). https://doi.org/10.1007/978-3-030-00928-1_44
3. Cootes, T.F., Taylor, C.J., Cooper, D.H., Graham, J.: Active shape models-their training and application. Comput. Vis. Image Underst. **61**(1), 38–59 (1995)
4. Durrleman, S., et al.: Morphometry of anatomical shape complexes with dense deformations and sparse parameters. NeuroImage **101**, 35–49 (2014)
5. Fischl, B.: Freesurfer. Neuroimage **62**(2), 774–781 (2012)
6. Frisoni, G.B., et al.: Mapping local hippocampal changes in Alzheimer's disease and normal ageing with MRI at 3 Tesla. Brain **131**(12), 3266–3276 (2008)
7. Gerardin, E., et al.: Multidimensional classification of hippocampal shape features discriminates Alzheimer's disease and mild cognitive impairment from normal aging. Neuroimage **47**(4), 1476–1486 (2009)
8. Goodfellow, I., et al.: Generative adversarial nets. In: Advances in Neural Information Processing Systems, pp. 2672–2680 (2014)
9. Goparaju, A., et al.: On the evaluation and validation of off-the-shelf statistical shape modeling tools: a clinical application. In: Reuter, M., Wachinger, C., Lombaert, H., Paniagua, B., Lüthi, M., Egger, B. (eds.) ShapeMI 2018. LNCS, vol. 11167, pp. 14–27. Springer, Cham (2018). https://doi.org/10.1007/978-3-030-04747-4_2
10. Gutiérrez-Becker, B., Wachinger, C.: Deep multi-structural shape analysis: application to neuroanatomy. In: Frangi, A.F., Schnabel, J.A., Davatzikos, C., Alberola-López, C., Fichtinger, G. (eds.) MICCAI 2018. LNCS, vol. 11072, pp. 523–531. Springer, Cham (2018). https://doi.org/10.1007/978-3-030-00931-1_60
11. Isola, P., Zhu, J.Y., Zhou, T., Efros, A.A.: Image-to-image translation with conditional adversarial networks. In: 2017 IEEE Conference on Computer Vision and Pattern Recognition (CVPR), pp. 5967–5976. IEEE (2017)
12. Jack, C.R., et al.: The Alzheimer's disease neuroimaging initiative (ADNI): MRI methods. J. Magn. Reson. Imaging **27**(4), 685–691 (2008)
13. Kendall, D.G.: A survey of the statistical theory of shape. Stat. Sci. **4**(2), 87–99 (1989)

14. Kingma, D.P., Welling, M.: Auto-encoding variational bayes. arXiv preprint arXiv:1312.6114 (2013)
15. Litjens, G., et al.: A survey on deep learning in medical image analysis. Med. Image Anal. **42**, 60–88 (2017)
16. Miller, M.I., Younes, L., Trouvé, A.: Diffeomorphometry and geodesic positioning systems for human anatomy. Technology **2**(01), 36–43 (2014)
17. Ng, B., Toews, M., Durrleman, S., Shi, Y.: Shape analysis for brain structures. In: Li, S., Tavares, J.M.R.S. (eds.) Shape Analysis in Medical Image Analysis. LNCVB, vol. 14, pp. 3–49. Springer, Cham (2014). https://doi.org/10.1007/978-3-319-03813-1_1
18. Pizer, S.M., et al.: Nested sphere statistics of skeletal models. In: Breuß, M., Bruckstein, A., Maragos, P. (eds.) Innovations for Shape Analysis. MATHVISUAL, pp. 93–115. Springer, Heidelberg (2013). https://doi.org/10.1007/978-3-642-34141-0_5
19. Qi, C.R., Su, H., Mo, K., Guibas, L.J.: PointNet: deep learning on point sets for 3D classification and segmentation. In: Proceedings of Computer Vision and Pattern Recognition (CVPR), vol. 1, no. 2, p. 4. IEEE (2017)
20. Rubner, Y., Tomasi, C., Guibas, L.J.: The earth mover's distance as a metric for image retrieval. Int. J. Comput. Vis. **40**(2), 99–121 (2000)
21. Shakeri, M., Lombaert, H., Tripathi, S., Kadoury, S.: Deep spectral-based shape features for Alzheimer's disease classification. In: Reuter, M., Wachinger, C., Lombaert, H. (eds.) SeSAMI 2016. LNCS, vol. 10126, pp. 15–24. Springer, Cham (2016). https://doi.org/10.1007/978-3-319-51237-2_2
22. Sohn, K., Lee, H., Yan, X.: Learning structured output representation using deep conditional generative models. In: Advances in Neural Information Processing Systems, pp. 3483–3491 (2015)
23. Wachinger, C., Golland, P., Kremen, W., Fischl, B., Reuter, M.: BrainPrint: a discriminative characterization of brain morphology. Neuroimage **109**, 232–248 (2015)
24. Wachinger, C., Rieckmann, A., Reuter, M.: Latent processes governing neuroanatomical change in aging and dementia. In: Descoteaux, M., Maier-Hein, L., Franz, A., Jannin, P., Collins, D.L., Duchesne, S. (eds.) MICCAI 2017. LNCS, vol. 10435, pp. 30–37. Springer, Cham (2017). https://doi.org/10.1007/978-3-319-66179-7_4

Manifold Exploring Data Augmentation with Geometric Transformations for Increased Performance and Robustness

Magdalini Paschali[1(✉)], Walter Simson[1], Abhijit Guha Roy[1,2], Rüdiger Göbl[1], Christian Wachinger[2], and Nassir Navab[1,3]

[1] Computer Aided Medical Procedures, Technische Universität München, Munich, Germany
magda.paschali@tum.de

[2] Department of Child and Adolescent Psychiatry, Psychosomatic and Psychotherapy, Ludwig-Maximilian-University, Munich, Germany

[3] Computer Aided Medical Procedures, Johns Hopkins University, Baltimore, USA

Abstract. In this paper we propose a novel augmentation technique that improves not only the performance of deep neural networks on clean test data, but also significantly increases their robustness to random transformations, both affine and projective. Inspired by ManiFool, the augmentation is performed by a line-search manifold-exploration method that learns affine geometric transformations that lead to the misclassification on an image, while ensuring that it remains on the same manifold as the training data.

This augmentation method populates any training dataset with images that lie on the border of the manifolds between two-classes and maximizes the variance the network is exposed to during training. Our method was thoroughly evaluated on the challenging tasks of fine-grained skin lesion classification from limited data, and breast tumor classification of mammograms. Compared with traditional augmentation methods, and with images synthesized by Generative Adversarial Networks our method not only achieves state-of-the-art performance but also significantly improves the network's robustness.

Keywords: Manifold learning · Deep learning · Data augmentation · Skin lesion classification · Breast tumor classification

1 Introduction

Recently, medical imaging tasks such as classification, segmentation and registration have been successfully carried out with state-of-the-art performance by

© Springer Nature Switzerland AG 2019
A. C. S. Chung et al. (Eds.): IPMI 2019, LNCS 11492, pp. 517–529, 2019.
https://doi.org/10.1007/978-3-030-20351-1_40

deep learning models, which have found their way into a plethora of Computer Assisted Diagnosis and Intervention (CAD/I) Systems which aid physicians. However, medical imaging datasets utilized to train such models are often characterized by large class variability, severe class imbalance, outliers, inter-observer variability, ambiguity and most prominently limited data. The aforementioned problems hinder the training of neural networks and lead to sub-optimal and overfit solutions. Moreover, deep learning models deployed by physicians in a CAD/I system must be thoroughly evaluated, with respect to not only their generalizability, i.e. performance on data originating from a given test set, but also their behavior on data corrupted by noise, unknown transformations and outliers, which can be described by the term robustness. Data augmentation describes the act of increasing the size and variance of a given dataset to train a machine learning model, in order to achieve better generalizability and capture a better understanding of the underlying distribution of the training data. The manifold of a class learned by a classifier can be perceived as the space that represents the distribution of the training data.

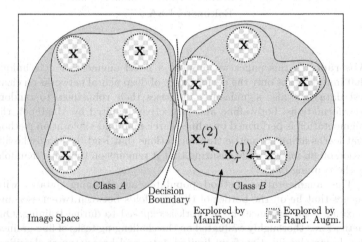

Fig. 1. Schematic representation of proposed augmentation: the proposed augmentation scheme based on ManiFool explores the present classes towards the decision boundaries, thus adding more relevant training samples $\mathbf{x}_\tau^{(i)}$ than random augmentation (checkerboard pattern) which explores the space around the original training samples $\mathbf{x}$ locally. Additionally, it is ensured that samples from ManiFool Augmentation originate from the ground truth class.

In this work our contribution is two-fold: We propose a novel data augmentation technique, utilizing an exhaustive manifold-exploration method that increases the performance of a deep learning model on the provided test set, and significantly improves its robustness to random geometric transformations. Furthermore, we provide quantitative measures to assess a classifier's robustness. Such a measure provides a significant step towards a thorough evaluation of machine learning models; a highly valuable step towards the safe and success-ful deployment of trained models by physicians in real-world scenarios involving patient diagnosis and treatment.

ManiFool Augmentation is performed by populating the training dataset for a given task with samples transformed with optimized affine geometric transfor-mations. The method is outlined in Fig. 1, where it is contrasted with traditional data augmentation performed with random transformations. The algorithm uti-lized to craft samples leveraged for data augmentation is inspired by ManiFool [1] (discussed in Sect. 2) and the intuition behind it is rather simple: Move an image via affine geometric transformations iteratively towards a classifier's decision boundary by following the direction that maximizes the gradient. After every step, project the calculated movement back onto the original training manifold of the class of the image being transformed. This process is repeated iteratively until either a transformation is found that causes the network to misclassify the transformed sample or a pre-defined maximum amount of steps is reached. In case of misclassification, we have crossed the decision boundary and stepped on the manifold of another class. We then backtrack to the manifold of the origi-nal class and use this calculated transformation for data augmentation during training.

Contrary to traditional augmentation methods with random transformations, ManiFool Augmentation ensures that the space explored by the network during training is not limited to the local vicinity of a training sample. Instead, aug-mentations are found globally up to the edges of each class-manifold for the whole training set as can be seen in Fig. 1. An effective augmentation technique should be able to ensure that the samples leveraged to increase the population of the training dataset originate from the same manifold as the original data. Aug-menting the training dataset with samples from a different distribution would not necessarily facilitate the model with learning a better embedding for each of the classes, but would rather encourage it, to map the same class to two different sub-spaces, one for each training manifold.

Exhaustive experimentation on two challenging medical datasets showcases that the proposed augmentation technique does not only increase the robustness of a model to geometric transformations, but it also significantly improves its performance on the original test data. This is additionally highlighted by cross-dataset testing, where networks trained with ManiFool Augmentation were able to better capture the underlying distribution of the training data.

Related Work. Many have taken steps in addressing the problem of limited data in deep learning applications in order to improve model accuracy without carrying the burden of costly data acquisition. Approaches range from elastic transformations [2], noise generation in a learned features space [3], to repeat, rotate and infill approaches whereby a known sample is scaled and rotated in a grid pattern, and background consistency is ensured [4]. Fawzi et al. proposed an algorithm for augmentation which can be integrated into the process of stochastic gradient decent and seeks an augmented sample with the greatest loss within a constrained exploration space or "trust region" [5].

Data augmentation has also been extensively formulated as a learning task. [6] shows significant improvement in accuracy of hand-written-digit classification with a method deploying DAGAN. AutoAugment, formulates the augmentation task as a discrete search problem in which the search algorithm itself is based on a reinforcement learning approach that strives to "learn" how to maximize the total classification accuracy via augmentation [7].

Specifically in the field of medical deep learning applications, creative augmentation approaches are necessary to combat the extreme lack of annotated data. [8] employed generated augmented samples and annotations via GANs to improve CT brain segmentation under severe lack of training data. [9] reported improved accuracy for liver segmentation by employing DCGANs for data augmentation.

2 Method

ManiFool [1] is an iterative algorithm that can be applied to any differentiable classifier f. In this Section we will discuss the mathematical operations that generate a geometrically transformed example leveraged for data augmentation.

Movement Direction. For an image $\mathbf{x}$ with ground truth label l and a binary classifier f an iterative process of i steps is initialized and the original image can be defined as $\mathbf{x}^{(0)}$. Initially, ManiFool finds the movement direction $\mathbf{u}$ towards the decision boundary of f, by following the opposite of the gradient, $-\nabla f(\mathbf{x})$. The gradient at the step i for the image $\mathbf{x}^{(i)}$ is the projection of $\nabla f(\mathbf{x}^{(i)})$ onto the tangent space and can be calculated utilizing the pseudoinverse operation:

$$\mathbf{u} = -\mathbf{J}_{\mathbf{x}^{(i)}}^{+} \nabla f(\mathbf{x}^{(i)}) = -(\mathbf{J}_{\mathbf{x}^{(i)}}^{\mathbf{T}} \mathbf{J}_{\mathbf{x}^{(i)}})^{-1} \mathbf{J}_{\mathbf{x}^{(i)}}^{\mathbf{T}} \nabla f(\mathbf{x}^{(i)}). \tag{1}$$

$\mathbf{J}_{\mathbf{x}^{(i)}}$ is the Jacobian matrix and the calculated $\mathbf{u}$ is the direction towards the decision boundary for step i.

To improve the accuracy and convergence speed during the calculation of $\mathbf{u}$ a manifold optimization technique similar to [10] has been adopted:

$$\mathbf{u}^{(i)} = -\lambda_i \frac{\mathbf{J}_{\mathbf{x}^{(i)}}^{+} \nabla f(\mathbf{x}^{(i)})}{||\mathbf{J}_{\mathbf{x}^{(i)}}^{+} \nabla f(\mathbf{x}^{(i)})||} + \gamma \mathbf{u}^{(i-1)}, \tag{2}$$

where λ_i is the calculated step size of the iteration and γ is a constant momentum.

Mapping Onto the Original Manifold. After the movement direction $\mathbf{u}$ is calculated it is mapped back onto the manifold $\mathcal{M}$ of the ground truth class. Following [1], this mapping is performed using retraction $R_{\mathbf{x}^{(i)}}(\mathbf{u}) = \mathbf{x}_{\tau_i}^{(i)}$, where τ_i is the affine transformation calculated as:

$$\tau_i = \exp\left(\sum_j u_j Gj\right). \tag{3}$$

G_j are the basis vectors of the Lie Group $\mathcal{T}$ of the calculated affine geometric transformation. There are two conditions for the termination of the algorithm, namely the misclassification of the calculated transformed image by the model or reaching the maximum number of allowed iterations $i_{\max}$. After i steps the accumulative affine transformations applied to $\mathbf{x}^{(0)}$ to generate the ManiFool sample are given by:

$$\hat{\tau} = \tau_0 \circ \tau_1 \circ \ldots \tau_i. \tag{4}$$

Multi-class Classifiers. The extension of the method from binary to multi-class classifiers is straightforward: We generate a ManiFool sample for each of the remaining classes, starting from the ground truth and based on the geodesic distance l of the transformed to the original image we leverage the sample with the smallest transformation $\tau_{l_{\min}}$. The class with the smallest geodesic distance between the transformations can be found by:

$$l_{\min} = \arg\min_{l \neq l_x} \tilde{d}_{\mathbf{x}^{(0)}}(e, \tau_l). \tag{5}$$

In the following subsections we discuss how the distance $\tilde{d}_{\mathbf{x}^{(0)}}$ is calculated and the significant role it plays as a measure of robustness for neural networks.

2.1 Invariance to Geometric Transformations

Geodesic Distance Between Transformations. The geodesic distance $d_{\mathbf{x}^{(i)}}$ between two transformations τ_1 and τ_2 is the length L of the shortest curve γ between τ_1 and τ_2. However, since the metric space of the manifold of the training data is unknown we have to acquire a metric in the Riemannian space by mapping the Lie group $\mathcal{T}$ to the differentiable image manifold of $\mathbf{x}_{\tau_1}^{(i)}$ and $\mathbf{x}_{\tau_2}^{(i)}$, which inherits the Riemannian metric from L_2 [11,12]. After this mapping, the geodesic distance between τ_1 and τ_2 is equal to the shortest path connecting $\mathbf{x}_{\tau_1}^{(i)}$ and $\mathbf{x}_{\tau_2}^{(i)}$, formulated as:

$$d_{\mathbf{x}^{(i)}}(\tau_1, \tau_2) = \min L(\gamma). \tag{6}$$

Geodesic Distance Between Original and ManiFool Samples. Having explained how to calculate the distance between two transformations and two transformed images, we can now show how to measure the geodesic distance between the original samples of our training dataset and the ones generated with ManiFool. The initial untransformed image $\mathbf{x}^{(0)}$ can be considered the initial point of the aforementioned γ curve if we define its transformation e as the identity one. Thus, the distance between the original sample $\mathbf{x}_e^{(0)}$ and $\mathbf{x}_{\tau_i}^{(i)}$, can be calculated by the distance between the identity transformation e and the final aggregated one τ_i:

$$\tilde{d}_{\mathbf{x}^{(i)}}(e, \tau_i) = \frac{d_{\mathbf{x}^{(i)}}(e, \tau)}{||\mathbf{x}^{(i)}||_{L^2}}. \tag{7}$$

Normalization of the distance by the norm of the image is crucial, to ensure generalizability of the distance measure.

Robustness to Geometric Transformations. Since every computed Mani-Fool example originates from the edge of a class manifold, measuring the afore-mentioned distance $\tilde{d}_{\mathbf{x}^{(i)}}$ between an original image and its respective trans-formed sample can act as a measure for the robustness of a classifier. Specifically networks that have learned a high-dimensional embedding space characterized by high class compactness and maximized distance between decision boundaries will require a larger average $\tilde{d}$ to transform a class from one class to another. In this work we compute the average distance $\tilde{\rho}_\tau$ of all the ManiFool samples as:

$$\tilde{\rho}_\tau(f) = \frac{1}{m} \sum_{j=1}^{m} \tilde{d}_{\mathbf{x}_j^{(i)}}(e, \tilde{\tau}), \tag{8}$$

where m is the number of crafted samples. $\tilde{\rho}_\tau$ acts as a quantitative measure of robustness of a neural network to geometric transformations, that can be used to compare the robustness of different deep model architectures or models trained with different augmentation techniques.

Another measure to quantify the robustness of classifier f is r_τ, given by Eq. 9. r_τ assesses a model's performance when it's evaluated on randomly trans-formed images. Specifically, for a range of given geodesic distances r we craft samples transformed with random transformations and measure misclassifica-tion rate of f.

$$r_\tau(f) = \min r \text{ s.t. } \mathbb{P}(f(\mathbf{x}_\tau^{(i)}) \neq f(\mathbf{x}^{(i)}) \mid d_{\mathbf{x}_\tau^{(i)}}(e, \tau) = r) \geq 0.5, \tag{9}$$

where 0.5 is a user defined threshold. A robust model can maintain higher classi-fication accuracy for images that have larger geodesic distance from the originals.

2.2   ManiFool Augmentation

A significant difference in our approach to the original ManiFool work is that our purpose is not to fool a deep neural network and craft an adversarial example [13], but rather to utilize the transformed images for data augmentation. Therefore, once we compute the affine transformation τ_i that crosses the decision boundary and fools f, we backtrack onto the original class manifold $\mathcal{M}$ via an iterative reduction of the final step size. Initially, for all the images in the training set of the given dataset, we create ManiFool Augmentation samples that reside around the edges of the class manifolds with an independent black-box classifier f. Afterwards, we mix the generated samples with the original data in an equal ratio and train a model from scratch. An alternative approach would have been to utilize all the geometrically transformed images at every step i towards the decision boundary for data augmentation. However, it was crucial to maintain an equal ratio of transformed and original samples in the final dataset, so that models utilizing it for training would not be biased to geometrically transformed images, due to an imbalanced amount of samples. Hence, we only utilized the transformed samples in the vicinity of the decision boundary, to provide the maximum possible variance to the models during training. Samples crafted with ManiFool Augmentation are presented in Fig. 2.

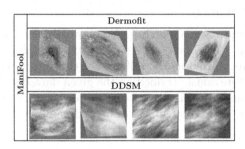

Fig. 2. Examples generated with ManiFool Augmentation for the two datasets, namely dermofit and DDSM.

3   Experimental Setup

Datasets. ManiFool Augmentation has been validated on two challenging, public, medical imaging classification datasets, namely, Digital Database for Screening Mammography (DDSM) [14,15] and Dermofit [16]. DDSM consists of 11.617 expert selected regions of interest (ROI) of mammograms from 1861 patients annotated as normal, benign or malignant by radiologists. Dermofit is an image library consisting of 1300 high-quality dermatoscopic images, with histologically validated fine-grained expert annotations (10 classes). Both datasets were split at patient-level with non-overlapping folds (70% training and 30% testing).

Model Training. Three state-of-the-art architectures, namely ResNet18 [17], VGG16 [18] and InceptionV3 [19], were used for the evaluation. All networks were initialized with ImageNet weights, therefore appropriate resizing and normalization of the input were performed. The loss function selected for the aforementioned classification problems was weighted Cross Entropy, since the selected datasets are characterized by severe class imbalance. Class weights were computed with median frequency balancing, as described in [20]. The models were optimized with Adam optimizer with an initial learning rate of 0.001 across the board. The experiments were implemented in the deep learning framework PyTorch [21] and an NVIDIA Titan Xp was used to train the models for 50 epochs.

Baseline Methods. To validate the proposed contributions we perform not only ablative studies but also comparison against other widely used augmentation techniques. ManiFool Augmentation was compared with models trained without any augmentation (referred to as "None" in the following Section) and models trained with traditional random augmentation ("Random"), i.e. rotation and horizontal flipping. The proposed method (noted as "ManiFool" in the tables of results) was also evaluated against augmentation techniques including Random Erasing [22] ("Erasing"), a commonly used and fast augmentation technique that replaces random patches of the image with Gaussian noise, and data augmentation with images synthesized by GANs ("DCGAN"), following the method described in [9].

ManiFool Augmentation Crafting. A noteworthy implementation detail is that for the crafting of the ManiFool Augmentation samples, black-box state-of-the-art models were utilized as the differential classifier f described in Sect. 2. Those models were previously trained on the given datasets but are not utilized in the evaluation phase of this work, to avoid any bias and to ensure that the dataset is previously unseen by all the evaluated models.

Table 1. Comparative evaluation of models trained on dermofit using different augmentation techniques and ManiFool Augmentation.

		None	Random	Erasing	ManiFool
ResNet	Original test	0.7379	0.7859	0.7867	**0.8126**
	Random affine	0.6515	0.6962	0.6573	**0.7900**
	Random projective	0.4373	0.4817	0.4555	**0.6263**
VGG	Original test	0.7526	0.8080	0.7924	**0.8258**
	Random affine	0.6993	0.7387	0.6751	**0.8011**
	Random projective	0.4319	0.5140	0.5071	**0.6200**
Inception	Original test	0.7303	0.8051	0.7898	**0.8275**
	Random affine	0.5544	0.7063	0.7123	**0.7883**
	Random projective	0.2149	0.4388	0.4630	**0.5376**

4   Results and Discussion

In this Section the detailed results of the ablative evaluation, as well as the baseline comparisons will be discussed, along with the effects of the proposed method to the performance and robustness of the models.

Performance improvement with ManiFool Augmentation. Tables 1 and 2 report the results of the ablative and baseline evaluation of the proposed ManiFool Augmentation method for the Dermofit and DDSM Datasets. Initially, it can be observed that the performance of models without any augmentation is significantly lower, due to overfitting and limited manifold exploration. Random Augmentation provides an improvement in performance but offers no guarantee regarding the increase in the variance that the model is exposed to during training. Moreover, random augmentation can result in out-of-distribution samples, which could hinder model training. Augmented samples created by ManiFool are guaranteed to originate from the same distribution as the original training data, a trait particularly crucial in the setting of medical applications, where misclassifications can have severe and undesired outcomes. Furthermore, Manifool Augmentation, with its improved exploration capabilities, increases the accuracy by 2%–3% across both datasets and model architectures. Additionally, ManiFool Augmentation consistently outperforms Random Erasing, Random Augmentation and GAN Augmentation by approximately 2% across datasets and models.

Table 2. Comparative evaluation of models trained on DDSM using different augmentation techniques and ManiFool Augmentation.

		None	Random	Erasing	DCGAN	ManiFool
ResNet	Original test	0.8321	0.8254	0.8294	0.8228	**0.8426**
	Random affine	0.7225	0.6849	0.6073	0.6964	**0.7970**
	Random projective	0.2483	0.2078	0.3245	0.2657	**0.3245**
VGG	Original test	0.7914	0.8381	0.8377	0.8405	**0.8443**
	Random affine	0.2444	0.6547	0.7194	0.7371	**0.8094**
	Random projective	0.1901	0.2046	0.2388	0.2279	**0.2733**
Inception	Original test	0.8438	**0.8454**	0.8424	0.8414	0.8451
	Random affine	0.4854	0.6423	0.6006	0.6980	**0.7330**
	Random projective	0.1954	0.2164	0.2019	0.1980	**0.2356**

Limitations of Augmentation with GANs. Generating synthetic images utilizing GANs is a task widely investigated recently as was discussed earlier in Sect. 1. However, limitations occur regarding GANs for medical imaging: In most cases the resolution of the synthetic images is low leading to a substantial loss of information and quality. Furthermore, GANs trained on the entire dataset do not provide the ground truth label of the generated samples. Therefore in order to use synthetic images for data augmentation with their respective label we have to train n conditional GANs [23], where n represents the number of classes. This is both time consuming and sometimes, unachievable due to limited data. For example, some classes of the Dermofit dataset only have 23 samples for training, making training a conditional GAN on 23 images extremely challenging, if at all possible. Attempts have been made to solve the GAN labelling problem in the medical context [8], by generating Brain CT scans along with a paired segmentation label map. However, this approach does not offer any guarantee on the correctness of the label maps and though the performance increase on the test set looks promising, mislabeling could induce ambiguity during training and jeopardize the robustness of the model.

Additionally, compared to Manifool Augmentation, augmentation with GANs does not guarantee increase in the variance to which the model is exposed, since images are sampled randomly from the training data distribution and not from the outer regions of the manifold as can be seen in Fig. 1.

Robustness to Random Geometric Transformations. A noteworthy finding highlighted in Tables 1 and 2 is the significant increase in the robustness of models trained with ManiFool Augmentation to random transformations. The improvement is not only impressive, because it ranges from 7% to 15%, but also because even though the proposed augmentation exclusively utilized affine transformations, the robustness to projective ones was drastically improved as well. The remaining evaluated augmentation techniques, i.e. Random Erasing and GAN augmentation, provided much lower, if any, improvement in the robustness of the networks in comparison to the standard random augmentation.

Another experiment evaluating the effect of the ManiFool Augmentation in the robustness of the trained models is shown in Fig. 3. As described in Sect. 2, Eq. 9 evaluates the misclassification rate of a classifier for samples transformed with random affine transformations for a given range of geodesic distances. In Fig. 4 we show images generated within a range of $G \in [1, 5]$ for Dermofit and $G \in [1, 3]$ that were used to evaluate the misclassification rates of the evaluated models. As can be seen in Fig. 3, the models trained with ManiFool Augmentation achieve significantly lower misclassification rates for larger values of the geodesic distance G.

Fig. 3. Robustness of models with different augmentation methods to random transformations with increasing geodesic distance.

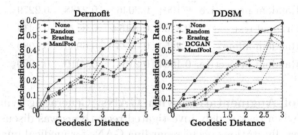

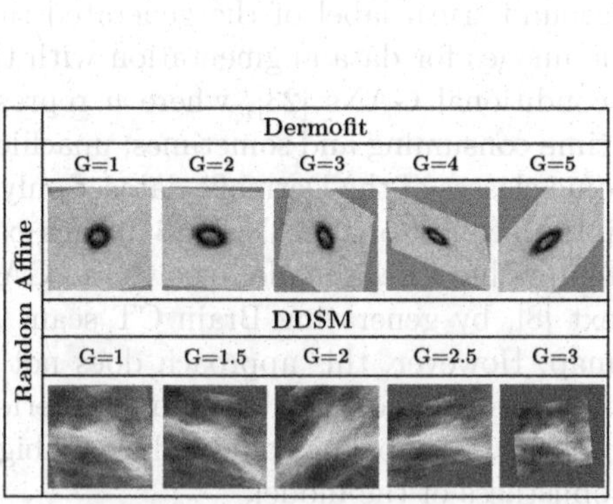

Fig. 4. Examples generated with random affine transformations for dermofit [16] and DDSM [14] for a specific range of Geodesic Distances G.

Effect on Cross-Dataset Performance. In order to showcase the improved robustness provided by the ManiFool Augmentation, we perform cross-dataset evaluation between Dermofit and HAM10000 [24], which consists of 10.000 skin lesion images and there are 7 overlapping classes between the two datasets. Notably all models trained with the proposed method, achieve 1% − 5% higher accuracy on the unseen dataset, as can be observed in Table 3. This validates the hypothesis that ManiFool Augmentation improves the model's understanding of the underlying data distribution and leads to the increase of the model's robustness not only on geometric transformations, but also on unseen test samples.

Table 3. Comparative evaluation of models trained on dermofit with different augmentation methods and deployed on HAM10k, an unseen skin lesion classification dataset.

	None		Random		Erasing		ManiFool	
	Dermofit	HAM10k	Dermofit	HAM10k	Dermofit	HAM10k	Dermofit	HAM10k
ResNet	0.7379	0.1983	0.7859	0.3847	0.7867	0.1699	**0.8136**	**0.3854**
VGG	0.7526	0.1911	0.8080	0.3101	0.7924	0.1947	**0.8238**	**0.3419**
Inception	0.7303	0.2798	0.8051	0.2520	0.7898	0.2140	**0.8275**	**0.3009**

Table 4. Reported average robustness measure score defined in Eq. 8 for different state-of-the-art architectures.

	Geodesic distance		
	ResNet	VGG	Inception
Dermofit	2.128	2.660	**3.391**
DDSM	**1.510**	1.240	1.242

Robustness of Different Architectures. After we utilize a classifier f to craft ManiFool Augmentation samples, we can calculate the average geodesic distance between the original and transformed samples (Eq. 8). This measure can quantify the robustness of a machine learning model, since it implicitly measures the distance between the learned decision boundaries. Therefore, models that achieve higher robustness will be characterized by a larger geodesic distance between classes. In previous works, such as [25], attempts have been made to evaluate the robustness of a classifier utilizing adversarial examples. However, such examples cannot appear naturally and no quantitative measures have been given regarding the robustness. In this work, after we generated the ManiFool Augmentation samples we calculated the robustness scores for the given classifiers, as can be seen in Table 4. This experiment showcases how the robustness of different architectures can fluctuate according to the given dataset. Therefore, it is not sufficient to utilize a state-of-the-art architecture, based on its results on an independent dataset, since its robustness can significantly vary. In our case, InceptionV3 was the most robust model for the Dermofit dataset, while ResNet18 achieved the highest robustness score for DDSM.

5 Conclusion

In this paper we proposed a novel data augmentation technique based on affine geometric transformations and quantified the robustness of machine learning classifiers. Experiments on challenging medical imaging tasks, namely fine grained skin lesion classification and mammogram tumor classification showcased the advantages of the proposed ManiFool Augmentation. On one hand the performance achieved by the evaluated models increased for the original test set and outperformed other commonly used data augmentation techniques. On the other hand, the robustness of the models trained with the proposed augmentation scheme was increased both for random affine and projective transformations but also cross-datasets, in an unseen test scenario. Furthermore, a qualitative measure for the robustness of machine learning classifiers was calculated and showcased the variations in the robustness of state-of-the-art models for different datasets. Future work includes extension of the ManiFool Augmentation to a wider range or transformations for a variety of medical imaging tasks.

References

1. Kanbak, C., Moosavi-Dezfooli, S.-M., Frossard, P.: Geometric robustness of deep networks: analysis and improvement. In: CVPR (2017)
2. Wong, S.C., Gatt, A., Stamatescu, V., McDonnell, M.D.: Understanding data augmentation for classification: when to warp? In: DICTA (2016)
3. Devries, T., Taylor, G.W.: Dataset augmentation in feature space. CoRR abs/1702.05538 (2017)
4. Okafor, E., Schomaker, L., Wiering, M.A.: An analysis of rotation matrix and colour constancy data augmentation in classifying images of animals. J. Inf. Telecommun. **2**(4), 465–491 (2018)
5. Fawzi, A., Samulowitz, H., Turaga, D., Frossard, P.: Adaptive data augmentation for image classification. In: IEEE International Conference on Image Processing (ICIP) (2016)
6. Antoniou, A., Storkey, A., Edwards, H.: Data augmentation generative adversarial networks. CoRR abs/1711.04340 (2017)
7. Cubuk, E.D., Zoph, B., Mané, D., Vasudevan, V., Le, Q.V.: AutoAugment: learning augmentation policies from data. CoRR abs/1805.09501 (2018)
8. Bowles, C., et al.: GAN augmentation: augmenting training data using generative adversarial networks. CoRR abs/1810.10863 (2018)
9. Frid-Adar, M., Klang, E., Amitai, M., Goldberger, J., Greenspan, H.: Synthetic data augmentation using GAN for improved liver lesion classification. In: IEEE International Symposium on Biomedical Imaging (ISBI) (2018)
10. Absil, P.-A., Mahony, R., Sepulchre, R.: Optimization Algorithms on Matrix Manifolds. Princeton University Press, Princeton (2008)
11. Kokiopoulou, E., Frossard, P.: Minimum distance between pattern transformation manifolds: algorithm and applications. IEEE Trans. Pattern Anal. Mach. Intell. (TPAMI) **31**(7), 1225–1238 (2009)
12. Tu, L.W.: Differential Geometry. GTM, vol. 275. Springer, Cham (2017). https://doi.org/10.1007/978-3-319-55084-8
13. Szegedy, C., et al.: Intriguing properties of neural networks (2014)

14. Heath, M., Bowyer, K., Kopans, D., Moore, R., Kegelmeyer, W.P.: The digital database for screening mammography. In: Yaffe, M.J. (ed) International Workshop on Digital Mammography, pp. 212–218. Medical Physics Publishing (2001)
15. Heath, M., et al.: Current status of the digital database for screening mammography. In: Digital Mammography, pp. 457–460. Kluwer Academic Publishers (1998)
16. Ballerini, L., Fisher, R.B., Aldridge, R.B., Rees, J.: A color and texture based hierarchical K-NN approach to the classification of non-melanoma skin lesions. In: Celebi, M., Schaefer, G. (eds.) Color Medical Image Analysis. LNCVB, vol. 6, pp. 63–86. Springer, Dordrecht (2013). https://doi.org/10.1007/978-94-007-5389-1_4
17. He, K., Zhang, X., Ren, S., Sun, J.: Deep residual learning for image recognition. In: IEEE Conference on Computer Vision and Pattern Recognition (CVPR) (2016)
18. Simonyan, K., Zisserman, A.: Very deep convolutional networks for large-scale image recognition. CoRR abs/1409.1556 (2014)
19. Szegedy, C., Vanhoucke, V., Ioffe, S., Shlens, J., Wojna, Z.: Rethinking the inception architecture for computer vision. In: CVPR (2016)
20. Roy, A.G., Conjeti, S., Sheet, D., Katouzian, A., Navab, N., Wachinger, C.: Error corrective boosting for learning fully convolutional networks with limited data. In: Descoteaux, M., Maier-Hein, L., Franz, A., Jannin, P., Collins, D.L., Duchesne, S. (eds.) MICCAI 2017. LNCS, vol. 10435, pp. 231–239. Springer, Cham (2017). https://doi.org/10.1007/978-3-319-66179-7_27
21. Paszke, A., et al.: Automatic differentiation in PyTorch. In: 31st Conference on Neural Information Processing Systems (NeurIPS) (2017)
22. Zhong, Z., Zheng, L., Kang, G., Li, S., Yang, Y.: Random erasing data augmentation. CoRR abs/1708.04896 (2017)
23. Radford, A., Metz, L., Chintala, S.: Unsupervised representation learning with deep convolutional generative adversarial networks. In: 4th International Conference on Learning Representations (ICLR) (2016)
24. Tschandl, P., Rosendahl, C., Kittler, H.: The HAM10000 dataset, a large collection of multi-source dermatoscopic images of common pigmented skin lesions. Sci. Data 5 (2018)
25. Paschali, M., Conjeti, S., Navarro, F., Navab, N.: Generalizability vs. robustness: investigating medical imaging networks using adversarial examples. In: Frangi, A.F., Schnabel, J.A., Davatzikos, C., Alberola-López, C., Fichtinger, G. (eds.) MICCAI 2018. LNCS, vol. 11070, pp. 493–501. Springer, Cham (2018). https://doi.org/10.1007/978-3-030-00928-1_56

Multifold Acceleration of Diffusion MRI via Deep Learning Reconstruction from Slice-Undersampled Data

Yoonmi Hong, Geng Chen, Pew-Thian Yap[✉], and Dinggang Shen[✉]

Department of Radiology and BRIC, University of North Carolina at Chapel Hill,
Chapel Hill, NC, USA
{ptyap,dgshen}@med.unc.edu

Abstract. Diffusion MRI (dMRI), while powerful for characterization of tissue microstructure, suffers from long acquisition time. In this paper, we present a method for effective diffusion MRI reconstruction from slice-undersampled data. Instead of full diffusion-weighted (DW) image volumes, only a subsample of equally-spaced slices need to be acquired. We show that complementary information from DW volumes corresponding to different diffusion wavevectors can be harnessed using graph convolutional neural networks for reconstruction of the full DW volumes. The experimental results indicate a high acceleration factor of up to 5 can be achieved with minimal information loss.

Keywords: Diffusion MRI · Accelerated acquisition ·
Super resolution · Graph CNN · Adversarial learning

1 Introduction

Diffusion MRI (dMRI) is a unique imaging technique for in vivo measurement of tissue microstructural properties. However, in contrast to structural MRI, dMRI typically requires longer acquisition times for sufficient coverage of the diffusion wavevector space (i.e., q-space). Each point in q-space corresponds to a diffusion-weighted (DW) image, and sufficient DW images are typically required for accurate characterization of the white matter neuronal architecture, such as fiber crossings and intra-/extra-cellular compartments [16,26,27]. To improve acquisition speed, we introduce in this paper a super-resolution (SR) reconstruction technique that only requires a subsample of slices for each DW volume.

In-plane and through-plane resolutions are determined by different factors. The former is affected by gradient strength, receiver bandwidth, phase encoding steps, and the number of readout points. The latter is determined by hardware limitations coupled with pulse sequence timing, and slice selection [8]. Fast and high-resolution reconstruction schemes can be designed by customizing MR

This work was supported in part by NIH grants (NS093842, EB022880, and EB006733).

A. C. S. Chung et al. (Eds.): IPMI 2019, LNCS 11492, pp. 530–541, 2019.
https://doi.org/10.1007/978-3-030-20351-1_41

acquisition and reconstruction. For example, SR reconstruction can be carried out with sub-voxel shifted scans in the in-plane [18] and slice-select [8] dimensions. Scherrer and his colleagues [21] proposed an SR method to reconstruct each DW volume from multiple anisotropic orthogonal scans, which they extended in [20] for estimation of tissue microstructural properties using diffusion compartment imaging. Ning et al. [17] proposed a compressed-sensing SR reconstruction framework that increases the spatio-angular resolution of dMRI data by using multiple overlapping thick-slice datasets with undersampling in q-space [17]. In [25], high-resolution diffusion parameters are estimated from a set of DW images with arbitrary slice orientation and diffusion gradient directions. Shi et al. [22] proposed a 4D low-rank and total variation regularized method for SR reconstruction. SR reconstruction based on a generative adversarial network is proposed in [1].

In this paper, we will introduce an SR reconstruction method for multifold acceleration of dMRI. We will show that, for each DW volume, only a subsample of slices in the slice select direction are needed to reconstruct the full 3D volumes, yielding an acceleration factor that is proportional to the subsampling factor. Each DW volume is subsampled with a different slice offset so that the volume captures complementary information that can be used to improve the reconstruction of other DW volumes. The non-linear mapping from the subsampled to full DW images is learned using a graph convolutional neural network (GCNN) [3,11], which generalizes CNNs to high-dimensional, irregular, and non-Euclidean domains. Such generalization is necessary in our framework since the sampling points in the q-space are not necessarily Cartesian. For improving perceptual quality, the GCNN is employed as the generator in a generative adversarial network (GAN) [7].

2 Methods

2.1 Formulation

A method overview is illustrated in Fig. 1. Each of the N DW volumes $\{X_n, n = 1, \cdots, N\}$ is undersampled in the slice-select direction by a factor of R:

$$\tilde{X}_n(\cdot, \cdot, z) := X_n(\cdot, \cdot, Rz + s_n), \tag{1}$$

where $s_n \in \{0, 1, \cdots, R-1\}$ is the slice offset for X_n. Our objective is to predict the full DW volumes from the undersampled data by learning a non-linear mapping function f such that

$$(X_1, \cdots, X_N) = f(\tilde{X}_1, \cdots, \tilde{X}_N). \tag{2}$$

Instead of reconstructing each DW volume individually, we reconstruct all DW volumes jointly by considering neighborhoods in the spatial and diffusion wavevector domains. The mapping function in (2) f is learned using GCNN.

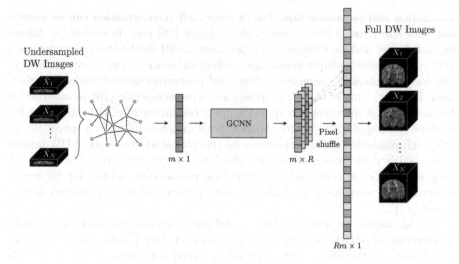

Fig. 1. Method overview.

2.2 Graph Representation

The dMRI sampling domain can be represented by a graph where each node represents a spatial location in physical space (x-space) and a diffusion wavevector in q-space. This graph is encoded using a weighted symmetric adjacency matrix W. The graph Laplacian is defined as $L = D - W$, where D is a diagonal degree matrix. L can be normalized via $L = I - D^{-1/2}WD^{-1/2}$, where I is an identity matrix. The eigenvectors of L define a graph Fourier basis that allows filtering to be performed in the spectral domain [5].

2.3 Spectral Filtering

According to Parseval's theorem [2], a filter is localized in the spatial domain if and only if it is smooth in the spectral domain [3]. This can be achieved by approximating and parameterizing filters by polynomials [2]. Spectral filters approximated by the K-th order polynomials of the Laplacian are exactly K-localized in the graph [9]. In this work, we employ the Chebyshev polynomial approximation and define the graph convolutional operation from input x to output y as

$$y = g_\theta(x) = \sum_{k=0}^{K} \theta_k T_k(\tilde{L})x, \tag{3}$$

where $\tilde{L}$ is the scaled Laplacian $\tilde{L} = 2L/\lambda_{\max} - I$ with $\lambda_{\max}$ being the maximal eigenvalue of L and $T_k(\cdot)$ is the Chebyshev polynomial of order k. Chebyshev polynomials $\{T_k(\cdot)\}$ form an orthogonal basis on $[-1, 1]$ and have recurrence relation

$$T_k(\lambda) = 2\lambda T_{k-1}(\lambda) - T_{k-2}(\lambda), \quad T_1(\lambda) = \lambda, \quad T_0(\lambda) = 1. \tag{4}$$

The graph convolutional layers in the GCNN can be written as

$$\boldsymbol{\Phi}^{(l)} = \xi\left(\sum_{k=0}^{K} \theta_k^{(l)} T_k(\tilde{L})\boldsymbol{\Phi}^{(l-1)}\right), \tag{5}$$

where $\boldsymbol{\Phi}^{(l)}$ denotes the feature map at the l-th layer, $\theta_k^{(l)}$ is a vector of Chebyshev polynomial coefficients to be learned at the l-th layer, and ξ is a non-linear activation function.

2.4 Adjacency Matrix

The adjacency matrix is defined by considering spatio-angular neighborhoods. Let each node be represented by a spatial location $\mathbf{x}_i \in \mathbb{R}^3$ and a normalized wave-vector $\mathbf{g}_j \in \mathbb{R}^3$. Inspired by the local neighborhood matching technique [4], we define an adjacency matrix W with weights $\{w_{i,j;i',j'}\}$:

$$w_{i,j;\,i',j'} := \exp\left(-\frac{\|\mathbf{x}_i - \mathbf{x}_{i'}\|_2^2}{\sigma_x^2}\right) \exp\left(-\frac{1 - \langle\mathbf{g}_j, \mathbf{g}_{j'}\rangle^2}{\sigma_g^2}\right), \tag{6}$$

where σ_x and σ_g are the parameters used to control the contributions of the spatial and angular distances, respectively. We note that, in (6), the numerators of the arguments of the exponential functions are normalized to $[0, 1]$.

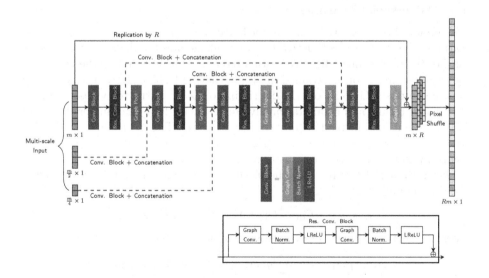

Fig. 2. The proposed graph CNN architecture.

2.5   Graph Convolutional Neural Networks

The proposed architecture is illustrated in Fig. 2. A residual convolutional block is employed to ease training since it can mitigate the vanishing gradient problem [10]. To increase the receptive field, a U-Net [19] structure with symmetric contraction paths for encoding and expansion paths for decoding is employed. Pooling and unpooling, realized using graph coarsening and uncoarsening, are applied respectively for each encoding and decoding step. As in [5], we adopt the Graclus multi-scale clustering algorithm [6] for graph coarsening. The diffusion signals corresponding to the nodes of the graph are rearranged via index permutation to form a vector. The uncoarsening operation is achieved via a one-dimensional upsampling operation followed by an inverse permutation of indices. We employ the transposed convolution filter [13] for upsampling.

Multi-scale graphs, obtained via graph coarsening, are fed as features via graph convolutions to each level of the contraction path. The skip connection at each level in the U-Net consists of a transformation module (graph convolutions and concatenation) for boosting the low-level features to complement the high-level features, as proposed in [15]. The transformation model narrows the gap between low- and high-level features.

The upsampling operation in slice direction is realized by a standard convolution in the low-resolution space followed by pixel shuffling [23]. The pixel-shuffling operation maps R feature maps of size $m \times 1$ to an output of size $Rm \times 1$, where m is the number of nodes in the input graph.

2.6   Adversarial Learning

We employ the adversarial learning for better perceptual quality. In adversarial learning, the generator estimates the target image and the discriminator distinguishes the target image from the estimated one. During training, the generator and the discriminator are trained in an alternating fashion. Here, the generator G is the proposed GCNN, and the discriminator D is constructed via patch-GAN [12] as it is robust and computationally efficient with fewer parameters by using fully-convolutional instead of fully-connected layers. The discriminator classifies whether each local patch is real or fake. In the generator and discriminator, we use leaky ReLU (LReLU) activation with a negative slope of 0.2.

For adversarial learning, for the input source $\mathbf{x}$ and the target $\mathbf{y}$, we define the discriminator loss as

$$\mathcal{L}_D(\mathbf{x}, \mathbf{y}) = \mathcal{L}_{\mathrm{BCE}}(D(\mathbf{y}), 1) + \mathcal{L}_{\mathrm{BCE}}(D(G(\mathbf{x})), \mathbf{0}), \qquad (7)$$

where $\mathcal{L}_{\mathrm{BCE}}$ is the binary cross-entropy function defined as

$$\mathcal{L}_{\mathrm{BCE}}(\mathbf{p}, \mathbf{q}) := -\sum_i [q_i \log p_i + (1 - q_i) \log (1 - p_i)]. \qquad (8)$$

In (8), $\mathbf{q}$ consists of 1's for a real target image and 0's for a generated image, and $\mathbf{p}$ is the probability given by the discriminator. The generator loss is defined as

$$\mathcal{L}_{G_{ADV}}(\mathbf{x}, \mathbf{y}) = \lambda_g \|G(\mathbf{x}) - \mathbf{y}\|_1 + \lambda_{ADV} \mathcal{L}_{\mathrm{BCE}}(D(G(\mathbf{x})), \mathbf{1}) \qquad (9)$$

so that the generator G can produce a more realistic output to fool the discriminator D.

3   Experimental Results

3.1   Material

We randomly selected 16 subjects from the Human Connectome Project (HCP) database [24] and divided them into 12 for training and 4 for testing using 4-fold cross-validation. For each subject, 90 DW images (voxel size: $1.25 \times 1.25 \times 1.25\,\mathrm{mm}^3$) with $b = 2000\,\mathrm{s/mm}^2$ were used for evaluation. The images were retrospectively undersampled by factors $R = 3, 4$, and 5. Specifically, the set of DW images was divided into R groups, where the diffusion wavevectors were uniformly distributed in each group. For each group, the source images were generated by undersampling the original images with a slice offset.

3.2   Implementation Details

All DW images were normalized by their corresponding non-DW image (b_0). We set the controlling parameters $\sigma_x^2 = 0.1$ and $\sigma_g^2 = 1.0$ in (6) for joint consideration of spatial and angular neighborhoods. We set $K = 3$ for the Chebyshev polynomials. For the loss functions, we set $\lambda_g = 1.0$, and $\lambda_{\mathrm{ADV}} = 0.01$. The proposed method was implemented using TensorFlow 1.12.0 and trained using the ADAM optimizer with initial learning rates of 0.0001 and 0.00001 respectively for the generator and the discriminators.

3.3   Results

We compared our method with two upsampling methods: bilinear interpolation and bicubic interpolation, for three undersampling factors $R = 3, 4$, and 5. We measured the reconstruction accuracy by computing the peak signal-to-noise ratio (PSNR) of generalized fractional anisotropy (GFA) images, structural similarity

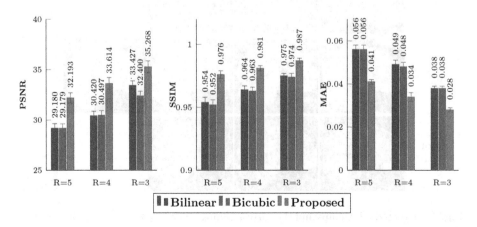

Fig. 3. Quantitative comparison using PSNR, SSIM, and MAE.

Table 1. Quantitative comparison of SH coefficients.

R	Bilinear	Bicubic	Proposed
3	0.128 ± 0.003	0.132 ± 0.003	**0.073 ± 0.003**
4	0.163 ± 0.004	0.169 ± 0.004	**0.096 ± 0.005**
5	0.191 ± 0.004	0.198 ± 0.004	**0.101 ± 0.004**

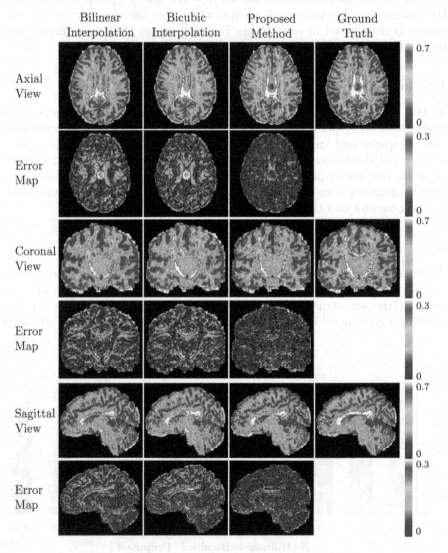

Fig. 4. Predicted GFA maps and the corresponding error maps shown in multiple views $(R = 4)$.

index (SSIM), and mean absolute error (MAE). The quantitative results are summarized in Fig. 3. The normalized root-mean-square errors (RMSE) in terms of spherical harmonic (SH) coefficients up to order 8 are summarized in Table 1.

Representative reconstruction results for GFA for a fixed undersampling factor $R = 4$, shown in Fig. 4, indicate that the proposed method recovers the details more accurately when compared with the two interpolation methods. Figure 5 shows the representative DW images and the RMSE maps of the SH coefficients. Figure 6 shows the reconstruction results with respect to various undersampling factors. Our method consistently produces more accurate details, even for a large R.

Figure 7 shows that our method yields fiber orientation distribution functions (ODFs) that are closer to the ground truth with less partial volume effects. We also extracted three representative tract bundles from whole brain tractography using the multi-ROI approach described in [14]. We extracted the forceps major (FMajor) using ROIs drawn in the occipital cortex and corpus callosum, and also the forceps minor (FMinor) using ROIs drawn in the prefrontal cortex and corpus callosum. For the corticospinal tract (CST), ROIs are drawn in precentral gyrus and posterior limb of the internal capsule. Figure 8 shows that our method yields richer fiber tracts that better resemble the ground truth.

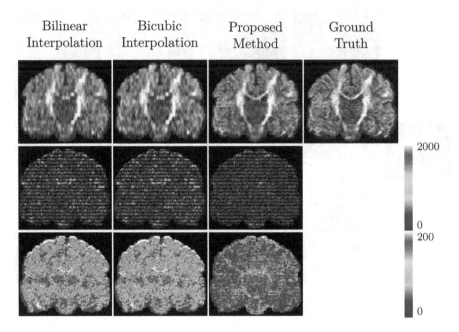

Fig. 5. Predicted DW images (top row), the corresponding error maps (middle row), and RMSE maps of SH coefficients (bottom row) ($R = 4$).

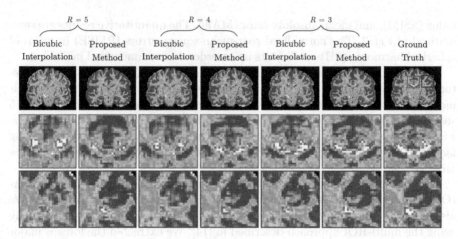

Fig. 6. Predicted GFA maps (top row) and their close-up views (middle and bottom rows).

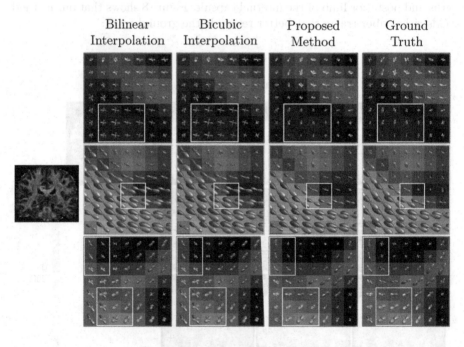

Fig. 7. Representative fiber ODFs.

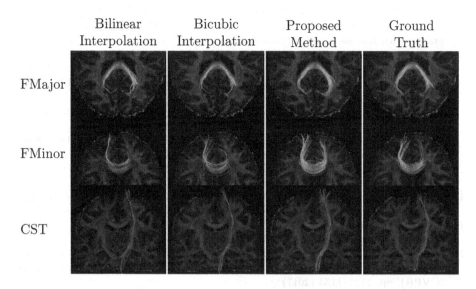

Fig. 8. Representative tractography results.

4 Conclusion

We have proposed to employ slice-undersampling for acceleration of dMRI. Each DW image is undersampled with a different slice offset and the missing slices are reconstructed by exploiting neighborhood information in the spatial and angular domains. The non-linear mapping from slice-undersampled DW images to full DW images is learned using GCNN. Spatio-angular relationship is jointly considered when constructing the graph for the GCNN. The experimental results demonstrate that the proposed method outperforms two commonly used interpolation methods.

References

1. Albay, E., Demir, U., Unal, G.: Diffusion MRI spatial super-resolution using generative adversarial networks. In: Rekik, I., Unal, G., Adeli, E., Park, S.H. (eds.) PRIME 2018. LNCS, vol. 11121, pp. 155–163. Springer, Cham (2018). https://doi.org/10.1007/978-3-030-00320-3_19
2. Bronstein, M.M., Bruna, J., LeCun, Y., Szlam, A., Vandergheynst, P.: Geometric deep learning: going beyond Euclidean data. IEEE Sig. Process. Mag. **34**(4), 18–42 (2017)
3. Bruna, J., Zaremba, W., Szlam, A., LeCun, Y.: Spectral networks and locally connected networks on graphs. arXiv preprint arXiv:1312.6203 (2013)
4. Chen, G., Dong, B., Zhang, Y., Shen, D., Yap, P.-T.: Neighborhood matching for curved domains with application to denoising in diffusion MRI. In: Descoteaux, M., Maier-Hein, L., Franz, A., Jannin, P., Collins, D.L., Duchesne, S. (eds.) MICCAI 2017. LNCS, vol. 10433, pp. 629–637. Springer, Cham (2017). https://doi.org/10.1007/978-3-319-66182-7_72

5. Defferrard, M., Bresson, X., Vandergheynst, P.: Convolutional neural networks on graphs with fast localized spectral filtering. In: Advances in Neural Information Processing Systems (NIPS), pp. 3844–3852 (2016)
6. Dhillon, I.S., Guan, Y., Kulis, B.: Weighted graph cuts without eigenvectors a multilevel approach. IEEE Trans. Pattern Anal. Mach. Intell. **29**(11), 1944–1957 (2007)
7. Goodfellow, I., et al.: Generative adversarial nets. In: Advances in Neural Information Processing Systems (NIPS), pp. 2672–2680 (2014)
8. Greenspan, H., Oz, G., Kiryati, N., Peled, S.: MRI inter-slice reconstruction using super-resolution. Magn. Reson. Imaging **20**(5), 437–446 (2002)
9. Hammond, D.K., Vandergheynst, P., Gribonval, R.: Wavelets on graphs via spectral graph theory. Appl. Comput. Harmon. Anal. **30**(2), 129–150 (2011)
10. He, K., Zhang, X., Ren, S., Sun, J.: Deep residual learning for image recognition. In: Computer vision and pattern recognition (CVPR), pp. 770–778 (2016)
11. Henaff, M., Bruna, J., LeCun, Y.: Deep convolutional networks on graph-structured data. arXiv preprint arXiv:1506.05163 (2015)
12. Isola, P., Zhu, J.Y., Zhou, T., Efros, A.A.: Image-to-image translation with conditional adversarial networks. In: Computer Vision and Pattern Recognition (CVPR), pp. 1125–1134 (2017)
13. Long, J., Shelhamer, E., Darrell, T.: Fully convolutional networks for semantic segmentation. In: Computer Vision and Pattern Recognition (CVPR), pp. 3431–3440 (2015)
14. Mori, S., Crain, B.J., Chacko, V.P., Van Zijl, P.C.: Three-dimensional tracking of axonal projections in the brain by magnetic resonance imaging. Ann. Neurol. **45**(2), 265–269 (1999)
15. Nie, D., Wang, L., Adeli, E., Lao, C., Lin, W., Shen, D.: 3-D fully convolutional networks for multimodal isointense infant brain image segmentation. IEEE Trans. Cybern. **49**(3), 1123–1136 (2019)
16. Ning, L., et al.: Sparse reconstruction challenge for diffusion MRI: validation on a physical phantom to determine which acquisition scheme and analysis method to use? Med. Image Anal. **26**(1), 316–331 (2015)
17. Ning, L., et al.: A joint compressed-sensing and super-resolution approach for very high-resolution diffusion imaging. NeuroImage **125**, 386–400 (2016)
18. Peled, S., Yeshurun, Y.: Superresolution in MRI: application to human white matter fiber tract visualization by diffusion tensor imaging. Magn. Reson. Med. **45**(1), 29–35 (2001)
19. Ronneberger, O., Fischer, P., Brox, T.: U-Net: convolutional networks for biomedical image segmentation. In: Navab, N., Hornegger, J., Wells, W.M., Frangi, A.F. (eds.) MICCAI 2015. LNCS, vol. 9351, pp. 234–241. Springer, Cham (2015). https://doi.org/10.1007/978-3-319-24574-4_28
20. Scherrer, B., Afacan, O., Taquet, M., Prabhu, S.P., Gholipour, A., Warfield, S.K.: Accelerated high spatial resolution diffusion-weighted imaging. In: Ourselin, S., Alexander, D.C., Westin, C.-F., Cardoso, M.J. (eds.) IPMI 2015. LNCS, vol. 9123, pp. 69–81. Springer, Cham (2015). https://doi.org/10.1007/978-3-319-19992-4_6
21. Scherrer, B., Gholipour, A., Warfield, S.K.: Super-resolution reconstruction to increase the spatial resolution of diffusion weighted images from orthogonal anisotropic acquisitions. Med. Image Anal. **16**(7), 1465–1476 (2012)
22. Shi, F., Cheng, J., Wang, L., Yap, P.-T., Shen, D.: Super-resolution reconstruction of diffusion-weighted images using 4D low-rank and total variation. In: Fuster, A., Ghosh, A., Kaden, E., Rathi, Y., Reisert, M. (eds.) Computational Diffusion MRI. MV, pp. 15–25. Springer, Cham (2016). https://doi.org/10.1007/978-3-319-28588-7_2

23. Shi, W., et al.: Real-time single image and video super-resolution using an efficient sub-pixel convolutional neural network. In: Computer Vision and Pattern Recognition (CVPR), pp. 1874–1883 (2016)
24. Sotiropoulos, S.N., et al.: Advances in diffusion MRI acquisition and processing in the human connectome project. NeuroImage **80**, 125–143 (2013)
25. Van Steenkiste, G., et al.: Super-resolution reconstruction of diffusion parameters from diffusion-weighted images with different slice orientations. Magn. Reson. Med. **75**(1), 181–195 (2016)
26. Yap, P.T., Zhang, Y., Shen, D.: Multi-tissue decomposition of diffusion MRI signals via ℓ_0 sparse-group estimation. IEEE Trans. Image Process. **25**(9), 4340–4353 (2016)
27. Ye, C., Zhuo, J., Gullapalli, R.P., Prince, J.L.: Estimation of fiber orientations using neighborhood information. Med. Image Anal. **32**, 243–256 (2016)

Riemannian Geometry Learning
for Disease Progression Modelling

Maxime Louis[1,2(✉)], Raphaël Couronné[1,2], Igor Koval[1,2], Benjamin Charlier[1,3],
and Stanley Durrleman[1,2]

[1] Sorbonne Universités, UPMC Univ Paris 06, Inserm, CNRS,
Institut du cerveau et de la moelle (ICM), Paris, France
maxime.louis.x2012@gmail.com
[2] Inria Paris, Aramis Project-Team, 75013 Paris, France
[3] Institut Montpelliérain Alexander Grothendieck CNRS, Univ. Montpellier,
Montpellier, France

Abstract. The analysis of longitudinal trajectories is a longstanding problem in medical imaging which is often tackled in the context of Riemannian geometry: the set of observations is assumed to lie on an a priori known Riemannian manifold. When dealing with high-dimensional or complex data, it is in general not possible to design a Riemannian geometry of relevance. In this paper, we perform Riemannian manifold learning in association with the statistical task of longitudinal trajectory analysis. After inference, we obtain both a submanifold of observations and a Riemannian metric so that the observed progressions are geodesics. This is achieved using a deep generative network, which maps trajectories in a low-dimensional Euclidean space to the observation space.

Keywords: Riemannian geometry · Longitudinal progression ·
Medical imaging

1 Introduction

The analysis of the longitudinal aspects of a disease is key to understand its progression as well as to design prognosis and early diagnostic tools. Indeed, the time dynamic of a disease is more informative than static observations of the symptoms, especially for neuro-degenerative diseases whose progression span over years with early subtle changes. More specifically, we tackle in this paper the issue of disease modelling: we aim at building a time continuous reference of disease progression and at providing a low-dimensional representation of each subject encoding his position with respect to this reference. This task must be achieved using longitudinal datasets, which contain repeated observations of clinical measurements or medical images of subjects over time. In particular, we aim at being able to achieve this longitudinal modelling even when dealing with very high-dimensional data.

© Springer Nature Switzerland AG 2019
A. C. S. Chung et al. (Eds.): IPMI 2019, LNCS 11492, pp. 542–553, 2019.
https://doi.org/10.1007/978-3-030-20351-1_42

The framework of Riemannian geometry is well suited for the analysis of longitudinal trajectories. It allows for principled approaches which respect the nature of the data - e.g. explicit constraints- and can embody some a priori knowledge. When a Riemannian manifold of interest is identified for a given type of data, it is possible to formulate generative models of progression on this manifold directly. In [3,10,14], the authors propose a mixed-effect model which assumes that each subject follows a trajectory which is parallel to a reference geodesic on a Riemannian manifold. In [16], a similar approach is constructed with a hierarchical model of geodesic progressions. All these approaches make use of a predefined Riemannian geometry on the space of observations.

A main limitation of these approaches is therefore the need of this known Riemannian manifold to work on. It may be possible to coin a relevant Riemannian manifold in low-dimensional cases and with expert knowledge, but it is nearly impossible in the more general case of high-dimensional data or when multiple modalities are present. Designing a Riemannian metric is in particular very challenging, as the space of Riemannian metrics on a manifold is vastly large and complex. A first possibility, popular in the literature, is to equip a submanifold of the observation space with the metric induced from a metric on the whole space of observations – e.g. ℓ^2 on images. However, we argue here that this choice of larger metric is arbitrary and has no reason to be of particular relevance for the analysis at hand. Another possibility is to consider the space of observations as a product of simple manifolds, each equipped with a Riemannian metric. This is only possible in particular cases, and even so, the product structure constrains the shapes of the geodesics which need to be geodesics on each coordinate. Other constructions of Riemannian metrics exist in special cases, but there is no simple general procedure. Hence, there is a need for data-driven metric estimation.

A few Riemannian metric learning approaches do exist in the litterature. In [6], the authors propose to learn a Riemannian metric which is defined by interpolation of a finite set of tensors, and they optimize the tensors so as to separate a set of data according to known labels. This procedure is intractable as the dimension of the data increases. In [1] and in [17], the authors estimate a Riemannian metric so that an observed set of data maximizes the likelihood of a generative model. Their approaches use simple forms for the metric. Finally, in [12], the authors show how to use transformation of the observation space to pull-back a metric from a given space back to the observation space, and give a density criterion for the obtained metric and the data.

We propose in this paper a new approach to learn a smooth manifold and a Riemannian metric which are adapted to the modelling of disease progression. We describe each subject as following a straight line trajectory parallel to a reference trajectory in a low-dimensional latent space $\mathcal{Z}$, which is mapped onto a submanifold of the observation space using a deep neural network Ψ, as seen in [15]. Using the mapping Ψ, the straight line trajectories are mapped onto geodesics of the manifold $\Psi(\mathcal{Z})$ equipped with the push-forward of the Euclidean metric on $\mathcal{Z}$. After inference, the neural network parametrizes a manifold which is close to the set of observations and a Riemannian metric on this manifold which is such that subjects follow geodesics on the obtained Riemannian manifold, which are all parallel to a common reference geodesic in the sense of [14]. This construction is motivated by the theorem proven in Appendix giving mild conditions under which there exists a Riemannian metric such that a family of curves are geodesics. Additionally, this particular construction of a Riemannian geometry allows very fast computations of Riemannian operations, since all of them can be done in closed form in $\mathcal{Z}$.

Section 2 describes the Riemannian structure considered, the model as well as the inference procedure. Section 3 shows the results on various features extracted from the ADNI data base [7] and illustrates the advantages of the method compared to the use of predefined simple Riemannian geometries.

2   Propagation Model and Deep Generative Models

2.1   Push-Forward of a Riemannian Metric

We explain here how to parametrize a family of Riemannian manifolds. We use deep neural networks, which we view as non-linear mappings, since they have the advantage of being flexible and computationally efficient.

Let $\Psi_w : \mathbf{R}^d \mapsto \mathbf{R}^D$ be a neural network function with weights w, where $d, D \in \mathbf{N}$ with $d < D$. It is shown in [15] that if the transfer functions of the neural network are smooth monotonic and the weight matrices of each layer are of full rank, then Ψ is differentiable and its differential is of full rank d everywhere. Consequently, $\Psi(\mathbf{R}^d) = \mathcal{M}_w$ is locally a d-dimensional smooth submanifold of the space $\mathbf{R}^D$. It is only locally a submanifold: M_w could have self intersections since Ψ_w is in general not one-to-one. Note that using architectures as in [8] would ensure by construction the injectivity of Ψ_w.

A Riemannian metric on a smooth manifold is a smoothly varying inner product on the manifold tangent space. Let g be a metric on $\mathbf{R}^d$. The push-forward of g on $\mathcal{M}_w$ is defined by, for any smooth vector fields X, Y on $\Psi_w(\mathbf{R}^d)$:

$$\Psi_w^*(g)(X, Y) := g((\Psi_w)_*(X), (\Psi_w)_*(Y))$$

where $(\Psi_w)_*(X)$ and $(\Psi_w)_*(Y)$ are the pull-back of X and Y on $\mathbf{R}^d$ defined by $(\Psi_w)_*(X)(f) = X(f \circ \Psi_w^{-1})$ for any smooth function $f : \mathbf{R}^d \to \mathbf{R}$, and where Ψ_w^{-1} is a local inverse of Ψ_w, which exists by the local inversion theorem.

By definition, Ψ_w is an isometry mapping a geodesic in $(\mathbf{R}^d, g)$ onto a geodesic in $(\mathcal{M}_w, \Psi_w^*(g))$. Note that the function Ψ_w parametrizes both a submanifold $\mathcal{M}_w$ of the space of observations and a metric $\Psi_w^*(g)$ on this submanifold. In particular, there may be weights w_1, w_2 for which the manifolds $\mathcal{M}_{w_1}, \mathcal{M}_{w_2}$ are the same, but the metrics $\Psi_{w_1}^*(g), \Psi_{w_2}^*(g)$ are different.

In what follows, we denote $g_w = \Psi_w^*(g)$ the push-forward of the Euclidean metric g. Since $(\mathbf{R}^d, g)$ is flat, so is $(\mathcal{M}_w, g_w)$. This neither means that $\mathcal{M}_w$ is flat for the induced metric from the Euclidean metric on $\mathbf{R}^D$ nor that the obtained manifold is Euclidean (ruled surfaces like hyperbolic paraboloid are flat still non euclidean). A study of the variety of Riemannian manifolds obtained under this form would allow to better understand how vast or limiting this construction is.

2.2   Model for Longitudinal Progression

We denote here $(y_{ij}, t_{ij})_{j=1,...,n_i}$ the observations and ages of the subject i, for $i \in \{1, ..., N\}$ where $N \in \mathbf{N}$ is the number of subjects and $n_i \in \mathbf{N}$ is the number of observation of the i-th subject. The observations lie in a D-dimensional space $\mathcal{Y}$. We model each individual as following a straight trajectory in $\mathcal{Z} = \mathbf{R}^d$ with $d \in \mathbf{N}$:

$$l_i(t) = e^{\eta_i}(t - \tau_i)e_1 + \sum_{j=2}^{d} b_i^j e_j \tag{1}$$

where $(e_1, ..., e_d)$ is the canonical basis of $\mathbf{R}^d$.

With this writing, on average, the subjects follow a trajectory in the latent space given by the direction e_1. To account for inter-subject differences in patterns of progression, each subject follows a parallel to this direction in the direction $\sum_{j=2}^{d} b_i^j e_j$. Finally, we reparametrize the velocity of the subjects in the e_1 direction using η_i which encodes for the pace of progression and τ_i which is a time shift. This writing is so that $l_i(\tau_i)$ is in $\text{Vec}(e_2, ..., e_d)$, the set of all possible states at the time τ_i. Hence, after inference, all the subjects progression should be aligned with similar values at $t = \tau_i$. We denote, for each subject i, $\varphi_i = (\eta_i, \tau_i, b_i^2, ..., b_i^d) \in \mathbf{R}^{d+1}$. φ_i is a low-dimensional vector which encodes the progression of the subject.

As shown above, we map $\mathcal{Z}$ to $\mathcal{Y}$ using a deep neural network Ψ_w. The subject reconstructed trajectories $t \mapsto y_i(t) = \Psi_w(l_i(t))$ are geodesics in the submanifold $(\mathcal{M}_w, g_w)$. The geodesics are parallel in the sense of [14] and [16]. Note that the apparently constrained form of latent space trajectories (1) is not restrictive: the family of functions parametrized by the neural network Ψ_w allows to curve and move the image of the latent trajectories in the observation space, and for example to align the direction e_1 with any direction in $\mathcal{Y}$.

2.3   Encoding the Latent Variables

To predict the variables φ for a given subject, we use a recurrent neural-network (RNN), which is to be thought as an encoder network. As noted in [4,5], the use of a recurrent network allows to work with sequences which have variable lengths. This is a significant advantage given the heterogeneity of the number of visits in medical longitudinals studies. In practice, the observations of the subject are not regularly spaced in time. To allow the network to adapt to this, we provide the ages of the visit at each update of the RNN.

We use an Elman network, which has a hidden state $h \in \mathbf{R}^H$ with $H \in \mathbf{N}$, initialized to $h_0 = 0$ and updated along the sequence according to $h_k = \rho_h(W_h y_{ik} + U_h h_{k-1} + b_h)$ and the final value predicted by the network after a sequence of length $f \in \mathbf{N}$ is $\varphi = W_\varphi \rho_\varphi(h_f) + b_z$ where ρ_φ and ρ_h are activation functions and $W_h, U_h, W_\varphi, b_h, b_\varphi$ are the weights and biases of the network. We denote $\theta = (W_h, U_h, W_\varphi, b_\varphi)$ the parameters of the encoder.

When working with scalar data, we use this architecture directly. When working with images, we first use a convolutional neural network to extract relevant features from the images which are then fed to the RNN. In this case, both the convolutional network and the recurrent network are trained jointly by back-propagation. Figure 1 summarizes the whole procedure.

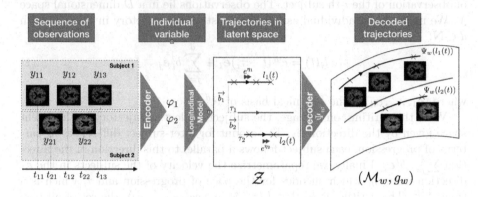

Fig. 1. The observed sequences are encoded into latent trajectories, which are then decoded into geodesics on a submanifold of the observation space.

2.4   Regularization

To impose some structure in the latent space $\mathcal{Z}$, we impose a regularization on the individual variables $\varphi_i = (\eta_i, \tau_i, b_i^2, \ldots, b_i^d)$. The regularization cost used is:

$$r(\eta, \tau, b^2, \ldots, b^d) = \frac{(\eta - \overline{\eta})^2}{\sigma_\eta^2} + \frac{(\tau - \overline{\tau})^2}{\sigma_\tau^2} + \sum_{j=2}^{d}(b^j)^2 \qquad (2)$$

This regularization requires the individual variables η and τ to be close to mean values $\overline{\tau}, \overline{\eta}$. The parameters $\overline{\eta}$, $\overline{\tau}$ are estimated during the inference. $\sigma_\eta > 0$ is fixed but the estimation of $\overline{\eta}$ allows to adjust the typical variation of η with respect to the mean pace $\overline{\eta}$, while the neural network Ψ_w adjusts accordingly the actual velocity in the observation space in the e_1 direction. σ_τ is set to the empirical standard deviation of the time distribution $(t_{ij})_{ij}$, meaning that we expect the delays between subjects to be of the same order as the standard deviation of the visit ages.

2.5   Cost Function and Inference

Overall, we optimize the cost function:

$$c(\theta, w, \overline{\eta}, \overline{\tau}) = \sum_i \sum_j \frac{\|y_i(t_{ij}) - y_{ij}\|_2^2}{\sigma^2} + \sum_i r(\varphi_i) \qquad (3)$$

where $\sigma > 0$ is a parameter controlling the trade-off reconstruction/regularity.

The first term contains the requirements that the geometry $(\mathcal{M}_w, g_w)$ be adapted to the observed progressions since it requires geodesics $y_i(t)$ to be good reconstructions of the individual trajectories. As shown in the Appendix, there exists solutions to problems of this kind: under mild conditions there exists a metric on a Riemannian manifold that the subjects progressions are geodesics. But this is only a partial constraint: there is a whole class of metrics which have geodesics in common (see [13] for the analysis of metrics which have a given family of trajectories as geodesics).

We infer the parameters of the model by stochastic gradient descent using the Adam optimizer [9]. After each batch of subjects B, we balance regularity and reconstruction by imposing a closed-form update on σ:

$$\sigma^2 = \frac{1}{N_B D} \sum_{i \in B} \sum_{j=1}^{N_i} \|\Psi_w(l_i(t_{ij})) - y_{ij}\|_2^2 \tag{4}$$

where $N_B = \sum_{i \in B} N_i$ is the total number of observations in the batch b. This automatic update of the trade-off criterion σ is inspired from Bayesian generative models which estimate the variance of the residual noise, as in e.g. [14,20].

3 Experimental Results

The neural network architectures and the source code for these experiments is available at gitlab.icm-institute.org/maxime.louis/unsupervised_geometric _longitudinal, tag IPMI 2019. For all experiments, the ages of the subjects are first normalized to have zero mean and unit variance. This allows the positions in the latent space to remain close to 0. We set $\sigma_\eta = 0.5$ and initialize $\bar{\eta}$ to 0.

3.1 On a Synthetic Set of Images

To validate the proposed methodology, we first perform a set of experiments on a synthetic data set. We generate 64×64 gray level images of a white cross on a black background. Each cross is described by the arms length and angles. We prescribe a mean scenario of progression for the arm lengths and sample the arm angles for each subject from a zero-centered normal distribution. Figure 2 shows subjects generated along this procedure. Note that with

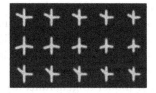

Fig. 2. Each row represents a synthetic subject.

this setting, an image varies smoothly with respect to the arms lengths and angles and hence the whole set of generated images is a smooth manifold.

We generate 10 training sets of 150 subjects and 10 test sets of 50 subjects. The number of observation of each subject is randomly sampled from a Poisson distribution with mean 5. The times at which the subject are observed are equally spaced within a randomly selected time window. We add different level of white noise on the images. We then run the inference on the 10 training sets for each level of noise. We set the dimension of the latent space $\mathcal{Z}$ to 3 for all the experiments.

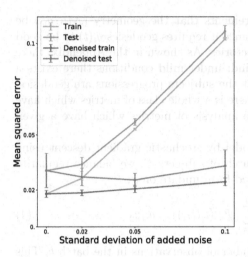

Fig. 3. Reconstruction error on train and test sets and on denoised train and test sets, unseen during training.

For each run, we estimate the reconstruction error on both training set and test set, as well as the reconstruction error to the de-noised images, which were not seen during training. Results are shown on Fig. 3. The model generalizes well to unseen data and successfully denoises the images, with a reconstruction error on the denoised images which does not vary with the scale of the added white noise. This means that the generated manifold of images is close to the manifold on which the original images lie. Besides, as shown on Fig. 4, the scenario of progression along the e_1 direction is well captured, while orthogonal directions e_2, e_3 allow to change the arm positions. Finally, we compare the individual variables (b_i^2, b_i^3) to the known arms angles which were used to generate the images. Figure 5 shows the results: the latent space is structured in a way that is faithful to the original arm angles.

3.2   On Cognitive Scores

We use the cognitive scores grading the subjects memory, praxis, language and concentration from the ADNI database as in [14]. Each score is renormalized to vary between 0 and 1, with large values indicating poor performances for the task. Overall, the data set consists of 223 subjects observed 6 times on average over 2.9 years. We perform a 10-fold estimation of the model. The measured mean squared reconstruction error is $0.079 \pm 1.1e-3$ on the train sets, while it is of $0.085 \pm 1.5e-3$ for the test sets. Both are close to the uncertainty in the estimation of these cognitive scores [18]. This illustrates the ability of the model to generalize to unseen observations. First, this indicates that M_w is a submanifold which is close to all the observations. Second, it indicates how relevant the learned Riemannian metric is, since unobserved subject trajectories are very close to geodesics on the Riemannian manifold.

Figure 6 shows obtained average trajectories $t \mapsto \Psi_w(e^{\bar{\eta}} e_0(t - \bar{\tau}))$ for a 10-fold estimation of the model on the data set, with $\mathcal{Z}$ dimension set to 2. All of these trajectories are brought back to a common time reference frame using the estimated $\bar{\tau}$ and $\bar{\eta}$. All average trajectories are very similar, underlining the stability of the proposed method. Note that despite the small average observation time of the subjects, the method proposed here allows to robustly obtain a mean scenario of progression over 30 years. Hence, despite all the flexibility that is provided through the different neural networks and the individual parameters, the model still exhibits a low variance.

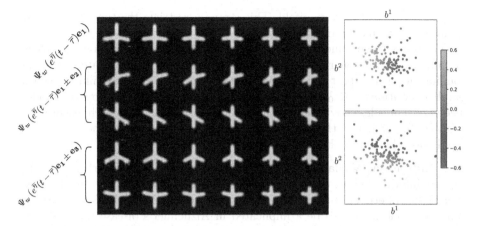

Fig. 4. First row is $t \mapsto \Psi_\theta(e_1 t)$. Following rows are $t \mapsto \Psi_\theta(e_1 t + e_i)$ for $i \in \{2, 3\}$. These parallel directions of progression show the same arm length reduction with different arm positions.

Fig. 5. Individual variables b_i^1 and b_i^2 colored by left (top) and right (bottom) arm angle. (Color figure online)

We compare the results to the mean trajectory estimated by the model [14], which is shown on Fig. 8. Both cases recover the expected order of onset of the different cognitive symptoms in the disease progression. Note that with our model the progression of the concentration score is much faster than the progression of the memory score, although it starts later: this type of behaviour is not allowed with the model described in [14] where the family of possible trajectories is much narrower. Indeed, because it is difficult to craft a relevant Riemannian metric for the data at hand, the authors modelled the data as lying on a product Riemannian manifold. In this case, a geodesic on the product manifold is a prod-

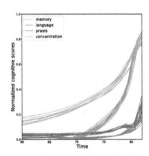

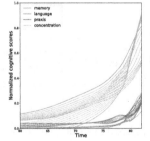

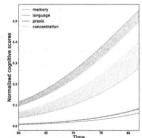

Fig. 6. Learned main progression of the cognitive scores, for the 10-fold estimation.

Fig. 7. Mean geodesic of progression and parallel variations $t \mapsto \Psi(e^{\overline{\eta}} e_0(t - \overline{\tau}) + \lambda e_1)$ for varying λ.

Fig. 8. Mean geodesic of progression and parallel variations for the model with user-defined metric.

uct of geodesics of each manifold. This strongly restricts the type of dynamics spanned by the model and hence gives it a high bias.

The use of the product manifold also has an impact on the parallel variations around the mean scenario: they can only delay and slow/accelerate one of the component with respect to another, as shown on Fig. 8. Figure 7 illustrates the parallel variations $\Psi(\overline{\alpha}e_0(t - \overline{\tau}) + e_1)$ one can observe with the proposed model. The variation is less trivial since complex interactions between each features are possible. In particular, the concentration score varies more in the early stages of the disease than in the late stages.

The Individual Variables φ. To show that the individual variables φ_i did capture information regarding the disease progression, we compare the distribution of the τ_i between subjects who have at least one APOE4 allele of the APOE gene -an allele known to be a implicated in Alzheimer's disease- and subjects which have no APOE4 allele of this gene. We perform a Mann-Whitney test on the distributions to see if they differ. For all folds, a p-value lower than 5% is obtained. For all folds, carriers have a larger τ meaning that they have an earlier disease onset than non-carriers. This is in accordance with [2]. Similarly, women have on average an earlier disease onset for all folds, in accordance with [11].

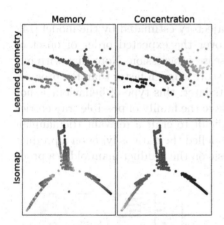

Fig. 9. Top (resp. bottom) latent positions (resp. isomap embedding) of the observations colored by memory and concentration score. (Color figure online)

A Closer Look at the Geometry. We look at the obtained Riemannian geometry by computing the latent position best mapped onto each of the observation by Ψ_w. We then plot the obtained latent positions to look at the structure of the learned Riemannian manifold. We compare the obtained structure with a visualisation of the structure induced by the ℓ^2 on the space of observations produced by Isomap [19]. Isomap is a manifold learning technique which attempts to reconstruct in low dimensions the geodesic distances computed from a set of observations. The results are shown on Fig. 9. The geometry obtained after inference is clearly much more suited for disease progression modelling. Indeed, the e_1 direction does correspond to typical increases in the different scores. The induced metric is not as adapted. This highlights the relevance of the learned geometry for disease modelling.

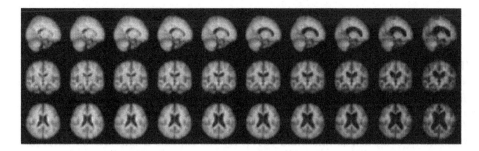

Fig. 10. $t \mapsto \Psi_\theta(e_0 t)$ on the MRI dataset. The growth of the ventricles, characteristic of aging and Alzheimer's disease is clearly visible.

3.3   On Anatomical MRIs

We propose here an estimation of the model on 3D MRIs preprocessed from the ADNI database, to check the behaviour of the proposed method in high dimension. We select subjects which ultimately convert to Alzheimer's disease. We obtain 325 subjects and a total of 1996 MRIs which we affinely align on the Colin-27 template and resample to $64 \times 64 \times 64$. We run a 5-fold estimation of the model with $\dim \mathcal{Z} = 10$, using a GPU backend. We obtain a train mean squared error of $0.002 \pm 1e - 5$ and a test mean squared error of $0.0024 \pm 3e - 5$. Figure 10 shows one of the learned mean trajectory.

Once the model is estimated, we compare the distributions of the pace of progressions η_i between the individuals who have at least one APOE4 allele of the APOE gene and the individuals who have no APOE4 allele. For all 5 folds, the distributions of the paces of progression significantly differ, with p-values lower than 5% and in each case, the APOE4 carriers have a greater pace of progression, in accordance with [2]. The same analysis between the individuals who have two APOE4 allele versus the individuals which have at maximum one APOE4 allele shows a significative difference for all folds for the τ variable: the APOE4 carriers have an earlier disease onset, as shown in [11]. This analysis further shows the value of the individual variables φ_i learned for each subject.

4   Conclusion

We presented a way to perform Riemannian geometry learning in the context of longitudinal trajectory analysis. We showed that we could build a local Riemannian submanifold of the space of observations which is so that each subject follows a geodesic parallel to a main geodesic of progression on this manifold. We illustrated how the encoding of each subject into these trajectories is informative of the disease progression. The latent space $\mathcal{Z}$ built in this process is a low-dimensional description of the disease progression. There are several possible continuations of this work. First, there is the possibility to conduct the same analysis on multiple modalities of data simultaneously. Then, after estimation, the latent space $\mathcal{Z}$ could be useful to perform classification and prediction tasks.

A   Existence of a Riemannian Metric Such that a Family of Curves Are Geodesics

Theorem 1. *Let $\mathcal{M}$ be a smooth manifold and $(\gamma_i)_{i \in \{1,\ldots,n\}}$ be a family of smooth regular injective curves on $\mathcal{M}$ which do not intersect. There exists a Riemannian metric g such that γ_i is a geodesic on $(\mathcal{M}, g)$ for all $i \in \{1, \ldots, n\}$.*

Proof. Open Neighborhood of the Curves. Let $i \in I$. Since γ_i is injective and regular, $\gamma_i([0, 1])$ is a submanifold of $\mathcal{M}$. By the tubular neighborhood theorem, there exists a vector bundle E_i on $\gamma_i([0, 1])$ and a diffeomorphism Φ_i from a neighborhood U_i of the 0-section in E_i to a neighborhood V_i of $\gamma_i([0, 1])$ in $\mathcal{M}$ such that $\Phi_i \circ 0_{E_i} = i_i$ where i_i is the embedding of $\gamma_i([0, 1])$ in $\mathcal{M}$. Without loss of generality, we can suppose $\gamma_j([0, 1]) \cap U_i = \emptyset$ for all $j \neq i$.

Riemannian Metric on the Neighborhoods. To do so, we use the fact that E_i is diffeomorphic to the normal bundle on the segment $[0, 1] \in \mathbf{R}$ which is trivial and which we denote N. Let $\Psi_i : E_i \mapsto N$ be such a diffeomorphism. Now N can be equipped with a Riemannian metric h_i such that $[0, 1]$ is a geodesic. Using Ψ_i and Φ_i, we can push-forward the metric h_i to get a metric g_i on U which is so that γ_i is a geodesic on (U_i, g_i).

Stitching the Metrics with a Partition of Unity. For each $i \in \{1, \ldots, n\}$, pick an open subset V_i such that $V_i \subset \overline{V_i} \subset U_i$ and which contains $\gamma_i([0, 1])$, and set $O = \mathcal{M} \backslash (\cup_i \overline{V_i})$. O is open so that $\mathcal{C} = \{O, U_1, \ldots, U_n\}$ is an open cover of $\mathcal{M}$. O can be equipped with a metric g_O (there always exists a Riemannian metric on a smooth manifold). Finally, we use a partition of the unity $\rho_O, \rho_1, \ldots, \rho_n$ on $\mathcal{C}$ and set $g = \rho_O g_O + \sum_i \rho_i g_i$. g is a Riemannian metric on $\mathcal{M}$ as a positive combination of Riemannian metrics. Each γ_i is a geodesic on $(\mathcal{M}, g)$ by construction. $\square$

In [13], the authors deal with a more general case but obtain a less explicit existence result. This theorem motivates our approach even if in Eq. (3) we ask for more: we want the existence a system of coordinates adapted to the progression.

References

1. Arvanitidis, G., Hansen, L.K., Hauberg, S.: A locally adaptive normal distribution. In: Advances in Neural Information Processing Systems, pp. 4251–4259 (2016)
2. Bigio, E., Hynan, L., Sontag, E., Satumtira, S., White, C.: Synapse loss is greater in presenile than senile onset Alzheimer disease: implications for the cognitive reserve hypothesis. Neuropathol. Appl. Neurobiol. **28**(3), 218–227 (2002)
3. Bône, A., Colliot, O., Durrleman, S.: Learning distributions of shape trajectories from longitudinal datasets: a hierarchical model on a manifold of diffeomorphisms. arXiv preprint arXiv:1803.10119 (2018)
4. Cui, R., Liu, M., Li, G.: Longitudinal analysis for Alzheimer's disease diagnosis using RNN. In: 2018 IEEE 15th International Symposium on Biomedical Imaging, ISBI 2018, pp. 1398–1401. IEEE (2018)

5. Gao, L., Pan, H., Liu, F., Xie, X., Zhang, Z., Han, J.: Brain disease diagnosis using deep learning features from longitudinal MR images. In: Cai, Y., Ishikawa, Y., Xu, J. (eds.) APWeb-WAIM 2018. LNCS, vol. 10987, pp. 327–339. Springer, Cham (2018). https://doi.org/10.1007/978-3-319-96890-2_27

6. Hauberg, S., Freifeld, O., Black, M.J.: A geometric take on metric learning. In: Advances in Neural Information Processing Systems, pp. 2024–2032 (2012)

7. Jack Jr., C.R., et al.: The Alzheimer's disease neuroimaging initiative (ADNI): MRI methods. J. Magn. Reson. Imaging Off. J. Int. Soc. Magn. Reson. Med. **27**(4), 685–691 (2008)

8. Jacobsen, J.H., Smeulders, A., Oyallon, E.: i-RevNet: deep invertible networks. arXiv preprint arXiv:1802.07088 (2018)

9. Kingma, D.P., Ba, J.: Adam: a method for stochastic optimization. arXiv preprint arXiv:1412.6980 (2014)

10. Koval, I., et al.: Statistical learning of spatiotemporal patterns from longitudinal manifold-valued networks. In: Descoteaux, M., Maier-Hein, L., Franz, A., Jannin, P., Collins, D.L., Duchesne, S. (eds.) MICCAI 2017. LNCS, vol. 10433, pp. 451–459. Springer, Cham (2017). https://doi.org/10.1007/978-3-319-66182-7_52

11. Lam, B., Masellis, M., Freedman, M., Stuss, D.T., Black, S.E.: Clinical, imaging, and pathological heterogeneity of the Alzheimer's disease syndrome. Alzheimer's Res. Ther. **5**(1), 1 (2013)

12. Lebanon, G.: Learning riemannian metrics. In: Proceedings of the Nineteenth Conference on Uncertainty in Artificial Intelligence, pp. 362–369. Morgan Kaufmann Publishers Inc. (2002)

13. Matveev, V.S.: Geodesically equivalent metrics in general relativity. J. Geom. Phys. **62**(3), 675–691 (2012)

14. Schiratti, J.B., Allassonniere, S., Colliot, O., Durrleman, S.: Learning spatiotemporal trajectories from manifold-valued longitudinal data. In: Advances in Neural Information Processing Systems, pp. 2404–2412 (2015)

15. Shao, H., Kumar, A., Fletcher, P.T.: The riemannian geometry of deep generative models. arXiv preprint arXiv:1711.08014 (2017)

16. Singh, N., Hinkle, J., Joshi, S., Fletcher, P.T.: Hierarchical geodesic models in diffeomorphisms. Int. J. Comput. Vis. **117**(1), 70–92 (2016)

17. Sommer, S., Arnaudon, A., Kuhnel, L., Joshi, S.: Bridge simulation and metric estimation on landmark manifolds. In: Cardoso, M.J., et al. (eds.) GRAIL/MFCA/MICGen -2017. LNCS, vol. 10551, pp. 79–91. Springer, Cham (2017). https://doi.org/10.1007/978-3-319-67675-3_8

18. Standish, T.I., Molloy, D.W., Bédard, M., Layne, E.C., Murray, E.A., Strang, D.: Improved reliability of the standardized Alzheimer's disease assessment scale (SADAS) compared with the Alzheimer's disease assessment scale (ADAS). J. Am. Geriatr. Soc. **44**(6), 712–716 (1996)

19. Tenenbaum, J.B., De Silva, V., Langford, J.C.: A global geometric framework for nonlinear dimensionality reduction. Science **290**(5500), 2319–2323 (2000)

20. Zhang, M., Fletcher, T.: Probabilistic principal geodesic analysis. In: Advances in Neural Information Processing Systems, pp. 1178–1186 (2013)

Semi-supervised Brain Lesion Segmentation with an Adapted Mean Teacher Model

Wenhui Cui[1], Yanlin Liu[2], Yuxing Li[2], Menghao Guo[1], Yiming Li[3], Xiuli Li[3,4], Tianle Wang[5], Xiangzhu Zeng[6], and Chuyang Ye[2(✉)]

[1] School of Computer Science and Technology, Xidian University, Xi'an, China
[2] School of Information and Electronics, Beijing Institute of Technology, Beijing, China
chuyang.ye@bit.edu.cn
[3] Deepwise AI Lab, Beijing, China
[4] Peng Cheng Laboratory, Shenzhen, China
[5] Department of Radiology, The People's Hospital of Nantong, Nantong, China
[6] Department of Radiology, Peking University Third Hospital, Beijing, China

Abstract. Automated brain lesion segmentation provides valuable information for the analysis and intervention of patients. In particular, methods that are based on *convolutional neural networks* (CNNs) have achieved state-of-the-art segmentation performance. However, CNNs usually require a decent amount of annotated data, which may be costly and time-consuming to obtain. Since unannotated data is generally abundant, it is desirable to use unannotated data to improve the segmentation performance for CNNs when limited annotated data is available. In this work, we propose a *semi-supervised learning* (SSL) approach to brain lesion segmentation, where unannotated data is incorporated into the training of CNNs. We adapt the mean teacher model, which is originally developed for SSL-based image classification, for brain lesion segmentation. Assuming that the network should produce consistent outputs for similar inputs, a loss of segmentation consistency is designed and integrated into a self-ensembling framework. Self-ensembling exploits the information in the intermediate training steps, and the ensemble prediction based on the information can be closer to the correct result than the single latest model. To exploit such information, we build a student model and a teacher model, which share the same CNN architecture for segmentation. The student and teacher models are updated alternately. At each step, the student model learns from the teacher model by minimizing the weighted sum of the segmentation loss computed from annotated data and the segmentation consistency loss between the teacher and student models computed from unannotated data. Then, the teacher model is updated by combining the updated student model with the historical information of teacher models using an exponential moving average strategy. For demonstration, the proposed approach was evaluated on ischemic stroke lesion segmentation. Results indicate that the proposed method improves stroke lesion segmentation with the incorporation of unannotated data and outperforms competing SSL-based methods.

© Springer Nature Switzerland AG 2019
A. C. S. Chung et al. (Eds.): IPMI 2019, LNCS 11492, pp. 554–565, 2019.
https://doi.org/10.1007/978-3-030-20351-1_43

Keywords: Semi-supervised learning · Brain lesion segmentation ·
Mean teacher model

1   Introduction

Automated segmentation of brain lesions in *magnetic resonance images* (MRIs)
provides valuable information for the analysis and intervention of patients [6].
Deep learning based approaches have been developed for the segmentation of
different types of brain lesions, such as stroke lesions [6,7] and brain tumors [4,
10,15]. Various architectures of *convolutional neural networks* (CNNs) have been
proposed and have achieved state-of-the-art segmentation performance. Deep
learning based approaches usually involve a huge number of parameters and
thus require a decent amount of annotated data, so that the parameters can be
properly learned [14]. However, manual annotation of brain lesions is costly and
time-consuming, whereas unannotated data is often abundant. Therefore, it is
desirable to exploit the unannotated data when there is limited annotated data
for training.

Semi-supervised learning (SSL) techniques have emerged as means to combine the limited annotated data and the abundant unannotated data to improve
the training process [16]. Several methods have been proposed for medical image
segmentation [1,14]. For example, the consistency of feature embedding between
annotated and unannotated data is enforced in [1], where a consistency loss is
incorporated into the loss function and provides regularization for training the
CNN. A similar idea is developed in [5], where the consistency of feature embedding is ensured with an adversarial learning strategy. Note that although the
approach in [5] is originally developed for transfer learning, it can be applied
to SSL as well. Another approach in [14] aims to achieve similar quality of segmentation on the annotated and unannotated data. The similarity is encouraged
with a deep adversarial network model, which consists of a segmentation network
and an evaluation network. These approaches have achieved promising results
when limited annotated data is available. However, the development of SSL techniques for CNN-based brain lesion segmentation is still an open problem, where
improved segmentation performance is desired.

In this work, we explore the integration of SSL into CNN-based brain lesion
segmentation. Inspired by the success of the *mean teacher* (MT) model [11] for
SSL-based image classification, we propose an adapted MT model for brain lesion
segmentation, where both annotated and unannotated data can be exploited to
boost segmentation performance.

We assume that the segmentation should be consistent for similar input
data [8], and define a segmentation consistency loss, which is computed for a
pair of inputs that are obtained by adding noises to the same unannotated
sample. In this way, unannotated data can be incorporated into the learning
process and provide regularization information. Note that unlike in previous
works [1,14] that measure the consistency between annotated data and unannotated data, here the consistency is computed between two noisy versions of the

same unannotated data. Since it is observed in [8] and [11] that self-ensembling could lead to better classification models, we apply a similar strategy to brain lesion segmentation and integrate the segmentation consistency loss into the self-ensembling framework. Specifically, we build a teacher model and a student model, which share the same network architecture. In this work we select the DeepMedic architecture [6] for the two models, because it has achieved state-of-the-art performance in brain lesion segmentation [9]. Self-ensembling is based on the observation that the ensemble prediction combining the network information after each step is more accurate than the current output [8,11]. Thus, the teacher model records the information at each step, and the student model learns from the teacher model by minimizing the loss of segmentation accuracy for annotated data and the consistency loss with respect to the outputs of the teacher model for unannotated data. Then, the teacher model is updated by combining the historical information of teacher models and the current student model with an *exponential moving average* (EMA) strategy. The student and teacher models are updated alternately, and the final teacher model is used for segmentation on test samples.

For demonstration, the proposed approach was evaluated on ischemic stroke lesion segmentation. Results indicate that the proposed method improves the segmentation quality by incorporating unannotated data and outperforms competing SSL-based segmentation strategies.

2   Methods

In this section, we first introduce the backbone CNN architecture shared by the teacher and student models. Then, we describe how unannotated data is used by the teacher and student models to regularize the model training. Finally, implementation details are given.

2.1   Backbone CNN Architecture

Due to its superior segmentation performance, the DeepMedic model [6] is used as our backbone network structure, which is shared by the teacher and student models. Specifically, DeepMedic is a dual pathway, 11-layer deep, three-dimensional CNN, and it performs multi-scale processing via parallel convolutional pathways. A graphical illustration of DeepMedic is shown in Fig. 1, and the parameters of each layer are summarized in Table 1. Note that the two pathways use the same settings of convolutional layers 1–8 in Table 1. DeepMedic takes image patches at two different resolutions as input. The two patches are centered at the same image location. The upper pathway in Fig. 1 takes normal resolution image patches as input, whereas the bottom pathway in Fig. 1 operates on downsampled patches (by a factor of three). Before the final segmentation, the multi-scale features are concatenated and fed into 1^3 convolutional layers. For more details about DeepMedic, we refer readers to [6].

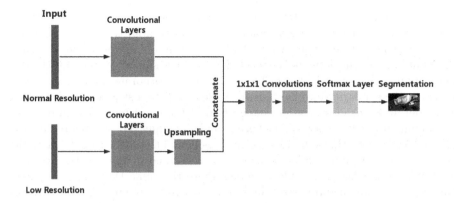

Fig. 1. The DeepMedic model proposed in [6].

Table 1. The specification of layers in DeepMedic.

Layer	Parameters
Convolutional layer 1	30 filters, 3^3
Convolutional layer 2	30 filters, 3^3
Convolutional layer 3	40 filters, 3^3
Convolutional layer 4	40 filters, 3^3
Convolutional layer 5	40 filters, 3^3
Convolutional layer 6	40 filters, 3^3
Convolutional layer 7	50 filters, 3^3
Convolutional layer 8	50 filters, 3^3
1^3 Convolution	250 filters, 1^3
1^3 Convolution	250 filters, 1^3

2.2 Semi-supervised Lesion Segmentation with an Adapted MT Model

To leverage the abundant unannotated data for lesion segmentation, we propose to use an SSL strategy. Our strategy is inspired by the MT model [11], which is developed for SSL-based image classification. Like in the MT model, we assume that CNN models should favor functions that produce consistent outputs for similar inputs. Pairs of similar input samples are generated by adding noises to the same unannotated data. In this way, unannotated data can be used to provide regularization for training the network. Note that unlike MT, we need to measure the consistency of segmentation instead of classification. Thus, we adapt the MT strategy by defining a segmentation consistency loss. The segmentation consistency loss is then integrated into a self-ensembling framework, which is motivated by the observation that the ensemble prediction based on the combined information after each step can be more accurate than the current output [11]. The detailed description of the proposed approach is given below.

For an unannotated input X_u, we add noises η and η' sampled from the same distribution, and the network is expected to produce similar outputs for the two noisy inputs. Although it is possible to directly incorporate a consistency loss based on the similarity into DeepMedic, which leads to a strategy similar to the Π model in [8] for classification, integration of the consistency loss into a self-ensembling framework can lead to better model training [11]. Therefore, like the original MT approach, we build a teacher model and a student model, where the student model attempts to learn the targets generated by the teacher model.

Both the teacher and student models share the same DeepMedic architecture [6]. Note that the proposed framework is not restricted to a specific segmentation network, and can be applied to other backbone segmentation architectures as well, such as 3D U-Net [2]. The two noisy inputs associated with η and η' are then fed into the student model and the teacher model, respectively. Since the student and teacher models share the same architecture, we denote their output for the noisy input as $f(X_u, \eta, \theta)$ and $f(X_u, \eta', \theta')$, respectively. Here, θ and θ' are the weights in the network of the student model and the teacher model, respectively.

The teacher model is initialized with the DeepMedic network trained with annotated data. Then, the teacher and student models are updated alternately. At each step, the student model learns from the teacher model by minimizing the weighted sum of the consistency loss $\mathcal{L}_c$ of unannotated data and segmentation loss $\mathcal{L}_s$ of annotated data. Specifically, we define $\mathcal{L}_c$ as the soft Dice loss between the predicted probability maps of the student and teacher models based on their corresponding noisy inputs

$$\mathcal{L}_c = 1 - \mathbb{E}_{X_u, \eta, \eta'} \left[\frac{1}{K} \sum_{i=1}^{K} \frac{\sum_{v=1}^{V} 2 f_v^i(X_u, \eta, \theta) f_v^i(X_u, \eta', \theta')}{\sum_{v=1}^{V} f_v^i(X_u, \eta, \theta) + \sum_{v=1}^{V} f_v^i(X_u, \eta', \theta')} \right] \qquad (1)$$

where $f_v^i(\cdot)$ represents the $f(\cdot)$ value that is at the v-th voxel and takes the i-th label, K represents the total number of possible labels, and V denotes the total number of voxels in the input. With the loss defined in Eq. (1), the output of the teacher model can also be considered a target label for the student model to learn. As in DeepMedic [6], $\mathcal{L}_s$ is the cross entropy loss between the predictions $f(X_a, \theta)$ (no noise η is applied) of the student model for the annotated input X_a and the corresponding annotation Y

$$\mathcal{L}_s = -\mathbb{E}_{X_a, Y} \left[\frac{1}{V} \sum_{v=1}^{V} \sum_{i=1}^{K} Y_v^i \log \left(f_v^i(X_a, \theta) \right) \right], \qquad (2)$$

where Y_v^i represents the value of Y at the v-th voxel with label i.

Then, the total loss function $\mathcal{L}$ of our model is

$$\mathcal{L} = \mathcal{L}_s + \beta \mathcal{L}_c, \qquad (3)$$

where β is an adaptive weighting coefficient. As suggested in [11], different β is used at different steps. Specifically, $\beta = \exp\left(-5(1 - \frac{S}{L})^2\right)$ (when $S \leq L$), where S is the current training step and L is called the ramp-up length; when $S > L$, β is set to one. In our experiment, we empirically set $L = 400$. Such an adaptive setting of β keeps the effect of consistency down in early steps, because the teacher model may not generate reasonable target labels at the beginning [11].

With the parameters θ_t of the student model at step t, we perform the EMA of weights to aggregate information in training steps as in the original MT model [11]. Specifically, we update the teacher model as follows

$$\theta'_t = \alpha\theta'_{t-1} + (1 - \alpha)\theta_t, \tag{4}$$

where α is the EMA decay. Compared with other ensembling strategies [8], EMA better prevents overfitting, especially when a large number of model parameters are learned from limited training data [11]. Following the MT method [11], we used $\alpha = 0.99$ in the first L steps (the ramp-up phase), and $\alpha = 0.999$ for the rest of the training. This strategy facilitates the teacher model to (1) forget the old inaccurate student weights quickly and (2) benefit from a longer memory when the student improvement slows down after the ramp-up phase. The final teacher model is used to perform lesion segmentation for test samples.

2.3 Implementation Details

The proposed method is implemented using TensorFlow (https://www.tensorflow.org). In the training of student models, we followed the settings in [6] and minimized the loss with an RMSProp optimizer [12], where the learning rate is 0.0001 and the decay rate is 0.9. The batch size is 16, which consists of eight annotated and eight unannotated samples. Both the annotated and unannotated training patches were sampled from the lesion region and healthy tissue with equal probability, which mitigates class imbalance [6]. Note that since the lesion region is unknown for unannotated data, it is approximated by the DeepMedic prediction.

The noise injection for the proposed method was applied as follows. We applied Gaussian noises to the inputs of the student and teacher models. Noise η consists of two different types: the additive noise η_s and the multiplicative noise η_m. Both are sampled from Gaussian distributions. At each voxel of the input patch, noise was applied independently, and the noisy intensity I' is computed from the original intensity I as follows

$$I' = (I + \eta_s) \times \eta_m. \tag{5}$$

3 Experiments

3.1 Data Description

For demonstration, the proposed method was evaluated on a task of ischemic stroke lesion segmentation. A total number of 246 *diffusion weighted images* (DWIs) of ischemic stroke patients were acquired on a 3T Siemens Verio scanner, where a b-value of 1000 s/mm^2 was applied and a $b0$ image (the image without diffusion weighting) was also acquired. The image resolution is 0.96 mm × 0.96 mm × 6.5 mm and the image dimension is 240 × 240 × 21. Manual delineations of stroke lesions were performed by an experienced radiologist on 50 DWIs, and the rest 196 DWIs are unannotated.

The image intensities were normalized for each scan. Specifically, a brain mask was extracted with the Dipy software [3]. Then, the mean and standard deviation of the intensity in the brain were computed. The mean was subtracted from the intensity at each voxel in the skull-stripped image and the resulting intensities were further divided by the standard deviation. The patch sizes for the normal resolution and downsampled pathways are 37 × 37 × 21 and 23 × 23 × 18, respectively, so that the multi-scale features can be concatenated. The additive noise was sampled from a Gaussian distribution which has a zero mean and a standard deviation of 0.05, whereas the multiplicative noise was sampled from a Gaussian distribution which has a mean of 1.0 and a standard deviation of 0.01.

3.2 Training Phase

We randomly selected 20 annotated subjects as training scans, and used the rest 30 annotated data as test scans. The 196 unannotated scans were included in the training process of the proposed approach as well. The training was performed on an NVIDIA GeForce GTX 1080Ti GPU, and it took about 12 h. The training process was evaluated and the Dice coefficients of the training data are shown for the student and teacher models in Fig. 2. We can see that both models better fit the training data as the training continues and become stable in the end. In addition, the teacher model consistently achieves higher Dice coefficients than the student model, until it is close to the end of the ramp-up phase (400 steps), where the two Dice coefficients are close. These observations are consistent with the assumption in self-ensembling and the settings of the EMA decay.

3.3 Evaluation of Lesion Segmentation

Then, we evaluated the segmentation results of the proposed method. The proposed method was compared with three methods. The DeepMedic approach [6] was included as the baseline method that does not use unannotated data for training. The strategy used by [14] was also integrated with DeepMedic for comparison, which performs SSL-based image segmentation. This strategy assumes that the segmentation of unannotated data should follow a distribution that is similar to that of annotated data. Such similarity is enforced by a separate evaluation network with adversarial learning. We replaced the segmentation network in [14] with DeepMedic for lesion segmentation. Due to the use of an evaluation network, this strategy is referred to as DeepMedic-EN. The network in [5] for unsupervised domain adaptation was also considered, because although it is originally developed for transfer learning, it can be directly used for SSL. This strategy applies an idea that is similar to [14], where adversarial learning is

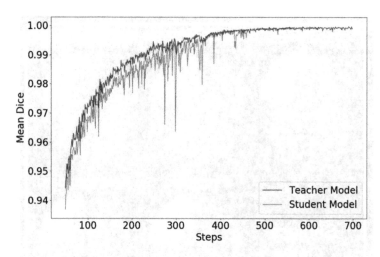

Fig. 2. The mean Dice coefficients of the training data for the teacher model and the student model after each training step.

applied so that the features extracted from the source (annotated) and target (unannotated) data follow similar distributions. Since the deep network in [5] is based on the DeepMedic architecture, we used the structure directly, and the method is referred to as DeepMedic-UDA, where UDA stands for unsupervised domain adaptation as described by [5].

We first qualitatively evaluated the proposed method. Cross-sectional views of the segmentation results overlaid on DWIs are shown in Fig. 3 for two representative test subjects with different sizes of lesions. The gold standard of the manual delineation and the results of the competing methods are also shown for comparison. It can be seen that the proposed method produced segmentation that better agrees with the gold standard.

Next, the proposed method was quantitatively evaluated. We computed the Dice coefficients on the test scans for the proposed and competing methods, and the results are summarized in Table 2. Here, the means and standard deviations of the Dice coefficients computed from the 30 test subjects are listed. The proposed method has the highest mean Dice coefficients, which indicates its better segmentation quality than the competing methods. In addition, the results were compared between the proposed method and each competing method with a paired Student's t-test. In all cases, the difference is significant ($p < 0.05$). Note that DeepMedic-EN and DeepMedic-UDA have smaller mean Dice coefficients than the baseline DeepMedic. This is possibly due to the limited number of training scans, which cannot adequately represent the distribution of annotated data. Thus, the adversarial learning in DeepMedic-EN and DeepMedic-UDA may incorrectly modify the segmentation result.

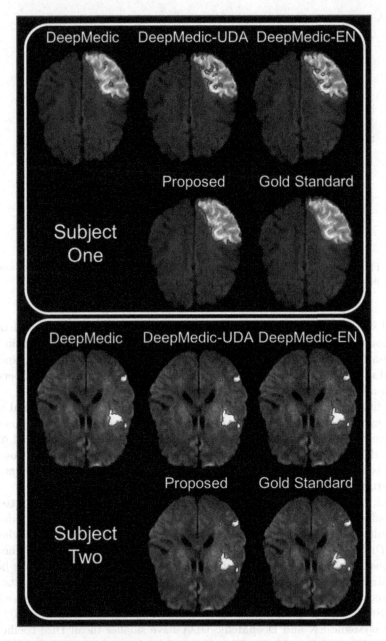

Fig. 3. Cross-sectional views of the segmentation results overlaid on DWIs for two representative test subjects with different sizes of lesions.

Table 2. Means and standard deviations of the Dice coefficients on test scans when 20 annotated scans were used for training. Best results are highlighted in bold font. Asterisks (*) indicate that the difference between the proposed method and the competing method is statistically significant ($p < 0.05$) using a paired Student's t-test.

DeepMedic	DeepMedic-UDA	DeepMedic-EN	Proposed
$0.6312 \pm 0.2617^*$	$0.6096 \pm 0.2819^*$	$0.6236 \pm 0.2577^*$	$\mathbf{0.6676 \pm 0.2392}$

Table 3. Means and standard deviations of the Dice coefficients on test scans when 10 and 30 annotated scans were used for training. Best results are highlighted in bold font. Asterisks (*) indicate that the difference between the proposed method and the competing method is statistically significant ($p < 0.05$) using a paired Student's t-test.

	10 annotated training scans	30 annotated training scans
DeepMedic	$0.5912 \pm 0.2243^*$	$0.6551 \pm 0.2514^*$
DeepMedic-UDA	$0.5562 \pm 0.2878^*$	$0.6627 \pm 0.2208^*$
DeepMedic-EN	$0.5684 \pm 0.2873^*$	$0.6503 \pm 0.2650^*$
Proposed	$\mathbf{0.6518 \pm 0.2484}$	$\mathbf{0.6879 \pm 0.2334}$

3.4 Impact of the Amount of Training Data

Lastly, we investigated the impact of the number of training scans. Specifically, we investigated two additional cases, where 10 and 30 randomly selected annotated scans were included in training and the rest annotated data were used for testing. For SSL-based methods, all the unannotated data were also included in training. The results are shown in Table 3, where the means and standard deviations of the Dice coefficients are listed. In all cases, the proposed approach has higher mean Dice coefficients than the competing methods, and the difference is significant using a paired Student's t-test. These results indicate that the proposed method outperforms the competitors.

4 Discussion

The original MT model is developed for semi-supervised image classification, and its consistency loss is simply the difference between class predictions. In our task, however, the consistency needs to be enforced for segmentation. Thus, we have adapted the MT model by defining the consistency loss based on the Dice coefficient. The results indicate that the adaption can be successfully applied to semi-supervised image segmentation.

We have performed experiments with different numbers of training scans. As expected, a greater number of training scans leads to more accurate segmentation for all the methods considered in the experiment. In addition, when the number of training scans is small, the SSL-based approaches DeepMedic-EN and DeepMedic-UDA perform even worse than the baseline DeepMedic model.

It is possibly due to the small number of training scans, which cannot adequately represent the distribution of desired features and segmentation. Thus, the adversarial learning strategy in DeepMedic-EN and DeepMedic-UDA cannot enforce proper regularization based on the unannotated data, where it is very likely that the segmentation or the extracted feature of unannotated data does not resemble that of the annotated data. As the number of training scans increases, the margin between the baseline DeepMedic and DeepMedic-EN or DeepMedic-UDA becomes smaller, possibly because the annotated data can better represent the distribution of expected features and segmentation. With 30 training scans, DeepMedic-UDA is able to outperform the baseline DeepMedic.

Unlike DeepMedic-EN and DeepMedic-UDA, the proposed approach relies on the assumption that similar inputs should produce consistent outputs, and the use of such consistency is further improved with a self-ensembling strategy. In contrast to the adversarial learning strategies in DeepMedic-EN and DeepMedic-UDA, the adapted MT model in the proposed work is less affected by the limited number of training scans, because it does not require the comparison between annotated data and unannotated data. This is confirmed by the results, where the propose approach is robust to the decrease in the number of training scans.

We have also observed that with only 10 annotated training scans, the proposed method outperforms the baseline DeepMedic model trained by 20 annotated scans and performs comparably to the baseline DeepMedic model trained by 30 annotated scans. This highlights the importance of the incorporation of unannotated data for training CNNs. It can potentially greatly reduce the annotation cost or increase the segmentation quality with existing annotated data.

We applied Gaussian noise to the input samples to generate a pair of similar inputs for the student and teacher models. Other strategies for generating pairs of similar inputs are possible. For example, dropout provides a convenient way for noise injection [13]. Future works may explore additional approaches to enforcing the consistency regularization to more efficiently use unannotated data.

5   Conclusion

We have proposed an SSL-based approach to brain lesion segmentation. A teacher model and a student model are constructed and updated alternately. By minimizing the segmentation loss computed from annotated data and segmentation consistency loss computed from unannotated data, the student model learns from the teacher model at each step. The teacher model is then updated with an EMA strategy, and the final teacher model performs lesion segmentation on test samples. The proposed method was applied to ischemic stroke lesion segmentation, and the results demonstrate the benefit of incorporating unannotated data using the proposed method.

Acknowledgement. This work is supported by the National Natural Science Foundation of China (61601461), Beijing Natural Science Foundation (7192108), and Beijing Institute of Technology Research Fund Program for Young Scholars.

References

1. Baur, C., Albarqouni, S., Navab, N.: Semi-supervised deep learning for fully convolutional networks. In: Descoteaux, M., Maier-Hein, L., Franz, A., Jannin, P., Collins, D.L., Duchesne, S. (eds.) MICCAI 2017. LNCS, vol. 10435, pp. 311–319. Springer, Cham (2017). https://doi.org/10.1007/978-3-319-66179-7_36

2. Çiçek, Ö., Abdulkadir, A., Lienkamp, S.S., Brox, T., Ronneberger, O.: 3D U-Net: learning dense volumetric segmentation from sparse annotation. In: Ourselin, S., Joskowicz, L., Sabuncu, M.R., Unal, G., Wells, W. (eds.) MICCAI 2016. LNCS, vol. 9901, pp. 424–432. Springer, Cham (2016). https://doi.org/10.1007/978-3-319-46723-8_49

3. Garyfallidis, E., et al.: Dipy, a library for the analysis of diffusion MRI data. Front. Neuroinformatics **8**(8), 1–17 (2014)

4. Havaei, M., et al.: Brain tumor segmentation with deep neural networks. Med. Image Anal. **35**, 18–31 (2017)

5. Kamnitsas, K., et al.: Unsupervised domain adaptation in brain lesion segmentation with adversarial networks. In: Niethammer, M., et al. (eds.) IPMI 2017. LNCS, vol. 10265, pp. 597–609. Springer, Cham (2017). https://doi.org/10.1007/978-3-319-59050-9_47

6. Kamnitsas, K., et al.: Efficient multi-scale 3D CNN with fully connected CRF for accurate brain lesion segmentation. Med. Image Anal. **36**, 61–78 (2017)

7. Kuang, H., Najm, M., Menon, B.K., Qiu, W.: Joint segmentation of intracerebral hemorrhage and infarct from non-contrast CT images of post-treatment acute ischemic stroke patients. In: Frangi, A.F., Schnabel, J.A., Davatzikos, C., Alberola-López, C., Fichtinger, G. (eds.) MICCAI 2018. LNCS, vol. 11072, pp. 681–688. Springer, Cham (2018). https://doi.org/10.1007/978-3-030-00931-1_78

8. Laine, S., Aila, T.: Temporal ensembling for semi-supervised learning. In: International Conference on Learning Representations (2016)

9. Maier, O., et al.: ISLES 2015-a public evaluation benchmark for ischemic stroke lesion segmentation from multispectral MRI. Med. Image Anal. **35**, 250–269 (2017)

10. Pereira, S., Pinto, A., Alves, V., Silva, C.A.: Brain tumor segmentation using convolutional neural networks in MRI images. IEEE Trans. Med. Imaging **35**(5), 1240–1251 (2016)

11. Tarvainen, A., Valpola, H.: Mean teachers are better role models: weight-averaged consistency targets improve semi-supervised deep learning results. In: Advances in Neural Information Processing Systems, pp. 1195–1204 (2017)

12. Tieleman, T., Hinton, G.: Lecture 6.5-RMSProp, coursera: neural networks for machine learning. University of Toronto, Technical Report (2012)

13. Wager, S., Wang, S., Liang, P.S.: Dropout training as adaptive regularization. In: Advances in Neural Information Processing Systems, pp. 351–359 (2013)

14. Zhang, Y., Yang, L., Chen, J., Fredericksen, M., Hughes, D.P., Chen, D.Z.: Deep adversarial networks for biomedical image segmentation utilizing unannotated images. In: Descoteaux, M., Maier-Hein, L., Franz, A., Jannin, P., Collins, D.L., Duchesne, S. (eds.) MICCAI 2017. LNCS, vol. 10435, pp. 408–416. Springer, Cham (2017). https://doi.org/10.1007/978-3-319-66179-7_47

15. Zhao, X., Wu, Y., Song, G., Li, Z., Zhang, Y., Fan, Y.: A deep learning model integrating FCNNs and CRFs for brain tumor segmentation. Med. Image Anal. **43**, 98–111 (2018)

16. Zhou, Z.H.: A brief introduction to weakly supervised learning. Nat. Sci. Rev. **5**(1), 44–53 (2017)

Shrinkage Estimation on the Manifold of Symmetric Positive-Definite Matrices with Applications to Neuroimaging

Chun-Hao Yang[1] and Baba C. Vemuri[2(✉)]

[1] Department of Statistics, University of Florida, Gainesville, FL, USA
[2] Department of CISE, University of Florida, Gainesville, FL, USA
vemuri@ufl.edu

Abstract. The James-Stein shrinkage estimator was proposed in the field of Statistics as an estimator of the mean for samples drawn from a Gaussian distribution and shown to dominate the maximum likelihood estimator (MLE) in terms of the risk. This seminal work lead to a flurry of activity in the field of shrinkage estimation. However, there has been very little work on shrinkage estimation for data samples that reside on manifolds. In this paper, we present a novel shrinkage estimator of the Fréchet Mean (FM) of manifold-valued data for the manifold, P_n, of symmetric positive definite matrices of size 'n'. We choose to endow P_n with the well known Log-Euclidean metric for its simplicity and ease of computation. With this choice of the metric, we show that the shrinkage estimator can be derived in an analytic form. Further, we prove that the shrinkage estimate of FM dominates the MLE of the FM in terms of the risk. We present several synthetic data examples with noise along with performance comparisons to estimated FM using other non-shrinkage estimators. As an application of shrinkage FM-estimation to real data, we compute the average motor sensory area (M1) tract from diffusion MR brain scans of controls and patients with Parkinson Disease (PD). We first show the dominance of the shrinkage FM estimator over the MLE of FM in this setting and then perform group testing to show differences between PD and controls based on the M1 tracts.

1 Introduction

In medical imaging, data taking the form of symmetric positive-definite (SPD) matrices are quite commonly encountered, for example, diffusion tensors, Cauchy deformation tensors, conductance tensors, etc. In such cases, data processing methods must perform geometry-aware computations, i.e., employ methods that take into account the nonlinear geometry of the data space. In medical imaging and many other domains, it is quite common to compute summary statistics from the data to characterize population groups. The most common and simple summary statistic is the mean. When the data space is nonlinear such as in the case of non-flat Riemannian manifolds, sample Fréchet mean (FM) is

© Springer Nature Switzerland AG 2019
A. C. S. Chung et al. (Eds.): IPMI 2019, LNCS 11492, pp. 566–578, 2019.
https://doi.org/10.1007/978-3-030-20351-1_44

the statistic we seek to compute. Sample FM is defined as the minimizer of the sum of squared geodesic distances from the data samples to the unknown center. This minimization is solved traditionally using the Riemannian gradient descent. Recently however, provably convergent and efficient recursive algorithms have been presented for computing the sample FM on a variety of Riemannian manifolds [4,10,17,22]. In the Euclidean space $\mathbb{R}^n$ with the usual metric, the sample FM is simply the sample mean of the observations and the James-Stein estimator [11], or a shrinkage estimator, is an estimator that is well known to be uniformly better (in terms of risk) than the sample mean when the observations are assumed to be normally distributed. Hence, the goal of this paper is to develop a novel shrinkage estimator for data residing on the space of SPD matrices.

The James-Stein estimator originated from the following problem. Given $X_i \overset{ind}{\sim} \mathcal{N}\left(\mu_i, \sigma^2\right)$, $i = 1, \ldots, p$ where $p > 2$ and σ^2 is known, what is a good estimator for μ_i under a quadratic loss? An intuitive answer would be the MLE X_i. However, Stein [20] proved that the MLE is inadmissible, and provided a class of estimators that dominate the MLE. Later, James and Stein [11] further sharpened the result and proposed the following estimator,

$$\left(1 - \frac{(p-2)\sigma^2}{\|X\|^2}\right) X_i \tag{1}$$

for μ_i, where $X = [X_1, \ldots, X_p]^T$. This estimator is referred to as the James-Stein estimator or the shrinkage estimator.

Ever since then, researchers have been trying to generalize this shrinkage phenomenon and apply it to different problems. For example, authors of [14] and [5] report a shrinkage estimator for a covariance matrix and authors of [3] and [24] generalized the shrinkage estimator to other family of distributions. From an applications perspective, authors of [15] developed a James-Stein version of Kalman filter which yielded robust parameter estimates in the presence of outliers in the data. In [16], authors proposed a shrinkage estimator to estimate the mean function in the Reproducing Kernel Hilbert space (RKHS). Shrinkage estimators for multi-task averaging problems was addressed recently in [7]. In [8], authors presented an interesting application of James-Stein estimation to the problem of geodesic regression in the space of diffeomorphisms to fit a generative model to images acquired over time. They showed that the shrinkage estimator of the momentum parameter estimated from cross-sectional scans and used to regularize the individual geodesic model improves prediction of the individual generative model. In all of the works cited above, the domain of the data has invariably been a vector space and as mentioned earlier, many applications naturally encounter data residing in non-Euclidean spaces. Hence, generalizing the shrinkage estimator to non-Euclidean spaces is a worthwhile pursuit. In this work, we focus on one such generalization of shrinkage estimation to the Riemannian manifold of SPD matrices.

In this paper, we derive a shrinkage estimator on the space of SPD matrices using a Bayesian framework for developing shrinkage estimators presented in

Xie et al. [25] and show that the proposed estimator is asymptotically optimal. We design synthetic experiments to demonstrate that the proposed estimator is better (in terms of risk) than the widely used Riemannian gradient descent based estimator and the recently developed inductive/recursive FM estimator in [10]. Further, we also apply the shrinkage estimator to find group differences between patients with Parkinson Disease and Controls.

Rest of this paper is organized as follows. In Sect. 2, we will present relevant background material about the space of SPD matrices and shrinkage estimation. The main result is presented in Sect. 3. Synthetic and real data experiments depicting the dominance of our shrinkage estimator of FM over MLE of FM are presented in Sect. 4. Finally, we conclude in Sect. 5.

2 Preliminaries

This section contains a review of some background differential geometry and statistics material that will be needed in the rest of the paper.

2.1 Geometry of P_n

We now present basic Riemannian geometry of symmetric positive definite (SPD) matrices denoted by P_n and refer the reader to [9,23] for details. The manifold P_n of $n \times n$ SPD matrices is defined as, $P_n = \{X = (x_{ij})_{1 \le i,j \le n} | X = X^T, \forall v \in \mathbb{R}^n, v \ne 0, v^T X v > 0\}$. The most commonly encountered example of SPD matrices is the covariance matrix (with non-zero eigenvalues), which is widely used in medical imaging, statistics, finance, computer vision and other fields. On P_n, the most widely used Riemannian metric is given by

$$\langle U, V \rangle_X = tr(X^{-1/2} U X^{-1} V X^{-1/2}) \tag{2}$$

for $X \in P_n$, $U, V \in T_X P_n$. The most important property of this metric the GL-invariance, i.e. for $g \in GL(n)$, $\langle U, V \rangle_X = \langle gUg^T, gVg^T \rangle_{gXg^T}$. Hereafter we refer this metric as GL-invariant metric to avoid confusion. With the GL-invariant metric, the induced geodesic distance between $X, Y \in P_n$ is given by (see [23])

$$d_{GL}(X, Y) = \sqrt{tr((\log(X^{-1}Y))^2)} \tag{3}$$

where log is the matrix logarithm. Since this distance is induced from the GL-invariant metric in Eq. (2), it is naturally GL-invariant i.e. $d_{GL}(X, Y) = d_{GL}(gXg^T, gYg^T)$.

More than a decade ago, Arsigny et al. [1] proposed the Log-Euclidean metric on the manifold P_n. This metric makes P_n a flat Riemannian manifold. The geodesic distance $d_{LE} : P_n \times P_n \to \mathbb{R}$ induced by the Log-Euclidean metric has a particularly simple form,

$$d_{LE}(X, Y) = \|\log X - \log Y\|_F.$$

Since for $X \in P_n$, $\log X \in \mathsf{Sym}(n) = \{X \in GL(n) | X = X^T\}$ and $\mathsf{Sym}(n)$ is isomorphic to $\mathbb{R}^{\frac{n(n+1)}{2}}$, it is convenient to use the map $vecd : \mathsf{Sym}(n) \to \mathbb{R}^{\frac{n(n+1)}{2}}$ defined in [19]. For $Y \in \mathsf{Sym}(n)$,

$$vecd(Y) = \left[y_{11}, ..., y_{nn}, \sqrt{2}(y_{ij})_{i<j} \right]^T.$$

For example,

$$Y = \begin{bmatrix} y_{11} & y_{12} & y_{13} \\ y_{12} & y_{22} & y_{23} \\ y_{13} & y_{23} & y_{33} \end{bmatrix}, vecd(Y) = \begin{bmatrix} y_{11} & y_{22} & y_{33} & \sqrt{2}y_{12} & \sqrt{2}y_{13} & \sqrt{2}y_{23} \end{bmatrix}^T.$$

To simplify the notation, for $X \in P_n$, we denote $\widetilde{X} = vecd(\log X) \in \mathbb{R}^{\frac{n(n+1)}{2}}$. From the definition of $vecd$, it is easy to see that $d_{LE}(X, Y) = \|\widetilde{X} - \widetilde{Y}\|$.

Given $X_1, \ldots, X_N \in P_n$, we denote the sample FM with respect to the two geodesic distances given above by,

$$\bar{X}_N^{GL} = \arg\min_{M \in P_n} \frac{1}{N} \sum_{i=1}^{N} d_{GL}^2(X_i, M) \text{ and} \tag{4}$$

$$\bar{X}_N^{LE} = \arg\min_{M \in P_n} \frac{1}{N} \sum_{i=1}^{N} d_{LE}^2(X_i, M) = \exp\left(\frac{1}{N} \sum_{i=1}^{N} \log X_i \right). \tag{5}$$

2.2   The Log-Normal Distribution on P_n

To model observations residing directly on P_n, Schwartzman [18] proposed the Log-Normal distribution which can be viewed as a generalization of the Log-Normal distribution on $\mathbb{R}^+$ to P_n.

Definition 1. *Let X be a P_n-valued random variable. We say X follows a Log-Normal distribution with mean $M \in P_n$ and covariance matrix $\Sigma \in P_{n(n+1)/2}$, or $X \sim LN(M, \Sigma)$ if*

$$\widetilde{X} \sim N(\widetilde{M}, \Sigma)$$

Important properties for this distribution are studied in [19]. The following proposition from [19] will be useful subsequently in this work. The proof of this proposition is straightforward and hence omitted.

Proposition 1. *Let $X_1, \ldots, X_N \overset{i.i.d}{\sim} LN(M, \Sigma)$. Then MLEs of M and Σ are $\hat{M}^{MLE} = \bar{X}_N^{LE}$ and $\hat{\Sigma}^{MLE} = \frac{1}{N} \sum_i \left(\widetilde{X}_i - \widetilde{\hat{M}^{MLE}} \right) \left(\widetilde{X}_i - \widetilde{\hat{M}^{MLE}} \right)^T$. The MLE of M is the sample FM under the Log-Euclidean metric.*

2.3   Bayesian Formulation of the Shrinkage Estimation in R^n

The shrinkage estimator arose from a simultaneous estimation problem namely: estimate μ_i given $X_i \overset{ind.}{\sim} N(\mu_i, \sigma^2)$, where $i = 1, \ldots, p$, $p > 2$, σ^2 is known. The seminal work of James and Stein [11] showed that the information contained in X_j, $j \neq i$ can help to improve the estimation of μ_i. Later on, Efron and Morris [6] formulated the same problem using a Bayesian model and gave an empirical Bayes interpretation to the shrinkage estimator. The corresponding Bayesian hierarchical model is given below:

$$X_i | \theta_i \overset{ind}{\sim} N(\theta_i, A), i = 1, \ldots, p$$
$$\theta_i \overset{i.i.d}{\sim} N(\mu, \lambda)$$

where, A is known and μ and λ are unknown. The maximum a posteriori (MAP) estimate for θ_i is given by,

$$\hat{\theta}_i^{\lambda, \mu} = \frac{\lambda}{\lambda + A} X_i + \frac{A}{\lambda + A} \mu. \tag{6}$$

The unknown parameters λ and μ can be estimated by empirical Bayes MLE (EBMLE) or an empirical Bayes method of moments (EBMOM). For the special case of $\mu = 0$, the EBMLE and EBMOM produce the same estimator which is the James-Stein estimator (1). A natural question would then arise: is there an optimal shrinkage estimator, i.e. how to estimate λ and μ such that they are optimal within such a class of estimators. The optimality here is defined in terms of the risk function, or the expected value of the loss function $R(\hat{\theta}, \theta) = E_\theta L(\hat{\theta}(X), \theta)$, where $\hat{\theta}(X)$ is an estimator of θ based on the observation X. An estimator $\hat{\theta}$ of θ is said to be optimal if $R(\hat{\theta}, \theta) \leq R(\hat{\theta}^\star, \theta)$ for all θ. Hence, the optimal choice of λ and μ are given by,

$$\hat{\lambda}^{\text{opt}}, \hat{\mu}^{\text{opt}} = \arg\min_{\lambda, \mu} R(\hat{\theta}^{\lambda, \mu}, \theta).$$

where, $\theta = [\theta_1, \ldots, \theta_p]^T$ and $\hat{\theta}^{\lambda, \mu} = [\hat{\theta}_1^{\lambda, \mu}, \ldots, \hat{\theta}_p^{\lambda, \mu}]^T$. However, since $R(\hat{\theta}^{\lambda, \mu}, \theta)$ involves θ, this problem is ill-posed. Motivated by Stein's unbiased risk estimate (SURE) [21], we minimize the unbiased risk estimate $\text{SURE}(\lambda, \mu)$ instead of the risk where,

$$E_\theta [\text{SURE}(\lambda, \mu)] = R(\hat{\theta}^{\lambda, \mu}, \theta).$$

Hence,

$$\hat{\lambda}^{\text{SURE}}, \hat{\mu}^{\text{SURE}} = \arg\min_{\lambda, \mu} \text{SURE}(\lambda, \mu)$$

This approach has been used to derive estimators for different models. For example, Xie et al. [25] derived the (asymptotically) optimal shrinkage estimator for heteroscedastic hierarchical model and their result is further generalized by [12] and [13].

3   Theory

We are now ready to present the main theoretical results of this paper involving a Bayesian formulation of the shrinkage estimator of M, the FM of Log-Normal distribution on P_n and a theorem on the dominance of our shrinkage estimator over the MLE of M on P_n endowed with the Log-Euclidean metric. The choice of Log-Euclidean metric here over other metrics is dictated by (i) computational efficiency of this metric over other choices and (ii) the existence of a closed form expression for the shrinkage estimator (to be derived here).

We model the data in this work as follows:

$$X_{ij}|M_i \overset{ind}{\sim} \mathrm{LN}(M_i, A_i I), j = 1, \ldots, N$$

$$M_i \overset{i.i.d}{\sim} \mathrm{LN}(\boldsymbol{\mu}, \lambda I), i = 1, \ldots, p$$

where A_i's are known and $\boldsymbol{\mu}$ and λ are unknown. Our goal in this paper is to develop a shrinkage estimator for M_i which is better than the MLE, $\bar{X}_i^{LE} = \exp(N^{-1} \sum_j \log X_{ij})$, in terms of risk. Given the above model, the MAP estimate for M_i is given by,

$$\hat{M}_i^{\lambda,\mu} = \exp\left(\frac{\lambda}{\lambda + A_i} \log \bar{X}_i^{\mathrm{LE}} + \frac{A_i}{\lambda + A_i} \log \boldsymbol{\mu}\right). \tag{7}$$

Let $\boldsymbol{M} = [M_1, \ldots, M_p]$ and $\hat{\boldsymbol{M}}^{\lambda,\mu} = [\hat{M}_1^{\lambda,\mu}, \ldots, \hat{M}_p^{\lambda,\mu}]$. Using the loss function, $l(\hat{\boldsymbol{M}}^{\lambda,\mu}, \boldsymbol{M}) = \frac{1}{p} \sum_i d_{\mathrm{LE}}^2(\hat{M}_i^{\lambda,\mu}, M_i)$, the risk function becomes,

$$R(\hat{\boldsymbol{M}}^{\lambda,\mu}, \boldsymbol{M}) = E\left[\frac{1}{p} \sum_{i=1}^p d_{\mathrm{LE}}^2(\hat{M}_i^{\lambda,\mu}, M_i)\right]$$

$$= \frac{1}{p} \sum_{i=1}^p \frac{A_i}{(\lambda + A_i)^2}\left(A_i \|\log \boldsymbol{\mu} - \log M_i\|^2 + \frac{q\lambda^2}{N}\right)$$

where $q = n(n+1)/2$. Since λ and $\boldsymbol{\mu}$ are unknown, our goal is to find the optimal λ and $\boldsymbol{\mu}$ in the sense that the risk is the smallest for all $\boldsymbol{M}$. Using the formalism given in Sect. 2.3 for approximating the risk function by SURE, we have,

$$\mathrm{SURE}(\lambda, \boldsymbol{\mu}) = \frac{1}{p} \sum_{i=1}^p \frac{A_i}{(\lambda + A_i)^2}\left(A_i \|\log \bar{X}_i^{\mathrm{LE}} - \log \boldsymbol{\mu}\|^2 + \frac{q(\lambda^2 - A_i^2)}{N}\right).$$

Hence, the choices of λ and $\boldsymbol{\mu}$ would be

$$\hat{\lambda}^{\mathrm{SURE}}, \hat{\boldsymbol{\mu}}^{\mathrm{SURE}} = \arg\min_{\lambda,\mu} \mathrm{SURE}(\lambda, \boldsymbol{\mu})$$

$$= \arg\min_{\lambda,\mu} \frac{1}{p} \sum_{i=1}^p \frac{A_i}{(\lambda + A_i)^2}\left(A_i \|\log \bar{X}_i^{\mathrm{LE}} - \log \boldsymbol{\mu}\|^2 + \frac{q(\lambda^2 - A_i^2)}{N}\right).$$

The proposed shrinkage estimator, SURE-FM, for M_i is

$$\hat{M}_i^{\text{SURE}} = \exp\left(\frac{\hat{\lambda}^{\text{SURE}}}{\hat{\lambda}^{\text{SURE}} + A_i}\log \bar{X}_i^{\text{LE}} + \frac{A_i}{\hat{\lambda}^{\text{SURE}} + A_i}\log \hat{\mu}^{\text{SURE}}\right). \tag{8}$$

Since $\hat{\lambda}^{\text{SURE}}$, $\hat{\mu}^{\text{SURE}}$ are the minimizers of $\text{SURE}(\lambda, \mu)$ instead of $R(\hat{M}^{\lambda,\mu}, M) = E\left[l(\hat{M}^{\lambda,\mu}, M)\right]$, we show in Theorem 1 that $\text{SURE}(\lambda, \mu)$ is a good approximation of $l(\hat{M}^{\lambda,\mu}, M)$.

Theorem 1. *Assume that,*

(A) $\limsup_{p\to\infty} \frac{1}{p}\sum_i A_i^2 < \infty$
(B) $\limsup_{p\to\infty} \frac{1}{p}\sum_i A_i\|\log M_i\|^2 < \infty$
(C) $\limsup_{p\to\infty} \frac{1}{p}\sum_i \|\log M_i\|^{2+\delta} < \infty$ *for some* $\delta > 0$.

Then,

$$\sup_{\lambda>0, \|\log\mu\|<\max_i \|\log \bar{X}_i^{LE}\|} |SURE(\lambda, \mu) - l(\hat{M}^{\lambda,\mu}, M)| \to 0$$

in probability as $p \to \infty$.

Proof. Let $\tilde{X}_i^{\text{LE}} = vecd(\log \bar{X}_i^{\text{LE}})$, $\tilde{\mu} = vecd(\log \mu)$, $\widetilde{M}_i^{\lambda,\mu} = vecd(\log \hat{M}_i^{\lambda,\mu})$, $\widetilde{M}_i = vecd(\log M_i)$. Then,

$$\text{SURE}(\lambda, \mu) = \sum_{j=1}^{q}\frac{1}{p}\sum_{i=1}^{p}\frac{A_i}{(\lambda + A_i)^2}\left(A_i\left((\tilde{X}_i^{\text{LE}})_j - (\tilde{\mu})_j\right)^2 + \frac{\lambda^2 - A_i^2}{N}\right) = \sum_{j=1}^{q}\text{SURE}_j(\lambda, (\tilde{\mu})_j)$$

and

$$l(\hat{M}^{\lambda,\mu}, M) = \sum_{j=1}^{q}\frac{1}{p}\sum_{i=1}^{p}\left((\widetilde{M}_i^{\lambda,\mu})_j - (\widetilde{M}_i)_j\right)^2 = \sum_{j=1}^{q}l_j.$$

Hence by Theorem 5.1 in [25] we have,

$$\sup_{\lambda>0, \|\log\mu\|<\max_i \|\log \bar{X}_i^{LE}\|} |SURE(\lambda, \mu) - l(\hat{M}^{\lambda,\mu}, M)|$$

$$\leq \sum_{j=1}^{q}\sup_{\lambda>0, \|\log\mu\|<\max_i \|\log \bar{X}_i^{LE}\|} |SURE_j(\lambda, (\tilde{\mu})_j) - l_j| \to 0$$

in probability as $p \to \infty$. $\qquad\square$

In next theorem, we will show that our proposed shrinkage estimator is asymptotically optimal in the sense that its risk is asymptotically smaller than any other estimator of the form (7).

Theorem 2. *Assume that (A), (B), (C) in Theorem 1 hold. Then,*

$$\lim_{p \to \infty} [R(\hat{\boldsymbol{M}}^{SURE}, \boldsymbol{M}) - R(\hat{\boldsymbol{M}}^{\lambda,\mu}, \boldsymbol{M})] \leq 0$$

Proof. Since

$$
\begin{aligned}
l(\hat{\boldsymbol{M}}^{SURE}, \boldsymbol{M}) - l(\hat{\boldsymbol{M}}^{\lambda,\mu}, \boldsymbol{M}) = {} & l(\hat{\boldsymbol{M}}^{SURE}, \boldsymbol{M}) - \text{SURE}(\hat{\lambda}^{SURE}, \hat{\boldsymbol{\mu}}^{SURE}) \\
& + \text{SURE}(\hat{\lambda}^{SURE}, \hat{\boldsymbol{\mu}}^{SURE}) - \text{SURE}(\lambda, \boldsymbol{\mu}) \\
& - l(\hat{\boldsymbol{M}}^{\lambda,\mu}, \boldsymbol{M}) + \text{SURE}(\lambda, \boldsymbol{\mu}) \\
& \leq 2 \sup |\text{SURE}(\lambda, \boldsymbol{\mu}) - l(\hat{\boldsymbol{M}}^{\lambda,\mu}, \boldsymbol{M})|,
\end{aligned}
$$

from Theorem 1, we have

$$\lim_{p \to \infty} \left[l(\hat{\boldsymbol{M}}^{SURE}, \boldsymbol{M}) - l(\hat{\boldsymbol{M}}^{\lambda,\mu}, \boldsymbol{M}) \right] \leq 0.$$

Hence,

$$\lim_{p \to \infty} \left[R(\hat{\boldsymbol{M}}^{SURE}, \boldsymbol{M}) - R(\hat{\boldsymbol{M}}^{\lambda,\mu}, \boldsymbol{M}) \right] = \lim_{p \to \infty} E \left[l(\hat{\boldsymbol{M}}^{SURE}, \boldsymbol{M}) - l(\hat{\boldsymbol{M}}^{\lambda,\mu}, \boldsymbol{M}) \right] \leq 0.$$

□

4   Experiments

In this section, we present both synthetic and real data experiments to show that the SURE-FM is better than the MLE of the FM on P_n in terms of risk.

4.1   Synthetic Data Experiments

In this subsection, we will demonstrate the dominance of the SURE-FM over MLE of the FM of Log-Normal distribution on P_n using synthetically generated data. We compare the performance of the three different estimators namely, (i) SURE-FM, (ii) MLE of FM, denoted FM.LE and (iii) sample FM using the GL-invariant metric (using the recursive algorithm in [10]), denoted FM.GL. We use the following loss function in our comparisons of accuracy, $l(\hat{M}, M) = d^2_{\text{LE}}(\hat{M}, M)$. The lower the loss, the better the estimator. The procedure is shown in Algorithm 1 and in all of our experiments we set $m = 1000$.

Algorithm 1. Procedure for synthetic data experiment on P_3.

Input: sample size N, variance λ, dimension p
Output: R^{LE}, R^{GL}, R^{SURE}

1 **for** $k = 1$ **to** m **do**
2 $\quad$ Generate $M_1, ..., M_p \overset{i.i.d}{\sim} \mathrm{LN}(I, \lambda I)$
3 $\quad$ Generate $A_1, ..., A_p \sim \mathrm{Uniform}(1, 5)$
4 $\quad$ Generate $X_{ij} \sim \mathrm{LN}(M_i, A_i I)$, $j = 1, ..., n$, $i = 1, ..., p$
5 $\quad$ Compute $\bar{X}_i^{GL}$, $\bar{X}_i^{LE}$, and $\hat{M}_i^{\mathrm{SURE}}$ in (4), (5), and (8)
6 $\quad$ Compute the loss $l_k^{\mathrm{LE}} = l(\bar{X}^{\mathrm{LE}}, M)$, $l_k^{\mathrm{GL}} = l(\bar{X}^{\mathrm{GL}}, M)$, and
   $\quad\quad$ $l_k^{\mathrm{SURE}} = l(\hat{M}^{\mathrm{SURE}}, M)$.
7 Compute $R^{\mathrm{LE}} = \frac{1}{m}\sum_k l_k^{\mathrm{LE}}$, $R^{\mathrm{GL}} = \frac{1}{m}\sum_k l_k^{\mathrm{GL}}$, and $R^{\mathrm{SURE}} = \frac{1}{m}\sum_k l_k^{\mathrm{SURE}}$.

In our experiments, we chose $\lambda = 1, 2, 4$, $n = 3, 5, 10, 20$, and $p = 50, 100, 150, 200$ to see how the performance changes under varying parameter values. The results are shown in Fig. 1. The percentages of improvement range from 20% to 40% under varying conditions. It is evident that the SURE-FM yields smaller average loss compared to the other two estimates of FM in most of the cases. In Fig. 2, we show the computational cost for different estimators. As discussed in [1], the Log-Euclidean metric based sample FM computation is much more efficient than the GL-invariant based sample FM computation. The SURE-FM is slightly slower than the FM.LE computation because of an extra optimization step that is involved.

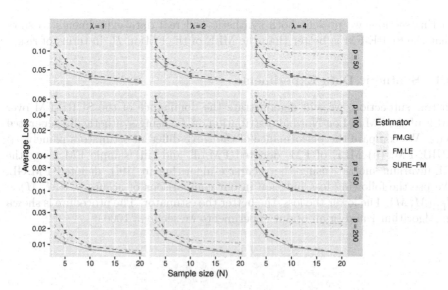

Fig. 1. The average loss for the three different estimators. Results for λ variation are shown across the columns and varying dimension p are shown across the rows.

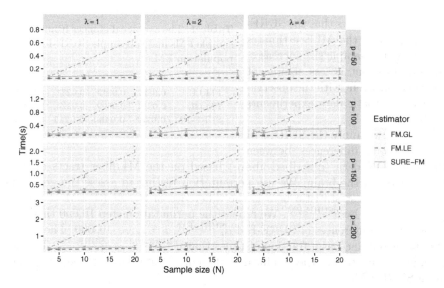

Fig. 2. The average time (on a log scale) taken for computing the three different estimators. Results for λ variation are shown across the columns and varying dimension p are shown across the rows.

4.2 Real Data Experiments

For the real data experiments, we test the performance of SURE-FM on the diffusion MRI datasets. The data consists of 50 patients with Parkinsons disease (PD) and 44 control cases (CON). The parameters of the diffusion image acquisition sequence were as follows: repetition time $= 7748\,\text{ms}$, echo time $= 86\,\text{ms}$, flip angle $= 90$, # of diffusion gradients: 64, field of view $= 224\,224\,\text{mm}$, in-plane resolution $= 2\,\text{mm}$ isotropic, slice-thickness $= 2\,\text{mm}$, SENSE factor $= 2$.

We extract the motor sensory area fiber tracts (M1 fiber tracts) from each member of the two groups (PD and CON) using the FSL software [2] and each tract here spans across 33 voxels for the left hemisphere tract and 34 voxels for the right hemisphere tract respectively. We then fit diffusion tensors to each voxel along each of the tracts to obtain 33 (34) (3×3) SPD matrices. We then compute the FM tract for each group (CON and PD). The FM tract here also has 33 (34) diffusion tensors along the tract. We will use these FMs computed from the full population of each group as the 'ground truth'. Then, we randomly draw a subsample of size $N = 3, 5, 10, 20$ from each group (PD and CON) and compute the FM.LE, FM.GL, and SURE-FM of each group for the aforementioned subsample. We compare the performance of different estimators by the distance between the estimator and the 'ground truth' FMs. We repeat the experiment for $m = 1000$ random draws of subsamples and report the average distances. The results are shown in Table 1.

The result shows that the SURE-FM dominates the MLE estimates of FM. As the sample size increases, the improvement is less significant which is consistent with the observations on synthetic data experiments in Sect. 4.1.

Finally, we apply the SURE-FM to find group differences between PD and CON data (described above) based on the M1 fiber tracts on both hemispheres of the brain. We use permutation testing to assess the group differences. The test statistic here is the difference of the SURE-FM of the two groups denoted by $d^{\text{SURE-FM}}$. We repeat the permutation step 10,000 times and recorded the differences of SURE-FM $d_i^{\text{SURE-FM}}$, $i = 1, \ldots, 10,000$. The p-value of 0.042 is obtained as a fraction of times that $d^{\text{SURE-FM}} < d_i^{\text{SURE-FM}}$. This low p-value is indicative of the significant difference found between the two groups using SURE-FM.

Table 1. The average distances from the subsample FMs and subsample SURE-FM to the population FM.

N	3	5	10	20
FM.LE	0.0827	0.0519	0.0231	0.0097
FM.GL	0.0814	0.0509	0.0224	0.0094
SURE-FM	**0.0738**	**0.0466**	**0.0211**	**0.0092**

5   Discussion and Conclusions

In this paper, we presented a Bayesian formulation to generalize shrinkage estimation from $\mathbb{R}^n$ to the manifold of SPD matrices and proved that it dominates the MLE of the FM in terms of risk The shrinkage factor and the shrinkage target are obtained by minimizing the Stein's unbiased risk estimate (SURE). Our theoretical results were derived using the Log-Euclidean metric, which is easy to compute and easy to manipulate formulae in our quest for the shrinkage estimator on P_n. We showed experimentally on synthetic and real data that SURE-FM is better than the sample FM estimates computed using the Log-Euclidean and the GL-invariant metrics respectively. The experiments depicted the dominance of the SURE-FM over MLE estimates as expected in the small sample size scenarios. This scenario is very pertinent to the medical imaging domain where one is faced with small sample population size but very high dimensional feature spaces. Thus, we envision that the research reported here can prove to be quite useful for statistical inference in such settings.

As is well known, the Log-Euclidean metric is not affine invariant and in some applications, such a property might be useful. However, from our preliminary attempts, we found it to be very challenging and almost intractable to derive a closed form solution for the estimator. Our future efforts will therefore focus on using symbolic manipulation tools to explore the possibility of tackling this problem. In parallel, we are also exploring formulations of shrinkage estimators for other manifolds commonly encountered in medical imaging applications.

Acknowledgements. This research was in part funded by the NSF grants IIS-1525431 and IIS-1724174 to BCV.

References

1. Arsigny, V., Fillard, P., Pennec, X., Ayache, N.: Geometric means in a novel vector space structure on symmetric positive-definite matrices. SIAM J. Matrix Anal. Appl. **29**(1), 328–347 (2007)
2. Behrens, T.E., Berg, H.J., Jbabdi, S., Rushworth, M.F., Woolrich, M.W.: Probabilistic diffusion tractography with multiple fibre orientations: what can we gain? Neuroimage **34**(1), 144–155 (2007)
3. Brandwein, A.C., Strawderman, W.E.: Stein estimation for spherically symmetric distributions: recent developments. Stat. Sci. **27**(1), 11–23 (2012)
4. Chakraborty, R., Vemuri, B.C.: Recursive fréchet mean computation on the grassmannian and its applications to computer vision. In: Proceedings of the IEEE International Conference on Computer Vision, pp. 4229–4237 (2015)
5. Daniels, M.J., Kass, R.E.: Shrinkage estimators for covariance matrices. Biometrics **57**(4), 1173–1184 (2001)
6. Efron, B., Morris, C.: Stein's estimation rule and its competitorsan empirical Bayes approach. J. Am. Stat. Assoc. **68**(341), 117–130 (1973)
7. Feldman, S., Gupta, M.R., Frigyik, B.A.: Revisiting stein's paradox: multi-task averaging. J. Mach. Learn. Res. **15**(1), 3441–3482 (2014)
8. Fleishman, G.M., Fletcher, P.T., Gutman, B.A., Prasad, G., Wu, Y., Thompson, P.M.: Geodesic refinement using james-stein estimators. Math. Found. Comput. Anat. **60**, 60–70 (2015)
9. Helgason, S.: Differential Geometry, Lie Groups and Symmetric Spaces. American Mathematical Society, Providence (2001)
10. Ho, J., Cheng, G., Salehian, H., Vemuri, B.: Recursive Karcher expectation estimators and geometric law of large numbers. In: Artificial Intelligence and Statistics, pp. 325–332 (2013)
11. James, W., Stein, C.: Estimation with quadratic loss. In: Proceedings of the Fourth Berkeley Symposium on Mathematical Statistics and Probability, vol. 1, pp. 361–379 (1961)
12. Jing, B.Y., Li, Z., Pan, G., Zhou, W.: On sure-type double shrinkage estimation. J. Am. Stat. Assoc. **111**(516), 1696–1704 (2016)
13. Kong, X., Liu, Z., Zhao, P., Zhou, W.: Sure estimates under dependence and heteroscedasticity. J. Multivar. Anal. **161**, 1–11 (2017)
14. Ledoit, O., Wolf, M.: A well-conditioned estimator for large-dimensional covariance matrices. J. Multivar. Anal. **88**(2), 365–411 (2004)
15. Manton, J.H., Krishnamurthy, V., Poor, H.V.: James-stein state filtering algorithms. IEEE Trans. Sig. Process. **46**(9), 2431–2447 (1998)
16. Muandet, K., Sriperumbudur, B., Fukumizu, K., Gretton, A., Schölkopf, B.: Kernel mean shrinkage estimators. J. Mach. Learn. Res. **17**(1), 1656–1696 (2016)
17. Salehian, H., Chakraborty, R., Ofori, E., Vaillancourt, D., Vemuri, B.C.: An efficient recursive estimator of the fréchet mean on a hypersphere with applications to medical image analysis. Math. Found. Comput. Anat. **3**, 143–154 (2015)
18. Schwartzman, A.: Random ellipsoids and false discovery rates: statistics for diffusion tensor imaging data. Ph.D. thesis, Stanford University (2006)
19. Schwartzman, A.: Lognormal distributions and geometric averages of symmetric positive definite matrices. Int. Stat. Rev. **84**(3), 456–486 (2016)
20. Stein, C.: Inadmissibility of the usual estimator for the mean of a multivariate normal distribution. In: Proceedings of the Third Berkeley Symposium on Mathematical Statistics and Probability, 1954–1955, vol. 1, pp. 197–206. University of California Press, Berkeley (1956)

21. Stein, C.M.: Estimation of the mean of a multivariate normal distribution. Ann. Stat. **9**(6), 1135–1151 (1981)
22. Sturm, K.T.: Probability measures on metric spaces of nonpositive. In: Heat Kernels and Analysis on Manifolds, Graphs, and Metric Spaces. Lecture Notes from a Quarter Program on Heat Kernels, Random Walks, and Analysis on Manifolds and Graphs, 16 April–13 July 2002, vol. 338, p. 357. Emile Borel Centre of the Henri Poincaré Institute, Paris (2003)
23. Terras, A.: Harmonic Analysis on Symmetric Spaces and Applications II. Springer Science & Business Media, New York (2012)
24. Xie, X., Kou, S.C., Brown, L.: Optimal shrinkage estimation of mean parameters in family of distributions with quadratic variance. Ann. Stat. **44**(2), 564 (2016)
25. Xie, X., Kou, S., Brown, L.D.: Sure estimates for a heteroscedastic hierarchical model. J. Am. Stat. Assoc. **107**(500), 1465–1479 (2012)

Simultaneous Spatial-Temporal Decomposition of Connectome-Scale Brain Networks by Deep Sparse Recurrent Auto-Encoders

Qing Li[1], Qinglin Dong[2], Fangfei Ge[2], Ning Qiang[3], Yu Zhao[2],
Han Wang[4], Heng Huang[5], Xia Wu[1(✉)], and Tianming Liu[2(✉)]

[1] Beijing Normal University, Beijing, China
wuxia@bnu.edu.cn
[2] The University of Georgia, Athens, GA, USA
tliu@cs.uga.edu
[3] Shaanxi Normal University, Xi'an, China
[4] Zhejiang University, Hangzhou, China
[5] Northeastern Polytechnic University, Xi'an, China

Abstract. Exploring the spatial patterns and temporal dynamics of human brain activities has long been a great topic, yet development of a unified spatial-temporal model for such purpose is still challenging. To better understand brain networks based on fMRI data and inspired by the success in applying deep learning for brain encoding/decoding, we propose a novel deep sparse recurrent auto-encoder (DSRAE) in an unsupervised spatial-temporal way to learn spatial and temporal patterns of brain networks jointly. The proposed DSRAE has been validated on the publicly available human connectome project (HCP) fMRI datasets with promising results. To our best knowledge, the proposed DSRAE is among the early unified models that can extract connectome-scale spatial-temporal networks from 4D fMRI data simultaneously.

Keywords: Task-based fMRI · Recurrent neural network · Auto-encoder

1 Introduction

Exploring and understanding brain function and its dynamics has been one of the most important topics in modern neuroscience [1, 2]. Mounting evidence has shown that the brain keeps undergoing noisy, massive and complex neural processes that are highly correlated both spatially and temporally [3–5], which suggests that it is desirable to model spatial and temporal information at the same time while analyzing fMRI data. To characterize and analyze the complex spatial-temporal functional states of human brain, a variety of data-driven models have been proposed to apply on fMRI data, such as sparse dictionary learning (SDL) [6], deep belief network (DBN) [7, 8], convolutional neural network (CNN) [9], and recurrent neural network (RNN) [10]. These frameworks can be generally classified into two categories: spatial approaches and temporal

---

Q. Li and Q. Dong—Co-first authors.

© Springer Nature Switzerland AG 2019
A. C. S. Chung et al. (Eds.): IPMI 2019, LNCS 11492, pp. 579–591, 2019.
https://doi.org/10.1007/978-3-030-20351-1_45

approaches. For example, some studies based on spatial approaches usually focused on the spatially decomposed components decoded from fMRI data and typically ignored temporal dynamics analysis [6, 7, 11, 12]. On the contrary, other studies based on temporal approaches mostly focused on temporal features modeling while spatial information is overlooked [8, 9]. Notably, a recent study based on deep spatial-temporal convolutional neural network (ST-CNN) tried to take the advantages of both spatial and temporal domains [13], yet their temporal features were derived from the spatial features inherently. In short, these previous studies focused on either spatial or temporal perspective of fMRI data and rarely modeled both domains simultaneously.

To bridge the above-mentioned gap and better understand brain networks, a novel deep sparse recurrent auto-encoder (DSRAE) is designed in this paper. The DSRAE is a unified spatial-temporal data-driven approach that can jointly characterize and recover the embedded spatial and temporal information from 4D fMRI data. To our best knowledge, our proposed model is among the early unified spatial-temporal models on 4D fMRI data in the literature, and it can be applied on both task fMRI (tfMRI) and resting fMRI (rfMRI) since the whole training process is completely unsupervised. To evaluate the performance of our model, two validation experiments were performed on two tfMRI datasets from human connectome project (HCP). Our experiment results showed that the DSRAE model can learn effective representations of both spatial patterns and temporal dynamics, which offers novel insights into the mysterious brain.

2 Materials and Methods

2.1 Overview

Figure 1 summarizes the architecture of our proposed DSRAE model, as well as the two validation experiments. After data preprocessing (Sect. 2.2), the fMRI data in each subject is extracted and normalized. With the fMRI data, inspired by RNN (Sect. 2.3) the DSRAE model is trained in an unsupervised manner (Sect. 2.4). Particularly, the activation of each hidden node represents a typical functional brain state, and its hidden response to specific stimulus represents the temporal activities of the brain states.

2.2 Data Description and Pre-processing

In this paper, HCP [14] grayordinate tfMRI data was used, as it is publicly available on https://db.humanconnectome.org. In total, 791 healthy adult participants that executed all tasks were used in this study. The HCP grayordinate data model the gray matter as combined cortical surface vertices and subcortical voxels across subjects in the standard MNI space. The preprocessing steps of the fMRI dataset include spatial smoothing, temporal filtering, nuisance regression, and motion censoring, which were all implemented with FreeSurfer Software [15]. The fMRI data of subjects who performed two tasks were used in our experiments and the task design information is shown in Table 1. In language task, there are two stimulations: story and math where the math blocks were designed to provide a comparison task that was attentional

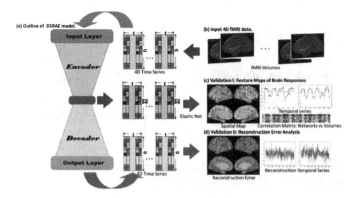

Fig. 1. Illustration of DSRAE model and the two validation experiments. (a) The outline of DSRAE model, in which the input and output layers are both fMRI time series, and the latent layer features are the networks with temporal information. (b) The input of DSRAE is the 4D fMRI data, which is a series of 3D brain volumes acquired in each task session. (c) Validation I: spatial maps are derived from latent layer time series via Elastic Net, which will be compared with benchmark maps via GLM; the time series will be validated by the task design ground truth; and the correlation matrix will be calculated between the obtained networks and original volumes to detect the brain states. (d) Validation II: The signal reconstruction error analysis based on Pearson correlation between reconstructed output and original input.

Table 1. Properties of HCP task-fMRI datasets.

Parameters	Task	
	Language	Working memory
# of frames	316	405
Duration (min)	3:57	5:01
# of task blocks	8	8

demanding [16]. In working memory task, a version of the N-back task was used to assess working memory capability [17]. It was reported that the associated brain activations were reliable across subjects [17] and time [18].

2.3   Basics of Recurrent Neural Network (RNN)

It has been shown that recurrent neural network (RNN) can use the internal state (memory) to process sequences of inputs. For each recurrent neural network layer, it can be unfolded as a deep feedforward network along temporal series, as illustrated in Fig. 2a. However, because of the vanishing gradient problem, the traditional basic RNN is difficult to train in complex data situation. To overcome this problem, Long Short-Term Memory (LSTM) units [19], with the "forget gate", were specifically designed and have become one of the most widely-used RNN architectures.

The internal memory, which stores information from previous time points, is in a cell state of each LSTM unit. As shown in Fig. 2b, there are gates in each unit to

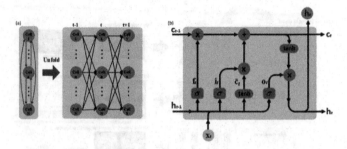

Fig. 2. A schematic illustration of LSTM cell model. (a) The interconnections in a common recurrent hidden layer. (b) LSTM memory unit.

control the contents of the cell states c_t and determine the outputs h_t based on the inputs x_t. The cell state of an LSTM unit is defined as follows:

$$c_t = f_t * c_{t-1} + i_t * \widetilde{c}_t \tag{1}$$

$$f_t = \sigma(U_f h_{t-1} + W_f x_t + b_f) \tag{2}$$

$$i_t = \sigma(U_i h_{t-1} + W_i x_t + b_i) \tag{3}$$

$$\widetilde{c}_t = tanh(U_c h_{t-1} + W_c x_t + b_c) \tag{4}$$

where f_t and i_t are the forget gate and input gate activities respectively, $\widetilde{c}_t$ are auxiliary variables, U_f, U_i, U_c and W_f, W_i, W_c are the corresponding weights, and b_f, b_i, b_c are the biases. The cell states c_t maintain information about the previous time points, the forget gates control what or if the previous information will be discarded from the cell states, and the input gates control what new information will be stored in the cell states.

Then, based on the cell state definition, the states of an LSTM unit are defined as follows:

$$h_t = o_t * tanh(c_t) \tag{5}$$

$$o_t = \sigma(U_o h_{t-1} + W_o x_t + b_o) \tag{6}$$

where o_t are the output of gate activity. After the output gate, the final outputs h_t could be derived.

2.4   Deep Sparse Recurrent Auto-Encoder (DSRAE)

Previous literature study has demonstrated the efficiency of RNN in modeling tfMRI data while preserving memories of previous state information and capturing the temporal dependences of input fMRI volumes [10]. However, considering the nature of weakly-labeled fMRI data, which has noise, intrinsic component networks and inter-subject variability, letting alone that the common resting state fMRI does not provide any volume-wise labels, the previous study [10] is conceived to have two limitations when modeling fMRI data. First, RNN heavily relies on strong supervision and the lack of volume-wise labels would simply hamper RNN's training and convergence. Second, since the RNN must be trained with task labels, the features learned are limited to task-related, possibly leaving out those resting-state functional intrinsic networks. Therefore, learning the intrinsic spatial-temporal structure of fMRI data without using explicitly provided labels is in great need and much desired.

To overcome these limitations, we proposed a novel LSTM-based deep sparsity recurrent auto-encoder (DSRAE), which is a deep generative sequential neural network framework to model connectome-scale functional brain networks based on fMRI data. As shown in Fig. 3, the proposed DSRAE is an eight-layer deep neural network model and it is composed of two parts: encoder and decoder. The encoder part encodes the input into high level features and is comprised of the first four layers: one input layer, one fully-connected layer, and two recurrent layers. The decoder part reconstructs the input and is comprised of the last four layers: two recurrent layers, one fully-connected layer, and one output layer. Specifically, the node number decreases from 59,421 (the number of voxels for each volume) to 128 in the fully-connected layer, then down to 64 in the first recurrent layer, and then down to 32 in the second recurrent layer. For the decoding component, there is a reverse way for node numbers, eventually increasing to 59,421 (the length of input) by layers.

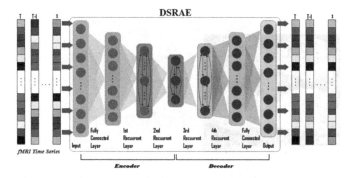

Fig. 3. The architecture of DSRAE. The DSRAE contains eight layers, in which, the first four layers are encoding layers, and the last four layers are decoding layers. One input layer, one fully-connected layer, two recurrent layers included in encoding layers; two recurrent layers, one fully-connected layer, and one output layer correspondingly included in decoding layers.

The DSRAE models were trained on 791 subjects with tfMRI dataset of both language task and working memory task. For each task, we set the LSTM see-back step as the length of the scan volumes, 316 and 405 separately. And all the other hyper-parameters are same for these two tasks: the learning rate is set as 0.01, the epoch is set as 5 based on convergence, and due to the memory restriction of the GPU, the batch size is set as 1. Notably, during the training or DSRAE, we empirically use the L1-regulation (10e−7) and L2-regulation (10e−4) at the same time to make our model more robust.

3   Experiment Results

We investigated the proposed DSRAE models on both task datasets to ensure the effectiveness and robustness across different tasks. The results have shown consistently good performance in terms of inferring and characterizing both task-evoked and spontaneous brain networks at the connectome scale, demonstrating that the DSRAE model is effective and robust.

3.1   DSRAE Reconstruction Error Analysis

To quantitatively evaluate and validate the signal reconstruction accuracy by DSRAE, the Pearson correlation coefficients between original tfMRI signals and reconstructed signals were calculated. As shown in Fig. 4a, the reconstruction result of DSRAE in spatial dimension is illustrated, in which DSRAE has good reconstruction performance, that is, all the correlations are larger than 0.9. Specifically, 4 voxels were randomly selected to show the reconstruction error in temporal dimension, in which the reconstruction time series (blue curve) have remarkably high correlation with the original fMRI data time series (orange curve) (as shown in Fig. 4b). The high correlations between the original signals and reconstructed signals indicate that our DSRAE model can encode good spatial-temporal representations and reconstruct the input data.

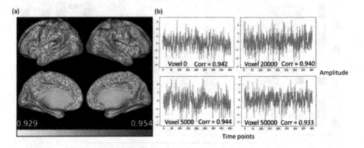

Fig. 4. The performance of DSRAE in reconstructing the fMRI signals. (a) The Pearson correlation coefficients between the reconstructed signals by DSRAE and the original signals in spatial dimension. (b) Temporal fluctuation comparison of the reconstructed voxels and original voxels. Blue curves are the reconstruction time series. Orange curves are the time series of original fMRI data. (Color figure online)

3.2   Interpreting Feature Maps of Brain Responses via DSRAE Model

To interpret the complex feature maps obtained by DSRAE, we treated the task paradigm via General Linear Model (GLM) as the benchmark event block map, which is a common practice in the fMRI field. For each task, we totally obtained 32 networks via DSRAE. Figures 5, 6 and 7 show the estimated outputs activated by language task, and Figs. 8, 9 and 10 show the estimated outputs activated by working memory task and their comparison results. As shown in Fig. 5, the resulted spatial and temporal patterns predicted by DSRAE model are consistent with the GLM-derived benchmark patterns and task design ground truth. There are two different stimulations within language task (story and math). Figure 5a is the estimated output map activated by story stimulation, which is the 6th network out of 32 networks. Comparing this brain network with the benchmark event block map via GLM, it is easy to recognize close match between them (as shown in Fig. 5b). Figure 5c shows the temporal fluctuation tendency of network #6 with the time series, in which the predicted time series (orange curve) has a very high similarity (the highest correlation coefficient is 0.8 among the 4 randomly selected subjects) with the ground truth of story stimulation (blue curve). Although all the subjects we showed here have similar high correlation coefficients, the temporal time series vary among different subjects, which suggests the unique activations of different individuals. Since our DSRAE model is an unsupervised architecture, there are some other similar spatial maps that can be detected during the activation of story stimulation (shown in Fig. 5d). Based on the time series compared with ground truth and the corresponding correlation coefficients (correlation coefficients are 0.745 and 0.683 separately), it can be observed that network #17 and #22 are both story activation maps, which indicates that the brain states would vary during time sessions even under the same stimulation, and the dynamic fluctuations would not change in a transient way.

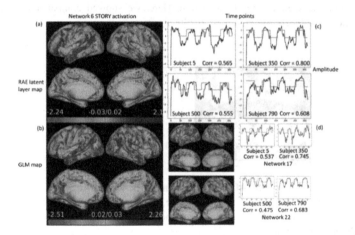

Fig. 5. The comparison between DSRAE and GLM outputs of story stimulation specific maps in language task. (a) The spatial activation map predicted by DSRAE, the 6th network of the total 32 networks. (b) The spatial benchmark activation map predicated by GLM. (c) The temporal fluctuation of network #6 and ground truth. Here, we showed the comparison results of four randomly selected subjects. Blue curves are ground truth. Orange curves are DSRAE temporal outputs. (d) Several other similar spatial maps of story activation and their temporal fluctuation. Here, we showed the comparison results of two randomly selected subjects for each map. (Color figure online)

Figure 6 shows the specific maps of math stimulation, which is the control experiment of story, the comparison with the task block GLM benchmark map, and task ground truth. Though the math stimulation is similar in auditory and phonological

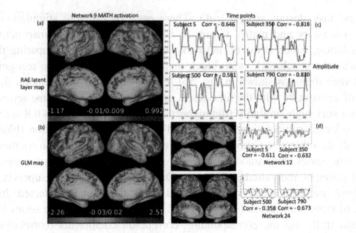

Fig. 6. The comparison between DSRAE and GLM-derived benchmark outputs of math stimulation specific maps in language task. (a) The activation map predicted by DSRAE, and the 9th network of the total 32 networks. (b) The activation map predicated by GLM. (c) The fluctuation of network #9 with time series. Here, 4 subjects were randomly selected. Blue curves are ground truth. Orange curves are DSRAE temporal outputs. (d) Several other similar maps as math activation and their temporal fluctuation. Here, we showed comparison results of two randomly selected subjects for each map. (Color figure online)

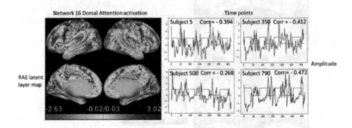

Fig. 7. New map found by DSRAE in language task. The Dorsal Attention Network activation (network #16), and its temporal fluctuation. Here, we showed the comparison results of four randomly selected subjects. Blue curves are ground truth. Orange curves are DSRAE temporal outputs. (Color figure online)

input, the spatial activated maps are quite different from that of story stimulation (as shown in Fig. 6a and b). In Fig. 6c, there is a quite high negative correlation of network #9 (the math specific state) with the story stimulation (versus with math stimulation). Here, the greater the negative correlation coefficient is, the more relevant the network is with the math stimulation. For subject #790, the absolute value of the correlation coefficient can even reach up to 0.830, which indicates that the network predicted by DSRAE is quite meaningful. Besides, in Fig. 6d, there are several similar networks as the math activation, which also have good correlation with the task design ground truth.

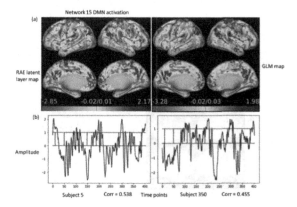

Fig. 8. The comparison between DSRAE and GLM benchmark outputs of cue period specific maps of working memory task. (a) The activation map predicted by DSRAE, the 15th network of the total 32 networks, and the benchmark activation map predicated by GLM. (b) The fluctuation of network #15 with time series, 2 subjects were randomly selected. Green curves are cue period ground truth. Blue curves are 2-back memory test. Orange curves are 0-back memory test. Red curves are DSRAE temporal outputs. (Color figure online)

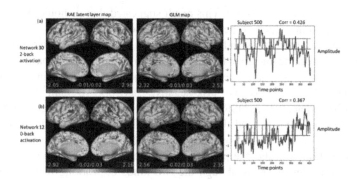

Fig. 9. The comparison between DSRAE and GLM outputs of working memory tasks specific maps. (a) The activation map of 2-back memory test predicted by DSRAE, the 30th network of the total 32 networks, the corresponding activation map predicated by GLM, and the time series of network #30. Here for simplicity, one subject was randomly selected for each spatial map. Green curves are cue period ground truth. Blue curves are 2-back memory test. Orange curves are 0-back memory test. Red curves are DSRAE temporal outputs. (b) The activation map of 0-back memory test predicted by DSRAE, the 12th network of the total 32 networks, the correspondent activation map predicated by GLM, and the time series of network #12. (Color figure online)

Since the DSRAE models were trained in an unsupervised training way, the features are not limited to task-related networks. In this way, the Dorsal Attention Network (DAN) can be detected via DSRAE model, which is a common distinct control network in language task. Figure 7 shows the spatial map of activation of DAN and its time series, where the DAN is negatively correlated with the story stimulation

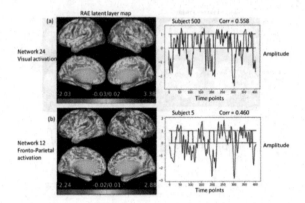

Fig. 10. New maps found by DSRAE in working memory task. (a) The Visual Network activation (network #24), and its temporal fluctuation. Here, we showed 1 randomly selected subject's comparison result with task design ground truth. Green curves are cue period ground truth. Blue curves are 2-back memory test. Orange curves are 0-back memory test. Red curves are DSRAE temporal outputs. (b) The Fronto-Parietal Network activation (network #12), and its fluctuation tendency. (Color figure online)

(correlation coefficient is − 0.472). This result suggested that it should be activated by the math stimulation, which is the control stimulation of story.

To evaluate the robustness and efficiency of our DSRAE model, we also tested the architecture on working memory task dataset. Two stimulations, 0-back memory test and 2-back memory test, and cue period were embedded. Firstly, in the cue period relevant network, which is the task-negative network, Default Mode Network (DMN) has been detected via DSRAE. Figure 8a shows the DMN (network #15 out of 32 networks) from DSRAE and that from GLM. To be more specific, here two subjects' time series of network #15 are shown in Fig. 8b, where the time series have high positive correlation with the cue period (correlation coefficient is 0.538).

For the task-relevant maps, though the two kinds of working memory tests have very similar activation maps, we still obtained the task-specific spatial maps, as shown in Fig. 9. In Fig. 9a, the 2-back relevant spatial map via DSRAE is shown (network #30), which is similar to that benchmark derived from GLM. And the time series also exhibited a stronger correlation between network #30 and the 2-back test (correlation coefficient is 0.426) than that between network #30 and the 0-back test. The 0-back test always has less memory loaded on the brain, so it is difficult to detect the specific network. Here, in Fig. 9b, network #12 has shown strong relevance to the 0-back test (correlation coefficient is 0.367).

Interestingly, via the unsupervised DSRAE model, the Visual Network (network #30) and Fronto-Parietal Network (network #12) have also been detected, as shown in Fig. 10. Because the working memory task needed the subjects to look at the screen to finish the test during the task, the Visual Network could be activated. And as shown in Fig. 10a, network #30 has a positive correlation (correlation coefficient is 0.558) with the working memory tasks, which may indicate that the subjects paid strong attention to the screen during the task performances. The connectivity of Fronto-Parietal Network which has been known to be important for subserving working memory was also derived from DSRAE, as shown in Fig. 10b. And the time series have a positive correlation (correlation coefficient is 0.46) with the working memory tasks.

3.3 Decoding Brain States During Task Periods

To detect what functional state the brain is in during the task period more specifically, we investigated the correlation of the input fMRI volumetric data and the learned feature networks via Pearson correlation, which is conceptually similar to the volumetric convolution operation used in the literature [13]. Essentially, both of these two metrics quantitatively measure how good the learned network map represents the original fMRI volume image [13]. In the correlation matrix, each row or column represents each network or original volume separately, which could show the relationship between each network and each original volume. Figure 11 shows the correlation matrix of 32 networks and the original volumes of two randomly selected subjects. Network #6 and network #9 are distinctive networks from story and math stimulation. No matter in which subject, the network #6 has the positive relevance during the story period, while network #9 has the negative relevance, which indicates that the networks predicted by DSRAE are stable and robust across all subjects we studied. Figure 12 shows the correlation matrix between brain networks and original volumes of working memory task, which has shown a similar result as that in language task. For example, network #15 is DMN and it has high relevance with the cue period, which could be an evidence that DMN could be suppressed during task period. In Figs. 11 and 12, there are some volumes which have high positive correlation or negative correlation with some networks, which suggests that the brain is in such states at those time points. However, some volumes have low correlation with all networks, which might indicate that the brain stays in multiple states at the same time. In general, our DSRAE model has revealed interesting patterns of spatial-temporal brain network dynamics that needs extensive future interpretation studies.

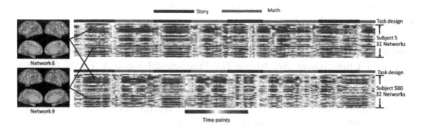

Fig. 11. The correlation matrix of the networks derived by DSRAE and the fMRI volumes of language task. 2 randomly selected subjects are shown.

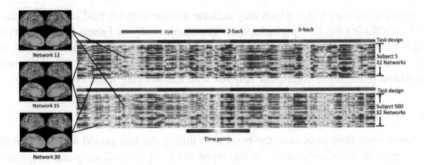

Fig. 12. The correlation matrix of the networks derived by DSRAE and the fMRI volumes of working memory task. 2 randomly selected subjects are shown.

4 Discussion and Conclusion

In this work, we proposed a novel deep sparse recurrent auto-encoder model to identify and characterize connectome-scale functional networks from the spatial-temporal 4D fMRI data in an unsupervised way. We used the HCP language and working memory tasks as our experiment testbed in this study and obtained promising results. To our best knowledge, the proposed DSRAE is among the early unified spatial-temporal deep learning models that can infer large-scale brain networks from 4D fMRI data directly in an unsupervised way. By analyzing the feature maps of the brain responses, we confirmed that the feature maps are robust and meaningful. Besides, some latent networks have been identified and compared with the benchmark from classic GLM, and the results confirmed the effectiveness of the DSRAE model. The DSRAE model also revealed the complex patterns of temporal brain network dynamics. For instance, DSRAE can detect some volumes that are highly correlated with one of the networks, which is expected. But for some volumes with low correlation, there might be some more subtle states that need to be further decoded. In our future work, we will conduct more interpretations into the feature networks learned by DSRAE to provide neuroscientific insights into the DSRAE. In addition, we will also consider applying the DSRAE framework on rfMRI datasets to potentially investigate the altered brain network states in brain disorders.

Acknowledgment. Q. Li was supported by the General Program of National Natural Science Foundation of China (Grant No. 61876021), Fundamental Research Funds for the Central Universities (Grant No. 2017EYT36) and the program of China Scholarships Council (No. 201806040083). T. Liu was partially supported by National Institutes of Health (DA033393, AG042599) and National Science Foundation (IIS-1149260, CBET1302089, BCS-1439051 and DBI-1564736). We thank the HCP projects for sharing their valuable fMRI datasets.

References

1. Logothetis, N.K.: What we can do and what we cannot do with fMRI. Nature **453**, 869–878 (2008)
2. Luiz, P.: Understanding brain networks and brain organization. Phys. Life Rev. **11**, 400–435 (2014)
3. Friston, K.J.: Transients, metastability, and neuronal dynamics. Neuroimage **5**, 164–171 (1997)
4. Shimony, J.S., et al.: Resting state spontaneous fluctuations in brain activity: a new paradigm for presurgical planning using fMRI **16**, 578 (2009)
5. Smith, S.M., et al.: Temporally-independent functional modes of spontaneous brain activity. Proc. Natl. Acad. Sci. **109**, 3131–3136 (2012)
6. Lv, J., et al.: Holistic atlases of functional networks and interactions reveal reciprocal organizational architecture of cortical function. IEEE TBME **62**, 1120–1131 (2015)
7. Plis, S.M., et al.: Deep learning for neuroimaging: a validation study. Front. Neurosci. **8**, 1–11 (2014)
8. Hu, X., et al.: Latent source mining in FMRI via restricted Boltzmann machine. Hum. Brain Mapp. **39**, 2368–2380 (2018)
9. Huang, H., et al.: Modeling task fMRI data via deep convolutional autoencoder. IEEE Trans. Med. Imaging **37**, 1551–1561 (2018)
10. Wang, H., et al.: Recognizing brain states using deep sparse recurrent neural network. IEEE Trans. Med. Imaging **38**, 1058 (2018)
11. Jiang, X., et al.: Sparse representation of HCP grayordinate data reveals novel functional architecture of cerebral cortex. Hum. Brain Mapp. **36**, 5301–5319 (2015)
12. Zhang, W., et al.: Experimental comparisons of sparse dictionary learning and independent component analysis for brain network inference from fMRI Data. IEEE Trans. Biomed. Eng. **66**, 289 (2018)
13. Zhao, Yu., et al.: Modeling 4D fMRI data via spatio-temporal convolutional neural networks (ST-CNN). In: Frangi, A.F., Schnabel, J.A., Davatzikos, C., Alberola-López, C., Fichtinger, G. (eds.) MICCAI 2018. LNCS, vol. 11072, pp. 181–189. Springer, Cham (2018). https://doi.org/10.1007/978-3-030-00931-1_21
14. Barch, D.M., et al.: Function in the human connectome: task-fMRI and individual differences in behavior. Neuroimage **80**, 169–189 (2013)
15. Glasser, M.F., et al.: The minimal preprocessing pipelines for the Human Connectome Project. Neuroimage **80**, 105–124 (2013)
16. Binder, J.R., et al.: Mapping anterior temporal lobe language areas with fMRI: a multicenter normative study. Neuroimage **54**, 1465–1475 (2011)
17. Drobyshevsky, A., Baumann, S.B., Schneider, W.: A rapid fMRI task battery for mapping of visual, motor, cognitive, and emotional function. Neuroimage **31**, 732–744 (2006)
18. Caceres, A., et al.: Measuring fMRI reliability with the intra-class correlation coefficient Alejandro. Neuroimage **45**, 758–768 (2009)
19. Hochreiter, S., Urgen, J.J.: Long short-term memory. Neural Comput. **9**(8), 1735–1780 (1997)

Ultrasound Image Representation Learning by Modeling Sonographer Visual Attention

Richard Droste[1]([✉]), Yifan Cai[1], Harshita Sharma[1], Pierre Chatelain[1],
Lior Drukker[2], Aris T. Papageorghiou[2], and J. Alison Noble[1]

[1] Department of Engineering Science,
University of Oxford, Oxford, UK
richard.droste@eng.ox.ac.uk
[2] Nuffield Department of Women's and Reproductive Health,
University of Oxford, Oxford, UK

Abstract. Image representations are commonly learned from class labels, which are a simplistic approximation of human image understanding. In this paper we demonstrate that transferable representations of images can be learned without manual annotations by modeling human visual attention. The basis of our analyses is a unique gaze tracking dataset of sonographers performing routine clinical fetal anomaly screenings. Models of sonographer visual attention are learned by training a convolutional neural network (CNN) to predict gaze on ultrasound video frames through visual saliency prediction or gaze-point regression. We evaluate the transferability of the learned representations to the task of ultrasound standard plane detection in two contexts. Firstly, we perform transfer learning by fine-tuning the CNN with a limited number of labeled standard plane images. We find that fine-tuning the saliency predictor is superior to training from random initialization, with an average F1-score improvement of 9.6% overall and 15.3% for the cardiac planes. Secondly, we train a simple softmax regression on the feature activations of each CNN layer in order to evaluate the representations independently of transfer learning hyper-parameters. We find that the attention models derive strong representations, approaching the precision of a fully-supervised baseline model for all but the last layer.

Keywords: Representation learning · Gaze tracking ·
Fetal ultrasound · Self-supervised learning · Saliency prediction ·
Transfer learning · Convolutional neural networks

1 Introduction

When interpreting images, humans direct their attention towards semantically informative regions [17]. This allocation of visual attention is typically quantified via the distribution of gaze points, which can be recorded with gaze tracking.

© Springer Nature Switzerland AG 2019
A. C. S. Chung et al. (Eds.): IPMI 2019, LNCS 11492, pp. 592–604, 2019.
https://doi.org/10.1007/978-3-030-20351-1_46

There has been great interest in developing models of human visual attention that, given an image, predict the likelihood that each pixel is fixated upon, hereafter referred to as *visual saliency map*. Currently, convolutional neural networks (CNNs) are the most effective visual attention models (VAMs) due to their ability to learn complex feature hierarchies through end-to-end training [2]. Here, we explore the following question: *To what extent can models of human visual attention transfer to tasks such as automatic image classification?*

We explore this question using the application of fetal anomaly ultrasound scanning. The scan is performed during mid-pregnancy in order to detect fetal anomalies that require prenatal treatment and to determine the place, time and mode of birth. Previous work related to this application has focused on detecting so-called ultrasound standard imaging planes through fully-supervised training of image classifiers [1,3,15]. Here, in contrast, we aim to learn transferable representations of the scan data without manual supervision by modeling sonographer visual attention. To this end, we acquire the gaze of sonographers in real-time through unobtrusive gaze tracking alongside anomaly scan recordings.

Sonographer visual attention is modeled by training a CNN to predict gaze on random video frames. We consider this to be *self-supervised representation learning* since it does not require any manual annotations and gaze data is acquired fully automatically. We extract high-resolution image features by introducing dilated convolutions [10,19] into a recently proposed image classification architecture [8]. Two methods for training the model for gaze prediction are evaluated: (i) *Visual saliency prediction:* Ground truth visual saliency maps are generated and used as training targets [2]. (ii) *Gaze-point regression:* The approach of gaze-point regression [14] is much less explored in the literature but is simpler since it does not require explicit modeling of foveal vision for ground truth saliency map generation. An existing mathematically differentiable method is based on a fully-connected layer [14] which does not scale well to high-resolution feature maps due to the exponentially increasing number of learnable parameters. Here, we propose a method based on the soft-argmax algorithm by Levine et al. [11] with no additional learnable parameters compared to saliency prediction.

The learned representations are evaluated on the task of standard plane detection in two contexts. (1) *Transfer learning:* We fine-tune the weights of the entire CNN with a limited number of training samples, thereby assessing the transferability of the learned representations in a realistic scenario. (2) *Softmax regression:* We fix the weights of the CNN and train a simple softmax regression on the spatially average-pooled feature activations of each layer. This procedure determines the generality of the representations independently of any transfer learning hyper-parameters.

Related Work. Visual saliency predictors have previously been employed to aid computer vision tasks. Cornia et al. [5] use a pre-trained saliency predictor as an attention module within an image captioning architecture. However, no representations are shared between the saliency predictor and the task-specific architecture. Cai et al. [3] show that saliency prediction can aid fetal abdominal standard plane detection. The authors fine-tune an existing standard plane detector

[1] with manually labeled data, using saliency prediction as an auxiliary task and as an attention module. In contrast, we show that transferable representations can be learned without manual annotations via visual attention modeling only. Moreover, we evaluate our framework on full-length freehand clinical fetal anomaly scans instead of short sequences (sweeps) of the fetal abdomen.

Within the field of unsupervised representation learning, our method is most closely related to *self-supervised learning*. The general idea is to exploit "free" supervision signals, i.e., supervision signals that can be extracted from the data itself without any manual annotation, which is comparable to our approach of using automatically acquired gaze for supervision. Specifically, representations are learned by either altering the data and inferring the alteration (e.g., spatial and color transformations [7]) or by predicting certain properties of the data that are withheld (e.g., the relative position of image patches [6] or the order of video frames [13]). However, all existing methods design artificial tasks that yield transferable representations as a "by-product". Human gaze, in contrast, is inherently a strong prior for semantic information [17].

Contributions. Our contributions are three-fold: (1) We propose an original framework for self-supervised image representation learning by modeling human visual attention. The method does not require manual annotations, is generic, and has the potential to be applied in any setting where gaze tracking and image data can be acquired simultaneously. To the best of our knowledge, this is the first attempt to study human visual attention modeling in the context of self-supervised representation learning; (2) we propose a method to regress gaze point coordinates via the soft-argmax algorithm, which is significantly simpler and more computationally efficient than the existing method by Ngo et al. [14]; (3) finally, we evaluate the attention models on the exemplary task of fetal anomaly ultrasound standard plane detection, both for transfer learning and as fixed feature extractors, thus demonstrating the applicability to a challenging real-world medical imaging task. The framework is illustrated in Fig. 1(a).

2   Representation Learning by Modeling Visual Attention

In this section we describe our method of learning image representations from video and gaze data in general terms. Let $\mathcal{X} \subset \mathbb{R}^{N_c \times H \times W}$ be the set of video frames with width W, height H and N_c channels and let $\mathcal{P} = [0, W] \times [0, H]$ be the set of all valid gaze points. Each frame $\mathbf{X} \in \mathcal{X}$ has a corresponding gaze point set $G = \{\mathbf{p}_i \mid \mathbf{p}_i \in \mathcal{P}\}_{i=1}^{N_G}$ with $N_G \geq 1$. The dataset $\mathcal{D} = \left\{ \left(\mathbf{X}^{(t)}, G^{(t)}\right) \right\}_{t=1}^{N_x}$ consists of N_x pairs of video frames and gaze point sets.

Let $\boldsymbol{f}_\theta : \mathcal{X} \rightarrow \mathbb{R}^{N_f \times \frac{1}{2^d} H \times \frac{1}{2^d} W}$ be a CNN with N_f feature channels, 2^d-fold spatial down-sampling and learnable parameters θ. The final, classification-specific operations (global pooling, fully-connected layers and softmax layers) are removed from the network at this stage. In our experiments we use the SE-ResNeXt [8] model, but any similar feed-forward CNN is suitable. Since

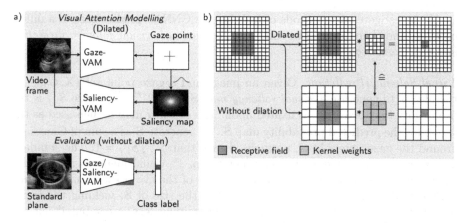

Fig. 1. (a) Illustration of our framework for learning and evaluating visual attention models (VAMs). (b) The upper part illustrates a dilated convolution after removed down-sampling operation. When the down-sampling operation is reintroduced for classification as shown in the lower part, the dilation is removed from the kernel without changing the learned kernel weights. The receptive field of the corresponding output neurons is unchanged and the operation is reversible.

such models are designed for image classification, they perform strong down-sampling in order to increase the receptive field of the higher-level neurons and to reduce computational complexity. In contrast, for visual attention modeling, it is desirable to preserve spatial information throughout the network. Consequently, we remove the last N_D down-sampling operations, i.e., max-pooling or strided convolutions. However, this modification reduces the receptive field of the subsequent neurons. If the down-sampling operations were reintroduced to restore the original architecture and use the representations for classification tasks, the learned weights would be invalid. Therefore, the 3×3 convolutions after the removed down-sampling operations are replaced with *dilated* 3×3 convolutions [19] such that each convolutional kernel maintains the same receptive field as in the original architecture, as illustrated in Fig. 1(b). Formally, given a matrix $\mathbf{M}$ and the kernel $k : [-r, r]^2 \cap \mathbb{Z}^2 \to \mathbb{R}$ of size $(2r + 1)^2$, the l-fold dilated convolution operator $*_l$ is defined as:

$$(\mathbf{M} *_l k)_{i,j} = \sum_{n=-r}^{r} \sum_{m=-r}^{r} \mathbf{M}_{i+ln,j+lm}\, k(n, m) \tag{1}$$

The resulting dilated CNN $f_\theta^\oplus$ has the increased output resolution of $(H_D, W_D) := (\frac{1}{2^{d-N_D}}H, \frac{1}{2^{d-N_D}}W)$. Next, we want to reduce the high-dimensional feature activations to a single probability map that can be used to model visual attention. Hence, a series of *adaptation layers* consisting of a 7×7 depthwise convolution and several 1×1 convolutions is appended that outputs a single activation map $\mathbf{A} \in \mathbb{R}^{H_D \times W_D}$. A probability map $\hat{\mathbf{S}}$ is then computed by applying a *softmax* across the activations with $\hat{S}_{i,j} = e^{A_{i,j}} / \sum_{i,j} e^{A_{i,j}}$.

We investigate two methods of training the CNN to predict gaze in a differentiable, and therefore end-to-end trainable, manner: *visual saliency prediction* and *gaze-point regression*.

Visual Saliency Prediction. Given an image and a gaze point set $(\mathbf{X}, G) \in \mathcal{D}$, the idea is to generate a *visual saliency map* $\mathbf{S} \in [0,1]^{H \times W}$, where $S_{i,j}$ is the probability that pixel $X_{i,j}$ is fixated upon. The saliency map is then used as the target for the predicted probability map $\hat{\mathbf{S}}$. We generate $\mathbf{S}$ as a sum of Gaussians around the gaze points in G, normalized such that $\sum_{i,j} S_{i,j} = 1$. The standard deviation of the Gaussians is equivalent to ca. $1°$ visual angle to account for the radius of visual acuity and the uncertainty of the eye tracker measurements [4]. Next, the saliency map is downscaled to the size of $\hat{\mathbf{S}}$, yielding the training target $\mathbf{S}^* \in [0,1]^{H_D \times W_D}$. Finally, the training loss is computed via the Kullback-Leibler divergence (KLD) between the predicted and the downscaled true distribution:

$$\mathcal{L}_s(\mathbf{S}^*, \hat{\mathbf{S}}) = D_{\mathrm{KL}}(\mathbf{S}^* \| \hat{\mathbf{S}}) = \sum_{i,j} S_{i,j}^* \cdot (log(S_{i,j}^*) - log(\hat{S}_{i,j})) \qquad (2)$$

Gaze-Point Regression. We propose a method for reducing $\hat{\mathbf{S}}$ to a single gaze point in order to compare it to the true gaze points. This eliminates the need to model the probability distribution of gaze points via a visual saliency map. First, $\hat{\mathbf{S}}$ is transformed into image coordinates via the soft-argmax algorithm [11]. With $g(i,j) := \left(\frac{j-0.5}{W_D} W, \frac{i-0.5}{H_D} H\right)$ as the function that maps entry (i,j) of $\hat{\mathbf{S}}$ to its corresponding point on the image plane, the predicted gaze point $\hat{\mathbf{p}}$ is computed as the expected value of the probability mass function defined by $\hat{\mathbf{S}}$:

$$\hat{\mathbf{p}} = \sum_{i,j} \hat{S}_{i,j}\, g(i,j) \qquad (3)$$

Next, the target gaze point $\mathbf{p}^*$ is obtained from the gaze point set G via the geometric median:

$$\mathbf{p}^* = \arg\min_{\mathbf{p}^* \in [0,W] \times [0,H]} \sum_{p_i \in G} \|\mathbf{p}_i - \mathbf{p}^*\|_2 \qquad (4)$$

This reduction is justified by the fact that the gaze points on each frame tend to be highly localized due to the short frame period (ca. 33 ms). Finally, the training loss is obtained as $\mathcal{L}_g(\mathbf{p}^*, \hat{\mathbf{p}}) = \|\mathbf{p}^* - \hat{\mathbf{p}}\|_2$, i.e., the Euclidean distance between the predicted and the target gaze point.

3   Experiments

Data. We acquired a novel dataset of clinical fetal ultrasound exams with real-time sonographer gaze tracking data. The exams are performed on a GE Voluson E8 scanner (General Electric, USA) while the video signal of the machine's

Table 1. SE-ResNeXt-50 (half-width) [18] and SonoNet-64 [1] (variant of VGG-16 [16]) architectures. Convolutional layers are denoted as 'conv <kernel-size>, <output-channels>[, <$C = cardinality$>]', where cardinality is the number of grouped convolutions. SE modules are denoted as 'fc' followed by the dimensions of the corresponding fully-connected layers. Scales in parentheses correspond to the dilated networks for attention modeling. The lower part of the table shows the heads for attention modeling and classification, respectively.

Layer name	SE-ResNeXt-50 (half-width, 7.4M parameters)		SonoNet-64 (14.9M parameters)	
	Scale	Layers	Scale	Layers
Layer 1	224×288	conv, 7×7, 64, stride 2	224×288	[conv, 3×3, 64] $\times 2$
	112×144	max pool, 3, stride 2		
Layer 2	56×72	$\begin{bmatrix} \text{conv, } 1 \times 1, 64 \\ \text{conv, } 3 \times 3, 64, C = 16 \\ \text{conv, } 1 \times 1, 128 \\ fc, [8, 128] \end{bmatrix} \times 3$	112×144	[conv, 3×3, 128] $\times 2$
Layer 3	28×36	$\begin{bmatrix} \text{conv, } 1 \times 1, 128 \\ \text{conv, } 3 \times 3, 128, C = 16 \\ \text{conv, } 1 \times 1, 256 \\ fc, [16, 256] \end{bmatrix} \times 4$	56×72	[conv, 3×3, 256] $\times 3$
Layer 4	14×18 (28×36)	$\begin{bmatrix} \text{conv, } 1 \times 1, 256 \\ \text{conv, } 3 \times 3, 256, C = 16 \\ \text{conv, } 1 \times 1, 512 \\ fc, [32, 512] \end{bmatrix} \times 6$	28×36	[conv, 3×3, 512] $\times 3$
Layer 5	7×9 (28×36)	$\begin{bmatrix} \text{conv, } 1 \times 1, 512 \\ \text{conv, } 3 \times 3, 512, C = 16 \\ \text{conv, } 1 \times 1, 1024 \\ fc, [64, 1024] \end{bmatrix} \times 3$	14×18	[conv, 3×3, 512] $\times 3$
Adaptation (attention)	28×36	conv $7 \times 7, 1024, C = 1024$ [conv $1 \times 1, 256 \times 2$] conv $1 \times 1, 1$	—	—
Adaptation (classification)	7×9	conv $1 \times 1, 256$ conv $1 \times 1, N_C$ avg. pool and softmax	14×18	conv $1 \times 1, 256$ conv $1 \times 1, N_C$ avg. pool and softmax

monitor is recorded lossless at 30 Hz. Gaze is simultaneously recorded at 90 Hz with a Tobii Eye Tracker 4C (Tobii, Sweden). Ethics approval was obtained for data recording and data are stored according to local data governance rules. For our experiments, we use 135 fetal anomaly scans, which are randomly split into three equally sized subsets for cross-validation.

CNN Architecture. Recent empirical evidence suggests that ImageNet performance is strongly correlated with performance on other vision tasks [9]. Therefore, we base our CNN on SE-ResNeXt [8], a ResNet-style model with aggregated convolutions and channel recalibration (*squeeze-and-excitation*, short *SE*) modules, which won the 2017 ImageNet classification competition. For attention modeling, layers 4 and 5 are dilated as described in Sect. 2. In preliminary

Table 2. Results of visual saliency prediction and gaze-point regression compared to static baselines (mean ± standard deviation). Next to the training loss (KLD), the Saliency-VAM is evaluated on the metrics normalized scanpath saliency (NSS), AUC-Judd, Pearson's correlation coefficient (CC) and histogram intersection (SIM) (for references see [2]). Best values are marked bold.

	Saliency-VAM					Gaze-VAM
	KLD	NSS	AUC [%]	CC [%]	SIM [%]	ℓ_2-norm
Static	3.41 ±0.02	1.39 ±0.05	85.9 ±0.3	14.9 ±0.4	8.5 ±0.1	54.4 ±0.6
Learned	**2.43** ±0.03	**4.03** ±0.05	**96.7** ±0.2	**31.6** ±0.3	**18.5** ±0.2	**27.4** ±0.4

experiments we found that halving the number of feature channels (except for layer 0) greatly reduced the computational cost without performance losses on our dataset. The resulting architecture is summarized in column 1 of Table 1. Column 2 shows SonoNet-64 [1], which we use as a reference for standard plane detection since the authors published network weights trained on over 22k standard plane images.

3.1 Visual Attention Modeling

Experimental Methods. Two visual attention models (VAMs) were trained on the ultrasound video and gaze data as described in Sect. 2, namely a visual saliency predictor (*Saliency-VAM*) and a gaze-point regressor (*Gaze-VAM*). For pre-processing, all video frames that did not correspond to 2D B-mode live scanning (e.g., Doppler, 3D/4D or frozen frames) or without gaze data were discarded. Further, all but every 8th frame were discarded to reduce temporal redundancy, resulting in a total of 403070 video frames. Next, the frames were cropped down to the region of the actual ultrasound image. Data augmentation was performed by uniformly sampling sub-crops of 70–90% side length that contained the gaze points, random horizontal flipping, and varying gamma and brightness by ±25%. Finally, the frames were down-sampled to a size of 224 × 288 pixels and normalized to zero-mean and unit-variance.

Both attention models were trained via stochastic gradient descent (SGD) with momentum of 0.9, weight decay of 10^{-4} and mini-batch size of 32. The Saliency-VAM was trained for 8 epochs at a learning rate (LR) of 0.1 while the Gaze-VAM converged more slowly and was trained for 10 epochs at a LR of 0.01. In each case, the LR was decayed by a factor of 10 for the final two epochs. All experiments were implemented in the PyTorch framework. Each training run was performed in 9–16 h on a single Nvidia GTX 1080 Ti.

Results. Table 2 summarizes the quantitative evaluation of the attention models. The static baseline for the Saliency-VAM is the normalized sum of all ground truth saliency maps. The baseline for the Gaze-VAM is the geometric median of all gaze points. The learned models clearly outperform the static baselines

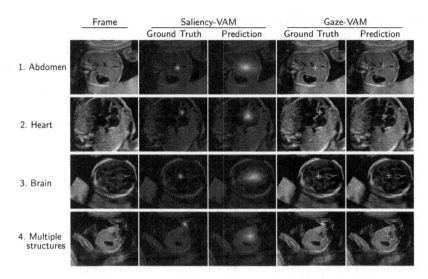

Fig. 2. Visual saliency and gaze point predictions with corresponding ground truths for representative validation set frames.

on every metric. Figure 2 shows visual saliency and gaze point predictions for four representative frames from the validation set. Frames 1.-3. each contain one anatomical structure and show examples of accurate prediction. Frame 4. contains several structures, which creates ambiguity.

3.2 Fetal Anomaly Standard Plane Detection

Experimental Methods. For comparison with Baumgartner et al. [1], we consider the same 13 standard plane classes and "background" class, except that our data contains the three vessels and trachea view (3VT) which is similar to their three-vessel view (3VV). From the available 135 anomaly scans, we obtained a total of 1129 standard plane frames with 62 to 148 samples per class (a plane may be acquired twice or may be skipped in a scan). Moreover, we sampled 1127 background frames in the vicinity of the standard planes. The same scan-level three-fold cross-validation split as for attention modeling was applied. For pre-processing, frames were cropped to the ultrasound image region as for attention modeling. The images were then augmented by random horizontal flipping, rotation by ±10°, varying the aspect-ratio by ±10%, sampling a sub-crop of 95–100% side length, and varying gamma and brightness by ±25%. As before, the images were down-sampled and normalized.

The trained visual attention models were fine-tuned (FT) on the standard plane detection task, yielding *Saliency-FT* and *Gaze-FT*. Moreover, two baselines were generated: A SE-ResNeXt model trained from random initialization and a fine-tuned SonoNet-64 (*SonoNet-FT*). Each epoch consisted of 1024 randomly sampled images. Analogous to Baumgartner et al., we overcome the class

Table 3. Standard plane detection results after fine-tuning (mean ± standard deviation [%]). *Rand. Init.* denotes the SE-ResNeXt model trained from scratch. The best score among the first three models is marked in bold. Scores of the fine-tuned SonoNet that exceed all three models are marked in bold as well. The literature SonoNet scores are given in parenthesis.

	Rand. Init	Gaze-FT	Saliency-FT	Δ(Saliency, Rand. Init.)	SonoNet-FT (Lit. value [1])
Precision	70.4 ± 2.3	67.2 ± 3.4	**79.5 ± 1.7**	9.1 ± 2.1	**82.3 ± 1.3 (81)**
Recall	64.9 ± 1.6	57.3 ± 4.5	**75.1 ± 3.4**	10.2 ± 1.9	**87.3 ± 1.1 (86)**
F1-score	67.0 ± 1.3	60.7 ± 3.9	**76.6 ± 2.6**	9.6 ± 2.1	**84.5 ± 0.9 (83)**
F1-scores per class:				↓	
RVOT	37.9 ± 3.8	30.4 ± 4.9	**58.7 ± 2.7**	20.8 ± 5.5	**71.2 ± 2.8**
LVOT	30.3 ± 4.7	25.8 ± 5.9	**48.6 ± 3.3**	18.4 ± 7.3	**69.9 ± 5.3**
4CH	43.1 ± 6.7	33.5 ± 8.5	**57.3 ± 10.8**	14.2 ± 11.9	**75.7 ± 9.1**
Kidneys	71.4 ± 5.5	68.5 ± 12.1	**84.7 ± 6.3**	13.3 ± 5.7	81.0 ± 5.0
Profile	77.5 ± 7.2	61.7 ± 7.7	**87.2 ± 7.5**	9.7 ± 3.7	**88.1 ± 4.5**
Lips	76.7 ± 2.6	74.2 ± 7.3	**85.6 ± 4.5**	8.8 ± 6.7	**92.9 ± 0.8**
Brain (Cb.)	84.9 ± 7.0	83.2 ± 1.5	**93.7 ± 4.6**	8.8 ± 2.3	92.8 ± 1.1
3VT	50.4 ± 1.9	47.1 ± 7.1	**58.3 ± 7.1**	7.9 ± 5.6	**77.9 ± 1.6**
Brain (Tv.)	86.1 ± 7.7	88.8 ± 2.8	**92.9 ± 5.0**	6.8 ± 2.8	92.1 ± 4.5
Spine (cor.)	72.9 ± 3.6	57.2 ± 2.8	**79.0 ± 3.7**	6.1 ± 6.2	**90.3 ± 4.9**
Abdominal	67.9 ± 5.1	60.8 ± 6.7	**72.9 ± 2.9**	5.0 ± 3.7	**85.0 ± 1.4**
Spine (sag.)	86.5 ± 3.5	80.2 ± 2.5	**89.1 ± 2.1**	2.7 ± 5.2	**91.6 ± 2.5**
Femur	85.7 ± 2.0	77.7 ± 0.1	**87.6 ± 1.3**	1.9 ± 1.5	**89.5 ± 1.8**
Background	85.2 ± 0.9	83.3 ± 0.7	**89.0 ± 0.4**	3.8 ± 1.2	**90.3 ± 0.4**

RVOT: right ventricular outflow tract; LVOT: left ventricular outflow tract; 4CH: four chamber view; 3VT: three vessel and trachea view; Brain (Cb.): brain cerebellum sub-occipitobregmatic plane; Brain (Tv.): brain transventricular plane; Cor.: Coronal plane; Sag.: Sagittal plane.

imbalance problem by sampling images from each standard plane class with the same frequency and sampling one background image per standard plane image. Fine-tuning was performed via SGD with momentum of 0.9, weight decay of 5×10^{-4}, mini-batch size of 16 and a cross-entropy loss. The attention models were fine-tuned for 50 epochs with a LR of 0.01, decayed by a factor of 10 at epochs 20 and 35. For the randomly initialized model, the LR was increased by a factor of 4. The SonoNet model was initialized with pre-trained weights published by the authors and fine-tuned for 25 epochs with a LR of 0.01, decayed at epochs 10 and 20. Longer training or higher learning rates led to overfitting for the latter two models due to the relatively small number of training samples. Due to the class imbalance, the overall precision, recall and F1-scores were computed as *macro-averages*, i.e., the average of the scores per standard plane.

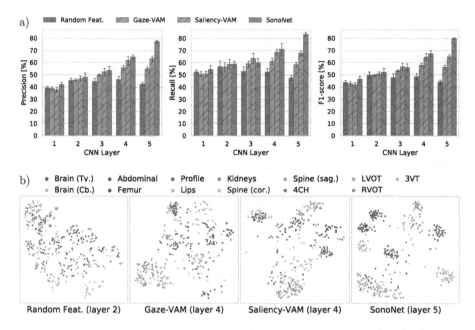

Fig. 3. (a) Results of the regression analysis of the fixed-weight attention models, and baselines. (b) t-SNE visualization of the feature embeddings at the respective layers with the highest F1-score (Background class omitted for legibility). Best viewed in color.

Besides fine-tuning, we trained a multinomial logistic regression (softmax regression) on the spatially average-pooled feature activations of each layer of the attention models and two baselines: an SE-ResNeXt model with random weights and the pre-trained SonoNet model. For each regression, the entire respective training set was sampled without augmentation. The classifier was trained with the L-BFGS solver and balanced class weights. The L2 regularization parameter was selected for each regression from a range of 16 logarithmically spaced values from 10^{-5} to 10^1 based on the validation F1-score.

Results. A quantitative evaluation of the fine-tuned attention models is shown in Table 3. The Saliency-FT model improves standard plane detection compared to the model trained from random initialization on every metric and for each standard plane. The largest improvement per anatomy is observed for the right ventricular outflow tract (RVOT) with an average 20.8% increase in F1-score, followed by the left ventricular outflow tract (LVOT) and the four chamber view (4CH). Further, the average F1-score of Saliency-FT exceeds that of SonoNet on 3/14 classes. The Gaze-FT model under-performs compared to training from random initialization. In general, the average precision, recall and F1-score of SonoNet-FT are in good agreement with the literature values. The authors do not provide per-anatomy scores for SonoNet-64.

The results of the regression analysis are shown in Fig. 3(a). The scores of both attention models monotonously increase up to layer 4 and stagnate at layer 5, peaking at F1-scores of $58.0 \pm 1.5\%$ for the Gaze-VAM and $64.9 \pm 1.5\%$ for the Saliency-VAM. The scores of the Saliency-VAM and SonoNet are at similar levels up to layer 4, while the Gaze-VAM achieves lower scores. For SonoNet the scores continue to increase at layer 5, reaching an F1-score of $79.9 \pm 0.6\%$. In general, the scores of the random features are comparable to those of the other models at layers 0 and 1 but decline afterwards, peaking at an F1-score of $49.5 \pm 2.7\%$.

The differences between the feature embeddings are illustrated for selected layers in Fig. 3(b) via t-SNE [12], a non-linear dimensionality reduction algorithm that visualizes high-dimensional neighborhoods. Compared to random features, a separation of the different standard plane classes emerges in the embeddings of the visual attention models. However, a large overlap remains among the two brain views and the cardiac views, respectively. Moreover, the views of coronal spine, kidneys, profile and lips are not well localized. In the embedding of SonoNet, most classes are well-separated with overlap remaining among the cardiac views.

4   Discussion and Conclusion

The evaluations have shown that the visual attention models have learned meaningful representations of ultrasound image data, which was the main goal of this work. In the transfer learning context, the Saliency-FT model clearly outperforms the model trained from random initialization. The largest benefit is observed for the cardiac views with an average increase in F1-score of 15.3%. In fact, the performance of Saliency-FT is closer to that of SonoNet-FT, although the latter had been pre-trained with over 22k labeled standard plane images, while the attention models are pre-trained only with sonographer gaze on unlabeled video frames. Since fine-tuning is performed with 753 standard plane images on average, this is a 30-fold reduction in the amount of manually annotated training data. Gaze-FT did not yield an improvement, indicating that visual saliency prediction is better suited to learn transferable representations.

Even without fine-tuning, the high-level features of the attention models are predictive for fetal anomaly standard plane detection, outperforming the baseline with random weights for softmax regression on the feature activations. Up to last network layer, the features of the Saliency-VAM are almost as predictive as those of SonoNet, even though it had received no explicit information about the concept of standard planes during training. This confirms our hypothesis, motivated by Wu et al. [17], that gaze is a strong prior for semantic information. At the last layer, the attention models fall behind SonoNet, indicating the task-specificity of that layer. The qualitative analysis through t-SNE confirms that some standard plane classes are well-separated in the respective feature spaces of the attention models, with overlap remaining for standard planes with similar appearance such as the brain views and the cardiac views, respectively. It should be noted that we did not compare our models to a recently proposed variation of SonoNet [15] with multi-layer attention-gating due to the added complexity of that architecture.

The results for both visual saliency prediction and gaze-point regression indicate successful learning of sonographer visual attention. This is supported by the fact that the scores on the key metrics of AUC and NSS are higher than the scores reported by Cai et al. [3] and than typical scores on the public MIT Saliency Benchmark of natural images (saliency.mit.edu). However, our scores on the CC, SIM and KLD metrics are worse compared to these sources and in general, the comparability is very limited since the maximum attainable values are dataset-dependent. For gaze-point regression, the proposed method based on the soft-argmax algorithm was found to be an effective solution.

In conclusion, we have shown that visual attention modeling is a promising method to learn image representations without manual supervision. The trained CNNs generalize well to the task of fetal anomaly standard plane detection, both for transfer learning and as fixed feature extractors. We have evaluated two methods for visual attention modeling, visual saliency prediction and gaze-point regression, and found that the representations learned with the former method generalize better. The representation learning framework presented herein is generic and therefore has the potential to be applied in many settings where gaze and image data can be readily acquired.

Acknowledgements. This work is supported by the ERC (ERC-ADG-2015 694581, project PULSE) and the EPSRC (EP/R013853/1 and EP/M013774/1). AP is funded by the NIHR Oxford Biomedical Research Centre.

References

1. Baumgartner, C.F., et al.: SonoNet: real-time detection and localisation of fetal standard scan planes in freehand ultrasound. IEEE Trans. Med. Imaging **36**(11), 2204–2215 (2017)
2. Borji, A.: Saliency prediction in the deep learning era: an empirical investigation. arXiv:1810.03716 (2018)
3. Cai, Y., Sharma, H., Chatelain, P., Noble, J.A.: Multi-task SonoEyeNet: detection of fetal standardized planes assisted by generated sonographer attention maps. In: Frangi, A.F., Schnabel, J.A., Davatzikos, C., Alberola-López, C., Fichtinger, G. (eds.) MICCAI 2018. LNCS, vol. 11070, pp. 871–879. Springer, Cham (2018). https://doi.org/10.1007/978-3-030-00928-1_98
4. Chatelain, P., Sharma, H., Drukker, L., Papageorghiou, A.T., Noble, J.A.: Evaluation of gaze tracking calibration for longitudinal biomedical imaging studies. IEEE Trans. Cybern. **99**, 1–11 (2018)
5. Cornia, M., Baraldi, L., Serra, G., Cucchiara, R.: Visual saliency for image captioning in new multimedia services. In: ICMEW (2017)
6. Doersch, C., Gupta, A., Efros, A.A.: Unsupervised visual representation learning by context prediction. In: ICCV (2015)
7. Dosovitskiy, A., Fischer, P., Springenberg, J.T., Riedmiller, M., Brox, T.: Discriminative unsupervised feature learning with exemplar convolutional neural networks. In: NIPS (2014)

8. Hu, J., Shen, L., Sun, G.: Squeeze-and-excitation networks. In: CVPR (2017)
9. Kornblith, S., Shlens, J., Le, Q.V.: Do better imagenet models transfer better? arXiv:1805.08974 (2018)
10. Kruthiventi, S.S.S., Ayush, K., Babu, R.V.: DeepFix: a fully convolutional neural network for predicting human eye fixations. IEEE Trans. Image Process. **26**(9), 4446–4456 (2015)
11. Levine, S., Finn, C., Darrell, T., Abbeel, P.: End-to-end training of deep visuomotor policies. J. Mach. Learn. Res. **17**(1), 1334–1373 (2015)
12. van der Maaten, L., Hinton, G.: Visualizing data using t-SNE. J. Mach. Learn. Res. **9**(Nov), 2579–2605 (2008)
13. Misra, I., Zitnick, C.L., Hebert, M.: Shuffle and learn: unsupervised learning using temporal order verification. In: Leibe, B., Matas, J., Sebe, N., Welling, M. (eds.) ECCV 2016. LNCS, vol. 9905, pp. 527–544. Springer, Cham (2016). https://doi.org/10.1007/978-3-319-46448-0_32
14. Ngo, T., Manjunath, B.S.: Saccade gaze prediction using a recurrent neural network. In: ICIP (2017)
15. Schlemper, J., et al.: Attention-gated networks for improving ultrasound scan plane detection. In: MIDL (2018)
16. Simonyan, K., Zisserman, A.: Very deep convolutional networks for large-scale image recognition. In: ICLR (2015)
17. Wu, C.C., Wick, F.A., Pomplun, M.: Guidance of visual attention by semantic information in real-world scenes. Front. Psychol. **5**, 54 (2014)
18. Xie, S., Girshick, R., Dollár, P., Tu, Z., He, K.: Aggregated residual transformations for deep neural networks. In: CVPR (2017)
19. Yu, F., Koltun, V.: Multi-scale context aggregation by dilated convolutions. In: ICLR (2016)

A Coupled Manifold Optimization Framework to Jointly Model the Functional Connectomics and Behavioral Data Spaces

Niharika Shimona D'Souza[1]([✉]), Mary Beth Nebel[2,3], Nicholas Wymbs[2,3], Stewart Mostofsky[2,3,4], and Archana Venkataraman[1]

[1] Department of Electrical and Computer Engineering, Johns Hopkins University, Baltimore, USA
`Shimona.Niharika.Dsouza@jhu.edu`
[2] Center for Neurodevelopmental Medicine and Research, Kennedy Krieger Institute, Baltimore, USA
[3] Department of Neurology, Johns Hopkins School of Medicine, Baltimore, USA
[4] Department of Pediatrics, Johns Hopkins School of Medicine, Baltimore, USA

Abstract. The problem of linking functional connectomics to behavior is extremely challenging due to the complex interactions between the two distinct, but related, data domains. We propose a coupled manifold optimization framework which projects fMRI data onto a low dimensional matrix manifold common to the cohort. The patient specific loadings simultaneously map onto a behavioral measure of interest via a second, non-linear, manifold. By leveraging the kernel trick, we can optimize over a potentially infinite dimensional space without explicitly computing the embeddings. As opposed to conventional manifold learning, which assumes a fixed input representation, our framework directly optimizes for embedding directions that predict behavior. Our optimization algorithm combines proximal gradient descent with the trust region method, which has good convergence guarantees. We validate our framework on resting state fMRI from fifty-eight patients with Autism Spectrum Disorder using three distinct measures of clinical severity. Our method outperforms traditional representation learning techniques in a cross validated setting, thus demonstrating the predictive power of our coupled objective.

1 Introduction

Steady state patterns of co-activity in resting state fMRI (rs-fMRI) are believed to reflect the intrinsic functional connectivity between brain regions [4]. Hence, there is increasing interest to use rs-fMRI as a diagnostic tool for studying neurological disorders such as autism, schizophrenia and ADHD. Unfortunately, the well reported confounds of rs-fMRI, coupled with patient heterogeneity makes the task of jointly analyzing rs-fMRI and behavior extremely challenging.

© Springer Nature Switzerland AG 2019
A. C. S. Chung et al. (Eds.): IPMI 2019, LNCS 11492, pp. 605–616, 2019.
https://doi.org/10.1007/978-3-030-20351-1_47

Behavioral Prediction from Neuroimaging Data. Joint analysis of rs-fMRI and behavioral data typically follows a two stage pipeline. Stage 1 is a feature selection or a representation learning step, while Stage 2 maps the learned features onto behavioral data through a statistical or machine learning model. Some notable examples of the Stage 1 feature extraction include graph theoretic measures which aggregate the associative relationships in the connectome, and dimensionality reduction techniques [5], which explain the variation in the data. From here, popular Stage 2 algorithms include Support Vector Machine (SVMs), kernel ridge regression [5]. This pipelined approach has been successful at classification for identifying disease subtypes and distinguishing between patients and healthy controls. However, there has been limited success in terms of predicting dimensional measures, such as behavioral severity from neuroimaging data.

The work of [3] develops a generative-discriminative basis learning framework, which decomposes the rs-fMRI correlation matrices into a group and patient level term. The authors use a linear regression to estimate clinical severity from the patient representation, and jointly optimize the group average, patient coefficients, and regression weights. In this work, we pose the problem of combining the neuroimaging and behavioral data spaces as a dual manifold optimization. Namely, we represent the each patient's fMRI data using a low rank matrix decomposition to project it onto a common vector space. The projection loadings are simultaneously used to construct a high dimensional non-linear embedding to predict a behavioral manifestation. We jointly optimize both representations in order to capture the complex relationship between the two domains.

Manifold Learning for Connectomics. Numerous manifold learning approaches have been employed to study complex brain topologies, especially in the context of disease classification. For example, the work of [11] used graph kernels on the spatio-temporal fMRI time series dynamics to distinguish between the autistic and healthy groups. Going one step further, [9] used higher order morphological kernels to classify ASD subpopulations.

While these methods are computationally efficient and simple in formulation, their generalization power is limited by the input data features. Often, subtle individual level changes are overwhelmed by group level confounds. We integrate the feature learning step directly into our framework by simultaneously optimizing both the embeddings and the projection onto the behavioral space. This optimization is also coupled to the brain basis, which helps us model the behavioral and neuroimaging data space jointly, and reliably capture individual variability. We leverage the kernel trick to provide both the representational flexibility and computational tractability to outperform a variety of baselines.

2   A Coupled Manifold Optimization (CMO) Framework

Figure 1 presents an overview of our Coupled Manifold Optimization (CMO) framework. The blue box represents our neuroimaging term. We group voxels into P ROIs, yielding the $P \times P$ input correlation matrices $\{\mathbf{\Gamma}_n\}_{n=1}^N$ for N patients. As seen, the correlation matrices are projected onto a low rank subspace

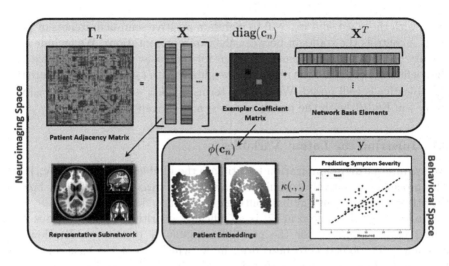

Fig. 1. Joint model for the functional connectomics and behavioral data. **Blue Box:** Matrix manifold representation **Gray Box:** Non-linear kernel ridge regression (Color figure online)

spanned by the group basis. The loadings are related to severity via a non-linear manifold and the associated kernel map, as indicated in the gray box.

Notice that $\mathbf{\Gamma}_n$ is positive semi-definite by construction. We employ a patient specific low rank decomposition $\mathbf{\Gamma}_n \approx \mathbf{Q}_n\mathbf{Q}_n^T$ to represent the correlation matrix. Each rank R factor $\{\mathbf{Q}_n \in \mathcal{R}^{P \times R}\}$, where $R \ll P$, projects onto a low dimensional subspace spanned by the columns of a group basis $\mathbf{X} \in \mathcal{R}^{P \times R}$. The vector $\mathbf{c}_n \in \mathcal{R}^{R \times 1}$ denotes the patient specific loading coefficients as follows:

$$\mathbf{\Gamma}_n \approx \mathbf{Q}_n\mathbf{Q}_n^T = \mathbf{X}\mathbf{diag}(\mathbf{c}_n)\mathbf{X}^T \tag{1}$$

where $\mathbf{diag}(\mathbf{c}_n)$ is a matrix with the entries of $\mathbf{c}_n$ on the leading diagonal, and the off-diagonal elements as 0. Equation (1) resembles a joint eigenvalue decomposition for the set $\{\mathbf{\Gamma}_n\}$ and was also used in [3]. The bases $\mathbf{X}_r \in \mathcal{R}^{P \times 1}$ capture co-activation patterns common to the group, while the coefficient loadings $\mathbf{c}_{nr}$ capture the strength of basis column r for patient n. Our key innovation is to use these coefficients to predict clinical severity via a non-linear manifold. We define an embedding map $\phi(\cdot) : \mathcal{R}^R \rightarrow \mathcal{R}^M$, which maps the native space representation of the coefficient vector $\mathbf{c}$ to an M dimensional embedding space, i.e. $\phi(\mathbf{c}) \in \mathcal{R}^{M \times 1}$. If $\mathbf{y}_n$ is the clinical score for patient n, we have the non-linear regression:

$$\mathbf{y}_n \approx \phi(\mathbf{c}_n)^T\mathbf{w} \tag{2}$$

with weight vector $\mathbf{w} \in \mathcal{R}^{M \times 1}$. Our joint objective combines Eqs. (1) and (2)

$$\mathcal{J}(\mathbf{X}, \{\mathbf{c}_n\}, \mathbf{w}) = \sum_n \left[||\mathbf{\Gamma}_n - \mathbf{X}\mathbf{diag}(\mathbf{c}_n)\mathbf{X}^T||_F^2 + \lambda ||\mathbf{y}_n - \phi(\mathbf{c}_n)^T\mathbf{w}||_2^2 \right] \tag{3}$$

along with the constraint $c_{nr} \geq 0$ to maintain positive semi-definiteness of $\{\Gamma_n\}$. Here, λ controls the trade-off between the two representations. We include an ℓ_1 penalty on $\mathbf{X}$ to promote sparse solutions for the basis. We also regularize both the coefficients $\{c_n\}$ and the regression weights $\mathbf{w}$ with ℓ_2 penalties to ensure that the objective is well posed. We add the terms $\gamma_1||\mathbf{X}||_1 + \gamma_2\sum_n ||c_n||_2^2 + \gamma_3||\mathbf{w}||_2^2$ to $\mathcal{J}(\cdot)$ in Eq. (3) with the penalties γ_1, γ_2 and γ_3 respectively.

2.1   Inferring the Latent Variables

We use alternating minimization to estimate the hidden variables $\{\mathbf{X}, \{c_n\}, \mathbf{w}\}$. This procedure iteratively optimizes each unknown variable in Eq. (3) by holding the others constant until global convergence is reached.

Proximal gradient descent [7] is an efficient algorithm which provides good convergence guarantees for the non-differentiable ℓ_1 penalty on $\mathbf{X}$. However, it requires the objective to be convex in $\mathbf{X}$, which is not the case due to the bi-quadratic Frobenius norm expansion in Eq. (1). Hence, we introduce N constraints of the form $\mathbf{V}_n = \mathbf{X}\mathrm{diag}(c_n)$, similar to the work of [3]. We enforce these constraints using the Augmented Lagrangians $\{\Lambda_n\}$:

$$\mathcal{J}(\mathbf{X}, \{c_n\}, \mathbf{w}, \{\mathbf{V}_n\}, \{\Lambda_n\}) = \sum_n ||\Gamma_n - \mathbf{V}_n\mathbf{X}^T||_F^2 + \lambda\sum_n ||\mathbf{y}_n - \phi(c_n)^T\mathbf{w}||_2^2$$

$$+ \sum_n \left[\mathrm{Tr}\left[\Lambda_n^T(\mathbf{V}_n - \mathbf{X}\mathrm{diag}(c_n))\right] + \frac{1}{2}||\mathbf{V}_n - \mathbf{X}\mathrm{diag}(c_n)||_F^2 \right] \quad (4)$$

with $c_{nr} \geq 0$ and $\mathrm{Tr}(\mathbf{M})$ denoting the trace operator. The additional terms $||\mathbf{V}_n - \mathbf{X}\mathrm{diag}(c_n)||_F^2$ regularize the trace constraints. Equation (4) is now convex in both $\mathbf{X}$ and the set $\{\mathbf{V}_n\}$, which allows us to optimize them via standard procedures. We iterate through the following four update steps till global convergence:

Proximal Gradient Descent on $\mathbf{X}$: The gradient of $\mathcal{J}$ with respect to $\mathbf{X}$ is:

$$\frac{\partial \mathcal{J}}{\partial \mathbf{X}} = \sum_n 2\left[\mathbf{X}\mathbf{V}_n^T - \Gamma_n\right]\mathbf{V}_n - \mathbf{V}_n\mathrm{diag}(c_n) + \mathbf{X}\mathrm{diag}(c_n)^2 - \Lambda_n\mathrm{diag}(c_n)$$

With a learning rate of t, the proximal update with respect to $||\mathbf{X}||_1$ is given by:

$$\mathbf{X}^k = \mathrm{prox}_{||\cdot||_1}\left[\mathbf{X}^{k-1} - \left[\frac{t}{\gamma_1}\right]\frac{\partial \mathcal{J}}{\partial \mathbf{X}}\right] \quad s.t. \quad \mathrm{prox}_t(\mathbf{L}) = \mathrm{sgn}(\mathbf{L}) \circ (\max(|\mathbf{L}| - t, \mathbf{0}))$$

Where $\circ$ denotes the Hadamard product. Effectively, this update performs an iterative shrinkage thresholding on a locally smooth quadratic model of $||\mathbf{X}||_1$.

Kernel Ridge Regression for $\mathbf{w}$: We denote $\mathbf{y}$ as the vector of the clinical severity scores and stack the patient embedding vectors i.e. $\phi(c_n) \in \mathcal{R}^{M \times 1}$ into a matrix $\Phi(\mathbf{C}) \in \mathcal{R}^{M \times N}$. The portion of $\mathcal{J}(\cdot)$ that depends on $\mathbf{w}$ is:

$$\mathcal{F}(\mathbf{w}) = \lambda||\mathbf{y} - \Phi(\mathbf{C})^T\mathbf{w}||_2^2 + \gamma_3||\mathbf{w}||_2^2 \quad (5)$$

Setting the gradient of Eq. (5) to 0, and applying the matrix inversion lemma, the closed form solution for $\mathbf{w}$ is similar to kernel ridge regression:

$$\mathbf{w} = \boldsymbol{\Phi}(\mathbf{C})\left[\boldsymbol{\Phi}(\mathbf{C})^T\boldsymbol{\Phi}(\mathbf{C}) + \frac{\gamma_3}{\lambda}\mathcal{I}_N\right]^{-1}\mathbf{y} = \boldsymbol{\Phi}(\mathbf{C})\boldsymbol{\alpha} = \sum_j \alpha_j\phi(\mathbf{c}_j) \qquad (6)$$

where $\mathcal{I}_N$ is the identity matrix. Let $\kappa(\cdot,\cdot) : \mathcal{R}^M \times \mathcal{R}^M \to \mathcal{R}$ be the kernel map for ϕ, i.e. $\kappa(\mathbf{c},\hat{\mathbf{c}}) = \phi(\mathbf{c})^T\phi(\hat{\mathbf{c}})$. The dual variable $\boldsymbol{\alpha}$ can be expressed as $\boldsymbol{\alpha} = (\mathbf{K} + \frac{\gamma_3}{\lambda}\mathcal{I}_N)^{-1}\mathbf{y}$, where $\mathbf{K} = \boldsymbol{\Phi}(\mathbf{C})^T\boldsymbol{\Phi}(\mathbf{C})$ is the Gram matrix for the kernel $\kappa(\cdot,\cdot)$. Equation (6) implies that $\mathbf{w}$ lies in the span of the coefficient embeddings defining the manifold. We use the form of $\mathbf{w}$ in Eq. (6) to update the loading vectors in the following step, without explicitly parametrizing the vector $\phi(\mathbf{c}_n)$.

Trust Region Update for $\{\mathbf{c}_n\}$***:*** The objective function for each patient loading vector $\mathbf{c}_n$ decouples as follows when the other variables are fixed:

$$\mathcal{F}(\mathbf{c}_n) = \lambda||\mathbf{y}_n - \phi(\mathbf{c}_n)^T\mathbf{w}||_2^2 + \gamma_2||\mathbf{c}_n||_2^2 + \text{Tr}\left[\boldsymbol{\Lambda}_n^T(\mathbf{V}_n - \mathbf{X}\text{diag}(\mathbf{c}_n))\right]$$
$$+ \frac{1}{2}||\mathbf{V}_n - \mathbf{X}\text{diag}(\mathbf{c}_n)||_F^2 \quad s.t. \quad c_{nr} \geq 0 \quad (7)$$

We now substitute this form into Eq. (7) and use the kernel trick, to write:

$$||\mathbf{y}_n - \phi(\mathbf{c}_n)^T\mathbf{w}||_2^2 = ||\mathbf{y}_n - \sum_j \phi(\mathbf{c}_n)^T\phi(\hat{\mathbf{c}}_j)\alpha_j||_2^2 = ||\mathbf{y}_n - \sum_j \kappa(\mathbf{c}_n, \hat{\mathbf{c}}_j)\alpha_j||_2^2$$

where $\{\hat{\mathbf{c}}_n\}$ denotes the coefficient vector estimates from the previous step to compute $\mathbf{w}$. Notice that the kernel trick buys a second advantage, in that we only need to optimize over the first argument of $\kappa(\cdot,\cdot)$. Since kernel functions typically have a nice analytic form, we can easily compute the gradient $\nabla\kappa(\mathbf{c}_n, \hat{\mathbf{c}}_j)$ and hessian $\nabla^2\kappa(\mathbf{c}_n, \hat{\mathbf{c}}_j)$ of $\kappa(\mathbf{c}_n, \hat{\mathbf{c}}_j)$ with respect to $\mathbf{c}_n$.

Given this, the gradient of $\mathcal{F}(\cdot)$ with respect to $\mathbf{c}_n$ takes the following form:

$$\mathbf{g}_n = \frac{\partial\mathcal{F}}{\partial\mathbf{c}_n} = \mathbf{c}_n \circ \left[\left[\mathcal{I}_R \circ (\mathbf{X}^T\mathbf{X})\right]\mathbf{1}\right] - \left[\mathcal{I}_R \circ (\boldsymbol{\Lambda}_n^T\mathbf{X} + \mathbf{V}_n^T\mathbf{X})\right]\mathbf{1} + 2\gamma_2\mathbf{c}_n$$
$$-\lambda\sum_i \alpha_i\left[2\nabla\kappa(\mathbf{c}_n, \hat{\mathbf{c}}_i)y_i - \sum_k \alpha_k\left[\kappa(\mathbf{c}_n, \hat{\mathbf{c}}_i)\nabla\kappa(\mathbf{c}_n, \hat{\mathbf{c}}_k) + \kappa(\mathbf{c}_n, \hat{\mathbf{c}}_k)\nabla\kappa(\mathbf{c}_n, \hat{\mathbf{c}}_i)\right]\right]$$

where $\mathbf{1}$ is the vector of all ones. Notice that the top line of the gradient term is from the matrix decomposition and regularization terms, and the bottom line corresponds to the kernel regression. The Hessian $\mathbf{H}_n = \partial^2\mathcal{F}/\partial\mathbf{c}_n^2$ can be similarly computed. Due to space limitations, we have omitted its explicit form.

Given the low dimensionality of $\mathbf{c}_n$, we derive a trust region optimizer for this variable. The trust region algorithm provides guaranteed convergence, like the popular gradient descent method, with the speedup of second-order procedures. The algorithm iteratively updates $\mathbf{c}_n$ according to the descent direction $\mathbf{p}_k$, i.e. $\mathbf{c}_n^{(k+1)} = \mathbf{c}_n^{(k)} + \mathbf{p}_k$. The vector $\mathbf{p}_k$ is computed via the following quadratic objective, which is a second order Taylor expansion of $\mathcal{F}$ around $\mathbf{c}_n^k$:

$$\mathbf{p} = \arg\min_{\mathbf{p}} \mathcal{F}(\mathbf{c}_n^k) + \mathbf{g}_n^k(\mathbf{c}_n^k)^T \mathbf{p} + \frac{1}{2}\mathbf{p}^T \mathbf{H}_n^k(\mathbf{c}_n^k)\mathbf{p} \quad s.t. \ \|\mathbf{p}\|_2 \le \delta_k, \ \mathbf{c}_{nr}^k + \mathbf{p}_r \ge 0$$

where $\mathbf{g}_n(\cdot)$ and $\mathbf{H}_n(\cdot)$ are the gradient and Hessian referenced above evaluated at the current iterate $\mathbf{c}_n^k$. We recursively search for a suitable trust region radius δ_k such that we are guaranteed sufficient decrease in the objective at each iteration. This algorithm has a lower bound on the function decrease per update, and with an appropriate choice of the δ_k, converges to a local minimum of $\mathcal{F}$ [12].

Augmented Lagrangian Update for $\mathbf{V}_n$ and $\mathbf{\Lambda}_n$: Each $\{\mathbf{V}_n\}$ has a closed form solution, while the dual variables $\{\mathbf{\Lambda}_n\}$ are updated via gradient ascent:

$$\mathbf{V}_n = (\mathrm{diag}(\mathbf{c}_n)\mathbf{X}^T + 2\mathbf{\Gamma}_n\mathbf{X} - \mathbf{\Lambda}_n)(\mathcal{I}_R + 2\mathbf{X}^T\mathbf{X})^{-1} \tag{8}$$

$$\mathbf{\Lambda}_n^{k+1} = \mathbf{\Lambda}_n^k + \eta_k(\mathbf{V}_n - \mathbf{X}\mathrm{diag}(\mathbf{c}_n)) \tag{9}$$

We cycle through the updates in Eqs. (8–9) to ensure that the proximal constraints are satisfied with increasing certainty at each step. We choose the learning rate parameter η_k for the gradient ascent step of the Augmented Lagrangian to guarantee sufficient decrease for every iteration of alternating minimization.

Prediction on Unseen Data: We use the estimates $\{\mathbf{X}^*, \mathbf{w}^*, \{\mathbf{c}_j^*\}\}$ obtained from the training data to compute the loading vector $\bar{\mathbf{c}}$ for an unseen patient. We must remove the data term in Eq. (4), as the corresponding value of $\bar{\mathbf{y}}$ is unknown for the new patient. Hence, the kernel terms in the gradient and hessian disappear. We also assume that the conditions for the proximal operator hold with equality; this eliminates the Augmented Lagrangians in the computation. The objective in $\bar{\mathbf{c}}$ reduces to the following quadratic form:

$$\frac{1}{2}\bar{\mathbf{c}}^T \bar{\mathbf{H}}\bar{\mathbf{c}} + \bar{\mathbf{f}}^T\bar{\mathbf{c}} \quad s.t. \ \bar{\mathbf{A}}\bar{\mathbf{c}} \le \bar{\mathbf{b}} \tag{10}$$

Note that the formulation is similar to the trust region update we used previously. For an unseen patient, the parameters from Eq. (10) are:

$$\bar{\mathbf{H}} = 2(\mathbf{X}^T\mathbf{X}) \circ (\mathbf{X}^T\mathbf{X}) + 2\gamma_2\mathcal{I}_R$$

$$\bar{\mathbf{f}} = -2\mathcal{I}_R \circ (\mathbf{X}^T\mathbf{\Gamma}_n\mathbf{X})\mathbf{1}; \quad \bar{\mathbf{A}} = -\mathcal{I}_R \quad \bar{\mathbf{b}} = \mathbf{0}$$

The Hessian $\bar{\mathbf{H}}$ is positive definite, which leads to an efficient quadratic programming solution to Eq. (10). The severity score for the test patient is estimated by $\bar{\mathbf{y}} = \phi(\bar{\mathbf{c}})^T\mathbf{w}^* = \sum_j \kappa(\bar{\mathbf{c}}, \mathbf{c}_j^*)\alpha_j^*$, where $\alpha^* = \left[\mathbf{\Phi}(\mathbf{C}^*)^T\mathbf{\Phi}(\mathbf{C}^*) + \frac{\gamma_3}{\lambda}\mathcal{I}_N\right]^{-1}\mathbf{y}$.

2.2   Baseline Comparison Methods

We compare our algorithm with the standard manifold learning pipeline to predict the target severity score. We consider two classes of representation learning techniques motivated from the machine learning and graph theoretic literature. From here, we construct a non-linear regression model similar to our manifold learning term in Eq. (3). Our five baseline comparisons are as follows:

1. Principal Component Analysis (PCA) on the stacked $\frac{P \times (P-1)}{2}$ correlation coefficients followed by a kernel ridge regression (kRR) on the projections
2. Kernel Principal Component Analysis (kPCA) on the correlation coefficients followed by a kRR on the embeddings
3. Node Degree computation (D_N) based on the thresholded correlation matrices followed by a kRR on the P node features
4. Betweenness Centrality (C_B) on the thresholded correlation matrices followed by a kRR on the P node features
5. Decoupled Matrix Decomposition (Eq.(3)) and kRR on the loadings $\{c_n\}$.

Baseline 5 helps us evaluate and quantify the advantage provided by our joint optimization approach as opposed to a pipelined prediction of clinical severity.

3   Experimental Results:

rs-fMRI Dataset and Preprocessing. We validate our method on a cohort of 58 children with high-functioning ASD (Age: 10.06 ± 1.26, IQ: 110 ± 14.03). rs-fMRI scans were acquired on a Phillips 3T Achieva scanner using a single-shot, partially parallel gradient-recalled EPI sequence with TR/TE = 2500/30 ms, flip angle = $70°$, res = $3.05 \times 3.15 \times 3$ mm, having 128 or 156 time samples. We use a standard pre-processing pipeline, consisting of slice time correction, rigid body realignment, normalization to the EPI version of the MNI template, Comp Corr [1], nuisance regression, spatial smoothing by a 6 mm FWHM Gaussian kernel, and bandpass filtering between 0.01–0.1 Hz. We use the Automatic Anatomical Labeling (AAL) atlas to define 116 cortical, subcortical and cerebellar regions. We subtract the contribution of the first eigenvector from the regionwise correlation matrices because it is roughly constant and biases the predictions. The residual correlation matrices, $\{\Gamma_n\}$, are used as inputs for all the methods.

We consider three separate measures of clinical severity quantifying different impairments associated with ASD. The Autism Diagnostic Observation Schedule (ADOS) [8] captures social and communicative deficits of the patient along with repetitive behaviors (dynamic range: 0–30). The Social Responsiveness Scale (SRS) [8] characterizes impaired social functioning (dynamic range: 70–200). Finally, the Praxis score [2] quantifies motor control, tool usage and gesture imitation skills in ASD patients (dynamic range: 0–100).

Characterizing the Non-linear Patient Manifold: Based on simulated data, we observed that the standard exponential kernel provides a good recovery performance in the lower part of the dynamic range, while polynomial kernels are more suited for modeling the larger behavioral scores, as shown in Fig. 2. Thus, we use a mixture of both kernels to capture the complete behavioral characteristics:

$$\kappa(\mathbf{c}_i, \mathbf{c}_j) = \exp\left[-\frac{\|\mathbf{c}_i - \mathbf{c}_j\|_2^2}{\sigma^2}\right] + \frac{\rho}{l}\left(\mathbf{c}_j^T \mathbf{c}_i + 1\right)^l$$

We vary the kernel parameters across 2 orders of magnitude and select the settings: ADOS $\{\sigma^2 = 1, \rho = 0.8, l = 2.5\}$, SRS $\{\sigma^2 = 1, \rho = 2, l = 1.5\}$ and

Praxis $\{\sigma^2 = 1, \rho = 0.5, l = 1.5\}$. The varying polynomial orders reflect the differences in the dynamic ranges of the scores.

Predicting ASD Clinical Severity. We evaluate every algorithm in a ten fold cross validation setting, i.e. we train the model on a 90% split of our data, and report the performance on the unseen 10%. The number of components was fixed at 15 for PCA and at 10 for k-PCA. For k-PCA, we use an RBF kernel with the coefficient parameter 0.1. There are two free parameters for the kRR, namely, the kernel parameter C and ℓ_2 parameter β. We obtain the best performance for the following settings: ADOS $\{C = 0.1, \beta = 0.2\}$, SRS $\{C = 0.1, \beta = 0.8\}$, and Praxis $\{C = 0.01, \beta = 0.2\}$. For the graph theoretic baselines, we obtained the best performance by thresholding the entries of $\{\mathbf{\Gamma}_n\}$ at 0.2. We fixed the parameters in our CMO framework using a grid search for $\{\lambda, \gamma_1, \gamma_2, \gamma_3\}$. The values were varied between $(10^{-3} - 10)$. The performance is insensitive to λ and γ_3, which are fixed at 1. The remaining parameters were set at $\{\gamma_1 = 10, \gamma_2 = 0.7, \gamma_3 = 1\}$ for all the scores. We fix the number of networks, R, at the knee point of the eigenspectrum of $\{\mathbf{\Gamma}_n\}$, i.e. $(R = 8)$.

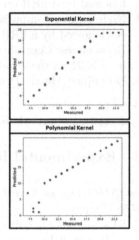

Fig. 2. Recovery **Top:** Exponential **Bottom:** Polynomial kernel

Performance Comparison. Figures 3, 4, and 5 illustrate the regression performance for ADOS, SRS, and Praxis respectively. The bold $\mathbf{x} = \mathbf{y}$ line indicates ideal performance. The red points denote the training fit, while the blue points indicate testing performance. Note that baseline testing performance tracks the mean value of the data (indicated by the horizontal black line). In comparison, our method not only consistently fits the training set more faithfully, but also generalizes much better to unseen data. We emphasize that even the pipelined treatment using the matrix decomposition in Eq. (3), followed by a kernel ridge regression on the learnt projections fails to generalize. This finding makes a strong case for coupling the two representation terms in our CMO strategy. We conjecture that the baselines fail to capture representative connectivity patterns that explain both the functional neuroimaging data space and the patient behavioral heterogeneity. On the other hand, our CMO framework leverages the underlying structure of the correlation matrices through the basis manifold representation. At the same time, it seeks those embedding directions that are predictive of behavior. As reported in Table 1, our method quantitatively outperforms the baselines approaches, in terms of both the Median Absolute Error (MAE) and the Mutual Information (MI) metrics.

Clinical Interpretation. Figure 6 illustrates the subnetworks $\{\mathbf{X}_r\}$ trained on ADOS. The colorbar indicates subnetwork contributions to the AAL regions.

Table 1. Performance evaluation using **Median Absolute Error (MAE)** & **Mutual Information (MI)**. Lower MAE & higher MI indicate better performance.

Score	Method	MAE train	MAE test	MI train	MI test
ADOS	PCA & kRR	1.29	3.05	1.46	0.87
	k-PCA & kRR	1.00	2.94	1.48	0.38
	C_B & kRR	2.10	2.93	1.03	0.95
	D_N & kRR	2.09	3.03	0.97	0.96
	Decoupled	2.11	3.11	0.82	1.24
	CMO Framework	**0.035**	**2.73**	**3.79**	**2.10**
SRS	PCA & kRR	7.39	19.70	2.78	3.30
	k-PCA & kRR	5.68	18.92	2.85	1.74
	C_B & kRR	11.00	17.72	2.32	3.66
	D_N & kRR	11.46	17.79	2.24	3.60
	Decoupled	15.9	18.61	2.04	3.71
	CMO Framework	**0.09**	**13.28**	**5.28**	**4.36**
Praxis	PCA & kRR	5.33	12.5	2.50	2.68
	k-PCA & kRR	4.56	11.15	2.56	1.51
	C_B & kRR	8.17	12.61	1.99	3.05
	D_N & kRR	8.18	13.14	2.00	3.20
	Decoupled	10.11	13.33	3.28	1.53
	CMO Framework	**0.13**	**9.07**	**4.67**	**3.87**

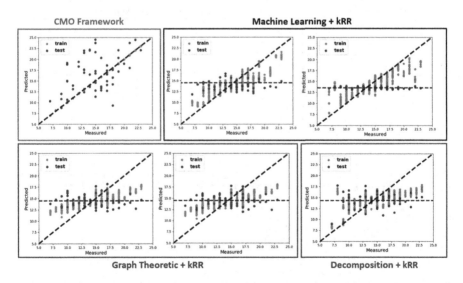

Fig. 3. Prediction performance for the ADOS score for **Red Box:** CMO framework. **Black Box: (L)** PCA and kRR **(R)** k-PCA and kRR, **Green Box: (L)** Node degree centrality and kRR **(R)** Betweenness centrality and kRR **Blue Box:** Matrix decomposition from Eq. (3) followed by kRR (Color figure online)

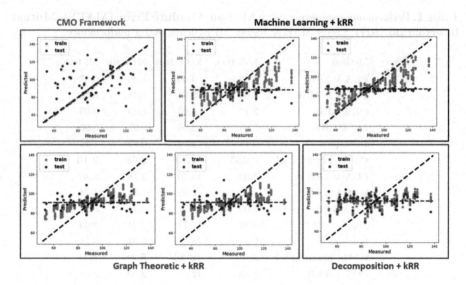

Fig. 4. Prediction performance for the SRS score for **Red Box:** CMO framework. **Black Box:** (**L**) PCA and kRR (**R**) k-PCA and kRR, **Green Box:** (**L**) Node degree centrality and kRR (**R**) Betweenness centrality and kRR **Blue Box:** Matrix decomposition from Eq. (3) followed by kRR (Color figure online)

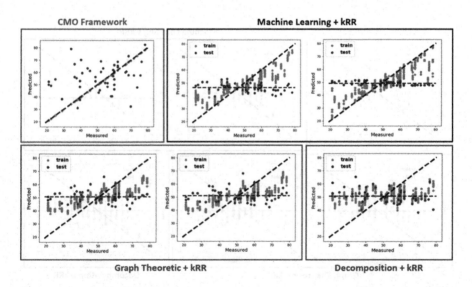

Fig. 5. Prediction performance for the Praxis score for **Red Box:** CMO framework. **Black Box:** (**L**) PCA and kRR (**R**) k-PCA and kRR, **Green Box:** (**L**) Node degree centrality and kRR (**R**) Betweenness centrality and kRR **Blue Box:** Matrix decomposition from Eq. (3) followed by kRR (Color figure online)

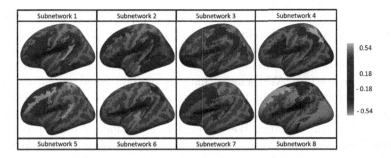

Fig. 6. Eight subnetworks identified by our model from the prediction of ADOS. The blue & green regions are anticorrelated with the red & orange regions. (Color figure online)

Regions storing negative values are anticorrelated with positive regions. From a clinical standpoint, Subnetwork 4 includes the somatomotor network (SMN) and competing i.e. anticorrelated contributions from the default mode network (DMN), previously reported in ASD [6]. Subnetwork 8 comprises of the SMN and competing contributions from the higher order visual processing areas in the occipital and temporal lobes. These findings are in line with behavioral reports of reduced visual-motor integration in ASD [6]. Though not evident from the surface plots, Subnetwork 5 includes anticorrelated contributions from subcortical regions, mainly, the amygdala and hippocampus, believed to be important for socio-emotional regulation in ASD. Finally, Subnetwork 6 has competing contributions from the central executive control network and insula, which are critical for switching between self-referential and goal-directed behavior [10].

Figure 7 compares Subnetwork 2 obtained from ADOS, SRS and Praxis prediction. There is a significant overlap in the bases subnetworks obtained by training across the different scores. This strengthens the hypothesis that our method is able to identify representative, as well as predictive connectivity patterns.

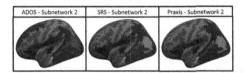

Fig. 7. Subnetwork 2 obtained from **L:** ADOS **M:** SRS and **R:** Praxis prediction

4   Conclusion

We have introduced a Coupled Manifold Optimization strategy that jointly analyzes data from two distinct, but related, domains through its shared projection. In contrast to conventional manifold learning, we optimize for the relevant embedding directions that are predictive of clinical severity. Consequently, our method captures representative connectivity patterns that are important for quantifying and understanding the spectrum of clinical severity among ASD patients. We would like to point out that our framework makes very few assumptions about the data and can be adapted to work with different similarity matrices and clinical scores. We believe that our method could potentially be an important diagnostic tool for the cognitive assessment of various neuropsychiatric disorders. We are working on a multi-score extension which jointly analyses different behavioral domains. We will explore extensions of our representation that simultaneously integrate functional, structural and behavioral information.

Acknowledgements. This work was supported by the National Science Foundation CRCNS award 1822575, National Science Foundation CAREER award 1845430, the National Institute of Mental Health (R01 MH085328-09, R01 MH078160-07, K01 MH109766 and R01 MH106564), the National Institute of Neurological Disorders and Stroke (R01NS048527-08), and the Autism Speaks foundation.

References

1. Behzadi, Y., et al.: A component based noise correction method (CompCor) for BOLD and perfusion based fMRI. Neuroimage **37**(1), 90–101 (2007)
2. Dowell, L.R., et al.: Associations of postural knowledge and basic motor skill with dyspraxia in autism: implication for abnormalities in distributed connectivity and motor learning. Neuropsychology **23**(5), 563 (2009)
3. D'Souza, N.S., Nebel, M.B., Wymbs, N., Mostofsky, S., Venkataraman, A.: A generative-discriminative basis learning framework to predict clinical severity from resting state functional MRI data. In: Frangi, A.F., Schnabel, J.A., Davatzikos, C., Alberola-López, C., Fichtinger, G. (eds.) MICCAI 2018. LNCS, vol. 11072, pp. 163–171. Springer, Cham (2018). https://doi.org/10.1007/978-3-030-00931-1_19
4. Fox, M.D., et al.: Spontaneous fluctuations in brain activity observed with functional magnetic resonance imaging. Nat. Rev. Neurosci. **8**(9), 700 (2007)
5. Murphy, K.P.: Machine learning: a probabilistic perspective (2012)
6. Nebel, M.B., et al.: Intrinsic visual-motor synchrony correlates with social deficits in autism. Biol. Psych. **79**(8), 633–641 (2016)
7. Parikh, N., Boyd, S., et al.: Proximal algorithms. Found. Trends® Opt. **1**(3), 127–239 (2014)
8. Payakachat, N., et al.: Autism spectrum disorders: a review of measures for clinical, health services and cost-effectiveness applications. Exp. Rev. Pharmacoeconomics Outcomes Res. **12**(4), 485–503 (2012)
9. Soussia, M., Rekik, I.: High-order connectomic manifold learning for autistic brain state identification. In: Wu, G., Laurienti, P., Bonilha, L., Munsell, B.C. (eds.) CNI 2017. LNCS, vol. 10511, pp. 51–59. Springer, Cham (2017). https://doi.org/10.1007/978-3-319-67159-8_7
10. Sridharan, D., et al.: A critical role for the right fronto-insular cortex in switching between central-executive and default-mode networks. Proc. Natl. Acad. Sci. **105**(34), 12569–12574 (2008)
11. Thiagarajan, J.J., et al.: Multiple kernel sparse representations for supervised and unsupervised learning. IEEE Trans. Image Process. **23**(7), 2905–2915 (2014)
12. Wright, S., et al.: Numerical optimization. Springer Sci. **35**(67–68), 7 (1999)

A Geometric Framework for Feature Mappings in Multimodal Fusion of Brain Image Data

Wen Zhang[1]([✉]), Liang Mi[1], Paul M. Thompson[2], and Yalin Wang[1]

[1] School of Computing, Informatics, and Decision Systems Engineering,
Arizona State University, Tempe, AZ, USA
wzhan139@asu.edu
[2] Imaging Genetics Center, Institute for Neuroimaging and Informatics,
University of Southern California, Los Angeles, CA, USA

Abstract. Fusing multimodal brain image features to empower statistical analysis has attracted considerable research interest. Generally, a feature mapping is learned in the fusion process so the cross-modality relationship in the multimodal data can be more effectively extracted in a common feature space. Most of the prior work achieve this goal by data-driven approaches without considering the geometry properties of the feature spaces where the data are embedded. It results in a huge sacrifice of untapped information. Here, we propose to fuse the multimodal brain images through a novel geometric approach. The key idea is to encode various brain image features with the local metric change on brain shapes, such that the feature mapping can be efficiently solved by some geometric mapping functions, i.e., quasiconformal and harmonic mappings. We approach our multimodal fusion framework (MFRM) in two steps: surface feature mapping and volumetric feature mapping. For each of them, we design an informative Riemannian metric based on distinct brain anatomical features and achieve image fusion via diffeomorphic maps. We evaluate our proposed method on two brain image cohorts. The experimental results reveal the effectiveness of our proposed framework which yields better statistical performances than state-of-the-art data-driven methods.

Keywords: Multimodal fusion · Riemannian metric ·
Quasiconformal mapping · Harmonic mapping · structural MRI ·
diffusion MRI

1 Introduction

The proliferation of multimodal brain image data helps researchers better understand the neurobiology of psychiatric and neurological disorders than learning from a single modality. Generally, multimodal neuroimaging data may contain images with different resolutions and dimensions, thus it is natural to design the

© Springer Nature Switzerland AG 2019
A. C. S. Chung et al. (Eds.): IPMI 2019, LNCS 11492, pp. 617–630, 2019.
https://doi.org/10.1007/978-3-030-20351-1_48

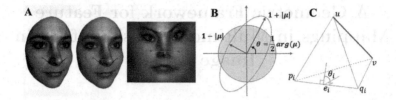

Fig. 1. A. The black curve is the geodesic curve between two points (left). After we update its Riemannian metric to one that induces a fattened surface, the geodesic curve is the green line between these two points (right). B. Quasi-conformal mapping. C. Volumetric string constant. (Color figure online)

feature mappings from different modality data to a common feature space. The cross-modality relationship is thus extracted and projected to that latent space during the feature mapping and later can be fed to the statistical analysis. The widely applied multimodal fusion methods, such as mutual information [17], independent component analysis (ICA) [4], multiple kernel learning [19], etc., use either information theory or machine learning techniques in the data-driven fashion to build feature mappings. However, these methods ignore the intrinsic structural relationship between brain image data sources, e.g. geometric properties of brain shapes. It results in a huge sacrifice of untapped information. Hence, developing effective computational frameworks to transform multimodal multidimensional neuroimaging data into integrated, informative biological knowledge remains an open problem.

Fusing multimodal imaging data to improve statistical analysis calls for a feature mapping to a common latent feature space. For example, a typical strategy is to find a canonical parameter space, e.g. a chosen shape template, and compute the intermediate mappings to that parameter space [1]. However, due to the diversity of multimodal features, e.g., structural features such as cortical thickness or white matter integrity, it is non-trivial to search for such a common feature space. Inspired by research in [9], we integrate imaging features from different modalities by using a concept from geometry research, i.e. Riemannian metrics, and construct a common feature space. In Riemannian geometry, the Riemannian metric is a family of positive definite inner products defined on a differentiable manifold. A manifold could have an infinite number of Riemannian metrics representing specific geometric functions. For example, Fig. 1(A) shows how different Riemannian metrics determine different geodesic curves on a human facial surface. Our main idea is as follows. First, we adjust the Riemannian metrics defined on the original mesh to obtain the feature embeddings. In the end, we pursue physically natural and geometrically intrinsic harmonic map solutions to register the feature-encoded metrics to the same canonical space (i.e., a unit ball domain). The multimodal fusion problem thereby can be solved by geometry registration approaches.

In this paper, we are interested in fusing two magnetic resonance imaging (MRI) modalities, i.e., structural MRI (sMRI) and diffusion MRI (dMRI). The sMRI provides the morphometric information on grey matter (GM) on the cortical surface whereas dMRI provides additional information to model white matter (WM) integrity in the interior of the brain. The GM geometry and WM integrity play vital roles during brain developmental and pathological processes [2,5] and they are the anatomical foundation of brain cognitive functions. There are a few attempts to model the high-level relationship between these two modalities. Tozer *et al.* [15] developed a methodology to find correspondences between WM fiber tracts and the GM regions linked by these fiber tracts. Savadjiev *et al.* [12] integrated multi-scale geometric properties of WM and cortical surface by using mutual information. However, the aforementioned studies are more interested in GM regions which are anatomically connected by WM fibers but did not aim to deal with the whole brain anatomical fusion, in general.

Here, we propose to adopt the Riemannian metric to model the intrinsic relationship between GM and WM anatomical features. We develop a practical algorithm to compute quasiconformal and harmonic maps under designed metrics carrying information from sMRI and dMRI data. In the experiments, we apply our algorithm to classify patients of Alzheimer's disease (AD), mild cognitive impairment (MCI) and Schizophrenia (SCZ) from normal control subjects and the results demonstrate considerable promise. Our main contributions are as follows. (1) Our work shows that the multimodal fusion problem for volumetric neuroimaging data can be tackled using geometry methods with defined Riemannian metrics. (2) We design a unified multimodal fusion framework that maps both surface and volume features to a shared parameterization domain. (3) We validate the effectiveness of our framework on different datasets and achieve significantly better performance than some state-of-the-art methods.

2   Theoretical Background

2.1   Surface Quasiconformal Mapping

A diffeomorphism $\phi : (M_1, \mathbf{g}_1) \to (M_2, \mathbf{g}_2)$ is a *conformal mapping* between two Riemannian manifolds if it preserves the first fundamental form of M_1, up to a scaling factor. Every conformal mapping is an angle-preserving mapping that preserves the local geometry of the surface. One generalization of a conformal mapping is a *quasiconformal map*, which is an orientation-preserving diffeomorphism between Riemann surfaces with bounded conformality distortion [10]. Its first order approximations takes small circles to small ellipses of bounded eccentricity [7]. Mathematically, given a mapping ϕ, and z and w to be the local conformal parameters of manifolds $(M_1, \mathbf{g}_1)$ and $(M_2, \mathbf{g}_2)$, respectively, such that $\mathbf{g}_1 = e^{2u_1} dz d\bar{z}, \mathbf{g}_2 = e^{2u_2} dw d\bar{w}$, then we say ϕ is quasi-conformal if it satisfies the Beltrami equation:

$$\frac{\partial \phi}{\partial \bar{z}} = \mu(z) \frac{\partial \phi}{\partial z}, \tag{1}$$

for complex valued functions $\mu(z)$ satisfying $\| \mu \|_\infty < 1$. μ is called *Beltrami coefficient* (BC). The ratio between two axes of the ellipse is called *dilation* given by $K = \frac{1+|\mu(z)|}{1-|\mu(z)|}$ and the orientation of the axis is $arg(\mu(z))$. Thus, the BC μ gives us important information about the properties of the map. Figure 1(B) shows a quasiconformal map from a circle to an ellipse. Given a BC $\mu : \mathbb{C} \to \mathbb{C}$ with $\| \mu \|_\infty < 1$, there is always a quasiconformal mapping from a complex plane $\mathbb{C}$ onto itself which satisfied Eq. 1 [7]. The following theory provides computation of quasiconformal mapping with designed Riemannian metric.

Theorem 1 ([18]). *Suppose $f : (M, \mathbf{g}_m) \to (N, \mathbf{g}_n)$ is a quasiconformal mapping associated with the BC μ. $\mathbf{g}_m = \sigma(z)dzd\bar{z}$ and $\mathbf{g}_n = \rho(w)dwd\bar{w}$. There is a well defined auxiliary Riemannian metric on M: $\tilde{\mathbf{g}}_m = e^{\sigma(z)}|dz + \mu d\bar{z}|^2$ such that the mapping $\tilde{f} : (M, \tilde{\mathbf{g}}_m) \to (N, \mathbf{g}_n)$ is a conformal mapping.*

2.2   Volumetric Harmonic Map

Suppose M is a simplicial complex, and $g : |M| \to \mathbb{R}^3$ a function that embeds $|M|$ in $\mathbb{R}^3$, then (M, g) is called a mesh. For a 3-simplex, it is a tetrahedral mesh, Te, and for a 2-simplex, it is a triangular mesh, Tr. The boundary of a tetrahedral mesh is a triangular mesh, $Tr = \partial Te$.

Definition 1 (Discrete Harmonic Energy). *Suppose a piecewise linear function $f \in C^{PL}(M)$, the discrete harmonic energy is defined as:*

$$E(f) = <f, f> = \sum_{[u,v] \in K} k(u, v) \| f(u) - f(v) \|^2. \tag{2}$$

Suppose that edge $e_{u,v} = [u, v]$ is shared by n tetrahedrons, the string constant [16] is formulated as:

$$k(u, v) = \frac{1}{12} \sum_{i=1}^{n} l_i \cot(\theta_i), \tag{3}$$

where l_i is the length of edge e_i to which edge $e_{u,v}$ is against and θ_i is the dihedral angles associate with the edge e_i (Fig. 1(C)). By changing $k(u, v)$ in Eq. 2, we can define different volumetric harmonic maps.

3   Algorithms

Figure 2 shows our multimodal brain image fusion framework (MFRM). Mathematically, given a brain volumetric mesh, M, where its surface is ∂M and interior is $M \backslash \partial M$, we want to compute a feature mapping $f_M = \{f_{\partial M}, f_{M \backslash \partial M}\} \to \mathbb{D}$ to a common feature domain $\mathbb{D}$, i.e., a unit ball. It can be divided into two steps: (1) surface feature mapping $f_{\partial M}$ for the cortical morphometric features, and (2) the volumetric feature mapping $f_{M \backslash \partial M}$ for WM anatomical features.

In the first part, we have a spherical surface feature mapping

$$f_{\partial M}(v) : \tau_{surf}(\mathbf{g}_{\partial M}, F_{\partial M}(v)) \to \mathbb{S}^2. \tag{4}$$

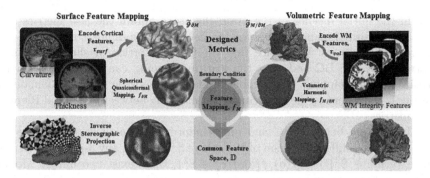

Fig. 2. Multimodal brain image fusion framework (MFRM). The left panel depicts surface feature mapping and the right panel depicts volumetric feature mapping. Multimodal imaging features are encoded in designed Riemannian metric. The framework produces feature mappings to a common space (a unit ball) where the vertex-wise correspondence is found through the geometric resampling.

We encode the vertex-wise surface features $F_{\partial M}(v)$, e.g. Gaussian curvature and cortical thickness, to the initial Riemannian metric $g_{\partial M}$ by using an feature embedding function $\tau_{surf}(.)$ and obtain a new metric $\tilde{g}_{\partial M}$. Then, a conformal mapping is computed to get the spherical ($\mathbb{S}^2$) parameterization of $\tilde{g}_{\partial M}$. Here, $\tau_{surf}(.)$ is learned with the optimized BC. Therefore, the variations of BC make the conformal mapping, i.e. spherical conformal mapping, to be the quasiconformal mapping. Details about BC variations in $\tau_{surf}(.)$ can be found in Algorithm 1.

The second part of the proposed framework is a volumetric feature mapping,

$$f_{M\backslash\partial M}(v) : \tau_{vol}(\mathbf{g}_{M\backslash\partial M}, F_{M\backslash\partial M}(v)) \to \mathbb{S}^3, \quad s.t. \quad f_{\partial M}. \tag{5}$$

In this mapping, the spherical parameterization in the surface feature mapping, i.e. $f_{\partial M}$ is the boundary constraint. Thus, the two steps of feature mapping in our framework are geometrically associated together. By changing the edge weights in the string constant $k(u,v)$ in Eq. 3, we are able to embed the volumetric feature, e.g. white matter integrity, to the initial metric on tetrahedron meshes. We then learn the volumetric parameterization through the harmonic mapping to a unit ball domain ($\mathbb{S}^3$). Details are shown in Algorithm 2.

3.1 Surface Feature Mapping

As outlined in Theorem 1, we model the surface feature fusion with quasiconformal mappings. Commonly, in geometry registration, with spherical conformal mapping, the source and target brain cortical surfaces are both mapped to a sphere and then we search for the point-wise correspondence on the sphere domain. This process relies on Riemannian metrics on the source and target surface. Here, we extend the idea of geometric mapping to the feature mapping where we design the new metrics accounting for the brain imaging features. We deform the initial metrics of the brain shapes to obtain the new metrics such that the conformal mapping between the new metrics minimizes the vertex-wise difference of features. We notice that the local distortion or shrinkage can be controlled by the BC and thus the feature mapping can be solved with the quasiconformal mapping. The conformal mapping between the new Riemannian metrics is equivalent to the quasiconformal mapping between the initial Riemannian metrics.

The relation between BC and quasiconformal mapping is unique. Let $f : \mathbb{S}^2 \to \mathbb{S}^2$ be any diffeomorphism of the sphere $\mathbb{S}^2$. Picking any 3-point correspondence $\{a, b, c \in \mathbb{S}^2\} \leftrightarrow \{f(a), f(b), f(c) \in \mathbb{S}^2\}$, there exist two unique Möbius transformations ϕ_1 and ϕ_2 that map $\{a, b, c\}$ and $\{f(a), f(b), f(c)\}$ to $0, 1, \infty$ respectively. Then, the composition map $\tilde{f} := \phi_2 \circ f \circ \phi_1^{-1}$ is a diffeomorphism of $\mathbb{S}^2$ that fix $0, 1, \infty$. There is a one-to-one correspondence between the set of diffeomorphisms $\{f^{(t)}\}$ of $\mathbb{S}^2$ fixing $0, 1, \infty$ and the set of BCs $\{\mu^{(t)}\}$ on $\mathbb{S}^2$ with $\| \mu \|_\infty < 1$. Given a diffeomorphism f of $\mathbb{S}^2$ with the fixed point correspondence, we can represent f uniquely by a BC.

Theorem 2 ([3]). *Let $\{\mu^{(t)}(z)\}$ be the set of BCs at point $z \in \mathbb{C}$ depending on a real or complex parameter t. The variation of $\mu^{(t)}(z)$ can be written as:*

$$\mu^{(t)}(z) = \mu(z) + t\nu(z) + t\sigma^{(t)}(z). \tag{6}$$

When $t \to 0$, $\| \sigma^{(t)} \|_\infty \to 0$. Then for all $w \in \mathbb{C}$, we can formulate the variation of the diffeomorphism f as:

$$f^{\mu^{(t)}}(w) = f^\mu(w) + tV(f^\mu, \nu)(w) + o(| t |), \tag{7}$$

locally uniformly on $\mathbb{C}$ as $t \to 0$, where

$$V(f^\mu, \nu)(w) = -\frac{f^\mu(w)(f^\mu(w) - 1)}{\pi} \times \int_\mathbb{C} \frac{\nu(z)(f_z^\mu(z))^2}{f^\mu(z)(f^\mu(z) - 1)(f^\mu(z) - f^\mu(w))} dz. \tag{8}$$

We further reformulate Eq. 8 as:

$$V(f^\mu, \nu)(w) = A(\mu(\omega)) \int_\mathbb{C} \left(\frac{G_1\nu_1 + G_2\nu_2}{G_3\nu_1 + G_4\nu_2} \right) dz, \tag{9}$$

where $\nu = \nu_1 + i\nu_2$ and G_1, G_2, G_3, G_4 are real-valued functions defined on $\mathbb{C}$. In this paper, we use $\binom{a}{b}$ to indicate complex value $a + ib$. Equation 7 links the variation of the BC, $\mu^{(t)}$, with the variation of the diffeomorphism $f^{\mu^{(t)}}$. In other words, the quasiconformal mapping can be conveniently solved by adjusting the BC values with a variational formula.

Given any energy function $E(f)$ defined on the space of surface diffeomorphisms f, we re-define it as $E(\mu)$ on the parameter domain of a sphere, which is an extended complex plane obtained by using the stereographic projection. We

---

Algorithm 1. Surface Feature Mapping

Input : Brain surfaces S_1 and S_2 with computed vertex-wise features, e.g. Gaussian curvature and cortical thickness. Step length dt and energy difference threshold ϵ.

Output: Quasiconformal diffeomorphism $f : S_1 \to S_2$

1 **Parameterize** the original surface to the spherical domain via the spherical harmonic mapping, denoted as $\phi_1 : S_1 \to \mathbb{S}^2$ and $\phi_2 : S_2 \to \mathbb{S}^2$;

2 **Initialize** mapping $\tilde{f}^0 := \mathbf{Id} : \mathbb{S}^2 \to \mathbb{S}^2$ and resample S_2 based on the parameterization $\phi_1(S_1)$ and $\phi_2(S_2)$. Set n=0;

3 **do**

4 $\quad$ Compute the Beltrami coefficient μ^n of $\tilde{f}^n$ via Eq. 1;

5 $\quad$ Update μ^{n+1} via Eq. 14;

6 $\quad$ Compute $V^n(\tilde{f}^n, \mu^{n+1} - \mu^n)$ via Eq. 9 and update $\tilde{f}^{n+1} = \tilde{f}^n + V^n$;

7 $\quad$ Update $f^{n+1} = \phi_2^{-1} \circ \tilde{f} \circ \phi_1$ and compute $\delta E = \mid E(\mu^{n+1}) - E(\mu^n) \mid$. Set $n = n + 1$;

8 **while** $\delta E > \epsilon$;

9 $\quad$ Return f^{n+1};

---

first formulate an energy function defined on the space of BC over the conformal parameter domain C, as:

$$E(\mu) = \int_C (F(\omega) - \tilde{F}(f^\mu(\omega)))^2 + \mid \mu(\omega) \mid^2 d\omega. \tag{10}$$

The optimization of minimizing $E(\mu)$ can be approximated by the gradient descent approach. We derived the Euler-Lagrange equation based on Eqs. 7 and 9, as follow:

$$\frac{d}{dt}\mid_{t=0} E(\mu + t\nu) = - \int_C 2(F - \tilde{F}(f^\mu))\nabla\tilde{F}(f^\mu)\frac{d}{dt}\mid_{t=0} f^{\mu+t\nu} - 2\mu \cdot \nu d\omega$$

$$= - \int_C \left[A \cdot \int_D G(z, \nu, \omega, \mu) \cdot \nu(z)dz - 2\mu(\omega) \cdot \nu(\omega) \right] d\omega \tag{11}$$

$$= - \int_C \left[\int_D \left(\begin{array}{c} G_1 a_1 + G_3 a_2 \\ G_2 a_1 + G_4 a_2 \end{array} \right) d\omega - 2\mu(z) \right] \cdot \nu(z)dz,$$

where $A = a_1 + ia_2 = 2(F - \tilde{F}(f^\mu))\nabla\tilde{F}(f^\mu)$. Therefore, we could derive the descent direction for μ as follow:

$$\frac{d\mu(\omega)}{dt} = \int_C \left(\begin{array}{c} G_1 a_1 + G_3 a_2 \\ G_2 a_1 + G_4 a_2 \end{array} \right) dz - 2\mu. \tag{12}$$

We note that this is a general quasiconformal mapping framework. In this study, we design our energy function by considering two important geometric features on the cortex of the human brain, i.e., curvature $F_1(\omega)$ and cortical thickness $F_2(\omega)$. The final energy function is:

$$E(\mu) = \alpha \int_C (F_1 - \tilde{F}_1(f^\mu))^2 + \beta \int_C (F_2 - \tilde{F}_2(f^\mu))^2 + \mid \mu(\omega) \mid^2 d\omega \tag{13}$$

and update μ to optimize $\min E(\mu)$ as:

$$\mu^{n+1} - \mu^n = dt \int_C \left(\begin{bmatrix} G_1 \ G_3 \\ G_2 \ G_4 \end{bmatrix} \cdot \begin{bmatrix} \alpha a_1 + \beta b_1 \\ \alpha a_2 + \beta b_2 \end{bmatrix} \right) dz - 2(\alpha + \beta)\mu, \qquad (14)$$

where $a_1 + ia_2 = 2(F_1 - \tilde{F}_1(f^\mu))\nabla \tilde{F}_1(f^\mu)$ and $b_1 + ib_2 = 2(F_2 - \tilde{F}_2(f^\mu))\nabla \tilde{F}_2(f^\mu)$. The detailed computational algorithm is summarized in Algorithm 1.

3.2   Volumetric Feature Mapping

With the surface quasiconformal mapping in the previous part as the boundary condition, we further design a volumetric feature mapping by using volumetric harmonic map. We first create a tetrahedral mesh based on the cortical surface to model geometry of the brain interior. Then the voxel-wise geometric features computed from dMRI are projected onto the mesh vertexes. In this study, we use three important features, i.e., *FA* (fractional anisotropy), *MD* (mean diffusivity) and *B0* (raw T2 signal with no diffusion weighting), which are widely applied in dMRI-based neuroimaging analyses [8]. Given a vertex v in the tetrahedral mesh M, we define a feature vector $F(v) = [FA(v), MD(v), B0(v)]$ and each element is scaled independently by the largest value of this feature among voxels in a brain. Recall the harmonic energy defined on a tetrahedral mesh:

$$E(f) = \sum_{[u,v] \in K} \tilde{k}(u,v) \|f(u) - f(v)\|^2. \qquad (15)$$

By changing the string constants $k(u,v)$ in Eq. 3, we can define different string energies. For the proposed vertex-wise DTI feature, we design a new metric based on the cosine similarity to evaluate feature difference and adopt it into the original string constant as:

$$\hat{k}(u,v) = e^{D_{Ang}(F(u),F(v))} k(u,v), \qquad (16)$$

where $D_{Ang}(F(u), F(v)) = \frac{1}{\pi}cos^{-1}(\frac{F(u) \cdot F(v)}{\|F(u)\|_2 \|F(v)\|_2})$. If features of two vertexes are similar, the new string parameter $\hat{k}(u,v) = k(u,v)$. If their features are totally distinct, $\hat{k}(u,v) = ek(u,v)$.

Lemma 1. *A volumetric harmonic map with the new harmonic energy defined with Eqs. 15 and 16 induces diffeomorphism.*

Proof. As the newly defined harmonic energy has a string constant bounded by $k(u,v) < \tilde{k}(u,v) < ek(u,v)$ where $k(u,v)$ is strictly positive due to acute dihedral angles in every tetrahedron, the energy defined with Eq. 15 is a harmonic energy. Since the spherical boundary induces a convex boundary, a harmonic map using Eqs. 15 and 16 has a global minimum which induces diffeomorphism between source and target volumes [13]. $\qquad \square$

Algorithm 2. Volumetric Feature Mapping

Input   : Volumetric tetrahedral meshes M_1 and M_2, computed dMRI
features, *FA*, *MD*, and *B0*, step length dt and energy difference
threshold δE

Output: Feature mapping $h : M_1 \to \mathbb{R}^3$

1 Extract the boundary surface S_1 and S_2 as $S_1 = \partial M_1$ and $S_2 = \partial M_2$. ;

2 Compute the feature mapping f on surface via Alg. 1 and get the spherical
parameterization of S_1 as $\phi(S_1) = f \circ \phi_1$, where ϕ_1 is the conformal
parameterization of S_2 ;

3 **Initialization.** For each boundary vertex, $v \in S_1$, let $g(v) = \phi(v_1)$. For each
interior vertex, $v \in M_1/\partial M_1$, let $g(v) = (0,0,0)$;

4 For every edge $e \in M_1$, compute the string parameters $\hat{k}(e)$ via Eq. 16 and
harmonic energy E_0 via Eq. 15;

5 **do**

6   For each interior vertex, $v \in M_1/\partial M_1$, compute its derivative $Dg(v)$ as in
Eq. 17 and update $g(v) = g(v) - dtDg(v)$;

7   Compute the harmonic energy E_n;

8 **while** $\mid E_n - E_{n-1} \mid > \delta E$;

9 Return $h = g$;

Suppose a mapping $f : M \to \mathbb{R}^3$ minimize the given string energy $E(f)$, it
can be solved with the steepest descent method by iteratively updating along
the direction

$$\frac{df(t)}{dt} = -\triangle f(t), t \in M. \tag{17}$$

$\triangle f(t)$ is the tangential component of the piecewise Laplacian of f, $\triangle_{PL}(f)$.

Definition 2. *The piecewise Laplacian is the linear operator $\triangle_{PL} : C^{PL} \to C^{PL}$ on the space of piecewise linear functions f on M, defined by the formula*

$$\triangle_{PL}(f) = \sum_{\{u,v\}\in K} k(u,v)(f(v) - f(u)). \tag{18}$$

For a map $f : M \to \mathbb{R}^3$, the piecewise Laplacian of $f = (f_1, f_2, f_3)$ is $\triangle_{PL}(f) = (\triangle_{PL}(f_1), \triangle_{PL}(f_2), \triangle_{PL}(f_3))$.

The detailed volumetric feature mapping algorithm is summarized in Algorithm 2.

4 Experiments

4.1 Datasets and Experimental Setting

To evaluate the effectiveness of our MFRM framework, we conduct disease classifications on two independent datasets which contain subjects from AD study and

SCZ study, respectively. Dataset 1 is a subset of Alzheimer's Disease Neuroimaging Initiative (ADNI), the second stage of the Northern American ADNI (http://adni.loni.usc.edu). There are 120 subjects, including 42 normal controls (NCs), 46 MCIs and 32 AD patients. Dataset 2 contains the multimodal data for SCZ studies collected by COBRE (http://cobre.mrn.org/). It contains 100 subjects, 50 of them are SCZ sufferers and the rest are matched NCs. In both datasets, brain images with sMRI and dMRI modalities are provided. We extract cortical surfaces from sMRI images by using FreeSurfer toolbox (https://surfer.nmr.mgh.harvard.edu) and then compute the vertex-wise structural features such as the cortical thickness and curvatures on the extracted GM/WM boundary. The dMRI images were processed using the FSL toolbox (https://fsl.fmrib.ox.ac.uk/fsl/fslwiki) and WM integrity features, e.g. FA, MD and B0, are measured. The cortical and WM structural features are then mapped to the FreeSurfer space for consistency. The hyper-parameters α and β in Eq. 13 are both empirically chosen to be 10. We apply linear SVM in Statistics and Machine Learning Toolbox of MATLAB (http://www.mathworks.com) as the classifier to perform disease classifications. Experiment results of accuracy, F1 scores and ROC curves with 5-fold cross validation are reported.

We compare the performance of our proposed framework with some state-of-the-art multimodal fusion methods as well as the variant of our model: **RawFA**: It is the non-fusion model. Raw individual FA features have been aligned to the template. Then PCA works on the new FA maps for feature dimension reduction. **PCA+jICA** [4]: It is the state-of-the-art method for data-driven fusion of multimodal data. FA, MD, B0 and T1 maps are fused with this method after being registered to the same space. **mCCA+jICA** [14]: Another state-of-the-art method uses canonical correlation analysis and ICA to extract both shared and distinct properties across modalities. **pFused**: A variant version of our method that fuses cortical features without considering the feature mapping between WM structures. It is the partial fusion model which is merely based on the mapping from cortical surface fusion. **HPvol**: Measures of the hippocampal volume which is an ROI feature typically used in AD prediction. In our MFRM method, we map FA volume images to the template based on the feature mapping and recompute the distribution of FA values. Thus each subject eventually obtains a point-wise FA feature map as the new representation.

4.2   Results

On Dataset 1, we conduct 2 kinds of classifications, i.e. binary classification and multilabel classification, to distinguish AD, MCI and NC. Statistical validation results are given in Table 1 and Fig. 3. MFRM reaches 85% accuracy in AD vs. NC, 79% accuracy in AD vs. MCI, 66% accuracy in MCI vs. NC and 62% accuracy in AD vs. MCI vs. NC. Compared to the state-of-the-art methods, our method has the relatively better performance. For example, in AD vs. NC classification, MFRM boosts the accuracy of performance by around 16% compared to PCA+jICA and 29% compared to mCCA+jICA. The similar trends

Table 1. Classification performance comparison on Dataset 1 (AD).

Methods	AD vs NC		AD vs MCI		MCI vs NC		AD vs MCI vs NC	
	Acc	F1	Acc	F1	Acc	F1	Acc	F1
RawFA	51.35%	0.4375	58.97%	**0.7419**	52.27%	**0.6866**	38.33%	0.5542
PCA+jICA	68.92%	0.6102	61.54%	0.7059	53.28%	0.5714	35.0%	0.3276
mCCA+jICA	58.11%	0.5373	56.41%	0.6600	48.86%	0.5545	39.17%	0.4146
pFused	77.03%	0.7119	73.08%	0.6316	62.50%	0.6292	56.67%	0.5439
HPvol	78.40%	0.7241	60.30%	0.2791	64.80%	0.6353	51.70%	0.4660
MFRM	**85.14%**	**0.8070**	**79.49%**	0.7037	**65.91%**	0.6739	**62.5%**	**0.5946**

are observed in other binary classification tasks. Moreover, MFRM yields significant improvements over the non-fused model (RawFA) by raising the accuracy nearly 34% in classifying AD and NC. It is also better than the partial fusion model (pFused) with an accuracy increase of around 8%. It is consistent with discoveries of previous research that disease-related brain structural alterations are partially represented by cortical or WM geometry properties [2]. Generally, performance on MCI classification tasks is worse than that on AD classification but our method still achieves superior accuracy compared with other methods. On Dataset 2, we carry out a binary classification task for Schizophrenia disease and shows the performance of all the compared methods on Table 2. Similar to AD results, MFRM significantly outperforms other competing methods. Features learned from MFRM increase the accuracy as opposed to the partial fusion model by 7% and to the state-of-the-art methods by 15%. Together with the results on dataset 1, the proposed multimodal fusion framework beats other methods with significant improvements in performance on brain disease classification.

Table 2. Classification performance comparison on Dataset 2 (SCZ).

Methods	SCZ vs NC	
	Accuracy	F1
RawFA	52%	0.4894
PCA+jICA	61%	0.6061
mCCA+jICA	62%	0.6346
pFused	70%	0.6591
MFRM	**77%**	**0.7294**

The above results suggest that, after the feature mapping, raw features from the same group become closer to each other and those from different groups are driven away from each other. We further confirm this observation by comparing the pair-wise similarities among the ADNI cohort. We compute the earth mover's distances (EMD) [6] between the fused features of each two subjects and compare

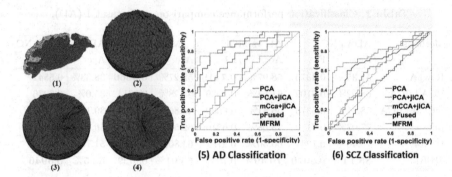

Fig. 3. Visualization of MFRM results and ROC curves for classification tasks ((5) for AD, (6) for SCZ). (1) is the raw volumetric data and (2) is the corresponding spherical volumetric harmonic map without feature encoding. (3) and (4) is the result of feature mapping (to a unit ball domain) of NC and AD, respectively. As we can see, compared to (3), (4) has the reduced anisotropy (more uniformly diffusive) which is consistent to the clinical discoveries [11].

the result with those from unfused features. Figure 4 shows the distance matrices. After the MFRM fusion, intra-class features indeed become relatively closer to each other and inter-class features become far away from each other.

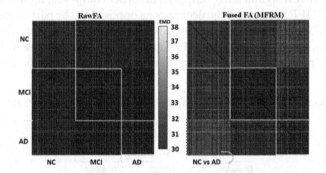

Fig. 4. Similarity matrix for Dataset 1 before (left) and after (right) feature fusion. The orange box marks the similarity between NC and AD, where is significantly brighter than the diagonal blocks (has the larger EMD values). (Color figure online)

5   Conclusion and Future Work

This paper describes a geometric framework for solving a multimodal brain images fusion problem. By varying Riemannian metrics to encode multimodal brain imaging features, we build the feature mapping efficiently with geometric registration methods, i.e., quasiconformal mapping and harmonic mapping.

There are several interesting directions for the future work. For example, we can apply the idea of changing Riemannian metrics for feature mapping to the analysis in brain ROIs. Besides, the variational framework designed on top of the Riemannian metrics in the Euclidean space can be extended to metrics in other geometric spaces, e.g., the hyperbolic space. Lastly, some other modalities, such as functional MR images or electroencephalography, can be the additional information sources to brain structural data and fused features derived from these modalities may contribute to the exploration of sensitive disease-related biomarkers.

Acknowledgement. This work was supported by the grants from NIH (R21AG-049216, RF1AG051710, R01EB025032, R01HL128818, U54EB020403).

References

1. Ashburner, J.: Computational anatomy with the SPM software. Magn. Reson. Imaging **27**(8), 1163–1174 (2009)
2. Assaf, Y., Pasternak, O.: Diffusion tensor imaging (DTI)-based white matter mapping in brain research: a review. J. Mol. Neurosci. **34**(1), 51–61 (2008)
3. Bojarski, B.: Homeomorphic solutions of Beltrami systems. In: Dokl. Akad. Nauk. SSSR, vol. 102, pp. 661–664 (1955)
4. Calhoun, V., Adali, T., Liu, J.: A feature-based approach to combine functional MRI, structural MRI and EEG brain imaging data. In: 28th Annual International Conference of the IEEE, EMBS 2006, pp. 3672–3675. IEEE (2006)
5. De Stefano, N., et al.: Evidence of early cortical atrophy in MS relevance to white matter changes and disability. Neurology **60**(7), 1157–1162 (2003)
6. Flamary, R., Courty, N.: Pot python optimal transport library (2017). https://github.com/rflamary/POT
7. Gardiner, F.P., Lakic, N.: Quasiconformal Teichmüller Theory, no. 76, American Mathematical Society, Providence (2000)
8. Jones, D.K., Leemans, A.: Diffusion tensor imaging. In: Magnetic Resonance Neuroimaging: Methods and Protocols, pp. 127–144 (2011)
9. Koehl, P., Hass, J.: Automatic alignment of genus-zero surfaces. IEEE Trans. Pattern Anal. Mach. Intell. (2013, in Press)
10. Lui, L.M., et al.: Optimization of surface registrations using Beltrami holomorphic flow. J. Sci. Comput. **50**(3), 557–585 (2012)
11. Nir, T.M., et al.: Effectiveness of regional DTI measures in distinguishing Alzheimer's disease, MCI, and normal aging. NeuroImage: Clin. **3**, 180–195 (2013)
12. Savadjiev, P., et al.: Fusion of white and gray matter geometry: a framework for investigating brain development. Med. Image Anal. **18**(8), 1349–1360 (2014)
13. Schoen, R., Yau, S.T.: Lectures on Differential Geometry. International Press, Vienna (1994)
14. Sui, J., et al.: Discriminating schizophrenia and bipolar disorder by fusing fMRI and DTI in a multimodal CCA+ joint ICA model. Neuroimage **57**(3), 839–855 (2011)
15. Tozer, D.J., et al.: Linking white matter tracts to associated cortical grey matter: a tract extension methodology. NeuroImage **59**(4), 3094–3102 (2012)
16. Wang, Y., Gu, X., Yau, S.T.: Volumetric harmonic map. Commun. Inf. Syst. **3**(3), 191–202 (2003)

17. Wells, W.M., Viola, P., Atsumi, H., Nakajima, S., Kikinis, R.: Multi-modal volume registration by maximization of mutual information. Med. Image Anal. **1**(1), 35–51 (1996)
18. Zeng, W., Lui, L.M., Luo, F., Chan, T.F.C., Yau, S.T., Gu, D.X.: Computing quasi-conformal maps using an auxiliary metric and discrete curvature flow. Numerische Mathematik **121**(4), 671–703 (2012)
19. Zhang, D., Wang, Y., Zhou, L., Yuan, H., Shen, D.: Multimodal classification of Alzheimer's disease and mild cognitive impairment. NeuroImage **55**(3), 856–867 (2011)

A Hierarchical Manifold Learning Framework for High-Dimensional Neuroimaging Data

Siyuan Gao[1(✉)], Gal Mishne[2], and Dustin Scheinost[3]

[1] Department of Biomedical Engineering, Yale University, New Haven, CT, USA
siyuan.gao@yale.edu
[2] Department of Mathematics, Yale University, New Haven, CT, USA
[3] Department of Radiology and Biomedical Imaging, Yale School of Medicine, New Haven, CT, USA

Abstract. Better understanding of large-scale brain dynamics with functional magnetic resonance imaging (fMRI) data is a major goal of modern neuroscience. In this work, we propose a novel hierarchical manifold learning framework for time-synchronized fMRI data for elucidating brain dynamics. Our framework—labelled 2-step diffusion maps (2sDM)—is based on diffusion maps, a nonlinear dimensionality reduction method. First, 2sDM learns the manifold of fMRI data for each individual separately and then learns a low-dimensional group-level embedding by integrating individual information. We also propose a method for out-of-sample extension within our hierarchical framework. Using 2sDM, we constructed a single manifold structure based on 6 different task-based fMRI (tfMRI) runs. Results on the tfMRI data show a clear manifold structure with four distinct clusters, or brain states. We extended this to embedding resting-state fMRI (rsfMRI) data by first synchronizing across individuals using an optimal orthogonal transformation. The rsfMRI data from the same individuals cleanly embedded onto the four clusters, suggesting that rsfMRI is a collection of different brains states. Overall, our results highlight 2sDM as a powerful method to understand brain dynamics and show that tfMRI and rsfMRI data share representative brain states.

1 Introduction

Recent studies of functional magnetic resonance imaging (fMRI) are beginning to quantify moment-to-moment changes in brain activity or connectivity [1–3]. A main goal of these works is to find representative brain states—or distinct, repeatable patterns of brain activity or connectivity—as a way of quantifying these brain dynamics. However, due to the high-dimensional nature of these brain patterns, assigning time points to specific brain states or even estimating the number of brain states remain unsolved problems. Moreover, the underlying network structure of the brain generates high degree of correlation in activation patterns across multiple brain regions. To convert brain dynamics into a

© Springer Nature Switzerland AG 2019
A. C. S. Chung et al. (Eds.): IPMI 2019, LNCS 11492, pp. 631–643, 2019.
https://doi.org/10.1007/978-3-030-20351-1_49

computational tractable problem, dimensionality reduction methods are used to project the fMRI time series into lower-dimensional space, consisting of only a few (*e.g.*, < 6) brain states [4,5]. While previous works have used a range of supervised or unsupervised methods, linear dimensionality reduction methods, such as principal component analysis (PCA), are the most widely used [1,2,5]. For example, brain states estimated from PCA were moderately correlated with the underlying working memory task, providing evidence that the observed brain states represent underlying neurobiology [2]. However, these patterns were insufficient to classify between several task states. As brain patterns exhibit nonlinear behavior and the number of observed states is small compared to the dimension of the data, nonlinear dimensionality reduction methods are more appropriate to estimate the large-scale brain state manifolds for a rich repertoire of tasks.

In this work, we propose a hierarchical, nonlinear manifold learning framework based on diffusion maps [6] for time-synchronized fMRI data. In contrast to linear embedding methods (*e.g.*, PCA), nonlinear methods focus on discovering the underlying manifold structure of the data by integrating local similarities into a global representation. By focusing on local similarities rather than global similarities, diffusion maps can better capture complex information in noisy high-dimensional data. To uncover the shared and unique features of different tasks, we applied our approach to 6 task fMRI (tfMRI) scans from the Human Connectome Project (HCP) dataset [7], and calculated a single brain state manifold that includes all 6 different task types. The embedded time points of the fMRI data naturally clustered into four brain states: fixation, transition, lower-level cognition, and higher-level cognition. We further summarized the characteristics of different tasks with task-specific temporal trajectories that were confined to the manifold. Finally, we propose a corresponding out-of-sample extension (OOSE) framework to embed new fMRI time series data. Combining this OOSE framework with BrainSync [8] to synchronize different individuals' resting-state fMRI (rsfMRI) data, we embedded rsfMRI into the tfMRI manifold. The rsfMRI embedding traverses all four brain states, suggesting that rsfMRI contains multiple states rather than a single monolithic state. Overall, our framework provides a novel way to reconstruct a brain state manifold from fMRI data and to quantify moment-to-moment changes in brain states.

2   2-Step Diffusion Maps (2sDM)

2.1   Diffusion Maps

Diffusion maps [6] is part of a broad class of manifold learning algorithms. Specifically, diffusion maps provides a global description of the data by considering only local similarities and is robust to noise perturbation. The new nonlinear representation provided by diffusion maps reveals underlying intrinsic parameters governing the data [9]. Here we develop a new framework utilizing diffusion maps to detect repeatable brain states in fMRI data.

The diffusion maps algorithm is as follows. The input is a pairwise similarity matrix $\mathbf{S}$, which can be computed using the Gaussian kernel $w_\epsilon(x, y) =$

Algorithm 1. Diffusion Maps

Input: $\mathbf{X} \in \mathbb{R}^{N \times P}$ - N instances with P features
   d - number of dimensions to keep in the embedding
   t - diffusion time parameter
Output: $\mathbf{\Psi} \in \mathbb{R}^{N \times d}$ - d-dimensional embedding
   function DM($\mathbf{X}, d, t$)
      Step 1: Build similarity matrix $\mathbf{L}$ using Gaussian kernel $w_\epsilon(x, y) = e^{-||x-y||^2/\epsilon}$
      Step 2: Normalize the matrix $\mathbf{L}$ to approximate the Laplace–Beltrami operator $\tilde{\mathbf{L}} = \mathbf{D}^{-1}\mathbf{L}\mathbf{D}^{-1}$, where D is a diagonal matrix and $D_{ii} = \sum_j L_{ij}$
      Step 3: Form the normalized random walk matrix $\mathbf{M} = \tilde{\mathbf{D}}^{-1}\tilde{\mathbf{L}}$, where $\tilde{\mathbf{D}}$ is a diagonal matrix and $\tilde{D}_{ii} = \sum_j \tilde{L}_{ij}$
      Step 4: Compute the largest d eigenvalues λ_i of $\mathbf{M}$ and the corresponding eigenvectors ψ_i, $\mathbf{\Psi}(\mathbf{X}) = (\lambda_1^t\psi_1, \lambda_2^t\psi_2, \ldots, \lambda_d^t\psi_d)$

$\exp(-||x-y||^2/\epsilon)$ between pairs of data points x and y. Then the rows of the similarity matrix are normalized by $\mathbf{P} = \mathbf{D}^{-1}\mathbf{S}$, where $D_{ii} = \sum_j S_{ij}$. This creates a random walk matrix on the data with entries set to $p(x, y) = w_\epsilon(x, y)/d(x)$. Taking powers of the matrix is equivalent to running the Markov chain forward. The kernel $p_t(\cdot, \cdot)$ can be interpreted as the transition probability between two points in t time steps. The matrix $\mathbf{P}$ has a complete sequence of bi-orthogonal left and right eigenvectors ϕ_i, ψ_i, respectively, and a corresponding sequence of eigenvalues $1 = \lambda_0 \geq |\lambda_1| \geq |\lambda_2| \geq \ldots$. Diffusion maps is a nonlinear embedding of the data points into a low-dimensional space, where the mapping is defined as $\mathbf{\Psi}(x) = (\lambda_1^t\psi_1(x), \lambda_2^t\psi_2(x), \ldots, \lambda_k^t\psi_k(x))$, where t is the diffusion time. Note that ψ_0 is neglected because it is a constant vector.

A diffusion distance $D_t^2(x, y)$ between two data points x, y is defined as:

$$D_t^2(x, y) = \sum_z \frac{(p_t(x, z) - p_t(y, z))^2}{\phi_0(y)}$$

where ϕ_0 represents the stationary distribution. This measures the similarity of two points by the evolution in the Markov chain. Two points are closer if there are more short paths connecting them. It is thus robust to noise as it considers all the possible paths between two points.

Proposition 1 (Coifman & Lafon). *Diffusion maps $\mathbf{\Psi}$ embeds data points into a Euclidean space $\mathbb{R}^k$ where the Euclidean distance approximates the diffusion distance:*

$$D_t^2(x, y) = ||\mathbf{\Psi}(x) - \mathbf{\Psi}(y)||_2^2$$

A detailed proof using the spectral theorem in Hilbert space can be found in [6]. In practice, eigenvalues of $\mathbf{P}$ typically exhibit a spectral gap such that the first few eigenvalues are close to one with all additional eigenvalues much smaller than one. Then the diffusion distance can be well approximated by only these first few eigenvectors [9]. Thus, we obtain a low-dimensional representation of the data by considering only the first few eigenvectors of the diffusion maps (See Algorithm 1). Intuitively, diffusion maps embeds data points closer when it is hard for the points to escape the local region within time t.

To remove dependence on the density of the data, the Gaussian similarity weights $w_\epsilon(\cdot, \cdot)$ are renormalized by the estimated density. This renormalization step leads to an anisotropic diffusion process and enables the algorithm to better recover the manifold structure so that it does not depend on the distribution of the points. The eigenvectors of the new random walk matrix now approximate the Laplace-Beltrami operator [9].

2.2   2-Step Diffusion Maps

Based on diffusion maps, we propose a hierarchical manifold learning framework for multi-individual fMRI BOLD time series. Under the assumption that individuals' fMRI responses are time-synchronized, we represent each individual's fMRI data as $\mathbf{X}_{i,,.} \in \mathbb{R}^{T \times V}, i = 1, \ldots, M$. Here T is the number of repetition time (TR) in the scan, V is the number of voxels or brain regions, and M is the total number of individuals. We label this framework 2-step diffusion maps (2sDM). Note that 2sDM can be applied to either domains of the data, resulting in a lower-dimensional representation of either time, individuals or brain regions. Here we illustrate the framework by embedding time into a lower-dimensional space. Reducing the other two domains just requires trivial adaptation.

First we apply diffusion maps to the fMRI time series of every single individual i to obtain the embedding $\boldsymbol{\Psi}_i \in \mathbb{R}^{T \times d_1}$, thus reducing each individual's V voxels or brain regions to a d_1-dimensional Euclidean space. Then, we concatenate the new representations of all individuals to a single matrix $\boldsymbol{\Psi}^{(1)} \in \mathbb{R}^{T \times (M d_1)}$. From this concatenated matrix, we can perform a second-step diffusion maps to further reduce the dimensionality of every time-frame to d_2. The final time-frame representation matrix with multi-individual similarity is $\boldsymbol{\Psi}^{(2)} \in \mathbb{R}^{T \times d_2}$. Our framework is presented in Algorithm 2. As the first-step diffusion maps produces a cleaner representation of the fMRI data, the reasoning of performing an embedding based on the results of the first-step embedding can be seen from the following proposition,

Proposition 2. *The distance between two frames u, v in $\boldsymbol{\Psi}^{(1)}$ equals the total diffusion distance for all individuals.*

Proof. By Proposition 1, $||\boldsymbol{\Psi}(x) - \boldsymbol{\Psi}(y)||_2 = D_t(x, y)$. Therefore

$$||\boldsymbol{\Psi}^{(1)}(u) - \boldsymbol{\Psi}^{(1)}(v)||_2^2 = \sum_{i=1}^{M} ||\boldsymbol{\Psi}_i(u) - \boldsymbol{\Psi}_i(v)||_2^2 = \sum_{i=1}^{M} D_t^2(\mathbf{X}_{i,u,.}, \mathbf{X}_{i,v,.}),$$

where $D_t^2(\mathbf{X}_{i,u,.}, \mathbf{X}_{i,v,.})$ is the diffusion distance of time points u and v for individual i with diffusion time t. $\square$

As such, if two concatenated vectors have relatively small Euclidean distance, it suggests that, on average, for all of the individuals there is small diffusion

---

Algorithm 2. 2-step Diffusion Maps

Input: $\mathbf{X} \in \mathbb{R}^{M \times T \times V}$ - M individuals' fMRI time series with T TRs and V regions
  d_1 - number of dimensions to keep for each individual
  d_2 - number of dimensions to keep in the final embedding
  t - diffusion time parameter
Output: $\mathbf{\Psi}^{(2)} \in \mathbb{R}^{T \times d_2}$ - lower-dimensional embedding for the second dimension
  function 2sDM($\mathbf{X}, d_1, d_2, t$)
    for each individual $\mathbf{X}_{i,\cdot,\cdot}$ **do**
      $\mathbf{\Psi}_i$=DM($\mathbf{X}_{i,\cdot,\cdot}, d_1, t$)
    $\mathbf{\Psi}^{(1)} = (\mathbf{\Psi}_1, \mathbf{\Psi}_2, \dots, \psi_M)$
    $\mathbf{\Psi}^{(2)}$=DM($\mathbf{\Psi}^{(1)}, d_2, t$)

---

distance between the two time points. Additionally, no functional alignment between individuals is needed as the similarity between time points is calculated in each individual's own embedding space separately and aggregated through the sum of diffusion distances.

2.3 Out-of-Sample Extension Framework

To embed new time points to the existing temporal manifold, we use out-of-sample extension (OOSE) for new time series data. The reason to use OOSE here is twofold: *(i)* OOSE enables to embed new data points without reapplying the eigendecomposition on the entire dataset, and *(ii)* OOSE keeps the existing manifold structure unaffected and makes it easier to interpret new time points in an unsupervised setting. The OOSE framework for time-synchronized fMRI data works in a similar hierarchical way, using two Nyström extension steps (a non-parametric OOSE method, described in Algorithm 3).

Algorithm 3. Nyström Out-of-sample Extension

Input: $\mathbf{X} \in \mathbb{R}^{N \times P}$ - training data
  $\mathbf{\Psi} \in \mathbb{R}^{N \times d}$ - d-dimensional embedding result for $\mathbf{X}$
  $\mathbf{X}' \in \mathbb{R}^{N' \times P}$ - N' new data points
Output: $\hat{\mathbf{\Psi}} \in \mathbb{R}^{N' \times d}$ - approximated low-dimensional embedding for $\mathbf{X}'$
  function OOSE($\mathbf{X}', \mathbf{X}, \mathbf{\Psi}$)
    $\hat{\psi}_l(x') = \frac{1}{\lambda_l} \sum_{j=1}^m p(x', x_j) \psi_l(x_j), l = 1, \dots, d$
    $\hat{\mathbf{\Psi}}(\mathbf{X}') = (\lambda_1^t \hat{\psi}_1, \lambda_2^t \hat{\psi}_2, \dots, \lambda_d^t \hat{\psi}_d)$

Given new time-synchronized fMRI data $\mathbf{X}'_{i,\cdot,\cdot} \in \mathbb{R}^{T' \times V}, i = 1, ..., M$ for the same group of individuals, we first approximate eigenvectors $\hat{\mathbf{\Psi}}_i^{(1)}$ for each individual. Then we concatenate all the individuals' eigenvectors $\hat{\mathbf{\Psi}}_i^{(1)}$ as the new data points and approximate its eigenvectors $\hat{\mathbf{\Psi}}^{(2)}$ as the final representation. The 2-step OOSE framework is described in Algorithm 4.

Algorithm 4. 2-step Out-of-sample Extension

Input: $\mathbf{X} \in \mathbb{R}^{M \times T \times V}$ - M individuals' fMRI time series with T TRs and V regions
   $\mathbf{\Psi}^{(1)} \in \mathbb{R}^{T \times M \times d_1}$ - first-step diffusion maps result for $\mathbf{X}$
   $\mathbf{\Psi}^{(2)} \in \mathbb{R}^{T \times d_2}$ - second-step diffusion maps result for $\mathbf{\Psi}^{(1)}$
   $\mathbf{X}' \in \mathbb{R}^{M \times T' \times V}$ - M individuals' new fMRI time series with T' TRs and V regions
Output: $\hat{\mathbf{\Psi}}^{(2)} \in \mathbb{R}^{T' \times d_2}$ - approximated low-dimensional embedding for $\mathbf{X}'$
   function 2-STEP OOSE($\mathbf{X}', \mathbf{\Psi}^{(1)}, \mathbf{\Psi}^{(2)}, \mathbf{X}$)
      for each individual $\mathbf{X}'_{i,\cdot,\cdot}$ do
         $\hat{\mathbf{\Psi}}_i^{(1)}(\mathbf{X}'_{i,\cdot,\cdot}) = $OOSE($\mathbf{X}'_{i,\cdot,\cdot}, \mathbf{X}_{i,\cdot,\cdot}, \mathbf{\Psi}^{(1)}_{\cdot,i,\cdot}$)
      $\hat{\mathbf{\Psi}}^{(1)}(\mathbf{X}') = (\hat{\mathbf{\Psi}}_1^{(1)}(\mathbf{X}'_{1,\cdot,\cdot}), \hat{\mathbf{\Psi}}_2^{(1)}(\mathbf{X}'_{2,\cdot,\cdot}), \ldots, \hat{\mathbf{\Psi}}_M^{(1)}(\mathbf{X}'_{M,\cdot,\cdot}))$
      $\hat{\mathbf{\Psi}}^{(2)}(\mathbf{X}') = $OOSE($\hat{\mathbf{\Psi}}^{(1)}, \mathbf{\Psi}^{(1)}, \mathbf{\Psi}^{(2)}$)

---

fMRI data that is not time-synchronized across individuals (*e.g.*, rsfMRI) needs to be synchronized across individuals before an out-of-sample application of the existing 2sDM embedding can be used. We used Brainsync [8] to temporally synchronize the rsfMRI data. Brainsync synchronizes one individual's time series data $\mathbf{Y} \in \mathbb{R}^{T \times V}$ to a reference individual's time series $\mathbf{X} \in \mathbb{R}^{T \times V}$ by finding an optimal orthogonal transformation $\mathbf{O}^s$ for $\mathbf{Y}$ to minimize the squared error: $\mathbf{O}^s = \arg \min_{\mathbf{O} \in \mathbf{O}(T)} ||\mathbf{X} - \mathbf{O}\mathbf{Y}||^2$. The problem can be solved by the Kabsch algorithm [10]. The $T \times T$ cross-correlation matrix $\mathbf{X}\mathbf{Y}^t$ is first formed and its singular value decomposition can be calculated as $\mathbf{X}\mathbf{Y}^t = \mathbf{U}\mathbf{\Sigma}\mathbf{V}^t$. The optimal $\mathbf{O}^s$ can be found by $\mathbf{O}^s = \mathbf{U}\mathbf{V}^t$ and $\mathbf{Y}$ can be synchronized to $\mathbf{X}$ by $\mathbf{O}^s\mathbf{Y}$.

3   Experiments

We assessed the performance of 2sDM using tfMRI and rsfMRI data from the Human Connectome Project (HCP) dataset. In this dataset, individuals performed 7 distinct tfMRI scans: Working memory (WM), Emotion, Gambling, Motor, Social, Relational, and Language. Each task had interleaved blocks of various conditions (*e.g.*, fixation, cue, 0-back, 2-back for the WM task). Most of the individuals had the same task block order and, thus, had synchronized fMRI time series. However, the Language task was excluded for analysis due to variable block timings, which caused non-synchronized time series between individuals. 390 individuals from the HCP dataset were retained after removing individuals for high motion, different task block orders, or incomplete data. We performed standard preprocessing, including motion correction, registration to common space, and regression of nuisance signals. For initial data reduction, a whole-brain functional atlas [11] was used to extract 268 time series from the fMRI data. Time series were z-scored to make them comparable across scans. Diffusion time $t = 1$ is used in all the experiments.

3.1   Task fMRI Manifold

Instead of embedding each task independently, we constructed a single manifold structure based on all the available tfMRI to discover the shared and unique features of different cognitive tasks. Specifically, every individual had two scans for the 6 tasks (corresponding to the left-right (LR) and right-left (RL) phase encoding direction), where the task block orders were different for the two scans. As our framework does not rely on the temporal structure, we concatenated all the tfMRI time series (including LR and RL scans) for each individual. In total, each concatenated time series has a length of 3020 time points, consisting of 17 different task block types. While the concatenation increases the number of time points to be used in the embedding, it requires our algorithm to be robust to noise differences across the different conditions and acquisitions.

We present the 1st three non-trivial coordinates of the embedding in 3D space in Fig. 1a. Visual inspection reveals a triangular structure from the first two coordinates. In this triangle, the lower right corner contains task blocks that require *higher-level cognition* (*e.g.*, 2-back, social, relation). The upper right corner contains the cue blocks and the immediately following time points. We label this corner as a *transition state*, where individuals are transitioning between different tasks. On the left corner of the triangle, most of fixation time frames clustered together with other time frames at the end of the task block (before the next fixation block). We identify this corner as the *fixation state*. When adding the third coordinate, a final state—labeled the *lower-level cognition state*—becomes apparent. The *lower-level cognition state* contains task blocks like motor, emotion, and 0-back. Given the 4 observable clusters, we applied k-means clustering ($k = 4$) on the tfMRI manifold to explicitly assign tfMRI time frames with a single brain state. While ψ_1 and ψ_2 focus more on the general difference (cognitive involvement), ψ_3 provides more localized information, separating between different tasks. Thus, 2sDM learns both the shared and distinct features of different tasks, revealing them in a hierarchical way in different coordinates.

Another perspective of looking at this multi-task structure is by "*temporal trajectories*". Prior work on high-dimensional neuronal data has suggested identifying low-dimensional trajectories as a compact representation of the neural activity that evolves over time [12]. By calculating the average temporal trajectory for each task block type across multiple blocks, we get a single representative trajectory for each block type. Plotting these trajectories (Fig. 1b) demonstrates that all the task blocks start near the task cues (*i.e.*, *transition state*) and progressively enter the task state and finally converge near the fixation state.

3.2   Resting-State fMRI Manifold

As rsfMRI data is not time-synchronized across individuals, the BrainSync procedure was applied to transform rsfMRI into time-synchronized data in reference to a given individual. One minor application difference from the original Brain-Sync paper, is that we used parcellated fMRI data instead of voxel-level data. Thus, $T > V$. In this case, the transformation matrix $\mathbf{O}$ will not be unique due

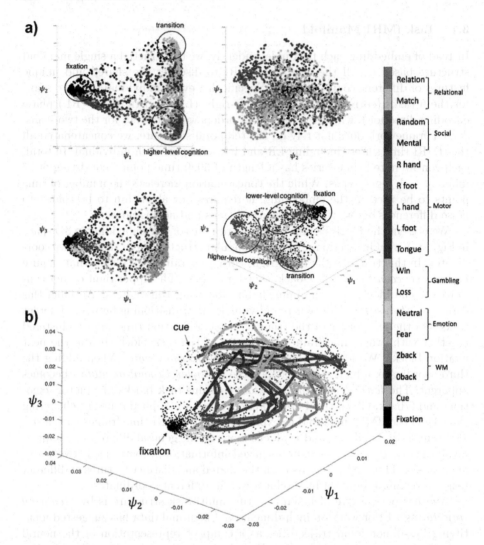

Fig. 1. (a) Manifold of tfMRI. (b) Temporal trajectories of tfMRI. Each point represents a time frame and the point or trajectory is colored by the task block type.

to repeated singular values. Nevertheless, all the solutions will still result in the same correlations and the solution would be still valid. In fact, the rank of the correlation matrices $\mathbf{X}\mathbf{Y}^t$ is much smaller than V or T. RsfMRI data from both phase encoding runs were used, resulting in 2400 time points per individual.

For validation, we examine whether BrainSync synchronizes the rsfMRI data across individuals. Before BrainSync, mean rsfMRI time series correlation between individuals is 0.0014 ± 0.00087. After applying BrainSync, the

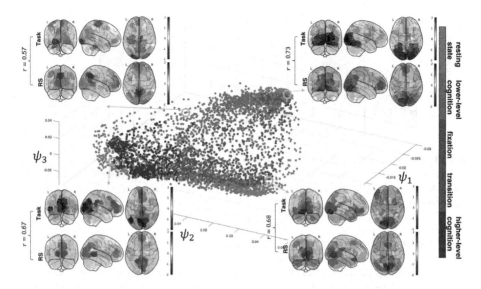

Fig. 2. Out-of-sample extension of rsfMRI onto the task manifold. Individual that has the lowest BrainSync squared error to all the other individuals is used as reference. The task manifold is colored by the k-means clustering results, representing our 4 brain states. Representative brain states for each cluster and its neighbors' average rsfMRI are also shown. Highly correlated brain activation is found between tfMRI and rsfMRI.

mean correlation is 0.75 ± 0.017. This mean is taken by using each individual as the reference individual and correlating all other individuals with the reference individual.

After synchronizing the rsfMRI data, we used our OOSE framework to embed the rsfMRI time frames onto the tfMRI manifold. The OOSE result (Fig. 2), shows that the rsfMRI spreads out over the four identified brain states. To further investigate the underlying brain dynamics in resting-state, we find the 10 nearest tfMRI neighbors for each extended rsfMRI time frame, and set it to be in the state that most of the neighbors are in. This assigns each time frame a single brain state. We can first calculate the dwell time distribution of the four states for rsfMRI (Fig. 3a). Fixation and transition states have the highest proportion while both lower-level and higher-level cognitive states have low proportion. Moreover, to actually see how the brain shifts between different states, we calculated the Markov matrix of rsfMRI (Fig. 3b). To validate and visualize the brain activity in different states, we chose one representative tfMRI time frame for each brain state and also the nearest rsfMRI time frame in the low-dimensional embedding space. We then averaged the brain activity across individuals in the chosen time frame and compared between tfMRI and rsfMRI. Highly correlated brain activities are found between tfMRI and rsfMRI (Fig. 2).

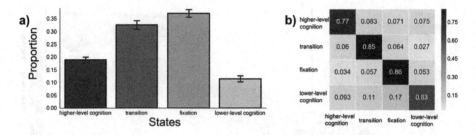

Fig. 3. **(a)** RsfMRI dwell times for brain states. Mean and standard deviation for different individual's dwell time are shown. Fixation is the most frequent state; while, lower-level cognition state is the least frequent. **(b)** Transition matrix of the identified brain states.

3.3   Method Validation and Comparison

First, we validated that 2sDM aggregates single individual's information into a multi-individual manifold that cannot be reconstructed from any single individual. We applied the diffusion maps embedding onto each single individual's tfMRI. Overall the embeddings for all the individuals look similar and here we show a randomly chosen individual's embedding (Fig. 4a). No clear structure was identified from any of the individuals.

Next, we compared our framework with PCA to investigate whether our manifold learning framework discovers structure that linear methods cannot recover. To have a fair comparison and considering the fact that our framework is modular, we used a similar 2-step PCA framework. By projecting tfMRI time frames into 3D space using the 1st three coordinates of PCA, no clear structure is shown from the embedding (Fig. 4b). The fact that 2sDM discovered the manifold structure, while PCA cannot, validates the usage of manifold learning.

Finally, we used the tfMRI data to cross-validate the accuracy of the OOSE framework. Using leave-one-task-out cross-validation, a single task session was held out when generating the tfMRI manifold. The left-out task was then embedded in the new tfMRI manifold using our OOSE framework and compared with the original tfMRI embedding created using all tfMRI. If the held-out task's extended coordinates are similar to the coordinates of the original embedding, it suggests that the OOSE framework is accurate. In Fig. 4c, we plot the extension of WM task's LR session. The 2-back and 0-back task blocks go to the correct higher-level cognition or lower-level cognition state respectively, while the fixation and cue time frames are also located in the correct brain states. The correlation between the extended coordinates and the coordinates from original embedding was highly significant, $r = 0.939, p < 0.001$. We also held out one session from all the other tasks, which produced similar results as the WM task.

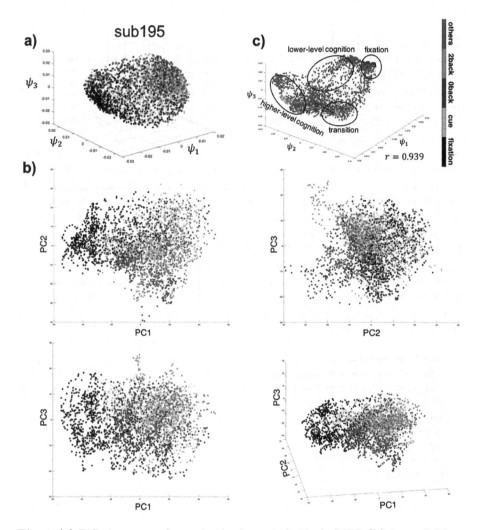

Fig. 4. (**a**) Diffusion maps of a randomly chosen individual tfMRI. (**b**) 2-step PCA on tfMRI. (**c**) OOSE with WM held out. Colormaps of (a) and (b) are the same as Fig. 1.

4   Conclusion

We proposed a hierarchical framework for learning a manifold for time-synchronized fMRI data, labelled 2sDM, based on diffusion maps. First, 2sDM learns the manifold of fMRI data for each individual separately and, then, learns a low-dimensional group-level embedding by integrating these individual manifolds. To embed additional fMRI data in an existing embedding, we also proposed a corresponding OOSE framework. Using 2sDM, a clear brain state manifold is discovered from our framework with four distinct states easily identified. In comparison, a similar 2-step PCA approach did not reveal a clear low-dimensional structure, suggesting our non-linear 2sDM is better able to capture brain states than previously used linear approaches [1,2,5]. Additionally, using our OOSE framework, rsfMRI data was embedded into all four distinct brain states identified from tfMRI data. These results suggest that rsfMRI is better represented by a collection of different brains states derived from many different tasks rather than a single, monolithic state.

Reconstructing low-dimensional manifolds from neural population activity is an active area of research in other areas of neuroscience, such as electrophysiology. Previous data provides a possible shift from neuron-centric to manifold-centric view of neural activity that fosters an important advance in understanding our brain [13]. Additionally, previous work have only performed these embeddings using specific task [13,14]. Our work extends these ideas from electrophysiology data to fMRI data. In addition, we highlight that clear manifold structures can be observed from a collections of different tasks, suggesting a shared low-dimensional structure across different tfMRI data.

In conclusion, our framework provides a novel way to reconstruct a brain state manifold from fMRI data and to quantify moment-to-moment changes in brain states. Overall, our results highlight 2sDM as a promising method to understand brain dynamics using manifold learning and show that tfMRI and rsfMRI data share representative brain states.

Acknowledgements. Data were provided in part by the Human Connectome Project, WU-Minn Consortium (Principal Investigators: David Van Essen and Kamil Ugurbil; U54 MH091657) funded by the 16 NIH Institutes and Centers that support the NIH Blueprint for Neuroscience Research; and by the McDonnell Center for Systems Neuroscience at Washington University. GM is supported by the US-Israel BSF, by the NSF (grant no. 2015582), and by the NIH (grant no. R01 NS100049).

References

1. Allen, E.A., Damaraju, E., Plis, S.M., Erhardt, E.B., Eichele, T., Calhoun, V.D.: Tracking whole-brain connectivity dynamics in the resting state. Cereb. Cortex **24**(3), 663–676 (2014)
2. Monti, R.P., Lorenz, R., Hellyer, P., Leech, R., Anagnostopoulos, C., Montana, G.: Decoding time-varying functional connectivity networks via linear graph embedding methods. Front. Comput. Neurosci. **11**, 14 (2017)
3. Lindquist, M.A., Xu, Y., Nebel, M.B., Caffo, B.S.: Evaluating dynamic bivariate correlations in resting-state fMRI: a comparison study and a new approach. NeuroImage **101**, 531–546 (2014)
4. Venkatesh, M., Jaja, J., Pessoa, L.: Brain dynamics and temporal trajectories during task and naturalistic processing. NeuroImage (2018)
5. Shine, J.M., et al.: The dynamic basis of cognition: an integrative core under the control of the ascending neuromodulatory system (2018)
6. Coifman, R.R., Lafon, S.: Diffusion maps. Appl. Comput. Harmonic Anal. **21**(1), 5–30 (2006)
7. Van Essen, D.C., et al.: The WU-Minn human connectome project: an overview. Neuroimage **80**, 62–79 (2013)

8. Joshi, A.A., Chong, M., Li, J., Choi, S., Leahy, R.M.: Are you thinking what i'm thinking? Synchronization of resting fMRI time-series across subjects. NeuroImage **172**, 740–752 (2018)
9. Nadler, B., Lafon, S., Coifman, R.R., Kevrekidis, I.G.: Diffusion maps, spectral clustering and reaction coordinates of dynamical systems. Appl. Comput. Harmonic Anal. **21**(1), 113–127 (2006)
10. Kabsch, W.: A solution for the best rotation to relate two sets of vectors. Acta Crystallogr. Sect. A Crystal Phy. Diffr. Theoret. Gen. Crystallogr. **32**(5), 922–923 (1976)
11. Shen, X., Tokoglu, F., Papademetris, X., Todd Constable, R.: Groupwise whole-brain parcellation from resting-state fMRI data for network node identification. Neuroimage **82**, 403–415 (2013)
12. Gao, P., et al.: A theory of multineuronal dimensionality, dynamics and measurement. BioRxiv, p. 214262 (2017)
13. Gallego, J.A., Perich, M.G., Miller, L.E., Solla, S.A.: Neural manifolds for the control of movement. Neuron **94**(5), 978–984 (2017)
14. Ganmor, E., Segev, R., Schneidman, E.: A thesaurus for a neural population code. Elife **4**, e06134 (2015)

A Model for Elastic Evolution on Foliated Shapes

Dai-Ni Hsieh[1]([✉]), Sylvain Arguillère[2], Nicolas Charon[1], Michael I. Miller[3], and Laurent Younes[1]

[1] Department of Applied Mathematics and Statistics, Johns Hopkins University, Baltimore, MD 21218, USA
dnhsieh@jhu.edu
[2] Institut Camille Jordan, Villeurbanne, France
[3] Department of Biomedical Engineering, Johns Hopkins University, Baltimore, MD 21218, USA

Abstract. We study a shape evolution framework in which the deformation of shapes from time t to $t+dt$ is governed by a regularized anisotropic elasticity model. More precisely, we assume that at each time shapes are infinitesimally deformed from a stress-free state to an elastic equilibrium as a result of the application of a small force. The configuration of equilibrium then becomes the new resting state for subsequent evolution. The primary motivation of this work is the modeling of slow changes in biological shapes like atrophy, where a body force applied to the volume represents the location and impact of the disease. Our model uses an optimal control viewpoint with the time derivative of force interpreted as a control, deforming a shape gradually from its observed initial state to an observed final state. Furthermore, inspired by the layered organization of cortical volumes, we consider a special case of our model in which shapes can be decomposed into a family of layers (forming a "foliation"). Preliminary experiments on synthetic layered shapes in two and three dimensions are presented to demonstrate the effect of elasticity.

1 Introduction

Understanding changes in anatomical shapes is an essential problem for the analysis of many diseases, and more specifically for their tracking over time. While a large variety of shape analysis methods have been successful in cross-sectional problems, in which one exhibits differences in some shape spaces between two populations, a longitudinal analysis of shape changes in a single subject requires a careful modeling of the process, including the structure of the deforming material and the process causing the changes.

Our interest is more specifically in the modeling of dynamical changes in biological tissues that typically occur over long periods of time (such as the progressive atrophy of an organ along the years of a disease) thus resulting in sequences

Laurent Younes partially supported by NIH 1R01DC016784-01.

A. C. S. Chung et al. (Eds.): IPMI 2019, LNCS 11492, pp. 644–655, 2019.
https://doi.org/10.1007/978-3-030-20351-1_50

of slow alterations in the material properties. Unlike several past approaches for longitudinal analysis based on generic deformation analysis pipelines [7,16], this work constitutes a step towards a model that could explain morphological variations through more physically interpretable features, while also enabling the estimation of the potential source location and severity of the pathology.

The setting we introduce in this paper is in part inspired from elastic models describing slow changes in biological shapes [1,6,13,18,19]. We propose a shape evolution framework in which the transition between time t and $t+dt$ is governed by a regularized anisotropic elasticity model in which shapes at rest (or stress free) at time t find a new elastic equilibrium at time $t+dt$ as a result of the application of a small force dF, reaching a configuration that becomes their new resting state for subsequent evolution.

The paper is organized as follows. Section 2 introduces a general mathematical setting for the shape evolution process, while Sect. 3 details the specific laminar elastic model used in our experiments. Section 4 provides some numerical illustrations of the method, focusing, so far, on synthetic data. We conclude the paper in Sect. 5.

2   Shape Evolution Paradigm

We first introduce a general shape evolution model which we shall make specific to layered elastic materials in the next section. Given an initial shape M_0 which we take as a compact domain of $\mathbb{R}^3$, we consider deformed shapes $t \mapsto \varphi(t, M_0)$ in which φ is a time-dependent diffeomorphism obtained as the flow of a time-dependent velocity field $t \mapsto v(t)$ satisfying the system:

$$\begin{cases} \partial_t \varphi(t) = v(t, \varphi(t)), \ \varphi(0) = id \\ L_{\varphi(t)} v(t) = j(t)\, dp \end{cases}. \tag{1}$$

We shall assume that each $v(t)$ belongs to V, a reproducing kernel Hilbert space (RKHS) of vector fields on $\mathbb{R}^3$, continuously embedded in the space $C_0^2(\mathbb{R}^3, \mathbb{R}^3)$, which denotes the Banach space of C^2 vector fields on $\mathbb{R}^3$ such that u, Du, and D^2u vanish at infinity, equipped with the norm defined by $\|u\|_{2,\infty} = \|u\|_\infty + \|Du\|_\infty + \|D^2u\|_\infty$. ($Du$ denotes the derivative of u.) Also, in (1), L_φ is a certain linear operator from V to V^*, $j(t)$ is a vector field on $\mathbb{R}^3$ supported by $\varphi(t, M_0)$, and $j(t)\, dp$ is its associated element in V^*. In the rest of the paper, for any generic function $(t, x) \mapsto f(t, x)$, we adopt the convention of writing $f(t)$ instead of $f(t, \cdot)$.

Our objective consists in estimating $j(t)$ given an observed initial shape M_0 and an observed target shape M_1, under the evolution model expressed in (1). In this general setting, such an inverse problem is typically formulated as an optimal control problem by adding either regularization penalties or constraints on j for well-posedness.

In spite of the fact that $\varphi(t)$ is a diffeomorphism obtained as the flow of a vector field, the important difference between this approach and standard registration of volumetric data in diffeomorphic frameworks such as [2] is that the evolution here is not controlled directly by the velocity v. Instead, v is implicitly determined by j through the operator L_φ. The definition of L_φ thus considerably affects the nature and properties of optimal solutions. In the next section, we define L_φ for layered structures based on anisotropic linear elasticity.

3   Elastic Evolution of Layered Shapes

We build the operator L_φ step by step. First, for a fixed elastic shape with elastic tensor Λ, we define the operator $\mathcal{L}_\Lambda$ such that the solution of $\mathcal{L}_\Lambda u = F\,dp$ characterizes, up to a small regularization, the elastic displacement from resting state to equilibrium when a force density F is applied. Next, we define an elastic tensor Λ in the special case of layered shapes. We then specify how the elastic tensor is transformed to Λ^φ when a diffeomorphism φ acts on layered shapes, which is needed to keep track of the configuration as it gets progressively deformed.

By our assumption that the deformed shapes are at rest at each time, the infinitesimal displacement at each time is given by $\mathcal{L}_{\Lambda^\varphi}\delta u = \delta F\,dp$ for some infinitesimal force density δF. After normalization by δt, we finally obtain the elastic operator for layered shapes as $L_\varphi = \mathcal{L}_{\Lambda^\varphi}$ such that $\mathcal{L}_{\Lambda^\varphi}v = j\,dp$.

3.1   Linear Elastic Model for Small Deformation

Let $M \subset \mathbb{R}^3$ be a compact domain, which is assumed to represent an elastic material at rest. When applying a small force F to M, the displacement field u of the small deformation $\psi = id + u$ can be obtained based on the minimum total potential energy principle, in which u minimizes

$$U_\Lambda(u) - \int_M F(p)^\top u(p)\,dp,$$

where $U_\Lambda(u)$ is the linear elastic energy resulting from the displacement u on M, and Λ is the elastic tensor describing elastic properties of the material. The exact expression of $U_\Lambda(u)$ is detailed below. Here, we assume that only a body force "inside the volume," i.e., a force density, affects the material, but that no pressure acts on its boundary.

In order to ensure, eventually, a diffeomorphic evolution of the shape when passing to a time-dependent model, we add a regularization term to the total potential energy and look for a regularized response u to the force F given by

$$u = \arg\min_{u' \in V} \left(\frac{\delta}{2}\|u'\|_V^2 + U_\Lambda(u') - \int_M F(p)^\top u'(p)\,dp \right), \tag{2}$$

in which $\delta > 0$ is a small regularization parameter.

Following [4,10,14], we now specify the definition of the elastic energy and characterize the solution of (2). For a displacement field u on M, we denote the linear strain tensor by

$$\varepsilon(u) = \frac{1}{2}\left(Du + Du^\top\right).$$

Let $\varepsilon_p(u)$ denote the evaluation of $\varepsilon(u)$ at a point $p \in M$. The linear elastic energy corresponding to u can then be written as

$$U_\Lambda(u) = \int_M \Lambda_p(\varepsilon_p(u)) \, dp,$$

where the elastic tensor $p \mapsto \Lambda_p$ is a mapping from M to the set of non-negative quadratic forms over the space of 3 by 3 symmetric matrices. The function Λ encodes the elastic properties of the material. For example, in an isotropic linear elastic material, one has $\Lambda_p(\varepsilon) = \frac{\lambda}{2} \left(\sum_{i=1}^3 \varepsilon_{ii} \right)^2 + \mu \sum_{i,j=1}^3 \varepsilon_{ij}^2$ for all $p \in M$, where λ and μ are the Lamé parameters.

If we further assume that $p \mapsto \|\Lambda_p\|$ is integrable over M, then there exists a linear operator $\mathcal{A}_\Lambda : C_0^1(\mathbb{R}^3, \mathbb{R}^3) \to C_0^1(\mathbb{R}^3, \mathbb{R}^3)^*$ defined by

$$U_\Lambda(u) = \frac{1}{2} \left(\mathcal{A}_\Lambda u \mid u \right),$$

where $(\alpha \mid u)$ denotes the application of a linear form α to a vector u. Since $V \hookrightarrow C_0^2(\mathbb{R}^3, \mathbb{R}^3)$, $\mathcal{A}_\Lambda$ can also be seen as an operator from V to V^*. Letting $L : V \to V^*$ denote the duality operator on V such that $(Lv \mid w) = \langle v, w \rangle_V$, one can define the operator $\mathcal{L}_\Lambda : V \to V^*$ by $\mathcal{L}_\Lambda = \delta L + \mathcal{A}_\Lambda$ and then write

$$\frac{1}{2} \left(\mathcal{L}_\Lambda u \mid u \right) = \frac{\delta}{2} \|u\|_V^2 + U_\Lambda(u).$$

As a result, the solution of (2) is given by u such that $\mathcal{L}_\Lambda u = F \, dp$.

3.2   Layered Shapes and Tangential Isotropic Elasticity

Beside being elastic, we assume that M comes with a layered structure as illustrated in Fig. 1 and that the elastic behavior of M is "isotropic tangentially to layers." This is defined precisely below by specifying the particular form of Λ in this configuration. One motivating example for such a construction is that of the cerebral cortex and its organization along cortical layers and columns.

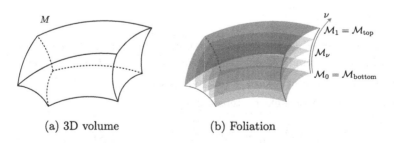

(a) 3D volume   (b) Foliation

Fig. 1. Shapes are assumed to have a layered foliation.

For the compact domain $M \subset \mathbb{R}^3$, we assume that there are two surfaces $\mathcal{M}_{\text{bottom}}$, the bottom layer, $\mathcal{M}_{\text{top}}$, the top layer, included in ∂M. Moreover, we assume that the top layer is obtained from a diffeomorphism $\Phi : [0, 1] \times \mathcal{M}_{\text{bottom}} \to M$, such that $\Phi(0) = id$ and $\Phi(1, \mathcal{M}_{\text{bottom}}) = \mathcal{M}_{\text{top}}$. We let S denote the vector field defined by $S(\Phi(\nu, p)) = \partial_\nu \Phi(\nu, p)$, and we assume that S is continuously differentiable.

Define intermediate layers as $\mathcal{M}_\nu = \Phi(\nu, \mathcal{M}_{\text{bottom}})$, so that $\{\mathcal{M}_\nu\}_{\nu \in [0,1]}$ forms a foliation of M to which S is *transversal*. Algorithms building such foliations of volumes have been introduced in brain imaging in order to estimate thickness, see e.g., [5,11,17]. Given such a transversal vector field S and layers $\{\mathcal{M}_\nu\}_{\nu \in [0,1]}$, we now define an elastic tensor Λ which is consistent with this layered structure and "isotropic on layers." For $p \in M$, let $\{T_1(p), T_2(p)\}$ be any orthonormal basis of $T_p \mathcal{M}_\nu$ (the tangent plane to $\mathcal{M}_\nu$ at p). We define the skew linear change of coordinates at p as the 3 by 3 matrix $C_p = \left[T_1(p) \; T_2(p) \; \frac{S(p)}{|S(p)|} \right]$. Now we consider Λ of the form $\Lambda_p(\varepsilon) = \bar{\Lambda}(C_p^\top \varepsilon C_p)$, where

$$\bar{\Lambda}(\xi) = \frac{1}{2} \mu_{\text{tan}} (\xi_{11} + \xi_{22})^2 + \frac{1}{2} \lambda_{\text{tan}} (\xi_{11}^2 + \xi_{22}^2 + 2\xi_{12}^2) + \frac{1}{2} \lambda_{\text{tsv}} \xi_{33}^2$$
$$+ \lambda_{\text{ang}} (\xi_{13}^2 + \xi_{23}^2). \tag{3}$$

$\bar{\Lambda}$ is independent of the position p if the parameters μ_{tan}, λ_{tan}, λ_{tsv}, and λ_{ang} are fixed, which is assumed in the following. Letting $\xi = C_p^\top \varepsilon C_p$, we note that ξ_{11}, ξ_{22} measure the stretches along tangential directions $T_1(p), T_2(p)$ respectively, and ξ_{33} measures the stretch along the transversal direction, which explains the particular form we take for $\bar{\Lambda}$.

Let $\{T_1'(p), T_2'(p)\}$ be another orthonormal basis of $T_p \mathcal{M}_\nu$. Then we have

$$C_p' = \left[T_1'(p) \; T_2'(p) \; \frac{S(p)}{|S(p)|} \right] = \left[T_1(p) \; T_2(p) \; \frac{S(p)}{|S(p)|} \right] \begin{bmatrix} G(p) & 0 \\ 0 & 1 \end{bmatrix},$$

where $G(p)$ is a 2 by 2 orthogonal matrix. It follows that $\text{tr}(\xi)$, $\text{tr}(\xi^2)$, and $\xi_{11}^2 + \xi_{22}^2 + 2\xi_{12}^2$ are invariant under this transformation, so Λ_p does not depend on the choice of orthonormal basis of $T_p \mathcal{M}_\nu$. Λ can thus be thought as "isotropic on $T_p \mathcal{M}_\nu$" for all $p \in M$.

Remark. One can make the same construction for a 2D domain M, with a foliation $\{\mathcal{M}_\nu\}_{\nu \in [0,1]}$ made of curves, instead of surfaces. One can then describe $T_p \mathcal{M}_\nu$ by a single unit vector $T(p)$ and define $C_p = \left[T(p) \; \frac{S(p)}{|S(p)|} \right]$, a 2 by 2 matrix. In this case, the elastic tensor simplifies to

$$\bar{\Lambda}(\xi) = \frac{1}{2} \lambda_{\text{tan}} \xi_{11}^2 + \frac{1}{2} \lambda_{\text{tsv}} \xi_{22}^2 + \lambda_{\text{ang}} \xi_{12}^2.$$

3.3   Boundary Condition

As the elastic energy is insensitive to the effect of rigid motions, one usually needs to specify certain boundary conditions in order to ensure that the displacement

u resulting from F is well-defined. Here, we impose boundary conditions on u such as, for example, $u = 0$ on some subset of M (typically the bottom layer $\mathcal{M}_{\text{bottom}}$). Going back to the case of cortical volumes, this is consistent with the typical assumption that grey matter atrophy is balanced mainly by expansion of the cerebrospinal fluid (CSF) region [12], which in our case corresponds the top layer of M. The bottom layer represents the gray/white matter boundary and should remain, in first approximation, relatively stable.

In the context of reproducing kernel Hilbert spaces, this boundary condition corresponds to replacing V by its closed subspace

$$V_0 = \{u \in V : u|_{\mathcal{M}_{\text{bottom}}} \equiv 0\},$$

which contains smooth vector fields that do not move $\mathcal{M}_{\text{bottom}}$. Under the constraint, the displacement response u to a force F is now given by

$$u = \underset{u' \in V_0}{\arg\min} \left(\frac{\delta}{2} \|u'\|_V^2 + \frac{1}{2} \left(\mathcal{A}_\Lambda u' \mid u' \right) - \left(F dp \mid u' \right) \right).$$

Because V_0 is a closed subspace of V, the induced norm makes it into an RKHS. Note that $\mathcal{A}_\Lambda$ can then be restricted as an operator from V_0 to V_0^*, so the same formal analysis applies, leading to an operator from V_0 to V_0^* that we still denote by $\mathcal{L}_\Lambda$.

3.4   Action of Diffeomorphisms

If the volume M is transformed by a diffeomorphism φ to $\varphi(M)$, the deformed layered structure can be specified by

$$\widetilde{\Phi} : [0,1] \times \varphi(\mathcal{M}_{\text{bottom}}) \to \varphi(M), \quad (\nu, \widetilde{p}) \mapsto \varphi(\Phi(\nu, \varphi^{-1}(\widetilde{p}))).$$

In particular, the transversal vector field S becomes $\widetilde{S}$ such that $\widetilde{S}(\varphi(p)) = D\varphi(p) S(p)$. Let $\widetilde{\mathcal{M}}_\nu = \varphi(\mathcal{M}_\nu)$ and $\{\widetilde{T}_1(\widetilde{p}), \widetilde{T}_2(\widetilde{p})\}$ be an orthonormal basis of $T_{\widetilde{p}}\widetilde{\mathcal{M}}_\nu$. One can then define a skew linear transformation $\widetilde{C} = \left[\widetilde{T}_1, \widetilde{T}_2, \frac{\widetilde{S}}{|\widetilde{S}|} \right]$ and the transformed elastic tensor Λ^φ given by $\Lambda_{\widetilde{p}}^\varphi(\varepsilon) = \bar{\Lambda}(\widetilde{C}_{\widetilde{p}}^\top \varepsilon \, \widetilde{C}_{\widetilde{p}})$ with $\bar{\Lambda}$ unchanged. This directly provides operators $\mathcal{A}_{\Lambda^\varphi}$ and $\mathcal{L}_{\Lambda^\varphi} = L_\varphi$.

3.5   Evolution Model for Large Deformation

We now have all required elements in place to operate the large deformation model of (1) for the particular operator L_φ defined in the previous sections. The connection between the small deformation model and the evolution equations can be made by considering that, at a given time t, the displacement δu resulting from an infinitesimal force density δF is given by $L_\varphi \, \delta u = \delta F \, dp$. The resulting velocity is $v = \frac{\delta u}{\delta t}$, and letting $j = \frac{\delta F}{\delta t}$ yields $L_\varphi v = j \, dp$.

The regularization in Eq. (2) ensures that $v(t)$ is smooth enough such that, under some conditions controlling the size of the control $j(t)$, it generates a flow of diffeomorphisms. This approach is inspired by methods in image and shape registration that use similar regularization, such as the large deformation diffeomorphic metric mapping algorithm [2, 20].

4   Numerical Results

In this section, we showcase several numerical experiments as applications of our model. In all these experiments, we consider a simplified case where j is of the form $j(t, \varphi(t, x)) = D\varphi(t, x) j_0(x)$, that is, j is completely specified by its value j_0 at time zero. We describe in the next section a low-dimensional model for j_0, specified by a small number of parameters. We then consider the inverse problem of estimating these parameters based on the observation of the original and deformed shapes.

4.1   Force Model

As a simple model of atrophy, we assume that j_0 is the gradient of a curved Gaussian which is defined by

$$g(p; c, h, \sigma_{\tan}, \sigma_{\text{tsv}}) = h \exp\left(-\frac{d_{\tan}^2(p, c)}{2\sigma_{\tan}^2} - \frac{d_{\text{tsv}}^2(p, c)}{2\sigma_{\text{tsv}}^2}\right),$$

where

$$d_{\tan}(p, c) = \frac{1}{2}\left(\text{length}(\gamma_\nu) + \text{length}(\gamma_{\nu'})\right)$$

and

$$d_{\text{tsv}}(p, c) = \frac{1}{2}\left(\text{length}(\alpha_c) + \text{length}(\alpha_p)\right).$$

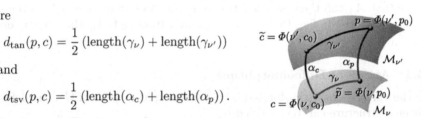

As shown in Fig. 2, γ_ν and $\gamma_{\nu'}$ are geodesics on $\mathcal{M}_\nu$ and $\mathcal{M}_{\nu'}$ joining c, $\tilde{p}$ and $\tilde{c}$, p respectively, and α_c and α_p are integral curves joining c, $\tilde{c}$ and $\tilde{p}$, p respectively.

Fig. 2. The four curves γ_ν, $\gamma_{\nu'}$, α_c, and α_p in the definition of curved Gaussian.

4.2   Inverse Problem

We assume that $\sigma_{\tan}$ and σ_{tsv} are known parameters and that the center of Gaussian c is constrained on the middle layer $\mathcal{M}_{\frac{1}{2}}$. This assumption is partially motivated by the case of Alzheimer's disease in which histological observations suggest that tau protein accumulation preceding the onset occurs in internal cortical layers [3]. Under all these assumptions, the control j, and, as a consequence, the entire evolution, is completely determined by the location of c and the height of peak h. Given an undeformed shape M_0 and a target shape M_1, the inverse problem can now be stated as minimizing

$$J(c, h) = d(\varphi(1, M_0), M_1) \text{ subject to } \begin{cases} \partial_t \varphi(t) = v(t, \varphi(t)) \\ \mathcal{L}_{\Lambda^{\varphi(t)}} v(t) = j(t) \, dp \\ j(t) = (D\varphi(t) j_0) \circ \varphi(t)^{-1} \\ j_0 = \nabla g \\ c \in \mathcal{M}_{\frac{1}{2}}, \; h > 0 \end{cases}.$$

We use in our experiments

$$d(M, M') = \text{volume}(M \triangle M') = \int_{\mathbb{R}^3} (\mathbb{1}_M - \mathbb{1}_{M'})^2 \, dx,$$

which computes the volume of non-overlapping region of two shapes. This does not require the layered structure of the target shape M_1 to be known since the information of layers is not included in the discrepancy measure d.

Since the constraint $c \in \mathcal{M}_{\frac{1}{2}}$ burdens an optimization algorithm, we consider the coordinate representation of J in c. In other words, let (U, ψ) be a local chart of $c \in \mathcal{M}_{\frac{1}{2}}$. We define $\widehat{J} : \psi(U) \times \mathbb{R}_+ \to \mathbb{R}$ by $\widehat{J}(\widehat{c}, h) = J(\psi^{-1}(\widehat{c}), h)$. Instead of minimizing the objective function J, we minimize equivalently its coordinate representation $\widehat{J}$. By moving the domain of the objective function from the curved space $\mathcal{M}_{\frac{1}{2}} \times \mathbb{R}_+$ to the Euclidean space, we can then utilize a derivative-free optimization algorithm with only box constraints.

Remark. Following the terminology introduced in [9], our model specifies a "deformation module." Such modules provide a deformation mechanism (here represented by j_0) that both drives the shape evolution and is advected by it (see [9] for more details). The free parameters for these modules are the control variables (c, h) with additional geometric parameters $\theta_f = (\sigma_{\text{tan}}, \sigma_{\text{tsv}})$ for the force and $\theta_e = (\delta, \mu_{\text{tan}}, \lambda_{\text{tan}}, \lambda_{\text{tsv}}, \lambda_{\text{ang}})$ for the elastic properties of the volume. One can also relate our construction to that provided in [8], in which our choice for j_0 provides what is called a "sink" in the referenced paper.

4.3 Discretization

Recall the layered structure $\mathcal{M}_\nu = \Phi(\nu, \mathcal{M}_{\text{bottom}})$ where Φ is a diffeomorphism. We use a discrete set of layers (hence letting ν be an integer) with consistent triangulations. More precisely, we assume that vertices in $\mathcal{M}_\nu$ are $(p_1^\nu, \ldots, p_N^\nu)$ (with N independent of ν) and faces (which are triples of integers in $\{1, \ldots, N\}$) are also independent of ν. We also define transverse edges between p_k^ν and $p_k^{\nu+1}$ and let $S(p_k^\nu) = p_k^{\nu+1} - p_k^\nu$ represent the discrete version of the transversal vector field (such a representation is provided, for example, by the algorithm introduced in [17]). This provides a decomposition of the volume M into triangular prisms. Without adding vertices, we further decompose the prisms into a consistent tetrahedral mesh using a method similar to that introduced in [15].

For the evaluation of the objective function, we use Dijkstra's algorithm to compute the length of geodesics needed to define the curved Gaussian map. Discretizing $j \, dp$ as a weighted sum of Dirac functions supported by vertices, one can show that the solution of $\mathcal{L}_{\Lambda^\varphi} v = j \, dp$ is uniquely specified by the values of v at vertices. This results in a large linear system (including the constraint that $v = 0$ on the bottom layer), which is solved using conjugate gradient.

4.4   Simulated Deformation

Figures 3b–d display the deformed shapes $\varphi(1, M_0)$ after applying the same j_0 to M_0, which is shown in Fig. 4a. The colors of landmarks from blue to red represent the values of curved Gaussian from low to high. The force parameters are $c = (0,0)$, $h = 3$, $(\sigma_{\text{tan}}, \sigma_{\text{tsv}}) = (0.1, 0.05)$. We used three different sets of elasticity parameters, that we call "tangent easy," "transverse easy," and "angle easy." All three simulations are done with V associated to a Matérn kernel of order three and width 0.01, $\delta = 10^{-6}$, $(\lambda_{\text{tan}}, \lambda_{\text{tsv}}, \lambda_{\text{ang}}) = (1,3,3)$, $(3,1,3)$ and $(3,3,1)$ in the tangent-easy, transverse-easy, and angle-easy cases, respectively.

The different elastic parameters produce different responses to the same j_0: in Fig. 3b, the landmarks mainly move tangentially; in Fig. 3c, they mainly move transversely; while in Fig. 3d, we see the least movement due to the constraint on the change of lengths between landmarks. Recall that in all cases the bottom layer is kept fixed by our model.

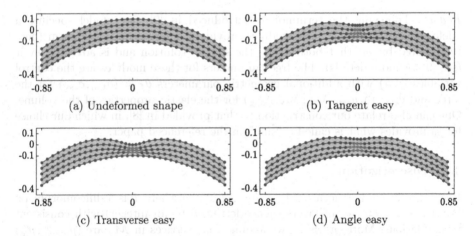

Fig. 3. Effects of different elastic parameters on shape deformations. (Color figure online)

4.5   Simulated Inverse Problem

We now present 2D and 3D simulated inverse problems, in which we first generated deformed targets using curved Gaussian, and then attempted to retrieve the parameters c and h. In our experiments, we used the `surrogateopt` function in Matlab to find a minimizer.

Two-dimensional results are shown in Figs. 4 and 5. We used a regular shape in Fig. 4, while Fig. 5 was created to resemble a lateral cut of cerebral cortex. The initial shapes are given in Figs. 4a and 5a, and the simulated targets are shown in Figs. 4b and 5b, in which the dashed curves indicate the positions of the initial shapes. (Recall that the inverse problem only uses the volume enclosed by the target shape, and that the pointwise displacement inside this volume is

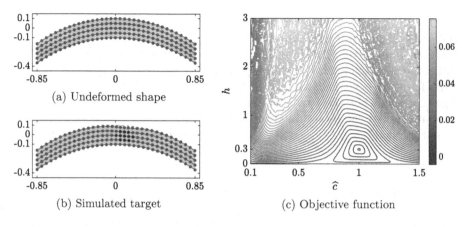

(a) Undeformed shape

(b) Simulated target

(c) Objective function

Fig. 4. 2D simulated experiment with the true solution at $(\widehat{c}, h) = (1, 0.3)$ (Color figure online)

considered as unobserved.) We used a very small force in both cases for the purpose of demonstration. Recall that c is restricted on the middle layer, and therefore only has one degree of freedom. We use the arc length from the leftmost landmark in both cases as the coordinate representation $\widehat{c}$. The level curves of the objective function $\widehat{J}(\widehat{c}, h)$ are presented in Figs. 4c and 5c, which demonstrate that the global minimizers are very close to the force parameters generating the targets, even though the deformation is small. Figure 5c also suggests that the optimization problem could be challenging for a highly curved shape. For example, if a gradient descent-like algorithm starts at $(\widehat{c}, h) = (1, 1)$, it would be difficult to locate the minimizer around $(2.2, 0.3)$.

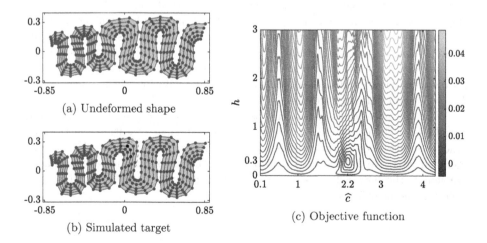

(a) Undeformed shape

(b) Simulated target

(c) Objective function

Fig. 5. 2D simulated experiment with the true solution at $(\widehat{c}, h) = (2.2, 0.3)$

Our 3D experiments are done on the initial shape shown in Fig. 6, which is a synthetic cerebral cortex. Table 1 compares the estimated parameters $(\widehat{c}, h)$ with the ground truth for a series of simulated deformations. Again, we see that the true solution for a simulated target can be accurately retrieved by our method.

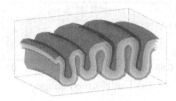

Fig. 6. A 3D synthetic folded shape.

Table 1. Estimated force parameters compared to their ground truth.

$(\widehat{c}_{\text{true}}, h_{\text{true}})$	(1.60, 0.50, 0.30)	(2.20, 0.50, 0.30)	(1.60, 0.65, 0.30)	(2.20, 0.65, 0.30)
$(\widehat{c}, h)$	(1.60, 0.50, 0.31)	(2.21, 0.49, 0.29)	(1.60, 0.65, 0.32)	(2.21, 0.65, 0.29)
$(\widehat{c}_{\text{true}}, h_{\text{true}})$	(1.60, 0.50, 0.35)	(2.20, 0.50, 0.35)	(1.60, 0.65, 0.35)	(2.20, 0.65, 0.35)
$(\widehat{c}, h)$	(1.60, 0.49, 0.36)	(2.20, 0.50, 0.34)	(1.60, 0.65, 0.36)	(2.21, 0.65, 0.34)

5   Discussion

We have presented in this paper a new model describing shape evolution where the control can be interpreted as the derivative of a body force density in the deforming volume. We also have provided a preliminary set of experiments, using simulated data, and based on derivative-free optimization methods.

Current and future work include applying this approach to medical imaging data, and in particular to the study of atrophy due to neurodegenerative diseases. This will require a more general definition of the force field than the single sink model we have used, and an interesting problem will be to maintain parametric identifiability for such models, by injecting suitable biological priors. Using more sophisticated optimization methods will require being able to explicitly compute gradients, which, even though formally feasible, represent serious numerical challenges, probably involving a solution of the linear system $L_\varphi v = j\, dp$ on parallel hardware.

We have not discussed in this paper any theoretical result on the well-posedness of the considered problems, such as sufficient conditions on the existence of solutions of (1), or consistency of the discretization schemes. We however included what we believe to be suitable smoothness assumptions regarding, in particular, the RKHS V. Such results are under investigation and will be published in the near future.

References

1. Amar, M.B., Goriely, A.: Growth and instability in elastic tissues. J. Mech. Phys. Solids **53**(10), 2284–2319 (2005)
2. Beg, M.F., Miller, M.I., Trouvé, A., Younes, L.: Computing large deformation metric mappings via geodesic flows of diffeomorphisms. Int. J. Comput. Vis. **61**(2), 139–157 (2005)
3. Braak, H., Braak, E.: Neuropathological stageing of Alzheimer-related changes. Acta Neuropathol. **82**(4), 239–259 (1991)
4. Ciarlet, P.G.: Three-Dimensional Elasticity, vol. 20. Elsevier, North Holland (1988)
5. Das, S.R., Avants, B.B., Grossman, M., Gee, J.C.: Registration based cortical thickness measurement. Neuroimage **45**(3), 867–879 (2009)
6. DiCarlo, A., Quiligotti, S.: Growth and balance. Mech. Res. Commun. **29**(6), 449–456 (2002)
7. Durrleman, S., Pennec, X., Trouvé, A., Braga, J., Gerig, G., Ayache, N.: Toward a comprehensive framework for the spatiotemporal statistical analysis of longitudinal shape data. Int. J. Comput. Vis. **103**(1), 22–59 (2013)
8. Grenander, U., Srivastava, A., Saini, S.: A pattern-theoretic characterization of biological growth. IEEE Trans. Med. Imaging **26**(5), 648–659 (2007)
9. Gris, B., Durrleman, S., Trouvé, A.: A sub-riemannian modular approach for diffeomorphic deformations. In: Nielsen, F., Barbaresco, F. (eds.) GSI 2015. LNCS, vol. 9389, pp. 39–47. Springer, Cham (2015). https://doi.org/10.1007/978-3-319-25040-3_5
10. Gurtin, M.E.: The linear theory of elasticity. In: Truesdell, C. (ed.) Linear Theories of Elasticity and Thermoelasticity, pp. 1–295. Springer, Heidelberg (1973). https://doi.org/10.1007/978-3-662-39776-3_1
11. Jones, S.E., Buchbinder, B.R., Aharon, I.: Three-dimensional mapping of cortical thickness using Laplace's equation. Hum. Brain Mapp. **11**(1), 12–32 (2000)
12. Khanal, B., Lorenzi, M., Ayache, N., Pennec, X.: A biophysical model of brain deformation to simulate and analyze longitudinal MRIs of patients with Alzheimer's disease. NeuroImage **134**, 35–52 (2016)
13. Lubarda, V.A., Hoger, A.: On the mechanics of solids with a growing mass. Int. J. Solids Struct. **39**(18), 4627–4664 (2002)
14. Marsden, J.E., Hughes, T.J.: Mathematical Foundations of Elasticity. Courier Corporation, North Chelmsford (1994)
15. Porumbescu, S.D., Budge, B., Feng, L., Joy, K.I.: Shell maps. ACM Trans. Graph. (TOG) **24**(3), 626–633 (2005)
16. Qiu, A., Albert, M., Younes, L., Miller, M.I.: Time sequence diffeomorphic metric mapping and parallel transport track time-dependent shape changes. NeuroImage **45**(1), S51–S60 (2009)
17. Ratnanather, J.T., Arguillère, S., Kutten, K.S., Hubka, P., Kral, A., Younes, L.: 3D normal coordinate systems for cortical areas. arXiv preprint arXiv:1806.11169 (2018)
18. Rodriguez, E.K., Hoger, A., McCulloch, A.D.: Stress-dependent finite growth in soft elastic tissues. J. Biomech. **27**(4), 455–467 (1994)
19. Tallinen, T., Chung, J.Y., Rousseau, F., Girard, N., Lefèvre, J., Mahadevan, L.: On the growth and form of cortical convolutions. Nat. Phys. **12**(6), 588 (2016)
20. Younes, L.: Shapes and Diffeomorphisms. AMS, vol. 171. Springer, Heidelberg (2010). https://doi.org/10.1007/978-3-642-12055-8

Analyzing Mild Cognitive Impairment Progression via Multi-view Structural Learning

Li Wang[1], Paul M. Thompson[2], and Dajiang Zhu[1]([✉])

[1] University of Texas at Arlington, Arlington, TX 76019, USA
dajiang.zhu@uta.edu
[2] University of Southern California, Los Angeles, CA 90033, USA

Abstract. Alzheimer's disease (AD), and its precursor, mild cognitive impairment (MCI), are progressive neurodegenerative conditions with a preclinical period that can last a decade or more. A variety of predictive models and algorithms have been developed to classify different clinical groups (e.g., elderly normal versus MCI) or predict conversion (e.g., from MCI to AD) based on longitudinal neuroimaging or other biomarker datasets. Even so, it is still unknown how brain structural and functional alterations jointly contribute to the MCI/AD progression process. Here we introduce a novel supervised multi-view structure learning framework to model the latent patterns of MCI/AD progression. Specifically, we learned and optimized a common data representation based on both structural and functional connectome data. Instead of determining patterns of abnormal structural and functional connectivity and their overlap, we create and analyze a common structure (graph) that can describe the entire process of disease progression. Different structural and functional connectome features contribute to this common structure simultaneously. The learned common structure reflects "a progression path" of MCI: it starts from elderly normal, proceeds through significant memory concern (SMC), early MCI and eventually ends with late MCI. As the common structure is learned from different structural and functional connectome features, it suggests that the connectome alterations related to MCI progression might happen in different structural and functional regions simultaneously.

Keywords: Alzheimer's disease · ADNI · Multi-view structure learning

1 Introduction

Alzheimer's disease (AD) is the only disorder in the top 10 causes of death in the United States that cannot be prevented, cured, or even slowed [1]. Unlike other brain diseases, the greatest known risk factor of AD is increasing age. AD is a progressive neurodegenerative disorder with a long preclinical period: around 50% of people with mild cognitive impairment (MCI) will convert to AD eventually and almost all AD patients experience the stage of MCI before developing AD. Therefore, it is extremely critical to establish a set of stable and objective biomarkers to examine how MCI patients progress. Measures of brain Aβ deposition (CSF Aβ42 and amyloid PET [2])

© Springer Nature Switzerland AG 2019
A. C. S. Chung et al. (Eds.): IPMI 2019, LNCS 11492, pp. 656–668, 2019.
https://doi.org/10.1007/978-3-030-20351-1_51

as well as markers of neurodegeneration (CSF tau [3]) or glucose metabolism (FDG PET [4]) are all widely-used AD biomarkers [5], but they can be invasive, costly and may not be readily available. Thus, further development of non-invasive markers from other imaging modalities - such as MRI - is of great interest. For example, structural MRI (T1-weighted and T2/FLAIR), diffusion imaging with tensor or more advanced models (dMRI) and resting state fMRI (rs-fMRI), are all powerful non-invasive neuroimaging techniques, poised to play an increasingly important role in the development of early imaging markers for MCI progression prediction.

There have been a variety of approaches proposed for early detection of AD or MCI and predicting the risk of disease progression, such as voxel-based morphometry (VBM) [6], the boundary shift integral (BSI) [7], tensor-based morphometry (TBM) [8], tract-based spatial statistics (TBSS for dMRI) [9] and multivariate analysis/machine learning-based algorithms [10]. Recently, deep learning methods such as convolution neural networks (CNN) [11] have also been proposed for classification. All these studies have shown that though the disease biomarkers might be most pronounced initially in specific brain regions, widespread alterations ensue, including changes in both structural and functional brain connectivity. Despite the tremendous advancements made by these computational methods, all of them have focused on classification, prediction or identification of statistical differences among different diagnostic groups (e.g., normal controls versus AD or MCI groups) or between clinically-defined stages of the disease (longitudinal studies). Given the continuous progression process of MCI, however, the intrinsic relations among different clinical groups and stages have been underexamined. As a consequence, we do not yet have an effective way to model the entire trajectory of MCI progression and how brain structural and functional alterations jointly contribute to the whole process.

In this work, we introduced a novel supervised multi-view structure learning framework to explore the latent patterns of MCI progression. Figure 1 illustrates the major steps: each hemisphere is labeled with 34 ROIs (regions of interest) using the Desikan-Killiany atlas [12]. Both structural and functional connectomes were reconstructed as the inputs for a multi-view structure learning algorithm. With domain knowledge (e.g., late MCI would be expected to be more similar to early MCI than to normal controls), we are able to learn a common structure that embeds the data and maximizes the differences among different clinical groups. Our method can successfully learn a common structure reflecting a "progression path" of MCI from both the structural and functional connectome: it starts from normal controls, proceeds through SMC (significant memory concern), EMCI (early MCI) and eventually ends with LMCI (late MCI). In comparison with existing methods, we did not focus on solving the group-wise difference and simple classification/prediction problem. Instead, we strive to learn a common structure representation (a graph) to describe the relations among multiple clinical groups. The common structure was learned and optimized by alternately training the model within a different space (structural view and functional view). Because different brain structural and functional connectivity may jointly contribute to the "progression path", our results suggest that the connectome alterations related to MCI progression might happen in different structural and functional regions simultaneously.

658   L. Wang et al.

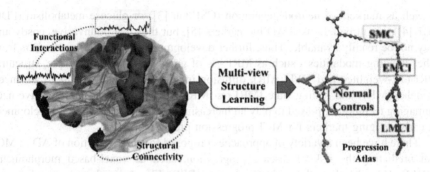

Fig. 1. Left: we adopted the Desikan-Killiany atlas [12] and each hemisphere was labeled with 34 ROIs. With linear registration, rsfMRI and diffusion tensor imaging (DTI) data were aligned within the same space. Both the structural and functional connectome were reconstructed as the inputs for multi-view structural learning. Middle: we developed a multi-view structure learning method to model and analyze the entire MCI progression process. Right: the learned common structure representation. Each color bubble represents the embedding point of a subject and the overall structure reflects a "progression path" of MCI. (Color figure online)

2 Method

2.1 Dataset

The dataset analyzed in this work was obtained from the Alzheimer's Disease Neuroimaging Initiative (ADNI3) [13]. Originally, we began with data from a total of 473 participants. Only 160 subjects (94 NC, 13 SMC, 24 EMCI and 29 LMCI participants) had data from all three MRI modalities including a T1-weighted volumetric image, DTI and rsfMRI at the time we conducted this analysis. The T1-weighted images had 1.0 mm isotropic voxels, TE = 2.98 ms, and TR = 2.3 s. For the DTI data, the number of gradient directions was 31 (18 subjects) and 55 (142 subjects), with 2.0 mm isotropic voxels, TE = 56 ms, TR = 7.2 ms. For rs-fMRI data, the range of image resolutions in X and Y dimensions was from 2.3 mm to 3.3 mm. The slice thickness was 3.31 mm, TE = 30 ms and TR ranged from 2.2 s to 3.1 s. There were 197 volumes for each participant.

Standard preprocessing procedures were applied including scalp removal and motion correction. For rsfMRI, we also applied spatial smoothing, temporal pre-whitening, slice time correction, global drift removal and band pass filtering (0.01–0.1 Hz). For DTI, we applied eddy current correction and fiber tracking (deterministic) via MedINRIA [14]. Then we registered both T1-weighted and rsfMRI images to the DTI space using FLIRT [15] and adopted the Desikan-Killiany atlas [12] for ROI labeling [16].

2.2 Generation of Structural and Functional Connectomes

By adopting the Desikan-Killiany atlas, each hemisphere was labeled with 34 ROIs. The brain's connectome can be represented using a graph, comprising a set of nodes

(ROIs) and the connecting edges (connectivity). In the structural connectome, the edge weight can be defined as the ratio of the number of DTI derived fibers (streamlines) connecting two ROIs to the total number of fibers. For the functional connectome, the edge is defined via the blood oxygen level dependent (BOLD) contrast signal correlation [17]. Thus, both structural and functional connectome can be represented as a 68×68 matrix. For the same pair of ROIs, it has two measures corresponding to structural and functional connectivity, respectively.

2.3 Relation Modeling Using Prior Knowledge

Traditional LDA

Linear discriminant analysis (LDA) [18] formulates the criterion of class separability using the scatter of data points computed in a projected space. Let $\{(x_i, y_i)\}_{i=1}^n$ be the given data, where $y_i \in \{1, 2, \cdots, c\}$ is the class of the ith data point $x_i \in \mathbb{R}^d$ in a d-dimensional space, c is the number of classes, and n is the number of data points. Denote $z_i \in \mathbb{R}^p$ as the projected point of x_i in a p-dimensional space by using a linear transformation $z = W^T x$, where the linear projection matrix is $W \in \mathbb{R}^{d \times p}$. Let $\delta(a, b)$ denote an indicator function such that $\delta(a, b) = 1$ if $a = b$ and $\delta(a, b) = 0$ otherwise. Accordingly, the number of data points of the rth class is $n_r = \sum_{i=1}^n \delta(r, y_i)$. In the projected space, we have the following statistics: the mean of all data points $\bar{z} = \frac{1}{n} \sum_{i=1}^n z_i$ and the mean of the rth class $\bar{z}_r = \frac{1}{n_r} \sum_{i=1}^n \delta(r, y_i) z_i$.

According to the definition of LDA, the *within-class scatter* is defined based on the scatter of samples belonging to the same class given by

$$J_w(W) = \sum_{i=1}^n \sum_{r=1}^c \delta(r, y_i) \|z_i - \bar{z}_r\|^2, \tag{1}$$

which is the sum of pairwise distances between any point and the mean of points having the same class as the given point. And, the *between-class scatter* is defined based on the sum of pairwise distances between the mean $\bar{z}_r, \forall r$, of the data points of the same class and the mean $\bar{z}$ of the data given by

$$J_b(W) = \sum_{i=1}^n \sum_{r=1}^c \delta(r, y_i) \|\bar{z}_r - \bar{z}\|^2, \tag{2}$$

By reformulating the above two objective functions in the form of matrices, we have

$$J_w(W) = \text{trace}(W^T S_w W), \quad J_b(W) = \text{trace}(W^T S_b W),$$

where the *within-class scatter* matrix S_w and the *between-class scatter* matrix S_b are respectively defined as

$$S_w = \sum_{i=1}^{n} \sum_{r=1}^{c} \delta(r, y_i)(x_i - \bar{x}_r)(x_i - \bar{x}_r)^T, \tag{3}$$

$$S_b = \sum_{r=1}^{c} n_r(\bar{x}_r - \bar{x})(\bar{x}_r - \bar{x})^T. \tag{4}$$

In order to obtain an optimal W for class separability, LDA aims to solve the following optimization problem

$$\max_W \text{trace}(W^T S_b W) : \text{s.t. } W^T S_w W = I, \tag{5}$$

which is solved by the generalized eigen-decomposition method.

Reweighting the Class Dependency Using Prior Information

LDA is proposed for class separability, so that projected points from different classes should be as distant as possible. In this work, to discover the relationships among the data across all classes, we further explore the *between-class scatter* objective: We propose a new objective function based on the *between-class scatter* by incorporating the relationships of class means in the projected space as the prior information.

Based on the evidence $\bar{z} = \frac{1}{n} \sum_{r=1}^{c} n_r \bar{z}_r$, we can rewrite Eq. (2) in terms of the sample size and the class means given by

$$J_b(W) = \frac{1}{2} \sum_{r=1}^{c} \sum_{r'=1}^{c} \frac{n_r n_{r'}}{n} \| \bar{z}_r - \bar{z}_{r'} \|^2 . \tag{6}$$

Maximizing Eq. (6) implies that LDA prefers the large pairwise distance between centers of two classes in the projected space if $n_r n_{r'}$ is large. This further verifies the class separability assumption used in LDA. Let $A \in \mathbb{R}^{c \times c}$ with the (r, r') th entry $A_{r,r'} = \frac{n_r n_{r'}}{n}$ and $\bar{Z} = [\bar{z}_1, \cdots, \bar{z}_c] \in \mathbb{R}^{p \times c}$. With simple matrix manipulations, we can reformulate $J_b(W)$ in a matrix form as

$$J_b(W) = \text{trace}\left(\bar{Z} \left(\text{diag}(A1) - A\right) \bar{Z}^T\right). \tag{7}$$

The equality (7) holds due to the property of the graph Laplacian matrix over the matrix A as the matrix representation of a weighted graph [19] (e.g., the adjacency matrix of a graph). As a result, LDA simply defines the similarity $A_{r,r'}$ between means of two classes, $\bar{z}_r$ and $\bar{z}_{r'}$ using only the cluster sizes.

In this work, we introduce two sources of prior knowledge into the traditional LDA model. First, the progression of MCI and AD is a continuous process [20]. Thus, an evolutionary tree structure is a good representation of the path of MCI development by learning information from multiple clinical groups. However, LDA cannot be used to capture this relationship over classes since A does not encode any meaningful distance/similarity information between classes. To address this limitation, we introduce C as a similarity matrix for encoding the similarities among classes and $L_C = \text{diag}(C1) - C$ as the graph Laplacian matrix over C. We formulate a new objective function in order to capture the class relationships in the data, given by

$$J_b(W) = \text{trace}\left(W^T \bar{X} L_C \bar{X}^T W\right), \tag{8}$$

where $\bar{X} = [\bar{x}_1, \cdots, \bar{x}_c] \in \mathbb{R}^{d \times c}$. Now, the objective function (8) encodes the relationship between classes, which is different from (7) since the prior information between class means is used as the prior for the class similarities not the cluster sizes. In order to preserve the relationships between classes in the projected space, we propose to solve the following optimization problem

$$\min_W \text{trace}\left(W^T(S_w + \alpha \bar{X} L_C \bar{X}^T)W\right) : \text{s.t. } W^T W = I, \tag{9}$$

where $\alpha > 0$ is the tradeoff parameter and I is the identity matrix of size p × p. It is worth noting that S_b is replaced by $\bar{X} L_C \bar{X}^T$ to capture the class relationships, instead of being considered as constraints in (5). This is because minimizing (8) can reach the goal that two class means $\bar{x}_r$ and $\bar{x}_{r'}$ are close if they have high similarity $C_{r,r'}, \forall r, r'$. In addition, this solves the degeneration problem faced by LDA using the generalized eigen-decomposition solver due to the singularity of matrix S_w when the number of features is larger than the number of data points.

The second source of prior knowledge is that data at different stages of MCI/AD progression possess certain ordering information [21]. For example, EMCI is believed to be a clinical stage between SMC and LMCI. To capture this order dependency information, we can define the following similarity matrix C as

$$C_{r,r'} = \begin{cases} 1, & r = r' + 1 \text{ or } r' + 1 = r \\ 0, & \text{otherwise.} \end{cases}$$

The proposed problem (9) can readily capture the sequential dependency among classes by incorporating the above similarity matrix. Here, problem (9) has an analytical solution, that is, the optimal W consists of eigen-vectors corresponding to the top p smallest eigen-values of matrix $S_w + \alpha \bar{X} L_C \bar{X}^T$.

2.4 Learning Latent Graph Structures from Data

In Sect. 2.3, we develop a novel supervised relation model by leveraging pairwise similarity among classes using external prior information. However, the graph structure over all projected points is still unknown. Here, we propose a novel method to learn a latent structure over the embedded points in the projected space so that embedded points are separated as much as possible and the relationships between classes can still be preserved.

Here, we adopt the reversed graph embedding strategy [22] to uncover graph structure from the high-dimensional data. The basic idea of the reversed graph embedding is to assume that a graph structure resides in a low-dimensional space, and the vertices of the graph are the points in the space. A function f projecting the observed data into a low-dimensional point is learned by jointly minimizing the following objective function with respect to f and the graph $G = \left[g_{i,j} \right] \in R^{n \times n}$ with the $(i, j)^{th}$ entry as $g_{i,j}$:

$$\min_{f, G} \sum_{i=1}^{n} \sum_{j=1}^{n} g_{i,j} \| f(x_i) - f(x_j) \|^2.$$

In general, the reversed graph embedding approach can efficiently learn the graph structure by introducing the regularization term. In addition, it can preserve the relative distance between two embedded points in the low dimensional space as the distance becomes small if the similarity of their corresponding points in the observed space is high. Let $M = S_w + \alpha \bar{X} L_C \bar{X}^T$. By combining (9) and the reversed graph embedding, we propose the following joint optimization problem with respect to the projection matrix W and the graph G over all the projected points given by

$$\min_{W, G} \operatorname{trace}\left(W^T M W \right) + \frac{\gamma}{2} \sum_{i=1}^{n} \sum_{j=1}^{n} g_{i,j} \| W^T (x_i - x_j) \|^2$$
$$\text{s.t. } W^T W = I, \ G = \left[g_{i,j} \right] \in G_g, \tag{10}$$

where $\gamma > 0$ is a regularization parameter for controlling the graph structure learned from data, $g_{i,j}$ is the $(i, j)^{th}$ entry of G, and G_g is the set of specific graphs. For example, a spanning tree over n points can be applied. With simple matrix manipulations, we can reformulate the above problem as

$$\min_{W, G} \operatorname{trace}\left(W^T \left(M + \gamma X (\operatorname{diag}(G1) - G) X^T \right) W \right)$$
$$\text{s.t. } W^T W = I, \ G = \left[g_{i,j} \right] \in G_g. \tag{11}$$

Alternating structure optimization can be used to solve problem (11): we first partition variables into two groups W and G, and then solve each subproblem iteratively until convergence is achieved. Specifically, given G, the analytical solution W can be obtained by solving (11) with respect to W, which is similar to solving problem (9) but the eigen-decomposition is applied to matrix $M + \gamma X (\operatorname{diag}(G1) - G) X$. Given W, problem (11) with respect to G can be rewritten as the problem of learning the graph structure given the pairwise distance defined by the given projection matrix W:

$$\min_{G \in G_g} \sum_{i=1}^{n} \sum_{j=1}^{n} g_{i,j} \| W^T (x_i - x_j) \|^2. \tag{12}$$

2.5   Multi-view Structure Learning

In this work, each pair of ROIs has both structural and functional connectivity that characterize different aspects of the edge. The motivation to conduct multi-view structure learning is to investigate if a common structure (a graph) can be learned by a set of structural and functional connectivity together. In other words, structural and functional connectomes might change in different ways as MCI progresses, but they jointly contribute to the learned progression structure in some way.

Model (10) is built on a single view of data for learning the latent graph structure. Therefore, we need to extend it accordingly: Let $\{ (x_i^{(1)}, \cdots, x_i^{(v)}, y_i) \}_{i=1}^n$ be the given data with v views, where $x_i^{(u)} \in \mathbb{R}^{d_u}$ is denoted as the uth view with the dimension of d_u for $u = 1, \cdots, v$. Our goal is to learn a unified structure G from v views even though they might have different latent spaces and associated latent points as the vertexes of the graph G. Based on this criterion, we propose to solve the following problem:

$$\min_{\{W^{(u)}\}_{u=1}^v, G} \sum_{u=1}^v \text{trace}\left(W^{(u)^T} M^{(u)} W^{(u)} \right) + \frac{\gamma}{2} \sum_{i=1}^n \sum_{j=1}^n g_{i,j} \left\| W^{(u)^T} \left(x_i^{(u)} - x_j^{(u)} \right) \right\|^2 \tag{13}$$
$$\text{s.t. } W^{(u)^T} W^{(u)} = I, \forall u, G \in G_g,$$

where $W^{(u)} \in \mathbb{R}^{d_u \times p}$ be the projection matrix for the uth view of data. Following the same derivations in Sects. 2.3–2.4, we have the following definitions of various matrices for the uth view as:

$$M^{(u)} = S_w^{(u)} + \alpha \bar{X}^{(u)} L_C \bar{X}^{(u)^T},$$
$$S_w^{(u)} = \sum_{i=1}^n \sum_{r=1}^c \delta(r, y_i) \left(x_i^{(u)} - \bar{x}_r^{(u)} \right) \left(x_i^{(u)} - \bar{x}_r^{(u)} \right)^T,$$
$$\bar{X}^{(u)} = \left[\frac{1}{n_1} \sum_{i=1}^n \delta(y_i, 1) x_i^{(u)}, \cdots, \frac{1}{n_c} \sum_{i=1}^n \delta(y_i, c) x_i^{(u)} \right]$$

Problem (13) can also be solved by alternating structure optimization. It is worth noting that given G, subproblems with respect to $W^{(u)}$ are decoupled, that is, for each u, the subproblem can be rewritten as

$$\min_{W^{(u)}} \text{trace}\left(W^{(u)^T} (M^{(u)} + \gamma \left(X^{(u)} (\text{diag}(G1) - G) X^{(u)^T} \right)) W^{(u)} \right) \tag{14}$$
$$\text{s.t. } W^{(u)^T} W^{(u)} = I.$$

As a result, problem (14) is similar to the optimization problem (11) for learning embedded points by using the uth view only.

3 Result

3.1 Progression Atlas for MCI

Given the structural and functional connectome (Sect. 2.2), we conducted multi-view structure learning proposed in Sects. 2.3–2.5. As mentioned before, instead of focusing on the distance/similarity between each pair of classes, here we tried to explore a common structure that can describe the latent relations among multiple clinical groups simultaneously: given the label information and domain knowledge including the preference of class-class similarity and order information, every sample can be projected onto the learned structure and their relative locations encode the potential relations among different clinical groups. Figure 2 shows the learned common structure representation in 3D space. Different colors represent different clinical groups including NC (*green*), SMC (*yellow*), EMCI (*orange*) and LMCI (*pink*). Each colored bubble represents an individual subject. The learned structure displays a virtual path of MCI progression: it starts from normal controls (*green*), goes through SMC (*yellow*), EMCI (*orange*) and eventually ends with LMCI (*pink*). Hence, we call it a "progression atlas" of MCI. We note that the "progression atlas" was learned by cross-sectional data from different clinical diagnostic groups instead of multiple clinical stages of the same group of participants (as could be defined from longitudinal data, if enough data were available).

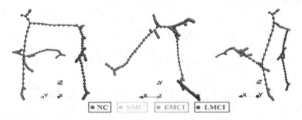

Fig. 2. The learned common structure from multiple clinical groups including NC, SMC, EMCI and LMCI. (Color figure online)

In this work, our multi-view structure learning problem was formulated as learning a unified structure G (not consistent structural and functional connectivity) from v views (e.g., from structural or functional view) that might possess different latent spaces. That is, for a specific ROI pair, its structural and functional connectivity might contribute to this learned common structure in a different way. We ordered structural and functional connectivity separately according to their contribution (via Laplacian score) to the learned structure. Figure 3 shows the top 5, 10 and 20 connectivity features that have the most contribution. In each sub-figure, the first row shows the brain regions (ROIs) involved in the connectivity. The second row shows the connectivity and the corresponding regions are represented as bubbles. The size of bubble indicates how many connectivity it involves. For example, the region highlighted with

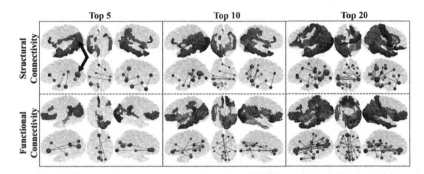

Fig. 3. Top connectivity that contribute most to the learned common structure. In each sub-figure, the top and bottom rows display the involved brain regions and connectivity, respectively. The size of bubble indicates how many connectivity it involves.

the black arrow is the right inferior parietal [12] region, and its bubble is larger because it is involved in two connectivity.

There are two interesting observations: first, the top structural connectivity tend to be the ones connecting different hemispheres, whereas the top functional connectivity incline to related different lobes, e.g. frontal and occipital lobes. Second, considering the same number of connectivity that have the most contribution to the learned structure, there are more brain regions involved in functional connectivity than structural ones. Even though there are more overlaps of structural and functional connectivity if we consider more contributors, all of these suggest that during MCI progression, brain structural and functional changes might show a complicated coupled pattern.

3.2 Reproducibility of Multi-view Structure Learning

In the proposed method, there are two parameters that can influence the multi-view structure learning results. The first is α - a tradeoff parameter to leverage the effects of the similarity within-class and between classes. Note that the similarity between classes was replaced by the external knowledge (Eq. 9) that encodes the preference of different clinical groups. That is, larger α means more weight is given to the external knowledge. The second parameter, γ, is a regularization parameter controlling the graph structure learned from data. Similar to α, γ is also a tradeoff parameter to ensure both the projection accuracy and the smoothness of the learned structure. Figure 4 shows the learned structures under different settings of α/γ and the results of convergence are also shown above as well. In general, given a wide range of α and γ, our method can always successfully learn a meaningful structure displaying a progression path of MCI. The overall structures are very consistent, in that NC and LMCI are located at the two ends and SMC, EMCI are in the middle. An interesting point is that though the shape of each clinical group might change, the patterns of the branches tend to be stable. That suggests the derived structure embedded similarity metric has the potential to be a reliable biomarker for monitoring the entire MCI progression process.

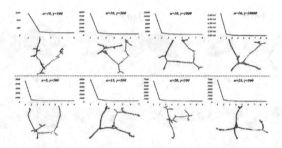

Fig. 4. Multi-view structure learning results under different settings of α and γ. Convergence results are also displayed within each sub-figure. X and Y axis represent the number of iterations and optimization loss, respectively.

3.3   Multi-view Structure Learning with Two Groups

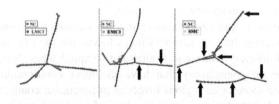

Fig. 5. Multi-view structure learning results based on input data from only two groups.

We showed how the learned structure from our method can reflect MCI progression process based on data from multiple clinical groups. Next, we are consider the case of learning using only two clinical groups, such as NC and one other diagnostic group, and the results are shown in Fig. 5. When we use input data from NC and LMCI groups only, the learned structure displayed a clearly separable pattern: NC is located at one end with five branches, and LMCI is at the other end. For NC and EMCI, the overall pattern of the structure is still separable, but we can see two mixing points - which means that two NC subjects were projected to the locations close to EMCI subjects. When the learning was conducted between NC and SMC, the two clinical groups are totally mixed together on the learned structure. There are no obvious patterns for either of the two groups; the black arrows highlight the locations of SMC subjects. Since the number of SMC is less than NC, more balanced samples might improve these results. However, given the similar number of LMCI, EMCI individuals, and their separable structures, our results suggest that NC and SMC might possess high similarity as two specific clinical groups.

4   Discussion

In this work, we aim to examine the entire MCI progression process by developing a multi-view structure learning method to explore the latent structure from both brain structural and functional connectomes. To effectively model the relations among different clinical groups, we introduce external knowledge and alternately conduct a structure learning approach in brain structural and functional space. The derived common structure is called an "MCI progression atlas" as it reflects a virtual path of MCI progression. Instead of pursuing the connectivity displaying both structural and functional alterations, our goal is to learn a unified graph representing MCI progression. This common graph can be derived from different structural and functional connectivity. Our results also show that the involved connectivity with the most contribution are not necessarily consistent in the brain structural and functional perspectives. On the other hand, compared to the 'single-view' method that considers structural and functional connectome separately, our multi-view approach did have higher overlaps. Table 1 summarizes the number of consistent connectivity in structural and functional domain when considering top N connectivity contributing to the learned structure.

Table 1. Comparison of the number of consistent connectivity when performing structure learning using single-view versus multi-view approaches.

Top N connectivity (having most contribution)	Single-view	Multi-view
100	4	**8**
200	10	**23**
300	37	**44**
400	67	**84**
500	108	**115**

References

1. Alzheimer's Association: Alzheimer's facts and figures report. Alzheimer's Association. https://www.alz.org/alzheimers-dementia/facts-figures
2. Villemagne, V.L., et al.: Longitudinal assessment of Aβ and cognition in aging and Alzheimer disease. Ann. Neurol. **69**, 181–192 (2011)
3. Shaw, L.M., et al.: Alzheimer's disease neuroimaging initiative: cerebrospinal fluid biomarker signature in Alzheimer's disease neuroimaging initiative subjects. Ann. Neurol. **65**, 403–413 (2009)
4. Jagust, W.J., et al.: Alzheimer's disease neuroimaging initiative: the Alzheimer's disease neuroimaging initiative positron emission tomography core. Alzheimers. Dement. **6**, 221–229 (2010)
5. Jack, C.R., et al.: Tracking pathophysiological processes in Alzheimer's disease: an updated hypothetical model of dynamic biomarkers. Lancet Neurol. **12**, 207–216 (2013)

6. Ashburner, J., Friston, K.J.: Voxel-based morphometry—the methods. Neuroimage **11**, 805–821 (2000)
7. Jack, C.R., et al.: Comparison of different MRI brain atrophy rate measures with clinical disease progression in AD. Neurology **62**, 591–600 (2004)
8. Thompson, P.M., Apostolova, L.G.: Computational anatomical methods as applied to ageing and dementia. Br. J. Radiol. **80**, S78–S91 (2007)
9. Smith, S.M., et al.: Tract-based spatial statistics: voxelwise analysis of multi-subject diffusion data. Neuroimage **31**, 1487–1505 (2006)
10. Vemuri, P., et al.: Alzheimer's disease diagnosis in individual subjects using structural MR images: validation studies. Neuroimage **39**, 1186–1197 (2008)
11. Liu, M., Cheng, D., Wang, K., Wang, Y.: Multi-modality cascaded convolutional neural networks for Alzheimer's disease diagnosis. Neuroinformatics **16**, 295–308 (2018)
12. Desikan, R.S., et al.: An automated labeling system for subdividing the human cerebral cortex on MRI scans into gyral based regions of interest. Neuroimage **31**, 968–980 (2006)
13. ADNI: Alzheimer's Disease Neuroimaging Initiative. http://adni.loni.usc.edu/
14. Medinria. https://med.inria.fr/
15. Jenkinson, M., Bannister, P., Brady, M., Smith, S.: Improved optimization for the robust and accurate linear registration and motion correction of brain images. Neuroimage **17**, 825–841 (2002)
16. FreeSurfer. https://surfer.nmr.mgh.harvard.edu/
17. Brier, M.R., et al.: Functional connectivity and graph theory in preclinical Alzheimer's disease. Neurobiol. Aging **35**, 757–768 (2014)
18. Fukunaga, K.: Introduction to Statistical Pattern Recognition. Academic Press, San Diego (1990)
19. Chung, F.: Spectral Graph Theory. Published for the Conference Board of the Mathematical Sciences by the American Mathematical Society (1996)
20. Corrada, M.M., Brookmeyer, R., Paganini-Hill, A., Berlau, D., Kawas, C.H.: Dementia incidence continues to increase with age in the oldest old: The 90+ study. Ann. Neurol. **67**, 114–121 (2010)
21. Swinford, C.G., Risacher, S.L., Charil, A., Schwarz, A.J., Saykin, A.J.: Memory concerns in the early Alzheimer's disease prodrome: regional association with tau deposition. Alzheimer's Dement. Diagn. Assess Dis. Monit. **10**, 322–331 (2018)
22. Wang, L., Mao, Q.: Probabilistic dimensionality reduction via structure learning. IEEE Trans. Pattern Anal. Mach. Intell. **41**(1), 205–219 (2019)

New Graph-Blind Convolutional Network for Brain Connectome Data Analysis

Yanfu Zhang[1] and Heng Huang[1,2(✉)]

[1] Electrical and Computer Engineering, University of Pittsburgh, Pittsburgh, USA
heng.huang@pitt.edu
[2] JD Digits, Mountain View, USA

Abstract. Human connectome provides essential insights in diagnosing many psychiatric disorders. Though machine learning methods in predicting clinical scores have been successfully applied, it is still challenging to capture the complex relation and exploit the graph structure of brain networks. In this paper, we proposed a method to address the problem by extracting the graph embeddings using graph convolutional network (GCN), and using multi-layer perceptron for the regression. Particularly, previous GCN explicitly requires pre-defined graph structures which is not clearly defined in brain connectome. To address this problem, we showed that with naive complete graph structure, GCN can get meaningful results. Meanwhile, an effective algorithm was proposed to learn the graph structure from the data, via generating random graph during training based on the small-world model. Also, the advantages of GCN over multi-layer perceptron was discussed. The experiments demonstrate that the proposed method outperform related baselines significantly on predicting depression scores.

Keywords: Brain connectome · Graph convolutional network · Random graph

1 Introduction

Connetome describes the neural connection within a brain [19]. Utilizing state-of-the-art neuroimaging techniques including functional resting state magnetic resonance imaging (rs-fMRI) [5] and structural diffusion tensorfimaging (DTI) [13], it is possible to capture the connectome at macro-scopic scale, which refers to the scenario involving anatomically segregated brain regions and inter-regional pathways. By graph based analysis, the information encoded by the connectome can promote critical understanding on how the brain manages cognition, what signals the connections convey and how these signals affect brain regions [9]. It has been discovered to be helpful in the early diagnosis of several neurological disorders, including epilepsy, Alzheimer's disease, and autism [10,15,23,25]. Across depressed patients and normal subjects, functional brain connectomes

© Springer Nature Switzerland AG 2019
A. C. S. Chung et al. (Eds.): IPMI 2019, LNCS 11492, pp. 669–681, 2019.
https://doi.org/10.1007/978-3-030-20351-1_52

derived from rs-fMRI also display distinct patterns [21, 26, 28], and some computational methods have been proposed to study the relation, for example linear support vector machine (SVM) [27], partial least square (PLC) [26]. Deep learning methods, which are successful on many tasks, are exploited as well. In [24], convolution neural network for classification is applied to brain networks with nodes reordered using a spectral clustering method.

Although meaningful clinical representations can be obtained from brain networks through previous methods, some issues still exists. The human connectome has sophisticated and non-linear structure, which may not be well captured by shallow linear models. Meanwhile, deep learning methods suffer from the enormous parameter sizes, which is both difficult for training and vulnerable to overfitting potentially. Besides, many methods do not make good use or even fail to preserve the graph structure. Thus, a concise graph based deep learning method is preferred on the task to discover the relation between human connectome and clinical scores. In the studies on graph data, great efforts are spent on node embeddings, with the majority of which are based on graph spectral properties and random walk techniques [3, 11, 17, 22]. Recently, several convolutional neural network methods for graph data are proposed [1]. Particularly, the graph convolution network (GCN) [6] based on spectral graph theory and its variants [12] are flexible in both graph and node analysis. However, GCN explicitly requires a known graph structure, which is typically not available in brain connectome. To address this challenge, in this paper we studied the GCN with *unknown* graph structure. In detail, we showed that GCN without given graph structure is applicable, by using a naive complete graph. Meanwhile, a method was propose to learn the graph structure from data to improve the performance of GCN, by generating random graph with small-world property for model training. The experiments demonstrates that the proposed method outperforms related baselines in the prediction of clinical depression scores, and the learned graph is superior to the naive complete graph settings.

The rest of this paper is organized as follow. Section 2 provides the preliminary and describes the detail of the proposed method. Section 3 shows the experiments and the results. Section 4 concludes the paper.

2 Methodology

To address the problem of predicting clinical depression scores, we proposed a two-stage regression method. The first stage is to obtain the embeddings of a single connectome, involving a graph convolution network that can be applied to data without predefined precise graph structure; the second stages is merely a standard MLP, for regression based on the embeddings. We introduced the preliminary on GCN in Sect. 2.1, and considered the GCN formulation without predefined graph structure in Sect. 2.2. In Sect. 2.3 the entire algorithm is given and some details are discussed.

2.1 Preliminary

A graph can be represented as $\{V, E, W\}$, with $V = \{v_1, v_2, \cdots, v_n\}$ the set of n vertices, $E \subseteq V \times V$ the set of m edges, and W the weighted adjacency matrix of the graph. The adjacency matrix $W \in \mathcal{R}^{n \times n}$, and W_{ij} encodes the relation between v_i and v_j if there is an edge, and 0 otherwise. The degree matrix of a graph can be expressed with diagonal matrix $D \in \mathcal{R}^{n \times n}$, with the diagonal entries $d_{ii} = \sum_j w_{i,j}$, representing the degree of node i. Graph Laplacian is an essential operation in spectral graph analysis, typically defined as $L_c = D - W$ in combinatorial form and $L_n = I_n - D^{-1/2} W D^{-1/2}$ in normalized form, with I_n a identity matrix. Graph convolutional network (GCN) [6] is designed to analysis the signals on nodes, with a given graph structure. As the name indicates, GCN is an extension of convolutional neural network (CNN). Convolution on 2D matrices, for example images, is well defined, serving as the basic building block in CNN. Graph convolution, however, is difficult to perform directly in spatial domains, due to the irregularity of neighbors of distinct nodes. One strategy is to conduct the operation in frequency domain using graph Laplacian, which is feasible according to the convolution theorem [16]. By definition, Laplacian matrix is positive semi definite, such that the eigenvalue decomposition exists, $L = U^T \Lambda U$, and $U = [u_0, u_1, \cdots, u_{n-1}]$ specifies a Fourier basis. The graph Fourier transform [18] is then defined as $\hat{x} = U^T x$, with $x \in \mathcal{R}^n$ the signal, and the inverse transform $x = U\hat{x}$. The spectral representation of node signals, $\hat{x}$, allows the fundamental filtering operation for graphs.

One potential problem in the above formulations is that in spectral domain, the filter is not naturally localized. Polynomial parametrization for localized filters [6] is proposed to tackle this challenge, through learning the coefficients Θ_K of a K-order Chebyshev polynomial. In detail, the filter is defined as $g_\theta(\Lambda) = \sum_{k=0}^{K-1} \theta_k T_k(\Lambda)$, and the graph convolution is defined as $y = U g_\theta(\Lambda) U^T x$, with y the filtered signal, θ_k the trainable parameters and $T_k(\Lambda)$ the polynomials. By the stable recurrence relation of Chebyshev polynomial, the costly multiplication in Fourier transform can also be reduced. Parallel to CNN, pooling operation in graph settings is accomplished by the graph coarsening [7] procedure.

The above method is suitable for graph classification, which is extended to node classification later [12]. By truncating the Chebyshev polynomial to only first order, GCN model can be reformulated similar to multi-layer perceptron, with each layer defined as $y = \sigma(\tilde{D}^{-1/2} \tilde{A} \tilde{D}^{-1/2} x\Theta)$, with $\tilde{A} = A + I_n$, $\tilde{D}$ accordingly defined as D, Θ the trainable parameters, and $\sigma(\cdot)$ an activation function. In the proposed method we will adopt the first order approximation version of GCN as the first stage to obtain embeddings for a graph, then use a MLP in the second stage for the regression task.

2.2 Graph Convolutional Network Without Pre-defined Graph Structure

Standard GCN, as well as its variants, defines the graph convolution based on a known adjacency matrix A. However, in our task we only know human connectomes are equipped with graph structure, while the precise graph is never provided. In this section we attempt to answer three questions: (1) can we apply GCN to graph data without predefined graph structure? (2) how can we find a "good" graph structure based on the task and the data? and (3) is GCN preferred compared to naive neural network?

Can We Apply GCN to Graph Data Without Predefined Graph Structure? The answer to the first question establishes the foundation of the solvability of the task. we will give the problem formulation and show that GCN is applicable under such formulation.

For a standard perceptron layer,

$$vec(y) = \sigma(vec(x)W) \simeq \sigma(vec(x)(\tilde{L}_g \otimes \tilde{\Theta})^T) = \tilde{L}_g x \tilde{\Theta}, \tag{1}$$

where $vec(\cdot)$ is vectorization operator, $x \in \mathcal{R}^{n \times n}$, $W \in \mathcal{R}^{n \times c}$ with c the channels of output y, $\otimes$ Kronecker product, and $\tilde{L}_g$ and $\tilde{\Theta}$ the decomposition of W. If the eigenvalue decomposition of $\tilde{L}_g$ exists,

$$\tilde{L}_g = U_g^T \tilde{\Lambda}_g U_g, \tag{2}$$

then $y = \sigma(U_w^T \Lambda_w U_w x)$ is identical with GCN [12] by their form, thus

$$\tilde{\Lambda}_g = \theta_0 + \theta_1(\frac{2}{\lambda_{max}}\Lambda_g - I_n), \tag{3}$$

where Λ_g is the eigenvalues of the underlying graph Laplacian L_g, and the graph Laplacian shares the same eigenvectors as $\tilde{L}_g$, thus $L_g = U_g^T \Lambda_g U_g$. Equation (3) implies that given a perceptron, an equivalent GCN layer can be induced. Essentially if L_g is given, we are inserting priors on the weight matrix W in perceptron, and the parameters of the model can be greatly reduced to merely θ_0 and θ_1.

Following the above argument, we can formulate L_g by selecting meaningful priors if it is not given. Here we show a naive choice, which is effective in denoising sense. The input connectome is $x = [x_1, x_2, \cdots, x_n]$, and We treat the column $x_i \in \mathcal{R}^n$ as the signals for the corresponding node i. Assume the collected connectome data are noisy,

$$x = x_0 + \sigma_0, \tag{4}$$

where σ_0 is a random noise matrix with entry-independent Gaussian distribution, and x_0 is the clean graph. For single layer GCN,

$$y = (\theta_0 - \theta_1)x - \frac{2\theta_1}{\lambda_{max}}L_g x, \tag{5}$$

the first term is 0 is we choose $\theta_0 - \theta_1 = 0$, making no contribution to the output. For the second term, we want to select the L_g that minimizes the effect of noise σ_0,

$$L_g = \arg\min_{L_g} E_{\sigma_0} \left(\left\| \frac{2\theta_1}{\lambda_{max}} L_g \sigma_0 \right\|_F^2 \right), \tag{6}$$

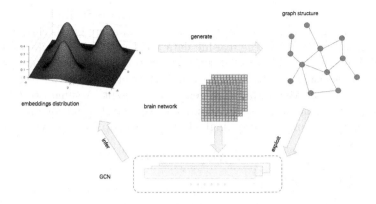

Fig. 1. The iterative procedure of random graph generation, GCN training, and embeddings inference.

where $\|\cdot\|_F$ is the Frobenius norm and $E_{\sigma_0}(\cdot)$ is the expectation over σ_0. Let $\frac{2\theta_1}{\lambda_{max}} \simeq 1$. The decomposition $L_g = U_g^T \Lambda_g U_g$ still exists. U_g is an orthogonal matrix and σ_0 is Gaussian, thus $U_g \sigma_0$ is still Gaussian. Let $U_g \sigma_0 = [\sigma_1, \sigma_2, \cdots, \sigma_n]$,

$$
\begin{aligned}
L_g &= \arg\min_{L_g} E_{\sigma_0}\left(tr\left(\sum_i \lambda_i^2 \sigma_i^T \sigma_i\right)\right) \\
&= \arg\min_{L_g} \sum_i \lambda_i^2 E_{\sigma_i}\left(n \times tr\left(\sigma_i^T \sigma_i\right)\right) \qquad (7) \\
&= \arg\min_{L_g} \|L_g\|_F^2 n E_{\sigma_i}\left(tr\left(\sigma_i^T \sigma_i\right)\right) = \arg\min_{L_g} \|L_g\|_F^2,
\end{aligned}
$$

To this end we just need to choose the L_g with minimum Frobenius norm,

$$
\begin{aligned}
\|L_g\|_F^2 &= tr((I_n - D^{-1/2}AD^{-1/2})^2) \\
&= tr(I_n - 2D^{-1/2}AD^{-1/2} + D^{-1/2}AD^{-1}AD^{-1/2}) \qquad (8) \\
&\geq tr(I_n) = n,
\end{aligned}
$$

because $tr(D^{-1/2}AD^{-1/2}) = 0$ and $tr(D^{-1/2}AD^{-1}AD^{-1/2}) \geq 0$. Let $L_g^* = I_n - \frac{1}{n-1}$, then the minimum is attained. L_g^* provides the best denoising effect, given Gaussian noise. Not surprisingly, such a L_g corresponds to a complete graph, which is a naive choice of graph structure. Intuitively, it indicates that if nothing is known about the potential node relations, we can just assume all node are related equivalently.

Moreover, the above result also minimizes the kernel norm,

$$
\arg\min_{L_g} E_{\sigma_0}\left(\left\|\frac{2\theta_1}{\lambda_{max}} L_g \sigma_0\right\|_*\right) \equiv \arg\min_{L_g} E_{\sigma_0}\left(\left\|\frac{2\theta_1}{\lambda_{max}} L_g \sigma_0\right\|_F\right), \qquad (9)
$$

which further strengthens the advantages of the naive complete graph choice.

How Can We Find a "Good" Graph Structure for Brain Connectome?
Although the naive as well as intuitive choice of complete graph is sufficient for
alleviating Gaussian noise, the real-life data are sophisticated and more flexible
methods are expected. This boils down to the importance of the second problem.

When different graph Laplacian is used, the obtained GCN will has different parameters and the outputs are generally different. Assume two GCNs are
trained on the same data using L_1 and L_2 respectively, and for one layer the
parameters are Θ_1 and Θ_2 accordingly, to make the two GCNs to yield the same
outputs, we need,

$$L_1 X \Theta_1 = L_2 X \Theta_2, \tag{10}$$

which can be re-formulated as,

$$L_2^{-1} L_1 X - X \Theta_2 \Theta_1^{-1} = \mathbf{0}, \tag{11}$$

the equation is a Sylvester function with fixed $L_2^{-1} L_1$ and $\Theta_2 \Theta_1^{-1}$, and the solution set X is the data. To fit the data $L_2^{-1} L_1$ and $\Theta_2 \Theta_1^{-1}$ must have common eigenvalues, which is possible only when the network is wide, namely
$\Theta_1, \Theta_2 \in \mathcal{R}^{d \times c}$, and $c \geq d$. This usually will not happen in realistic models.
Therefore, selecting graph structure is necessary.

A "good" graph structure is supposed to have two properties: ideally it should
reflect the structure of data; also, it should be stable, in the sense that networks
with similar graph structures should share similar parameters and outputs. Intuitively, we can initialize the graph Laplacian with high correlations in brain
connectomes, and update the network in order to exploit the data structure.
However, the naive back-propagation method in training neural networks is not
applicable, because unlike normal neural network parameters, graph Laplacian is
a structural matrix, satisfying some particular properties. Instead of solving the
complex constraint optimization problem, we propose a random generated graph
Laplacian using small-world model during the training, to infer the underlying
data structure.

In the proposed method GCN is used to extract the embeddings of connectomes, on which a popular assumption is that its prior distribution is known.
Further, we assume distributions are associated with the graph structure. For
simplicity, we assume the underlying model is known, and our target is to obtain
embeddings characterizing both the dependent variables and the graph structure.
Therefore we can apply a loop structure during training, which is illustrated in
Fig. 1: novel random graph is iterative generated, used as the graph structure
training the current model; meanwhile, the latent embeddings are optimized
with the evolving of the random graph. The training ultimately yields stable
embeddings, and we use the expectation of the generated random graph in the
inference, which can be viewed as a "good" graph structure, because it integrates
the average results of the embeddings.

In this paper, we use the small-world network to relate the latent embeddings
to the graph structure. In this model, the distance between most nodes are a
small number of hops or steps, and nodes with common neighbors are more likely
to be directly connected. Meanwhile, human brains are also found to display some

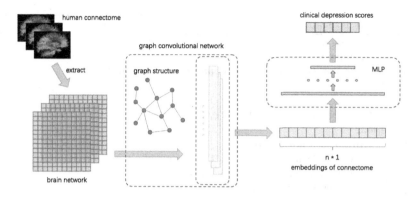

Fig. 2. The structure of the proposed method. Brain connectome is transformed into embeddings using GCN and MLP is used for regression successively.

properties of this model [2,4], which provides an intuitive interpretation: ROIs commutes information through small-world like networks, whose behaviors are simulated by the GCN. The embeddings of connectome are $h \in \mathcal{R}^n$, and the probability of the existence of an edge between node i and j is [14],

$$p_{e_{ij}} = \frac{\epsilon_p}{|h_i - h_j|^{\delta_p} + \epsilon_p}, \tag{12}$$

here δ_p and ϵ_p are hyper parameters. During training random graph structure is generated using Eq. (12), meanwhile the graph parameters are adjusted according to the embeddings. We apply K-means algorithm to cluster the clinical depression scores and obtain the centers of the embeddings for each cluster during the loop. The random graph is then generated by sampling these centers. The cluster of each subject is called "pseudo-label" and kept unchanged throughout.

Is GCN Preferred Compared to Naive Neural Network? Exploiting neural network in node classification has been actively studied. The extension to multi-task regression problem on graph data thus is natural. Naive neural network methods flatten the graph data into vectors and build a multi-layer perceptron for the regression task, which involves enormous amounts of parameters: the dimension of a single input is n^2, and the hidden units are decided accordingly. In the proposed model, the parameter sizes are significantly reduced. Meanwhile, the number of hidden units for both stages can be drastically decreased. Though over-parameterization has some potential benefits [8], it makes the model difficult for training, particularly in our task with limit data.

Sparsity is highly effective in solving high-dimension machine learning tasks. Unfortunately utilizing sparsity structure is not trivial in neural network models. The first-stage of the proposed method, in which the graph data is reduced to vector embeddings, can be viewed as dimension reductions. Particularly,

---

Algorithm 1. Training GCN without pre-defined graph structure

---

Input: training set x, validation set x_v, clinical depression scores y, hyper
      parameters δ_p, σ_p.
Output: the embedding of the graph and the trained model
1   Initialization;
2   **for** k **do**
3 | K-Means, generate pseudo labels c, $w.r.t$ y;
4 | **repeat**
5 | **while** *epoch not end* **do**
6 | Obtain embeddings h, *i.e.* the output of GCN;
7 | Estimate center for each cluster;
8 | Generate a random graph $w.r.t.$ Eq. (12);
9 | Train GCN and MLP $w.r.t.$ Eq. (13);
10 | **end**
11 | Generate expected graph laplacian;
12 | **until** *converge*;
13 **end**
14 Choose best model on validation set.

---

unlike "black-box" encoder models with elusive representations, the connectome embeddings are explicit connected to the graph structure of human brains, and clustered according to the depression scores, which is more explainable.

2.3 Pseudo-label

To this end we achieve approval answers on the three questions and in this section the entire method is given. The proposed method is composed of two stages. In the first stage a GCN is used to extract the embeddings of a connectome, and in the second stage a MLP is used for the regression using the embeddings. The model's structure is illustrated in Fig. 2.

The proposed method is straight-forward if the naive complete graph is used in the GCN. If the graph structure is to be learned, the proposed method explicitly requires data "labels" for inferring the graph structure. In this paper we use K-Means to generate the pseudo data "labels" based on the dependent variables during training. The objective is,

$$\mathcal{L} = \|\hat{Y} - Y\|_F + \lambda_1 \|W\|_2 + \lambda_2 \|\hat{H} - H\|, \tag{13}$$

where $\hat{Y}$ and Y are estimated and ground truth clinical depression scores respectively, W is the model parameter, $\hat{H}$ and H are estimated and ground truth connectome pseudo-labels respectively, and λ_1 and λ_2 is a tunable parameter. The optimization generally follows the procedure of EM algorithm, because the embeddings are sufficient statistics for inferring the graph structure. The algorithm involving learning the graph structure is summarized in Algorithm 1.

K-Means method is known to be sensitive to parameters and converges only to local minimum. In our experiments we found that with fixed k and random initialization occasionally the graph structure converge to unsatisfactory results. To achieve the best performance, we can use multiple starts with different k in the K-Means step and choose the best model with regard to validation data.

3   Experiments

3.1   Data Description

We conducted the experiments to predict clinical depression scores using the Human Connectome Project (HCP) data (www.humanconnectomeproject.org). The fMRI measurements were obtained on a 3T GE Signa HDx scanner with a 2D EP/GR. The subjects were asked to not take psychotropic drugs before experiments. The images were acquired when they laid down with eyes open, kept awake and thought of nothing, after-while processed following SPM8 standard procedures. Different brain regions with different resolutions were defined based on voxels, according to the automatic anatomical labeling atlas [20]. Between each pair of regions, functional connectivity were computed using the cross correlation of the corresponding time-series.

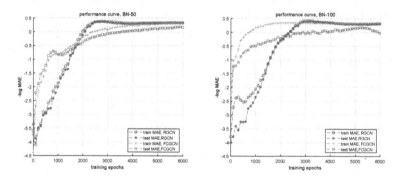

Fig. 3. Comparison of training curves of FCGCN and RGCN.

The rs-FMRI signals involving 1000 subjects are obtained with different ROI resolutions. Through our experiment, we use the connectome with resolution of 50 and 100 node graphs. For all subjects, eight measures of clinical depression scores are used as the dependent variables, including *ASR Anxious/Depressed, ASR Thought Problems, ASR Attention Problems, ASR Aggressive Behavior, ASR Rule Breaking Behavior, ASR DSM Depressive Problems, ASR DSM Anxiety Problems* and *ASR DSM Antisocial Personality Problems Raw Scores.* In the pre-processing, we normalized the depression scores to zero mean and unit variance, and randomly split subjects to the training, validation, and test sets, respectively using 70%, 10%, and 20% of the data. We repeated the allocation 5 times and reported the mean and standard error of mean absolute error (MAE).

Table 1. Quantitative comparison of baselines and the proposed method. Both the mean and the standard error are given, and the best results are bold faced. Metrics without significant difference between baselines and FCGCN are denoted with ⋆; the metric without significant difference between FCGCN and kGCN/RGCN is denoted with ◇.

Methods	MAE, BN-50	MAE, BN-100
RL	1.1176 ± 0.1723	1.2510 ± 0.1625
LASSO	0.9996 ± 0.1783	1.0078 ± 0.1025
EN	0.9538 ± 0.1616	0.9476 ± 0.0773
MLP	$0.8202 \pm 0.1258^{\star}$	$0.7690 \pm 0.0339^{\star}$
FCGCN	0.8176 ± 0.1656	0.7704 ± 0.0220
kGCN	$0.8397 \pm 0.0864^{\circ}$	$0.7449 \pm 0.0516^{\circ}$
RGCN	$\mathbf{0.7372 \pm 0.0684}$	$\mathbf{0.7226 \pm 0.0579}^{\circ}$

3.2   Experiment Setting

We compare the proposed method with several other regression methods: multivariate Ridge Regression (RR), Least Absolute Shrinkage and Selection Operator (LASSO), Elastic Net (EN), which is the combination of L_1 and L_2 norm, and Multi-Layer Perceptron (MLP). For RR, LASSO, and EN, the hyper-parameter was tuned on validation data. For MLP, we used a two layer structure and kept the hidden layers of the size with the embeddings of the proposed method. Through the paper, the proposed method is adapted from the fast GCN using first-order approximation. In this section, we provide both the results using Fully-Connected Graph Convolution Network (FCGCN), and Random generated Graph Convolution Network (RGCN). Besides, we also provide the results of simple sparse graph (kGCN), keeping top 50% strongest edges of the average correlations. In RGGCN, we use a two layer GCN in the first stage, with 10 hidden units, and also a two layer MLP in the second stage, with 20 hidden units. Leaky ReLU is exploited as the activation function. For the random graph, we use $\delta_p = 2$ and $\sigma_P = 0.01$, and run six independent K-Means with k ranging from 3 to 8, respectively. The results are reported based on the validation set. The RMSProp optimization algorithm is used with learning rate of 0.001. For FCGCN and kGCN, identical parameter settings are utilized, except that the graph structure is fixed as a complete graph or a simple sparse graph.

3.3   Performance Comparison

The results of the proposed method using both complete graph and learned graph are listed in Table 1. From the table we can find that the proposed method constantly outperform linear baselines on all scales. This results imply that non-linear models are potentially more suitable for our task. Particularly, FCGCN yields comparable results with MLP, using much less parameters, which demonstrates the advantages of GCN models. kGCN shows improvements against

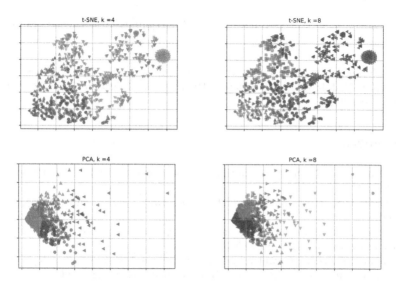

Fig. 4. Visualization of clustering of clinical depression scores using t-SNE and PCA respectively, from a random start. The clustering is obtained through K-Means with $K = 4$ and 8

FCGCN w.r.t. MAE, but worsens MSE. Meanwhile, the proposed method using trainable graph structure has better performance than complete graph case, showing the importance of graph structure selection and the effectiveness of the proposed algorithm.

We also want to mention that with the random generated graph structure, the training of the proposed method actually is faster than the fixed scenario. The training curve is illustrated in Fig. 3, in which RGCN provides a higher prediction ability and a smaller generalization error. This results further demonstrate that the learned structure fits the data better thus yields better performances.

In this paper we use K-Means as the clustering algorithm, which, though serves solid functions in our experiments, may not be stable. To depict this phenomenon, we present the clustering results by dimension reductions using both t-SNE and principle component analysis, and the results are listed in Fig. 4. Apparently, the clustering may not be intuitively preferable. That explains the necessity to improve the robustness of the proposed method through multiple start K-Means.

4   Conclusion

In this paper we proposed a novel method to predict the clinical scores using brain connectomes. We demonstrate that GCN can be applied to graph data even without pre-defined graph structure, and proposed an effective algorithm to learn the graph structure from the data. The experiments show the proposed method outperform standard methods, and particularly the learned graph structure yields a better results than the naive complete graph assumption.

Acknowledgement. This work was partially supported by U.S. NSF IIS 1836945, IIS 1836938, DBI 1836866, IIS 1845666, IIS 1852606, IIS 1838627, IIS 1837956, and NIH R01 AG049371.

References

1. Atwood, J., et al.: Diffusion-convolutional neural networks. In: NeurIPS, pp. 1993–2001 (2016)
2. Bassett, D.S., et al.: Small-world brain networks. Neuroscientist **12**(6), 512–523 (2006)
3. Belkin, M., et al.: Laplacian eigenmaps and spectral techniques for embedding and clustering. In: NeurIPS, pp. 585–591 (2002)
4. Bullmore, E., et al.: Complex brain networks: graph theoretical analysis of structural and functional systems. Nat. Rev. Neurosci. **10**(3), 186 (2009)
5. Craddock, R.C., et al.: Disease state prediction from resting state functional connectivity. Magn. Reson. Med. **62**(6), 1619–1628 (2009)
6. Defferrard, M., et al.: Convolutional neural networks on graphs with fast localized spectral filtering. In: NeurIPS, pp. 3844–3852 (2016)
7. Dhillon, I.S., et al.: Weighted graph cuts without eigenvectors a multilevel approach. IEEE TPAMI **29**(11), 1944–1957 (2007)
8. Du, S.S., et al.: Gradient descent finds global minima of deep neural networks. arXiv preprint arXiv:1811.03804 (2018)
9. Fornito, A., et al.: Graph analysis of the human connectome: promise, progress, and pitfalls. Neuroimage **80**, 426–444 (2013)
10. Gao, H., et al.: Identifying connectome module patterns via new balanced multigraph normalized cut. In: Navab, N., Hornegger, J., Wells, W.M., Frangi, A.F. (eds.) MICCAI 2015. LNCS, vol. 9350, pp. 169–176. Springer, Cham (2015). https://doi.org/10.1007/978-3-319-24571-3_21
11. Grover, A., et al.: Node2vec: scalable feature learning for networks. In: ACM SIGKDD, pp. 855–864. ACM (2016)
12. Kipf, T.N., et al.: Semi-supervised classification with graph convolutional networks. arXiv preprint arXiv:1609.02907 (2016)
13. Le Bihan, D., et al.: Diffusion tensor imaging: concepts and applications. J. Magn. Reson. Imaging **13**(4), 534–546 (2001)
14. Li, C., et al.: From which world is your graph. In: Guyon, I., et al. (eds.) Advances in Neural Information Processing Systems, vol. 30, pp. 1469–1479. Curran Associates, Inc. (2017). http://papers.nips.cc/paper/6745-from-which-world-is-your-graph.pdf
15. Luo, D., et al.: New probabilistic multi-graph decomposition model to identify consistent human brain network modules. In: ICDM, pp. 301–310 (2016)
16. Mallat, S.: A wavelet tour of signal processing. Elsevier, San Diego (1999)
17. Perozzi, B., et al.: DeepWalk: online learning of social representations. In: ACM SIGKDD, pp. 701–710. ACM (2014)
18. Shuman, D.I., et al.: The emerging field of signal processing on graphs: extending high-dimensional data analysis to networks and other irregular domains. IEEE Sig. Process. Mag. **30**(3), 83–98 (2013)

19. Sporns, O., et al.: The human connectome: a structural description of the human brain. PLoS Comput. Biol. **1**(4), e42 (2005)
20. Tzourio-Mazoyer, N., et al.: Automated anatomical labeling of activations in SPM using a macroscopic anatomical parcellation of the MNI MRI single-subject brain. Neuroimage **15**(1), 273–289 (2002)
21. Veer, I.M., et al.: Whole brain resting-state analysis reveals decreased functional connectivity in major depression. Front. Syst. Neurosci. **4**, 41 (2010)
22. Wang, D., et al.: Structural deep network embedding. In: ACM SIGKDD, pp. 1225–1234. ACM (2016)
23. Wang, D., et al.: Human connectome module pattern detection using a new multi-graph minmax cut model. In: Golland, P., Hata, N., Barillot, C., Hornegger, J., Howe, R. (eds.) MICCAI 2014. LNCS, vol. 8675, pp. 313–320. Springer, Cham (2014). https://doi.org/10.1007/978-3-319-10443-0_40
24. Wang, S., et al.: Structural deep brain network mining. In: ACM KDD, pp. 475–484. ACM (2017)
25. Yahata, N., et al.: A small number of abnormal brain connections predicts adult autism spectrum disorder. Nat. Commun. **7**, 11254 (2016)
26. Yoshida, K., et al.: Prediction of clinical depression scores and detection of changes in whole-brain using resting-state functional MRI data with partial least squares regression. PloS One **12**(7), e0179638 (2017)
27. Zeng, L.L., et al.: Identifying major depression using whole-brain functional connectivity: a multivariate pattern analysis. Brain **135**(5), 1498–1507 (2012)
28. Zhang, X., et al.: Can depression be diagnosed by response to mother's face? A personalized attachment-based paradigm for diagnostic fMRI. PloS One **6**(12), e27253 (2011)

CIA-Net: Robust Nuclei Instance Segmentation with Contour-Aware Information Aggregation

Yanning Zhou[1]([✉]), Omer Fahri Onder[2], Qi Dou[3], Efstratios Tsougenis[2], Hao Chen[1,2]([✉]), and Pheng-Ann Heng[1,4]

[1] Department of Computer Science and Engineering,
The Chinese University of Hong Kong, Hong Kong, Hong Kong SAR, China
{ynzhou,hchen}@cse.cuhk.edu.hk
[2] Imsight Medical Technology, Co., Ltd., Hong Kong, Hong Kong SAR, China
[3] Department of Computing, Imperial College London, London, UK
[4] Guangdong Provincial Key Laboratory of Computer Vision and Virtual Reality Technology, Shenzhen Institutes of Advanced Technology,
Chinese Academy of Sciences, Shenzhen, China

Abstract. Accurate segmenting nuclei instances is a crucial step in computer-aided image analysis to extract rich features for cellular estimation and following diagnosis as well as treatment. While it still remains challenging because the wide existence of nuclei clusters, along with the large morphological variances among different organs make nuclei instance segmentation susceptible to over-/under-segmentation. Additionally, the inevitably subjective annotating and mislabeling prevent the network learning from reliable samples and eventually reduce the generalization capability for robustly segmenting unseen organ nuclei. To address these issues, we propose a novel deep neural network, namely Contour-aware Informative Aggregation Network (CIA-Net) with multi-level information aggregation module between two task-specific decoders. Rather than independent decoders, it leverages the merit of spatial and texture dependencies between nuclei and contour by bi-directionally aggregating task-specific features. Furthermore, we proposed a novel smooth truncated loss that modulates losses to reduce the perturbation from outliers. Consequently, the network can focus on learning from reliable and informative samples, which inherently improves the generalization capability. Experiments on the 2018 MICCAI challenge of Multi-Organ-Nuclei-Segmentation validated the effectiveness of our proposed method, surpassing all the other 35 competitive teams by a significant margin.

1 Introduction

Digital pathology is nowadays playing a crucial role for accurate cellular estimation and prognosis of cancer [18]. Specifically, nuclei instance segmentation

© Springer Nature Switzerland AG 2019
A. C. S. Chung et al. (Eds.): IPMI 2019, LNCS 11492, pp. 682–693, 2019.
https://doi.org/10.1007/978-3-030-20351-1_53

which not only captures location and density information but also rich morphology features, such as magnitude and the cytoplasmic ratio, is critical in tumor diagnosis and following treatment procedures [23]. However, automatically segmenting the nuclei at instance-level still remains challenging due to several reasons. First, the vast existence of nuclei occlusions and clusters can easily cause over or under-segmentation, which impedes accurate morphological measurements of nuclei instances. Second, the blurred border and inconsistent staining makes images inevitable to contain indistinguishable instances, and hence introduces subjective annotations and mislabeling, which is challenging to get robust and objective results [8]. Third, the variability in cell appearance, magnitude, and density among diverse cell types and organs requires the method to possess good generalization ability for robust analysis.

Most of the earlier methods are based on thresholding and morphological operations [3, 10], which fail to find reliable threshold in the complex background. While deep learning-based methods are generally more robust and have become the benchmark for medical image segmentation [11, 21, 25]. For example, Chen et al. [2] proposed a deep contour-aware network (DCAN) for the task of instance segmentation that firstly harnesses the complementary information of contour and instances to separate the attached objects. In order to utilize contour-specific features to assist nuclei prediction, BES-Net [17] directly concatenates the output contour features with nuclei features in decoders. However, it only learns complementary information in nuclei branch but ignores the potentially reversed benefits from nuclei to contour, which is more essential since contour appearance is more complicated and has larger intra-variance than that of nuclei.

Another challenge is to eliminate the effect from inevitably noisy and subjective annotations. Different training strategies and loss functions have been proposed [6, 9, 19, 24]. A bootstrapped loss [20] was proposed to rebalance the loss weight by taking the consistency between the label and reliable output into account. However, when dealing with noise labeling especially the mislabeling nuclei, the network tends to predict probability with a high confidence score, where the negative log-likelihood magnitude is non-trivial and cannot be appropriately adjusted by the consistent term. As we will show later (Sect. 2.3), these outliers overwhelm others in loss calculation and dominate the gradient.

To address the issues mentioned above, we have following contributions in this paper. (1) We propose an Information Aggregation Module (IAM) which enables the decoders to collaboratively refine details of nuclei and contour by leveraging the spatial and texture dependencies in bi-directionally feature aggregation. (2) A novel smooth truncated Loss is proposed to modulate the outliers' perturbation in loss calculation, which endows the network with the ability to robustly segment nuclei instances by focusing on learning informative samples. Moreover, eliminating outliers alleviates the network from overfitting on these noisy samples, eventually enabling the network with better generalization capability. (3) We validate the effectiveness of our proposed Contour-aware Information Aggregation Network (CIA-Net) with the advantages of pyramidal information aggregation and robustness on Multi-Organ Nuclei Segmentation (MoNuSeg)

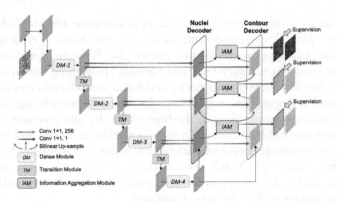

Fig. 1. An overview of our proposed CIA-Net for nuclei instance segmentation.

dataset with seven different organs, and achieved the 1st place on 2018 MICCAI Challenge, demonstrating the superior performance of the proposed approach.

2   Method

Figure 1 presents overview of the CIA-Net, which is a fully convolutional network (FCN) consisting of one densely connective encoder and two task-specific information aggregated decoders for refinement. To fully leverage the benefit of complementary information from highly correlated tasks, instead of directly concatenating task-specific features, our method conducts a hierarchical refinement procedure by aggregating multi-level task-specific features between decoders.

2.1   Densely Connected Encoder with Pyramidal Feature Extraction

To effectively train the deep FCN, dense connectivity is introduced in encoder [7]. In each Dense Module (DM), let x_i denotes the output of the i-th layer, dense connectivity can be described as $x_i = \mathcal{F}_i([x_1, x_2, \ldots, x_{i-1}], \mathcal{W}_i)$. It sets up direct connections from any bottleneck layer to all subsequent layers by concatenation, which not only effectively and efficiently reuses features but also benefits gradient back-propagation in the deep network. Transition Module (TM) is added after DM to reduce the spatial resolution and make the features more compact, which contains a 1×1 convolution layer and an average pooling layer with a stride of 2. Next, we hierarchically stack four DMs where each followed by a TM except the last one. For each DM, it consists of $\{6, 12, 24, 16\}$ bottleneck layers, respectively.

Inspired by feature pyramid network [13] which takes advantage of multi-scale features for accurate object detection, we propose to make full use of pyramidal features hierarchically by building multi-level lateral connections between encoder and decoders. In this way, localization and texture information from earlier layers can help the low-resolution while strong-semantic features refine the details. The encoder features with $\{1/2, 1/4, 1/8\}$ of original size are passed

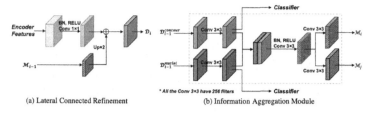

(a) Lateral Connected Refinement   (b) Information Aggregation Module

Fig. 2. Detail structure of (a) Lateral connected refinement and (b) Information aggregation module in proposed CIA-Net.

through the lateral connections by a 1×1 convolution to reduce feature map number and merged with the upsampled deeper features in decoders by summation operation, as shown in Fig. 2(a).

2.2 Bi-directional Feature Aggregation for Accurate Segmentation

Given that contour region encases the corresponding nuclei, it is intuitive that nuclei and contour have high spatial and contextual relevance, which is helpful for decoders to localize and focus on learning informative patterns. In other words, the neural response from the specific kernel in nuclei branch can be considered as an extra spatial or contexture cue for localizing contour to refine details and vice versa. In this regard, we proposed Information Aggregation Module (IAM) which aims at utilizing information from highly-correlated sub-tasks to bidirectionally aggregate the task-specific features between two decoders. Figure 2(b) shows the details of IAM structure, it takes features after lateral connection as inputs, and then selects and aggregates informative features for each sub-task.

To start the iteration, we attach a 3×3 convolution on the top of the encoder to generate the coarsest feature maps. For each decoder, the feature maps $\mathcal{M}_{i-1}$ from a higher level are upsampled by bilinear interpolation to double the resolution and added with high-resolution feature maps from encoder through lateral connections (see Fig. 2(a)). After that, the IAM takes the merged maps $\mathcal{D}_{i-1}$ as inputs and adds a 3×3 convolution without nonlinear activation to smoothen and eliminate the grid effects. Then the smooth features are fed into the classifier to predict multi-resolution score maps. Meanwhile, these task-specific features are concatenated along the channel dimension and then passed through two parallel convolution layers to select and integrate the complementary informative features $\mathcal{M}_i$ for further details refinement in the next iteration.

Besides, to prevent the network from relying on single level discriminative features, deep supervision mechanism [4] is introduced at each stage to strengthen learning of multi-level contextual information. This also benefits training of deeper network architectures by shortening the back-propagation path.

2.3 Smooth Truncated Loss for Robust Nuclei Segmentation

The existence of blurred edge and inconsistent staining makes images inevitably contain indistinguishable instances, which leads to subjective annotations such as

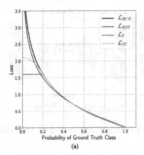 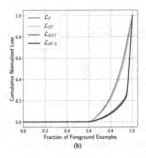

(a)   (b)

Fig. 3. Visualization of different loss functions (a) with $\gamma = 0.2$ and the cumulative loss functions of normalized loss from foreground regions (b).

mislabelled objects and inaccurate boundary. Additionally, to enhance the ability to split attached nuclei, conventional practice is to preprocess the training ground truth by subtracting the dilated contour mask, which is also suboptimal and has the risk of introducing noises. Both factors show that it is unavoidable for pixel-wise nuclei annotations to contain imperfect labels, which is harmful to network training from at least two aspects. Firstly, the inaccurate labeling encountered during training has the tendency to overwhelm other regions in loss calculation and dominate the gradients. This phenomenon is observed from the sorted cumulative distribution function of normalized loss in Fig. 3(b) using a converged model. Notice that top 10% samples account for more than 80% value of cross-entropy loss, which prevents network learning from informative samples during gradient back-propagation. Secondly, forcibly learning the subjective labeling would eventually push the network to particularly fit them and tend to overfitting, which is even more pernicious when predicting unseen organ nuclei. To handle the noisy and incomplete labeling, [20] proposed bootstrapped loss ($\mathcal{L}_{BST}$) to rebalance the loss weight by considering the consistency between the label and reliable output. However, as can be seen in Fig. 3(b), when faced with errors with low predicted probability, it cannot easily compensate for the loss with non-trivial magnitude.

To solve this problem, our insight is to reduce outliers' interference in training by modulating contribution in loss calculation. Under the premise of high credibility of network prediction, the majority of outliers will lie in low predicted probability regions and get large values of error. Inspired by Huber loss [5] for robust regression, which is quadratic for small values of error and linear for large values to decline the influence of outliers, we propose the prototype of loss function, namely Truncated Loss ($\mathcal{L}_T$), which reduces the contribution of outliers with high confidence prediction. Let p_t denotes the predicted probability of the ground truth, $p_t = p$ if $t = 1$ and $p_t = 1-p$ otherwise, in which $t \in \{0, 1\}$ specifies the ground truth label. Formally, the loss is truncated when the corresponding p_t is smaller than a threshold $\gamma \in [0, 0.5]$:

$$\mathcal{L}_T = -\max(\log(p_t), \log(\gamma)). \tag{1}$$

The truncated loss only clips outliers with $p_t < \gamma$, while preserves loss value for the other. Intuitively, this operation adds a constraint of maximum contribution in loss calculation from each pixel and hence can ease the gradient domination from outliers and benefit of learning the informative samples. However, in Eq. (1) the derivative of $\mathcal{L}_T$ at clipping point $p_t = \gamma$ is undefined. Meanwhile, the perturbation of low p_t prediction will not be reflected in loss calculation if we force the loss value larger than the threshold to a constant, therefore the smoothed version is preferred for optimization. In this regard, we propose Smooth Truncated Loss $\mathcal{L}_{ST}$:

$$\mathcal{L}_{ST} = \begin{cases} -\log(\gamma) + \frac{1}{2}(1 - \frac{p_t^2}{\gamma^2}), & p_t < \gamma \\ -\log(p_t), & p_t \geqslant \gamma \end{cases} \tag{2}$$

A quadratic function with the same value and derivative as negative log-likelihood at the truncated point γ is used to modulate the loss weight for outliers. By incorporating constraint for the loss magnitude, it reduces the contribution of outliers, where the smaller p_t, the more considerable modulation. This, in turn, let the network discard the indistinguishable parts and focus on informative and learnable regions. Furthermore, by reducing the influence of the outlier samples that interferences the network training, it encourages the network to predict with higher confidence scores and narrow the uncertain regions, which is helpful for alleviating over-segmentation.

2.4 Overall Loss Function

Based on the proposed Smooth Truncated Loss, we can derive the overall loss function. Note that the contour prediction is much more difficult than that of nuclei due to irregularly curved form. In this case, the primary component of regions with high loss is not by the outliers, but the inlier samples, and hence utilizing truncated loss may confuse the network. Instead, we use Soft Dice Loss to learn the shape similarity:

$$\mathcal{L}_{Dice} = 1 - \frac{2\sum_{i=1}^{n} p_i q_i}{\sum_{i=1}^{n} p_i^2 + \sum_{i=1}^{n} q_i^2}, \tag{3}$$

where p_i denotes the predicted probability of i-th pixel and q_i denotes the corresponding ground truth. In sum, the total loss function for proposed CIA-Net training is:

$$\mathcal{L}_{total} = \mathcal{L}_{ST} + \lambda \mathcal{L}_{Dice} + \beta \|\mathcal{W}\|_2^2, \tag{4}$$

where the first and second terms calculate error from contour and nuclei prediction respectively, and the third term is the weight decay. λ and β are hyperparameters to balance three components.

3   Experimental Results

3.1   Dataset and Evaluation Metrics

We validated our proposed method on MoNuSeg dataset of 2018 MICCAI challenge, which contains 30 images (size: 1000×1000) captured by The Cancer Genomic Atlas (TCGA) from whole slide images (WSIs) [12]. The dataset consists of breast, liver, kidney, prostate, bladder, colon and stomach containing both benign and malignant cases, which is then divided into training set (*Train*), test set1 from the same organs of training data (*Test1*) and test set2 from unseen organs (*Test2*) with 14, 8 and 6 images, respectively. The *Train* contains 4 organs - breast, kidney, liver and prostate with 4 images from each organ, the *Test1* includes 2 images from per organ mentioned in *Train*, and *Test2* contains 2 images from each unseen organ, i.e., bladder, colon and stomach.

We employed Average Jaccard Index (AJI) [12] for comparison, which considers an aggregated intersection cardinality numerator and an aggregated union cardinality denominator for all ground truth and segmented nuclei. Let $G = \{G_1, G_2, \ldots G_n\}$ denotes the set of instance ground truths, $S = \{S_1, S_2, \ldots S_m\}$ denotes the set of segmented objects and N denotes the set of segmented objects with none intersection to ground truth. $\text{AJI} = \dfrac{\sum_{i=1}^{n} G_i \bigcap S_j}{\sum_{i=1}^{n} G_i \bigcup S_j + \sum_{k \in N} S_k}$, where $j = \underset{k}{\arg\max} \dfrac{G_i \bigcap S_k}{G_i \bigcup S_k}$. F1-score $(F1 = \dfrac{2 \cdot Precision \cdot Recall}{Precision + Recall})$ [2] is used for nuclei instance detection performance evaluation and we also report it for reference.

3.2   Implementation Details

We implemented our network using Tensorflow (version 1.7.0). The default parameters provided at https://github.com/pudae/tensorflow-densenet is used in the Densenet backbone. Stain normalization method [16] was performed before training. Data augmentations including crop, flip, elastic transformation and color jitter were utilized. The outputs of nuclei and contour maps were first subtracted and then the connected components were detected get the final results. The network was trained on one NVIDIA TITAN Xp GPU with a mini-batch size of three. We utilized the pre-trained DenseNet model [7] from ImageNet to initialize the encoder. The hyper-parameters λ and β were set as 0.42 and 0.0001 to balance the loss and regularization. AdamW optimizer was used to optimize the whole network and learning rate was initialized as 0.001 and decayed according to cosine annealing and warm restarts strategy [15].

3.3   Evaluation and Comparison

Effectiveness of Contour-Aware Information Aggregation Architecture. Firstly, we conduct a series of experiments to compare different informative feature aggregation strategies in decoders: (1) *Cell Profiler* [1]: a python-based software for computational pathology employing intensity thresholoding method. (2) *Fiji* [22]: a Java-based software utilizing watershed transform nuclear segmentation method. (3) *CNN3* [12]: a 3-class FCN without deep dense connectivity. (4) *DCAN* [2]: a deep FCN with multi-task learning strategy for objects and contours. (5) *PA-Net* [14]: a modified path aggregation network by adding path augmentation in two independent decoders to enhance the instance segmentation performance. (6) *BES-Net* [17]: the original boundary-enhanced segmentation network which concatenated contour features with nuclei features to enhance learning in boundary region. (7) *CIA-Net w/o IAM*: the proposed network architecture with two independent decoders for nuclei and contour prediction respectively, but without Information Aggregation Module in decoders. (8) *Proposed CIA-Net*: Our Contour-aware Information Aggregation Network with Information Aggregation Module between nuclei and contour decoders. Notice that unless specified otherwise, we utilized the same encoder structure with pyramidal feature extraction strategy and loss functions to establish fair comparison (Table 1).

Table 1. Performance comparison of different methods on *Test1* (seen organ) and *Test2* (unseen organ).

	Method	AJI		F1-score	
		Test1	Test2	Test1	Test2
(1)	Cell profiler [1]	0.1549	0.0809	0.4143	0.3917
(2)	Fiji [22]	0.2508	0.3030	0.6402	0.6978
(3)	CNN3 [12]	0.5154	0.4989	0.8226	0.8322
(4)	DCAN [2]	0.6082	0.5449	0.8265	0.8214
(5)	PA-Net [14]	0.6011	0.5608	0.8156	0.8336
(6)	BES-Net [17]	0.5906	0.5823	0.8118	0.7952
(7)	CIA-Net w/o IAM	0.6106	0.5817	**0.8279**	0.8356
(8)	**Proposed CIA-Net**	**0.6129**	**0.6306**	0.8244	**0.8458**

It is observed that all CNN-based approaches achieved much higher results on all evaluation criterions than conventional approaches, highlighting the superiority of deep learning based methods for segmentation related tasks. Moreover, results from (4) to (8) have a striking improvement regarding the evaluation metric of AJI on both *Test1* and *Test2* compared with (3), validating the efficacy of dense connectivity structure, which is more powerful to leverage multilevel features and mitigate gradient vanishing in training deep neural network. While methods (4) to (7) achieved comparable performance on the evaluation performance of *Test1*, the results from *BES-Net* and proposed *CIA-Net w/o IAM* outperform others significantly on AJI of *Test2*, demonstrating the exploitation of high spatial and context relevance between nuclei and contour can generate task-specific features for assisting feature refinement between both tasks. This can help enhance the generalization capability to unseen data. Meanwhile, in comparison with *BES-Net* and proposed *CIA-Net w/o IAM*, our proposed network *CIA-Net* further outperforms these two methods consistently regarding the metric of AJI, achieving overall best performance and boosting results to 0.6306 on *Test2* and 0.6129 on *Test1*. Different from *BES-Net* which directly concatenates features in contour decoder to nuclei branch, the proposed *CIA-Net* with IAM bi-directionally aggregating the task-specific features and passing them through parallel convolutions to iteratively aggregate informative features in decoders. Therefore, it is a learnable procedure for network to find favorable features, which mutually benefits two sub-tasks. Compared with the improvement on AJI, the improvement on F1-score is less significant, this is because AJI is a segment-based metric while F1-score is the detection-based metric.

Effectiveness of Proposed Smooth Truncated Loss. Toward the potential of clinical application, the proposed method should be robust under the numerous circumstances, especially for the diffused-chromatin and attached nuclei in unseen organs, which is evaluated in *Test2* set. We compare the results of our proposed CIA-Net with four different functions: (1) $\mathcal{L}_{BCE}$: Binary Cross-Entropy loss. (2) $\mathcal{L}_{BST}$: Soft Bootstrapped loss by rebalancing the loss weight. (3) $\mathcal{L}_T$: Proposed Truncated loss without smoothing around truncated point, i.e., Eq. (1). (4) $\mathcal{L}_{ST}$: Proposed Smooth Truncated loss which utilizes quadratic function as soft modulation, i.e., Eq. (2).

Table 2. Comparison of proposed CIA-Net with different loss functions.

Loss	AJI		F1-score	
	Test1	Test2	Test1	Test2
$\mathcal{L}_{BCE}$	0.6104	0.5934	0.8303	0.8433
$\mathcal{L}_{BST}$	0.6123	0.6058	**0.8415**	0.8260
$\mathcal{L}_T$	0.6133	0.6153	0.8377	0.8307
$\mathcal{L}_{ST}$	0.6129	**0.6306**	0.8244	**0.8458**

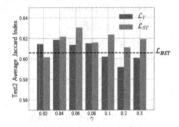

Fig. 4. Results of varying γ for $\mathcal{L}_T$ and $\mathcal{L}_{ST}$ on *Test2*.

As can be seen in Table 2, the improvement of $\mathcal{L}_{BST}$ compared to $\mathcal{L}_{BCE}$ is limited. Compared with first two rows, results from $\mathcal{L}_T$ and $\mathcal{L}_{ST}$ outperform others on *Test2* consisting of unseen organs by a large margin (nearly 2.5% for $\mathcal{L}_{ST}$ and 1% for $\mathcal{L}_T$) regarding the metric of AJI, and are analogous on *Test1*. The proposed $\mathcal{L}_{ST}$ achieved significant improvements in comparison with $\mathcal{L}_T$ on *Test2*, shows it is less sensitive on γ and has better generalization capability on different organ images. The proposed Smooth Truncated loss introduces one new hyper-parameter, the truncating parameter γ, which controls the starting point of down-weighting outliers. When $\gamma = 0$, the loss function degenerates into Binary Cross-entropy $\mathcal{L}_{BCE}$. As γ increases, more examples with p_t lower than γ are considered as outliers or less informative samples to down-weight in loss calculation. Figure 4 illustrates the influence of varying γ. We can see $\mathcal{L}_{ST}$ have

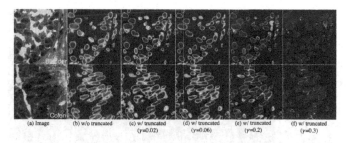

Fig. 5. Visualization of heatmaps in different γ values from $Test2$.

a striking overall improvement compared with $\mathcal{L}_{BST}$ and $\mathcal{L}_T$. More importantly, results from $\mathcal{L}_{ST}$ demonstrate less sensitivity for choosing different γ.

We visualize the nuclei heatmaps from setting different γ in $\mathcal{L}_{ST}$ (see Fig. 5) to give an intuitive understanding of our proposed method. It is observed that heatmaps trained by $\mathcal{L}_{BCE}$ (Fig. 5(b)) contain massive blur and noise, which is unfavorable for binarizing instances. As γ increases, the heatmaps turn to be more concrete with less uncertain areas, which is of great significance for instance segmentation to prevent over-segmentation. While setting too large γ increases the risk of under-segmentation, as can be seen in Fig. 5(f). This is because over suppressing low p_t region also penalties learning from informative inlier samples, especially boundary regions where the p_t is relatively small.

2018 MICCAI MoNuSeg Challenge Results. We employed above entire dataset for training and 14 additional images provided by organizer for independent evaluation with ground truth held out[1]. Top 20 results of 36 teams are shown in Fig. 6. Our submitted entry surpassed all the other methods, highlighting the strength of the proposed CIA-Net and Smooth Truncated loss.

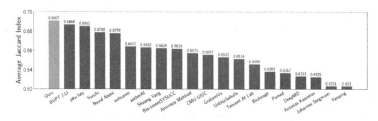

Fig. 6. The instance segmentation results of different methods in 2018 MICCAI multi-organ nuclei segmentation challenge (top 20 of 36 methods are shown in figure).

Qualitative Analysis. Figure 7 shows representative samples from $Test1$ and $Test2$ with challenging cases such as diffuse-chromatin nuclei and irregular shape. Notice that our proposed CIA-Net (Fig. 7(e)) can generate the segmentation results similar to the annotations of human experts, outperforming others with less over or under-segmentation on the prolific nuclei clusters and attached cases.

---

[1] https://monuseg.grand-challenge.org.

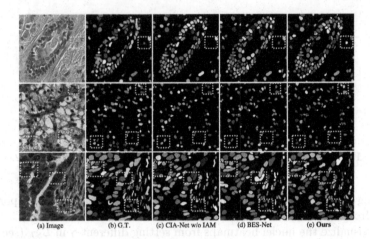

(a) Image   (b) G.T.   (c) CIA-Net w/o IAM   (d) BES-Net   (e) Ours

Fig. 7. Qualitative results of multi-organ nuclei (from top to bottom: breast, kidney, colon) on *Test1* and *Test2*. Yellow rectangles highlight the difference among predictions. (Color figure online)

4   Conclusion

Instance-level nuclei segmentation is the pivotal step for cell estimation and further pathological analysis. In this paper, we propose CIA-Net with the smooth truncated loss to tackle the challenges of prolific nuclei clusters and inevitable labeling noise in pathological images. Our method inherently can be adapted to a wide range of medical image segmentation tasks to boost the performance such as histology gland segmentation.

Acknowledgments. This work was supported by Hong Kong Innovation and Technology Fund (Project No. ITS/041/16), Guangdong province science and technology plan project (No. 2016A020220013).

References

1. Carpenter, A.E., et al.: Cellprofiler: image analysis software for identifying and quantifying cell phenotypes. Genome Biol. **7**(10), R100 (2006)
2. Chen, H., Qi, X., Yu, L., Dou, Q., Qin, J., Heng, P.A.: DCAN: deep contour-aware networks for object instance segmentation from histology images. Med. Image Anal. **36**, 135–146 (2017)
3. Cheng, J., Rajapakse, J.C., et al.: Segmentation of clustered nuclei with shape markers and marking function. IEEE Trans. Biomed. Eng. **56**(3), 741–748 (2009)
4. Dou, Q., et al.: 3D deeply supervised network for automated segmentation of volumetric medical images. Med. Image Anal. **41**, 40–54 (2017)
5. Friedman, J., Hastie, T., Tibshirani, R.: The Elements of Statistical Learning. Springer series in statistics, vol. 1. Springer, New York (2001). https://doi.org/10.1007/978-0-387-21606-5

6. Goldberger, J., Ben-Reuven, E.: Training deep neural-networks using a noise adaptation layer. In: ICLR 2017 (2017)
7. Huang, G., Liu, Z., Van Der Maaten, L., Weinberger, K.Q.: Densely connected convolutional networks. In: CVPR (2017)
8. Irshad, H., et al.: Crowdsourcing image annotation for nucleus detection and segmentation in computational pathology: evaluating experts, automated methods, and the crowd. In: Pacific Symposium on Biocomputing, pp. 294–305. World Scientific (2014)
9. Jiang, L., Zhou, Z., Leung, T., Li, L.J., Fei-Fei, L.: MentorNet: learning data-driven curriculum for very deep neural networks on corrupted labels. In: ICML (2018)
10. Jung, C., Kim, C.: Segmenting clustered nuclei using H-minima transform-based marker extraction andcontour parameterization. IEEE Trans. Biomed. Eng. **57**(10), 2600–2604 (2010)
11. Kazeminia, S., et al.: GANs for medical image analysis. arXiv preprint arXiv:1809.06222 (2018)
12. Kumar, N., Verma, R., Sharma, S., Bhargava, S., Vahadane, A., Sethi, A.: A dataset and a technique for generalized nuclear segmentation for computational pathology. IEEE Trans. Med. Imaging **36**(7), 1550–1560 (2017)
13. Lin, T.Y., Dollár, P., Girshick, R.B., He, K., Hariharan, B., Belongie, S.J.: Feature pyramid networks for object detection. In: IEEE CVPR (2017)
14. Liu, S., Qi, L., Qin, H., Shi, J., Jia, J.: Path aggregation network for instance segmentation. In: IEEE CVPR (2018)
15. Loshchilov, I., Hutter, F.: Fixing weight decay regularization in adam. arXiv preprint arXiv:1711.05101 (2017)
16. Macenko, M., et al.: A method for normalizing histology slides for quantitative analysis. In: IEEE ISBI (2009)
17. Oda, H., et al.: BESNet: boundary-enhanced segmentation of cells in histopathological images. In: Frangi, A.F., Schnabel, J.A., Davatzikos, C., Alberola-López, C., Fichtinger, G. (eds.) MICCAI 2018. LNCS, vol. 11071, pp. 228–236. Springer, Cham (2018). https://doi.org/10.1007/978-3-030-00934-2_26
18. Pantanowitz, L.: Digital images and the future of digital pathology. J. Pathol. Inform. **1**, 15 (2010)
19. Patrini, G., Rozza, A., Krishna Menon, A., Nock, R., Qu, L.: Making deep neural networks robust to label noise: A loss correction approach. In: IEEE CVPR (2017)
20. Reed, S., Lee, H., Anguelov, D., Szegedy, C., Erhan, D., Rabinovich, A.: Training deep neural networks on noisy labels with bootstrapping. arXiv preprint arXiv:1412.6596 (2014)
21. Ronneberger, O., Fischer, P., Brox, T.: U-Net: convolutional networks for biomedical image segmentation. In: Navab, N., Hornegger, J., Wells, W.M., Frangi, A.F. (eds.) MICCAI 2015. LNCS, vol. 9351, pp. 234–241. Springer, Cham (2015). https://doi.org/10.1007/978-3-319-24574-4_28
22. Schindelin, J., et al.: Fiji: an open-source platform for biological-image analysis. Nat. Methods **9**(7), 676 (2012)
23. Veta, M., et al.: Prognostic value of automatically extracted nuclear morphometric features in whole slide images of male breast cancer. Mod. Pathol. **25**(12), 1559 (2012)
24. Xue, C., Dou, Q., Shi, X., Chen, H., Heng, P.A.: Robust learning at noisy labeled medical images: applied to skin lesion classification (2019)
25. Yi, X., Walia, E., Babyn, P.: Generative adversarial network in medical imaging: a review. arXiv preprint arXiv:1809.07294 (2018)

Data-Driven Model Order Reduction for Diffeomorphic Image Registration

Jian Wang[1]([⊠]), Wei Xing[2], Robert M. Kirby[2], and Miaomiao Zhang[1]

[1] Computer Science and Engineering, Washington University in St. Louis,
St. Louis, MO, USA
jianw@wustl.edu
[2] Scientific Computing and Imaging Institute, University of Utah,
Salt Lake City, UT, USA

Abstract. This paper presents a data-driven model reduction algorithm to reduce the computational complexity of diffeomorphic image registration in the context of large deformation diffeomorphic metric mapping (LDDMM). In contrast to previous methods that repeatedly evaluate a full-scale regularization term governed by partial differential equations (PDEs) in the parameterized space of deformation fields, we introduce a reduced order model (ROM) to substantially lower the overall computational cost while maintaining accurate alignment. Specifically, we carefully construct the registration regularizer with a compact set of data-driven basis functions learned by proper orthogonal decomposition (POD), based on a key fact that the eigen spectrum decays extremely fast. This projected regularization in a low-dimensional subspace naturally leads to effective model order reduction with the underlying coherent structures well preserved. The iterative optimization involving computationally expensive PDE solvers is now carried out efficiently in a low-dimensional subspace. We demonstrate the proposed method in neuroimaging applications of pairwise image registration and template estimation for population studies.

1 Introduction

Diffeomorphic image registration has been successfully applied in the field of medical image analysis, as it maximally maintains the biological correctness of deformation fields in terms of object topology preservation. Examples of applications include alignment of functional data to a reference coordinate system [8,27], anatomical comparison across individuals [21,24], and atlas-based image segmentation [3,15]. The problem of image registration is often formulated as constrained optimization over the transformation that well aligns a source image and a target image. A plethora of transformation models to today fit into various categories of parameterizations, e.g., stationary velocity fields that remain constant over time [2], and time-varying velocity fields in the framework of LDDMM [6].

J. Wang and W. Xing—Authors contributed equally to the work.

A. C. S. Chung et al. (Eds.): IPMI 2019, LNCS 11492, pp. 694–705, 2019.
https://doi.org/10.1007/978-3-030-20351-1_54

We focus on the latter as it supports a distance metric in the space of diffeomorphisms that is critical for deformation-based statistical shape analysis, such as least squares mean estimator [15], geodesic regression [19,23], anatomical shape variability quantification [21], and groupwise geometrical shape comparison [24].

Despite the aforementioned advantages, one major challenge that hinders the widespread use of LDDMM is its high computational cost and large memory footprint [6,8,25]. The algorithm inference typically requires costly optimization, particularly on solving a full-scale regularization term defined on a dense image grid (e.g., a brain MRI with size of 128^3). Prior knowledge in the form of regularization is used to enforce the smoothness of transformation fields, also known as geodesic constraints in the space of diffeomorphisms, by solving a set of high-dimensional PDEs [17,25]. This makes iterative optimization approaches, such as gradient descent [6], BFGS [20], or the Gauss-Newton method [4], computationally challenging. While improved computational capabilities have led to a substantial run-time reduction, such solution of a single pairwise image registration still takes tens of minutes to finish on dense 3D image grids [23].

In this paper, we aim at an approximate inference method that significantly lowers the computational complexity with little to no impact on the alignment accuracy. Our solution is motivated by the observation that smooth vector fields in the tangent space of diffeomorphisms can be characterized by a low-dimensional geometric descriptor, including a finite set of control points [10], or Fourier basis functions representing low frequencies [28,29]. As a consequence, we hypothesize that the solution to high-dimensional PDE systems can be effectively approximated in a subspace with much lower dimensions. We develop a data-driven model reduction algorithm that constructs a low-dimensional subspace to approximate the original high-dimensional dynamic system for diffeomorphic image registration. We employ proper orthogonal decomposition (POD), a widely used technique for PDE systems, in which the approximating subspace is obtained from a discretized full-order model at selected time instances. A reduced-order model can then be constructed through Galerkin projection methods [9], where the PDEs are projected onto a compact set of POD eigenfunctions.

To the best of our knowledge, this method has not yet been applied to large systems of PDEs such as the one employed in diffeomorphic registration. While we focus on the context of LDDMM, the theoretical tools developed in this paper are broadly applicable to all PDE-constrained diffeomorphic registration models. To evaluate the proposed method, we perform image registration of real 3D MR images and show that the accuracy of our estimated results is comparable to the state of the art, while with drastically lower runtime and memory consumption. We also demonstrate this method in the context of brain atlas building (mean template estimation) for efficient population studies.

2   Background: PDE-Constrained Diffeomorphic Image Registration

In this section, we briefly review the LDDMM algorithm with PDE-constrained regularization [6,25]. Let S be the source image and T be the target image defined on a d-dimensional torus domain $\Gamma = \mathbb{R}^d/\mathbb{Z}^d$ ($S(x), T(x) : \Gamma \to \mathbb{R}$). The problem of diffeomorphic image registration is to find the shortest path to generate time-varying diffeomorphisms $\{\psi_t(x)\} : t \in [0,1]$ such that $S \circ \psi_1$ is similar to T, where $\circ$ is a composition operator that resamples S by the smooth mapping ψ_1. This is typically solved by minimizing an explicit energy function over the transformation fields ψ_t as

$$E(\psi_t) = \text{Dist}(S \circ \psi_1, T) + \text{Reg}(\psi_t), \tag{1}$$

where the distance function $\text{Dist}(\cdot, \cdot)$ measures the image dissimilarity. Commonly used distance functions include sum-of-squared difference of image intensities [6], normalized cross correlation [5], and mutual information [26]. The regularization term $\text{Reg}(\cdot)$ is a constraint that enforces the spatial smoothness of transformations, arising from a distance metric on the tangent space V of diffeomorphisms, i.e., an integral over the norm of time-dependent velocity fields $\{v_t(x)\} \in V$,

$$\text{Reg}(\psi_t) = \int_0^1 (Lv_t, v_t)\, dt, \quad \text{with} \quad \frac{d\psi_t}{dt} = -D\psi_t \cdot v_t, \tag{2}$$

where $L : V \to V^*$ is a symmetric, positive-definite differential operator that maps a tangent vector $v_t \in V$ into its dual space as a momentum vector $m_t \in V^*$. We typically write $m_t = Lv_t$, or $v_t = Km_t$, with K being an inverse operator of L. The notation $(\cdot, \cdot)$ denotes the pairing of a momentum vector with a tangent vector, which is similar to an inner product. Here, the operator D denotes a Jacobian matrix and $\cdot$ represents element-wise matrix multiplication.

A geodesic curve with a fixed end point is characterized by an extremum of the energy function (2) that satisfies the Euler-Poincaré differential (EPDiff) equation [1,17]

$$\frac{\partial v_t}{\partial t} = -K\left[(Dv_t)^T \cdot m_t + Dm_t \cdot v_t + m_t \cdot \text{div } v_t\right], \tag{3}$$

where div is the divergence. This process in Eq. (3) is known as *geodesic shooting*, stating that the geodesic path $\{\phi_t\}$ can be uniquely determined by integrating a given initial velocity v_0 forward in time by using the rule (3).

Therefore, we rewrite the optimization of Eq. (1) equivalently as

$$E(v_0) = \text{Dist}(S \circ \psi_1, T) + (Lv_0, v_0), \quad \text{s.t. Eq. (3)}. \tag{4}$$

As suggested in (4), solving the time-dependent and nonlinear registration problem requires a large number of time steps and iterations. A full-order model is not affordable in many-query or real-time context of clinical problems. For example, an image-guided navigation system that employs registration algorithms to identify residual brain tumor during the surgery [16].

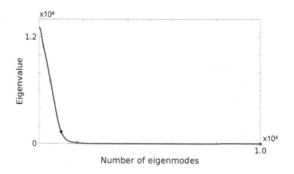

Fig. 1. An example eigenvalue plot of velocity fields generated from 2D synthetic data.

3 Our Model: Data-Driven Model Order Reduction of Diffeomorphic Image Registration

We develop a POD-based model order reduction algorithm, particularly for the registration regularization term governed by high-dimensional PDEs (EPDiff in Eq. (4)), to approximate a subspace via a given set of velocity fields in an optimal least-square sense. We then derive a Galerkin projection (orthogonal projection) of EPDiff equations onto the subspace to obtain a reduced-order model.

3.1 Low-Dimensional Subspace of Velocity Fields

Given a set of full-dimensional velocity fields $\{\mathbf{v}_t\} \in \mathcal{V}^q$, e.g., $q = 3 \times 128^3$ for a 3D discretized image grid with the size of 128^3, we are seeking an approximated subspace $\mathcal{U}^r = \mathrm{span}\{\mathbf{u}_1, \cdots, \mathbf{u}_r\} \subset \mathcal{V}^q$ ($r \ll q$), where $\mathbf{u}_i$ is the basis, to best characterize our data. A projection from such low-dimensional subspace to the original space can be effectively performed by $\mathbf{v}_t = \mathbf{U}\boldsymbol{\alpha}_t$, where $\mathbf{U}^{q \times r} = [\mathbf{u}_1, \cdots, \mathbf{u}_r]$ and $\boldsymbol{\alpha}_t$ is a r-dimensional vector representing factor coefficients. Here, we require the basis vectors to be orthonormal, i.e., $\mathbf{U}^T\mathbf{U} = \mathbf{I}$. The inverse projection can thus be written as $\boldsymbol{\alpha}_t = \mathbf{U}^T\mathbf{v}_t$. Our objective is to minimize the projection error defined in the tangent space of diffeomorphisms

$$\arg \min_{\mathbf{U}} \int (\mathbf{L}(\mathbf{v}_t - \mathbf{U}\boldsymbol{\alpha}_t), \mathbf{v}_t - \mathbf{U}\boldsymbol{\alpha}_t) \, dt. \tag{5}$$

where $\mathbf{L}$ is the discrete operator of L defined in Eq. (2). The minimization problem of Eq. (5), is the classic problem known as Karhunen-Loève decomposition or principal component analysis, and holds an equivalent solution to the following eigen decomposition problem of a covariance matrix $\mathbf{C}^{q \times q}$ [18,22],

$$\mathbf{C}\mathbf{u}_i = \lambda_i \mathbf{u}_i, \text{ with } \mathbf{C} = \int \mathbf{L}(\mathbf{v}_t - \bar{\mathbf{v}})(\mathbf{v}_t - \bar{\mathbf{v}})^T dt,$$

where $\bar{\mathbf{v}} = \int \mathbf{v}_t dt$ is the mean field, and the basis $\mathbf{u}_i, i \in \{1, \cdots, r\}$ corresponds to the i-th eigenvector of $\mathbf{C}$ with associated eigenvalue λ_i. In practice, the covariance is empirically computed by a finite set of M observations (snapshots) over the full-scale dynamic system of $\mathbf{v}_t$, i.e., $\mathbf{C} \approx \frac{1}{M} \sum_{t=1}^{M} \mathbf{L}(\mathbf{v}_t - \bar{\mathbf{v}})(\mathbf{v}_t - \bar{\mathbf{v}})^T$.

Due to a key fact that the spectrum of eigenvalues decays incredibly fast (as shown in Fig. 1), we propose to use an optimal set of eigen-functions to form the projected subspace of velocity fields. An explicit way thus to formulate the projection error in Eq. (5) is

$$\sum_{i=r+1}^{q} \lambda_i, \text{ with } \lambda_1 > \cdots > \lambda_r \cdots > \lambda_q.$$

This closed-form solution provides an elegant way to measure the projection loss $e = 1 - (\sum_{i=1}^{r} \lambda_i / \sum_{i=1}^{q} \lambda_i)$, where r is typically chosen such as $e < 0.01$ [12, 18].

3.2 Reduced-Order Regularization via Galerkin Projection

As introduced in the previous section, we developed a method to estimate a low-dimensional subspace of velocity fields that uniquely determines the geodesics of diffeomorphisms. We are now ready to construct a reduced-order model of image registration, subject to complex regularizations governed by high-dimensional PDEs (i.e., EPDiff). This procedure is known as *Galerkin projection* and has been widely used to reduce the high computational complexity of PDEs, or ODEs [12, 13, 18].

Consider the EPDiff in Eq. (3), we characterize a velocity field $\mathbf{v}_t$ by projecting it onto a finite-dimensional subspace $\mathcal{U}^r$ with much compact basis $\{\mathbf{u}_1, \cdots, \mathbf{u}_r\}$. To simplify the notation, we drop the time index t of velocity fields in remaining sections. A discretized formulation of EPDiff equation in terms of matrix multiplication is

$$\frac{\partial \mathbf{v}}{\partial t} = -\mathbf{K} \left(\mathrm{diag}(\mathbf{Lv})\mathbf{D}^T\mathbf{v} + \mathrm{diag}(\mathbf{v})\mathbf{D}(\mathbf{Lv}) + \mathrm{diag}(\mathbf{Lv}) \, \mathrm{div} \, \mathbf{v} \right),$$

$$= -\mathbf{K} \sum_{i=1}^{q} \left(\mathrm{diag}(\mathbf{l}_i)v_i\mathbf{D}^T\mathbf{v} + v_i\mathbf{DLv} + \mathrm{diag}(\mathbf{l}_i)v_i \, \mathrm{div} \, \mathbf{v} \right),$$

$$= -\mathbf{K} \sum_{i=1}^{q} \left(\mathrm{diag}(\mathbf{l}_i)\mathbf{D}^T + \mathbf{DL} + \mathrm{diag}(\mathbf{l}_i) \, \mathrm{div} \right) v_i\mathbf{v}, \tag{6}$$

where $\mathbf{v}$ is a q-dimensional vector, and $\mathrm{diag}(\cdot)$ converts a vector to a diagonal matrix. The matrices $\mathbf{L}^{q \times q}$, $\mathbf{K}^{q \times q}$, $\mathbf{D}^{q \times q}$, and $\mathbf{div}^{q \times q}$ denote discrete analogs of the differential operator L with its inverse K, Jacobian matrix D, and divergence div obtained by finite difference schemes respectively. Here, $\mathbf{l}_i$ is the i-th column of the matrix $\mathbf{L}$ and v_i is the i-th element of vector $\mathbf{v}$.

By defining a composite operator $\mathbf{A}_i^{q \times q} \triangleq \mathbf{K}(\mathrm{diag}(\mathbf{l}_i)\mathbf{D}^T + \mathbf{DL} + \mathrm{diag}(\mathbf{l}_i) \, \mathbf{div})$, we write Eq. (6) as

$$\frac{\partial \mathbf{v}}{\partial t} = \sum_{i=1}^{q} \mathbf{A}_i v_i \mathbf{v}. \tag{7}$$

Next, we derive a reduced-order model of EPDiff via Galerkin projection by plugging $\mathbf{v} = \mathbf{U}^{q \times r} \boldsymbol{\alpha}$ into Eq. (7). We then have

$$\frac{\partial \mathbf{U} \boldsymbol{\alpha}}{\partial t} = \sum_{i=1}^{q} \mathbf{A}_i (\mathbf{U} \boldsymbol{\alpha})_i \mathbf{U} \boldsymbol{\alpha},$$

$$\frac{\partial \boldsymbol{\alpha}}{\partial t} = \mathbf{U}^T \sum_{i=1}^{q} \mathbf{A}_i (\sum_{j=1}^{r} \mathbf{U}_{ij} \alpha_j) \mathbf{U} \boldsymbol{\alpha} = \sum_{j=1}^{r} \sum_{i=1}^{q} \mathbf{U}^T \mathbf{A}_i \mathbf{U} \mathbf{U}_{ij} \alpha_j \boldsymbol{\alpha} \triangleq \sum_{j=1}^{r} \tilde{\mathbf{A}}_j \alpha_j \boldsymbol{\alpha}, \quad (8)$$

where $\mathbf{U}_{ij}$ the element of $\mathbf{U}$ in the i-th row and j-th column. Here, we define $\tilde{\mathbf{A}}_j^{r \times r} = \sum_{i=1}^{q} \mathbf{U}^T \mathbf{A}_i \mathbf{U} \mathbf{U}_{ij}$ as a reduced-order model operator of A_j. It is worthy to mention that the computation of $\tilde{\mathbf{A}}_i$ is a one-time cost accomplished offline. No further update is needed once a proper subspace is sought. Solution to this reduced-order model can be found by employing commonly used temporal differential schemes, e.g., Euler or Runge-Kutta Method, with an initial condition $\boldsymbol{\alpha}_0 = \mathbf{U}^T \mathbf{v}_0$.

4   ROM for Diffeomorphic Image Registration

In this section, we present a reduced-order model of LDDMM algorithm with geodesic shooting for diffeomorphic image registration. We run gradient descent on a projected initial velocity, represented by the loading coefficient $\boldsymbol{\alpha}_0$, entirely in a low-dimensional subspace. A geodesic path consequently generates a flow of diffeomorphisms by Eq. (2) after constructing the time-dependent velocity fields back in its original space using $\mathbf{v}_t = \mathbf{U} \boldsymbol{\alpha}_t$.

The redefined energy function of LDDMM in Eq. (4) with sum-of-squared dissimilarity between images is

$$E(\boldsymbol{\alpha}_0) = \frac{1}{2\sigma^2} \|S \circ \psi_1 - T\|_2^2 + (\mathbf{L} \boldsymbol{\alpha}_0, \boldsymbol{\alpha}_0), \quad s.t. \text{ Eq. (8)}. \quad (9)$$

Here, we adopt a commonly used Laplacian operator $\mathbf{L} = (-\beta \Delta + \mathbf{I})^c$, where β is a positive weight parameter, c controls the level of smoothness, and $\mathbf{I}$ is an identity matrix.

Analogous to solving the optimal control problems in [28], we compute the gradient term by using a forward-backward sweep scheme. Below are the general steps for gradient computation (please refer to Algorithm 1 for more details):

(i) Compute the gradient $\nabla_{\boldsymbol{\alpha}_1} E$ of the energy (9) at $t = 1$ by integrating both the diffeomorphism ψ_t and the projected velocity field α_t forward in time, i.e.,

$$\nabla_{\boldsymbol{\alpha}_1} E = \mathbf{K} \left(\frac{1}{\sigma^2} (S \circ \psi_1 - T) \cdot \nabla(S \circ \psi_1) \right). \quad (10)$$

(ii) Bring the gradient $\nabla_{\boldsymbol{\alpha}_1} E$ back to $t = 0$. We obtain $\nabla_{\boldsymbol{\alpha}_0} E$ by integrating reduced adjoint Jacobi field equations [7] backward in time as

$$\frac{d\hat{\alpha}}{dt} = -\text{ad}_\alpha^\dagger \hat{h}, \quad \frac{d\hat{h}}{dt} = -\hat{\alpha} - \text{ad}_\alpha \hat{h} + \text{ad}_{\hat{h}}^\dagger \alpha, \quad (11)$$

where ad† is an adjoint operator and $\hat{h}, \hat{\alpha} \in V$ are introduced adjoint variables with an initial condition $\hat{h} = 0, \hat{\alpha} = \nabla_{\boldsymbol{\alpha}_1} E$ at $t = 1$.

Algorithm 1. Optimization of Reduced order model for diffeomorphic image registration

---

Input: source image S, target image T
/* Online optimization */
1   Initialize $\boldsymbol{\alpha}_0 = 0$;
2   **repeat**
    /* Forward shooting of $\boldsymbol{\alpha}_0$ */
3 | forward integrate the reduced-order model of EPDiff equation (8) to generate $\{\boldsymbol{\alpha}_t\}$ at discrete time points;
    /* Compute the diffeomorphic transformations ψ_t */
4 | integrate the transformation fields ψ by using (2) after constructing velocity fields back to the original space via $\mathbf{v}_t = \mathbf{U}^T \boldsymbol{\alpha}_t$;
    /* Compute gradient at time point $t = 1$ */
5 | compute the gradient $\nabla_{\boldsymbol{\alpha}_1} E$ by (10);
    /* Propagate gradient back to time point $t = 0$ */
6 | integrate the reduced adjoint Jacobi field equations (11) backward in time to obtain $\nabla_{\boldsymbol{\alpha}_0} E$.
7 | Update $\boldsymbol{\alpha}_0 \leftarrow \boldsymbol{\alpha}_0 - \varepsilon \nabla_{\boldsymbol{\alpha}_0} E$, where ε is the step size;
8   **until** *convergence*;

---

5   Experimental Evaluation

To demonstrate the effectiveness of our proposed model, we compare its performance with the state-of-the-art vector momentum LDDMM [23] in applications of pairwise image registration and atlas building. For fair comparison, we use $\beta = 3, c = 6$ for the L operator, and $\sigma = 0.01$ with 10 time-steps for Euler integration across all baseline algorithms.

Data. We applied the algorithm to 3D brain MRI scans from a public released resource Open Access Series of Imaging Studies (OASIS) for Alzheimer's disease [11]. The data includes fifty healthy subjects as well as disease, aged 60 to 96. To better evaluate the estimated transformations, we employed another fifty 3D brain MRI scans with manual segmentations from Alzheimer's Disease Neuroimaging Initiative(ADNI) [14]. All MRIs are of dimension $128 \times 128 \times 128$ with the voxel size of $1.25 \,\mathrm{mm}^3$. The images underwent downsampling, skull-stripping, intensity normalization, bias field correction and co-registration with affine transformation.

Experiments. We first tested our algorithm for pairwise image registration at different levels of projected dimension $r = 4^3, 8^3, 12^3, 20^3$ and compared the total energy formulated in Eq. (9). In order to find an optimal basis, we ran parallel programs of the full-scale EPDiff equation in (3) and generated a collection of snapshots to perform POD effectively. Since the learning process of basis functions were conducted offline with one-time cost for all experiments, we only focused on the exact runtime, memory consumption, and convergence rate of our model after the fact.

We validated registration results by examining the accuracy of propagated delineations for cortex (Cor), caudate (Caud), and corpus collusum (CC). After aligning all volumes to a reference image, we transformed the manual segmentation from the reference to other volumes by using the estimated deformations. We evaluated dice similarity coefficient (volume overlap) between the propagated segmentation and the manual segmentation for each structure.

We also ran both our method and the baseline algorithm to build an atlas from a set of 3D brain MRIs. We initialized the template image as an average of image intensities, and set the projected dimension as $r = 20^3$ as that was shown to be optimal in our eigen plots. In this experiment, we used a message passing interface (MPI) parallel programming implementation for all methods, and distributed data on four processors in total.

Results. Figure 2 reports the total energy in formulation (9) averaged over 10 random selected pairs of test images for different values of projected dimensions. Our method arrives at the same solution at $r = 12^3$ and higher, which indicates that the estimated subspace has fairly recovered the result of full-scale registration algorithms. Figure 2 also provides runtime and memory consumption across all three methods, including the baseline algorithm vector momemtum LDDMM. Our algorithm has substantially lower computational cost than vector momentum LDDMM performed in a full-dimensional space.

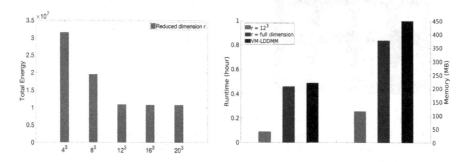

Fig. 2. Left: average total energy for different values of projected dimensions $r = 4^3, 8^3, 12^3, 16^3, 20^3$. Right: exact runtime and memory consumption for all methods.

Figure 3 reports segmentation volume overlap on different brain structures, estimated from both our method and the baseline algorithm. It show that our algorithm is able to achieve comparable results, while offering significant improvements in computational efficiency. The right panel of Fig. 3 illustrates results for an example case from the study. We observe that the delineations

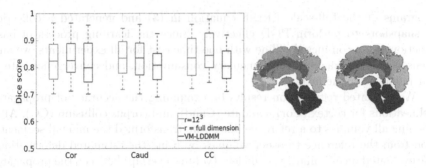

Fig. 3. Left: volume overlap between manual segmentations and propagated segmentations of three important regions cortex (Cor), caudate (Caud), and corpus collusum (CC); Middle: example ground truth segmentation; Right: propagated segmentation with three structures obtained by our method. 2D slices are shown for visualization only, all computations are carried out fully in 3D.

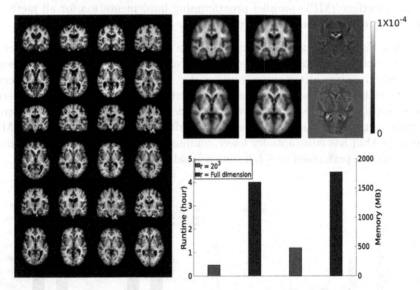

Fig. 4. Left: axial view and coronal view of twelve example brain MRIs selected from dataset. Right top: atlas images estimated by our method and vector momentum LDDMM with difference map shown by side. Right bottom: a comparison of exact runtime and memory consumption.

achieved by transferring manual segmentations from the reference frame to the coordinate system of the target frame align fairly well with the manual segmentations. The left panel of Fig. 4 shows the axial and coronal slices from 12 of the selected 3D MRI dataset. The right panel demonstrates the atlas image estimated by our algorithm, followed by the atlas estimated by vector momenta LDDMM. The difference image between the two atlas results shows that our

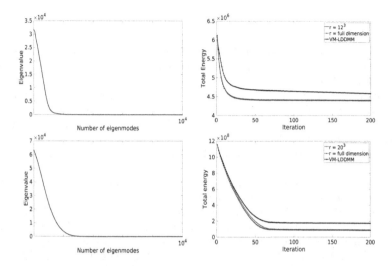

Fig. 5. Top to bottom: results of pairwise image registration vs. atlas building. Left to right: eigenvalue spectrum of velocity fields vs. total energy with an optimal projected dimension, a full dimension of our method, and vector momemtum LDDMM.

algorithm generated a very similar atlas to vector momenta LDDMM, but at a fraction of the time and memory cost (as illustrated on the right bottom panel of Fig. 4).

Figure 5 shows the eigenvalue spectrum and convergence plot for both image registration (top) and atlas building (bottom). It is clear to see that our method conducted in a low-dimensional space is able to arrive at the same solution as the full dimensional scenario. We outperform the baseline algorithm vector momentum LDDMM, i.e., lower energy at the optimal solution.

6   Conclusion

We presented a data-driven model reduction algorithm for diffeomorphic image registration in the context of LDDMM with geodesic shooting. Our method is the first to simulate the high-dimensional dynamic system of diffeomorphisms in an approximated subspace via proper orthogonal decomposition and Galerkin projection. This approach substantially reduces the computational cost of diffeomorphic registration algorithms governed by high-dimensional PDEs, while preserving comparative accuracy. The theoretical tools developed in this paper are broadly applicable to all PDE-constrained diffeomorphic registration models with gradient-based optimization.

Acknowledgments. This work is supported by DARPA TRADES HR0011-17-2-0016.

References

1. Arnol'd, V.I.: Sur la géométrie différentielle des groupes de Lie de dimension infinie et ses applications à l'hydrodynamique des fluides parfaits. Ann. Inst. Fourier **16**, 319–361 (1966)
2. Arsigny, V., Commowick, O., Pennec, X., Ayache, N.: A Log-Euclidean framework for statistics on diffeomorphisms. In: Larsen, R., Nielsen, M., Sporring, J. (eds.) MICCAI 2006. LNCS, vol. 4190, pp. 924–931. Springer, Heidelberg (2006). https://doi.org/10.1007/11866565_113
3. Ashburner, J., Friston, K.J.: Unified segmentation. Neuroimage **26**(3), 839–851 (2005)
4. Ashburner, J., Friston, K.J.: Diffeomorphic registration using geodesic shooting and gauss-newton optimisation. NeuroImage **55**(3), 954–967 (2011)
5. Avants, B.B., Epstein, C.L., Grossman, M., Gee, J.C.: Symmetric diffeomorphic image registration with cross-correlation: evaluating automated labeling of elderly and neurodegenerative brain. Med. Image Anal. **12**(1), 26–41 (2008)
6. Beg, M.F., Miller, M.I., Trouvé, A., Younes, L.: Computing large deformation metric mappings via geodesic flows of diffeomorphisms. Int. J. Comput. Vis. **61**(2), 139–157 (2005)
7. Bullo, F.: Invariant affine connections and controllability on lie groups. Technical report, technical Report for Geometric Mechanics, California Institute of Technology (1995)
8. Christensen, G.E., Rabbitt, R.D., Miller, M.I.: Deformable templates using large deformation kinematics. IEEE Trans. Image Process. **5**(10), 1435–1447 (1996)
9. Cockburn, B., Shu, C.W.: TVB Runge-Kutta local projection discontinuous Galerkin finite element method for conservation laws. II. General framework. Math. Comput. **52**(186), 411–435 (1989)
10. Durrleman, S., Prastawa, M., Gerig, G., Joshi, S.: Optimal data-driven sparse parameterization of diffeomorphisms for population analysis. In: Székely, G., Hahn, H.K. (eds.) IPMI 2011. LNCS, vol. 6801, pp. 123–134. Springer, Heidelberg (2011). https://doi.org/10.1007/978-3-642-22092-0_11
11. Fotenos, A.F., Snyder, A., Girton, L., Morris, J., Buckner, R.: Normative estimates of cross-sectional and longitudinal brain volume decline in aging and AD. Neurology **64**(6), 1032–1039 (2005)
12. Hajek, B., Wong, E.: Stochastic processes in information and dynamical systems (1989)
13. Holmes, P., Lumley, J.L., Berkooz, G., Rowley, C.W.: Turbulence, Coherent Structures, Dynamical Systems and Symmetry. Cambridge University Press, Cambridge (2012)
14. Jack Jr., C.R., et al.: The Alzheimer's disease neuroimaging initiative (ADNI): MRI methods. J. Magn. Reson. Imaging: Official J. Int. Soc. Magn. Reson. Med. **27**(4), 685–691 (2008)
15. Joshi, S., Davis, B., Jomier, M., Gerig, G.: Unbiased diffeomorphic atlas construction for computational anatomy. NeuroImage **23**, S151–S160 (2004)
16. Luo, J., et al.: A feature-driven active framework for ultrasound-based brain shift compensation. arXiv preprint arXiv:1803.07682 (2018)
17. Miller, M.I., Trouvé, A., Younes, L.: Geodesic shooting for computational anatomy. J. Math. Imaging Vis. **24**(2), 209–228 (2006). https://doi.org/10.1007/s10851-005-3624-0

18. Newman, A.J.: Model reduction via the Karhunen-Loeve expansion part I: an exposition. Technical report (1996)
19. Niethammer, M., Huang, Y., Vialard, F.-X.: Geodesic regression for image time-series. In: Fichtinger, G., Martel, A., Peters, T. (eds.) MICCAI 2011. LNCS, vol. 6892, pp. 655–662. Springer, Heidelberg (2011). https://doi.org/10.1007/978-3-642-23629-7_80
20. Polzin, T., Niethammer, M., Heinrich, M.P., Handels, H., Modersitzki, J.: Memory efficient LDDMM for lung CT. In: Ourselin, S., Joskowicz, L., Sabuncu, M.R., Unal, G., Wells, W. (eds.) MICCAI 2016. LNCS, vol. 9902, pp. 28–36. Springer, Cham (2016). https://doi.org/10.1007/978-3-319-46726-9_4
21. Qiu, A., Younes, L., Miller, M.I.: Principal component based diffeomorphic surface mapping. IEEE Trans. Med. Imaging **31**(2), 302–311 (2012)
22. Shah, A., Xing, W., Triantafyllidis, V.: Reduced-order modelling of parameter-dependent, linear and nonlinear dynamic partial differential equation models. Proc. Math. Phys. Eng. Sci. **473**(2200) (2017)
23. Singh, N., Hinkle, J., Joshi, S., Fletcher, P.T.: A vector momenta formulation of diffeomorphisms for improved geodesic regression and atlas construction. In: International Symposium on Biomedial Imaging (ISBI), April 2013
24. Vaillant, M., Miller, M.I., Younes, L., Trouvé, A.: Statistics on diffeomorphisms via tangent space representations. NeuroImage **23**, S161–S169 (2004)
25. Vialard, F.X., Risser, L., Rueckert, D., Cotter, C.J.: Diffeomorphic 3D image registration via geodesic shooting using an efficient adjoint calculation. Int. J. Comput. Vis. **97**(2), 229–241 (2012)
26. Wells, W., Viola, P., Atsumi, H., Nakajima, S., Kikinis, R.: Multi-modal volume registration by maximization of mutual information. Med. Image Anal. **1**, 35–51 (1996)
27. Zhang, M., Singh, N., Fletcher, P.T.: Bayesian estimation of regularization and atlas building in diffeomorphic image registration. In: Gee, J.C., Joshi, S., Pohl, K.M., Wells, W.M., Zöllei, L. (eds.) IPMI 2013. LNCS, vol. 7917, pp. 37–48. Springer, Heidelberg (2013). https://doi.org/10.1007/978-3-642-38868-2_4
28. Zhang, M., Fletcher, P.T.: Finite-dimensional lie algebras for fast diffeomorphic image registration. In: Ourselin, S., Alexander, D.C., Westin, C.-F., Cardoso, M.J. (eds.) IPMI 2015. LNCS, vol. 9123, pp. 249–260. Springer, Cham (2015). https://doi.org/10.1007/978-3-319-19992-4_19
29. Zhang, M., et al.: Frequency diffeomorphisms for efficient image registration. In: Niethammer, M., et al. (eds.) IPMI 2017. LNCS, vol. 10265, pp. 559–570. Springer, Cham (2017). https://doi.org/10.1007/978-3-319-59050-9_44

DGR-Net: Deep Groupwise Registration of Multispectral Images

Tongtong Che[1], Yuanjie Zheng[1,2](✉), Xiaodan Sui[1], Yanyun Jiang[1],
Jinyu Cong[1], Wanzhen Jiao[3], and Bojun Zhao[3]

[1] School of Information Science and Engineering, Shandong Normal University,
Jinan 250358, China
zhengyuanjie@gmail.com
[2] Key Lab of Intelligent Computing and Information Security
in Universities of Shandong, Shandong Provincial Key Laboratory
for Novel Distributed Computer Software Technology, Institute of Biomedical
Sciences, Shandong Normal University, Jinan 250358, China
[3] Department of Ophthalmology, Shandong Provincial Hospital,
Shandong University, Jinan 250021, China

Abstract. Groupwise registration of multispectral images (MSI) is clinically essential to facilitate accurate information fusion across different modalities. However, the groupwise registration of multispectral images is a challenging task because multiple different imaging modalities makes it difficult to jointly optimize the deformation. In this work, we propose an unbiased deep groupwise registration framework, DGR-Net, which takes a complete consideration of the information aggregated by calculating the deformation of the sequence image. Our framwork guided by principal component analysis (PCA) image. Network optimization is accelerated by combining internal smoothing and external correlation of the deformation fields. Experimental results have shown that, the proposed method can achieve promising accuracy and efficiency for the challenging multi-modality groupwise registration task and also outperforms the state-of-the-art approaches.

Keywords: Deep groupwise registration · Joint optimization ·
Principal component analysis · Multispectral images

1 Introduction

Image registration is a key stage in image fusion, change detection and super-resolution imaging, among others. The goal is to establish the best spatial correspondences between warped source image and target image. It is of great help to doctors diagnose the disease, both in terms of time and precision. In recent years, there is an increasing interest in simultaneously aligning more than two images using groupwise registration to provide more useful information. For example, MSI sequence images from different wavelengths contain different information.

A. C. S. Chung et al. (Eds.): IPMI 2019, LNCS 11492, pp. 706–717, 2019.
https://doi.org/10.1007/978-3-030-20351-1_55

However, the image-to-image spatial misalignment is caused by object movement during scanning. Computer-based groupwise registration algorithms can effectively align a set of images to help doctors diagnose.

There are many registration algorithms have been proposed in the past decades. Traditionally, feature-based methods [6] and area-based methods [1] have received much attention. However, computational complexity of these methods is higher with the increase of transformation complexity. Furthermore, the most of registration algorithms are performed by a pair of images, the source image is only one. Simultaneous registration of multiple images has become more and more popular in recent years because it can provide more useful information and make unbiased analysis of population data. In the research of group registration, a variety of groupwise registration algorithms have been proposed, including the method of template selection [11] which based on a single image in a group, the approach of the pairwise estimate [21] which accumulate all possible pairwise estimates of images in the group and the algorithm of average template [12] which iteratively calculate the group mean image and accumulate mean squared differences to compare every image in the group to the average image. However, these methods prone to introduce a bias towards the content of the selected template and lead to excessive computational load. Furthermore, most of these methods are only available for mono-modal images. In case of large inter-subject variations, it is difficult to register multiple faraway subjects with different anatomical structures.

Since recently, numerous researchers address image registration problems based on deep learning approaches. In deep learning-based registration, existing general methods can only solve pairwise registration. There are several deep registration approaches, including the supervised training approaches based on ground-truth deformation fields [14,22] and unsupervised training approaches [20] which learns to register images by directly optimizing a similarity metric between the template and the moving images. These methods solve the registration of a pair of mono-modal images. For multi-modal registration, some researchers have explored unsupervised network to learn similarity metrics [4,7]. Based on our previous research [19], unsupervised convolutional neural networks were used to achieve groupwise registration of mono/multi-modal sequence images from multispectral images (MSI). In this paper, this method is called DGR-Net1 as a variant of DGR-Net. Although this method achieves a good alignment of a set of images, it is easy to cause the aligned images to be biased and the convergence speed is slow. There are two factors that lead to this phenomenon. (1) The deformation fields corresponding to each image are independent. During the training, only the smoothness constraints inside the single deformation field are considered, and the correlation between the deformation fields is neglected. (2) Some high-dimensional features are lost when the deformation field is calculated based on the encoder-decoder. To overcome the above limitation, we use deep learning based method to optimize groupwise registration problem of MSI images which simultaneously aligning more than two images from different modalities.

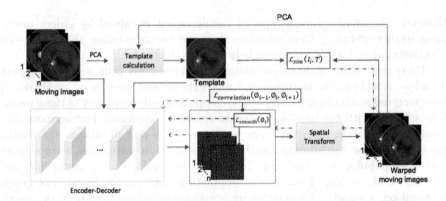

Fig. 1. Schematic illustration for our proposed DGR-Net. The network that does not use the correlation constraint (represented by the red box) between the deformation fields is called DGR-Net1. Conversely, it is called DGR-Net2. The input are N moving images $I_1, I_2 \ldots, I_N$ in a group and a template image which generated by PCA. The output are N warped images. (Color figure online)

In this paper, we propose a novel robust groupwise registration method, DGR-Net, based on joint optimization guided by PCA. This framework takes a group of moving images and template image based on PCA as inputs, and outputs warped moving images. Joint optimization of deformation field is employed to align all images in a group simultaneously. The proposed method is validated on MSI registration and the experimental results demonstrate that our method outperforms the conventional algorithm with remarkable speed and precision. The novelty of DGR-Net is that:

(1) In order to control the unbiased alignment of all images at the fastest convergence speed, we combine the internal smoothness constraints of the deformation field with the correlation between different deformation fields.
(2) We proposed a new end-to-end network based on ResNet and U-Net as encoder-decoder which effectively combine the features from shallow and deep layers through multi-path information confusion to optimize the deformation field quickly.
(3) To improve the speed and accuracy of groupwise registration, we use a deep unsupervised network to iteratively update representative template images based on PCA.

2   Methods

2.1   Problem Description

Suppose there are N images $\{I_1, I_2 \ldots, I_N\}$ to be registered in a group and the images come from different modalities. To register these images into a common coordinate frame, we can define a template image T which by PCA as common

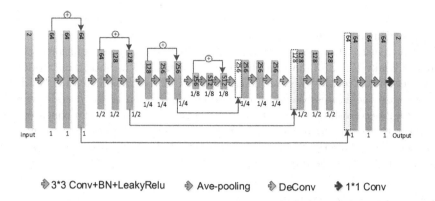

Fig. 2. The detailed network architecture of DGR-Net. The network with ResNet is called DGR-Net2, otherwise it is called DGR-Net1. Each blue box corresponds to a multi-channel feature map. The number of channels is denoted top of the box and the number below the box indicates the size of the feature map as a percentage of the input image. (Color figure online)

reference frame. The ultimate goal of this work is to propose a tractable deep framework for registering I_i with optimal deformation fields ϕ_i to warped moving images $I'_i = I_i \circ \phi_i$ by iteratively registering N images to the latest estimated template image T. Based on this method, the similarity of all images in the group is optimized at the fastest convergence speed possible.

2.2   The Architecture of DGR-Net

Figure 1 presents an overview of proposed DGR-Net which contains two variants, DGR-Net1 and DGR-Net2. The DGR-Net1 has been validated in previous work to simultaneously align N mono/multi-modal images with good registration accuracy. DGR-Net2 reduces time consumption and ensure unbiased registration of all images while improving registration accuracy. Given N scans, we initialize the template image by PCA and obtaining deformation fields based on encoder-decoder. Subsequently, update the representative template image iteratively until all the images are well aligned to the latest template image adaptively. In Fig. 1, the solid arrows indicate the forward propagation of the network. The dashed arrows denote the back propagation of the network that adjust the network parameters to update the deformation fields.

The network for deformation fields calculation is approximated as an encoder-decoder is not trained with known registration transformations, as shown in Fig. 2. It take a single input formed by concatenating a moving image I_i in a group and template image T. In more detail, the architecture of the proposed DGR-Net is based on Res-Net [8] and U-net [17]. In the encoder, we create a Res-Net-style network with 4 blocks of 3×3 convolutional layers which combine the features from shallow and deep layers by use the deformed residual unit of

ResNet. We exploit 2×2 average pooling operation with stride 2 for downsampling which reduce the spatial dimensions while preventing useless parameters from increasing time complexity. Furthermore, we apply convolutions followed by the Leaky ReLU [3] and batch normalization (BN) in both the encoder and decoder stage. Notably, we use the Leaky ReLU activations instead of ReLU [16] to increase the expressiveness of our model. Every step in the decoder consists of a 2×2 deconvolution layer, two 3×3 convolution layers and a concatenation connect the feature map extracted at the encoder to the new feature maps in the decoder to directly generate the registration. The output of the decoder, ϕ_i, is the same size as the input image.

2.3   Template Calculation

The focus of group registration is to deform each image to a common space which is the key to groupwise registration. Consider the superior performance of PCA in the center of all population data, thus obtaining a representative template image data dimensionality reduction. We combine PCA with deep learning to generate a template image containing the principal component information of N images in a group. We consider each pixel as a observation and the different images are taken as different variables. The PCA is used to reduce the dimension to a one-dimensional subspace. The eigenvector $V = (w_1, w_2, w_3 \ldots w_N)$ associated with the largest eigenvalue can serve as the weights w for the construction of the template image $T(x) = \sum_{i=1}^{N} w_i(I_i \circ \phi_i(x))$.

2.4   Transformation Optimization

The DGR-Net iteratively update deformation fields by maximizing similarity between warped moving image $I_i \circ \phi_i$ and current template image T. We transform I_i into the space of T by a differentiable spatial transformation operation which based on spatial transformer networks [9]. Explain further, deform image M_i into template T by composing the mapping $I'_i = I_i \circ \phi_i$. Additionally, for each pixel p, we compute a pixel location $\phi(p)$ in I_i. Bilinear interpolation is applied to spatial transformation and is defined as:

$$I'_i = I_i \circ \phi_i = \sum_{q \in \{p + \phi(p)\}} M_i(q) \prod_{d \in \{x,y\}} (1 - |\phi_d(p) - q_d|) \qquad (1)$$

Where $\{p + \phi(p)\}$ denote the 4-pixel neighborhood around the location $p + \phi(p)$. d indicates two directions in 2D image space. Since the spatial transformation operation we defined is differentiable, the registration parameters are optimized by backpropagation.

The target of DGR-Net is to calculate a common template image to transform the original moving images onto a correct template space. In order to guide the network to gradually become better during training, DGR-Net1 supervises training by maximizing the similarity L_{sim} between the current template image and the moving image and controlling the smoothness of the single deformation field L_{smooth}. The difference from DGR-Net1 is that DGR-Net2 constrains the correlation between different deformation fields while controlling the smoothness of a single deformation field. Based on this paradigm, joint optimization of all deformation fields is achieved to speed up convergence. Also, such constraint could guide the network to focus on the correct direction of deformation under all image, and help eliminate any possible paranoia. The objective function of loss layer is as follows:

$$L = -L_{sim}(T^{pca}, M_i \circ \phi_i) + L_{smooth}(\phi_i) + L_{correlation}(\phi_{i-1}, \phi_i, \phi_{i+1}) \quad (2)$$

Where the first term L_{sim} is a similarity metric quantifying the cost of the registration by deformation field ϕ_i. Particularly, the template image T^{pca} is computed by PCA of the current warped moving images in a group. The second term L_{smooth} is a smoothness constraint which constraining the deformation field. The last term $L_{correlation}(\phi_{i-1}, \phi_i, \phi_{i+1}$ denotes the correlation between the deformation fields corresponding to the N images which ensure joint optimization of the deformation fields. Since multispectral images are multimodal images, we embed mutual information (MI) into the DGR-Net to calculate the similarity. L_{sim} is defined as:

$$L_{sim} = argmax_{\phi_i, I_i}(H(T^{pca}) + H(I_i \circ \phi_i) - H(T^{pca}, I_i \circ \phi_i)) \quad (3)$$

Here, $H(T^{pca})$ and $H(I_i \circ \phi_i)$ refer to, respectively, the marginal entropy of template image and warped moving image. $H(T^{pca}, I_i \circ \phi_i)$ is the joint entropy of template image and warped moving image. A higher L_{sim} indicates a better alignment and we calculate L_{sim} efficiently using convolutional operations over $M_i \circ \phi_i$ and T^{pca}. Each warped moving image I' gradually to approximate iteratively optimized template image by maximizing the image similarity L_{sim}. The parameters of the encoder-decoder are continuously adjusted by the back-propagation dissimilarity $-L_{sim}$ between moving image and template image using stochastic gradient descent (SGD). Additionally, L_{smooth} constrain the smoothness of the deformation field ϕ_i is defined as:

$$L_{smooth} = \lambda_1 \|\nabla^2 \phi\|^2 + \lambda_2 \|\phi\|^2 \quad (4)$$

Where the two regularization parameters λ_1, λ_2 are empirically set to $\lambda_1 = 0.5$, $\lambda_1 = 0.01$ which control the internal smoothness of deformation field. Since the encoder-decoder outputs a plurality of independent deformation fields, it is prone to a certain deformation deviation. We set a constraint between different deformation fields which learn the correlation to supervise the correctness of each deformation. This correlation constraint is set to:

$$L_{correlation} = min(\phi_{i-1} + \phi_{i+1} - 2\phi_i) \quad (5)$$

Where $\phi_{i-1}, \phi_i, \phi_{i+1}$ are three deformation fields corresponding to three adjacent moving images, respectively, and $L_{correlation}$ is cycle-consistent $\phi_{i-1}, \phi_i, \phi_{i+1}$ for 3-cycle.

3   Dataset and Configuration

3.1   Data Description

We conducted multi-modal deformable groupwise registration experiments on a set of multispectral images taken from an Annidis RHA (Annidis Health Systems Corp Ottawa, Canada). RHA is based on multispectral imaging. The monochromatic LED source produces monochromatic slices at 11 wavelengths (550 nm to 850 nm) for comprehensive assessment of the retina from shallow to deep (RPE) and choroid. However, spatial misalignment of sequence images occurs due to the eye saccade movement being faster than the MSI image acquisition speed. This dataset consists of oculus dexter (OD) and oculus sinister (OS) from 40 healthy subjects and 100 patients with fundus lesions. The dataset adds 880 images compared to our previous work. In order to improve the robustness of the training model, we also made three rotate ($90°, 180°, 270°$) and two flipped (left-right, up-down) variants on the dataset for data enhancement. All images were resized from the original image size of 2048×2048 to 512×512 to accommodate network training. We split our dataset into 12320, 1540 and 1540 volumes for train, validation, and test sets, respectively. For all test images, the optic, vascular and significant points in MSI are manually labeled by ophthalmologist and used for final quantitative evaluation.

3.2   Experimental Settings

We initialize the template image based on a linear combination of a set of images resulting from PCA. Subsequently, N moving images are sequentially paired with the template image as input to DGR-Net. These moving images were anatomically corresponding slices from the same subject but acquired at different depths of the retina. We use PyTorch [13] with cuDNN library for deep learning to train the network. The learning rate was set to $1e^{-3}$ for the initial training stage and $1e^{-8}$ for the fine-tuning training stage. The network were trained on four NVIDIA Tesla V100 GPUs. Additionally, we train separate networks with different λ values until convergence. DGR-Net was eventually trained 5,000 iterations.

3.3   Evalution Metric

In this work, to evaluate the registration results of DGR-Net. We use three metrics, including (1) Dice Similarity Coefficient (DSC) [5], (2) Ratio of registration (Ratio) [23] and (3) Target Registration Error (TRE) [15].

DSC measures the overlap ratio between any two MSI corresponding retinal vessel maps in a group, and the final average Dice score of each structure is calculated over all subjects, defined as $DSC = \frac{2 \times \|V_{I'_i}^r \cap V_{I'_j}^r\|}{\|V_{I'_i}^r\| + \|V_{I'_j}^r\|}$. Here, $V_{I'_i}^r$ and $V_{I'_j}^r$ represent the set of pixels of anatomic structure r for two images after registration, while $\| \cdot \|$ denotes the cardinality of a set.

Ratio measures the average distance between manually-labeled points in each MSI image of after registration and the other images correspondence, defined as $Ratio = \frac{Q(d(I_i'(S_k)),(I_j'(S_k))<t)}{15C_N^2}$. It is worth noting that pathologist manually pick 15 points and then annotated them based on MRIcron [18] for each test image and the registration is considered to be correct when the average distance divided by the radius of the retinal (1035 pixels in our experiment) is below a threshold. Q denotes the number of points where the distance between the corresponding points between any two images is less than the threshold. $\{S_k|k \in [1,15]\}$ represents the set of manually labeled points.

TRE was used as a measure for the error of the registration with ground truth annotations of certain anatomical landmarks in the test images, defined as $TRE = \|I_{i,k}' - I_{j,k}'\|$. Here, $I_{i,k}', I_{j,k}'$ represents the kth anatomic structure from the ith image and the jth image, Respectively. Similar to DSC, the final average TRE value of each structure is calculated over all subjects.

4 Results and Analysis

4.1 Methods for Comparison

(1) We first compare our DGR-Net with two baseline methods. First, the group-wise registration is implemented by iteratively constructing the group mean image and estimating the deformation fields of all subjects towards the estimated tentative group mean image (AMI) [12]. We implement group mean image based to register each image to the latest estimated group mean image. Second, the groupwise registration is implemented by the individual template selection (ITS) based method. The MSI groupwise registration is implemented by ITS which exploit the MSI images acquired at 550 nm with the highest sharpness as the template image and register images acquired at other wavelengths to this template image. The experiments was implemented by DGR-Net without template calculation.

(2) Then we compare our method with three state-of-the-art pairwise registration methods, including two mainstream traditional registration algorithms Affine [10] and SyN [2] and a deep learning based registration algorithm DIRNet [20].

(3) In addition, we further compare DGR-Net with two variants, called DGR-Net1 and DGR-Net2, respectively. Specifically, DGR-Net1 without $L_{correlation}$ and ResNet block. That is, DGR-Net1 is actually using a simple U-Net in encoder-decoder and the Loss layer has no correlation between different deformation fields. DGR-Net2 uses both internal and external constraints to achieve joint optimization of the deformation fields. Furthermore, DGR-Net2 use a end-to-end network based on ResNet and U-Net for deformation field.

It is worth noting that, all of the above registration methods use mutual information (MI) as a metric of similarity metrics.

4.2   Performance Comparison

We evaluate the effectiveness of the proposed DGR-Net in groupwise registration experiments on the new large MSI dataset. In Table 1, we report the experimental results achieved by the proposed DGR-Net and five comparison methods. And Fig. 3 shows the mean image before and after registration by 7 different methods. The high precision and performance of the proposed DGR-Net can be analyzed from three perspectives.

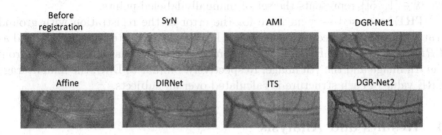

Fig. 3. Visualization results of MSI registration achieved by 7 different methods. These partial images denote mean image of all subjects after registration

Table 1. Evaluation result for groupwise registration of MSI. Comparison of Dice, Ratio and TRE of registration for these methods listed above and DGR-Net. For Ratio, the threshold values (t) are set to 0, 0.05, and 0.1, respectively.

Metric	Dice		Ratio			TRE	
	Optic	Vascular	$t=0$	$t=0.05$	$t=0.1$	Optic	Vascular
Affine	0.834 ± 0.072	0.412 ± 0.057	0.59	0.65	0.68	3.22 ± 0.31	4.13 ± 0.36
SyN	0.877 ± 0.051	0.653 ± 0.061	0.64	0.76	0.79	2.70 ± 0.37	3.61 ± 0.39
DIRNet	0.863 ± 0.035	0.658 ± 0.065	0.64	0.72	0.80	2.48 ± 0.28	3.10 ± 0.33
AMI	0.932 ± 0.031	0.726 ± 0.035	0.69	0.75	0.78	2.42 ± 0.24	3.12 ± 0.35
ITS	0.934 ± 0.049	0.729 ± 0.057	0.72	0.78	0.80	2.03 ± 0.21	2.60 ± 0.21
DGR-Net1	0.968 ± 0.032	0.734 ± 0.043	0.73	0.86	0.91	1.78 ± 0.19	2.49 ± 0.18
DGR-Net2	$\mathbf{0.971 \pm 0.029}$	$\mathbf{0.752 \pm 0.047}$	**0.76**	**0.88**	**0.92**	$\mathbf{1.73 \pm 0.14}$	$\mathbf{2.43 \pm 0.28}$

Template Evaluation. The core of group registration is to find an unbiased template image and register other images into the system space where the image resides. We compared DGR-Net2 based on PCA and group average image (AMI) as templates. The sharpness of the template during training is shown in the Fig. 4. We can see that PCA-based DGR-Net2 has far more clarity than AMI in 3000 iterations. This implies that our method begins with a clear PCA image as shown in the second row of Fig. 4, which is close to the population center. The slow convergence of the groupwise registration due to the lack of clear and consistent information from the fuzzy group mean image to guide the registration. Combined with Table 1, we found that the fuzzy group mean image fails to

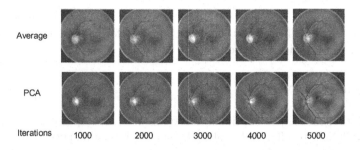

Fig. 4. In the group registration in which the template image is interpreted as PCA and the template image is interpreted as a group average image, the sharpness of the template image is compared during training.

provide clear guidance to the subsequent pairwise registrations and leads to the loss of anatomical details which can be hardly recovered from the initial fuzzy group mean image.

Deformation Constraint Analysis and Computational Cost. Although our previous work DGR-Net1 achieved group registration of MSI, compared to DGR-Net2, the loss layer has no correlation constraint between deformation fields. From Table 1, the performance of groupwise registration produced by DGR-Net2 outperforms DGR-Net1. This is because the correlation constraint between the deformation fields guides the correct calculation of all deformations and thus avoids any possible bias. Besides, we compared the computational time of DGR-Net2 with DGR-Net1 during training. The convergence of DGR-Net1 requires nearly 3,000 iterations, and DGR-Net2 converges in less than 1800 iterations. It is clear that DGR-Net2 achieved much faster convergence speed. There are two reasons for this. First, the correlation constraint can always control the moving image to be warped to the center of the set of images so as to quickly increase the convergence speed. Second, ResNet and U-Net based encoder-decoder can effectively prevent gradient degradation and make all deformation fields efficiently optimized.

Comparisons with State-of-the-Art Techniques. The registration results for vascular are very low due to the particularity of the vascular structure and the uneven distribution. The average Dice value of before registration is 0.236 ± 0.034. By comparing the results of our DGR-Net with other classic registration methods, we can make the following observations. First, the experimental results achieved by DGR-Net shows the best accuracy, which indicates that, joint alignment outperforms pairwise registration. Second, PCA-based groupwise registration is superior to the groupwise registration based on group average image and a single image in the group. As a major reason, the PCA image considers the principal component information of a set of MSI sequence images fairly and comprehensively. The visualization results implies that the proposed

DGR-Net improves the algorithm performance, by deep learning-based method iteratively updates the template image. Especially for DGR-Net2, the alignment of all images is particularly precise.

5 Conclusion

We have proposed a joint optimization framework of deep group-wise registration (DGR-Net) to effectively solve the spatial misalignments introduced into sequential MSI images. In order to improve the overall registration performance of the whole population, we construct an unbiased deep groupwise registration method based on PCA. Besides, DGR-Net contains two variants, DGR-Net1 and DGR-Net2. On the basis of DGR-Net1, DGR-Net2 adds the external smoothness constraint deformation fields (the correlation between deformation fields). Moreover, combining ResNet and U-Net to obtain effective deformation fields enable a robust registration model at the fastest convergence speed. Experimental results on 140 subjects with MSI from funds images suggest that DGR-Net is superior to several state-of-the-art methods in both registration precision and computational cost. In future work, we will extend DGR-Net to the 3D network architecture and use DGR-Net to solve image group registration problems in other areas (CT, MRI, remote sensing images, etc.).

References

1. Althof, R.J., Wind, M.G., Dobbins, J.T.: A rapid and automatic image registration algorithm with subpixel accuracy. IEEE Trans. Med. Imaging **16**(3), 308–316 (1997)
2. Avants, B.B., Epstein, C.L., Grossman, M., Gee, J.C.: Symmetric diffeomorphic image registration with cross-correlation: evaluating automated labeling of elderly and neurodegenerative brain. Med. Image Anal. **12**(1), 26–41 (2008)
3. Bing, X., Wang, N., Chen, T., Mu, L.: Empirical evaluation of rectified activations in convolutional network. Computer Science (2015)
4. Cao, X., Yang, J., Wang, L., Xue, Z., Wang, Q., Shen, D.: Deep learning based inter-modality image registration supervised by intra-modality similarity. In: Shi, Y., Suk, H.-I., Liu, M. (eds.) MLMI 2018. LNCS, vol. 11046, pp. 55–63. Springer, Cham (2018). https://doi.org/10.1007/978-3-030-00919-9_7
5. Dice, L.R.: Measures of the amount of ecologic association between species. Ecology **26**(3), 297–302 (1945)
6. Goshtasby, A., Stockman, G.C.: Point pattern matching using convex hull edges. IEEE Trans. Syst. Man Cybern. (5), 631–637 (1985)
7. Hanaizumi, N., Fujimur, S.: An automated method for registration of satellite remote sensing images. In: International Geoscience and Remote Sensing Symposium, IGARSS 1993, Better Understanding of Earth Environment, vol. 3, pp. 1348–1350 (1993)
8. He, K., Zhang, X., Ren, S., Jian, S.: Deep residual learning for image recognition. In: IEEE Conference on Computer Vision and Pattern Recognition (2016)
9. Jaderberg, M., Simonyan, K., Zisserman, A., Kavukcuoglu, K.: Spatial transformer networks, pp. 2017–2025 (2015)

10. Jenkinson, M., Smith, S.: A global optimisation method for robust affine registration of brain images. Med. Image Anal. **5**(2), 143–156 (2001)
11. Jia, H., Yap, P.T., Wu, G., Wang, Q., Shen, D.: Intermediate templates guided groupwise registration of diffusion tensor images. NeuroImage **54**(2), 928–939 (2011)
12. Joshi, S., Davis, B., Jomier, M.G.: Unbiased diffeomorphic atlas construction for computational anatomy. Neuroimage **23**(1), S151–S160 (2004)
13. Ketkar, N.: Introduction to PyTorch. In: Ketkar, N. (ed.) Deep Learning with Python, pp. 195–208. Apress, Berkeley (2017). https://doi.org/10.1007/978-1-4842-2766-4_12
14. Liao, R., et al.: An artificial agent for robust image registration (2016)
15. Polfliet, M., Klein, S., Huizinga, W., Paulides, M.M., Niessen, W.J., Vandemeulebroucke, J.: Intrasubject multimodal groupwise registration with the conditional template entropy. Med. Image Anal. **46**, 15–25 (2018)
16. Nair, V., Hinton, G.E.: Rectified linear units improve restricted Boltzmann machines. In: International Conference on International Conference on Machine Learning (2010)
17. Ronneberger, O., Fischer, P., Brox, T.: U-net: convolutional networks for biomedical image segmentation. In: Navab, N., Hornegger, J., Wells, W.M., Frangi, A.F. (eds.) MICCAI 2015. LNCS, vol. 9351, pp. 234–241. Springer, Cham (2015). https://doi.org/10.1007/978-3-319-24574-4_28
18. Rorden, C., Brett, M.: Stereotaxic display of brain lesions. Behav. Neurol. **12**(4), 191–200 (2000)
19. Che, T., et al.: Deep group-wise registration for multi-spectral images from fundus images. In: IEEE Access (2019)
20. de Vos, B.D., Berendsen, F.F., Viergever, M.A., Staring, M., Išgum, I.: End-to-end unsupervised deformable image registration with a convolutional neural network. In: Cardoso, M.J., et al. (eds.) DLMIA/ML-CDS -2017. LNCS, vol. 10553, pp. 204–212. Springer, Cham (2017). https://doi.org/10.1007/978-3-319-67558-9_24
21. Wachinger, C., Wein, W., Navab, N.: Three-dimensional ultrasound mosaicing. In: Ayache, N., Ourselin, S., Maeder, A. (eds.) MICCAI 2007. LNCS, vol. 4792, pp. 327–335. Springer, Heidelberg (2007). https://doi.org/10.1007/978-3-540-75759-7_40
22. Wulff, J., Black, M.J.: Efficient sparse-to-dense optical flow estimation using a learned basis and layers. In: Computer Vision and Pattern Recognition, pp. 120–130 (2015)
23. Zhao, B., et al.: Joint alignment of multispectral images via semidefinite programming. Biomed. Opt. Express **8**(2), 890 (2017)

Efficient Interpretation of Deep Learning Models Using Graph Structure and Cooperative Game Theory: Application to ASD Biomarker Discovery

Xiaoxiao Li[1](✉), Nicha C. Dvornek[2], Yuan Zhou[2], Juntang Zhuang[1], Pamela Ventola[3], and James S. Duncan[1,2,4,5]

[1] Biomedical Engineering, Yale University, New Haven, CT, USA
xiaoxiao.li@yale.edu
[2] Radiology and Biomedical Imaging, Yale School of Medicine, New Haven, CT, USA
[3] Child Study Center, Yale School of Medicine, New Haven, CT, USA
[4] Electrical Engineering, Yale University, New Haven, CT, USA
[5] Statistics and Data Science, Yale University, New Haven, CT, USA

Abstract. Discovering imaging biomarkers for autism spectrum disorder (ASD) is critical to help explain ASD and predict or monitor treatment outcomes. Toward this end, deep learning classifiers have recently been used for identifying ASD from functional magnetic resonance imaging (fMRI) with higher accuracy than traditional learning strategies. However, a key challenge with deep learning models is understanding just what image features the network is using, which can in turn be used to define the biomarkers. Current methods extract biomarkers, i.e., important features, by looking at how the prediction changes if "ignoring" one feature at a time. However, this can lead to serious errors if the features are conditionally dependent. In this work, we go beyond looking at only individual features by using Shapley value explanation (SVE) from cooperative game theory. Cooperative game theory is advantageous here because it directly considers the interaction between features and can be applied to any machine learning method, making it a novel, more accurate way of determining instance-wise biomarker importance from deep learning models. A barrier to using SVE is its computational complexity: 2^N given N features. We explicitly reduce the complexity of SVE computation by two approaches based on the underlying graph structure of the input data: (1) only consider the centralized coalition of each feature; (2) a hierarchical pipeline which first clusters features into small communities, then applies SVE in each community. Monte Carlo approximation can be used for large permutation sets. We first validate our methods on the MNIST dataset and compare to human perception. Next, to insure plausibility of our biomarker results, we train a Random Forest (RF) to classify ASD/control subjects from fMRI and compare SVE results to standard RF-based feature importance. Finally, we show initial results on ranked fMRI biomarkers using SVE on a deep learning classifier for the ASD/control dataset.

© Springer Nature Switzerland AG 2019
A. C. S. Chung et al. (Eds.): IPMI 2019, LNCS 11492, pp. 718–730, 2019.
https://doi.org/10.1007/978-3-030-20351-1_56

1   Introduction

Autism spectrum disorder (ASD) affects the structure and function of the brain. To better target the underlying roots of ASD for diagnosis and treatment, efforts to identify reliable biomarkers are growing [1]. Deep learning models have been used in fMRI analysis [2], which is used to characterize the brain changes that occur in ASD [3]. However, how the different brain regions coordinate on the deep convolutional neural network (DNN) has not been previously explored. When features are not independent, Shapley value explanation (SVE) is a useful tool to study each feature's contribution [4–6]. The methods are based on fundamental concepts from cooperative game theory [7], which assigns a unique distribution (among the players) of a total surplus generated by the coalition of all players in the cooperative game. However, if the interactive features' dimensions are high, SVE becomes computationally consuming (exponential time complexity).

The innovations of this study include: (1) We applied SVE on interactive features' prediction power analysis; (2) Our proposed method does not require retraining the classifier; (3) To handle the high dimensional inputs of the DNN classifier, we propose two methods to reduce the dimension of SVE testing features, once the underlying graph structure of features is defined; and (4) Different from kernel SHAP proposed in [4], as a model interpreter, our proposed methods do not require model approximation. In Sect. 2, we introduce the background on cooperative game theory. In Sect. 3, we propose the two approaches to approximate Shapley value. We also show the approximation is true under certain assumptions. Three experiments are given in Sect. 4 to show the feasibility and advantage of our proposed methods.

2   Background on Cooperative Game Theory

2.1   Shapley Value

Our approach to analyzing the contributions of individual nodes to the overall network is the assignment of Shapley values. The Shapley value is a means of fairly portioning the collective profit attained by a coalition of players, based on the relative contributions of the players in some game. Let $\mathcal{N} = \{1, 2, \ldots, N\}$ be the set of all the players, $S \subset \mathcal{N}$ be a subset of players forming a coalition within this game, and $v : 2^{\mathcal{N}} \to \mathbb{R}$ be the function that assigns a real numbered profit to the subset S of players. By definition, for any v, $v(\varnothing) = 0$, here $\varnothing$ is the empty set. A Shapley value is assigned by a Shapley function $\Phi : \mathcal{N} \to \mathbb{R}$, which associates each player in $\mathcal{N}$ with a real number and which is uniquely defined by the following axioms [7]: 1. *Efficiency*; 2. *Symmetry*; 3. *Dummy*; and 4. *Additivity*. In our context, we are interested in the brain regions that discriminate ASD and control subjects. Classification prediction score is the total value to be distributed, and each brain region is a player, which will be assigned a unique reward (i.e. importance score) by its contribution to the classifier.

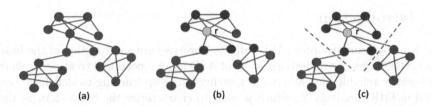

Fig. 1. (a) Toy visualization of graph structure of the input data. When estimating the contribution of feature r (yellow), (b) C-SVE considers r's directly connected neighbors (red) and (c) H-SVE considers the community (red) to which r belongs. (Color figure online)

2.2 Challenges of Using Shapley Value

While Shapley values give a more accurate interpretation of the importance of each player in a coalition, their calculation is expensive. When the number of features (i.e., players in the game) is a massive N, the computational complexity is 2^N, which is especially expensive if the model is slow to run. We propose addressing this computational challenge by utilizing the graph structure of the data. Consider the case when the underlying graph structure of the data is sparsely connected, e.g., the sparse brain functional network. Under this observation, we propose two approaches (Fig. 1) to simplify Shapley value calculation. *Method I* only considers the centralized coalition of each player to reduce the number of permutation cases by assigning weight 0 to features that rarely collaborate. *Method II* first applies community detection on the feature connectivity network to cluster similar features (forming different games and teams), then within the selected communities, assigns a feature's contribution by SVE.

3   Methods

In classification tasks, only certain features in a given input provide evidence for the classification decision. For a given prediction, the classifier assigns a relevance value to each input feature with respect to a class label $Y \in \mathcal{C}$. The probability of class Y for input $\boldsymbol{X} = (X_1, X_2, \ldots, X_N)$ is given by the predictive score of the DNN model $f : \mathcal{D} \to \mathbb{R}^{|\mathcal{C}|}$ where $\mathcal{D}$ is the domain for input X and each component of the output of f represents the conditional probability of assigning a class label, i.e. $p(Y|\boldsymbol{X})$.

The basic idea used in prediction difference analysis [8] is that the relevance of a feature x_i can be estimated by measuring how the prediction changes if the feature is unknown. Here we extend this setting by considering the interaction of a set of different features instead of examining the features one by one. Denote the image corrupted at a feature set $S \subseteq \mathcal{N}$ as $\boldsymbol{X}_{\mathcal{N} \setminus S}$. To calculate $p(Y|\boldsymbol{X}_{\mathcal{N} \setminus S})$, following [8], we marginalize out the corrupted feature set S:

$$p(Y|\boldsymbol{X}_{\mathcal{N} \setminus S}) = \mathbb{E}_{\boldsymbol{X}_S \sim p(\boldsymbol{X}_S | \boldsymbol{X}_{\mathcal{N} \setminus S})} p(Y|\boldsymbol{X}_{\mathcal{N} \setminus S}, \boldsymbol{X}_S). \tag{1}$$

Denote v_X the importance score evaluation function for input X. The prediction power for the rth feature is the weighted sum of all possible marginal contributions:

$$\Phi_r(v_X) = \frac{1}{|\mathcal{N}|} \sum_{S \subseteq \mathcal{N} \backslash \{r\}} \binom{|\mathcal{N}| - 1}{|S|}^{-1} (v_X(S \cup \{r\}) - v_X(S)). \qquad (2)$$

Similar to [5], we introduce the *importance score* of a feature set S

$$v_X(S) := \mathbb{E}_Y[-\log \frac{1}{p(Y|X)}|X] - \mathbb{E}_Y[-\log \frac{1}{p(Y|X_{\mathcal{N}\backslash S})}|X], \qquad (3)$$

which can be interpreted as the negative of the expected number of bits required to encode the output of the model based on the input $X_{\mathcal{N}\backslash S}$.

Theorem 1. $\langle \mathcal{N} = \{1, 2, \ldots, N\}, v_X \rangle$ *is a cooperative form game and* $\Phi(v_X) = (\Phi_1, \Phi_2, \ldots, \Phi_N)$ *corresponds to the game's Shapley value.*

The proof can be directly borrowed from [6] showing it has a unique solution and satisfies Axioms 1–4.

An illustrative example is Boolean logic expression, $\mathrm{OR}((x_1, x_2)) = 1$ when x_1 or x_2 is one and zero otherwise for $\mathcal{N} = \{1, 2\}$, $\mathcal{D} = \{0, 1\} \times \{0, 1\}$. Suppose $p(Y = 1|X) = \mathrm{OR}(X)$ and the base of the logarithm is 2. We aim to find the contributions of predicting 1 given input $X = (1, 1)$. If both values of X are unknown, one can predict that the probability of the result being 1 is $\frac{3}{4}$. We have $v_X(\varnothing) = 0 - (-\log \frac{1}{1}) = 0$, $v_X(\{1\}) = v_X(\{2\}) = 0 - (-\log(\frac{1}{1})) = 0$ and total value $v_X(\{1, 2\}) = 0 - (-\log \frac{4}{3}) = \log \frac{4}{3}$. Therefore the contributions of each feature are: $\Phi_1 = \frac{1}{2}[(v_X(\{1\}) - v_X(\varnothing)) + (v_X(\{1, 2\}) - v_X(\{2\}))] = \frac{1}{2}[(0 - 0) + (\log \frac{4}{3} - 0)] = \frac{1}{2} \log \frac{4}{3}$ and $\Phi_2 = \frac{1}{2}[(v_X(\{2\}) - v_X(\varnothing)) + (v_X(\{1, 2\}) - v_X(\{1\}))] = \frac{1}{2}[(0 - 0) + (\log \frac{4}{3} - 0)] = \frac{1}{2} \log \frac{4}{3}$. The generated contributions reveal that both features contribute the same amount towards the prediction being 1 given input $(1, 1)$. In addition, we can interpret there is coalition between the two players, since $v_X(\{1, 2\}) > v_X(\{1\}) + v_X(\{2\})$. However, we will get the myopic conclusion that both features are unimportant by only ignoring a single feature, because given one feature $X_i = 1$, $p = 1$ is for sure.

With the underlying structure of data, we have prior knowledge that some features of the data set are barely connected; in other words, there is very likely no coalition between these features. We define a connected graph $\mathcal{G} = (\mathcal{V}, \mathcal{E})$ with nodes $\mathcal{V}$ and edges $\mathcal{E}$. Given an adjacency matrix $\mathcal{A} = (a_{ij})$ of the undirected graph $\mathcal{G}$ (for example, the Pearson correlation of mean time series of brain regions), we use a threshold th to binarize a_{ij}, i.e. $a_{ij}^b = 1$ when $a_{ij} > th$ and zero otherwise, resulting in a sparsely connected graph.

3.1   Method I: Centralized Shapley Value Explanation (C-SVE)

For a given feature i, its 1-step connected *neighborhood* is defined by the set $\mathcal{N}_i := \{j \in \mathcal{V} | a_{ij}^b = 1\}$. As an approximation, we propose Centralized Shapley

Value Explanation (C-SVE), which only calculates the marginal contribution when a feature collaborates with its neighbors.

Definition 1. *Given classifier f and sample $\boldsymbol{X}$, the C-SVE assigns the prediction power on feature r by*

$$\hat{\Phi}_r^C(v_{\boldsymbol{X}}) = \frac{1}{|\mathcal{N}_r|} \sum_{S \subseteq \mathcal{N}_r \setminus \{r\}} \binom{|\mathcal{N}_r| - 1}{|S|}^{-1} (v_{\boldsymbol{X}}(S \cup \{r\}) - v_{\boldsymbol{X}}(S)). \tag{4}$$

The coefficients in front of the marginal contributions is a weighted transformation of the original SVE form (in Eq. (2)), where instead of assigning each permutation the same weight, sets not belonging to the *neighborhood* were assigned 0 weight. In practice, we can reject the non-coalition permutations and average the Shapley values for the remaining terms.

Theorem 2. *We have $\hat{\Phi}_{\boldsymbol{X}}^C(r) = \Phi_{\boldsymbol{X}}(r)$ almost surely if we have $X_r \perp \boldsymbol{X}_{\mathcal{N} \setminus \mathcal{N}_r} |$ $\boldsymbol{X}_U$ and $X_r \perp \boldsymbol{X}_{\mathcal{N} \setminus \mathcal{N}_r} | \boldsymbol{X}_U, Y$ for any $U \subset \mathcal{N}_r \setminus \{r\}$.*

The proof is shown in Appendix A. It is important to show that our proposed approximation is a good one. We can easily check the necessary condition that for $k \notin \mathcal{N}_r$, the angle between the average time series $\bar{X}_r$ in ROI r and $\bar{X}_k$ in ROI k satisfies $\cos(\bar{X}_r, \bar{X}_k) < \epsilon$, which corresponds to the small edge weight (~ 0) in the graph that we created using Pearson correlation.

3.2 Method II: Hierarchical Shapley Value Explanation (H-SVE)

In method II, we approximate the Shapley value by a hierarchical approach: (1) detect communities in the graph, then (2) apply SVE in each community individually.

Modularity-Based Community Detection. We use the same undirected graph architecture defined in *Method I*, but use *greedy modularity method* [9] to divide all the features into non-overlapping communities. Then the whole features sets can be expressed by a combination of non-overlapping communities $\mathcal{N} = A_1 \bigcup A_2 \bigcup \cdots \bigcup A_M$ and the features in one community only cooperate within the group, hence are independent to those in the different communities. Therefore we can define different Shapley value rules in the different communities, but the Shapley values are comparable within and across communities.

Shapley Value of Each Feature in the Community. With the assumption that different communities of players do not play in a game (rarely connect), we assume the communities of features are independent. In order to compare the feature importance in the whole brain, firstly we define the Shapley value for feature subset S in community A_i as

$$v_{\boldsymbol{X}}(S) := \mathbb{E}_Y[-\log \frac{1}{p(Y|\boldsymbol{X}_{A_i})} | \boldsymbol{X}_{A_i}] - \mathbb{E}_Y[-\log \frac{1}{p(Y|\boldsymbol{X}_{A_i \setminus S})} | \boldsymbol{X}_{A_i}]. \tag{5}$$

Algorithm 1. Approximating the prediction power of rth feature's value Φ_r

> **Input:** X, a given instance; m, number of samples; v, importance score function
> 1: $\Phi_r \leftarrow 0$
> 2: **for** $j = 1$ to m **do**
> 3:   choose a random permutation of features $O \in \pi(\mathcal{N}_r)$
> 4:   choose a random instance $\hat{X}$ from the training dataset
> 5: $v_1 \leftarrow v(\tau(X, \hat{X}, Pre^r(O) \bigcup \{r\}))$
> 6: $v_2 \leftarrow v(\tau(X, \hat{X}, Pre^r(O)))$
> 7: $\Phi_r \leftarrow \Phi_r + (v_1 - v_2)$
> 8: **end for**
> 9: $\Phi_r \leftarrow \frac{\Phi_r}{m}$
> (where $\mathcal{N}$ is the neighborhood of r in C-SVE or community of r in H-SVE)

Definition 2. *Suppose the features are clustered into* $\mathcal{N} = A_1 \bigcup A_2 \bigcup \cdots \bigcup A_M$. *The H-SVE assigns the prediction power of feature* r *in* A_i *by*

$$\hat{\Phi}_r^H(v_X) = \frac{1}{|A_i|} \sum_{S \subseteq A_i \setminus \{r\}} \binom{|A_i| - 1}{|S|}^{-1} (v_X(S \cup \{r\}) - v_X(S)). \qquad (6)$$

Theorem 3. *When* $X_{A_1} \perp X_{A_2} \perp \cdots \perp X_{A_M}$, *we have* $\hat{\Phi}_r^H(v_X) = \Phi_r(v_X)$ *almost surely.*

The proof is similar to the proof for *Theorem* 2.

3.3 Monte Carlo Approximation for Large Neighborhood

Although we simplify SVE by C-SVE or H-SVE methods, computation may still be challenging. For example: (1) in C-SVE, feature node r to be analyzed is densely connected with the other nodes and (2) in H-SVE, there exists large communities. Based on the alternative formulation of the Shapley value (Eq. (7)), let $\pi(\mathcal{N})$ be the set of all ordered permutations of $\mathcal{N}$. Let $Pre^r(O)$ be the set of players which are predecessors of player r in the order $O \in \pi(\mathcal{N})$, we have

$$\Phi_r(v_X) = \frac{1}{|\mathcal{N}|!} \sum_{O \in \pi(\mathcal{N})} (v_X(Pre^r(O) \cup \{r\}) - v_X(Pre^r(O))). \qquad (7)$$

We use the following Monte Carlo (MC) algorithm to approximate Eqs. (4) and (6). We define:

$$\tau(x, \hat{x}, S) = (z_1, z_2, \ldots, z_s), \quad z_i = \begin{cases} x_i; & i \in S \\ \hat{x}_i; & i \notin S \end{cases}. \qquad (8)$$

Then the unbiased MC approximation can be expressed as in Algorithm 1. Given m, if $2^{|\mathcal{N}(r)|} \gg m$, we will apply MC approximation.

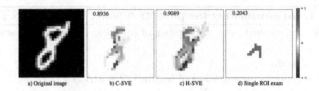

a) Original image   b) C-SVE   c) H-SVE   d) Single ROI exam

Fig. 2. The predictive power for identifying (a) the digit 8 by (b) C-SVE, (c) H-SVE, and (d) single ROI explanation. The prediction difference after corrupting the ROIs which contribute 90% in total are denoted on the left corner.

4   Experiments and Results

4.1   Validation on MNIST Dataset

In order to show the feasibility of the proposed two approaches, we test the explanation results on MNIST dataset [10], where we can compare to human judgment about the feature importance. We trained a convolutional network (Conv2D(32) → Conv2D(64) → Dense(128) → Dense(10)) achieving 97.32% accuracy. We parcellate the image into ROIs using *slic* [11] to mimic the setting of detecting saliency brain ROI for identifying ASD. Denoting the distance between the center of ROI i and ROI j as d_{ij}, we define the connection between ROI i and j as $a_{ij} = exp(-d_{ij}/2)$. Here we use $th = \frac{\sum_i \sum_j a_{ij}}{|\mathcal{E}|}$. The results are shown in Fig. 2, where we uniformly divided each ROI's importance score by the number of pixels in the ROI to mitigate dominance by large ROIs and divided by $\max_{i \in \mathcal{N}}(\Phi_i)$ for visualization. The interpretation results matched our human perception that the "*x cross*" shape in the center is important for recognizing digit 8. Compared with single ROI testing, our proposed methods assigned smoother and more widely distributed importance scores to more pixels. To examine the effect of important ROIs on prediction, we corrupted pixels whose importance power added up to 90% of the positive importance scores. We then compared the difference between the original prediction probability of digit 8 and the new prediction probability using the corrupted image. C-SVE and H-SVE could better fool the classifier, which decreased the prediction probability by 0.8939 and 0.9089 respectively, compared to only a 0.2043 decrease for the single ROI method. Some ROIs may not contribute to classification on their own but influence the results when combined with other regions. In the single ROI method, these ROIs will be assigned 0 importance score. However, by our proposed SVE method these ROIs can be discovered.

4.2   ASD Task-fMRI Dataset and Underlying Graph Structure

We tested our methods on a group of 82 children with ASD and 48 age and IQ-matched healthy controls used for training the classifiers to distinguish the two groups. Each subject underwent a biological motion perception task [3] fMRI scan (BOLD, TR = 2000 ms, TE = 25 ms, flip angle = 60°, voxel size

$3.44 \times 3.44 \times 4 \,\mathrm{mm}^3$) acquired on a Siemens MAGNETOM Trio TIM 3T scanner. We randomly split 80% of the data for training, 10% for validation of model parameters, and 10% for testing.

The Automated Anatomical Labeling (AAL) atlas [12] was used to parcellate the brain into 116 regions. For each subject, we computed the 116×116 adjacency matrix using Pearson correlation. We averaged the adjacency matrix over the patient subjects in the training data and binarized the edges based on whether its weight is larger than average weight (assigning 1) or not (assigning 0). For H-SVE method, we obtained the non-overlapping community clustering for each subject by greedy modularity method [13], which resulted in 10 communities.

4.3 Comparison with Random Forest-Based Feature Importance

As an additional "reality check" for our method, we apply a Random Forest (RF) strategy (1000 trees) to the same dataset (71.4% accuracy on testing set) and compare the results, using the RF-based feature importance (mean Gini impurity decrease) as a form of standard method for comparison. Instead of inputting the entire fMRI image, we input the node-weighted modularity, which is defined by $\mathcal{M}_i = \sum_{j \neq i} a_{ij}$ where a_{ij} is the partial correlation coefficient between ROI i and j. Therefore the inputs are 116×1 vectors. Based on axiom 4, we can treat each subject as a game and each ROI as a player, and then do group-based analysis by adding $\Phi(r)$ over the subjects to investigate ROI r's importance. For a fair comparison, like in RF, we used all of the training dataset. The interpretation results are shown in Fig. 3. Seven of the top 10 important ROIs discovered by C-SVE and H-SVE overlapped with RF interpretation.

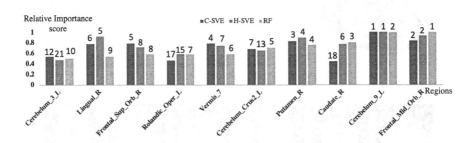

Fig. 3. The relative importance scores of the top 10 important ROIs assigned by Random Forest and their corresponding importance scores in C-SVE and H-SVE. The importance rank of each ROI is denoted on the bar.

Table 1. Prediction decrease after corrupting important ROIs for the DNN

	C-SVE	H-SVE	Single region
$\Delta prob$	0.720 (0.221)	0.693 (0.144)	0.335 (0.060)
Δacc	0.714	0.714	0.428

($\Delta prob$ = decrease in test prediction probability, Δacc = decrease in test accuracy)

4.4 Explaining the ASD Brain Biomarkers Used in Deep Convolutional Neural Network Classifier

Here we chose the deep neural network 2CC3D (Fig. 4) described in [14] using each voxel's mean and standard deviation as two channel input. We start with preprocessed 3D fMRI volumes downsampled to $32 \times 32 \times 32$. We defined the original fMRI sequence as $X(x, y, z, t)$, the mean-channel sequence as $\tilde{X}(x, y, z, t)$ and the standard deviation-channel as $\hat{X}(x, y, z, t)$. For any x, y, z in $\{0, 1, \cdots, 31\}$, $\tilde{X}(x, y, z, t) = \frac{1}{w} \sum_{\tau=t+1-w}^{t} X(x, y, z, \tau)$, $\hat{X}(x, y, z, t)^2 = \frac{1}{w-1} \sum_{\tau=t+1-w}^{t} [X(x, y, z, \tau) - \tilde{X}(x, y, z, t)]^2$, where w is the temporal sliding window size and $w = 3$ in our experiment, hereby we augment data to 18720 samples. Training, validation and testing data was split based on subjects. It achieved 85.7% classification accuracy by majority voting. Running on a workstation with a Nvidia 1080 Ti GPU, testing all 7 ASD subjects in the testing dataset took $21k$ s and $26k$ s for C-SVE and H-SVE, respectively, using 1000 samples for MC approximation, which converged to the stable ranks. As in the MNIST experiment, we divided $\Phi(r)$ by the number of voxels in ROI r, avoiding domination by large ROIs.

The contribution/prediction power of the regions (relative to the most important one) averaged over testing subjects are illustrated in Fig. 5 and listed in Fig. 6. There are 19 overlapping ROIs out of the top 20 important ROIs found

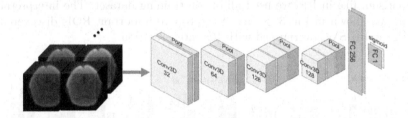

Fig. 4. 2CC3D network architecture

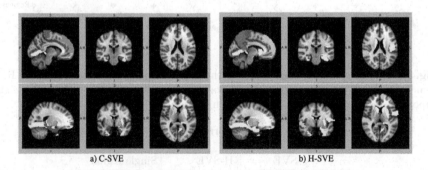

a) C-SVE   b) H-SVE

Fig. 5. Top 20 predictive biomarkers detected by (a) C-SVE and (b) H-SVE for the deep learning classifier. More yellow ROIs signify higher importance. (Color figure online)

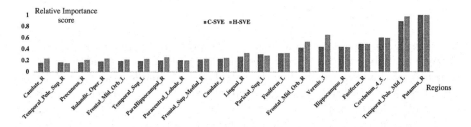

Fig. 6. The relative importance scores of the top 20 ROIs assigned by C-SVE and their corresponding importance scores in H-SVE for the deep learning model.

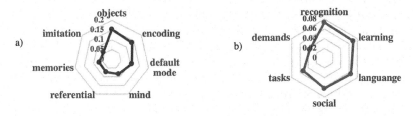

Fig. 7. (a) The top *positive* correlations and (b) the top *negative* correlations between deep learning model biomarkers and functional keywords.

by C-SVE and H-SVE, although the orders were different. The *Spearman rank-order correlation coefficient* [15] of the importance score ranks of all the ROIs explained by both methods was 0.58. These detected regions were consistent with the previous findings in the literature [2,3]. Also, we used Neurosynth [16] to decode the functional keywords associated with the overlapping biomarkers found by C-SVE and H-SVE (Fig. 7). These top regions are positively related to self-referential/perspective-taking concepts (higher level social communication) and negatively related to more basic social and language concepts (lower level skills). Using the manner described in Eq. (1), we corrupted the important ROIs (50% of the positive importance scores summing up in order) determined by C-SVE, H-SVE, and single region testing separately and calculated the average decrease in probability $\Delta prob$ (showing mean and standard deviation) and accuracy Δacc for the subjects in the testing set. The results are listed in Table 1.

Notice that the top 10 biomarkers we discovered using SVE in the RF model were different from the ones found in the 2CC3D model. Possible reasons are: (1) the inputs are different. 2CC3D used activation whereas RF used connectivity and 2CC3D used ASD subjects in testing set whereas RF used all the training set; (2) the prediction accuracy of RF model is much lower than 2CC3D; and (3) our proposed methods performed as a model interpreter rather than data interpreter, which may have different sensitivity response to the different models.

5   Conclusion and Future Work

Considering the interaction of features, we proposed two approaches (C-SVE and H-SVE) to analyze feature importance based on SVE, using the underlying graph structure of the data to simplify the calculation of Shapley value. C-SVE only considers the centralized interaction, while H-SVE uses a hierarchical approach to first cluster the feature communities, then calculate the Shapley value in each community. When a feature's neighborhood/community still contains a large number of features, we apply MC integration method for further approximation. Experiments on the MNIST dataset showed our proposed methods can capture more interpretable features. Comparing the results with Random Forest feature interpretation on the ASD task-fMRI dataset, we further validated the accuracy and feasibility of the proposed methods. When applying both methods on a deep learning model, we discovered similar possible brain biomarkers, which matched the findings in the literature and had meaningful neurological interpretation. The pipeline can be generalized to other feature importance analysis problems, where the underlying graph structure of features is available.

Our future work includes testing the methods on different atlases, graph building methods, and community clustering methods, etc. In addition, the interaction score is embedded in the proposed algorithms. It can be disentangled to understand the interaction between the features.

A   Appendix: Proof of Theorem 2

For any subset $A \subset \mathcal{N}$, we use the short notation $U_r(A) := A \cap \mathcal{N}_r$ and $V_r(A) := A \cap (\mathcal{N} \setminus \mathcal{N}_r)$, noting that $A = U_r(A) \cup V_r(A)$. Rewriting Eq. (2) as

$$\Phi_r(v_X) = \frac{1}{|\mathcal{N}|} \sum_{U \subseteq \mathcal{N}_r \setminus \{r\}} \sum_{A \subseteq \mathcal{N}, U_r(A)=U} \binom{|\mathcal{N}| - 1}{|A|}^{-1} (v_X(A \cup \{r\}) - v_X(A)),$$

and using

$$\sum_{A \subseteq \mathcal{N}, U_r(A)=U} \binom{|\mathcal{N}| - 1}{|A|}^{-1} = \frac{|\mathcal{N}|}{|\mathcal{N}_r|} \binom{|\mathcal{N}_r| - 1}{|U| - 1}^{-1},$$

the expected error between $\hat{\Phi}_r^C(v_X)$ and $\Phi_r(v_X)$ is

$$\mathbb{E}[|\hat{\Phi}_r^C(v_X) - \Phi_r(v_X)|] \leq \frac{1}{|\mathcal{N}|} \sum_{U \subseteq \mathcal{N}_r \setminus \{r\}} \sum_{A \subseteq \mathcal{N}, U_r(A)=U} \binom{|\mathcal{N}| - 1}{|A|}^{-1} \mathbb{E}[|\Delta_r^X(U, A)|]$$

where

$$\begin{aligned}
\Delta_r^X(U, A) &= (v_X(U \cup \{r\}) - v_X(U)) - (v_X(A \cup \{r\}) - v_X(A)) \\
&= \log \frac{p(Y|X_{\mathcal{N} \setminus U})}{p(Y|X_{\mathcal{N} \setminus (U \cup \{r\})})} - \log \frac{p(Y|X_{\mathcal{N} \setminus (U \cup V)})}{p(Y|X_{\mathcal{N} \setminus (U \cup V \cup \{r\})})},
\end{aligned}$$

with V short for $V_r(A)$. Let $W = \mathcal{N} \setminus (\mathcal{N}_r \cup V)$, $Z = \mathcal{N}_r \setminus (\{r\} \cup U)$. Then

$$\Delta_r^X(U, A) = \log \frac{p(Y|X_{W \cup V \cup Z \cup \{r\}})p(Y|X_{W \cup Z})}{p(Y|X_{W \cup V \cup Z})p(Y|X_{W \cup Z \cup \{r\}})}. \tag{9}$$

Since $X_r \perp X_V | X_Z$, we have $p(X_V | X_{W \cup Z \cup \{r\}}) = p(X_V | X_{W \cup Z})$, and

$$(\star) = \frac{p(X_{W \cup V \cup Z \cup \{r\}})p(X_{W \cup Z})}{p(X_{W \cup V \cup Z})p(X_{W \cup Z \cup \{r\}})} = \frac{p(X_{W \cup Z \cup \{r\}})p(X_V | X_{W \cup Z \cup \{r\}})p(X_{W \cup Z})}{p(X_{W \cup Z})p(X_V | X_{W \cup Z})p(X_{W \cup Z \cup \{r\}})} = 1.$$

We can multiply the quotient in Eq. (9) by $(\star)$,

$$\begin{aligned}
\Delta_r^X(U, A) &= \log \frac{p(Y|X_{W \cup V \cup Z \cup \{r\}})p(Y|X_{W \cup Z})}{p(Y|X_{W \cup V \cup Z})p(Y|X_{W \cup Z \cup \{r\}})} \frac{p(X_{W \cup V \cup Z \cup \{r\}})p(X_{W \cup Z})}{p(X_{W \cup V \cup Z})p(X_{W \cup Z \cup \{r\}})} \\
&= \log \frac{p(X_{W \cup V \cup \{r\}}|Y, X_Z)p(Y, X_Z)p(Y, X_Z)p(X_W|Y, X_Z)}{p(Y, X_Z)p(X_{W \cup V}|Y, X_Z)p(Y, X_Z)p(X_{W \cup \{r\}}|Y, X_Z)}.
\end{aligned}$$

We have $p(X_{W \cup V \cup \{r\}}|Y, X_Z) = p(X_{W \cup V}|Y, X_Z)p(X_r|Y, X_Z)$, since $X_{W \cup V} \perp X_r|Y, X_Z$. So

$$\Delta_r^X(U, A) = \log \frac{p(X_{W \cup V}|Y, X_Z)p(X_r|Y, X_Z)p(X_W|Y, X_Z)}{p(X_{W \cup V}|Y, X_Z)p(X_{W \cup \{r\}}|Y, X_Z)}.$$

Since $X_W \perp X_r|Y, X_Z$, we have $p(X_{W \cup \{r\}}|Y, X_Z) = p(X_W|Y, X_Z)p(X_r|Y, X_Z)$. Hence $\Delta_r^X(U, A) = \log 1 = 0$. Therefore we have $\mathbb{E}[|\hat{\Phi}_r^C(v_X) - \Phi_r(v_X)|] = 0$.

References

1. Goldani, A.A.S., Downs, S.R., Widjaja, F., Lawton, B., Hendren, R.L.: Biomarkers in autism. Front. Psychiatry **5**, 100 (2014)
2. Li, X., Dvornek, N.C., Zhuang, J., Ventola, P., Duncan, J.S.: Brain biomarker interpretation in ASD using deep learning and fMRI. In: Frangi, A.F., Schnabel, J.A., Davatzikos, C., Alberola-López, C., Fichtinger, G. (eds.) MICCAI 2018. LNCS, vol. 11072, pp. 206–214. Springer, Cham (2018). https://doi.org/10.1007/978-3-030-00931-1_24
3. Kaiser, M.D., et al.: Neural signatures of autism. Proc. Natl. Acad. Sci. **107**(49), 21223–21228 (2010)
4. Lundberg, S.M., Lee, S.-I.: A unified approach to interpreting model predictions. In: Advances in Neural Information Processing Systems, pp. 4765–4774 (2017)
5. Chen, J., Song, L., Wainwright, M.J., Jordan, M.I.: L-shapley and C-shapley: efficient model interpretation for structured data. arXiv preprint arXiv:1808.02610 (2018)
6. Kononenko, I., Strumbelj, E.: An efficient explanation of individual classifications using game theory. J. Mach. Learn. Res. **11**(Jan), 1–18 (2010)
7. Shapley, L.S.: A value for n-person games. Contrib. Theory Games **2**(28), 307–317 (1953)
8. Zintgraf, L.M., Cohen, T.S., Adel, T., Welling, M.: Visualizing deep neural network decisions: prediction difference analysis. arXiv preprint arXiv:1702.04595 (2017)

9. Clauset, A., Newman, M.E., Moore, C.: Finding community structure in very large networks. Phys. Rev. E **70**(6), 066111 (2004)
10. LeCun, Y., Bottou, L., Bengio, Y., Haffner, P.: Gradient-based learning applied to document recognition. Proc. IEEE **86**(11), 2278–2324 (1998)
11. Achanta, R., Shaji, A., Smith, K., Lucchi, A., Fua, P., Süsstrunk, S.: Slic superpixels compared to state-of-the-art superpixel methods. IEEE Trans. Pattern Anal. Mach. Intell. **34**(11), 2274–2282 (2012)
12. Tzourio-Mazoyer, N., et al.: Automated anatomical labeling of activations in SPM using a macroscopic anatomical parcellation of the MNI MRI single-subject brain. Neuroimage **15**, 273–289 (2002)
13. Newman, M.: Networks. Oxford University Press, Oxford (2018)
14. Li, X., et al.: 2-channel convolutional 3D deep neural network (2CC3D) for fMRI analysis: ASD classification and feature learning. In: 2018 IEEE 15th International Symposium on Biomedical Imaging (ISBI 2018), pp. 1252–1255. IEEE (2018)
15. Young, R.C., Biggs, J.T., Ziegler, V.E., Meyer, D.A.: A rating scale for mania: reliability, validity and sensitivity. Br. J. Psychiatry **133**(5), 429–435 (1978)
16. Yarkoni, T., Poldrack, R.A., Nichols, T.E., Van Essen, D.C., Wager, T.D.: Large-scale automated synthesis of human functional neuroimaging data. Nat. Methods **8**(8), 665 (2011)

Generalizations of Ripley's K-function with Application to Space Curves

Jon Sporring[1(✉)], Rasmus Waagepetersen[2], and Stefan Sommer[1]

[1] Department of Computer Science, University of Copenhagen,
Copenhagen, Denmark
{sporring,sommer}@di.ku.dk

[2] Department of Mathematical Sciences, Aalborg University, Aalborg, Denmark
rw@math.aau.dk

Abstract. The intensity function and Ripley's K-function have been used extensively in the literature to describe the first and second moment structure of spatial point sets. This has many applications including describing the statistical structure of synaptic vesicles. Some attempts have been made to extend Ripley's K-function to curve pieces. Such an extension can be used to describe the statistical structure of muscle fibers and brain fiber tracks. In this paper, we take a computational perspective and construct new and very general variants of Ripley's K-function for curves pieces, surface patches etc. We discuss the method from [3] and compare it with our generalizations theoretically, and we give examples demonstrating the difference in their ability to separate sets of curve pieces.

Keywords: Descriptive statistics · Point and curve processes · Ripley's K-function · Currents

1 Introduction

In this paper, we consider descriptive statistics of sets of curves and particularly whether or not there is a tendency for the curves to cluster or repel each other. In the human body, such curve structures appear in multiple places. Examples include skeletal muscles and fiber tracts in the human brain. We here aim to introduce descriptive statistics for the medical imaging community and discuss estimation methods for geometric data using medical imaging analysis techniques such as morphology and currents.

Ripley's K-function [7] is a well-established tool for describing the second moment structure of point sets [1], and some attempt has been made to generalize this function to curve pieces as described in [3].

For a homogeneous point point pattern $p_i \in \mathbb{R}^d$, $i = 1 \ldots n$ in an observation window W, the sample-based estimate of Ripley's K-function [7] measures the deviation from complete spatial randomness. Complete spatial randomness informally means that points occur uniformly in space and independently of

© Springer Nature Switzerland AG 2019
A. C. S. Chung et al. (Eds.): IPMI 2019, LNCS 11492, pp. 731–742, 2019.
https://doi.org/10.1007/978-3-030-20351-1_57

each other. More formally, the points are distributed according to a Poisson point process with constant intensity. An estimator of Ripley's K-function is,

$$K(r) = \frac{1}{n\lambda} \sum_{i \neq j} 1(\text{dist}(p_i, p_j) < r), \tag{1}$$

where n is the number of points, $\lambda = \frac{|W|}{n}$ is the sample intensity, and 1 is the indicator function. Deviations from homogeneity are identified by comparing $K(r)$ with the volume of a d-dimensional ball of radius r, i.e., if $K(r)$ is greater than or smaller than the volume of the said ball, then points tend to cluster or repel each other respectively at distances r.

For this article, we highlight the following algorithm for computing (1). Given a set of points $\{p_i\}$, we estimate Ripley's K-function by the following algorithm.

```
// Calculate the distance matrix
1. d_ij ← dist(p_i, p_j)
// Sort the non-diagonal values of d_ij in increasing order.
2. r_k ← sort(d_ij), for i ≠ j and k = 1, 2, ... (n² − n)
// Generate the set of pairs ordered by k
3. c ← {c_k = (r_k, k)}
// Remove duplicates of r_k keeping that with highest value of k
4. do
5.     del ← {(r_k, k)|∃(r'_k, k'), where r_k = r'_k and k < k')}
6.     c ← c \ del
7. until c = {}
// Assign values to estimator (non−uniformly sampled).
8. K(r_l) ← l
```

Listing 1. An algorithm for estimating Ripley's K-function by sorting

Examples of using this algorithm on different point sets in $\mathbb{R}^2$ are given in Fig. 1. The figure shows 4 different randomly generated point sets together with the estimated Ripley's K-function. The red squares denotes the observation window. In this article, we will not discuss boundary artifacts and for this reason, we include the blue points asymmetrically, such that when evaluating $\text{dist}(p_i, p_j)$, we let i iterate over all red points and j over all red and blue points except where $i = j$. The black curve is the theoretical value for Ripley's K-function under complete spatial randomness. In the figures, we see that for randomly and uniformly distributed points, as in Fig. 1a, the estimator tend to approximate the curve πr^2. For locally clustered points, as in Fig. 1b, the estimator lies above πr^2 for a range of distances approximately corresponding to the width of the local cluster. For noisy grid points Fig. 1c and grid points Fig. 1d, the estimator lies below πr^2.

Ripley's K-function may be extended to more general random sets of geometrical objects than point sets. A K-function for so-called fiber-processes is reviewed in [3].

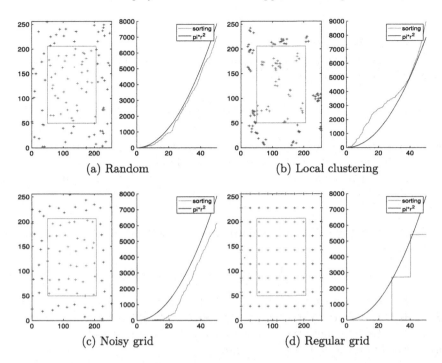

(a) Random   (b) Local clustering

(c) Noisy grid   (d) Regular grid

Fig. 1. Point sets and Ripley's K-function estimated by Listing 1 and compared with the theoretical function for complete spatial randomness. The red square denotes the observation window. The figures show the estimation for random point sets that are (a) independently and uniformly distributed, (b) randomly generated mother processes with independent and normally distributed children, (c) regular grid points perturbed by a normal distribution centered in the gridpoint, and (d) regular grid points. (Color figure online)

Related work is [5], where currents are used to define moments of sets of curves and other geometrical primitives. This allows the authors to visualize and build simplified models using the principal modes of the covariance structure.

In this article, we propose two extensions of Ripley's K-function for manifold pieces of any dimension, which includes the original definition for point sets, and compare [3] with our alternatives theoretically and on simple sets.

2 K-function for Fibers: K_f

In [3], is discussed a number of spatial descriptive statistics including a K-function for curve segments, coined fibers. A fiber process $\Phi \subseteq \mathbb{R}^d$ is a random union of fibers (or curve segments) γ where each γ satisfies that the length of $\gamma \cap B$ is well-defined and finite for all bounded $B \subset \mathbb{R}^d$. Moreover, for any bounded $B \subseteq \mathbb{R}^d$, the random total length $L(B)$ of fibers in $\Phi \cap B$ is finite. The current approach, e.g., reviewed in [3, Chapter 8] to statistically characterizing fiber processes is based on moment properties of the random variables $L(B)$ for bounded subsets $B \subset \mathbb{R}^d$.

Assuming that Φ is stationary (i.e. its distribution is invariant to translations), the intensity ρ of Φ is defined by

$$\rho = \frac{\mathbb{E}L(B)}{|B|}$$

where B is any subset of positive d-dimensional volume $|B|$. In other words, ρ is the expected length of fibers in a set of unit volume.

The second moment measure is defined via second order moments of the length variables:

$$\mu^{(2)}(A \times B) = \mathbb{E}[L(A)L(B)]$$

for bounded $A, B \subset \mathbb{R}^d$. By standard measure-theoretical results, $\mu^{(2)}$ can be decomposed as

$$\mu^{(2)}(A \times B) = \rho^2 \int_A \mathcal{K}(B - x)\mathrm{d}x$$

where $\mathcal{K}(\cdot)$ defined on subsets of $\mathbb{R}^d$ is called the reduced moment measure. Here $B - x$ is B translated by the vector $-x$ for $B \subset \mathbb{R}^d$ and $x \in \mathbb{R}^d$.

Letting $b(0, r)$ denote the d-dimensional ball of radius r and centered in the origo, we obtain the K-function for fibers

$$K_f(r) = \mathcal{K}(b(0, r)).$$

For each $r \geq 0$, $K_f(r)$ can be interpreted a the expected total fiber length in $b(u, r)$ conditional on that $u \in \Phi$ for $u \in \mathbb{R}^d$. Thus, given that a fiber intersects $u \in \mathbb{R}^d$, the K_f-function describes the tendency of further fibers in Φ to aggregate in or avoid the ball $b(u, r)$ centered around u.

2.1   Relation to Cox Process

Suppose we generate a point process Y by placing points on Φ according to a Poisson process. More specifically, for each fiber γ in Φ, a Poisson process of intensity λ is generated on γ. Then the intensity of Y becomes $\lambda \rho$. The second order factorial moment measure of Y is closely related to the second moment measure of Φ:

$$\alpha_Y^{(2)}(A \times B) = \mathbb{E} \sum_{u,v \in Y}^{\neq} 1[u \in A, v \in B] = \lambda^2 \mathbb{E} \int_\Phi \int_\Phi 1[u \in A, v \in B]\mathrm{d}u\mathrm{d}v$$

$$= \lambda^2 \mathbb{E}[\Phi(A)\Phi(B)] = \lambda^2 \mu^{(2)}(A \times B)$$

for bounded $A, B \subset \mathbb{R}^d$. Here and in the following $\int_\Phi$ should be interpreted as a curve integral along the fibers in Φ.

The usual point process K-function for Y is

$$K_Y(r) = \mathcal{K}_Y(b(0, r))$$

where $\mathcal{K}_Y(b(0,r))$ is defined by the equation

$$\alpha_Y^{(2)}(A \times B) = \lambda^2 \int_A \mathcal{K}_Y(B - x)\mathrm{d}x.$$

We thus obtain that the K-functions of Φ and Y coincide,

$$K_f(r) = K_Y(r)$$

and

$$\rho K_f(r) = \frac{1}{\rho|A|}\mathbb{E}\left[\int_\Phi \int_\Phi 1[u \in A, \|v - u\| \le r]\mathrm{d}v\mathrm{d}u\right]$$

$$= \mathbb{E}\left[\frac{1}{\rho|A|}\int_{\Phi \cap A} L(b(u,r))\mathrm{d}u\right].$$

It follows that $\rho K_f(r)$ can further be viewed as the expectation of a spatial average of lengths $L(b(u,r))$ for $u \in \Phi \cap A$.

2.2   Estimation of K_f

Suppose Φ is observed within a bounded observation window $W \subset \mathbb{R}^d$ and let $W \ominus r = \{x \in W | b(x,r) \subset W\}$ denote the erosion of W by the distance r. Then

$$\hat{K}_f(r) = \frac{1}{\rho^2|W \ominus r|}\int_{\Phi \cap W \ominus r} L(b(u,r))\mathrm{d}u$$

is an unbiased estimate of K_f. Alternatively, one can generate a point process Y on Φ as described in the previous section and estimate $K_f(r) = K_Y(r)$ by the usual estimator of point process K-functions as described in Sect. 1. This essentially corresponds to evaluating the integrals/lengths in $\hat{K}_f(r)$ by Monte Carlo integration. Figure 2a shows an illustration of this approximation. The figure shows a step in the process of estimating K_f: a ball has been placed around a point on a curve (thick line), and the contribution to the estimate for that radius and that point is the number of other points on the other lines.

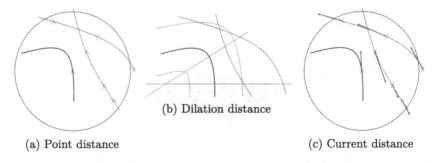

(a) Point distance   (b) Dilation distance   (c) Current distance

Fig. 2. Geometric comparison of three different K-estimators. (a) K_f discussed in Sect. 2.1, (b) K_m discussed in Sect. 3, and (c) K_c discussed in Sect. 4. (Color figure online)

2.3 K_f in Terms of Curve Segments

Let $\Phi = \cup_{i=1}^{\infty} \gamma_i$ where the γ_i represent the individual fibers/curve segments and let for a bounded A,

$$d_A(\gamma_i, \gamma_j) = \int_{\gamma_i \cap A} \int_{\gamma_j} 1[\|v - u\| \le r] dv du.$$

Thus, a large value of $d_A(\gamma_i, \gamma_j)$ indicates that $\gamma_i \cap A$ and γ_j are 'close' so that d_A is a kind of measure of association between γ_i and γ_j. Then

$$\rho K_f(r) = \frac{1}{\rho|A|} \mathbb{E}\left[\sum_{\gamma_i : \gamma_i \cap A \ne \emptyset} \sum_{\gamma_j} \int_{\gamma_i \cap A} \int_{\gamma_j} 1[\|v - u\| \le r] dv du \right]$$

$$= \frac{1}{\rho|A|} \mathbb{E}\left[\sum_{\gamma_i : \gamma_i \cap A \ne \emptyset} \sum_{\gamma_j} d_A(\gamma_i, \gamma_j) \right]$$

Thus, K_f can be viewed as a kind of average of $d_A(\gamma_i, \gamma_j)$ for pairs of distinct fibers γ_i and γ_j in Φ. In this paper, we exploit this point of view by investigating alternative measures of association between fibers.

2.4 Some Experiments with Random Curves and K_f

We will in the following motivate alternative definitions of K_f by presenting a number of comparable cases in two dimensions.

To generate random curves in $\mathbb{R}^2$, we draw a second-degree polynomial $f : \mathbb{R}^2 \to \mathbb{R}$ with random coefficients a_i, and we choose a distribution $p(x, y)$ of initial points. Then we draw n initial points and develop a curve along the gradient field of f. Thus, we consider curve pieces that extends beyond the observation window. Examples of this is shown in Fig. 3. A Cox process is generated by distributing a random number of points uniformly along each curve. In Fig. 4 we

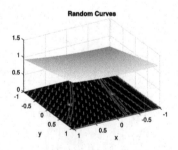

Fig. 3. An example of a randomly generated set of curves: a random surface is shown in gray hovering above the lines, its gradient field is shown as blue arrows, a distribution of starting points is shown as a gray image, and red lines are flow lines each passing through random starting point. (Color figure online)

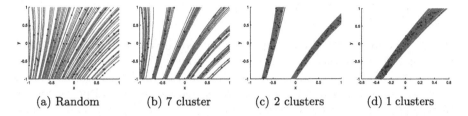

| (a) Random | (b) 7 cluster | (c) 2 clusters | (d) 1 clusters |

Fig. 4. Random curves and random points on curves. All curves are generated from the same vector field shown in Fig. 3.

show four sets of curves, which will be used as comparison cases throughout this paper. The curves were generated by the same vector field shown in Fig. 3, but where the distribution of initial points varies from being essentially uniform or distributed within 7, 2, or 1 localized region. 100 curves were randomly generated for each set. The blue dots show the sample points along the curves, and we use Listing 1 to estimate K_f for these points. The result of 10 experiments, where 100 points were sampled on the same set of curves is shown in Fig. 5. All estimates of K_f in these experiments seem to converge to 4 for large values of r. This is due to the identical sampling and observation window and that no boundary correction terms are included, thereby implying that there are no points outside the observation window. The estimated K_f for the wide and the narrow cluster (Fig. 5a and d) shows the expected behavior: For the wide initial set of curves, the K_f initially follows πr^2, while for the narrow set of curves, the estimated K_f is above πr^2. The estimates of K_f for 7 regions is disappointingly similar to the those of the wide cluster, indicating that K_f is not well suited to distinguish the clustering behavior of these 2 sets of curves. For clusters, there is some structure in the estimated K_f. Nevertheless, by these experiments we are motivated to investigate other functions that are similar to K_f, but with better descriptive power.

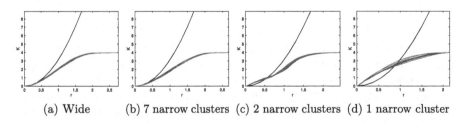

| (a) Wide | (b) 7 narrow clusters | (c) 2 narrow clusters | (d) 1 narrow cluster |

Fig. 5. Repeated estimates of K_f for randomly generated points on randomly generated curves. Black shows the theoretical curve for a Poisson process, and each red curve corresponds to an experiment. (Color figure online)

3   A K-function by Morphology: K_m

The K_f-function essentially measures aggregated curve length within neighborhoods and does not take into account the geometry of the curves. Below we present one of two algorithmically inspired alternatives: An essential part of Ripley's K-function is the distance function, and the statistical power for distinguishing various clustering or repulsion behavior may be increased by incorporating other distance or pseudo-distance measures in the construction of a K-function. Thus, for this article, we are less concerned with the measurement theoretic basis and more with the ability of the resulting functions to distinguish groups of curves. Our first alternative to K_f is to replace the point-wise ball of radius r with a dilation of curves with a ball of radius r.

Consider a smooth space curve in $c : \mathbb{R} \rightarrow \mathbb{R}^3$ and its length, $\text{len}(c) = \int \|c'(t)\| \, dt$, where c' is the tangent vector of c and $\|c'\|$ is its length. The intersection of a curve with a region of interest W may result in several disjoint curves c_i, and we introduce the intersection length as,

$$\text{len}_W(c) = \sum_i \int_{\Gamma_i} \|c'(t)\| \, dt, \tag{2}$$

where we sum over all intervals $\Gamma_i \subset \mathbb{R}$ for which the curve intersects W. We define a curve's r-neighborhood by dilation as the set

$$\mathcal{N}_{r,j} = \mathcal{N}_r(c_j) = c_j \oplus b(0, r), \tag{3}$$

for a ball of center 0 and radius r. Thus, $\mathcal{N}_{r,j}$ is the set of all points closer than r to the curve. For a set of curves c_j, $j = 1 \ldots n$, we generalize Ripley's K-function as,

$$K_m(r) = \frac{1}{n\rho} \sum_j \frac{1}{\text{len}_W(c_j)} \sum_{i \neq j} \text{len}_{W \cap \mathcal{N}_{r,j}}(c_i) \tag{4}$$

where ρ is the mean curve length per unit area.

The geometry is illustrated in Fig. 2b. Similarly to Fig. 2a, we consider the curve shown as a thick line. The stippled lines parallel to this denotes a dilation with a ball with radius r, and the length of the other lines intersection with the region between the two stippled parallel lines are the curve's contribution to K_m. Further, for straight parts of the thick line, the contribution will be close to counting how many neighboring lines there are within a distance r in the normal direction. However, when the thick line has curvature, then neighboring lines are 'counted' in a wedge shape, as illustrated by the two stippled straight lines perpendicular to the thick line.

3.1   Some Experiments with Random Curves and K_m

We have performed experiments on the same curves described in Sect. 2.4. We have performed 10 trials with 30 random curves, and the result is shown in Fig. 6. Note that in these experiments, we compare full curves with each other

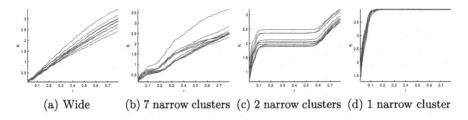

(a) Wide   (b) 7 narrow clusters (c) 2 narrow clusters (d) 1 narrow cluster

Fig. 6. K_m on randomly generated curves as demonstrated by Fig. 3.

instead of points on curves with each other. The spread of the estimates of the K_m-by-dilation functions is greater than in Fig. 5. This is to be expected since the estimates are based on fewer samples, 30 curves as compared to 100 points. In terms of the shape of K_m, we see that Fig. 6a is close to linear for all radii. The remaining experiments show a close to linear growth for $r \in [0, 0.1]$, which corresponds well with the width of each individual cluster of curves. Further, Fig. 6b shows a plateau for $r \in [0.1, 0.2]$, which corresponds well to the distances between its clusters. Similarly, Fig. 6c has a plateau for $r \in [0.1, 0.6]$, which again is in close relation with the distance between the two bundles. Finally, Fig. 6d plateaus for $r > 0.1$, which is to be expected, since no other clusters are present in the data. Thus, for these cases, K_m much better separates the different clustering behavior of our curves.

4   A K-function for Current Metrics: K_c

In this section, we will define the K_c by currents, where we replace the Euclidean distance in Listing 1 with that of currents for curves.

4.1   Currents

The theory of currents, see e.g. [4,6], embed geometric objects, here specifically curves, into vector spaces that appear as dual spaces to a set of test vector fields. This embedding allows structure from the vector space of test fields to be carried to the space of curves. Specifically, the currents representation inherits the metric structure of the vector space. We here briefly outline the currents construction referring to the above references for details.

Let $l : I \to \Omega$ denote a C^1 line in the domain $\Omega \subseteq \mathbb{R}^d$, and let v be a square integrable vector field on the domain. The assignment $l(v) := \int_l v(x)^T \dot{l}(x) d\lambda(x)$ produces a real number: It is the integral over the line of the inner product between the vector field and the derivative $\dot{l} = \frac{d}{dt} l(t)$ of the curve evaluated at the point $x \in \Omega$. The integral is with respect to the Lebesgue measure on the line. The use of the inner product makes the assignment linear in v. If we settle on a suitable space V to which v can belong, then the assignment allows l to be seen as a member of the dual space V^*. The currents construction is this embedding of l into V^*. Note that though any C^1 curve can be embedded in

V^* in this way, we cannot expect to find a curve representing e.g. an arbitrary linear combination of elements of V^*.

If V is a normed space, we can inherit from it a norm on V^* by setting $\|l\|_{V^*} = \sup_{v \in V, \|v\|=1} |l(v)|$. This gives a metric on the space of curves by setting $d(l_1, l_2) = \|l_1 - l_2\|_{V^*}$. To be more explicit, the currents construction assumes V is a reproducing kernel Hilbert space with reproducing kernel $G : \Omega \times \Omega \to \mathbb{R}^{d \times d}$. Then, for $p \in \Omega$ and $\alpha \in \mathbb{R}^d$, the map $G(\cdot, p)\alpha$ is a vector field on Ω, and elements of V appear as infinite linear combinations of such elements. The reproducing property implies that V has an inner product $\langle \cdot, \cdot \rangle_V$ and that

$$\langle G(p_1, \cdot)\alpha_1, G(p_2, \cdot)\alpha_2, \rangle_V = \alpha_1^T G(p_1, p_2)\alpha_2. \tag{5}$$

The inner product defines a norm $\| \cdot \|_V$ and metric d_V on V.

For currents, the interest is rather V^* than V. A special set of elements in V^*, the Dirac delta currents δ_p^α, take a role in V^* similar to the vector fields $G(\cdot, p)\alpha$ in V. Particularly, we can regard l as an infinite sum of such currents with the point $l(t)$ represented by $\delta_{l(t)}^{\dot{l}(t)}$. V^* inherits the inner product from V and $\langle \delta_{p_1}^{\alpha_1}, \delta_{p_2}^{\alpha_2} \rangle_{V^*} = \langle G(p_1, \cdot)\alpha_1, G(p_2, \cdot)\alpha_2, \rangle_V$. If we discretize l into a finite set of Dirac delta currents $l \approx \sum_{i=1}^n \delta_{l(t_i)}^{\dot{l}(t_i)}$, the current norm of l appears as $\|l\|^2 \approx \| \sum_{i=1}^n \delta_{l(t_i)}^{\dot{l}(t_i)} \|^2 = \sum_{i,j=1}^n \dot{l}(t_i)^T G(l(t_i), l(t_j)) \dot{l}(t_j)$. This norm is consistent when we pass to the limit using an infinite number of points to represent l. Note that the points here are oriented because each Dirac delta $\delta_{l(t_i)}^{\dot{l}(t_i)}$ carries the derivative of curve in the vector $\dot{l}(t_i)$. The currents can be seen as dual spaces to the set of differential m-forms for any m. The construction, therefore, applies as well to unoriented points ($m = 0$) and surfaces ($m = 2$).

The currents norm necessitate a choice of reproducing kernel Hilbert space structure on V. An often used choice is the Gaussian kernel $G(x, y) = \alpha e^{-\frac{\|x-y\|^2}{2\sigma^2}} \mathrm{Id}_d$ where Id_d is the identity matrix on $\mathbb{R}^d$ and $\alpha, \sigma \in \mathbb{R}$ the amplitude and variance of the kernel, respectively.

Distance between two discretized curves is defined by the inner product as,

$$d_c(c_1, c_2) = \left\| \sum_i G(p_{1i}, \cdot)\alpha_{1i} - \sum_j G(p_{2j}, \cdot)\alpha_{2j} \right\| \tag{6}$$

$$= \sqrt{\sum_i \sum_j \alpha_{1i}^T G(p_i, p_j)\alpha_{1j} + \sum_i \sum_j \alpha_{2i}^T G(p_i, p_j)\alpha_{2j} - 2\sum_i \sum_j \alpha_{1i}^T G(p_i, p_j)\alpha_{2j}}.$$

Finally, we define K_c as Listing 1 using $d(c_1, c_2) = \min(d_c(c_1, c_2), d_c(c_1, -c_2))$, where $-c_2$ is the curve with orientation opposite of c_2, see also the varifold representation [2].

The geometry is illustrated in Fig. 2c. Similarly to Fig. 2a, we consider a step in the process of estimating the K_c: a Gaussian, depicted as a ball, has been placed around the point on a curve (thick line) with its tangent vector at this point shown as a blue arrow. We then consider other points and their tangent vectors, and the dot product of the tangent at the origin and at the other points are in turn calculated and weighted by their distance according to G. As a consequence, the current distant measure emphasizes points on curves in a soft neighborhood that are close to parallel.

4.2 Some Experiments with Random Curves and K_c

We have performed experiments on the same curves as described in Sect. 2.4. As in Sect. 3.1 we performed 10 trials with 30 random curves from the same random set of curves described in Sect. 2.4. We have used the Gaussian kernel with $\sigma = 0.5$ to correspond with the expected size of statistical structures observed in the data. The result is shown in Fig. 7. As the experiments with K_m, all curves show a linear increase starting at $r = 0$, and superficially, the experiment with 7, 2, and 1 narrow cluster show a stepping like behavior similarly to K_m. However, interpretation of these curves is slightly more complicated, since they describe a mixture of pointwise distance and the dot product of their tangents. Curves that are parallel will have small values of (6), while curves that are perpendicular will have large distances.

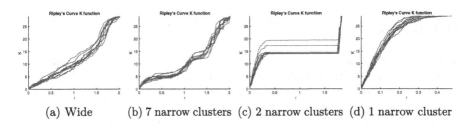

(a) Wide   (b) 7 narrow clusters (c) 2 narrow clusters (d) 1 narrow cluster

Fig. 7. K_c using $\sigma = 0.5$ and on curves as demonstrated by Fig. 3.

5 Discussion and Conclusion

In this article, we have considered Ripley's K-function for sets of points and a K-function, K_f, for curves, and we observed that the two definitions are very similar for a certain type of Cox processes. We also observed that the definition of K_f, given in [3], is not well suited to distinguish simple line patterns, as demonstrated on a small number of cases. This has motivated us to consider two alternative K-like functions: K_m, which uses mathematical morphology to define pseudo-distance between curves, and K_c, which defines distances by currents. Both give rise to K-functions that are more descriptive in terms of the simple examples presented. However, they differ in how they interpret the geometry of curves and their relations. Oversimplified examples may shed some light on their differences: Consider two infinite lines in an infinite two-dimensional space crossing at a right angle. The contribution for a point right at the center will for the three K-functions be: $K_f(r) = \mathcal{O}(r)$, $K_m(r) = \frac{r}{L}$, $K_c(r) = 0$. In contrast, for two infinite parallel lines at distance d, for a point on one of the lines, the three K-functions will be $K_f(r) = 0$ if $r < d$ else $\mathcal{O}(\sqrt{r^2 + d^2})$, $K_m(r) = 0$ if $r < d$ else 1, or $K_c(r) \simeq 0$ if $r < \sigma\sqrt{2\pi}\exp\frac{-d^2}{2\sigma^2}$ else 1. Thus, for orthogonal lines, K_f and K_m are similar, while for parallel lines, K_m and K_c are similar. All three K-functions are highly general, easily defined in higher dimensions and for manifold pieces of higher dimensions. However, it is expected that K_f will be the fastest to compute since it only depends on sampled points on manifold pieces. K_c is also fast to compute for rotational symmetric kernels, which likewise can be approximated by sample points and their tangent space. However, K_c has a free parameter, which require further investigation in order to properly set. The pseudo-distance measure used for K_m has geometrical appeal to these authors, and may have useful applications.

Our future work will focus on studying the relation between the (pseudo-) distance function used, the implied K-function, and the statistical problem to be solved.

Acknowledgments. This work was funded by the Villum Foundation through the Center for Stochastic Geometry and Advanced Bioimaging (http://csgb.dk).

References

1. Baddeley, A., Rubak, E., Turner, R.: Spatial Point Patterns: Methodology and Applications with R. Chapman and Hall/CRC, London/Boca Raton (2015)
2. Charon, N., Trouvé, A.: The varifold representation of nonoriented shapes for diffeomorphic registration. SIAM J. Imaging Sci. **6**(4), 2547–2580 (2013)
3. Chiu, S., Stoyan, D., Kendall, W., Mecke, J.: Stochastic Geometry and Its Applications. Wiley Series in Probability and Statistics. Wiley, Hoboken (2013)
4. Durrleman, S.: Statistical models of currents for measuring the variability of anatomical curves, surfaces and their evolution. Ph.D. thesis, de l'Université Nice - Sophia Antipolis, France (2010)
5. Durrleman, S., Pennec, X., Trouvé, A., Ayache, N.: Statistical models of sets of curves and surfaces based on currents. Med. Image Anal. **13**, 793–808 (2009)
6. Glaunès, J.: Transport Par Difféomorphismes de Points, de Mesures et de Courants Pour La Comparaison de Formes et l'anatomie Numérique. Ph.D. thesis, Université Paris 13, Villetaneuse, France (2005)
7. Ripley, B.D.: Modelling spatial patterns. J. R. Stat. Soc. Ser. B (Methodol.) **39**(2), 172–212 (1977)

Group Level MEG/EEG Source Imaging via Optimal Transport: Minimum Wasserstein Estimates

H. Janati[1,3(✉)], T. Bazeille[1], B. Thirion[1], M. Cuturi[2,3], and A. Gramfort[1]

[1] Inria, CEA Neurospin, Saclay, France
hicham.janati@inria.fr
[2] Google Brain, Paris, France
[3] CREST/ENSAE, Palaiseau, France

Abstract. Magnetoencephalography (MEG) and electroencephalography (EEG) are non-invasive modalities that measure the weak electromagnetic fields generated by neural activity. Inferring the location of the current sources that generated these magnetic fields is an ill-posed inverse problem known as source imaging. When considering a group study, a baseline approach consists in carrying out the estimation of these sources independently for each subject. The ill-posedness of each problem is typically addressed using sparsity promoting regularizations. A straightforward way to define a common pattern for these sources is then to average them. A more advanced alternative relies on a joint localization of sources for all subjects taken together, by enforcing some similarity across all estimated sources. An important advantage of this approach is that it consists in a single estimation in which all measurements are pooled together, making the inverse problem better posed. Such a joint estimation poses however a few challenges, notably the selection of a valid regularizer that can quantify such spatial similarities. We propose in this work a new procedure that can do so while taking into account the geometrical structure of the cortex. We call this procedure Minimum Wasserstein Estimates (MWE). The benefits of this model are twofold. First, joint inference allows to pool together the data of different brain geometries, accumulating more spatial information. Second, MWE are defined through Optimal Transport (OT) metrics which provide a tool to model spatial proximity between cortical sources of different subjects, hence not enforcing identical source location in the group. These benefits allow MWE to be more accurate than standard MEG source localization techniques. To support these claims, we perform source localization on realistic MEG simulations based on forward operators derived from MRI scans. On a visual task dataset, we demonstrate how MWE infer neural patterns similar to functional Magnetic Resonance Imaging (fMRI) maps.

Keywords: Brain · Inverse modeling · EEG/MEG source imaging

© Springer Nature Switzerland AG 2019
A. C. S. Chung et al. (Eds.): IPMI 2019, LNCS 11492, pp. 743–754, 2019.
https://doi.org/10.1007/978-3-030-20351-1_58

1 Introduction

Magnetoencephalography (MEG) measures the components of the magnetic field surrounding the head, while Electroencephalography (EEG) measures the electric potential at the surface of the scalp. Both can do so with a temporal resolution of less than a millisecond. Localizing the underlying neural activity on a high resolution grid of the cortex, a problem known as source imaging, is inherently an "ill-posed" linear inverse problem: Indeed, the number of potential sources is larger than the number of MEG and EEG sensors, which implies that, even in the absence of noise, different neural activity patterns could result in the same electromagnetic field measurements.

To limit the set of possible solutions, prior hypotheses on the nature of the source distributions are necessary. The minimum-norm estimates (MNE) for instance are based on ℓ_2 Tikhonov regularization which leads to a linear solution [11]. An ℓ_1 norm penalty was also proposed by [34], modeling the underlying neural pattern as a sparse collection of focal dipolar sources, hence their name "Minimum Current Estimates" (MCE). These methods have inspired a series of contributions in source localization techniques relying on noise normalization [6,28] to correct for the depth bias [1] or block-sparse norms [10,30] to leverage the spatio-temporal dynamics of MEG signals. While such techniques have had some success, source estimation in the presence of complex multi-dipole configurations remains a challenge. In this work we aim to leverage the anatomical and functional diversity of multi-subject datasets to improve localization results.

Related Work. This idea of using multi-subject information to improve statistical estimation has been proposed before in the neuroimaging literature. In [20] it is showed that different anatomies across subjects allow for point spread functions that agree on a main activation source but differ elsewhere. Averaging across subjects thereby increases the accuracy of source localization. On fMRI data, [35] proposed a probabilistic dictionary learning model to infer activation maps jointly across a cohort of subjects. A similar idea led [19] to introduce a Bayesian framework to account for functional intersubject variability. To our knowledge, the only contribution formulating the problem as a multi-task regression model employs a Group Lasso with an ℓ_{21} block sparse norm [21]. Yet this forces every potential neural source to be either active for all subjects or for none of them.

Contribution. The assumption of identical functional activity across subjects is clearly not realistic. Here we investigate several multi-task regression models that relax this assumption. One of them is the multi-task Wasserstein (MTW) model [15]. MTW is defined through an Unbalanced Optimal Transport (UOT) metric that promotes support proximity across regression coefficients. However, applying MTW to group level data assumes that the signal-to-noise ratio is the same for all subjects. We propose to build upon MTW and alleviate this problem by inferring estimates of both sources and noise variance for each subject. To do so, we follow similar ideas that lead to the concomitant Lasso [25,27,31] or the multi-task Lasso [24].

This paper is organized as follows. Section 2 introduces the multi-task regression source imaging problem. Section 3 presents some background on UOT metrics and explains how MWE are carried out. Section 4 presents the results of our experiments on both simulated and MEG datasets.

Notation. We denote by $\mathbb{1}_p$ the vector of ones in $\mathbb{R}^p$ and by $[\![q]\!]$ the set $\{1, \ldots, q\}$ for any integer $q \in \mathbb{N}$. The set of vectors in $\mathbb{R}^p$ with non-negative (resp. positive) entries is denoted by $\mathbb{R}^p_+$ (resp. $\mathbb{R}^p_{++}$). On matrices, log, exp and the division operator are applied elementwise. We use $\odot$ for the elementwise multiplication between matrices or vectors. If $\mathbf{X}$ is a matrix, $\mathbf{X}_{i.}$ denotes its ith row and $\mathbf{X}_{.j}$ its jth column. We define the Kullback-Leibler (KL) divergence between two positive vectors by $\text{KL}(\mathbf{x}, \mathbf{y}) = \langle \mathbf{x}, \log(\mathbf{x}/\mathbf{y}) \rangle + \langle \mathbf{y} - \mathbf{x}, \mathbb{1}_p \rangle$ with the continuous extensions $0 \log(0/0) = 0$ and $0 \log(0) = 0$. We also make the convention $\mathbf{x} \neq 0 \Rightarrow \text{KL}(\mathbf{x}|0) = +\infty$. The entropy of $\mathbf{x} \in \mathbb{R}^n$ is defined as $H(\mathbf{x}) = -\langle \mathbf{x}, \log(\mathbf{x}) - \mathbb{1}_p \rangle$. The same definition applies for matrices with an element-wise double sum.

2   Source Imaging as a Multi-task Regression Problem

We formulate in this section the inverse problem of interest in this paper, and recall how a multi-task formulation can be useful to carry out a joint estimation of all these parameters through regularization.

Source Modeling. Using a volume segmentation of the MRI scan of each subject, the positions of potential sources are constructed as a set of coordinates uniformly distributed on the cortical surface of the gray matter. Moreover, synchronized currents in the apical dendrites of cortical pyramidal neurons are thought to be mostly responsible for MEG signals [26]. Therefore, the dipole orientations are usually constrained to be normal to the cortical surface. We model the current density as a set of focal current dipoles with fixed positions and orientations. The purpose of source localization is to infer their amplitudes. The ensemble of possible candidate dipoles forms the *source space*.

Forward Modeling. Let n denote the number of sensors (EEG and/or MEG) and p the number of sources. Following Maxwell's equations, at each time instant, the measurements $\mathbf{B} \in \mathbb{R}^n$ are a linear combination of the current density $\mathbf{x} \in \mathbb{R}^p : \mathbf{B} = \mathbf{Lx}$. However, we observe noisy measurements $\mathbf{Y} \in \mathbb{R}^n$ given by:

$$\mathbf{Y} = \mathbf{B} + \varepsilon = \mathbf{Lx} + \varepsilon, \tag{1}$$

where ε is the noise vector. The linear forward operator $\mathbf{L} \in \mathbb{R}^{n \times p}$ is called the *leadfield* or *gain matrix*, and can be computed by solving Maxwell's equations using the Boundary element method [12]. Up to a whitening pre-processing step, ε can be assumed Gaussian distributed $\mathcal{N}(0, \sigma I_n)$.

Source Localization. Source localization consists in solving in $\mathbf{x}$ the inverse problem (1) which can be cast as a least squares problem:

$$\mathbf{x}^\star = \arg\min_{\mathbf{x}\in\mathbb{R}^p} \|\mathbf{Y} - \mathbf{L}\mathbf{x}\|_2^2. \tag{2}$$

Since $n \ll p$, problem (2) is ill-posed and additional constraints on the solution $\mathbf{x}^\star$ are necessary. When analyzing evoked responses, one can promote source configurations made of a few focal sources, e.g. using the ℓ_1 norm. This regularization leads to problem (3) called minimum current estimates (MCE), also known in the machine learning community as the Lasso [32], given a hyperparameter $\lambda > 0$:

$$\mathbf{x}^\star = \arg\min_{\mathbf{x}\in\mathbb{R}^p} \frac{1}{2n}\|\mathbf{Y} - \mathbf{L}\mathbf{x}\|_2^2 + \lambda\|\mathbf{x}\|_1, \tag{3}$$

Common Source Space. Here we propose to go beyond the classical pipeline and carry out source localization jointly for S subjects. First, dipole positions (features) must correspond to each other across subjects. To do so, the source space of each subject is mapped to a high resolution average brain using morphing where the sulci and gyri patterns are matched in an auxiliary spherical inflating of each brain surface [8]. The resulting leadfields $\mathbf{L}^{(1)}, \ldots, \mathbf{L}^{(S)}$ have therefore the same shape $(n \times p)$ with aligned columns.

Multi-task Framework. Jointly estimating the current density $\mathbf{x}^{(s)}$ of each subject s can be expressed as a multi-task regression problem where some coupling prior is assumed on $\mathbf{x}^{(1)}, \ldots, \mathbf{x}^{(S)}$ through a penalty Ω:

$$\min_{\mathbf{x}^{(1)},\ldots,\mathbf{x}^{(S)}\in\mathbb{R}^p} \frac{1}{2n}\sum_{s=1}^{S}\|\mathbf{Y}^{(s)} - \mathbf{L}^{(s)}\mathbf{x}^{(s)}\|_2^2 + \Omega(\mathbf{x}^{(1)},\ldots,\mathbf{x}^{(S)}). \tag{4}$$

Following the work of [15], we propose to define Ω using an UOT metric.

3   Minimum Wassertein Estimates

We start this section with background material on UOT. Consider the finite metric space (E, d) where each element of $E = \{1,\ldots,p\}$ corresponds to a vertex of the source space. Let $\mathbf{M}$ be the matrix where $\mathbf{M}_{ij}$ corresponds to the geodesic distance between vertices i and j. Kantorovich [16] defined a distance for normalized histograms (probability measures) on E. However, it can easily be extended to non-normalized measures by relaxing marginal constraints [4].

Marginal Relaxation. Let $\mathbf{a}, \mathbf{b}$ be two normalized histograms on E. Assuming that transporting a fraction of mass $\mathbf{P}_{ij}$ from i to j is given by $\mathbf{P}_{ij}\mathbf{M}_{ij}$, the total cost of transport is given by $\langle \mathbf{P}, \mathbf{M} \rangle = \sum_{ij} \mathbf{P}_{ij}\mathbf{M}_{ij}$. Minimizing this total cost with respect to $\mathbf{P}$ must be carried out on the set of feasible transport plans with marginals $\mathbf{a}$ and $\mathbf{b}$. The (normalized) Wasserstein-Kantorovich distance reads:

$$\mathrm{WK}(\mathbf{a}, \mathbf{b}) = \min_{\substack{\mathbf{P} \in \mathbb{R}_+^{p \times p} \\ \mathbf{P}\mathbb{1}=\mathbf{a}, \mathbf{P}^\top \mathbb{1}=\mathbf{b}}} \langle \mathbf{P}, \mathbf{M} \rangle. \tag{5}$$

In practice, if $\mathbf{a}$ and $\mathbf{b}$ are positive and normalized current densities, $\mathrm{WK}(\mathbf{a}, \mathbf{b})$ will quantify the geodesic distance between their supports along the curved geometry of the cortex. This property makes OT metrics adequate for assessing the proximity of functional patterns across subjects. To allow $\mathbf{a}, \mathbf{b}$ to be non-normalized, the marginal constraints in (5) can be relaxed using a KL divergence:

$$\min_{\mathbf{P} \in \mathbb{R}_+^{p \times p}} \langle \mathbf{P}, \mathbf{M} \rangle + \gamma \mathrm{KL}(\mathbf{P}\mathbb{1}|\mathbf{a}) + \gamma \mathrm{KL}(\mathbf{P}^\top \mathbb{1}|\mathbf{b}), \tag{6}$$

where $\gamma > 0$ is a hyperparameter that enforces a fit to the marginals.

Entropy Regularization. Entropy regularization was introduced by [5] to propose a faster and more robust alternative to the direct resolution of the linear programming problem (5). Formally, this amounts to minimizing $\langle \mathbf{P}, \mathbf{M} \rangle - \varepsilon H(\mathbf{P})$ where $\varepsilon > 0$ is a tuning hyperparameter. This penalized loss can be written: $\varepsilon \mathrm{KL}(\mathbf{P}, e^{-\frac{\mathbf{M}}{\varepsilon}})$ up to a constant [3]. Combining entropy regularization with the relaxation (6), we get the unbalanced Wasserstein distance as introduced by [4]:

$$W(\mathbf{a}, \mathbf{b}) = \min_{\mathbf{P} \in \mathbb{R}_+^{p \times p}} \varepsilon \mathrm{KL}(\mathbf{P}|e^{-\frac{\mathbf{M}}{\varepsilon}}) + \gamma \mathrm{KL}(\mathbf{P}\mathbb{1}|\mathbf{a}) + \gamma \mathrm{KL}(\mathbf{P}^\top \mathbb{1}|\mathbf{b}), \tag{7}$$

Generalized Sinkhorn. Problem (7) can be solved as follows. Let $\mathbf{K} = e^{-\frac{\mathbf{M}}{\varepsilon}}$ and $\psi = \gamma/(\gamma + \epsilon)$. Starting from two vectors $\mathbf{u}, \mathbf{v}$ set to $\mathbb{1}$ and iterating the scaling operations $\mathbf{u} \leftarrow (\mathbf{a}/\mathbf{K}\mathbf{v})^\psi$, $\mathbf{v} \leftarrow (\mathbf{b}/\mathbf{K}^\top \mathbf{u})^\psi$ until convergence, the minimizer of (7) can be computed as $P^\star = (\mathbf{u}_i \mathbf{K}_{ij} \mathbf{v}_j)_{i,j \in [\![p]\!]}$. This algorithm is a generalization of the Sinkhorn algorithm [18]. Since it involves matrix-matrix operations, it benefits from parallel hardware, such as GPUs.

Extension to $\mathbb{R}^p$. We extend next the Wasserstein distance to signed measures. We adopt a similar idea to what was suggested in [15,23,29] using a decomposition into positive and negative parts, $\mathbf{x}^{(s)} = \mathbf{x}^{(s)+} - \mathbf{x}^{(s)-}$ where $\mathbf{x}^{(s)+} = \max(\mathbf{x}^{(s)+}, 0)$ and $\mathbf{x}^{(s)-} = \max(-\mathbf{x}^{(s)+}, 0)$. For any vectors $\mathbf{a}, \mathbf{b} \in \mathbb{R}^p$, we define the generalized Wasserstein distance as:

$$\widetilde{W}(\mathbf{a}, \mathbf{b}) \stackrel{\text{def}}{=} W(\mathbf{a}^+, \mathbf{b}^+) + W(\mathbf{a}^-, \mathbf{b}^-). \tag{8}$$

Note that $W(\mathbf{0}, \mathbf{0}) = 0$ (see [15] for a proof), thus on positive measures $\widetilde{W} = W$. For the sake of convenience, we refer to $\widetilde{W}$ in (8) by the Wasserstein distance, even though it does not verify indiscernability. In practice, this extension allows to compare current dipoles across subjects according to their polarity which could be either towards the deep or superficial layers of the cortex.

Algorithm 1. MWE algorithm

Input: σ_0, $\mu, \epsilon, \gamma, \lambda$ and cost matrix **M**. data $(\mathbf{Y}^{(s)})_s (\mathbf{L}^{(s)})_s$.
Output: MWE: $(\mathbf{x}^{(s)})$, minimizers of (10).
repeat
    for $s = 1$ **to** S **do**
        Update $\mathbf{x}^{(s)+}$ with proximal coordinate descent to solve (12).
        Update $\mathbf{x}^{(s)-}$ with proximal coordinate descent to solve (12).
        Update $\sigma^{(s)}$ with (11).
    end for
    Update left marginals $\mathbf{m}^{(1)+}, \dots, \mathbf{m}^{(S)+}$ and $\bar{x}^+$ with generalized Sinkhorn.
    Update left marginals $\mathbf{m}^{(1)-} \dots, \mathbf{m}^{(S)-}$ and $\bar{x}^-$ with generalized Sinkhorn.
until convergence

The MTW Model. The multi-task Wasserstein model is the specific case of (4) with a penalty Ω promoting both sparsity and supports' proximity:

$$\Omega_{\text{MTW}}(\mathbf{x}^{(1)}, \dots, \mathbf{x}^{(S)}) \stackrel{\text{def}}{=} \mu \min_{\bar{x} \in \mathbb{R}^p} \frac{1}{S} \sum_{s=1}^{S} \widetilde{W}(\mathbf{x}^{(s)}, \bar{x}) + \lambda \|\mathbf{x}^{(s)}\|_1, \tag{9}$$

where $\mu, \lambda \geq 0$ are tuning hyperparameters. The OT term in (9) can be seen as a spatial variance. Indeed, the minimizer $\bar{x}$ corresponds to the Wasserstein barycenter with respect to the distance $\widetilde{W}$.

Minimum Wasserstein Estimates. One of the drawbacks of MTW is that λ is common to all subjects. Indeed, the loss considered in MTW implicitly assumes that the level of noise is the same across subjects. Following the work of [25] on the smoothed concomitant Lasso, we propose to extend MTW by inferring the specific noise standard deviation $\sigma^{(s)}$ along with the regression coefficient $\mathbf{x}^{(s)}$ of each subject. This allows to scale the weight of the ℓ_1 according to the level of noise. The Minimum Wasserstein Estimates (MWE) model reads:

$$\min_{\substack{\mathbf{x}^{(1)}, \dots, \mathbf{x}^{(S)} \in \mathbb{R}^p \\ \sigma^{(1)}, \dots, \sigma^{(S)} \in [\sigma_0, +\infty]}} \sum_{s=1}^{S} \frac{1}{2n\sigma^{(s)}} \|\mathbf{Y}^{(s)} - \mathbf{L}^{(s)}\mathbf{x}^{(s)}\|_2^2 + \frac{\sigma^{(s)}}{2} + \Omega_{\text{MTW}}(\mathbf{x}^{(1)}, \dots, \mathbf{x}^{(S)}),$$

$$\tag{10}$$

where σ_0 is a pre-defined constant. This lower bound constraint avoids numerical issues when $\lambda \to 0$ and therefore the standard deviation estimate also tends to 0. In practice σ_0 can be set for example using prior knowledge on the variance of the data or as a small fraction of the initial estimate of the standard deviation $\sigma_0 = \alpha \min_s \frac{\|\mathbf{Y}^{(s)}\|}{\sqrt{n}}$. In practice we adopt the second option and set $\alpha = 0.01$.

Algorithm. By combining (7), (8) and (10), we obtain an objective function taking as arguments $\big((\mathbf{x}^{(s)+})_s, (\mathbf{x}^{(s)-})_s, (\mathbf{P}^{(s)+})_s, (\mathbf{P}^{(s)-})_s, \bar{x}^+, \bar{x}^-, (\sigma^{(s)})_s\big)$. This function restricted to all parameters except $(\sigma^{(s)})_s$ is jointly convex [15]. Moreover, each $\sigma^{(s)}$ is only coupled with the variable $\mathbf{x}^{(s)}$. The restriction on every pair $(\mathbf{x}^{(s)}, \sigma^{(s)})$ is also jointly convex [25]. Thus the problem is jointly convex in all its variables. We minimize it by alternating optimization. To justify the convergence of such an algorithm, one needs to notice that the non-smooth ℓ_1 norms in the objective are separable [33]. The update with respect to each $\sigma^{(s)}$ is given by solving the first order optimality condition (Fermat's rule):

$$\sigma^{(s)} \leftarrow \frac{\|\mathbf{Y}^{(s)} - \mathbf{L}^{(s)}\mathbf{x}^{(s)}\|_2}{\sqrt{n}} \wedge \sigma_0, \tag{11}$$

which also corresponds to the empirical estimator of the standard deviation when the constraint is not active. To update the remaining variables, we follow the same optimization procedure laid out in [15] and adapted to MWE in Algorithm 1. Briefly, let $\mathbf{m}^{(s)+} \stackrel{\text{def}}{=} \mathbf{P}^{(s)+}\mathbb{1}$ (resp. $\mathbf{m}^{(s)+} \stackrel{\text{def}}{=} \mathbf{P}^{(s)+}\mathbb{1}$), when minimizing with respect to one $\mathbf{x}^{(s)+}$ (resp. $\mathbf{x}^{(s)-}$), the resulting problem can be written (dropping the exponents for simplicity):

$$\min_{\mathbf{x} \in \mathbb{R}_+^p} \frac{1}{2n}\|\mathbf{Y} - \mathbf{Lx}\|_2^2 + \frac{\mu\gamma}{S}(\langle \mathbf{x}, \mathbb{1} \rangle - \langle \log(\mathbf{x}), \mathbf{m} \rangle) + \lambda\sigma\|\mathbf{x}\|_1, \tag{12}$$

which can be solved using proximal coordinate descent [7]. The additional inference of a specific $\sigma^{(s)}$ for each subject allows to scale the Lasso penalty depending on their particular level of noise. The final update with respect to $((\mathbf{P}^{(s)+})_s, (\mathbf{P}^{(s)-})_s, \bar{\mathbf{x}}^+, \bar{\mathbf{x}}^-)$ can be cast as two Wasserstein barycenter problems, carried out using generalized Sinkhorn iterations [4]. Note that we do not compute the transport plans $P^{(s)}$ since inferring every source estimate $\mathbf{x}$ only requires the left marginal $\mathbf{m} = \mathbf{P}\mathbb{1}$ which does not require storing $\mathbf{P}$ in memory.

4 Experiments

Benchmarks: Dirty Models and Multi-level Lasso. As discussed in introduction, standard sparse source localization solvers are based on an ℓ_1 norm regularization, applied to the data of each subject independently. We use the independent Lasso estimator as a baseline. We compare MWE to the Group-Lasso estimator [2,37] which was proposed in this context to promote functional consistency across subjects [21]. It falls in the multi-task framework of (4) where the joint penalty is defined through an ℓ_{21} mixed norm $\|\mathbf{X}\|_{21} = \sum_{j=1}^p \sqrt{\sum_{s=1}^S \mathbf{x}_j^{(s)2}}$ where $\mathbf{X} = (\mathbf{x}_j^{(s)})_{(j,s)} \in \mathbb{R}^{p \times S}$. We also evaluate the performance of more flexible block sparse models where only a fraction of the source estimates are shared across all tasks: Dirty models [14] and the multivel lasso [22]. In Dirty models source estimates are written as a sum of two parts which are penalized with different norms. One common to all subjects (penalty ℓ_{21}) and one specific for each subject (penalty ℓ_1). The Multi-level Lasso (MLL) [22] applies the same idea using instead a product decomposition and a Lasso penalty on both parts. We also compare MWE with MTW to evaluate the benefits of inferring noise levels adaptively.

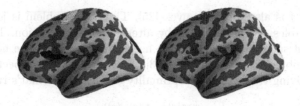

Fig. 1. Left: 3 labels from the aparc.a2009s parcellation. Right: Simulated activations for $S = 6$ subjects. Each color corresponds to a subject. Different radiuses are used to distinguish overlapping sources.

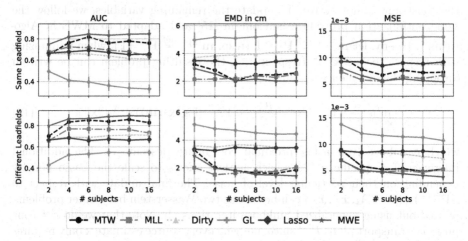

Fig. 2. Performance of different models over 30 trials in terms of AUC, EMD and MSE using the same leadfield for all subjects (randomly selected in each trial) (top) and specific leadfields (bottom).

Simulation Data and MEG/fMRI Datasets. We use the public dataset DS117 [36] which provides MEG, EEG and fMRI data of 16 healthy subjects to whom were presented images of famous, unfamiliar and scrambled faces. Using the MRI scan of each subject, we compute a source space and its associated leadfield comprising around 2500 sources per hemisphere [9]. Keeping only MEG gradiometer channels, we have $n = 204$ observations per subject.

For realistic data simulation, we use the actual leadfields from all subjects, yet restricted to the left hemisphere. We thus have 16 leadfields with $p = 2500$. We simulate an inverse solution $\mathbf{x}^s$ with q sources (q-sparse vector) by randomly selecting one source per label among q pre-defined labels using the *aparc.a2009s* parcellation of the Destrieux atlas. To model functional consistency, 50% of the subjects share sources at the same locations, the remaining 50% have sources randomly generated in the same labels (see Fig. 1). Their amplitudes are taken uniformly between 20 and 30 nAm. Their sign is taken at random with a Bernoulli distribution (0.5) for each label. We simulate $\mathbf{Y}$ using the forward model with a variance matrix σI_n. We set σ so as to have an average signal-to-noise ratio across

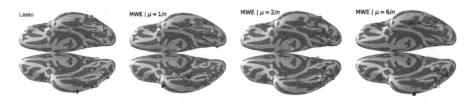

Fig. 3. Support of source estimates. Each color corresponds to a subject. Different radiuses are displayed for a better distinction of sources. The fusiform gyrus is highlighted in green. Increasing μ promotes functional consistency across subjects. (Color figure online)

subjects equal to 4 (SNR $\overset{\text{def}}{=} \sum_{s=1}^{S} \frac{\|\mathbf{L}^{(s)}\mathbf{x}^{(s)}\|}{S\sigma}$). We evaluate the performance of all models knowing the ground truth by comparing the best estimates in terms of three metrics: the mean squared error (MSE) to quantify accuracy in amplitude estimation, AUC and a generalized Earth mover distance (EMD) to assess supports estimation. We generalize the PR-AUC (Area under the curve Precision-recall) by defining $\text{AUC}(\hat{\mathbf{x}}, \mathbf{x}^\star) = \frac{1}{2}\text{PR-AUC}(\hat{\mathbf{x}}^+, \mathbf{x}^{\star+}) + \frac{1}{2}\text{PR-AUC}(\hat{\mathbf{x}}^-, \mathbf{x}^{\star-})$ where PR-AUC is computed between the estimated coefficients and the true supports. We compute EMD between normalized values of sources: $\text{EMD}(\hat{\mathbf{x}}, \mathbf{x}^\star) = \frac{1}{2}\text{WK}(\frac{\hat{\mathbf{x}}^+}{\hat{\mathbf{x}}^+\mathbb{1}}, \frac{\mathbf{x}^{\star+}}{\mathbf{x}^{\star+}\mathbb{1}}) + \frac{1}{2}\text{WK}(\frac{\hat{\mathbf{x}}^-}{\hat{\mathbf{x}}^-\mathbb{1}}, \frac{\mathbf{x}^{\star-}}{\mathbf{x}^{\star-}\mathbb{1}})$. Since $\mathbf{M}$ is expressed in centimeters, WK can be seen as an expectation of the geodesic distance between sources. The mean across subjects is reported for all metrics.

Simulation Results. We set the number of sources to 3 and vary the number of subjects under two conditions: (1) using one leadfield for all subjects, (2) using individual leadfields. Each model is fitted on a grid of hyperparameters and the best AUC/MSE/EMD scores are reported. We perform 30 different trials (with different true activations and noise, different common leadfield for condition (1)) and report the mean within a 95% confidence interval in Fig. 2.

Various observations can be made. The Group Lasso performs poorly – even compared to independent Lasso – which is expected since sources are not common for all subjects. Non-convexity allows MLL to be very effective with less than 2–4 subjects. Its performance yet degrades with more subjects. OT-based models (MWE and MTW) however benefit from the presence of more subjects by leveraging spatial proximity. They reduce the average error distance from 4 cm (Lasso) to less than 1 cm and reach an AUC of 0.9. The estimation of the noise standard deviation in the MTW model also does improve performance. Finally, we can appreciate the improvement of multi-task models when increasing the number subjects, especially when using different leadfield matrices. We argue that the different folding patterns of the cortex across subjects lead to different dipole orientations thereby increasing the chances of source identification.

Results on MEG/fMRI Data. The fusiform face area specializes in facial recognition and activates around 170ms after stimulus [13,17]. To study this response, we perform MEG source localization using Lasso and MWE. We pick the time point with the peak response for each subject within the interval 150–200 ms

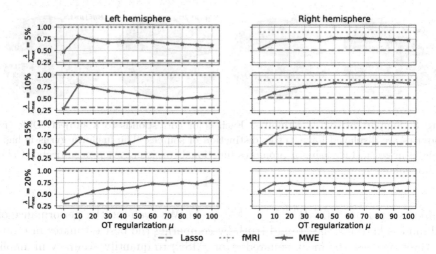

Fig. 4. Ratio of Maximum amplitudes: "in the fusiform gyrus"/"in the hemisphere". The mean across the 16 subjects is reported for different relative ℓ_1 norm regularization weights λ/λ_{max} (for $\lambda \geq \lambda_{max}$, all source estimates are null).

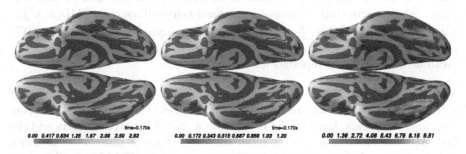

Fig. 5. Neural patterns of subject 2. Absolute amplitudes of MEG source estimates (in nAm) given by Lasso (Left) and MWE (Middle). Absolute values of fMRI Z-scores. (Right). The fusiform gyrus is highlighted in green. (Color figure online)

after visual presentation of famous faces. For both models, we select the smallest ℓ_1 tuning parameter λ for which less than 10 sources are active for each subject. Figure 3 shows how UOT regularization favors activation in the ventral pathway of the visual cortex. The Lasso solutions in Fig. 3 show significant differences between subjects. Since no ground truth exists, one could argue that MWE promotes consistency at the expense of individual signatures. To address this concern we compute the standardized fMRI Z-score of the conditions *famous vs scrambled faces*. We compare Lasso, MWE and fMRI by computing for each subject the ratio *largest value in fusiform gyrus/largest absolute value*. We report the mean across all subjects in Fig. 4. Note that for all subjects, the fMRI Z-score reaches its maximum in the fusiform gyrus, and that MWE regularization leads to more agreement between MEG and fMRI. Figure 5 shows MEG with MWE and fMRI results for subject 2.

5   Conclusion

We proposed in this work a novel approach to promote functional consistency through a convex model defined using an Unbalanced Optimal Transport regularization. Using a public MEG and fMRI dataset, we presented experiments demonstrating that MWE outperform multi-task sparse models in both amplitude and support estimation. We have shown in these experiments that MWE can close the gap between MEG and fMRI source imaging by gathering data from different subjects.

References

1. Ahlfors, S.P., Ilmoniemi, R.J., Hämäläinen, M.S.: Estimates of visually evoked cortical currents. Electroencephalogr. Clin. Neurophysiol. **82**(3), 225–236 (1992/2018)
2. Argyriou, A., Evgeniou, T., Pontil, M.: Multi-task feature learning. In: NIPS (2007)
3. Benamou, J., Carlier, G., Cuturi, M., Nenna, L., Peyré, G.: Iterative Bregman Projections For Regularized Transportation Problems. Society for Industrial and Applied Mathematics (2015)
4. Chizat, L., Peyré, G., Schmitzer, B., Vialard, F.X.: Scaling Algorithms for Unbalanced Transport Problems. arXiv:1607.05816 [math.OC] (2017)
5. Cuturi, M.: Sinkhorn distances: lightspeed computation of optimal transport. In: NIPS (2013)
6. Dale, A.M., et al.: Dynamic statistical parametric mapping. Neuron **26**(1), 55–67 (2000)
7. Fercoq, O., Richtárik, P.: Accelerated, parallel and proximal coordinate descent. SIAM J. Optim. **25**, 1997–2023 (2015)
8. Fischl, B., Sereno, M.I., Dale, A.M.: Cortical surface-based analysis: II: inflation, flattening, and a surface-based coordinate system. NeuroImage **9**, 195–207 (1999). Mathematics in Brain Imaging
9. Gramfort, A., et al.: MNE software for processing MEG and EEG data. NeuroImage **86**, 446–460 (2013)
10. Gramfort, A., Strohmeier, D., Haueisen, J., Hämäläinen, M., Kowalski, M.: Time-frequency mixed-norm estimates: sparse M/EEG imaging with non-stationary source activations. NeuroImage **70**, 410–422 (2013)
11. Hämäläinen, M.S., Ilmoniemi, R.J.: Interpreting magnetic fields of the brain: minimum norm estimates. Med. Biol. Eng. Comput. **32**(1), 35–42 (1994)
12. Hämäläinen, M.S., Sarvas, J.: Feasibility of the homogeneous head model in the interpretation of neuromagnetic fields. Phys. Med. Biol. **32**(1), 91 (1987)
13. Henson, R.N., Wakeman, D.G., Litvak, V., Friston, K.J.: A parametric empirical Bayesian framework for the EEG/MEG inverse problem: generative models for multi-subject and multi-modal integration. Front. Hum. Neurosci. **5**, 76 (2011)
14. Jalali, A., Ravikumar, P., Sanghavi, S., Ruan, C.: A dirty model for multi-task learning. In: NIPS (2010)
15. Janati, H., Cuturi, M., Gramfort, A.: Wasserstein regularization for sparse multi-task regression (2018)
16. Kantorovic, L.: On the translocation of masses. C.R. Acad. Sci. URSS (1942)
17. Kanwisher, N., McDermott, J., Chun, M.M.: The fusiform face area: a module in human extrastriate cortex specialized for face perception. J. Neurosci. **17**(11), 4302–4311 (1997)

18. Knopp, P., Sinkhorn, R.: Concerning nonnegative matrices and doubly stochastic matrices. Pac. J. Math. **1**(2), 343–348 (1967)
19. Kozunov, V.V., Ossadtchi, A.: Gala: group analysis leads to accuracy, a novel approach for solving the inverse problem in exploratory analysis of group MEG recordings. Front. Neurosci. **9**, 107 (2015)
20. Larson, E., Maddox, R.K., Lee, A.K.C.: Improving spatial localization in MEG inverse imaging by leveraging intersubject anatomical differences. Front. Neurosci. **8**, 330 (2014)
21. Lim, M., Ales, J., Cottereau, B.M., Hastie, T., Norcia, A.M.: Sparse EEG/MEG source estimation via a group lasso. PLOS (2017)
22. Lozano, A., Swirszcz, G.: Multi-level lasso for sparse multi-task regression. In: ICML (2012)
23. Mainini, E.: A description of transport cost for signed measures. J. Math. Sci. **181**(6), 837–855 (2012)
24. Massias, M., Fercoq, O., Gramfort, A., Salmon, J.: Generalized concomitant multi-task lasso for sparse multimodal regression. In: Proceedings of Machine Learning Research, vol. 84, pp. 998–1007. PMLR, 09–11 April 2018
25. Ndiaye, E., Fercoq, O., Gramfort, A., Leclère, V., Salmon, J.: Efficient smoothed concomitant lasso estimation for high dimensional regression. J. Phys.: Conf. Ser. **904**(1), 012006 (2017)
26. Okada, Y.: Empirical bases for constraints in current-imaging algorithms. Brain Topogr. **5**, 373–377 (1993)
27. Owen, A.B.: A robust hybrid of lasso and ridge regression. Contemp. Math. **443**, 59–72 (2007)
28. Pascual-Marqui, R.: Standardized low-resolution brain electromagnetic tomography (sLORETA): technical details. Methods Find Exp. Clin. Pharmacol. **24**, D:5–D:12 (2002)
29. Profeta, A., Sturm, K.T.: Heat flow with dirichlet boundary conditions via optimal transport and gluing of metric measure spaces (2018)
30. Strohmeier, D., Bekhti, Y., Haueisen, J., Gramfort, A.: The iterative reweighted mixed-norm estimate for spatio-temporal MEG/EEG source reconstruction. IEEE Trans. Med. Imaging **35**(10), 2218–2228 (2016)
31. Sun, T., Zhang, C.H.: Scaled sparse linear regression. Biometrika **99**, 879–898 (2012)
32. Tibshirani, R.: Regression shrinkage and selection via the lasso. J. R. Stat. Soc. **58**(1), 267–288 (1996)
33. Tseng, P.: Convergence of a block coordinate descent method for nondifferentiable minimization. J. Optim. Theory Appl. **109**(3), 475–494 (2001)
34. Uutela, K., Hämäläinen, M.S., Somersalo, E.: Visualization of magnetoencephalographic data using minimum current estimates. NeuroImage **10**(2), 173–180 (1999)
35. Varoquaux, G., Gramfort, A., Pedregosa, F., Michel, V., Thirion, B.: Multi-subject dictionary learning to segment an atlas of brain spontaneous activity. In: Székely, G., Hahn, H.K. (eds.) IPMI 2011. LNCS, vol. 6801, pp. 562–573. Springer, Heidelberg (2011). https://doi.org/10.1007/978-3-642-22092-0_46
36. Wakeman, D., Henson, R.: A multi-subject, multi-modal human neuroimaging dataset. Sci. Data **2**(150001) (2015)
37. Yuan, M., Lin, Y.: Model selection and estimation in regression with grouped variables. J. R. Stat. Soc. **68**(1), 49–67 (2006)

InSpect: INtegrated SPECTral Component Estimation and Mapping for Multi-contrast Microstructural MRI

Paddy J. Slator[1]([✉]), Jana Hutter[2,3], Razvan V. Marinescu[1], Marco Palombo[1], Alexandra L. Young[1], Laurence H. Jackson[2,3], Alison Ho[4], Lucy C. Chappell[4], Mary Rutherford[2], Joseph V. Hajnal[2,3], and Daniel C. Alexander[1]

[1] Centre for Medical Image Computing, Department of Computer Science, University College London, London, UK
p.slator@ucl.ac.uk
[2] Centre for the Developing Brain, King's College London, London, UK
[3] Biomedical Engineering Department, King's College London, London, UK
[4] Women's Health Department, King's College London, London, UK

Abstract. We introduce a novel algorithm for deriving meaningful maps from multi-contrast MRI experiments. Such experiments enable the estimation of multidimensional correlation spectra, in domains such as T1-diffusivity, T2-diffusivity, or T1-T2. These spectra combine information from complementary MR properties, and therefore have the potential for improved quantification of distinct tissue types compared to single-contrast analyses. However, spectral estimation is an ill-conditioned problem which is highly sensitive to noise and requires significant regularisation. We propose an Expectation-Maximisation based method - which we term InSpect - for unified analysis of multi-contrast MR images. The algorithm simultaneously estimates canonical spectra associated with distinct tissue types within an image, and produces maps quantifying the spatial distribution of these spectra. We test the algorithm's capabilities on simulated data, then apply to placental diffusion-relaxometry data. On placental data we identified significant within-organ and across-subject variation in T2*-ADC spectra - showing the potential of InSpect for detailed separation and quantification of distinct microstructural environments.

1 Introduction

Multidimensional magnetic resonance (MR) experiments simultaneously measure multiple MR properties, and hence promise more specific characterisation of tissue. Examples of multidimensional MR techniques include various types of correlation spectroscopy, such as relaxometry-relaxometry [6] and diffusion-relaxometry [12]. Several recent papers have leveraged recent advances in scanner hardware to extend these ideas into imaging, in the T1-diffusion [4], T2-diffusion [9,13], and T1-T2-diffusion [2] domains.

© Springer Nature Switzerland AG 2019
A. C. S. Chung et al. (Eds.): IPMI 2019, LNCS 11492, pp. 755–766, 2019.
https://doi.org/10.1007/978-3-030-20351-1_59

An attractive approach to analysing such data is continuum modelling. This assumes that spins have a distribution of values (e.g. relaxivity, diffusivity), which are quantified by a multidimensional spectrum. The exponential dependence on relaxation constants and diffusivity leads to a Laplace transform model on the MR signal; the spectrum can therefore be estimated using an inverse Laplace transform with regularisation [6].

However, fitting the spectrum requires high signal-to-noise ratio (SNR) data, which can make individual voxel fits - and hence the derivation of quantitative maps of spectral variation across an image - particularly problematic. In practice, this means that additional spatial regularisation is often necessary. This can mean averaging the signal over a region of interest (ROI), or also "spectrally integrating" within user-defined regions. This usually involves identifying canonical components in ROI-derived spectra, then integrating voxelwise spectra within the regions corresponding to these components, hence obtaining apparent spectral volume fraction estimates [2,9,10].

Recently, methods have been proposed for increasing robustness of voxelwise spectral fits, utilising marginal distributions [1] or spatial regularisation [9]. These methods can improve subsequent spatial mapping, yet there are inherent limitations to existing approaches which motivate this paper. Specifically, canonical spectral components require manual identification, and therefore may be ill-defined if estimated over inhomogeneous regions, and may not cover the full range of observations over the extent of an image.

In this paper we present a method - named InSpect - which addresses these problems in a data-driven way. Our algorithm automatically segments multidimensional MR images by clustering voxels with similar spectra, and simultaneously infers representative spectra for these clusters. This offers many potential advantages over voxelwise approaches. By averaging over similar voxels we reduce noise in canonical spectrum estimates. Additionally, the method is fully data-driven so is unlikely to miss any important spectral components that appear in the data. In short, the InSpect algorithm seeks a compact representation of the whole image that captures intrinsic variation in the data without overfitting.

The paper proceeds as follows: we first define the InSpect model, then derive an Expectation-Maximisation algorithm for its inference. We finally test the algorithm's utility on simulated and real multidimensional MRI data. We present a general form of InSpect in two dimensions, but emphasise that extension to higher dimensions is simple.

2   Methods

2.1   Multidimensional Spectrum Estimation

The standard approach for estimating the spectrum from a multidimensional MRI experiment proceeds as follows [6]; for a general 2D multi-contrast MRI experiment the signal, S, can be described by a continuum model

$$S(t_1, t_2) = \int \int F(\omega_1, \omega_2) K(t_1, t_2, \omega_1, \omega_2) \, d\omega_1 d\omega_2 \tag{1}$$

where t_1 and t_2 are experimental parameters which are varied to yield contrast in intrinsic MR properties ω_1 and ω_2, via the specific form of the kernel $K(t_1, t_2, \omega_1, \omega_2)$. $F(\omega_1, \omega_2)$ is the 2D spectrum of ω_1 and ω_2, i.e. the distribution of these values across all spins. Discretising onto a N_{ω_1} by N_{ω_2} grid yields

$$S(t_1, t_2) = \sum_{i=1}^{N_{\omega_1}} \sum_{j=1}^{N_{\omega_2}} F(\omega_1^{(i)}, \omega_2^{(j)}) K(t_1, t_2, \omega_1^{(i)}, \omega_2^{(j)}) \tag{2}$$

By choosing a suitable ordering of spectrum coordinates ω_1, ω_2, the signal for all MR encodings in the experiment can be written in matrix form

$$\mathbf{S} = \mathbf{KF} \tag{3}$$

where $\mathbf{S}$ is a column vector, length N_s of the signals at each encoding, K is an N_s by $N_{\omega_1} N_{\omega_2}$ matrix of discretised kernel values, and F is an $N_{\omega_1} N_{\omega_2}$ length column vector of spectrum values. The spectrum F can then be calculated as follows, including a non-negativity constraint and regularisation term

$$\mathbf{F} = \underset{\mathbf{F} \geq 0}{\arg \min} \, \|\mathbf{KF} - \mathbf{S}\|_2^2 + \alpha \|\mathbf{F}\|_2^2. \tag{4}$$

By solving the above equation with non-negative least squares regression the spectrum can be estimated within a single voxel. However, as mentioned earlier, low SNR can lead to noisy spectrum estimates and hence poor spatial maps. This is the case whether these maps are produced directly from the estimated spectra, or through picking canonical spectral regions and integrating the fitted voxelwise spectra within them. In the following section we describe our novel approach to this problem.

2.2   InSpect Model

We move from considering the signal from a single voxel, to an image (or volume) consisting of N voxels in total. We assume that the signal from each voxel, $\mathbf{S}_n$, is described by the continuum model of Eq. (1) as described in the previous section.

Rather than naively fitting spectra to each $\mathbf{S}_n$, we seek a data-driven lower dimensional representation of the spectral image. Thus, we assume a small number of voxel types each defined by a canonical spectrum. We then seek to simultaneously estimate the set of canonical spectra and the assignment of voxels to spectra. This has the effect of grouping voxels into clusters, so a byproduct is a segmentation of the image into distinct regions based on spectral properties.

We start from the assumption that there are M clusters of voxels, with each cluster having an associated spectrum $\mathbf{F}_m$, which we estimate from the data. In practice, we do not know each voxel's cluster a-priori and also need to estimate it. These cluster membership indices are hence model latent states, which we write as $z_n = m$ if voxel n belongs to cluster m. The set of latent states for the whole image is therefore $\mathbf{z} = \{z_n\}_{n=1}^{N}$, where $z_n \in \{1, ..., M\}$. The cluster membership probabilities are modelled with a categorical distribution, the parameters are the number of clusters, M, and the cluster probabilities $\{p_m\}_{m=1}^{M}$.

We consider a Gaussian model on the observed signal. For a voxel, n belonging to cluster m the expected value for each element of the observed signal vector, $\mathbf{S}_n$, is the corresponding $\mathbf{KF}_m$ term. We also assume that all observations in a voxel have the same variance σ_n^2. We write this as follows

$$\mathbf{S}_n \sim \mathcal{N}(\mathbf{KF}_m, \sigma_n^2). \tag{5}$$

Assuming that voxels are independent, the complete data model likelihood for an image given the parameters θ is therefore

$$\pi(\mathbf{D}, \mathbf{z}|\theta) = \pi(\mathbf{z}|\theta)\pi(\mathbf{D}|\mathbf{z}, \theta) = \prod_{n=1}^{N} p_{z_n} N(\mathbf{S}_n; \mathbf{KF}_{z_n}, \sigma_n^2) \tag{6}$$

where $N(\mathbf{S}_n; \mathbf{KF}_{z_n}, \sigma_n^2)$ refers to the product over the Normal PDFs of each measured signal value within the voxel, and we have denoted $\mathbf{D} = \{\mathbf{S}_n\}_{n=1}^{N}$ for notational simplicity. By summing over all possible clusterings we get the marginal likelihood

$$\pi(\mathbf{D}|\theta) = \sum_{\text{all } \mathbf{z}} \pi(\mathbf{D}, \mathbf{z}|\theta) = \sum_{m=1}^{M} \prod_{n=1}^{N} p_{z_n} N(\mathbf{S}_n; \mathbf{KF}_{z_n}, \sigma_n^2) \tag{7}$$

The maximum likelihood estimate (MLE) of θ is the value that maximises this. This calculation is intractable in practice, so we derive an Expectation-Maximisation (EM) algorithm [5]. The full set of model parameters is $\theta = \{p_1, ..., p_M, \mathbf{F}_1, ..., \mathbf{F}_M, \sigma_1^2, ..., \sigma_N^2\}$, but in practice we estimate the σ_n^2's by calculating the empirical variance of the observed data at each voxel, so do not consider this in the EM algorithm. We also need to choose the number of clusters M - ideally from the data. We do this by fitting the model for a range of reasonable M, then comparing model selection statistics - such as the Bayesian information criterion (BIC) and Akaike information criterion (AIC) - across this range.

2.3   Expectation-Maximisation Algorithm

To implement an EM algorithm we first calculate an expression for the expected value of $\log \pi(\mathbf{D}, \mathbf{z}|\theta)$ (complete data log-likelihood) with respect to $\pi(\mathbf{z}|\mathbf{D})$ (posterior probability of latent states given the data and current parameters). Using the notation of Bishop [3] we write this function as

$$Q(\theta, \theta^{(t-1)}) = \mathbb{E}_{\mathbf{z}|\mathbf{D}, \theta^{(t-1)}} \left[\log \pi(\mathbf{D}, \mathbf{z}|\theta)\right] = \sum_{\mathbf{z}} \pi(\mathbf{z}|\mathbf{D}, \theta^{(t-1)}) \log \pi(\mathbf{D}, \mathbf{z}|\theta) \tag{8}$$

where $\theta^{(t)}$ denotes the model parameters at step t of the algorithm. Marginalising over the clusters, applying the independence of voxels, substituting the likelihood

(Eq. (6)), and taking the log gives the final expression for Q

$$Q(\theta, \theta^{(t-1)}) = \sum_{n=1}^{N} \sum_{m=1}^{M} w_{nm} \left[\log p_m - \frac{N_s}{2} \log 2\pi\sigma_n^2 - \left\| \frac{\mathbf{S}_n - \mathbf{KF}_m}{\sqrt{2\sigma_n^2}} \right\|_2^2 \right] \quad (9)$$

where $w_{nm} = \pi(z_n = m|\mathbf{S}_n, \theta^{(t-1)})$. These w_{nm} terms are calculated (for all n and m) in the E-step, and the M-step maximises $Q(\theta, \theta^{(t-1)})$ with respect to the parameters θ.

E-step. For the E-step we first note the full posterior distribution for the model

$$\pi(\theta, \mathbf{z}|\mathbf{D}) \propto \pi(\mathbf{D}|\theta, \mathbf{z})\pi(\mathbf{z}, \theta) = \prod_{n=1}^{N} p_{z_n} N(\mathbf{S}_n; \mathbf{KF}_{z_n}, \sigma_n^2) \quad (10)$$

where we have assumed a uniform prior on both the latent states $\mathbf{z}$, and the parameters θ. The posterior distribution for each z_n - normalised across all clusters - is therefore

$$w_{nm} = \pi(z_n = m|\mathbf{S}_n, \theta^{(t-1)}) = \frac{p_m N(\mathbf{S}_n; \mathbf{KF}_m, \sigma_n^2)}{\sum_{i=1}^{M} p_i N(\mathbf{S}_n; \mathbf{KF}_i, \sigma_n^2)}. \quad (11)$$

M-step. In the M-step we optimise the parameters given the current cluster weights w_{nm}. In other words we solve

$$\theta = \arg\max_{\theta} Q(\theta, \theta^{(t-1)}) \quad (12)$$

sequentially for each parameter $\theta = \{p_1, ..., p_M, \mathbf{F}_1, ..., \mathbf{F}_M\}$. For $p_1, ...p_M$ maximising this equation, whilst implementing the constraint $\sum_{m=1}^{M} p_m = 1$ using a Lagrange multiplier (e.g. Bishop [3]), gives

$$p_m = \frac{1}{N} \sum_{n=1}^{N} w_{nm} \quad (13)$$

in other words the current mean cluster weight over all voxels.

For the canonical cluster-associated spectra, $\mathbf{F}_1, ...\mathbf{F}_M$, we have (ignoring constant terms, and swapping $\arg\max_{\mathbf{F}_m}$ for $\arg\min_{\mathbf{F}_m}$ due to the sign)

$$\mathbf{F}_m = \arg\min_{\mathbf{F}_m} \sum_{n=1}^{N} w_{nm} \left\| \frac{\mathbf{S}_n - \mathbf{KF}_m}{\sqrt{2}\sigma_n} \right\|_2^2 \quad (14)$$

Taking the derivative with respect to $\mathbf{F}_m$, setting equal to zero and rearranging gives

$$\mathbf{KF}_m = \frac{1}{W_m} \sum_{n=1}^{N} w_{nm} \mathbf{S}_n \quad (15)$$

where $W_m = \sum_{n=1}^{N} w_{nm}$. In other words, we need to minimise the difference between $\mathbf{KF}_m$ and the mean signal over all voxels normalised by cluster weights. This implies the following modification to Eq. (4) to calculate the spectrum associated with each cluster

$$\mathbf{F}_m = \underset{\mathbf{F}_m > 0}{\arg\min} \left\| \mathbf{KF}_m - \frac{1}{W_m} \sum_{n=1}^{N} w_{nm} \mathbf{S}_n \right\|_2^2 + \alpha \|\mathbf{F}_m\|_2^2 \qquad (16)$$

which we can solve with non-negative least squares regression as described earlier. By iterating E and M steps we therefore calculate the MLE of model parameters (cluster probabilities and cluster-associated spectra for each cluster), and posterior distribution of latent states (cluster weights for each voxel).

2.4   Application to Placenta Diffusion-Relaxometry Data

We applied our algorithm to data from combined diffusion-relaxometry experiments previously published by Slator et al. [11]. In this work the authors varied the b-value and echo time (TE) using a sequence called ZEBRA [8], yielding simultaneous diffusivity and T2* contrast. The sequence consists of 66 diffusion weightings (ranging from b = 5 to 1600 s mm^{-2}, including six b = 0 volumes) and 5 TEs (78, 114, 150, 186, 222 ms) for a total of 330 contrast-encodings. Other acquisition parameters were FOV = $300 \times 320 \times 84$ mm, TR = 7 s, SENSE = 2.5, halfscan = 0.6, resolution = 3 mm^3.

We fit InSpect to placental scans from 12 participants, of whom 9 were categorised as healthy controls, two had chronic hypertension in pregnancy, and one had pre-eclampsia (PE) with additional fetal growth restriction (FGR). One participant with chronic hypertension was scanned two times, four weeks apart, and developed superimposed pre-eclampsia by the second scan. A placenta and uterine wall region of interest (ROI) was manually segmented on all images.

There are multiple approaches possible when applying InSpect to a dataset with multiple participants: fit to each image independently and find separate canonical spectra and clusters for each; fit to all images simultaneously and estimate a common set of spectra; or any number of hybrid approaches. The best approach will depend on the specific application. One important consideration is the extent to which one wants to probe within-image heterogeneity, as opposed to across-image differences. In this paper our aim is to gain an initial idea of typical placental T2*-ADC spectra, and their spatial distributions, across healthy and unhealthy tissue. We therefore fit InSpect in two ways: first to each participant's scan individually for various values of M, to determine a parsimonious number of clusters from the data. Then, given this information, we fix the number of clusters and fit InSpect to the data from all patients simultaneously.

The number of clusters which best explained the data in individual image fits, as measured by the BIC and AIC, varied across participants. For the placentas of participants diagnosed with a pregnancy complication the typical number of clusters was three. For healthy placentas we tended to see BIC and AIC values levelling off at around eight clusters. Given this information, we fixed the number of clusters at eight when fitting InSpect to the data from all participants simultaneously.

We also also naively fit voxelwise T2*-ADC spectra to all scans by solving Eq. (4), and derived spectral volume fraction maps from these by integrating in six regions (defined later) of T2*-ADC space, mirroring the approach in references [2,9,10].

2.5   Application to Simulated Data

We performed simulations, using the same contrast encodings (i.e. b-value, TE pairs) as the placental data, to test InSpect. We constructed a minimal example by first creating a synthetic image of 1000 voxels, with the voxels split evenly between two clusters. Each cluster was next associated a simple one-component spectrum with a fixed T2* and ADC value. Given a voxel's T2* and ADC we simulated the signal with a simple joint model as follows

$$S(b, T_E) = \exp\left(-b\text{ADC}\right) \exp\left(-T_E/T_2^*\right) \tag{17}$$

adding Gaussian measurement noise with a realistic SNR level of 20 (e.g. [11]) in all voxels. We ran a total of 72 simulations by varying the properties of cluster-associated spectra (details in Fig. 1 caption). This allowed us to investigate how different cluster-associated spectra need to be for InSpect to distinguish them, and if this varies across regions of T2*-ADC space.

We first fit spectra in the standard voxelwise manner (using Eq. (4)) for all simulated images. We subsequently derived spectral volume fraction maps from the voxelwise fits, following the aforementioned integration approach (e.g. [2,9,10]). We defined the areas in which to spectrally integrate as two regions separated by the midpoint of the two cluster-associated spectra. We fit InSpect to all synthetic images separately with the number of clusters set to two, thereby automatically obtaining segmentations and canonical spectrum estimates.

2.6   Algorithm Implementation Details

For the voxelwise fits we set the value of α in Eq. (4) at 0.01 using the L-curve method [7]. We used the same α value in Eq. (16) for the InSpect fits. For all InSpect fits we initialised the cluster weights by sampling from a uniform random distribution. We estimate σ^2 voxelwise by calculating the empirical variance of the b = 0 volumes with the lowest TE. We determined convergence of the EM algorithm by manually checking for stationarity of parameters, 25 EM steps were typically sufficient for convergence. The EM algorithm output is robust over multiple runs from different random initialisations.

3   Results

Figure 1 shows that InSpect performs significantly better than voxelwise mapping by spectral integration; recovering the ground truth clusters in the majority of simulations. These results are not a complete characterisation of the ability of InSpect, but they do show that it works for various parameter combinations across the T2*-ADC domain under the same contrast encodings as the placental data. The limits of InSpect - under this acquisition sequence - were reached when T2* was low, especially for components with close ADC values. This reflects the fact that most signal has attenuated for these T2* values at the acquired TEs.

Figure 2 shows the InSpect fit to the placental data - with all 13 scans fit at once. The InSpect maps show clear structure - both within organ and across participants. The corresponding eight cluster-associated spectra show varying number of peaks, T2*, and ADC values.

We also compare InSpect mapping to spectral integration of voxelwise fits (Fig. 3). The voxelwise maps show similar features to InSpect maps, although they average over some small-scale features. Visualisation of these substructures may be possible from voxelwise fits given a sufficiently delicate partitioning of the spectral domain.

4   Discussion

We demonstrate InSpect, a data-driven method for mapping spectral components in multi-contrast microstructural MRI experiments. This is an alternative to mapping by spectral integration of voxelwise fits, which is inherently unstable because of high noise, and fails to exploit the likely low variation in underlying spectra across individual (or groups of) images. InSpect automatically maps the spectral components, whereas voxelwise integration requires user-defined choices of regions in the spectral domain. Another advantage of InSpect over voxelwise approaches is speed; the method avoids computationally heavy non-negative least squares fitting in every voxel.

On simulated data we show that InSpect significantly improves mapping based on spectral properties, even when the total number of voxels is relatively small compared to a typical clinical scan (Fig. 1). On placental diffusion-relaxometry MRI data InSpect segmented clear anatomically-linked structures (Fig. 2A). This suggests that InSpect maps provide insight into microstructure and microcirculation across the placenta. Clusters 8 and 6 likely represent the centre and periphery of placental lobules respectively. The spectra associated with these clusters both have very high T2*, potentially reflecting the high oxygen levels in healthy placentas. We also observed very clear differences in cluster assignments between scans of participants who were diagnosed with a pregnancy disorder compared to controls (Fig. 2C).

In fact, we observed a canonical spectrum type which appears solely in pathological cases (cluster 1 in Fig. 2). This demonstrates a significant advantage when fitting the model to the full data set - as we did for the placental data - as opposed to individual images. By sharing data across subjects we automatically quantify spectral differences between control and dysfunctional placentas. It also ensures consistent interpretation across all images in a data set, avoiding problems such as the matching of clusters across images. However, this comes at the expense

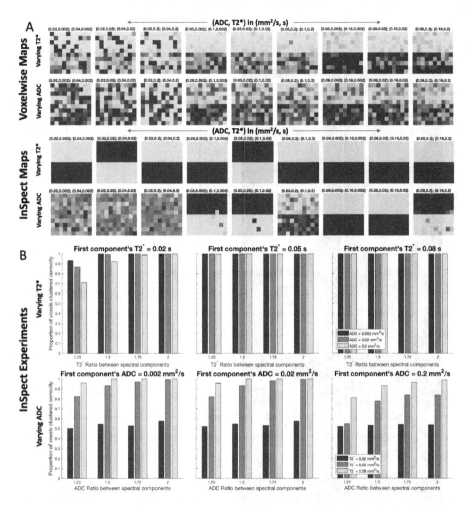

Fig. 1. InSpect applied to synthetic diffusion-relaxometry images. Each image comprises two clusters - located in the top and bottom halves of the image. Each cluster is associated with a one component T2*-ADC spectrum. Three quantities were varied across simulations: distance between the two cluster-associated spectral components (either in T2* space with ADC fixed, or vice versa, we used 4 distances between 1.25 and 4), value of the fixed parameter (3 in total), and value of the varying parameter (3 in total). There were hence a total of 72 simulations. SNR was set to 20 for all images. (A) Volume fraction maps obtained from spectral integration of voxelwise fits (e.g. [2,9,10]) in two domains delineated by the midpoint of the simulation components, and InSpect segmentation maps (posterior weights on clusters in each voxel). Note that in some cases where InSpect exactly infers the simulated ground truth the cluster labels are swapped. (B) Bar plots showing the proportion of voxels where InSpect successfully recovered the ground truth for various combinations of T2* and ADC characterising the two cluster-associated spectra.

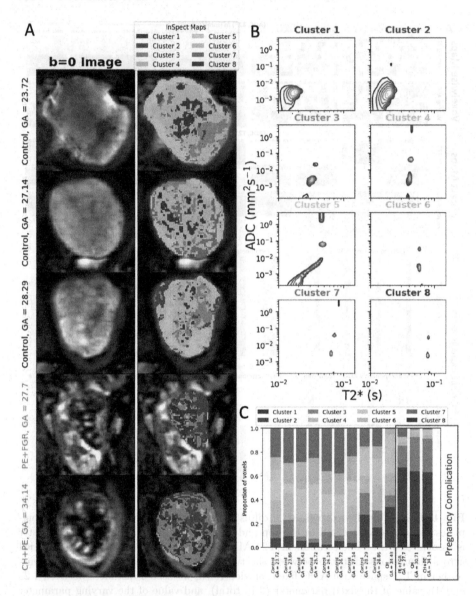

Fig. 2. InSpect simultaneously applied to 13 placental diffusion-relaxometry images. (A) InSpect maps and b = 0 images for five of the 13 participants, including two who had been diagnosed with a pregnancy complication at the time of the scan. (B) Corresponding T2*-ADC spectra for the eight clusters in (A). (C) Proportion of voxels assigned to each cluster for all participants.

of averaging inter-organ heterogeneity - within-participant fits may make sense in other contexts.

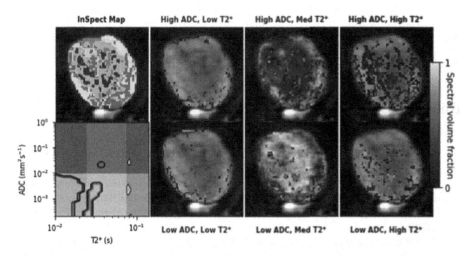

Fig. 3. Comparison between InSpect mapping (top left panel) and spectral integration of voxelwise fits for a single participant. Voxelwise maps (all but the top left panel) were obtained by the standard spectral integration approach (e.g. [2,9,10]) within the six regions displayed in the bottom left panel. The bottom left panel also outlines three inferred InSpect spectra (clusters 1, 5 and 8 in Fig. 2), each in a different color, for comparison.

An advantage of the voxelwise spectral integration approach over InSpect is that it implicitly considers partial volume effects. This observation implies a clear direction for future work - an extension of the discrete clustering approach we propose here to continuous spectral component mapping. This would have continuous latent states, rather than discrete, and therefore would better quantify partial voluming. These developments should work towards the ultimate aim of using multi-contrast MRI experiments to improve tissue microstructure measurements; enabling the quantification of tissue properties - both healthy and diseased - which cannot usually be separated by a single MR contrast. These methods have wide-ranging potential applications: spectroscopic imaging techniques are prominent in the brain and other organs; there many parameters other than T2* and ADC that could be exploited; and extending to higher dimensional spectra is straightforward.

5   Conclusion

We introduce the InSpect algorithm, which simultaneously undertakes two complementary tasks - multidimensional spectrum estimation and mapping - by sharing information across voxels. Although we applied InSpect to diffusion-relaxometry data, the method is immediately applicable to any multidimensional MR imaging experiment.

Acknowledgements. We thank all mothers, midwives, obstetricians, and radiographers who played a key role in obtaining the data sets. This work was funded by the NIH (Human Placenta Project, 1U01HD087202-01); Wellcome Trust (201374/Z/16/Z); EPSRC (N018702, M020533, EP/N018702/1); and NIHR (RP-2014-05-019).

References

1. Benjamini, D., Basser, P.J.: Use of marginal distributions constrained optimization (MADCO) for accelerated 2D MRI relaxometry and diffusometry. J. Magn. Reson. **271**, 40–45 (2016)
2. Benjamini, D., Basser, P.J.: Magnetic resonance microdynamic imaging reveals distinct tissue microenvironments. NeuroImage **163**, 183–196 (2017)
3. Bishop, C.M.: Pattern Recognition and Machine Learning. Springer, Heidelberg (2006)
4. De Santis, S., Barazany, D., Jones, D.K., Assaf, Y.: Resolving relaxometry and diffusion properties within the same voxel in the presence of crossing fibres by combining inversion recovery and diffusion-weighted acquisitions. Magn. Reson. Med. **75**(1), 372–380 (2016)
5. Dempster, A.P., Laird, N., Rubin, D.B., Rubin, D.: Maximum likelihood from incomplete data via the EM algorithm. J. Royal Stat. Soc. Ser. B (Methodol.) **39**(1), 1–38 (1977)
6. English, A.E., Whittall, K.P., Joy, M.L., Henkelman, R.M.: Quantitative two-dimensional time correlation relaxometry. Magn. Reson. Med. **22**(2), 425–434 (1991)
7. Hansen, P.C.: Analysis of discrete Ill-posed problems by means of the L-curve. SIAM Rev. **34**(4), 561–580 (1992)
8. Hutter, J., et al.: Integrated and efficient diffusion-relaxometry using ZEBRA. Sci. Rep. **8**(1), 15138 (2018)
9. Kim, D., Doyle, E.K., Wisnowski, J.L., Kim, J.H., Haldar, J.P.: Diffusion-relaxation correlation spectroscopic imaging: a multidimensional approach for probing microstructure. Magn. Reson. Med. **78**(6), 2236–2249 (2017)
10. Mackay, A., Whittall, K., Adler, J., Li, D., Paty, D., Graeb, D.: In vivo visualization of myelin water in brain by magnetic resonance. Magn. Reson. Med. **31**(6), 673–677 (1994)
11. Slator, P.J., et al.: Combined diffusion-relaxometry MRI to identify dysfunction in the human placenta. Magn. Reson. Med., 1–12 (2019)
12. Van Dusschoten, D., Moonen, C.T., De Jager, P.A., Van As, H.: Unraveling diffusion constants in biological tissue by combining Carr- Purcell-Meiboom-Gill imaging and pulsed field gradient NMR. Magn. Reson. Med. **36**(6), 907–913 (1996)
13. Veraart, J., Novikov, D.S., Fieremans, E.: TE dependent diffusion imaging (TEdDI) distinguishes between compartmental T2 relaxation times. NeuroImage **182**, 360–369 (2018)

Joint Inference on Structural and Diffusion MRI for Sequence-Adaptive Bayesian Segmentation of Thalamic Nuclei with Probabilistic Atlases

Juan Eugenio Iglesias[1,2,3]([✉]), Koen Van Leemput[2,4], Polina Golland[3],
and Anastasia Yendiki[2]

[1] Centre for Medical Image Computing, Department of Medical Physics and
Biomedical Engineering, University College London, London, UK
e.iglesias@ucl.ac.uk
[2] Athinoula A. Martinos Center for Biomedical Imaging,
Massachusetts General Hospital and Harvard Medical School, Boston, USA
[3] Computer Science and Artificial Intelligence Laboratory, MIT, Cambridge, USA
[4] Department of Health Technology, Technical University of Denmark,
Kongens Lyngby, Denmark

Abstract. Segmentation of structural and diffusion MRI (sMRI/dMRI) is usually performed independently in neuroimaging pipelines. However, some brain structures (e.g., globus pallidus, thalamus and its nuclei) can be extracted more accurately by fusing the two modalities. Following the framework of Bayesian segmentation with probabilistic atlases and unsupervised appearance modeling, we present here a novel algorithm to jointly segment multi-modal sMRI/dMRI data. We propose a hierarchical likelihood term for the dMRI defined on the unit ball, which combines the Beta and Dimroth-Scheidegger-Watson distributions to model the data at each voxel. This term is integrated with a mixture of Gaussians for the sMRI data, such that the resulting joint unsupervised likelihood enables the analysis of multi-modal scans acquired with any type of MRI contrast, b-values, or number of directions, which enables wide applicability. We also propose an inference algorithm to estimate the maximum-a-posteriori model parameters from input images, and to compute the most likely segmentation. Using a recently published atlas derived from histology, we apply our method to thalamic nuclei segmentation on two datasets: HCP (state of the art) and ADNI (legacy) – producing lower sample sizes than Bayesian segmentation with sMRI alone.

1 Introduction

Automated segmentation of MRI scans is a prerequisite for most human neuroimaging studies. Most of the algorithms commonly used for this task rely solely on structural MRI (sMRI) scans, and belong to one of three categories: Bayesian segmentation with a probabilistic atlas (e.g., [1,2]); multi-atlas segmentation [3];

© Springer Nature Switzerland AG 2019
A. C. S. Chung et al. (Eds.): IPMI 2019, LNCS 11492, pp. 767–779, 2019.
https://doi.org/10.1007/978-3-030-20351-1_60

and, more recently, convolutional neural networks (e.g., [4]). Typically, these techniques segment the brain into tissue types (i.e., gray matter, white matter, and cerebrospinal fluid), or into finer anatomical structures (e.g., hippocampus, ventricle). Bayesian methods drive the primary segmentation modules of the most widespread neuroimaging packages, like FreeSurfer [2], FSL [5], or SPM [1].

The aforementioned approaches rely mostly on T1 contrast to distinguish between gray and white matter. However, some boundaries between structures are nearly invisible in T1 (and other structural MR contrasts) due to insufficient difference in proton density and relaxation times. This is exacerbated by lower contrast-to-noise ratio in deep-brain structures, due to greater distance from the head coil. Two examples from the state-of-the-art Human Connectome Project (HCP) dataset [6] are shown in Fig. 1. In the first example, the lateral boundary of the thalamus appears very faint (Fig. 1a). In the second, the lateral boundary of the globus pallidus is visible thanks to the contrast with the neighboring putamen, but the medial boundary is not (Fig. 1c).

These issues create a need for fusing data from several MR modalities to better delineate structure boundaries. A natural complement to sMRI is diffusion MRI (dMRI), which may help discriminate between certain tissue types, despite its lower resolution. For example, in Fig. 1b, the lateral boundary of the thalamus is clearly discernible in the principal diffusion direction map obtained from dMRI. The diffusion data also complement the T1 scan in the pallidum, which can be delineated by combining contours obtained from the two modalities (medial from dMRI, lateral from sMRI, see Fig. 1d).

Most prior work on segmentation of dMRI focuses on delineating white matter structures, using tractography [7–9] or volumetric segmentation [10,11]. Tractography has also been used to subdivide subcortical structures (e.g., thalamus [12], amygdala [13]) based on long-range connections. Surprisingly, the literature on *joint* modeling of multimodal sMRI/dMRI is sparse. When sMRI and dMRI are used by the same tool, this is most often done serially, e.g., a segmentation derived from sMRI is used to analyze the dMRI (e.g., to derive priors for Bayesian tractography [9]). To the best of our knowledge, the only works analyzing sMRI and dMRI simultaneously have been on thalamic nuclei segmentation with random forests [14,15]. The main concern with such discriminative techniques is their generalization ability to other datasets, which is limited by differences in MRI acquisition. For sMRI segmentation, this problem can be ameliorated with data augmentation and pretraining [4]. However, this is harder to do in dMRI, where acquisition protocols are much less standardized.

The ability to generalize across datasets is critical when software is released publicly and few assumptions can be made on the acquisition. In such scenarios, Bayesian segmentation methods that automatically estimate appearance models from input images remain very popular, as they are agnostic to the MRI contrast of the input scan, and thus robust to acquisition differences. These methods are used for tissue segmentation by major neuroimaging packages (e.g., Unified Segmentation [1] in SPM, and FAST [16] in FSL). However, they can be inaccurate when segmenting structures with poor sMRI contrast (see Fig. 1).

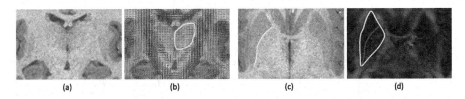

Fig. 1. (a) Coronal plane across the thalami of a T1 scan from the HCP. (b) Corresponding map of principal diffusion directions, and manual delineation of the left thalamus. (c) Axial plane of the T1 scan across the basal ganglia, and manual delineation of the boundary between the putamen and globus pallidus. (d) Corresponding principal diffusion directions (weighted by FA), with the joint boundary of the putamen and pallidum (in yellow, visible in this map) and the contour from the T1 (in red). (Color figure online)

Here we propose a sequence-adaptive Bayesian algorithm that uses a probabilistic atlas to segment sMRI and dMRI data *simultaneously*[1]. This is achieved via a novel dMRI likelihood term, which relies on a hierarchical model for the fractional anisotropy (FA) and principal diffusion orientation. Combined with a Gaussian likelihood for sMRI, this model of image intensities is flexible enough to produce accurate segmentations, while keeping dimensionality low. We also propose a novel inference algorithm to automatically segment scans by fitting the model to multi-modal sMRI/dMRI data. Thanks to unsupervised intensity modeling, applicability across a wide range of acquisition protocols is achieved, which is demonstrated experimentally on two considerably different datasets.

2 Methods

2.1 Forward Probabilistic Model

The graphical model of our framework is shown in Fig. 2a. The observed variables are a bias field corrected (possibly multispectral) sMRI scan $S = [s_1, \ldots, s_V]$ defined on V voxels, a dMRI scan $D = [d_1, \ldots, d_V]$ defined at the same voxel coordinates (which might require resampling), and a probabilistic atlas A, which provides the probabilities of observing one of C neuroanatomical classes at every location across a reference spatial coordinate system. The model is governed by three sets of deterministic hyperparameters specified by the user: γ^a, γ^s and γ^d.

At the top of the generative model we find the atlas A, along with a set of related parameters θ^a that deform this atlas into the space of the MRI data. These parameters are a sample of a distribution that regularizes the deformation field by penalizing, e.g., its bending energy. The strength of the regularization is controlled by the set of hyperparameters γ^a.

---

[1] Henceforth, we use "Bayesian segmentation" to refer to this specific family of Bayesian methods, using probabilistic atlases and unsupervised appearance modeling.

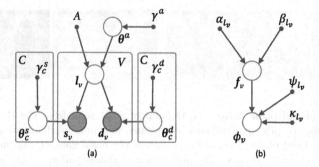

Fig. 2. (a) Graphical model of proposed framework. (b) Hierarchical model of dMRI likelihood. Circles represent random variables (open if hidden, shaded if observed). Smaller solid circles are deterministic parameters. Plates indicate replication.

Given the deformed atlas, a labeling (segmentation) $L = [l_1, \dots, l_V]$, with $l_v \in \{1, \dots, C\}$, is obtained by independently sampling the categorical distribution defined by the deformed atlas at each voxel location. Given L, the observed sMRI and dMRI data are assumed to be conditionally independent from each other and across voxels. The sMRI data s_v at v follows a distribution (typically a Gaussian) whose parameters θ_c^s depend on the corresponding label $c = l_v$. Any prior knowledge on these parameters is encoded in their priors, which are governed by hyperparameter vectors $\{\gamma_c^s\}$. Similarly, d_v is also assumed to be a mixture conditioned on the segmentation, described by parameters $\{\theta_c^d\}$ and hyperparameters $\{\gamma_c^d\}$, which yields a symmetric likelihood model (Fig. 2a). The joint probability density function (PDF) of the model is therefore:

$$p(S, D, L, \theta^a, \theta^s, \theta^d | A, \gamma^a, \gamma^s, \gamma^d)$$
$$= p(S|L, \theta^s)p(D|L, \theta^d)p(L|A, \theta^a)p(\theta^s|\gamma^s)p(\theta^d|\gamma^d)p(\theta^a|\gamma^a)$$
$$= \left(\prod_{v=1}^{V} p(s_v|\theta_{l_v}^s)p(d_v|\theta_{l_v}^d)p_v(l_v|A, \theta^a) \right) \left(\prod_{c=1}^{C} p(\theta_c^s|\gamma_c^s)p(\theta_c^d|\gamma_c^d) \right) p(\theta^a|\gamma^a), \quad (1)$$

where $\theta^s = \{\theta_c^s\}_{c=1,\dots,C}$, $\gamma^s = \{\gamma_c^s\}_{c=1,\dots,C}$, $\theta^d = \{\theta_c^d\}_{c=1,\dots,C}$, $\gamma^d = \{\gamma_c^d\}_{c=1,\dots,C}$.

2.2 Model Instantiation

Probabilistic Atlas: We follow the framework of the thalamic atlas [17] that we use in the experiments in Sect. 3, in which the atlas is encoded as a tetrahedral mesh. Deforming the mesh is penalized by a regularizer R, weighted by the mesh stiffness λ. The prior is given by (see further details in [18]):

$$p(\theta^a|\gamma^a) \propto \exp[-\lambda R(\theta^a)], \quad \text{and} \quad l_v \sim \text{Cat}[A_v(\theta^a)], \quad (2)$$

where $A_v(\theta^a) = [A_{v1}, \dots, A_{vc}]^t$ is simply the vector of C label probabilities provided by the atlas at voxel v when deformed with parameters θ^a; $\text{Cat}[\cdot]$ is the categorical distribution; and hyperparameters γ^a comprise just λ, i.e., $\gamma^a = \{\lambda\}$.

Likelihood of sMRI: In order to model the sMRI intensities given the segmentation L, we follow the Bayesian brain MR segmentation literature (e.g., [1,16,17]) and use Gaussian intensity distributions, such that $\theta_c^s = \{\mu_c, \Sigma_c\}$, i.e., the mean and covariance of the intensities of class c. We place a Normal Inverse Wishart (NIW) distribution on these parameters (i.e., the conjugate prior), with zero degrees of freedom for the covariance, as we found it difficult in practice to inform such parameter a priori. Therefore, we have: $\gamma_c^s = \{M_c, n_c\}$, where M_c is the hypermean and n_c is the scale. The sMRI likelihood is thus:

$$\mu_c, \Sigma_c \mid M_c, n_c \sim \text{NIW}(M_c, n_c, 0, 0I),$$
$$s_v \mid l_v, \{\mu_c\}, \{\Sigma_c\} \sim \mathcal{N}(\mu_{l_v}, \Sigma_{l_v}), \tag{3}$$

where $\mathcal{N}(\cdot, \cdot)$ is the Gaussian distribution and I is the identity matrix.

Likelihood of dMRI: We have two requirements for the likelihood function of the dMRI: low demands on gradient directions and b-values to accommodate legacy data; and low number of parameters to facilitate unsupervised clustering (yet sufficient to separate the classes). To satisfy the first requirement, we adopt the diffusion tensor imaging (DTI) model, which can be fit from virtually all available dMRI data. Rather than modeling the tensors directly (e.g., with a Wishart distribution, which we found in pilot experiments to fade too quickly from its mode), we use a hierarchical model (Fig. 2b) that only considers the FA f_v and the principal eigenvector ϕ_v at each voxel, i.e., $d_v = \{f_v, \phi_v\}$.

At the first level, we model the FA conditioned on the class, with Beta distributions parameterized by $\{\alpha_c, \beta_c\}$. We chose the Beta because it can model location and dispersion of signals defined on the $[0, 1]$ interval with two parameters. At the second level, we model the principal eigenvector with the Dimroth-Scheidegger-Watson (DSW) distribution, which is axial (i.e., antipodally symmetric), accommodating the directional invariance of dMRI [19]. This distribution is also rotationally symmetric around a mean direction ψ and its opposite $-\psi$ ($\|\psi\| = 1$), with a dispersion around the mean parameterized by a concentration κ. It has fewer parameters than other axial distributions, such as the (non rotationally symmetric) Bingham. Its PDF is given by [20]:

$$f(\phi; \psi, \kappa) = [Z(\kappa)]^{-1} \exp\left[\kappa(\psi^t \phi)^2\right], \tag{4}$$

with domain $\|\phi\| = 1$, and where the partition function is the Kummer function in 3D [20]: $Z\kappa = \int_0^1 \exp(\kappa t^2) dt$. We further assume that the concentration is modulated (multiplied) by the FA. This is a simple yet effective way of modeling the higher directional dispersion in voxels with low FA (e.g., in areas of unrestricted diffusion or fiber crossings), without having to resort to mixtures or additional parameters. The overall model for the dMRI likelihood is thus:

$$f_v \mid l_v, \{\alpha_c\}, \{\beta_c\} \sim \text{Beta}(\alpha_{l_v}, \beta_{l_v}),$$
$$\phi_v \mid l_v, f_v, \{\psi_c\}, \{\kappa_c\} \sim \text{DSW}(\psi_{l_v}, f_v \kappa_{l_v}), \tag{5}$$

and the set of parameters is thus: $\theta_c^d = \{\alpha_c, \beta_c, \psi_c, \kappa_c\}$, with $\|\psi_c\| = 1, \forall c$. We decided not to inform these parameters, such that $p(\theta_c^d) \propto 1$, and $\gamma_c^d = \emptyset$. We note that this likelihood model defines a PDF on the unit ball for vector $f_v \phi_v$.

2.3   Segmentation as Bayesian Inference

Within our joint generative model of sMRI and dMRI, we pose segmentation as an optimization problem, seeking to maximize the posterior probability of the labeling, given the known hyperparameters and observed input data:

$$\operatorname*{argmax}_{L} \int \int \int p(L|\theta^a, \theta^s, \theta^d, S, D, A) p(\theta^a, \theta^s, \theta^d | S, D, A, \gamma^a, \gamma^s) d\theta^a d\theta^s d\theta^d,$$

$$\approx \operatorname*{argmax}_{L} p(L|\hat{\theta}^a, \hat{\theta}^s, \hat{\theta}^d, S, D, A), \tag{6}$$

where we have made the standard approximation that the posterior distribution of the parameters is heavily peaked around point estimates $\hat{\theta}^a$, $\hat{\theta}^s$, $\hat{\theta}^d$ given by:

$$\{\hat{\theta}^a, \hat{\theta}^s, \hat{\theta}^d\} = \operatorname*{argmax}_{\{\theta^a, \theta^s, \theta^d\}} p(\theta^a, \theta^s, \theta^d | S, D, A, \gamma^a, \gamma^s). \tag{7}$$

Therefore, we segment a scan by first estimating the parameters with Eq. 7, and then obtaining the (approximate) most likely labeling with Eq. 6.

Applying Bayes rule to Eq. 7, marginalizing over the hidden segmentation L, and considering the structure of the model and our design choices, we obtain:

$$\{\hat{\theta}^a, \hat{\theta}^s, \hat{\theta}^d\} = \operatorname*{argmax}_{\{\theta^a, \theta^s, \theta^d\}} p(\theta^a | \gamma^a) p(\theta^s | \gamma^s) \sum_L p(S|L, \theta^s) p(D|L, \theta^d) p(L|\theta^a, A).$$

Expanding and taking logarithm, we obtain the following objective function:

$$O(\theta^a, \{\mu_c, \Sigma_c, \alpha_c, \beta_c, \psi_c, \kappa_c\}) = \log p(\theta^a | \gamma^a) + \sum_{c=1}^{C} \log p(\mu_c, \Sigma_c | M_c, n_c)$$

$$+ \sum_{v=1}^{V} \log \left[\sum_{c=1}^{C} p(s_v | \mu_c, \Sigma_c) p(f_v | \alpha_c, \beta_c) p(\phi_v | f_v, \psi_c, \kappa_c) p(l_v = c | A, \theta^a) \right]. \tag{8}$$

We maximize Eq. 8 with a Generalized Expectation Maximization (GEM) algorithm [21], iterating between expectation (E) and maximization (M) steps:

E step: In the E step, we use Jensen's inequality to build a lower bound for the objective function, which touches it at the current value of the parameters:

$$O \geq Q = \sum_{v=1}^{V} \sum_{c=1}^{C} w_{vc} \log \left[p(s_v | \mu_c, \Sigma_c) p(f_v | \alpha_c, \beta_c) p(\phi_v | f_v, \psi_c, \kappa_c) p(l_v = c | A, \theta^a) \right]$$

$$+ \log p(\theta^a | \gamma^a) + \sum_{c=1}^{C} \log p(\mu_c, \Sigma_c | M_c, n_c) - \sum_{v=1}^{V} \sum_{c=1}^{C} w_{vc} \log w_{vc}, \tag{9}$$

where $\{w_{vc}\}$ a soft segmentation according to the current parameter estimates:

$$w'_{vc} = p(s_v|\mu_c, \Sigma_c)p(f_v|\alpha_c, \beta_c)p(\phi_v|f_v, \psi_c, \kappa_c)p(l_v = c|A, \theta^a)$$

$$= |\Sigma_c|^{-1/2} \exp[-\frac{1}{2}(s_v - \mu_c)^t \Sigma_c^{-1}(s_v - \mu_c)]f_v^{\alpha_c-1}(1 - f_v)^{\beta_c-1}[B(\alpha_c, \beta_c)]^{-1}$$

$$\times [Z(f_v\kappa_c)]^{-1}\exp[f_v\kappa_c(\psi_c^t\phi_v)^2]A_{vc}(\theta^a), \text{ and } w_{vc} = w'_{vc}/\sum_{c'=1}^{C} w'_{vc'}, \qquad (10)$$

where B is the Beta function.

M step: In the generalized M step, we seek to improve the lower bound Q in Eq. 9. While optimizing the bound with respect to all parameters simultaneously is difficult, optimizing different subsets each time (coordinate ascent) is feasible.

Optimizing θ^a: Fixing all other parameters and switching signs, we obtain:

$$\underset{\theta^a}{\text{argmin}} \sum_{v=1}^{V}\sum_{c=1}^{C} w_{vc} \log[w_{vc}/A_{vc}(\theta^a)] + \lambda R(\theta^a). \qquad (11)$$

This is a registration problem combining the regularizer R with a data term: the Kullback–Leibler (KL) divergence between the deformed atlas and the current soft segmentation. We solve it numerically with the conjugate gradient method.

Optimizing $\{\mu_c, \Sigma_c\}$: Setting derivatives to zero yields a closed-form solution:

$$\mu_c = \frac{n_c M_c + \sum_{v=1}^{V} w_{vc}s_v}{n_c + \sum_{v=1}^{V} w_{vc}}, \qquad (12)$$

$$\Sigma_c = \frac{n_c(\mu_c - M_c)(\mu_c - M_c)^t + \sum_{v=1}^{V} w_{vc}(s_v - \mu_c)(s_v - \mu_c)^t}{1 + \sum_{v=1}^{V} w_{vc}}. \qquad (13)$$

Optimizing $\{\alpha_c, \beta_c\}$: Substituting the expression of the Beta distribution into Eq. 9, the problem decouples across classes:

$$\underset{\alpha_c, \beta_c}{\text{argmax}}(\alpha_c - 1)\sum_{v=1}^{V} w_{vc}\log f_v + (\beta_c - 1)\sum_{v=1}^{V} w_{vc}\log(1 - f_v) - \log B(\alpha_c, \beta_c)\sum_{v=1}^{V} w_{vc}.$$
$$(14)$$

This is a simple 2D optimization problem, which we solve with conjugate gradient. In the first iteration, we use the method of moments for initialization.

Optimizing $\{\psi_c\}$: This optimization can also be carried out one c at the time:

$$\underset{\psi_c:\|\psi_c\|=1}{\text{argmax}} \sum_v w_{vc}f_v(\psi_c^t\phi_v)^2 = \underset{\psi_c:\|\psi_c\|=1}{\text{argmax}} \psi_c^t\Big[\sum_v w_{vc}f_v\phi_v\phi_v^t\Big]\psi_c,$$

with closed-form solution given by the leading eigenvector of: $\sum_v w_{vc}f_v\phi_v\phi_v^t$.

Optimizing $\{\kappa_c\}$: This optimization problem also decouples across classes:

$$\underset{\kappa_c}{\text{argmax}} \; \kappa_c \sum_{v=1}^{V} w_{vc} f_v (\psi_c^t \phi_v)^2 - \sum_{v=1}^{V} w_{vc} \log Z(f_v \kappa_c), \tag{15}$$

which we solve with conjugate gradient, initializing $\kappa_c = 10$ in the first iteration.

Final Segmentation: It is straightforward to show that the approximate posterior probability of the segmentation from Eq. 6 factorizes across voxels and is given by $p(\boldsymbol{L} | \hat{\boldsymbol{\theta}}^a, \hat{\boldsymbol{\theta}}^s, \hat{\boldsymbol{\theta}}^d, \boldsymbol{S}, \boldsymbol{D}, \boldsymbol{A}, \boldsymbol{\gamma}^a, \boldsymbol{\gamma}^s) = \prod_{v=1}^{V} \hat{w}_{v,l_j}$, where $\hat{w}_{v,l_j}$ is obtained by evaluating Eq. 10 at the optimal parameter values $\hat{\boldsymbol{\theta}}^a, \hat{\boldsymbol{\theta}}^s, \hat{\boldsymbol{\theta}}^d$. Therefore, the optimal segmentation can be computed independently at each location v as:

$$\hat{l}_v = \underset{c}{\text{argmax}} \; \hat{w}_{vc}, \tag{16}$$

and the expected value of the volume of class c is given by: $\sum_{v=1}^{V} \hat{w}_{vc}$ (in voxels).

Implementation Details: Since GEM only requires *improving* the bound at each iteration, we follow a schedule in which all the model parameters except for θ^a are updated once in the M step. Since updating θ^a requires solving a more computationally expensive registration problem, we only update θ^a in the M step every five GEM iterations. The method is summarized in Algorithm 1.

In practice, we also force some parameters $\{\boldsymbol{\theta}_c^s\}$ and $\{\boldsymbol{\theta}_c^d\}$ to be shared across classes, for increased robustness of the algorithm. For the sMRI parameters ($\{\mu_c, \sigma_c^2\}$), we follow [17] and force parameter sharing across: cortex, hippocampus and amygdala; reticular nucleus and white matter; mediodorsal and pulvinar nuclei; rest of thalamic nuclei; and contralateral structures. For the FA, parameters $\{\alpha_c, \beta_c\}$ are shared across each of the six groups of thalamic nuclei in Table 2 of [17], and across contralateral structures. The same grouping – but without contralateral constraints – is used for the directional parameters $\{\psi_c, \kappa_c\}$.

3   Experiments and Results

3.1   Data

We evaluate our method with a recent probabilistic atlas of 25 thalamic nuclei and surrounding regions derived from histology [17]. The thalamus is an excellent target region, due to its faint lateral boundaries in sMRI (as explained in Sect. 1), and its set of nuclei with different connectivity. We use two considerably different datasets in evaluation: HCP (state of the art) and ADNI (legacy).

HCP: Isotropic T1 and dMRI scans from 100 healthy subjects (age 29.1 ± 3.3, 44 males), at 0.7 mm (T1) and 1.25 mm resolution (dMRI). We fit the DTI model to the $b = 1000$ s/mm^2 shell (180 directions) and 12 scans with $b = 0$ (details in [22]).

Algorithm 1. Bayesian segmentation with sMRI and dMRI

Require: $A, S, D, \gamma^a, \gamma^s, \{M_c, n_c\}$
Ensure: $\hat{\theta}^a, \{\hat{\mu}_c, \hat{\Sigma}_c, \hat{\alpha}_c, \hat{\beta}_c, \hat{\psi}_c, \hat{\kappa}_c\}$

  Initialize θ^a, with affine registration and mutual information
  Initialize $w_{vc} \leftarrow p(l_v = c | A, \theta^a), \forall v, c$
  Initialize $\kappa_c = 10, \forall c$
  Initialize α_c, β_c with method of moments, $\forall c$
  it $\leftarrow 0$
  while $\theta^a, \{\mu_c, \Sigma_c, \alpha_c, \beta_c, \psi_c, \kappa_c\}$ change AND it $\leq$ it$_{max}$ **do**
    it $\leftarrow$ it $+ 1$
    for $c = 1, \ldots, C$ **do**
      Update μ_c, Σ_c with Eqs. 12 and 13
      Update α_c, β_c by numerically optimizing Eq. 14 with conjugate gradient
      Update $\psi_c \leftarrow$ leading eigenvector of: $\sum_v w_{vc} f_v \phi_v \phi_v^t$
      Update κ_c by numerically optimizing Eq. 15 with conjugate gradient
    end for
    if mod(its,5)=0 **then**
      Update θ^a by numerically optimizing Eq. 11
    end if
    Update w_{vc} with Eq. 10, $\forall v, c$
  end while
  Compute final segmentation with Eq. 16.

ADNI: T1 and dMRI scans from 77 subjects from ADNI2: 39 Alzheimer's disease (AD) and 38 age-matched controls (74.1 ± 8.1 years; 40 females total). T1 resolution: $1.2 \times 1 \times 1$ mm (sagittal); dMRI resolution: $1.35 \times 1.35 \times 2.7$ mm (axial); 5 volumes with b $= 0$, 41 directions (b $= 1000$ s/mm^2; details at adni-info.org).

3.2 Experimental Setup

We evaluate three competing methods: *(i)* Segmentation of the whole thalamus with FreeSurfer [2]; *(ii)* Segmentation of thalamic nuclei using Bayesian segmentation on T1 only [17]; and *(iii)* Segmentation of thalamic nuclei with the full model, including dMRI. We compare these approaches in three experiments: *(i)* Qualitative assessment of segmentation and tractography in HCP; *(ii)* Correlation between thalamic and total intracranial volume (ICV) in HCP; and *(iii)* Ability to discriminate AD and control subjects based on volumes in ADNI. The sMRI and dMRI data are resampled to 0.5 mm isotropic in a bounding box around the thalami (DTI is interpolated in a log-euclidean framework [23]). We set $\lambda = 0.05$ as in [17], M_c to the median T1 intensity in class c according to the main FreeSurfer segmentation, and n_c to the volume of the class in mm^3.

3.3 Results

Figure 3 shows qualitative results on an HCP subject. FreeSurfer almost completely misses the left pallidum (yellow arrow in the figure) and oversegments the thalami. We test the effects of the latter on tractography by reconstructing the full dMRI data with generalized q-sampling [24], performing whole-brain tractography, and isolating the tracts that intersect the whole thalami, as automatically segmented by the three competing methods. The FreeSurfer thalamus yields many false positive tracts, mostly due to overlap with the internal capsule (red arrow). Aggregating the nuclei produced by Bayesian segmentation on the T1 produces a more accurate boundary, but still oversegments the anterior thalamus (white arrow), and undersegments the pulvinar nucleus (black arrow). Our multi-modal method yields less false positive tracts, and segments thalamic nuclei that are more homogeneous in terms of diffusion orientation and FA.

We also evaluate segmentation performance quantitatively on HCP, in an indirect fashion, by computing the correlation of total thalamic volume obtained by each method (left-right averaged) with the ICV estimated by FreeSurfer; noisy thalamic segmentations are expected to degrade this correlation. Scatter plots and regression lines are shown in Fig. 4. The FreeSurfer volumes are quite large on average, and their correlation with ICV is $\rho = 0.71$. Bayesian segmentation with T1 yields $\rho = 0.68$ (not significantly different, with $p = 0.37$ on a two-tailed Steiger test). The proposed algorithm produces fewer outliers than the other two, and yields the highest correlation ($\rho = 0.81$), significantly higher than those of FreeSurfer ($p = 0.006$) and T1-only segmentation ($p = 0.001$).

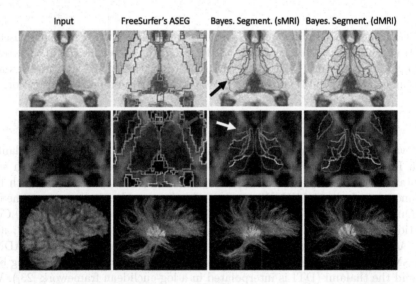

Fig. 3. Top two rows: axial slice of a T1 scan and principal diffusion directions of an HCP subject, with segmentations from FreeSurfer, Bayesian segmentation (T1 only), and the proposed method (T1+dMRI). Bottom row (left to right): Whole-brain tractography (25,000 tracts); subset of tracts going through the thalami (in yellow) as segmented by: FreeSurfer (2,602 tracts); Bayesian segmentation of T1 (2,193 tracts); and proposed method (1,676 tracts). See Sect. 3.3 for a description of the arrows. (Color figure online)

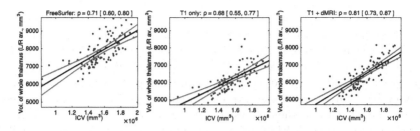

Fig. 4. Scatter plot for intracranial vs. whole thalamic volumes (left-right averaged), and regression lines (black) with 95% confidence intervals (in red). (Color figure online)

Finally, we evaluate the ability of the segmented volumes to classify the ADNI subjects into AD and controls. We use a simple linear discriminant analysis, whose performance is mostly determined by the quality of the volumes. We project the volumes (left-right averaged, corrected for ICV and age) onto the normal to the discriminant hyperplane in a leave-one-out fashion. We use the projections to compute the area under the ROC curve (AUC), accuracy at its elbow, and sample sizes ($\alpha = 0.05$, $\beta = 0.2$). Results are shown in Table 1. Our method yields a fair improvement compared with T1-only Bayesian segmentation (increase of 7 points in accuracy and AUC, and reduction of 6 samples). Compared with FreeSurfer, our algorithm reduces the sample size by 60%.

Table 1. AUC, accuracy at elbow, and sample size for the AD classification experiment.

Method	FreeSurfer (whole)	Bayes. Seg. T1	Proposed
AUC	60.3%	66.5%	73.6%
Accuracy at elbow	61.0%	67.5%	74.0%
Sample size	50	26	20

4 Conclusion

We have presented a Bayesian method for joint segmentation of sMRI and dMRI, which is robust to changes in acquisition platform and protocol – as shown with two substantially different datasets. Compared with Bayesian segmentation using sMRI alone, our method produces more accurate boundaries for subcortical structures, and yields smaller sample sizes in an AD classification task.

Future work at the methodological level will follow five main directions: *(i)* Modeling partial voluming in the dMRI, which may be important for smaller structures; *(ii)* Exploring other axial PDFs, as well as mixtures; *(iii)* Placing a prior on the dMRI likelihood parameters, e.g., to utilize prior knowledge on the FA; *(iv)* Modeling the bias field in the sMRI data, e.g., as in [1]; and *(v)* Adding connectivity derived from tractography to the dMRI likelihood, which may be challenging because tractography results depend largely on the MR acquisition.

We also plan to manually trace structures some of the HCP and AD data, with three purposes. First, to include white matter bundles in the atlas, as modeling the whole cerebral white matter with a single Beta-DSW is not realistic (not even within a bounding box). Second, to enable direct evaluation of our segmentations. And third, to help us explain discrepancies in AD classification accuracy between our results and those presented in [17], which may be due to the their larger dataset, their different ADNI sample, or some other factor.

As high-resolution dMRI becomes more common in neuroimaging, we believe that segmentation techniques that jointly model gray and white matter with sMRI and dMRI – like the one in this paper – will become increasingly important.

Acknowledgement. Supported by Horizon 2020 (ERC Starting Grant 677697, Marie Curie grant 765148), Danish Council for Independent Research (DFF-6111-00291), NIH (R21AG050122, P41EB015902), Wistron Corp., SIP, and AWS.

References

1. Ashburner, J., Friston, K.: Unified segmentation. Neuroimage **26**, 839–851 (2005)
2. Fischl, B., Salat, D.H., Busa, E., Albert, M., Dieterich, M., et al.: Whole brain segmentation: automated labeling of neuroanatomical structures in the human brain. Neuron **33**(3), 341–355 (2002)
3. Iglesias, J.E., Sabuncu, M.R.: Multi-atlas segmentation of biomedical images: a survey. Med. Im. Anal. **24**(1), 205–219 (2015)
4. Roy, A.G., Conjeti, S., Navab, N., Wachinger, C.: QuickNAT: segmenting MRI neuroanatomy in 20 seconds. NeuroImage **186**(1), 713–727 (2019)
5. Patenaude, B., Smith, S., Kennedy, D., Jenkinson, M.: A bayesian model of shape and appearance for subcortical brain segmentation. NeuroImage **56**, 907–922 (2011)
6. Van Essen, D.C., Smith, S.M., Barch, D.M., Behrens, T.E., Yacoub, E., et al.: The WU-Minn human connectome project: an overview. NeuroImage **80**, 62–79 (2013)
7. O'Donnell, L.J., Westin, C.F.: Automatic tractography segmentation using a high-dimensional white matter atlas. IEEE Trans. Med. Im. **26**(11), 1562–1575 (2007)
8. Wassermann, D., Bloy, L., Kanterakis, E., Verma, R., Deriche, R.: Unsupervised white matter fiber clustering and tract probability map generation: applications of a Gaussian process framework for white matter fibers. NeuroImage **51**, 228 (2010)
9. Yendiki, A., Panneck, P., Srinivasan, P., Stevens, A., Zöllei, L., et al.: Automated probabilistic reconstruction of white-matter pathways in health and disease using an atlas of the underlying anatomy. Front. Neuroinform. **5**, 23 (2011)
10. Awate, S.P., Zhang, H., Gee, J.C.: A fuzzy, nonparametric segmentation framework for DTI and MRI analysis: with applications to DTI-tract extraction. IEEE Trans. Med. Im. **26**(11), 1525–1536 (2007)
11. Hagler, D.J., Ahmadi, M.E., Kuperman, J., Holland, D., McDonald, C.R., et al.: Automated white-matter tractography using a probabilistic diffusion tensor atlas: application to temporal lobe epilepsy. Hum. Brain Map. **30**(5), 1535–1547 (2009)
12. Behrens, T.E., Johansen-Berg, H., Woolrich, M., Smith, S., Wheeler-Kingshott, C., et al.: Non-invasive mapping of connections between human thalamus and cortex using diffusion imaging. Nat. Neurosci. **6**(7), 750 (2003)

13. Saygin, Z.M., Osher, D.E., Augustinack, J., Fischl, B., Gabrieli, J.D.: Connectivity-based segmentation of human amygdala nuclei using probabilistic tractography. Neuroimage **56**(3), 1353–1361 (2011)
14. Stough, J.V., Glaister, J., Ye, C., Ying, S.H., Prince, J.L., Carass, A.: Automatic method for thalamus parcellation using multi-modal feature classification. In: Golland, P., Hata, N., Barillot, C., Hornegger, J., Howe, R. (eds.) MICCAI 2014. LNCS, vol. 8675, pp. 169–176. Springer, Cham (2014)
15. Glaister, J., Carass, A., Stough, J.V., Calabresi, P.A., Prince, J.L.: Thalamus parcellation using multi-modal feature classification and thalamic nuclei priors. Proc SPIE Int. Soc. Opt. Eng. **9784**, 97843J (2016)
16. Zhang, Y., Brady, M., Smith, S.: Segmentation of brain MR images through a hidden markov random field model and the expectation-maximization algorithm. IEEE Trans. Med. Im. **20**(1), 45–57 (2001)
17. Iglesias, J.E., Insausti, R., Lerma-Usabiaga, G., Bocchetta, M., Van Leemput, K., et al.: A probabilistic atlas of the human thalamic nuclei combining ex vivo MRI and histology. NeuroImage **183**, 314–326 (2018)
18. Van Leemput, K.: Encoding probabilistic brain atlases using bayesian inference. IEEE Trans. Med. Im. **28**(6), 822 (2009)
19. Zhang, H., Schneider, T., Wheeler-Kingshott, C.A., Alexander, D.C.: NODDI: practical in vivo neurite orientation dispersion and density imaging of the human brain. Neuroimage **61**(4), 1000–1016 (2012)
20. Mardia, K., Jupp, P.: Directional Statistics, vol. 494. Wiley, New York (2009)
21. Dempster, A.P., Laird, N.M., Rubin, D.B.: Maximum likelihood from incomplete data via the EM algorithm. J. R. Stat. Soc. B **39**, 1–38 (1977)
22. Sotiropoulos, S.N., Jbabdi, S., Xu, J., Andersson, J.L., Moeller, S., et al.: Advances in diffusion MRI acquisition and processing in the human connectome project. Neuroimage **80**, 125–143 (2013)
23. Arsigny, V., Fillard, P., Pennec, X., Ayache, N.: Log-euclidean metrics for fast and simple calculus on diffusion tensors. Magn. Reson. Med. **56**(2), 411–421 (2006)
24. Yeh, F.C., Wedeen, V.J., Tseng, W.Y.I.: Generalized q-sampling imaging. IEEE Trans. Med. Im. **29**(9), 1626–1635 (2010)

Learning-Based Optimization
of the Under-Sampling Pattern in MRI

Cagla Deniz Bahadir[1(✉)], Adrian V. Dalca[2,3], and Mert R. Sabuncu[1,4]

[1] Meinig School of Biomedical Engineering, Cornell University, Ithaca, USA
cagladeniz94@gmail.com
[2] Martinos Center for Biomedical Imaging, Massachusetts General Hospital,
HMS, Boston, USA
[3] Computer Science and Artificial Intelligence Lab, MIT, Cambridge, USA
[4] School of Electrical and Computer Engineering, Cornell University, Ithaca, USA

Abstract. Acquisition of Magnetic Resonance Imaging (MRI) scans can
be accelerated by under-sampling in k-space (i.e., the Fourier domain).
In this paper, we consider the problem of optimizing the sub-sampling
pattern in a data-driven fashion. Since the reconstruction model's performance depends on the sub-sampling pattern, we combine the two
problems. For a given sparsity constraint, our method optimizes the sub-
sampling pattern *and* reconstruction model, using an end-to-end learning
strategy. Our algorithm learns from full-resolution data that are under-
sampled retrospectively, yielding a sub-sampling pattern and reconstruction model that are customized to the type of images represented in the
training data. The proposed method, which we call LOUPE (Learning-
based Optimization of the Under-sampling PattErn), was implemented
by modifying a U-Net, a widely-used convolutional neural network architecture, that we append with the forward model that encodes the under-
sampling process. Our experiments with T1-weighted structural brain
MRI scans show that the optimized sub-sampling pattern can yield significantly more accurate reconstructions compared to standard random
uniform, variable density or equispaced under-sampling schemes. The
code is made available at: https://github.com/cagladbahadir/LOUPE.

Keywords: k-space under-sampling ·
Convolutional Neural Networks · Compressed sensing

1 Introduction

MRI is a non-invasive, versatile, and reliable imaging technique that has been
around for decades. A central difficulty in MRI is the long scan times that reduce
accessibility and increase costs. A method to speed up MRI is parallel imaging
that relies on simultaneous multi-coil data acquisition and thus has hardware
requirements. Another widely used acceleration technique is Compressed Sensing
(CS) [15], which does not demand changes in the MR hardware.

© Springer Nature Switzerland AG 2019
A. C. S. Chung et al. (Eds.): IPMI 2019, LNCS 11492, pp. 780–792, 2019.
https://doi.org/10.1007/978-3-030-20351-1_61

MRI measurements are spatial frequency transform coefficients, also known as k-space, and images are computed by solving the inverse Fourier transform that converts k-space data into the spatial domain. Medical images often exhibit considerable spatial regularity. For example, intensity values usually vary smoothly over space, except at a small number of boundary voxels. This regularity leads to redundancy in k-space and creates an opportunity for sampling below the Shannon-Nyquist rate [15]. Several Cartesian and non-Cartesian under-sampling patterns have been proposed in the literature and are widely used in practice, such as Random Uniform [5], Variable Density [25] and equispaced Cartesian [7] with skipped lines.

A linear reconstruction of under-sampled k-space data (i.e., a direct inverse Fourier) yields aliasing artifacts, which are challenging to distinguish from real image features for regular sub-sampling patterns. Stochastic sub-sampling patterns, on the other hand, create noise-like artifacts that are relatively easier to remove [15]. The classical reconstruction strategy in CS involves regularized regression, where a non-convex objective function that includes a data fidelity term and a regularization term is optimized for a given set of measurements. The regularization term reflects our *a priori* knowledge of regularity in natural images. Common examples include sparsity-encouraging penalties such as L1-norm on wavelet coefficients and total variation [16].

In regularized regression, optimization is achieved via iterative numerical strategies, such as gradient-based methods, which can be computationally demanding. Furthermore, the choice of the regularizer is often arbitrary and not optimized in a data-driven fashion. These drawbacks can be addressed using machine learning approaches, which enable the use of models that learn from data and facilitate very efficient and fast reconstructions.

1.1 Machine Learning for Under-Sampled Image Reconstruction

Dictionary learning techniques [9,18,20] have been used to implement customized penalty terms in regularized regression-based reconstruction. A common strategy is to project the images (or patches) onto a "sparsifying" dictionary. Thus, a sparsity-inducing norm, such as L1, on the associated coefficients can be used as a regularizer. The drawback of such methods is that they still rely on iterative numerical optimization, which can be computationally expensive.

Recently, deep learning has been used to speed up and improve the quality of under-sampled MRI reconstructions [13,17,19,23,26]. These models are trained on data to learn to map under-sampled k-space measurements to image domain reconstructions. For a new data point, this computation is often non-iterative and achieved via a single forward pass through the "anti-aliasing" neural network, which is computationally efficient. However, these machine learning-based methods are typically optimized for a specific under-sampling pattern provided by the user. Furthermore, there are also techniques that are optimizing the sub-sampling patterns for given reconstruction methods [27–30]. The reconstruction model's performance will depend significantly on the sub-sampling pattern. In this paper, we are interested in optimizing the sub-sampling pattern in a data-driven fashion. Therefore, our method optimizes the sub-sampling pattern *and* reconstruction model *simultaneously*, using an end-to-end learning strategy. We are able to achieve this thanks to the two properties of deep learning based reconstruction models: their speed and differentiable nature. These properties enable us to rapidly evaluate the effect of small changes to the sub-sampling pattern on reconstruction quality.

1.2 Optimization of the Sub-sampling Pattern

Some papers have proposed ways to optimize the sub-sampling pattern in compressed sensing MRI. The OEDIPUS framework [8] uses the information-theoretic Cramer-Rao bound to compute a deterministic sampling pattern that is tailored to the specific imaging context. Seeger et al. [22] present a Bayesian approach to optimize k-space sampling trajectories under sparsity constraints. The resulting algorithm is computationally expensive and does not scale well to large datasets. To alleviate this drawback, Liu et al. [14] propose a computationally more efficient strategy to optimize the under-sampling trajectory. However, this method does not consider a sophisticated reconstruction technique. Instead, they merely optimize for the simple method of inverse Fourier transform with zero-filling.

Below, we describe the proposed method, LOUPE, that computes the optimal probabilistic sub-sampling mask together with a state-of-the-art rapid neural network based reconstruction model. We train LOUPE using an end-to-end unsupervised learning approach with retrospectively sub-sampled images.

2 Method

2.1 Learning-Based Optimization of the Under-Sampling Pattern

In this section, we describe the details of our novel problem formulation and the approach we implement to solve it. We call our algorithm LOUPE, which stands for Learning-based Optimization of the Under-sampling Pattern. LOUPE considers the two fundamental problems of compressed sensing simultaneously: the optimization of the under-sampling pattern and learning a reconstruction model that rapidly solves the ill-posed anti-aliasing problem.

In LOUPE, we seek a "probabilistic mask" p that describes an independent Bernoulli (binary) random variable $\mathcal{B}$ at each k-space (discrete Fourier domain) location on the full-resolution grid. Thus, a probabilistic mask p is an image of probability values in k-space. A binary mask m has a value of 1 (0) that indicates that a sample is (not) acquired at the corresponding k-space point. We assume m is a realization of $M \sim \prod_i \mathcal{B}(p_i)$, where i is the k-space location index. Let x_j denote a full-resolution (e.g., 2D) MRI slice in the image (spatial) domain, where j is the scan index. While p, M, m and x_j are defined on a 2D grid (in k-space or image domain), we vectorize them in our mathematical expressions.

Our method is not constrained to 2D images and can be applied 3D sampling grids as well.

LOUPE aims to solve the following optimization problem:

$$\arg\min_{p,A} \mathbb{E}_{M \sim \prod_i \mathcal{B}(p_i)} \left[\lambda \sum_i M_i + \sum_j \|A(F^H \text{diag}(M)F x_j) - x_j\|_1 \right], \quad (1)$$

where F is the (forward) Fourier transform matrix, F^H is its inverse (i.e., Hermitian transpose of F), $A(\cdot)$ is an anti-aliasing (de-noising) function that we will parameterize via a neural network, $M_i \sim \mathcal{B}(p_i)$ is an independent Bernoulli, $\text{diag}(M)$ is a diagonal matrix with diagonal elements set to M, $\lambda \in \mathbb{R}^+$ is a hyper-parameter, and $\|\cdot\|_1$ denotes the L1-norm of a vector. While in our experiments x_j is real-valued, F and F^H are complex valued, and $A(\cdot)$ accepts a complex-valued input. We design A to output a real-valued image.

The first term in Eq. (1) is a sparsity penalty that encourages the number of k-space points that will be sampled to be small. The hyper-parameter λ controls the influence of the sparsity penalty, where higher values yield a more aggressive sub-sampling factor. We approximate the second term using a Monte Carlo approach. Thus the LOUPE optimization problem becomes:

$$\arg\min_{p,A} \lambda \sum_i p_i + \sum_j \frac{1}{K} \sum_{k=1}^{K} \|A(F^H \text{diag}(m^{(k)})F x_j) - x_j\|_1, \quad (2)$$

where $m^{(k)}$ is an independent binary mask realization of $M \sim \prod_i \mathcal{B}(p_i)$, and we use K samples. We further re-parameterize the second term of Eq. (2):

$$\arg\min_{p,A} \lambda \sum_i p_i + \sum_j \frac{1}{K} \sum_{k=1}^{K} \|A(F^H \text{diag}(u^{(k)} \le p)F x_j) - x_j\|_1, \quad (3)$$

where $u^{(k)}$ is a realization of a random vector of independent uniform random variables on $[0, 1]$, and $u^{(k)} \le p$ is a binary random vector where each entry is set to 1 if the inequality is satisfied, and 0 otherwise.

2.2 Implementation

We implement LOUPE using deep neural networks, which solve the learning problem via stochastic gradient descent. To make the loss function differentiable everywhere, we relax the thresholding operation in Eq. (3) via a sigmoid:

$$\arg\min_{p,\theta} \lambda \sum_i p_i + \sum_j \frac{1}{K} \sum_{k=1}^{K} \|A_\theta(F^H \text{diag}(\sigma_s(u^{(k)} - p))F x_j) - x_j\|_1, \quad (4)$$

where $\sigma_s(a) = \frac{1}{1+e^{-sa}}$, and A_θ denotes a neural network parameterized with weights θ. We set the slope for this sigmoid to be relatively steep to better approximate the thresholding step function.

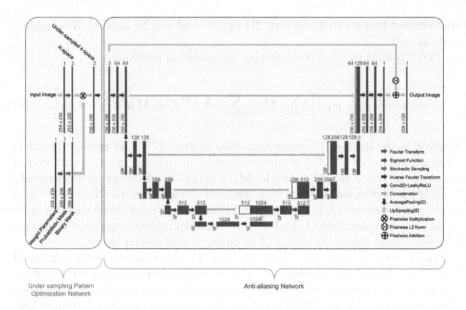

Fig. 1. The neural network architecture for LOUPE. Each vertical blue line represents a 2D image, with the number of channels indicated above and the size shown on the lower left side. The green line represents a 2D real-valued image of *weight* parameters, where one parameter is learned at each location, which is then passed through a sigmoid to yield the probability mask **p**. (Color figure online)

The anti-aliasing function A_θ is a fully-convolutional neural network that builds on the widely used U-Net architecture [21]. The input to A_θ is a two-channel 2D image, which correspond to the real and imaginary components. As in [13], the U-Net estimates the difference between the aliased reconstruction (i.e., the result of applying the inverse Fourier transform to the zero-filled under-sampled k-space measurements), and the fully-sampled ground truth image. Finally, the probabilistic mask p is formed by passing an unrestricted real-valued image through a sigmoid. Figure 1 illustrates the full architecture that combines all these elements. The red arrows represent 2D convolution layers with a kernel size 3×3, and a Leaky ReLU activation followed by Batch Normalization. The convolutions use zero-padding to match the input and output sizes. The gray arrows indicate skip connections, which correspond to concatenation operations. We also implement a stochastic sampling layer that draws uniform random vectors $u^{(k)}$. This is similar to the Monte Carlo strategy used in variational neural networks [11].

We train our model on a collection of full-resolution images $\{x_j\}$. Thus, LOUPE minimizes the unsupervised loss function (4) using an end-to-end learning strategy to obtain the probabilistic mask p and the weights θ of the anti-aliasing network A_θ. The hyper-parameter λ is set empirically to obtain the desired sparsity. We implement our neural network in Keras [2], with Tensor-

Flow [1] as the back-end and using layers from Neuron library [31]. The code is made available at: https://github.com/cagladbahadir/LOUPE. We use the ADAM [10] optimizer with an initial learning rate of 0.001 and terminate learning when validation loss plateaued. Our mini-batch size is 32 and $K = 1$. The input images are randomly shuffled.

3   Empirical Analysis

3.1   Data

In our analyses, we used 3D T1-weighted brain MRI scans from the multi-site ABIDE-1 study [3]. We used 100 high quality volumes, as rated by independent experts via visual assessment, for training LOUPE, while a non-overlapping set of fifty subjects were used for validation. For testing all methods, including LOUPE, we used ten held-out independent test subjects. All our experiments were conducted on 2D axial slices, which consisted of $1 \times 1\text{mm}^2$ pixels and were of size 256×256. We extracted 175 slices from each 3D volume, which provided full coverage of the brain - our central region of interest, and excluded slices that were mostly background.

3.2   Evaluation

During testing, we computed peak signal to noise ratio (PSNR) between the reconstructions of the different models and the full-resolution ground truth images for each volume. PSNR is a standard metric of reconstruction quality used in compressed sensing MRI [23]. Our quantitative results with other metrics (not included) were also consistent.

3.3   Benchmark Reconstruction Methods

The first benchmark method is ALOHA [12], which uses a low-rank Hankel matrix to impute missing k-space values. We employed the code distributed by the authors[1]. Since the default setting did not produce acceptable results on our data, we optimized the input parameters to minimize the MAE on a training subject.

The second benchmark reconstruction method we consider is a novel regularized regression technique that combines total generalized variation (TGV) and the shearlet transform. This method has been demonstrated to yield excellent accuracy in compressed sensing MRI [6]. We used the code provided by the authors[2].

---

[1] https://bispl.weebly.com/aloha-for-mr-recon.html.

[2] http://www.math.ucla.edu/~wotaoyin/papers/tgv_shearlet.html.

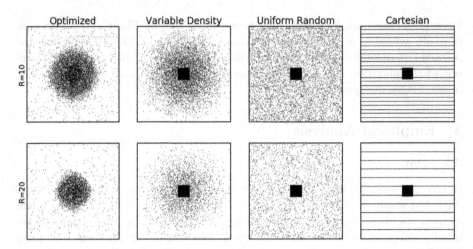

Fig. 2. Optimized and benchmark masks for two levels of sub-sampling rates: $R = 10$ and $R = 20$. Figures are in 2D k-space and black dots indicate the points at which a sample is acquired. Representative instantiations are visualized for the random masks.

Our third benchmark method is based on the Block Matching 3D (BM3D) method, which was recently shown to offer high quality reconstructions for under-sampled MRI data [4]. BM3D is an iterative method that alternates between a de-noising step and a reconstruction step. We employed the open source code[3].

Finally, we consider a U-Net based reconstruction method, similar to the recently proposed deep residual learning for anti-aliasing technique of [13]. This reconstruction model is the one we used in LOUPE, with an important difference: in the benchmark implementation, the anti-aliasing model is trained from scratch, for each sub-sampling mask, separately. In LOUPE, this model is trained *jointly* with the optimization of the sub-sampling mask.

3.4   Sub-sampling Masks

In this study, we consider three different sub-sampling patterns that are widely used in the literature: Random Uniform [5], Random Variable Density [25] and equispaced Cartesian [7] - all with a fixed 32×32 so-called "calibration region" in the center of the k-space. The calibration region is a fully sampled rectangular region around the origin, and has been demonstrated to yield better reconstruction performance [24]. We experimented with excluding the calibration region and sub-sampling over the entire k-space. However, reconstruction performance was no better than including the calibration region, so we omit these results.

The Uniform and Variable Density patterns were randomly generated by drawing independent Bernoulli samples. For Uniform, the probability value at each k-space point was the same and equal to the desired sparsity level. For

---

[3] http://web.itu.edu.tr/eksioglue/pubs/BM3D_MRI.htm.

Table 1. Average per volume run times (in sec) for different reconstruction methods. All except U-Net (GPU) were evaluated on a CPU - a dual Intel Xeon (E5-2640, 2.4 GHz).

ALOHA [12]	TGV [6]	BM3D [4]	U-Net [13] (CPU)	U-Net [13] (GPU)
498 ± 43.9	492 ± 33.8	1691.1 ± 216.4	55.9 ± 0.3	1.6 ± 0.4

Variable Density, the probability value at each k-space point was chosen from a Gaussian distribution, centered at the k-space origin. The proportionality constant was set to achieve the desired sparsity level. The Cartesian sub-sampling pattern is deterministic, and yields a k-space trajectory that is straightforward to implement. Figure 2 visualizes these masks. We consider two sparsity levels: 10% and 5%, which correspond to $R = 10$ and $R = 20$ sub-sampling rates.

4   Results

Table 1 lists run time statistics for the different reconstruction methods, computed on the test subjects. For the U-Net, we provide run-times for both GPU (NVidia Titan Xp) and CPU. The U-Net model is significantly faster than the other reconstruction methods, which are all iterative. This speed, combined with the fact that the neural network model is differentiable, enabled us to use the U-Net in the end-to-end learning of LOUPE, and optimize the sub-sampling pattern.

Figure 2 shows the optimized sub-sampling mask that was computed by LOUPE on T1-weighted brain MRI scans from 100 training subjects. The resulting mask has similarities with to the Variable Density mask. While it does not include a calibration region, it exhibits a denser sampling pattern closer to the origin of k-space. However, at high frequency values, the relative density of the optimized mask is much smaller than the Variable Density mask.

Figure 3 includes box plots for subject-level PSNR values of reconstructions obtained with four reconstruction methods, four different masks, and two sub-sampling rates. The Cartesian and Uniform masks overall yielded worse reconstructions than the Variable Density and Optimized masks. In all except a single scenario, the Optimized mask significantly outperformed other masks (FDR corrected $q < 0.01$ on paired t-tests). The only case where the Optimized mask was not the best performer was for the 10% sub-sampling rate, coupled with the BM3D reconstruction method [4]. Here, the PSNR values were slightly worse than the best-performing mask, that of Variable Density.

While the quantitative results give us a sense of overall quality, we found it very informative to visually inspect the reconstructions. Figures 4 and 5 show typical examples of reconstructed images. We observe that our optimized mask yielded reconstructions that capture much more anatomical detail than what competing masks yielded (highlighted with red arrows in the pictures). In particular, the cortical folding pattern and the boundary of the putamen – a subcortical structure – were much better discernible for our optimized mask. The

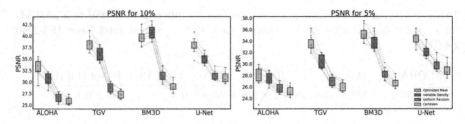

Fig. 3. Quantitative evaluation of reconstruction quality. For each plot, we show four reconstruction methods using four acquisition masks, including the Optimized Mask obtained using LOUPE in green. Each dot is the PSNR value for a single test subject across slices. For each box, the red line shows the median value, and the whiskers indicate the most extreme (non-outlier) data points. (Color figure online)

difference in reconstruction quality between the different methods can also be appreciated. Overall, U-Net and BM3D offer more faithful reconstructions that can be recognized in the zoomed-in views.

5   Discussion

We presented a novel learning-based approach to simultaneously optimize the sub-sampling pattern and reconstruction model. Our experiments on retrospectively under-sampled brain MRI scans suggest that our optimized mask can yield reconstructions that are of higher quality than those computed from other widely-used under-sampling masks.

There are several future directions we would like to explore. First, sampling associated cost is captured with an L1 penalty in our formulation. We are interested in exploring alternate metrics that would better capture the true cost of a k-space trajectory, which is constrained by hardware limitations. Second, in LOUPE we used L1 norm for reconstruction loss. This can also be replaced with alternate metrics, such as those based on adversarial learning or emphasizing subtle yet important anatomical details and/or pathology. Third, we will consider combining LOUPE with a multi-coil parallel imaging approach to obtain even higher levels of acceleration. Fourth, we plan to explore optimizing sub-sampling patterns for other MRI sequences and organ domains. More broadly, we believe that the proposed framework can be used in other compressed sensing and communication applications.

Acknowledgements. This work was supported by NIH R01 grants (R01LM012719 and R01AG053949), the NSF NeuroNex grant 1707312, and NSF CAREER grant (1748377). This work was also supported by the Fulbright Scholarship.

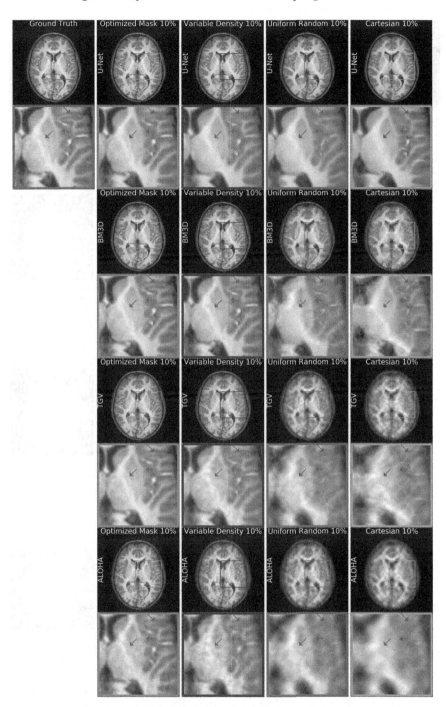

Fig. 4. Reconstructions for a representative slice and 10% sub-sampling. Each row is a reconstruction method. Each column corresponds to a sub-sampling mask. We observe that our optimized mask yields reconstructions that capture more anatomical detail. Red arrows highlight some nuanced features that were often missed in reconstructions. (Color figure online)

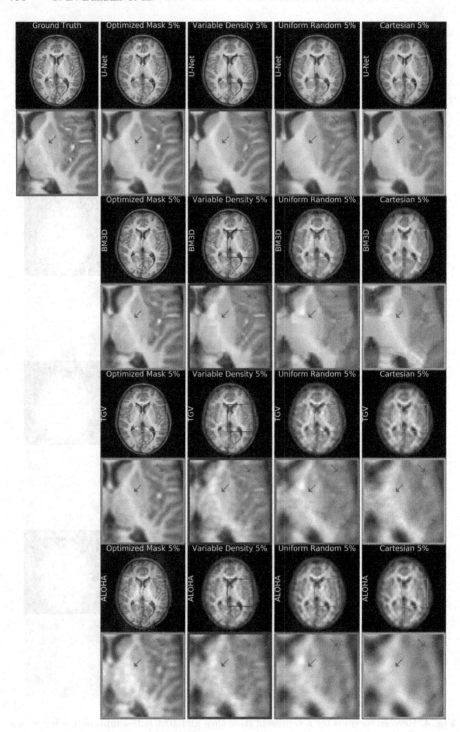

Fig. 5. Reconstructions for a representative slice and 5% sub-sampling. See caption of Fig. 4 and text for more detail. (Color figure online)

References

1. Abadi, M., et al.: Tensorflow: a system for large-scale machine learning. In: OSDI, vol. 16, pp. 265–283 (2016)
2. Chollet, F., et al.: Keras (2015)
3. Di Martino, A., et al.: The autism brain imaging data exchange: towards a large-scale evaluation of the intrinsic brain architecture in autism. Mol. Psychiatry 19(6), 659 (2014)
4. Eksioglu, E.M.: Decoupled algorithm for MRI reconstruction using nonlocal block matching model: BM3D-MRI. J. Math. Imaging Vis. 56(3), 430–440 (2016)
5. Gamper, U., Boesiger, P., Kozerke, S.: Compressed sensing in dynamic MRI. Magn. Reson. Med.: Official J. Int. Soc. Magn. Reson. Med. 59(2), 365–373 (2008)
6. Guo, W., Qin, J., Yin, W.: A new detail-preserving regularization scheme. SIAM J. Imaging Sci. 7(2), 1309–1334 (2014)
7. Haldar, J.P., Hernando, D., Liang, Z.P.: Compressed-sensing MRI with random encoding. IEEE Trans. Med. Imaging 30(4), 893–903 (2011)
8. Haldar, J.P., Kim, D.: OEDIPUS: an experiment design framework for sparsity-constrained MRI. arXiv preprint arXiv:1805.00524 (2018)
9. Huang, Y., Paisley, J., Lin, Q., Ding, X., Fu, X., Zhang, X.P.: Bayesian non-parametric dictionary learning for compressed sensing MRI. IEEE Trans. Image Process. 23(12), 5007–5019 (2014)
10. Kingma, D.P., Ba, J.: Adam: a method for stochastic optimization. arXiv preprint arXiv:1412.6980 (2014)
11. Kingma, D.P., Welling, M.: Auto-encoding variational bayes. arXiv preprint arXiv:1312.6114 (2013)
12. Lee, D., Jin, K.H., Kim, E.Y., Park, S.H., Ye, J.C.: Acceleration of MR parameter mapping using annihilating filter-based low rank hankel matrix (ALOHA). Magn. Reson. Med. 76(6), 1848–1864 (2016)
13. Lee, D., Yoo, J., Ye, J.C.: Deep residual learning for compressed sensing MRI. In: 2017 IEEE 14th International Symposium on Biomedical Imaging (ISBI 2017), pp. 15–18. IEEE (2017)
14. Liu, D.D., Liang, D., Liu, X., Zhang, Y.T.: Under-sampling trajectory design for compressed sensing MRI. In: 2012 Annual International Conference of the IEEE Engineering in Medicine and Biology Society (EMBC), pp. 73–76. IEEE (2012)
15. Lustig, M., Donoho, D.L., Santos, J.M., Pauly, J.M.: Compressed sensing MRI. IEEE Signal Process. Mag. 25(2), 72–82 (2008)
16. Ma, S., Yin, W., Zhang, Y., Chakraborty, A.: An efficient algorithm for compressed MR imaging using total variation and wavelets. In: IEEE Conference on Computer Vision and Pattern Recognition, CVPR 2008, pp. 1–8. IEEE (2008)
17. Mardani, M., et al.: Deep generative adversarial networks for compressed sensing automates MRI. arXiv preprint arXiv:1706.00051 (2017)
18. Qu, X., Hou, Y., Lam, F., Guo, D., Zhong, J., Chen, Z.: Magnetic resonance image reconstruction from undersampled measurements using a patch-based non-local operator. Med. Image Anal. 18(6), 843–856 (2014)
19. Quan, T.M., Nguyen-Duc, T., Jeong, W.K.: Compressed sensing MRI reconstruction using a generative adversarial network with a cyclic loss. IEEE Trans. Med. Imaging 37(6), 1488–1497 (2018)
20. Ravishankar, S., Bresler, Y.: MR image reconstruction from highly undersampled k-space data by dictionary learning. IEEE Trans. Med. Imaging 30(5), 1028 (2011)

21. Ronneberger, O., Fischer, P., Brox, T.: U-Net: convolutional networks for biomedical image segmentation. In: Navab, N., Hornegger, J., Wells, W.M., Frangi, A.F. (eds.) MICCAI 2015. LNCS, vol. 9351, pp. 234–241. Springer, Cham (2015). https://doi.org/10.1007/978-3-319-24574-4_28

22. Seeger, M., Nickisch, H., Pohmann, R., Schölkopf, B.: Optimization of k-space trajectories for compressed sensing by Bayesian experimental design. Magn. Reson. Med.: Official J. Int. Soc. Magn. Reson. Med. **63**(1), 116–126 (2010)

23. Sun, J., Li, H., Xu, Z., et al.: Deep ADMM-Net for compressive sensing MRI. In: Advances in Neural Information Processing Systems, pp. 10–18 (2016)

24. Uecker, M., et al.: ESPIRiT-an eigenvalue approach to autocalibrating parallel MRI: where sense meets grappa. Magn. Reson. Med. **71**(3), 990–1001 (2014)

25. Wang, Z., Arce, G.R.: Variable density compressed image sampling. IEEE Trans. Image Process. **19**(1), 264–270 (2010)

26. Yang, G., et al.: DAGAN: deep de-aliasing generative adversarial networks for fast compressed sensing MRI reconstruction. IEEE Trans. Med. Imaging **37**(6), 1310–1321 (2018)

27. Gozcu, B., et al.: Learning-based compressive MRI. IEEE Trans. Medical Imaging **37**(6), 1394–1406 (2018)

28. Baldassarre, L., Li, Y.H., Scarlett, J., Gozcu, B., Bogunovic, I., Cevher, V.: Learning-based compressive subsampling. IEEE J. Sel. Top. Sign. Process. **10**(4), 809–822 (2016)

29. Mahabadi, R.K., Lin, J., Cevher, V.: A learning-based framework for quantized compressed sensing. IEEE Signal Process. Lett. **26**(6), 883–887 (2019)

30. Mahabadi, R.K., Aprile, C., Cevher, V.: Real-time DCT learning-based reconstruction of neural signals. In: 2018 26th European Signal Processing Conference (EUSIPCO), pp. 1925–1929. IEEE (2018)

31. Dalca, A.V., Guttag, J., Sabuncu, M.R.: Anatomical priors in convolutional networks for unsupervised biomedical segmentation. In: The IEEE Conference on Computer Vision and Pattern Recognition CVPR (2018)

Melanoma Recognition via Visual Attention

Yiqi Yan$^{(\boxtimes)}$ ⓘ, Jeremy Kawahara ⓘ, and Ghassan Hamarneh ⓘ

Medical Image Analysis Lab, Simon Fraser University, Burnaby, BC, Canada
yiqiy@sfu.ca

Abstract. We propose an attention-based method for melanoma recognition. The attention modules, which are learned together with other network parameters, estimate attention maps that highlight image regions of interest that are relevant to lesion classification. These attention maps provide a more interpretable output as opposed to only outputting a class label. Additionally, we propose to utilize prior information by regularizing attention maps with regions of interest (ROIs) (e.g., lesion segmentation or dermoscopic features). Whenever such prior information is available, both the classification performance and the attention maps can be further refined. To our knowledge, we are the first to introduce an end-to-end trainable attention module with regularization for melanoma recognition. We provide both quantitative and qualitative results on public datasets to demonstrate the effectiveness of our method. The code is available at https://github.com/SaoYan/IPMI2019-AttnMel.

1 Introduction

Melanoma is one of the deadliest skin cancers in the world. The American Cancer Society reported that over 70% of skin cancer related deaths in the U.S. are associated with melanoma [19]. Fortunately, early diagnosis can facilitate proper treatment. However, accurate diagnosis of melanoma is non-trivial and requires expert human knowledge. Many automatic algorithms were proposed to classify melanoma from dermoscopy images. Particularly, deep learning based methods have been used in top-performing approaches [3,7].

Many deep learning methods turned to network or feature ensembles. Harangi et al. [8] trained an ensemble of AlexNet, VGGNet, and GoogLeNet, fusing their final features for a shared softmax classification layer. Codella et al. [2] trained an SVM using both deep convolutional features and sparse coding, which they later extended to an ensemble of 8 different features [4]. Similarly, Yu et al. [25,26] aggregated deep network features and fisher vector encoding. Training ensemble methods is time-consuming and is sensitive to how different models or feature extractors are tuned.

Other works trained a segmentation network to guide the classification. Yu et al. [24] designed a two-stage method. In the first step, a segmentation network was trained, which was used to detect and crop the lesion from the

ⓒ Springer Nature Switzerland AG 2019
A. C. S. Chung et al. (Eds.): IPMI 2019, LNCS 11492, pp. 793–804, 2019.
https://doi.org/10.1007/978-3-030-20351-1_62

entire image. Then a classification network was trained using the cropped images. Yang et al. and Chen et al. exploited the lesion segmentation in a parallel manner by applying a multi-task model that simultaneously tackled the problems of segmentation and classification [1,23]. When pixel-level annotations are not available, the training of these models becomes infeasible.

Although deep learning methods are widely used for skin lesion analysis, only a few efforts have been made to interpret which part of the image the model "concentrates" on. Van Molle et al. [21] visualized CNN features by rescaling the feature map to the input size and overlapping it with the input image. They attempted to gain insights into which image regions contribute to the results. They observed that the features seem to focus on specific characteristics, such as skin color, lesion border, hair, and artifacts, but there were no specific conclusions on how these features correlate with classification. A similar feature visualization was performed by Kawahara et al. [12]. Wu et al. [22] sought image biomarkers through *prediction difference analysis*. Specifically, a certain image region was corrupted each time, and the importance of that region was represented by the difference between the prediction scores based on the original and the corrupted images. Prediction difference analysis is a post-processing method designed to explain a fully trained network, while our model is trained end-to-end with learnable attention maps.

In this paper, we leverage attention mechanisms for melanoma recognition. A similar idea was presented by Ge et al. [6], who computed a class activation map (CAM) [27] as a saliency map to assign spatial weights to bilinear pooling features. CAM is a post-hoc analysis technique that requires extra computation based on a fully trained classification network. Similar to the works of Jetley et al. and Schlemper et al. [10,18], we propose an end-to-end solution via a trainable attention module. Our model extends the linear attention module proposed by Jetley et al. to more complex non-linear computations. Additionally, we propose to regularize the attention maps in order to train the model to focus on the expected regions of interest (ROIs). Our model not only yields state-of-the-art classification performance, but also produces attention maps indicating relevant image regions for classification. Our contributions are as follows:

- We incorporate end-to-end trainable attention modules for melanoma recognition. The attention maps automatically highlight image regions that are relevant to classification, which produces additional interpretable information as opposed to a mere class label. We perform a series of ablation studies to examine the effectiveness of attention.
- We introduce a method to efficiently utilize prior information via regularizing the attention maps with regions of interest (ROIs) (e.g., lesion segmentation, dermoscopic features). With prior information, the learned attention maps are refined and the classification performance is improved.
- The proposed regularization method can also be used to validate the effectiveness of ROI priors. For example, we show that regularizing using image background impedes the performance. This confirms that the model is properly

deeming the background less relevant to classification compared to the areas of skin lesion and dermoscopic features.

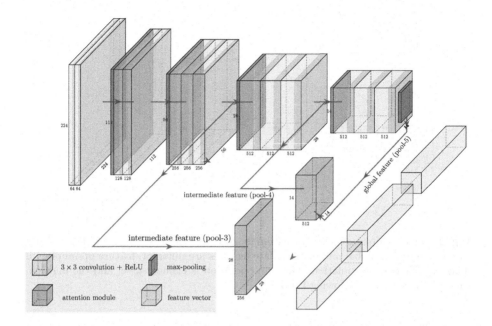

Fig. 1. The overall network architecture. The backbone network is VGG-16 (the yellow and red blocks) without any dense layers. Two attention modules (described in Fig. 2) are applied (the gray blocks). The three feature vectors (green blocks) are computed via global average pooling and are concatenated together to form the final feature vector, which serves as the input to the classification layer. The classification layer is not shown here. (Color figure online)

2   Proposed Method

2.1   Network Architecture

The human vision system focuses on objects in its field-of-view that are relevant to the task at hand. For example, when diagnosing skin cancer, dermatologists may focus more on the lesion rather than irrelevant areas such as background or hair. To imitate this visual exploration pattern, we use an attention module to estimate a spatial (pixel-wise) attention map. The proposed network architecture is illustrated in Fig. 1, with the attention modules shown as gray blocks. The inner details of the attention module are shown in Fig. 2.

We adopt VGG-16 [20], with all dense layers removed, as the backbone network of our model. We exploit intermediate feature maps (pool-3 and pool-4 in VGG-16) to infer attention maps. When computing the attention maps, the

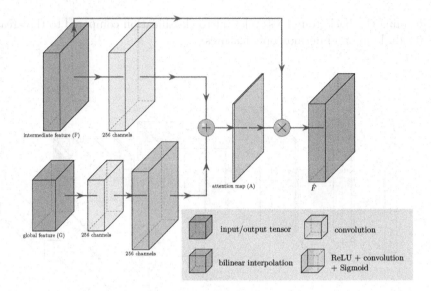

Fig. 2. Inner architecture of the attention module (i.e., the gray blocks in Fig. 1). When the spatial size of global and intermediate features are different, feature upsampling is done via bilinear interpolation. The sum operation is element-wise, and the multiplication is "pixel-wise" following Eq. 3

output of pool-5 serves as a form of "global guidance" (denoted as $\mathcal{G}$) because the last-stage feature contains the most compressed and abstracted information over the entire image. Let $\mathcal{F} = (\boldsymbol{f}_1, \boldsymbol{f}_2, \dots, \boldsymbol{f}_n)$ denote the intermediate feature, where $\boldsymbol{f}_i$ is the feature vector at the i-th spatial location. $\mathcal{F}$ and $\mathcal{G}$ are fed through an attention module (Fig. 2), yielding a one-channel response $\mathcal{R}$,

$$\mathcal{R} = \boldsymbol{W} \circledast \mathrm{ReLU}\big(\boldsymbol{W}_f \circledast \mathcal{F} + up(\boldsymbol{W}_g \circledast \mathcal{G})\big), \tag{1}$$

where $\circledast$ represents a convolutional operation, $\boldsymbol{W}_f$ and $\boldsymbol{W}_g$ are convolutional kernels with 256 filters, and the convolutional kernel $\boldsymbol{W}$ outputs a single channel. $up(\,\cdot\,)$ is bilinear interpolation that aligns the spatial size.

The attention map $\mathcal{A}$ is then calculated as the normalization of $\mathcal{R}$,

$$\mathcal{A} = Sigmoid(\mathcal{R}). \tag{2}$$

Each scalar element $a_i \in \mathcal{A}$ represents the degree of attention to the corresponding spatial feature vector in $\mathcal{F}$. The feature map with attention ($\hat{\mathcal{F}}$) is then computed by "pixel-wise" multiplication. That is, each feature vector $\boldsymbol{f}_i$ is multiplied by the attention element,

$$\hat{\boldsymbol{f}}_i = a_i \cdot \boldsymbol{f}_i. \tag{3}$$

Now that we have the attention version of pool-3 and pool-4 features ($\hat{\mathcal{F}}^{(3)}$, $\hat{\mathcal{F}}^{(4)}$), we obtain the final feature vector by concatenating the global average pooling of $\hat{\mathcal{F}}^{(3)}$, $\hat{\mathcal{F}}^{(4)}$, and $\mathcal{G}$ (green blocks in Fig. 1). A softmax classification layer is then formed based on this final feature. The whole network is trained end-to-end.

2.2 Regularization via Regions of Interest

Given binary maps of some specific ROIs, we incorporate these maps as prior information to guide the attention maps. To this end, we introduce a regularization term where these ROIs serve as a reference. Inspired by [11], we minimize a negative Sørensen-Dice-F1 loss,

$$\mathcal{L}_D(\mathcal{A}, \bar{\mathcal{A}}) = 1 - D(\mathcal{A}, \bar{\mathcal{A}}) = 1 - \frac{2 \cdot \sum_{i=1}^{n} (a_i \cdot \bar{a}_i)}{\sum_{i=1}^{n} (a_i + \bar{a}_i)}, \tag{4}$$

where $\bar{\mathcal{A}}$ is a reference binary map of ROIs. We do not compute $\mathcal{L}_D$ per image to avoid division-by-zero when there exists $\bar{\mathcal{A}}$ with no positive pixel labels. Instead, we treat one batch of data as a high dimensional tensor and calculate $\mathcal{L}_D$ using these two tensors. The overall loss with regularization becomes

$$\mathcal{L} = \mathcal{L}_{focal} + \lambda_1 \mathcal{L}_D(\mathcal{A}^{(3)}, \bar{\mathcal{A}}^{(3)}) + \lambda_2 \mathcal{L}_D(\mathcal{A}^{(4)}, \bar{\mathcal{A}}^{(4)}), \tag{5}$$

where $\mathcal{L}_{focal}$ is the focal loss [13], which is a modified cross-entropy loss designed to deal with imbalanced training data; $\mathcal{A}^{(3)}$, $\mathcal{A}^{(4)}$ are the attention maps corresponding to pool-3 and pool-4 with $\bar{\mathcal{A}}^{(3)}$, $\bar{\mathcal{A}}^{(4)}$ being their reference maps respectively. The original reference maps, which have the same size as the input image, are downsampled to the size of pool-3 and pool-4 before computing the loss. We fix $\lambda_1 = 0.001$, $\lambda_2 = 0.01$. λ_2 has a larger value as the features in the deeper layers should be more discriminative.

3 Experiments

3.1 Implementation Details

Data Preparation and Preprocessing. Our experiments are performed on ISIC 2016 [7] and ISIC 2017 [3]. ISIC 2016 contains two classes: benign and malignant (melanoma). While in ISIC 2017 there are three classes: melanoma, nevus, and seborrheic keratosis. Participants were tasked with two independent binary classification tasks: melanoma vs others, and seborrheic keratosis vs others. We focus on melanoma recognition, which is the harder task. For a fair comparison, we use the exact same training, validation, and test sets as were provided in the challenge. We preprocess the data by center-cropping the image to a squared size with the length of each side equal to $0.8 \times \min(Height, Width)$, and then resizing to 256×256.

Dealing with Imbalanced Data. The ISIC dataset is highly imbalanced. For example, there are 304 benign and 75 malignant samples in the training set of

ISIC 2016. Classifiers are prone to bias towards the more frequent label. We perform data oversampling in our experiments. Besides, we use focal loss [13] as the main classification loss term in Eq. 5, as it can automatically down-weight easy samples in the training set.

Table 1. Quantitative results on ISIC 2016 test set. The first ranking in terms of AP or AUC is highlighted in **bold**, and the second ranking is indicated in *italics*. **The proposed method (*AttnMel-CNN*) achieves state-of-the-art without using an ensemble of models or ground truth segmentations.** Notations: *AP*: average precision; *AUC*: the area under the ROC curve; *Lesion*: requires lesion segmentation or not; *Interp*: interpretable or not; *Ensemble*: ensemble method or not.

		AP	AUC	Lesion	Interp	Ensemble
#1	Yu et al. [24]	0.637	0.804	✓	✗	✗
#2	Codella et al. [4]	0.596	0.808	✗	✗	✓
#3	Yu et al. [25,26]	*0.685*	**0.852**	✗	✗	✓
#4	VGG-16	0.602	0.806	✗	✗	✗
#5	VGG-16-GAP	0.635	0.815	✗	✓	✗
#6	Mel-CNN	0.664	*0.844*	✗	✗	✗
#7	**AttnMel-CNN**	**0.693**	0.852	✗	✓	✗

Network Training. We implement our method using PyTorch [17]. The backbone network is initialized with VGG-16 pre-trained on ImageNet, and the attention modules are initialized using He's initialization [9]. The whole network is trained end-to-end for 50 epochs using stochastic gradient descent with momentum. The initial learning rate is 0.01 and is decayed by 0.1 every 10 epochs. We apply run-time data augmentation (random cropping, rotation, and flipping) via PyTorch transform modules.

Model Evaluation. The performance is evaluated over the test set based on the average precision (AP) and the area under the ROC curve (AUC)[1], as they were the official metrics used in the ISIC 2016 and 2017 challenge [3,7], respectively. We always pick the best epoch according to the area under the ROC curve (AUC) on the validation set, and report the final result on the test set.

3.2 Ablation Study

First, we train our model *without* regularization, i.e., only $\mathcal{L}_{focal}$ is used for training. We denote this model as *AttnMel-CNN*. We compare *AttnMel-CNN*

---

[1] We use APIs *average_precision_score* and *roc_auc_score* from scikit-learn toolbox (https://scikit-learn.org).

Table 2. Quantitative results on the ISIC 2017 test set. The highest rankings in terms of AP or AUC are highlighted in **bold**, and the second ranking is indicated in *italics*. **The proposed method with attention maps achieves comparable performance without external data, model ensembles, or any ground truth ROIs (*AttnMel-CNN*).** When ROIs are available, the performance is further improved. **Notation:** *AP*: average precision; *AUC*: the area under the ROC curve; *Lesion*: use lesion segmentation or not; *Dermo*: use dermoscopic features or not; *Interp*: interpretable or not; *Ensemble*: ensemble method or not; *External*: use external training data or not.

		AP	AUC	Lesion	Dermo	Interp	Ensemble	External
#1	ISIC 2017 Winner 1 [15]	–	0.868	✗	✗	✗	✓	✓
#2	ISIC 2017 Winner 2 [5]	–	0.856	✓	✓	✗	✗	✓
#3	ISIC 2017 Winner 3 [16]	–	*0.874*	✗	✗	✗	✓	✓
#4	Harangi et al. [8]	–	0.836	✗	✗	✗	✓	✗
#5	Mahbod et al. [14]	–	*0.873*	✗	✗	✗	✓	✓
#6	VGG-16	0.600	0.824	✗	✗	✗	✗	✗
#7	VGG-16-GAP	0.627	0.834	✗	✗	✓	✗	✗
#8	Mel-CNN	0.653	0.854	✗	✗	✗	✗	✗
#9	**AttnMel-CNN**	0.655	0.872	✗	✗	✓	✗	✗
#10	**AttnMel-CNN-Dermo**	*0.665*	0.864	✗	✓	✓	✗	✗
#11	**AttnMel-CNN-Lesion**	**0.672**	**0.883**	✓	✗	✓	✗	✗
#12	AttnMel-CNN-Bkg	0.647	0.849	✓	✗	✓	✗	✗

with three baselines (*VGG-16*, *VGG-16-GAP*, *Mel-CNN*) to verify the effectiveness of attention. Then we add regularization using different ROIs, yielding *AttnMel-CNN-Lesion* and *AttnMel-CNN-Dermo*. We also apply background (the inverse of lesion segmentation) as a "wrong" ROI to demonstrate how improper attention influence the performance. We discuss the details of each model in the following paragraphs.

Comparing with the Original VGG. The first baseline model is the original VGG network. We modify the last classification layer to have 2 output nodes, and the rest of the network parameters are initialized with ImageNet pre-training. We denote this baseline *VGG-16*. Note that even though our backbone network is based on the VGG network (Fig. 1), we remove the two dense layers and add our own attention modules. Since dense layers take nearly 90% of the parameters in *VGG-16*, our network is much more lightweight (around $100M$ fewer parameters). Referring to Table 1 (rows 4,7) and Table 2 (rows 6,9), *AttnMel-CNN* achieves better performance despite the large degree of parameter reduction.

Comparison with the Truncated VGG. The poor performance of the original *VGG-16* could be due to overfitting. For a fair comparison, we design another baseline, termed *VGG-16-GAP*, by replacing the dense layers with global average pooling. Note that this is also equivalent to our model without attention. Referring to Tables 1 and 2, *VGG-16-GAP* slightly outperforms the original *VGG-16*, but is surpassed by the proposed *AttnMel-CNN*. This demonstrates that overfitting can be reduced by removing the dense layers, but that further improvements come from the proposed architecture, which explicitly leverages the intermediate features.

Does Attention Help? After confirming the usefulness of intermediate features, one may ask whether it helps to assign attention maps to these features. In order to validate the effectiveness of attention modules themselves, we compute global average pooling on pool-3 and pool-4 instead of their attention versions. We denote this baseline *Mel-CNN*. According to Tables 1 and 2, this baseline yields worse performance than *AttnMel-CNN*. This is an expected result because shallow features are not well compressed and abstracted, and attention maps help rule out irrelevant information within shallow features.

How does the Regularization Influence the Model? We re-train the network using the loss proposed in Eq. 5 with three different reference maps ($\mathcal{A}$): (1) *AttnMel-CNN-Lesion* uses the whole lesion segmentation map (available from ISIC 2017 Task 1); (2) *AttnMel-CNN-Dermo* uses the union of four dermoscopic features[2] (available from ISIC 2017 Task 2); and (3) *AttnMel-CNN-Bkg* uses image background (the inverse of whole lesion segmentation). Table 2 shows that encouraging attention to lesion or dermoscopic features yields better performance, while improper attention (*AttnMel-CNN-Bkg*) harms the performance.

3.3   Visual Interpretability

In order to show whether better attention correlates with higher performance, we evaluate the learned attention maps both qualitatively and quantitatively.

Qualitative Analysis. We visualize the learned attention maps of *AttnMel-CNN*, *AttnMel-CNN-Lesion* and *AttnMel-CNN-Dermo* on the ISIC 2017 test data by upsampling $\mathcal{A}$ (Eq. 2) to align with the input image. The results are shown in Fig. 3. When comparing rows 2 and 3, we observe that the shallower layer (pool-3) tends to focus on more general and diffused areas, while the deeper layer (pool-4) is more concentrated, focusing on the lesion and avoiding irrelevant objects. Furthermore, rows 4–7 demonstrate that the models with additional regularization pay attention to more semantically meaningful regions, which accounts for the performance improvement illustrated in Table 2.

Quantitative Analysis. We quantify the "quality" of the learned attention map by computing its overlap with the ground truth lesion segmentation. First,

---

[2] We convert the superpixel labels to binary pixel labels in the same way as [11], and use the union across all the dermoscopic features.

Table 3. Jaccard index of (binarized) attention maps and class activation maps with respect to the ground truth lesion segmentations.

AttnMel-CNN		AttnMel-CNN-Dermo		AttnMel-CNN-Lesion		VGG-16-GAP
pool3	pool4	pool3	pool4	pool3	pool4	CAM
0.3105	0.3186	0.3621	0.4767	0.5533	0.6560	0.2825

we re-normalize each attention map to $[0, 1]$ and binarize it using a threshold of 0.5. Then we compute the Jaccard index with respect to the ground truth lesion segmentation. We also calculate the class activation map (CAM) [27] from *VGG-16-GAP* and follow the same procedure as above to compute the Jaccard index value. The results reported in Table 3 lead to several conclusions: (1) The proposed learnable attention module highlights the relevant image regions better than the post-processing-based attention (CAM). (2) The attention map of the deeper layer (pool-4) yields a higher Jaccard index value, demonstrating that the deeper layer learns more discriminative features than the shallower layer. (3) The regularization encourages the attention maps to concentrate more on relevant ROIs.

3.4 Comparison with Previous Methods

We summarize previous work in Table 1 rows 1–3 and Table 2 rows 1–5. Comparison with [1,23] is not feasible as separate results for melanoma classification are not reported. The advantages of our method are:

– Our method yields state-of-the-art performance for melanoma classification even without additional regularization (*AttnMel-CNN*), and produces further performance improvements when reference ROIs are available (*AttnMel-CNN-Lesion* and *AttnMel-CNN-Dermo*). Additionally, we achieve state-of-the-art performance without any external training data.
– Our method relies on a single model, avoiding complex model ensembles.
– Compared with other methods utilizing segmentation maps [1,5,23,24], our method is more robust and flexible in that: (1) One of our models (*AttnMel-CNN*), optimized using only the focal loss, performs well without any regions of interests, while network training in those competing works requires pixel-wise annotations. (2) The competing works can only utilize whole lesion segmentations, but our regularization method can efficiently use dermoscopic (*AttnMel-CNN-Dermo*). We note that in a fair number of images, no dermoscopic features occur, and our proposed model is improved through these "sparse" reference maps.

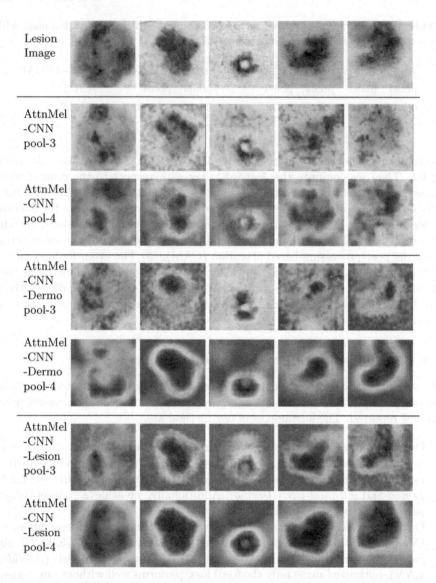

Fig. 3. Visualization of attention maps for different models. The deeper layer (pool-4) exhibits more concentrated attention to valid regions than the shallower layer (pool-3). The models with additional regularization (rows 4–7) produce more refined and semantically meaningful attention maps.

4   Conclusion and Discussion

In this paper, we proposed an attention-based network for melanoma recognition with a novel technique to regularize the attention maps with prior information. We achieve state-of-the-art performance for melanoma classification on two public datasets without external training data or complex model ensembles. One limitation of this work is that we only apply the model to a binary classification task. Future work would explore visual attention in more general skin lesion classification problems.

Acknowledgement. Partial funding for this project is provided by the Natural Sciences and Engineering Research Council of Canada (NSERC). The authors are grateful to the NVIDIA Corporation for donating a Titan X GPU used in this research. We use PlotNeuralNet (https://github.com/HarisIqbal88/PlotNeuralNet) for drawing the network diagrams in this paper.

References

1. Chen, S., Wang, Z., Shi, J., Liu, B., Yu, N.: A multi-task framework with feature passing module for skin lesion classification and segmentation. In: IEEE International Symposium on Biomedical Imaging, pp. 1126–1129 (2018)
2. Codella, N., Cai, J., Abedini, M., Garnavi, R., Halpern, A., Smith, J.R.: Deep learning, sparse coding, and SVM for melanoma recognition in dermoscopy images. In: Zhou, L., Wang, L., Wang, Q., Shi, Y. (eds.) MLMI 2015. LNCS, vol. 9352, pp. 118–126. Springer, Cham (2015). https://doi.org/10.1007/978-3-319-24888-2_15
3. Codella, N.C., et al.: Skin lesion analysis toward melanoma detection: a challenge at the 2017 international symposium on biomedical imaging (ISBI), hosted by the international skin imaging collaboration (ISIC). In: IEEE International Symposium on Biomedical Imaging, pp. 168–172 (2018)
4. Codella, N.C., et al.: Deep learning ensembles for melanoma recognition in dermoscopy images. IBM J. Res. Dev. **61**(4), 1–15 (2017)
5. Díaz, I.G.: Incorporating the knowledge of dermatologists to convolutional neural networks for the diagnosis of skin lesions. arXiv preprint arXiv:1703.01976 (2017)
6. Ge, Z., Demyanov, S., Chakravorty, R., Bowling, A., Garnavi, R.: Skin disease recognition using deep saliency features and multimodal learning of dermoscopy and clinical images. In: Descoteaux, M., Maier-Hein, L., Franz, A., Jannin, P., Collins, D.L., Duchesne, S. (eds.) MICCAI 2017. LNCS, vol. 10435, pp. 250–258. Springer, Cham (2017). https://doi.org/10.1007/978-3-319-66179-7_29
7. Gutman, D., et al.: Skin lesion analysis toward melanoma detection: a challenge at the international symposium on biomedical imaging (ISBI) 2016, hosted by the international skin imaging collaboration (ISIC). arXiv preprint arXiv:1605.01397 (2016)
8. Harangi, B., Baran, A., Hajdu, A.: Classification of skin lesions using an ensemble of deep neural networks. In: 40th Annual International Conference of the IEEE Engineering in Medicine and Biology Society, pp. 2575–2578. IEEE (2018)
9. He, K., Zhang, X., Ren, S., Sun, J.: Delving deep into rectifiers: surpassing human-level performance on imagenet classification. In: Proceedings of the IEEE International Conference on Computer Vision, pp. 1026–1034 (2015)
10. Jetley, S., Lord, N.A., Lee, N., Torr, P.H.: Learn to pay attention. In: International Conference on Learning Representation (2018)
11. Kawahara, J., Hamarneh, G.: Fully convolutional neural networks to detect clinical dermoscopic features. IEEE J. Biomed. Health Inform. **23**(2), 578–585 (2019)
12. Kawahara, J., Daneshvar, S., Argenziano, G., Hamarneh, G.: Seven-point checklist and skin lesion classification using multitask multimodal neural nets. IEEE J. Biomed. Health Inform. **23**(2), 538–546 (2019)

13. Lin, T.Y., Goyal, P., Girshick, R., He, K., Dollar, P.: Focal loss for dense object detection. In: 2017 IEEE International Conference on Computer Vision (ICCV), pp. 2999–3007. IEEE (2017)
14. Mahbod, A., Schaefer, G., Ellinger, I., Ecker, R., Pitiot, A., Wang, C.: Fusing fine-tuned deep features for skin lesion classification. Comput. Med. Imaging Graph. **71**, 19–29 (2018)
15. Matsunaga, K., Hamada, A., Minagawa, A., Koga, H.: Image classification of melanoma, nevus and seborrheic keratosis by deep neural network ensemble. arXiv preprint arXiv:1703.03108 (2017)
16. Menegola, A., Tavares, J., Fornaciali, M., Li, L.T., Avila, S., Valle, E.: Recod titans at isic challenge 2017. arXiv preprint arXiv:1703.04819 (2017)
17. Paszke, A., et al.: Automatic differentiation in pytorch. In: NIPS Workshop on Autodiff (2017)
18. Schlemper, J., et al.: Attention-gated networks for improving ultrasound scan plane detection. In: Medical Imaging with Deep Learning Conference (2018)
19. Siegel, R.L., Miller, K.D., Jemal, A.: Cancer statistics. CA: Cancer J. Clin. **67**(1), 7–30 (2017)
20. Simonyan, K., Zisserman, A.: Very deep convolutional networks for large-scale image recognition. In: International Conference on Learning Representation (2015)
21. Van Molle, P., De Strooper, M., Verbelen, T., Vankeirsbilck, B., Simoens, P., Dhoedt, B.: Visualizing convolutional neural networks to improve decision support for skin lesion classification. In: Stoyanov, D., et al. (eds.) MLCN/DLF/IMIMIC -2018. LNCS, vol. 11038, pp. 115–123. Springer, Cham (2018). https://doi.org/10.1007/978-3-030-02628-8_13
22. Wu, J., Li, X., Chen, E.Z., Jiang, H., Dong, X., Rong, R.: What evidence does deep learning model use to classify skin lesions? arXiv preprint arXiv:1811.01051 (2018)
23. Yang, X., Li, H., Wang, L., Yeo, S.Y., Su, Y., Zeng, Z.: Skin lesion analysis by multi-target deep neural networks. In: 2018 40th Annual International Conference of the IEEE Engineering in Medicine and Biology Society (EMBC), pp. 1263–1266. IEEE (2018)
24. Yu, L., Chen, H., Dou, Q., Qin, J., Heng, P.A.: Automated melanoma recognition in dermoscopy images via very deep residual networks. IEEE Trans. Med. Imaging **36**(4), 994–1004 (2017)
25. Yu, Z., Jiang, X., Wang, T., Lei, B.: Aggregating deep convolutional features for melanoma recognition in dermoscopy images. In: Wang, Q., Shi, Y., Suk, H.-I., Suzuki, K. (eds.) MLMI 2017. LNCS, vol. 10541, pp. 238–246. Springer, Cham (2017). https://doi.org/10.1007/978-3-319-67389-9_28
26. Yu, Z., et al.: Melanoma recognition in dermoscopy images via aggregated deep convolutional features. IEEE Trans. Biomed. Eng. **66**, 1006–1016 (2018)
27. Zhou, B., Khosla, A., Lapedriza, A., Oliva, A., Torralba, A.: Learning deep features for discriminative localization. In: Proceedings of the IEEE Conference on Computer Vision and Pattern Recognition. pp. 2921–2929 (2016)

Nonlinear Markov Random Fields
Learned via Backpropagation

Mikael Brudfors$^{(\boxtimes)}$, Yaël Balbastre, and John Ashburner

The Wellcome Centre for Human Neuroimaging, UCL, London, UK
{mikael.brudfors.15,y.balbastre,j.ashburner}@ucl.ac.uk

Abstract. Although convolutional neural networks (CNNs) currently dominate competitions on image segmentation, for neuroimaging analysis tasks, more classical generative approaches based on mixture models are still used in practice to parcellate brains. To bridge the gap between the two, in this paper we propose a marriage between a probabilistic generative model, which has been shown to be robust to variability among magnetic resonance (MR) images acquired via different imaging protocols, and a CNN. The link is in the prior distribution over the unknown tissue classes, which are classically modelled using a Markov random field. In this work we model the interactions among neighbouring pixels by a type of recurrent CNN, which can encode more complex spatial interactions. We validate our proposed model on publicly available MR data, from different centres, and show that it generalises across imaging protocols. This result demonstrates a successful and principled inclusion of a CNN in a generative model, which in turn could be adapted by any probabilistic generative approach for image segmentation.

1 Introduction

Image segmentation is the process of assigning one of several categorical labels to each pixel of an image, which is a fundamental step in many medical image analyses. Until recently, some of the most accurate segmentation methods were based on probabilistic mixture models [1]. These models define a probability distribution over an observed image ($\boldsymbol{X}$), conditioned on unknown class labels ($\boldsymbol{Z}$) and parameters ($\boldsymbol{\theta}$). Assuming a prior distribution over unknown variables, Bayes rule is used to form a posterior distribution:

$$p(\boldsymbol{Z}, \boldsymbol{\theta} \mid \boldsymbol{X}) \propto p(\boldsymbol{X} \mid \boldsymbol{Z}, \boldsymbol{\theta})\, p(\boldsymbol{Z}, \boldsymbol{\theta}), \tag{1}$$

which can be evaluated or approximated. Wells III *et al.* [2] introduced these types of models for brain segmentation from magnetic resonance (MR) images. By assuming that the log-transformed image intensities followed a normal distribution in the likelihood term $p(\boldsymbol{X} \mid \boldsymbol{Z}, \boldsymbol{\theta})$, they segmented the brain into three classes: grey matter (GM), white matter (WM) and cerebrospinal fluid (CSF).

As generative models require the data-generating process to be defined, they can be extended to more complex joint distributions than in [2], allowing for

© Springer Nature Switzerland AG 2019
A. C. S. Chung et al. (Eds.): IPMI 2019, LNCS 11492, pp. 805–817, 2019.
https://doi.org/10.1007/978-3-030-20351-1_63

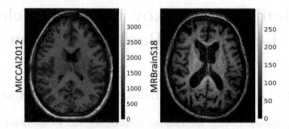

Fig. 1. T1-weighted MR images from two different, publicly available, datasets: MIC-CAI2012 and MRBrainS18 (on which we evaluate our method). It is evident that learning from one of these populations, and subsequently testing on the other is very challenging. The intensities are different by an order of magnitude, the bias is stronger in the MRBrainS18 subject. Additionally, age related change and pathology can be clearly seen, such as differences in ventricle size and white matter hyper-intensities, which further complicates the learning problem.

segmentation methods robust to, *e.g.*, slice thickness, MR contrast, field strength and scanner variability. Many of today's most widely used neuroimaging analysis software, such as SPM [3], FSL [4] and FreeSurfer [5], rely on these kinds of models, and have been shown to reliably segment a wide variety of MR data [6,7].

However, recent advances in convolutional neural networks (CNNs) have provided a new method for very accurate (and fast) image segmentation [8], circumventing the need to define and invert a potentially complex generative model. Discriminative CNNs learn a function that maps an input (*e.g.*, an MRI) to an output (*e.g.*, a segmentation) from training data, where the output is known. They typically contain many layers, which sequentially apply convolutions, pooling and nonlinear activation functions to the input data. Their parameters are optimised by propagating gradients backwards through the network (*i.e.*, backpropagation). For medical imaging, the U-net architecture [9] is the most popular and now forms the basis for most top performing entries in various medical imaging challenges aimed at segmenting, *e.g.*, tumours, the whole brain or white matter hyper-intensities[1]. The more classical segmentation frameworks based on probabilistic models seem to have met their match.

Challenges on medical image segmentation can be seen as lab experiments and – as with new medical therapies – there is a large gap to get *from bench to bedside*. CNNs excel in this context, factorising the commonalities in an image population of training data, which generalise to new data from the same population. They can struggle, however, when faced with new data that contain unseen features [10], *e.g.*, a different contrast (Fig. 1). This scenario usually requires the model being trained anew, on that unseen image contrast. In fact, even without considering inter-individual variability (age, brain shape, pathology, etc), a CNN-based segmentation software has yet to be presented that is agnostic to

---

[1] braintumorsegmentation.org, wmh.isi.uu.nl, mrbrains18.isi.uu.nl.

the great variability in MR data [11]. Lack of such software is largely due to the limited amount of labelled data available in medical imaging, which is a clear obstacle to their generalisability. Some methods have been developed to address this problem, *e.g.*, intensity normalisation [12], transfer learning [13] and batch normalisation [14]. Still, none of these methods are yet general enough to solve the task of segmenting across scanners and protocols. Recently, approaches based on realistic data augmentation have shown promising results [15, 16].

In this paper, we propose an approach to bridge between the classical, but robust, generative segmentation models and more recent CNN based methods. The link is in the prior term of (1), where we encode the unknown tissue distribution as drawn from a Markov random field (MRF). Using an MRF is in itself nothing new; they have been used successfully for decades in order to introduce spatial dependencies into generative segmentation models [17, 18], relaxing the independent voxels assumption. Here however, we instead model and learn the interactions among neighbouring pixels by a type of CNN. This allows us to parametrise the MRF by a more complex mathematical function than in the regular linear case, as well as cover a larger neighbourhood than a second-order one. The idea is that learning at the tissue level may generalise better than learning directly from the image intensities. We validate our approach on two publicly available datasets, acquired in different centres, and show favourable results when applying the model trained on one of these datasets to the other.

Related Work: Rather than reviewing the use of MRFs in image segmentation we will here briefly discuss two fairly recent additions to the computer vision field [19, 20], because they are closely related to the method we present in the subsequent section. The idea of both these papers is to cast the application and learning of a conditional random field (CRF) into a CNN framework. A CRF is a statistical modeling method that directly defines the posterior distribution in (1). To compute the CRF both papers apply a mean-field approximation, which they implement in the form of a CNN.

In contrast to the works described above, we are interested in defining the full generative model, whilst keeping the separation between likelihood and prior in (1). Modelling these two components separately allows us to include expert knowledge and image-intensity independent prior information over the segmentation labels. It also integrates easily with existing mixture-model-based approaches. Furthermore, modelling the prior as an MRF, without data-dependency in the neighbourhood model, may help in generalising among different image populations. Finally, our model allows an arbitrarily complex MRF distribution to be defined, including, *e.g.*, nonlinearities.

2   Methods

In this section we use the generative model defined by (1) to encode an MRF over the unknown labels. We show that computing this MRF term is analogous to the mathematical operations performed by a CNN. We then go on to formulate learning the MRF clique potentials as the training of a CNN. This allows us to introduce nonlinearities and increasing complexity in the MRF neighbourhood.

Generative Model: The posterior in (1) allows us to estimate the unknown tissue labels. For simplicity, we will from now on assume that all parameters ($\boldsymbol{\theta}$) are known; we therefore only want to infer the posterior distribution over categorical labels $\boldsymbol{Z} \in \{0,1\}^{I \times K}$, where I are the number of pixels in the image and K are the number of classes, conditioned on an observed image $\boldsymbol{X} \in \mathbb{R}^{I \times C}$, where C are the number of channels. Modelling multi-channel images allows the use of all acquired MR contrasts of the same subject. In practice, unknown parameters of, *e.g.*, class-wise intensity distributions would need inferring too. Variational Bayesian (VB) inference, along with a well-chosen mean-field approximation, allows any such model to fit within the presented framework [21].

Making use of the product rule, we may define the joint model likelihood $p(\boldsymbol{X}, \boldsymbol{Z})$ as the product of a data likelihood $p(\boldsymbol{X} \mid \boldsymbol{Z})$ and a prior $p(\boldsymbol{Z})$. In a mixture model, it is assumed that once labels are known, intensities are independent across pixels and all pixels with the same label k are sampled from the same distribution $p_k(\boldsymbol{x})$. This can be written as:

$$p(\boldsymbol{X} \mid \boldsymbol{Z}) = \prod_{i=1}^{I} \prod_{k=1}^{K} p_k(\boldsymbol{x}_i)^{z_{ik}}. \tag{2}$$

A common prior distribution for labels in a mixture model is the categorical distribution, which can be stationary ($p(\boldsymbol{z}_i) = \mathrm{Cat}\,(\boldsymbol{z}_i \mid \boldsymbol{\pi})$) or non-stationary ($p(\boldsymbol{z}_i) = \mathrm{Cat}\,(\boldsymbol{z}_i \mid \boldsymbol{\pi}_i)$) [22]. However, both these distributions assume conditional independence between pixels. MRFs can be introduced to model dependencies between pixels in a relatively tractable way by assuming that interactions are restricted to a finite neighbourhood:

$$p(\boldsymbol{z}_i \mid \{\boldsymbol{z}_j\}_{j \neq i}) = p(\boldsymbol{z}_i \mid \boldsymbol{z}_{\mathcal{N}_i}), \tag{3}$$

where $\mathcal{N}_i$ defines pixels whose cliques contain $\boldsymbol{z}_i$. We make the common assumption that this neighbourhood is stationary, meaning that it is defined by relative positions with respect to i: $\mathcal{N}_i = \{i + \delta \mid \delta \in \mathcal{N}\}$. Here, we assume that this conditional likelihood factorises over the neighbours and that each factor is a categorical distribution:

$$p(\boldsymbol{z}_i \mid \boldsymbol{z}_{\mathcal{N}_i}) = \prod_{\delta \in \mathcal{N}} \prod_{k=1}^{K} \prod_{l=1}^{K} (\pi_{k,l,\delta})^{z_{i,k} \cdot z_{i+\delta,l}}. \tag{4}$$

Mean-Field Inference: Despite the use of a relatively simple interaction model, the posterior distribution over labels is intractable. Therefore, our approach is to search for an approximate posterior distribution that factorises across voxels:

$$p(\boldsymbol{Z} \mid \boldsymbol{X}) \approx q(\boldsymbol{Z}) = \prod_{i=1}^{I} q(\boldsymbol{z}_i). \tag{5}$$

We use VB inference [21] to iteratively find the approximate posterior q that minimises its Kullback-Leibler divergence with the true posterior distribution. Let us assume a current approximate posterior distribution $q(\boldsymbol{Z}) = \prod_j \text{Cat}(\boldsymbol{z}_j \mid \boldsymbol{r}_j)$; each voxel follows a categorical distribution parameterised by $\boldsymbol{r}_j$, which is often called a *responsibility*. VB then gives us the optimal updated distribution for factor i by taking the expected value of the joint model log-likelihood, with respect to all other variables:

$$\ln q^\star(\boldsymbol{z}_i) = \sum_{k=1}^{K} z_{ik} \left(\ln p_k(\boldsymbol{x}_i) + \sum_{\delta \in \mathcal{N}} \sum_{l=1}^{K} r_{i+\delta,l} \ln \pi_{k,l,\delta} \right) + \text{const.} \qquad (6)$$

This distribution is again categorical with parameters:

$$r_{ik}^\star \propto \exp \left(\ln p_k(\boldsymbol{x}_i) + \sum_{\delta \in \mathcal{N}} \sum_{l=1}^{K} r_{i+\delta,l} \ln \pi_{k,l,\delta} \right). \qquad (7)$$

Implementation as a CNN: Under VB assumptions, posterior distributions should be updated one at a time, in turn. Taking advantage of the limited support of the neighbourhood, an efficient update scheme can be implemented by updating at once all pixels that do not share a neighbourhood[2]. Another scheme can be to update all pixels at once based on the previous state of the entire field. Drawing a parallel with linear systems, this is comparable to Jacobi's method, while updating in turn is comparable to the Gauss-Siedel method. In the Jacobi case, updating the labels' expected values can be implemented as a convolution, an addition and a softmax operation; three basic layers of CNNs:

$$\boldsymbol{R}^\star = f(\boldsymbol{R}) = \text{softmax}(\boldsymbol{C} + \boldsymbol{W} * \boldsymbol{R}). \qquad (8)$$

The matrix $\boldsymbol{C}$ contains the conditional log-likelihood terms $(\ln p_k(\boldsymbol{x}_i))$. The convolution weights $\boldsymbol{W} \in \mathbb{R}^{|\mathcal{N}| \times K \times K}$ are equal to the log of the MRF weights $(\ln \pi_{k,l,\delta})$ and, very importantly, their centre is always zero. We call such filters *MRF filters*, and the combination of softmaxing and convolving an *MRF layer*. These weights are parameters of the approximate posterior distribution $q^\star(\boldsymbol{Z})$. Note that multiple mean-field updates can be implemented by making the MRF layer recurrent, where the output is also the input [19].

Now, let us assume that we have a set of true segmentations $\hat{\boldsymbol{Z}}_{1...N}$, along with a set of approximate distributions with parameters $\boldsymbol{R}_{1...N}$. One may want to know the MRF parameters $\boldsymbol{W}$ that make the new posterior estimate $q^\star$ with parameters $\boldsymbol{R}^\star = f(\boldsymbol{R})$ the most likely to have generated the true segmentations. This reduces to the optimisation problem:

$$\boldsymbol{W}^\star = \underset{\boldsymbol{W}}{\text{argmax}} \sum_{n=1}^{N} \ln q^\star(\hat{\boldsymbol{Z}}_n \mid \boldsymbol{W}) = \underset{\boldsymbol{W}}{\text{argmax}} \sum_{i=1}^{I} \sum_{k=1}^{K} \hat{z}_{nik} \ln r_{nik}^\star, \qquad (9)$$

---

[2] When $\mathcal{N}$ contains four second-order neighbours, this corresponds to a checkerboard update scheme.

which is a maximum-likelihood (ML), or risk-minimisation, problem. Note that this objective function is the negative of what is commonly referred to as the categorical cross-entropy loss function in machine-learning. If the optimisation is performed by computing gradients from a subset of random samples, this is equivalent to optimising a CNN, with only one layer, by stochastic gradient descent.

Post-processing MRFs: MRFs are sometimes used to post-process segmentations, rather than as an explicit prior in a generative model. In this case, the conditional data term is not known, and the objective is slightly different: approximating a factorised label distribution $q(\boldsymbol{Z}) = \prod_{i=1}^{I} q(\boldsymbol{z}_i)$ that resembles the prior distribution $p(\boldsymbol{Z})$. This can be written as finding such distribution q that minimises the Kullback-Leibler divergence with the prior p:

$$q^{\star} = \underset{q}{\operatorname{argmin}} \operatorname{KL}(q\|p). \tag{10}$$

Again, assuming all other factors fixed with $q(\boldsymbol{z}_j) = \operatorname{Cat}(\boldsymbol{z}_j \mid \boldsymbol{r}_j)$, the optimal distribution for factor i is obtained by taking the expected value of the prior log-likelihood:

$$\ln q^{\star}(\boldsymbol{z}_i) = \sum_{k=1}^{K} z_{ik} \left(\sum_{\delta \in \mathcal{N}} \sum_{l=1}^{K} r_{i+\delta,l} \ln \pi_{k,l,\delta} \right) + \text{const}, \tag{11}$$

which is equivalent to dropping the conditional term in the generative case. Equation (8) is then written as $\boldsymbol{R}^{\star} = \operatorname{softmax}(\boldsymbol{W} * \boldsymbol{R})$.

Nonlinear MRF: The conditional prior distribution $p(\boldsymbol{z}_i \mid \boldsymbol{z}_{\mathcal{N}_i})$ that defines an MRF can, in theory, be any strictly positive probability distribution. However, in practice, they are usually restricted to simple log-linear functions, which are easy to implement and efficient to compute. On the other hand, deep neural networks allow highly nonlinear functions to be implemented and computed efficiently. Therefore, we propose a more complex layer based on multiple MRF filters and nonlinearities, that implements a nonlinear MRF density. To ensure that we implement a conditional probability, a constraint is that the input value of a voxel may not be used to compute its posterior density. Therefore, the first layer consists MRF filters that do not have a central weight, and subsequent layers are of size one to avoid reintroducing the centre value by deconvolution. We thus propose the first layer to be an MRF filter $\boldsymbol{W} \in \mathbb{R}^{|\mathcal{N}| \times K \times F}$, where F is the number of output features. Setting $F > K$ allows the information to be decoupled into more than the initial K classes and may help to capture more complex interactions. This first convolutional layer is followed by a ReLU activation function, 1D convolutions that keep the number of features untouched, and another ReLU activation function. This allows features to be combined together. A final 1D linear layer is used to recombine the information into K classes, followed by a softmax. Figure 2 shows our proposed architecture.

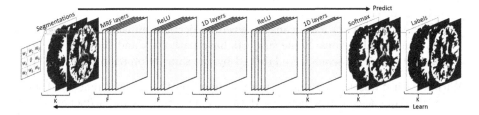

Fig. 2. An illustration of the architecture of our MRF CNN. Outlined are the operations performed for learning to predict the centre of a segmented pixel. The nonlinearities are introduced by the ReLU activations. By setting the number of MRF layers to K and keeping only the final softmax layer, the linear MRF model is obtained. The convolution kernel applied by the MRF filter is shown left of the segmentations, with its centre constrained to be zero.

Implementation and Training: In this work we set the number of MRF layers to $F = 16$, we use three by three convolutions and leaky ReLU activation functions with $\alpha = 0.1$. We optimise the CNN using the Adam optimiser. To reduce overfitting, we augment the data in two ways: (1) by simple left-right reflection; and (2), by sampling warps from anatomically feasible affine transformations, followed by nearest neighbour interpolation. Realistic affine transformations can be sampled by parametrising them by their 12 parameter Lie group (from which the transformation matrix can be constructed via an exponential mapping [23]) and then learning their mean and covariance from a large number of subjects' image headers.

3 Validation

This section aims to answer a series of questions: (1) does applying a linear MRF trained by backpropagation to the output segmentations of a generative model improve the segmentation accuracy? (2) does complexifying the MRF distribution using numerous filters and nonlinearities improve the segmentation accuracy compared to a linear MRF? (3) do the learnt weights generalise to new data from an entirely different dataset?

Datasets and Preprocessing: Our validation was performed on axial 2D slices extracted from two publicly available datasets[3]:

- **MICCAI2012:** T1-weighted MR scans of 30 subjects aged 18 to 96 years, (mean: 34, median: 25). The scans were manually segmented into 136 anatomical regions by Neuromorphometrics Inc. for the MICCAI 2012 challenge on multi-atlas segmentation.

---

[3] my.vanderbilt.edu/masi/workshops, mrbrains18.isi.uu.nl.

– **MRBrainS18:** Multi-sequence (T1-weighted, T1-weighted inversion recovery and T2-FLAIR) MR scans of seven subjects, manually segmented into ten anatomical regions. Some subjects have pathology and they are all older than 50 years. All scans were labelled by the same neuroanatomist.

Within each dataset, all subjects were scanned on the same scanner and with the same sequences, whilst between datasets, the scanners and sequences differ (Fig. 1). Both datasets have multiple labelled brain structures, such as cortical GM, cerebellum, ventricles, *etc.* We combined these so as to obtain the same three labels for each subject: GM, WM and OTHER $(1 - GM - WM)$. These labels were used as targets when training our model.

All T1-weighted MR scans were segmented with the algorithm implemented in the SPM12 software[4], which is based on the generative model described in [3]. In this model, the distribution over categorical labels is independent across voxels, non-stationary, and encoded by a probabilistic atlas deformed towards each subject. The algorithm generates soft segmentations, that is, parameters of the posterior categorical distribution over labels. We pulled the GM, WM and OTHER classes from these segmentations. Figure 3 shows the T1-weighted image of one subject from each dataset, with its corresponding target labels and SPM12 segmentations[5].

Model Training and Evaluation: We trained two different models: a regular, second-order MRF (*Lin*); and a second-order nonlinear MRF (*Net*). Figure 2 explains the differences in architecture between the two. For each subject and each class, we computed the Dice score of the ML labels obtained using SPM12 and those obtained after application of the linear MRF and the nonlinear MRF. Statistical significance of the observed changes was tested using two-sided Welch's t-tests between paired measures. Multiple comparisons were accounted for by applying the Bonferroni correction.

We first evaluated the learning abilities of the networks. To this end, we performed a 10-fold cross validation of the MICCAI2012 dataset, where groups of three images were tested using a model trained on the remaining 27 images. This yielded Dice scores for the entire MICCAI2012 dataset, which are shown in Fig. 4a. Next, we evaluated the generalisability of the networks, that is, what kind of performances are obtained when the models are tested on images from an entirely new dataset, with different imaging features. We randomly selected models trained on one of the MICCAI2012 folds and applied them to the images from the MRBrainS18 dataset. The results are shown in Fig. 4b.

Results: The 10-fold cross validation results in Fig. 4a show that the increase in Dice scores for both GM and WM is statistically significant after applying either of our two MRF CNN models. (Fig. 3 shows the results for a randomly selected

---

[4] www.fil.ion.ucl.ac.uk/spm/software/spm12.

[5] Besides disabling the final MRF clean-up, we used the default parameters of SPM12.

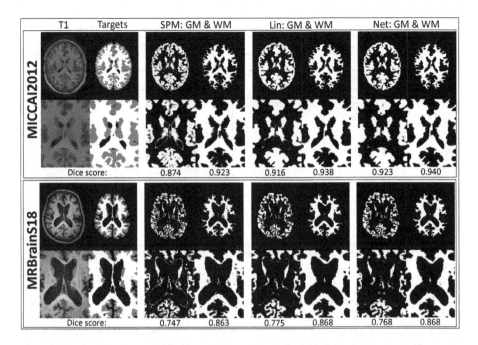

Fig. 3. Example training data and results. From left to right: T1-weighted MR image with target labels, SPM GM and WM segmentations, results of applying the linear MRF model to the SPM segmentations, results of applying the nonlinear MRF model to the SPM segmentations. Below each tissue class are the corresponding Dice scores, computed with the target labels as reference.

MICCAI2012 subject). With a mean Dice of {GM = 0.867, WM = 0.921} for SPM12, and {GM = 0.901, WM = 0.929} and {GM = 0.909, WM = 0.931} after applying the linear and nonlinear MRF, respectively. The results imply that the classical generative approach of SPM12, which currently ranks in the top 50 on the MRBrainS13 challenge website[6], could move up quite a few positions by application of our proposed model trained on the challenge data. As can be seen in Fig. 4a, for one of the subjects, all models perform substantially worse. On closer inspection, this subject suffers from major white matter hyper-intensities. This abnormality is currently not handled well by the MRF CNN models, which obtain lower Dice scores than the initial SPM12 segmentations.

Figure 4b shows results when applying the models to data from a different centre, not part of the training data (Fig. 3 shows the results for a randomly selected MRBrainS18 subject). Mean Dice scores are {GM = 0.722, WM = 0.816} for SPM12, and {GM = 0.761, WM = 0.831} and {GM = 0.755, WM = 0.829} after application of the linear and nonlinear MRF, respectively. Application of the MRF improves both GM and WM segmentations. The nonlinear MRF performs slightly worse than the linear version. This result could be due

---

[6] mrbrains13.isi.uu.nl/results.php.

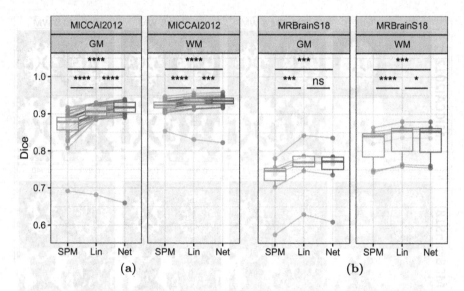

Fig. 4. Validation of our model on the MICCAI2012 (a) and MRBrainS18 (b) datasets. Dice scores were computed for known labels (GM and WM) and: SPM12 segmentations (SPM); and linear (Lin) and nonlinear (Net) 8-neighbour MRF applied to the SPM12 segmentations. Asterisks indicate statistical significance of paired t-tests after Bonferroni correction: 0.05 ($*$), 0.01 ($**$), 0.001 ($*\,*\,*$) & 0.0001 ($*\,*\,*\,*$).

to the nonlinear model – which possesses many more parameters than the linear model – overfitting to the training subjects of MICCAI2012. Additionally, the nonlinear MRF may struggle with the MRBrainS18 subjects that have pathology (*e.g.* white matter hyperintensities). Still, the fact that Dice scores improve when applying the model to new data shows that we can successfully improve segmenting images from different MR imaging protocols.

4   Discussion

In this paper, we introduced an image segmentation method that combines the robustness of a well-tuned generative model with some of the outstanding learning capability of a CNN. The CNN encodes an MRF in the prior term over the unknown labels. We evaluated the method on annotated MR images and showed that a trained model can be deployed on an unseen image population, with very different characteristics from the training population. We hope that the idea presented in this paper introduces to the medical imaging community a principled way of bringing together probabilistic modelling and deep learning.

In medical image analysis – where labelled training data is sparse and images can vary widely – generalisability across different image populations is one of the most important properties of learning-based methods. However, achieving this generalisability is made difficult by the limited amount of annotated data; the datasets we used in this paper contained, in total, only 37 subjects. This issue may be addressed by realistic, nonlinear data augmentation, which is able to capture changes due to ageing and disease. Learning this variability in shape from a large and diverse population could be a step in that direction [24]. On the other hand – manual segmentations suffer from both intra- and inter-operator variability, is it clinically meaningful to learn from these very imperfect annotations? Could automatic segmentations prove more anatomically informative than manual ones (*c.f.*, Fig. 3)? Semi-supervised techniques, leveraging both labelled and unlabelled data, could be an option for making our method less dependent on annotations (see *e.g.*, [25]).

We chose the architecture of our proposed MRF CNN with the idea of keeping the number of parameters low (to reduce overfitting), while still introducing a more complex neighbourhood than in regular MRF models. However, we did not extensively investigate different architectures, *e.g.*, activation functions and filter size. There is therefore a possibility of improved performance by design changes to the network. Such a change could be to hierarchically apply MRF filters of decreasing size, which could increase neighbourhood size without increased overfitting. Another potentially interesting idea would be to 'plug in' the MRF filters at the end of a segmentation network, such as a U-net, emulating MRF post-processing inside the network. Finally, we intend to integrate our model into a generative segmentation framework and then validate its performance by comparing it to other existing segmentation software.

Acknowledgements. JA was funded by the EU Human Brain Project's Grant Agreement No. 785907 (SGA2). YB was funded by the MRC and Spinal Research Charity through the ERA-NET Neuron joint call (MR/R000050/1).

References

1. Klauschen, F., Goldman, A., Barra, V., Meyer-Lindenberg, A., Lundervold, A.: Evaluation of automated brain MR image segmentation and volumetry methods. Hum. Brain Mapp. **30**(4), 1310–1327 (2009)
2. Wells III, W.M., Grimson, W.E.L., Kikinis, R., Jolesz, F.A.: Adaptive segmentation of MRI data. IEEE Trans. Med. Imaging **15**(4), 429–442 (1996)
3. Ashburner, J., Friston, K.J.: Unified segmentation. Neuroimage **26**(3), 839–851 (2005)
4. Zhang, Y., Brady, M., Smith, S.: Segmentation of brain MR images through a hidden Markov random field model and the expectation-maximization algorithm. IEEE Trans. Med. Imaging **20**(1), 45–57 (2001)
5. Fischl, B., et al.: Sequence-independent segmentation of magnetic resonance images. Neuroimage **23**, S69–S84 (2004)
6. Kazemi, K., Noorizadeh, N.: Quantitative comparison of SPM, FSL, and brainsuite for brain MR image segmentation. J Biomed. Phys. Eng. **4**(1), 13 (2014)
7. Heinen, R., Bouvy, W.H., Mendrik, A.M., Viergever, M.A., Biessels, G.J., De Bresser, J.: Robustness of automated methods for brain volume measurements across different MRI field strengths. PloS One **11**(10), e0165719 (2016)

8. Long, J., Shelhamer, E., Darrell, T.: Fully convolutional networks for semantic segmentation. In: Proceedings of the IEEE International Conference on Computer Vision, pp. 3431–3440 (2015)

9. Ronneberger, O., Fischer, P., Brox, T.: U-Net: convolutional networks for biomedical image segmentation. In: Navab, N., Hornegger, J., Wells, W.M., Frangi, A.F. (eds.) MICCAI 2015. LNCS, vol. 9351, pp. 234–241. Springer, Cham (2015). https://doi.org/10.1007/978-3-319-24574-4_28

10. Dolz, J., Desrosiers, C., Ayed, I.B.: 3D fully convolutional networks for subcortical segmentation in MRI: a large-scale study. NeuroImage **170**, 456–470 (2017)

11. Akkus, Z., Galimzianova, A., Hoogi, A., Rubin, D.L., Erickson, B.J.: Deep learning for brain MRI segmentation: state of the art and future directions. J. Digit. Imaging **30**(4), 449–459 (2017)

12. Han, X., Fischl, B.: Atlas renormalization for improved brain MR image segmentation across scanner platforms. IEEE Trans. Med. Imaging **26**(4), 479–486 (2007)

13. Van Opbroek, A., Ikram, M.A., Vernooij, M.W., De Bruijne, M.: Transfer learning improves supervised image segmentation across imaging protocols. IEEE Trans. Med. Imaging **34**(5), 1018–1030 (2015)

14. Karani, N., Chaitanya, K., Baumgartner, C., Konukoglu, E.: A Lifelong Learning Approach to Brain MR Segmentation Across Scanners and Protocols. arXiv preprint arXiv:1805.10170 (2018)

15. Jog, A., Fischl, B.: Pulse sequence resilient fast brain segmentation. In: Frangi, A.F., Schnabel, J.A., Davatzikos, C., Alberola-López, C., Fichtinger, G. (eds.) MICCAI 2018. LNCS, vol. 11072, pp. 654–662. Springer, Cham (2018). https://doi.org/10.1007/978-3-030-00931-1_75

16. Zhao, A., Balakrishnan, G., Durand, F., Guttag, J.V., Dalca, A.V.: Data augmentation using learned transforms for one-shot medical image segmentation. arXiv:1902.09383 (2019)

17. Van Leemput, K., Maes, F., Vandermeulen, D., Suetens, P.: Automated model-based tissue classification of MR images of the brain. IEEE Trans. Med. Imaging **18**(10), 897–908 (1999)

18. Agn, M., Puonti, O., Rosenschöld, P.M., Law, I., Van Leemput, K.: Brain tumor segmentation using a generative model with an RBM prior on tumor shape. In: Crimi, A., Menze, B., Maier, O., Reyes, M., Handels, H. (eds.) BrainLes 2015. LNCS, vol. 9556, pp. 168–180. Springer, Cham (2016). https://doi.org/10.1007/978-3-319-30858-6_15

19. Zheng, S., et al.: Conditional random fields as recurrent neural networks. In: Proceedings of the IEEE International Conference on Computer Vision, pp. 1529–1537 (2015)

20. Schwing, A.G., Urtasun, R.: Fully connected deep structured networks. arXiv preprint arXiv:1503.02351 (2015)

21. Bishop, C.M.: Pattern Recognition and Machine Learning. Springer, New York (2006)

22. Ashburner, J., Friston, K.: Multimodal image coregistration and partitioning—a unified framework. Neuroimage **6**(3), 209–217 (1997)

23. Ashburner, J., Ridgway, G.R.: Symmetric diffeomorphic modeling of longitudinal structural MRI. Front. Neurosci. **6**, 197 (2013)

24. Balbastre, Y., Brudfors, M., Bronik, K., Ashburner, J.: Diffeomorphic brain shape modelling using gauss-newton optimisation. In: Frangi, A.F., Schnabel, J.A., Davatzikos, C., Alberola-López, C., Fichtinger, G. (eds.) MICCAI 2018. LNCS, vol. 11070, pp. 862–870. Springer, Cham (2018). https://doi.org/10.1007/978-3-030-00928-1_97
25. Roy, A.G., Conjeti, S., Navab, N., Wachinger, C.: QuickNAT: a fullyconvolutional network for quick and accurate segmentation of neuroanatomy. NeuroImage **186**, 713–727 (2018)

Robust Biophysical Parameter Estimation with a Neural Network Enhanced Hamiltonian Markov Chain Monte Carlo Sampler

Thomas Yu[1](✉), Marco Pizzolato[1](✉), Gabriel Girard[2],
Jonathan Rafael-Patino[1], Erick Jorge Canales-Rodríguez[1,2,3,4],
and Jean-Philippe Thiran[1,2,5]

[1] Signal Processing Lab (LTS5), École Polytechnique Fédérale de Lausanne,
Lausanne, Switzerland
{thomas.yu,marco.pizzolato}@epfl.ch

[2] Department of Radiology, Centre Hospitalier Universitaire Vaudois (CHUV),
Lausanne, Switzerland

[3] FIDMAG Germanes Hospitalàries, Sant Boi de Llobregat, Barcelona, Spain

[4] Mental Health Research Networking Center (CIBERSAM), Madrid, Spain

[5] University of Lausanne, Lausanne, Switzerland

Abstract. Probabilistic parameter estimation in model fitting runs the gamut from maximum likelihood or maximum a posteriori point estimates from optimization to Markov Chain Monte Carlo (MCMC) sampling. The latter, while more computationally intensive, generally provides a better characterization of the underlying parameter distribution than that of point estimates. However, in order to efficiently explore distributions, MCMC methods ideally require generating uncorrelated samples while also preserving reasonable acceptance probabilities; this becomes particularly important in problematic regions of parameter space. In this paper, we extend a recently proposed Hamiltonian MCMC sampler parametrized by neural networks (L2HMC) by modifying the loss function to jointly optimize the distance between samples and the acceptance probability such that it is stable and efficient. We apply this enhanced sampler to parameter estimation in a recently proposed MRI model, the multi-echo spherical mean technique. We show that it generally outperforms the state of the art Hamiltonian No-U-Turn (NUTS) sampler, L2HMC, and a least squares fitting in terms of accuracy and precision, also enabling the generation of more informative parameter posterior distributions. This illustrates the potential of machine learning enhanced samplers for improving probabilistic parameter estimation for medical imaging applications.

Keywords: Markov Chain Monte Carlo ·
Hamiltonian MCMC sampler · Magnetic resonance imaging ·
Optimization · Parameter estimation

© Springer Nature Switzerland AG 2019
A. C. S. Chung et al. (Eds.): IPMI 2019, LNCS 11492, pp. 818–829, 2019.
https://doi.org/10.1007/978-3-030-20351-1_64

1   Introduction

Given a data vector $\mathbf{s} \in \mathbb{R}^d$ generated from varying an independent experimental variable $v \in \mathbb{R}$, and a model $M(\mathbf{x}, v) : \mathbb{R}^n \times \mathbb{R} \to \mathbb{R}$ with parameters $\mathbf{x} \in \mathbb{R}^n$ to explain the data, probabilistic parameter estimation constructs a probabilistic model for the data and views the problem as inferring the parameters of a probability distribution [17]. For example, one can define the likelihood of the data given fixed parameters by treating each data point as an independent sample from a Gaussian distribution with mean at the model evaluated at the corresponding $v, \mathbf{x}$ and with a variance coming from the measurement noise. Using Bayes' theorem, the posterior probability distribution of the parameters given the data is proportional to the product of the likelihood function and the priors on the parameters:

$$p(\mathbf{x}|\mathbf{s}) \propto p(\mathbf{s}|\mathbf{x})p(\mathbf{x}), \tag{1}$$

where,

$$p(\mathbf{s}|\mathbf{x}) = \mathcal{N}(M(\mathbf{x}, \mathbf{v}), \sigma^2) = \prod_{i=1}^{d} \frac{1}{\sqrt{2\pi\sigma^2}} \exp(\frac{(\mathbf{s}_i - M(\mathbf{x}, \mathbf{v}_i))^2}{2\sigma^2}), \tag{2}$$

and σ^2 denotes the noise variance. The prior distribution $p(\mathbf{x})$ encodes constraints such as sum constraints or upper/lower bounds through, for example, Dirichlet and uniform distributions [1]. An immediate candidate for a parameter estimate is then the maximum a posteriori (MAP) point estimate

$$\mathbf{x}^* = \arg \max_{\mathbf{x}} p(\mathbf{x}|\mathbf{s}). \tag{3}$$

This reduces the parameter estimation to an optimization problem. However, there are two potential problems with this point estimate. First, the general problems of uniqueness and feasibility of optimization, i.e. finding the MAP estimate. Second, the underlying assumption of this point estimate is that the mode is a good representation of the underlying probability distribution. Intuitively, we can see the truth of this assumption for many commonly used distributions in three or less dimensions e.g. normal or exponential. However, this assumption can fail as the dimensionality and complexity of the distribution increases due to the geometry of high dimensional spaces [3] and the concentration of measure phenomenon [3,14]. Hence, inferring the parameters of a probabilistic model of high dimension and/or complexity through a mode point estimate can lead to spurious results. One approach to handle these issues is to first characterize the posterior distribution with Markov Chain Monte Carlo (MCMC) techniques [9] by sampling from the posterior distribution. One can then, as an example, use the mode, mean, median, etc. of the marginal posterior distributions of the parameters for the parameter estimate. In this paper, we use the expectation of each parameter over its marginal posterior, approximated by

$$\mathbf{x}^* \approx \frac{1}{N} \sum_{i}^{N} \mathbf{x_i}, \tag{4}$$

where the subscript i denotes one of the N samples.

The contributions of this paper are, first, to extend a Hamiltonian MCMC sampler parametrized with neural networks proposed in [15]. We modify the loss function to balance acceptance probability and mixing such that both fast mixing and stable exploration of problematic regions of state space are possible. Second, we apply our extended sampler to estimate the parameters of a recently proposed MRI model and compare it to a least squares fitting and application of two state of the art Hamiltonian samplers.

2   Related Work

2.1   Hamiltonian Markov Chain Monte Carlo

In the following, we denote the posterior distribution from which we want to sample as $p(\mathbf{x})$ with $\mathbf{x} \in \mathbb{R}^n$ being the state variables. MCMC methods sample from the posterior by generating a sequence of samples where each new sample $\mathbf{x}_t$ is generated from the previous sample $\mathbf{x}_{t-1}$ according to a transition distribution $T(\mathbf{x}_t|\mathbf{x}_{t-1})$ [4]. In order for the posterior to be the unique distribution to which this sequence converges, the transition distribution must satisfy ergodicity, which can usually be safely assumed, and an invariance property which is usually shown by proving a property called detailed balance $p(\mathbf{x}_t)T(\mathbf{x}_{t-1}|\mathbf{x}_t) = p(\mathbf{x}_{t-1})T(\mathbf{x}_t|\mathbf{x}_{t-1})$.

One well known way to construct a transition satisfying detailed balance called the Metropolis-Hastings algorithm [9] is as follows: given a proposal distribution $q(\mathbf{x}'|\mathbf{x}_{t-1})$, sample a candidate $\mathbf{x}'$; then, accept $\mathbf{x}'$ with probability $A(\mathbf{x}'|\mathbf{x}_{t-1}) = min(1, \frac{p(\mathbf{x}')q(\mathbf{x}_{t-1}|\mathbf{x}')}{p(\mathbf{x}_{t-1})q(\mathbf{x}'|\mathbf{x}_{t-1})})$. If accepted, $\mathbf{x}_t = \mathbf{x}'$. If rejected, $\mathbf{x}_t = \mathbf{x}_{t-1}$. However, even if a sampler satisfies these properties, the convergence is only proven asymptotically [4]. The typical procedure is to first have a burn-in stage where the sampler is run for some amount of steps in order for it to converge. Then, the actual sampling begins, with the burn-in samples being discarded [4].

For efficient exploration, the samples should ideally be uncorrelated, which can be accomplished by large distances between samples in the sample space, i.e. mixing. Autocorrelation analysis using multiple chains of samples can be used as a rough measure of how many samples are necessary. We emphasize that a balance must be found between the acceptance probability and the mixing; acceptance probabilities which are very high can mean the samples are very close/correlated and large distances between samples can lead to only a small number of samples being accepted. One powerful MCMC method which scales with the dimensionality and complexity of the posterior is Hamiltonian MCMC (HMCMC) [6]. In HMCMC, one generates proposal samples by integrating along trajectories of a Hamiltonian dynamical system constructed from combining the posterior distribution of interest with a momentum distribution. This is then followed by the Metropolis acceptance step to yield a new sample. Formally a joint distribution is constructed with state variables $(\mathbf{x}, \mathbf{p})$:

$$p^H(\mathbf{x}, \mathbf{p}) \propto \exp(-U(\mathbf{x}) - K(\mathbf{p})), \tag{5}$$

$$p(\mathbf{x}) \propto \exp(-U(\mathbf{x})), \tag{6}$$

$$K(\mathbf{p}) = \frac{1}{2}\mathbf{p}^T\mathbf{p}, \tag{7}$$

where we omit a normalizing constant and $\mathbf{p}$ are the momentum variables which are added. This form is motivated from statistical physics by the canonical distribution of energy states of a system, where U and K denote the potential and kinetic energy respectively, and the Hamiltonian (total energy) is $H = U + K$ [6]. HMCMC samples from $p^H(\mathbf{x}, \mathbf{p})$, and we can obtain the marginal distribution of $\mathbf{x}$ from the samples. H defines a dynamical system, which is a set of differential equations used to evolve $\mathbf{x}, \mathbf{p}$ forward in time from an initial sample.

In practice, these equations are integrated numerically, characterized by a step size ϵ and a number of steps L such that $L\epsilon$ is the time period over which a sample trajectory is evolved. The most common numerical scheme is the leapfrog scheme, which we write below for one time step with initial condition $(\mathbf{x}, \mathbf{p})$ and result $(\mathbf{x}', \mathbf{p}')$.

$$\mathbf{p}^{\frac{1}{2}} = \mathbf{p} - \frac{\epsilon}{2}\partial_x U(\mathbf{x}), \ \mathbf{x}' = \mathbf{x} + \epsilon\mathbf{p}^{\frac{1}{2}}, \ \mathbf{p}' = \mathbf{p} - \frac{\epsilon}{2}\partial_x U(\mathbf{x}'). \tag{8}$$

Given an initial $\mathbf{x_0}$, an initial momentum $\mathbf{p_0}$ is sampled from a distribution, usually a standard Gaussian [4]. The proposed sample from running the dynamics, $(\mathbf{x}', \mathbf{p}')$, is then accepted in a Metropolis-Hastings step with probability $\alpha = min(1, \frac{\exp(-U(\mathbf{x}) - \frac{1}{2}\mathbf{p}^T\mathbf{p})}{\exp(-U(\mathbf{x_0}) - \frac{1}{2}\mathbf{p_0}^T\mathbf{p_0})})$. Ideally, this procedure is then repeated until the convergence of the samples to the distribution, with the output of each proposal becoming the new initial sample. The main advantage of HMCMC is that it generally proposes samples which are far away from the initial sample, thus efficiently exploring the posterior, while maintaining reasonable acceptance probabilities [4]. A state of the art HMCMC sampler called the No U Turn Sampler (NUTS) [10] improves on standard HMCMC by adaptively tuning L, ϵ to manage the distance between samples and acceptance probability. HMCMC can perform poorly in certain circumstances, in particular, in highly curved sample spaces such as those that might arise in the posteriors derived from parameter estimation of complex models [8].

2.2 L2HMC

Levy et al. [15] recently proposed a framework called L2HMC which parametrizes the standard HMCMC sampler with a neural network and maximizes the expected distance between samples through minimization of a loss function which rewards large expected squared distances between samples. Furthermore, the parametrization is carefully tailored to preserve detailed balance and have a tractable Jacobian for the correction of the acceptance probability due to the potential non-volume preserving dynamics. The algorithm of L2HMC is structurally similar to standard HMCMC, but modifications are made to the proposal stage. First, for each step t, $1 \leq t \leq L$, a random binary mask $m_t \in \{0,1\}^n$ is constructed such that approximately half of the entries of the mask are 1. The conjugate mask is denoted as m_t^c. Instead of updating $\mathbf{x}$ in one step according to the classical algorithm, the update is split into two steps each updating only the variables of $\mathbf{x}$ corresponding to m_t, m_t^c separately. These are denoted as $\mathbf{x}_{m_t} = \mathbf{x} \odot m_t$ and $\mathbf{x}_{m_t^c} = \mathbf{x} \odot m_t^c$ respectively, where $\odot$ is the component-wise multiplication operator. Each update equation is modified with scaling factors for each term depending on only variables which are not being updated. Concretely, let $\zeta_1 = (\mathbf{x}, \partial_x U(\mathbf{x}'), t)$. Then $\mathbf{p}$ is first updated according to

$$\mathbf{p}^{\frac{1}{2}} = \mathbf{p} \odot \exp(\frac{\epsilon}{2} S_p(\zeta_1)) - \frac{\epsilon}{2} \partial_x U(\mathbf{x}) \odot \exp(\epsilon Q_p(\zeta_1)) + T_p(\zeta_1), \qquad (9)$$

where $S_p, Q_p, T_p : \mathbb{R}^{2n+1} \to \mathbb{R}^n$ are scaling functions parameterized by a neural network. Let $\zeta_2 = (\mathbf{x}_{m_t^c}, \mathbf{p}, t)$ and $\zeta_3 = (\mathbf{x}_{m_t}^{\frac{1}{2}}, \mathbf{p}, t)$. Then $\mathbf{x}$ is updated according to

$$\mathbf{x}^{\frac{1}{2}} = \mathbf{x}_{m_t^c} + m_t \odot \left[\mathbf{x} \odot \exp(\epsilon S_x(\zeta_2)) + \epsilon(\mathbf{p}^{\frac{1}{2}} \odot \exp(\epsilon Q_x(\zeta_2)) + T_x(\zeta_2))\right], \quad (10)$$

$$\mathbf{x}' = \mathbf{x}_{m_t} + m_t^c \odot \left[\mathbf{x} \odot \exp(\epsilon S_x(\zeta_3)) + \epsilon(\mathbf{p}^{\frac{1}{2}} \odot \exp(\epsilon Q_x(\zeta_3)) + T_x(\zeta_3))\right], \quad (11)$$

where $S_x, Q_x, T_x : \mathbb{R}^{2n+1} \to \mathbb{R}^n$ are also scaling functions parameterized by a neural network. Finally, let $\zeta_4 = (\mathbf{x}', \partial_x U(\mathbf{x}'), t)$:

$$\mathbf{p}' = \mathbf{p}^{\frac{1}{2}} \odot \exp(\frac{\epsilon}{2} S_p(\zeta_4)) - \frac{\epsilon}{2} \partial_x U(\mathbf{x}') \odot \exp(\epsilon Q_p(\zeta_4)) + T_p(\zeta_4). \qquad (12)$$

These learned scaling functions, structured as a two layer neural network, can allow the sampler to learn, for example, how to carefully navigate regions of high curvature in the parameter space rather than having to manipulate ϵ and L to accomplish this. As in NUTS [10], the time reversed version of the above dynamics can also be used to propose samples, and L2HMC takes a random combination of the forward and backward dynamics proposal as the final proposal [15]. Let θ be the vector of parameters of the above functions. After each complete cycle of proposal and acceptance, the loss function is optimized using Adam [12]. Concretely, let $\xi = (x, p)$ be the initial sample, and $\xi' = (x', p')$ be the sample after the acceptance step. Let $\delta(\xi, \xi') = \|x - x'\|_2^2$ and $A(\xi', \xi)$ denote the acceptance probability. Then the loss function $\mathcal{L}(\theta)$ used is

$$\mathcal{L}(\theta) = \mathbb{E}_{p(\xi)}\left[-\frac{\delta(\xi, \xi') A(\xi', \xi)}{\lambda^2} + \frac{\lambda^2}{\delta(\xi, \xi') A(\xi', \xi)}\right], \qquad (13)$$

where the expectation is taken over the batch of samples over which the training is taking place. λ is the typical length scale of the distribution, which Levy et al. set in the case of a multivariate normal distribution, as the smallest standard deviation in the covariance matrix. For simplicity, in Eq. 13, we omit an additional term with identical form as above [15] designed to enhance burn-in by using an arbitrary proposal distribution. Figure 1 shows a flowchart of the algorithm of sampling with the neural network parametrization.

Neural Network Enhanced HMCMC

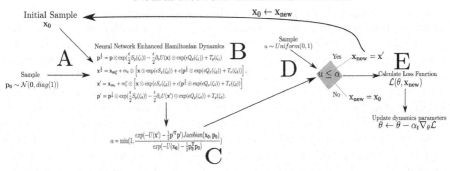

Fig. 1. Flowchart of the training algorithm for neural network parametrization of HMCMC. The components of the algorithm are very similar to standard HMCMC; however, the differences lie in the altered dynamics/proposal stage and the update of the neural network parameters after each step. When sampling, the network parameters are fixed at the last training values.

3   Methods

3.1   Neural Network Enhanced Hamiltonian MC (NNEHMC)

The first contribution of this paper is to extend L2HMC by augmenting the loss function to balance acceptance probability and the distance between samples. Let $A_{HMC}(\xi', \xi)$ denote the acceptance probability used in standard HMCMC. We introduce the loss function

$$\mathcal{L}^{NNEHMC}(\theta) = \mathbb{E}_{p(\xi)} \left[-\delta(\xi, \xi') A(\xi', \xi) - \beta A_{HMC}(\xi', \xi) \right]. \qquad (14)$$

We removed the reciprocal distance term as it did not meaningfully change the dynamics of the sampling in the distributions we considered. Further, we do not integrate the time reversed dynamics in our sampling. We argue that this form of loss function more faithfully and naturally enhances the desirable properties of Hamiltonian dynamics. In theory, Hamiltonian dynamics preserve energy along trajectories; hence, since the probability of a sample is proportional to $\exp(-H)$, the acceptance probability is always 1 [4]. However, the introduction of numerical integration causes violation of this property; nonetheless HMCMC still, generally, provides high acceptance rates, with additional tuning possible through changing ϵ or L. One can view this tuning as reducing the error of the leapfrog scheme such that the numerical integration gets closer and closer to the theoretical Hamiltonian dynamics with its property of preserving energy. However, the dynamics of L2HMC is no longer a numerical approximation of Hamiltonian dynamics due to the scaling terms. Hence, while it is valid as an MCMC sampler, there is no theoretical basis for the sampler to produce samples with high acceptance probabilities which are largely independent of the squared distance as in standard HMCMC.

As a way of both inducing the sampler to remain close to Hamiltonian dynamics and balancing the acceptance probability and mixing, we add the negative standard HMCMC acceptance probability in the loss function, with the parameter β enforcing the tradeoff between it and the negative expected squared distance. We argue that this loss function can lead to two desirable properties. First, it could lead to faster mixing and faster convergence than in L2HMC since, from the beginning, it can balance learning the standard, approximately energy preserving Hamiltonian dynamics with opportunities to move great distances. One can interpret the additional term as enforcing approximate conformity, in some sense, to Hamiltonian dynamics, mediated by β. Second, crucial for parameter estimation, we argue that this term helps to keep the sampler stable when exploring high curvature regions. In these regions, the acceptance probability can drop to zero easily due to large distance steps and numerical issues can develop [8]. The acceptance probability of the neural network parametrized sampler differs from the classical acceptance by the Jacobian of the new, scaled dynamics, which is identically 1 in the standard case. Hence, if the standard acceptance probability is the dominant term, it can still enforce high acceptance probabilities for the sampler. We thus treat the neural network as an enhancement that allows the sampler to learn "approximate" Hamiltonian dynamics which can balance and enhance the desirable properties of HMCMC while learning to minimize its weaknesses. We henceforth refer to our sampler as Neural Network Enhanced Hamiltonian MC (NNEHMC).

In the results, we compare the performance of NNEHMC and L2HMC on a toy distribution also tested in [15]. The distribution is a strongly correlated 2-D Normal distribution with mean zero, and a covariance matrix obtained from $diag(100, 0.1)$ rotated by $45°$. For both samplers, we use the same $\epsilon = 0.1, L = 10$, initialize with the same 200 samples, train in batches of 200 samples for 5000 steps, then fix the neural network parameters and sample 200 chains for 2000 steps using the trained sampler [15]. We tune β in NNEHMC by looking at the autocorrelation analysis and the acceptance probabilities. We set $\lambda = 0.1$ as is done in [15]. We compare the two samplers by the autocorrelation of the samples as well as the effective sample size derived from the autocorrelation, which can be seen as a measure of how many of the samples are "useful" for inference [4].

3.2   Biophysical Parameter Estimation

The second contribution of this paper to apply NNEHMC to biophysical parameter estimation in a recently proposed MRI model, the Multi Echo Spherical Mean Technique (MESMT) [5].

Multi Echo Spherical Mean Technique (MESMT). MRI Diffusometry and T_2 relaxometry can be combined into a multi-modal analysis which jointly estimates diffusivities, T_2's, and water volume fractions of different tissue compartments. The extended spherical mean technique (SMT) framework introduced by [5] is one example of this, generalizing the diffusion MRI model SMT [11] by including the effects of changing the echo time T_E in the acquisition on the MRI signal and using the additional information to simultaneously estimate the T_2's and diffusivities of the compartments in brain white matter. The model signal is a function of b and T_E. For given b, T_E

$$
\begin{aligned}
Model(T_E, b, \mathbf{x}) = {} & v_I \exp(\frac{-T_E}{T_2^I}) \frac{\sqrt{\pi} \operatorname{erf}(\sqrt{b\lambda_\parallel})}{2\sqrt{b\lambda_\parallel}} \\
& + v_E \exp(\frac{-T_E}{T_2^E}) \exp(-b\lambda_\perp) \frac{\sqrt{\pi} \operatorname{erf}(\sqrt{b(\lambda_\parallel - \lambda_\perp)})}{2\sqrt{b(\lambda_\parallel - \lambda_\perp)}} \\
& + v_{CSF} \exp(\frac{-T_E}{T_2^{csf}}) \exp(-bD_{csf}),
\end{aligned}
$$

where v_I, v_E, v_{CSF} are the volume fractions of the intra-axonal, extra-axonal, and cerebrospinal fluid (CSF) compartments respectively, $\lambda_\parallel, \lambda_\perp$ are the parallel and perpendicular diffusivities. The likelihood of this model is constructed as in the introduction. In the fitting, we fix the values of $T_2^{csf} = 2\,\mathrm{s}$ and $D_{csf} = 0.003\,\frac{\mathrm{mm}^2}{\mathrm{s}}$ at those of free water [11,16], but we allow v_{CSF} to be free.

Using our proposed sampler, we can bound the T_2's and diffusivities based on prior physical knowledge [11,16] so we use uniform priors as follows:
$T_2^I \sim \mathcal{U}(5\,\mathrm{ms}, 200\,\mathrm{ms})$, $T_2^E \sim \mathcal{U}(5\,\mathrm{ms}, 100\,\mathrm{ms})$, $\lambda_\parallel \sim \mathcal{U}(0.0005\,\frac{\mathrm{mm}^2}{\mathrm{s}}, 0.003\,\frac{\mathrm{mm}^2}{\mathrm{s}})$,
$\lambda_\perp \sim \mathcal{U}(0.0001\,\frac{\mathrm{mm}^2}{s}, 0.0005\,\frac{\mathrm{mm}^2}{\mathrm{s}})$.

Experimental Setup. We simulate three datasets using three different $T_E's = 50, 75, 100\,\mathrm{ms}$, with three $b = 300, 2150, 4000\,\mathrm{s/mm}^2$ values per dataset, and fit them simultaneously. The ground truth parameters are as follows: $v_I = 0.5, v_E = 0.3, v_{CSF} = 0.2, \lambda_\parallel = 0.0015\,\frac{\mathrm{mm}^2}{\mathrm{s}}, \lambda_\perp = 0.0002\,\frac{\mathrm{mm}^2}{\mathrm{s}}, T_2^I = 140\,\mathrm{ms}, T_2^E = 70\,\mathrm{ms}$. Since the volume fractions must sum to one, we use a 3D, symmetric Dirichlet prior for the volumes: $(v_I, v_E, v_{CSF}) \sim \mathbf{Dir}(1.0, 1.0, 1.0)$. We generated one hundred signals from the ground truth parameters by adding one hundred realizations of Gaussian noise with a standard deviation of $\sigma = \frac{1}{120}$. We simulated many instances of a typical diffusion acquisition using Dmipy [7] with a mean SNR of 20 on the b_0 data, then performed spherical averaging on each instance. The standard deviation of the resulting signals over the instances was estimated to be around $\frac{1}{120}$, which motivates our setting of σ. We then estimated the parameters over each signal using NUTS, L2HMC, and NNEHMC within the Bayesian framework described in Sect. 3.2. We also show a fitting using constrained least squares (LSQ). We imposed the same constraints in both the probabilistic and deterministic fittings. We initialize NUTS with a variational inference estimate [13], and use 1000 samples for burn-in and 1000 samples for inference. We initialize L2HMC and NNEHMC with the first 50 samples of the NUTS burn-in, train on batches of 50 samples for 1000 steps, then fix the parameters of the network and use the trained sampler to generate 1000 samples for inference. We set $\lambda = \sigma$, since it is roughly the length scale of the distribution. In the results, we report the relative absolute error as follows: letting g denote

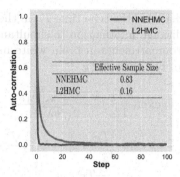

Fig. 2. Plot of the average autocorrelation of 200 chains of length 2000 for L2HMC and NNEHMC with the corresponding effective sample size. The autocorrelation and effective sample size are calculated as in [15]. We see that NNEHMC mixes faster in sampling steps and has a larger effective sample size.

the ground truth parameter and e as the estimate, the relative absolute error is computed as $|g - e|/g$. We note that we scale b by 10e$-$2 and the diffusivities by 10e2 in the sampling and results.

4   Results and Discussion

4.1   Strongly Correlated Gaussian

In Fig. 2, we show the average autocorrelation of the samples over 50 chains from sampling the strongly correlated Gaussian as a function of steps in the chain as well as a table with the effective sample sizes derived from the autocorrelation. We note that NNEHMC mixes faster and has an effective sample size almost eight times larger than that of L2HMC. Further, on the same computer, NNEHMC requires 179 s of computation time while L2HMC requires 1561 s. This is mostly because NNEHMC does not use the time reversed dynamics. In cases with tractable distributions and derivatives one can also speed up the sampling by using GPU computation [2].

4.2   Multi Echo Spherical Mean Technique (MESMT)

In Figs. 3, 4, we show the relative absolute error and an example of the marginal posterior probability distributions produced by the MCMC samplers.

We can see that, in general, the MCMC samplers are more accurate and precise than the least squares fitting. However, we see that NNEHMC and L2HMC significantly outperform NUTS in estimating volume fractions and $\lambda_\parallel$, even though they all start from the same initialization. Inspection of the probability distributions reveals that NUTS gives distributions biased away from the ground truth for these parameters. Furthermore, we note that NNEHMC generally outperforms L2HMC regarding the accuracy and variance of the estimates.

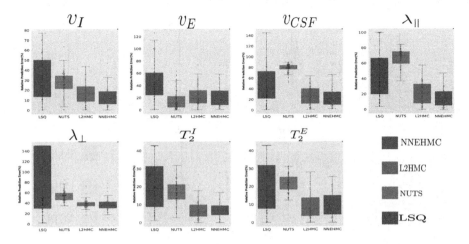

Fig. 3. Box plots of relative absolute errors from ground truth using least squares (blue), NUTS (orange), L2HMC (green), and NNEHMC (red). We note that in general, NNEHMC has the lowest mean error and variance. Further, NUTS has significant issues in the estimation of $\lambda_{\parallel}$ and the volume fractions, which is not observed in NNEHMC or L2HMC. (Color figure online)

Unlike in the toy example, where we knew the precise mean and variance of the distribution, we can only compute an approximate autocorrelation analysis in this case. We obtained an effective sample size of $1.5e-3$ for NNEHMC and $1.9e-3$ for L2HMC. However, the mean computation times for a single signal are $280\,\text{s}$ for NNEHMC and $443\,\text{s}$ for L2HMC.

Furthermore we emphasize that using L2HMC on this model is numerically unstable. By changing the random seed in our implementation, 18 out of the 100 trials with L2HMC either decline to and remain at zero acceptance probability for all chains by the end of training or encounter numerical errors (NaN, infinities). This can happen, for instance, if the proposal samples move too far away. NNEHMC was robust to such changes. We do not consider these results in the analysis since they are invalid for parameter estimation and would artificially bias the results for L2HMC negatively. In order for NUTS not to develop similar numerical issues, we had to set a desired acceptance probability of 99%. It is probable that the poor results of NUTS stem, in part, from inefficient sampling due to a highly curved parameter space which the adaptive tuning could not overcome. Thus, we can see that the parametrization with a neural network can enable efficient sampling of problematic regions in parameter space; however, regularization with an acceptance probability term is needed for stability.

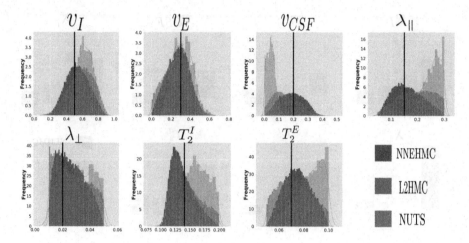

Fig. 4. Representative plots of the marginal probability distributions for each parameter, where the black vertical line denotes the ground truth value. We can see that NNEHMC provides informative posterior distributions from which inference seems justified, while NUTS provides quasi-uniform distributions and distributions biased towards the parameter bounds.

5   Conclusion

In this paper, we have proposed and tested a parametrization of Hamiltonian MCMC with a neural network (NNEHMC) which jointly optimizes sample acceptance probability and distances between successive samples in order to efficiently and stably sample probability distributions, particularly in regions of parameter space with high curvature. Such regions frequently occur in the probabilistic estimation of parameters in bio-physical models since the posterior distributions are parametrized, in part, by highly nonlinear models. We show on a recently proposed MRI model that the neural network enhancement provides parameter estimates which are more accurate and precise than those given by a least squares fitting and the state of the art NUTS and L2HMC samplers; in addition NNEHMC provides more numerically stable sampling than NUTS or L2HMC. Furthermore, we show that the neural network parametrization provides qualitatively different and more informative posterior distributions than those produced from NUTS; NNEHMC can produce posterior distributions which are Gaussian-like centered near the correct parameter values. This highlights the potential of augmenting MCMC methods with neural networks to improve probabilistic estimation of parameters in biophysical models.

Acknowledgements. Thomas Yu is supported by the European Union's Horizon 2020 program under the Marie Sklodowska-Curie project TRABIT (agreement No 765148). Marco Pizzolato is supported by the SNSF under Sinergia CRSII5_170873. This work is also supported by the Center for Biomedical Imaging (CIBM) of the

Universities of Geneva and Lausanne and the EPFL as well as the foundations of Leenaards and Louis-Jeantet.

References

1. Balakrishnan, N., Nevzorov, V.B.: A Primer on Statistical Distributions. Wiley, Hoboken (2004)
2. Beam, A.L., Ghosh, S.K., Doyle, J.: Fast Hamiltonian Monte Carlo using GPU computing. J. Comput. Graph. Stat. **25**(2), 536–548 (2016)
3. Betancourt, M.: A conceptual introduction to Hamiltonian Monte Carlo. arXiv preprint arXiv:1701.02434 (2017)
4. Brooks, S., Gelman, A., Jones, G., Meng, X.L.: Handbook of Markov Chain Monte Carlo. CRC Press, Boca Raton (2011)
5. Canales Rodriguez, E.J., et al.: Unified multi-modal characterization of microstructural parameters of brain tissue using diffusion MRI and multi-echo T2 data. In: Joint Annual Meeting ISMRM-ESMRMB (2018)
6. Duane, S., Kennedy, A.D., Pendleton, B.J., Roweth, D.: Hybrid Monte Carlo. Phys. Lett. B **195**(2), 216–222 (1987)
7. Fick, R., Wassermann, D., Deriche, R.: Mipy: an open-source framework to improve reproducibility in brain microstructure imaging. In: OHBM 2018-Human Brain Mapping, pp. 1–4 (2018)
8. Girolami, M., Calderhead, B.: Riemann manifold Langevin and Hamiltonian Monte Carlo methods. J. Roy. Stat. Soc. Ser. B (Stat. Methodol.) **73**(2), 123–214 (2011)
9. Hastings, W.K.: Monte Carlo sampling methods using Markov chains and their applications (1970)
10. Hoffman, M.D., Gelman, A.: The No-U-Turn sampler: adaptively setting path lengths in Hamiltonian Monte Carlo. J. Mach. Learn. Res. **15**(1), 1593–1623 (2014)
11. Kaden, E., Kelm, N.D., Carson, R.P., Does, M.D., Alexander, D.C.: Multicompartment microscopic diffusion imaging. NeuroImage **139**, 346–359 (2016)
12. Kingma, D.P., Ba, J.: Adam: a method for stochastic optimization. arXiv preprint arXiv:1412.6980 (2014)
13. Kucukelbir, A., Tran, D., Ranganath, R., Gelman, A., Blei, D.M.: Automatic differentiation variational inference. J. Mach. Learn. Res. **18**(1), 430–474 (2017)
14. Ledoux, M.: The Concentration of Measure Phenomenon. No. 89, American Mathematical Soc. (2001)
15. Levy, D., Hoffman, M.D., Sohl-Dickstein, J.: Generalizing Hamiltonian Monte Carlo with neural networks. arXiv preprint arXiv:1711.09268 (2017)
16. MacKay, A.L., Laule, C.: Magnetic resonance of myelin water: an in vivo marker for myelin. Brain Plast. **2**(1), 71–91 (2016)
17. Sengijpta, S.K.: Fundamentals of statistical signal processing: estimation theory (1995)

SHAMANN: Shared Memory Augmented Neural Networks

Cosmin I. Bercea[3], Olivier Pauly[4(✉)], Andreas Maier[2],
and Florin C. Ghesu[1,2(✉)]

[1] Digital Technology and Innovation, Siemens Healthineers, Erlangen, Germany
florin.ghesu@siemens-healthineers.com
[2] Pattern Recognition Lab, Friedrich-Alexander-Universität, Erlangen, Germany
[3] Robert Bosch GmbH, Corporate Research–Computer Vision, Hildesheim, Germany
[4] Google Cloud AI, Munich, Germany

Abstract. Current state-of-the-art methods for semantic segmentation use deep neural networks to learn the segmentation mask from the input image signal as an image-to-image mapping. While these methods effectively exploit global image context, the learning and computational complexities are high. We propose shared memory augmented neural network actors as a dynamically scalable alternative. Based on a decomposition of the image into a sequence of local patches, we train such actors to sequentially segment each patch. To further increase the robustness and better capture shape priors, an external memory module is shared between different actors, providing an implicit mechanism for image information exchange. Finally, the patch-wise predictions are aggregated to a complete segmentation mask. We demonstrate the benefits of the new paradigm on a challenging lung segmentation problem based on X-Ray images, as well as on two synthetic tasks based on MNIST. On the X-Ray data, our method achieves state-of-the-art accuracy with a significantly reduced model size, 3–5 times compared to reference methods. In addition, we reduce the number of failure cases by at least half.

1 Introduction

The automatic parsing of medical images represents a fundamental task that impacts the efficiency of the entire clinical workflow from diagnosis to intervention and follow-up investigations. An essential step is the semantic segmentation of anatomical structures which supports the radiologist to analyze the image content. Recent approaches, e.g., [14,25], apply fully convolutional neural networks to achieve state-of-the-art results on various segmentation problems. Usually, these methods use the entire image to directly predict the complete segmentation mask. While this allows the integration of valuable global image context, it also increases the learning complexity, requiring models to capture the entire

---

C. I. Bercea and O. Pauly—Contributed to this work during their time at Siemens Healthineers.

A. C. S. Chung et al. (Eds.): IPMI 2019, LNCS 11492, pp. 830–841, 2019.
https://doi.org/10.1007/978-3-030-20351-1_65

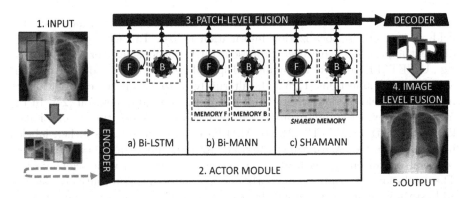

Fig. 1. Generic architecture overview with two SHAMANN actors denoted by F and B that traverse a series of local image patches sequentially in a forward, respectively backward manner and segment each patch. For completeness we also visualize two simplified alternatives, one in which the actors do not share their memory (Bi-MANN), and the other with no external memory (Bi-LSTM).

variability in the shape and appearance of objects. In addition, this strategy does not scale well to (volumetric) high resolution data due to memory limitations.

In this paper, we propose a new paradigm for semantic medical image segmentation based on a novel neural architecture called shared memory augmented neural network (SHAMANN). Based on a decomposition of the original image into a sequence of image subregions, e.g., local patches, we define different so called SHAMANN actors which traverse the sequence differently and segment each image subregion. An external memory module enables each actor to capture relations between different subregions within its sequence and increase the robustness of its predictions. In particular, this external module is shared among all actors and serves as a means to implicitly exchange local image context information in order to better capture global image properties, such as shape priors. Finally, the predictions of all actors are fused to obtain a semantic segmentation mask for the original image. See Fig. 1 for an overview.

Our contributions are: (i) SHAMANN - a memory efficient and dynamically scalabale alternative to end-to-end fully convolutional segmentation networks, that can also implicitly capture global image properties through a shared external memory module; and (ii) a comprehensive analysis of the method and comparison against state-of-the-art methods on a large chest X-Ray dataset.

2   Related Work

Segmentation. In the fields of computer vision and medical imaging, segmentation is a fundamental task for understanding the semantic content of an image. State-of-the-art results on different segmentation benchmarks have been achieved by using fully convolutional neural networks [6,15]. However, one limitation of such networks is the use of pooling layers. By down-sampling and increasing the field-of-view, precise localization information is lost. To tackle this issue, two different approaches have been proposed. First, encoder-decoder architectures, e.g., U-NET [14], recover the details and spatial dimension using de-convolutions and shortcut connections [1,25]. The alternative is to use dilated convolutions to increase the field-of-view without decreasing the spatial dimension [27]. In the medical context, a standard approach for medical segmentation is multi-atlas label propagation (MALP) [21]. In MALP, a collection of atlases, i.e., labeled images, is required. At runtime, one needs to perform expensive non-linear registration operations of each atlas to unseen data to achieve a segmentation. These solutions typically scale poorly and are inefficient. Alternatively, one can address the segmentation problem by using random forests [4], providing stronger unary predictions through joint class and shape regression. Milletari et al. [11] employed an additional patch-voting scheme to increase the robustness against outliers. Other approaches use linear shape models to incorporate prior information (SSM) [7]. In marginal space deep learning [3], SSMs have been coupled with deep learning for the segmentation of anatomical structures. While these methods provide good results and are relatively easy to train, they do not exploit global image information and are inefficient on large 3D data.

Memory Networks and Recurrent Models. Recently, neural networks have been augmented with an external memory module to decouple the memorization capacity from the network parameters, making these methods better suited for capturing long-range dependencies in sequential data. These networks have been used in the context of classification [18], meta-learning [16], reinforcement learning [13], graph problems [5] or question answering [17], to name a few. Close to our work are generative methods [12], which model the conditional probability of a pixel based on previous pixels, using long short term memory (LSTM) units [8]. In [2,22] a memory-based strategy is proposed for the task of machine translation. There, recurrent neural networks (RNN) are used to save encoded inputs in an external memory, which is then used for the final prediction. In contrast, our proposed method allows information exchange between SHAMANN actors while processing the input sequence, enabling each agent to gradually access global image context. Visin et al. [20] propose to use RNN models for semantic segmentation. We build upon their work and propose an extended framework based on the concept of shared memory networks. To the best of our knowledge, this is the first paper that proposes a method based on (shared) memory networks for the task of image segmentation.

3   Proposed Methods

In this section, we introduce the shared memory augmented neural networks (SHAMANN) architecture for semantic segmentation. In a standard bidirectional recurrent setup, information from different directions is not explicitly exchanged. We hypothesize that by sharing an external memory, we can implicitly enable this exchange and achieve an accurate segmentation.

3.1   Problem Formulation

In the following $\boldsymbol{x}$ and $\boldsymbol{x}^T$ will denote a row and column vector respectively, and $\boldsymbol{A}$ a matrix. The following formulations are focused on but not limited to 2D images. Formally, let us consider an input image $\boldsymbol{I} : \Omega \to \mathbb{R}^{H_I \times W_I \times C}$, with $\Omega \subset \mathbb{R}^2$ the image domain; H_I, W_I and C denoting the height, width and number of channels of the image signal. The goal of the segmentation task is to assign a label to every pixel/voxel $\boldsymbol{x}$ in the input image, considering a predefined set of K object classes $\{y_1, \ldots, y_K\}$. The segmentation result can be represented as a set of segmentation channels $\boldsymbol{Y} : \Omega \to \mathbb{R}^{H_I \times W_I \times K}$, where the value of a pixel (x, y) of a given channel k encodes the probability of observing the class y_k. A final segmentation mask can then be obtained by applying a softmax function along the different class-specific channels. In this work, we propose to reformulate the segmentation problem as a sequential learning task. Let us consider a sequence of T patches $P = \{\boldsymbol{P}_0, \ldots, \boldsymbol{P}_T\}$ covering the image domain, with $\boldsymbol{P}_t : \Omega \to \mathbb{R}^{H_p \times W_p \times C}$, where H_p, W_p are the height and width of the patch. For example, these patches may be extracted using uniform sampling. We propose to learn a function f that maps the sequence of input patches to a sequence of patch segmentation masks as $f(\boldsymbol{P}_t)_{t=0}^T = (\boldsymbol{\Phi}_t)_{t=0}^T$, with $f : \mathbb{R}^{T \times H_p \times W_p \times C} \to \mathbb{R}^{T \times H_p \times W_p \times K}$.

3.2   Architecture Overview

In this section, we introduce in more detail the components of our model (see Fig. 1). The encoder extracts a rich visual representation from the raw patch intensities. We model it as a function (e.g., a convolutional network), mapping the input to a d-dimensional feature space: $E(\boldsymbol{P}_t)_{t=0}^T = (\boldsymbol{\psi}_t)_{t=0}^T$, with $E : \mathbb{R}^{H_p \times W_p \times C} \to \mathbb{R}^d$. The actor module, defined as component 2, learns the sequence of input feature vectors $\Psi = \{\boldsymbol{\psi}_0, \ldots, \boldsymbol{\psi}_T\}$ and captures distal spatial dependencies. Each actor scans the input sequence Ψ differently, to produce an output sequence $H^J = \{\boldsymbol{h}_0^J, \ldots, \boldsymbol{h}_T^J\}$, with $\boldsymbol{h}^J \in \mathbb{R}^d$. Here, we use two actors, one scanning the input in the forward direction $(J := F)$, and the other in the backward direction $(J := B)$. The patch-level fusion step combines the outputs of the actors as $\sigma(H^F \oplus H^B) = H$, with $\sigma : \mathbb{R}^{2 \times d} \to \mathbb{R}^d$ and $\oplus$ the concatenation operator. The mapping σ could be a simple function, e.g., an average or a concatenation operation. In our work, we propose to explicitly learn how to combine the different outputs using a neural network with a single fully connected layer. The decoder maps the fused outputs of the actors to patch segmentation masks as $D(\boldsymbol{h}_t)_{t=0}^T = (\boldsymbol{\Phi}_t)_{t=0}^T$, with $D : \mathbb{R}^d \to \mathbb{R}^{H_p \times W_p \times K}$. In the final image-level fusion step (see component 4), all patch segmentation masks $\Phi = \{\boldsymbol{\Phi}_0, \ldots, \boldsymbol{\Phi}_T\}$ are aggregated over the full image domain to generate the final segmentation mask $\boldsymbol{Y}$. For fusion, we propose to use averaging [9].

3.3   Image Segmentation as a Sequential Learning Task

In the following, we show three different alternatives for the actor module: the bidirectional long-short term memory units (Bi-LSTM), the bidirectional

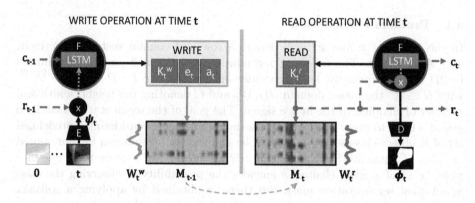

Fig. 2. Detailed illustration of a forward actor network that uses an external memory module to perform a sequential segmentation task. At the time iteration t, the actor updates its memory cell c_t using the previous memory cell c_{t-1} and the current encoded input patch ψ_t, concatenated with the previous information read from the memory r_{t-1}. The actor then writes to and reads from an external memory module and produces a segmentation mask Φ_t.

memory-augmented neural networks (Bi-MANN), and our proposed SHAMANN framework.

Bidirectional Long-Short Term Memory Networks: Bi-LSTM. One of the most common challenges in training a recurrent neural network is the vanishing gradient effect. To address this challenge, LSTM units have been proposed by [8]. These units have achieved high performance on real-world problems such as image captioning [19]. The core element of the LSTM unit is the memory cell c_t, which is an abstract representation of the previously observed input. The definition of the output h_t and c_t can be summarized as:

$$[h_t, c_t] = LSTM(\psi_t, h_{t-1}, c_{t-1}), \qquad (1)$$

where LSTM stands for the gated processing structure. The bidirectional LSTM processes the sequence data both in forward and backward directions with separate LSTM units. Thus, the forward LSTM unit will process the input sequence $\Psi^F = \{\psi_0, \ldots, \psi_T\}$ and produce the output sequence $H^F = \{h_0^F, \ldots, h_T^F\}$, while the backward LSTM cell will process the reverse input sequence $\Psi^B = \{\psi_T, \ldots, \psi_0\}$ and yield the output sequence $H^B = \{h_T^B, \ldots, h_0^B\}$. The final output of the Bi-LSTM is given by $H = \sigma(H^F \oplus H^B)$, where $\oplus$ denotes the concatenation operator.

Bidirectional Memory-Augmented Neural Networks: Bi-MANN. One limitation of Bi-LSTM is that the number of network parameters grows proportionally to the memorization capacity, making it unsuitable for sequences with long-range dependencies. These types of dependencies often occur in our formulation of the segmentation task, depending on the image content, the sequence length, and the patch size. One can alleviate this issue and increase the memorization capacity by making use of an external memory.

These networks called memory augmented neural networks (MANN) use a controller network, i.e., an LSTM, to access an external memory $M \in \mathbb{R}^{Q \times N}$, where N is the number of memory cells and Q is the dimension of each cell [5].

Following these principles, we propose to enhance each actor with an external memory capability. Figure 2 illustrates how a forward actor addresses such a memory module to perform a sequential segmentation task. At every time iteration t, the actor produces write and read heads to interact with a small portion of the memory constrained by weights associated with previous observations. The write operation uses the write weights $w_t^w \in \mathbb{R}^N$ to remove content from the memory with an erase vector $e_t \in [0,1]^Q$, then write the add vector $a_t \in \mathbb{R}^Q$: $M_t[i] \leftarrow (1 - w_t^w[i] \cdot e_t) \circ M_{t-1}[i] + w_t^w[i] \cdot a_t$, where $\circ$ and $\cdot$ denote the element-wise and scalar multiplication respectively and $1 \in \mathbb{R}^Q$ a vector of ones. Similarly, the output of a read operation using the read weights $w_t^r \in \mathbb{R}^N$ is the weighted sum over the memory locations: $r_t(M) = \sum_{i=1}^N w_t^r[i] \cdot M_t[i]$. We use content lookup to define the read weights, in which a key $k_t^r \in \mathbb{R}^Q$ emitted by the actor is compared to the content of each memory location. The attention score for a read operation at row i is the i-th value in the column vector $w_t^r = exp(F(k_t^r, M_t[i]))/\sum_{j=1}^N exp(F(k_t^r, M_t[j]))$, where F computes the similarity between two vectors, i.e., cosine similarity, and $[]$ is the row operator. The content lookup weights $\hat{w}_t^w \in \mathbb{R}^N$ allow the write operation to update content in the memory. In order to also allocate new memory slots, we extend the addressing with a mechanism that returns the most unused location $\tilde{w}_t^w \in \{0,1\}^N$ (as a one hot vector). At every iteration the write operation uses an allocation gate α to either update the content of a location, or write to a new, unused location: $w_t^w = \alpha \hat{w}_t^w + (1 - \alpha)\tilde{w}_t^w$. The read and write keys, erase and add vectors and the allocation gate are linear mappings of the memory cell of an actor.

We extend MANNs to a bidirectional formulation, where two actors, each with its individual external memory module, scan the input sequence in a forward $(J := F)$ and backward $(J := B)$ manner and produce the output and memory cell a time t as:

$$[g_t^J, c_t^J] = LSTM(\psi_t \oplus r_{t-1}(M^J), g_{t-1}^J, c_{t-1}^J), \tag{2}$$

where $g_t^J = W_g^J(h_t^J \oplus r_t(M^J)) + b_g^J$ are linear mappings of the concatenation of the output vectors and the currently read information from the memory module. The final output is: $H = \sigma(\{g_0^F, g_1^F, \ldots, g_T^F\} \oplus \{g_T^B, g_{T-1}^B, \ldots, g_0^B\})$.

Shared Memory-Augmented Neural Networks: SHAMANN. While the external memory module addresses the limited memorization capability of standard Bi-LSTM units, the sequence processing by the different actors remains suboptimal - in the sense that there is no active exchange of context information between them. The hypothesis is that through such an exchange, individual actors can observe more global context, leading to a more robust segmentation.

With this in mind, we propose to share the external memory module between actors. By reading and writing information to the same memory module, the

actors can interact in an implicit way. The output and memory cell for a time
iteration t are defined as follows:

$$[g_t^J, c_t^J] = LSTM(\psi_t \oplus r_{t-1}(M), g_{t-1}^J, c_{t-1}^J), \tag{3}$$

where $g_t^J = W_g^J(h_t^J \oplus r_t(M)) + b_g^J$ are linear mappings of the concatenation
of the output vectors and the current read information from the shared memory module. Note that the matrix M in Eq. 3 represents the memory module, which is shared by both the forward and backward actors. In contrast, in
Eq. 2, M^F and M^B denote different memory modules. The two actors write
and read alternatively from the memory, first the forward actor, then the backward actor. To ensure the correct allocation of free memory, the two actors
also share the usage vector. The final output of the SHAMANN framework is:
$H = \sigma(\{g_0^F, g_1^F, \ldots, g_T^F\} \oplus \{g_T^B, g_{T-1}^B, \ldots, g_0^B\})$. Our network is fully differentiable and can be trained end-to-end via back-propagation through time [24].

4   Experiments

We benchmarked our method on a large chest X-Ray dataset and compared it to
state-of-the-art deep learning methods [14,26]. Additionally, we conducted two
synthetic experiments on MNIST [10] with the goal of analyzing the memorization capacity of the different models and providing insights into the benefits of
sharing an external memory module.

4.1   Chest X-Ray Lung Segmentation

This is a fundamental preprocessing task towards automated diagnosis of lung
diseases [23]. The main challenges are the variability in shape and intensities of
the lungs, as well as reduced anatomy contrast. The chest X-Ray dataset consists
of 7083 images of 7083 patients from the public database ChestX-Ray8 [23], each
of size 1024×1024 pixels. Segmentation masks were provided by clinical experts.
We performed a random patient-based split into 5000 training, 583 validation
and 1500 test images. The patch size was set to 160×160 pixels with a stride
of 80×80, resulting in a sequence of 169 patches per image.

Table 1. Quantitative results.

Method	Dice (mean ± STD)	#params (millions)	High-res data	#failures
SHAMANN	**96.97 ± 1.36**	**6.2**	**Flexible**	**5**
U-NET [14]	96.92 ± 1.34	20.1	Memory limited	10
DRN(c26) [26]	96.95 ± 1.67	20.6	Memory limited	10
DRN(c42) [26]	96.78 ± 1.52	30.7	Memory limited	12

Table 1 shows quantitative results. We compute the dice score using the definition of true positive (TP), false positive (FP) and false negative (FN) as:

INPUT + LABEL	U-NET	DRN c26	DRN c42	SHAMANN

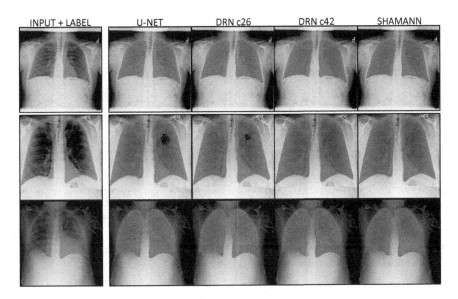

Fig. 3. Qualitative results. From left to right: input image with label, segmentation masks using the U-NET architecture [14], the DRN (c26 and c42) architectures [26] and SHAMANN. The last rows show the effectiveness of the SHAMANN method in capturing the global context. The groundtruth mask in shown in magenta, the prediction in turquoise and their overlap in blue. (Colour figure online)

$(2*TP)/(2*TP+FP+FN)$. The experiment demonstrates that, even though we use sequences of local patches, our algorithm reaches state-of-the-art performance – effectively capturing the global context through the shared memory. In particular, our model requires significantly less parameters in comparison to the reference methods. The combination of these two elements allows in theory a more (memory) efficient application to high-resolution (volumetric) data without the loss of global image context. Furthermore, in our formulation one can dynamically split the sequence length (both at training and testing time) and maintain global context in the shared memory to achieve an even higher degree of flexibility. We are investigating these benefits on large 3D/4D medical scans.

An additional important property of our method is the robustness on difficult cases, caused by, e.g., large scale variations between children and adults, different image artifacts and abnormalities, such as pleural effusion or large lesions. We manage to reduce the number of cases with large error, i.e., a dice score below 0.9, by at least half. Figure 3 shows qualitative results.

4.2   MNIST Image Completion: Memory Analysis

To investigate the benefits of extending neural networks with an external memory, we designed two synthetic tasks based on the MNIST dataset. First, we deleted the bottom half of the input images and trained our models to complete

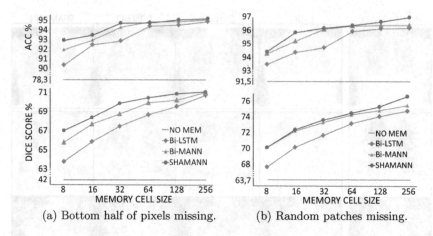

(a) Bottom half of pixels missing.   (b) Random patches missing.

Fig. 4. MNIST quantitative results. SHAMANN performs best both in terms of dice and classification accuracy for different cell state sizes.

the missing information. The goal of this experiment was to observe the networks' capacity to extrapolate the missing data based only on the first half of the image. In a second experiment, we removed random patches from the input images. Since in this case the location of the missing data is not deterministic, the networks have to adaptively learn a more complex strategy for the memorization and lookup of information to better extrapolate the missing data. For both experiments we used the original MNIST images as labels. The MNIST data consist of 70000 pictures of handwritten digits (55000 train, 5000 validation and 10000 test) and their associated label. We considered patches of size 8 × 8 with a stride of 4 × 4 resulting in a sequence of 49 patches per image.

For the quantitative evaluation we measured dice scores, as well as classification accuracy on the reconstructed digits. To measure the classification accuracy we trained a deep neural network classifier on the original MNIST dataset and used this network to evaluate the images reconstructed by our methods. The accuracy of this classifier on the original MNIST dataset was **99.23%**. On the altered test sets, without applying any completion, the accuracy was **56.14%** for the first and **67.8%** for the second experiment.

Figure 4 shows quantitative results. Using SHAMANN to perform image completion on the altered data, the classification accuracy was increased to **95.2%** for the first, and **96.9%** for the second experiment. In both experiments the networks augmented with memory outperform the Bi-LSTM network and especially the model without memory (called NO MEM). This demonstrates that more effective image completion strategies can be learned with the use of an external memory module, reaching best performance when the memory is shared. Note that as the capacity of the Bi-LSTM units increases, the difference in reconstruction performance to both Bi-MANN and SHAMANN reduces. As expected, given a large enough cell size, LSTM units can emulate the high memorization capacity of an external memory. In contrast, for the second experiment the differences

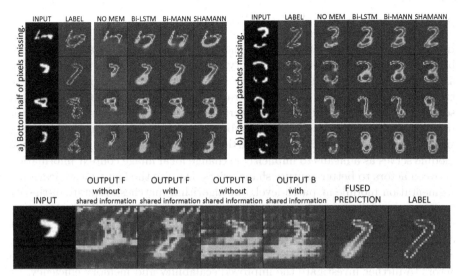

(c) Insights in the shared memory.

Fig. 5. Figures a and b show qualitative results. From left to right: altered input image, label, reconstructed images using actors with no memory, actors with internal memory, actors with individual external memory, and actors that share the memory module. Figure c illustrates the benefits of information exchange.

Table 2. Hyperparameters for both experiments.

	Encoder/decoder			Actor		Ext. memory	
	#layers	Shortcuts	#filters	Mem. cell	#read heads	N	Q
X-Ray	5	Yes	$\{8, 16, \ldots, 256\}$	128	32	400	128
MNIST	3	No	$\{16, 16, 16\}$	8-256	8	100	8-256

between the methods is considerably large, even at the largest cell size level. This indicates that for more complex problems the performance of the Bi-LSTM is limited, even for larger cell sizes.

Figures 5a and b show qualitative results. Different from SHAMANN, on these examples the other methods fail to extrapolate correctly the missing parts of the digits. The last row shows a failure case for all methods. However, considering the high difficulty in reconstructing these digits, one can argue that the output of the SHAMANN method is reasonable. Figure 5c shows the benefits of sharing the memory module, by comparing the prediction of individual actors with and without the information exchange via the shared memory.

Table 2 shows the system hyperparameters that were determined using a grid search strategy. For training we used the RMSProp optimizer with a learning rate of 10^{-3} and minimized the mean squared error on all experiments.

5   Conclusion and Future Work

In this paper, we presented a novel memory efficient segmentation approach based on sequence learning and memory augmented neural networks. Based on a decomposition of the original image into a sequence of image patches, we trained two SHAMANN actors that traverse the sequence bidirectionally and segment each image subregion. An external memory module enables each actor to capture relations between different subregions within its sequence and increase the robustness of its predictions. In particular, the shared nature of the external module serves as a means to implicitly exchange local image context information between actors to better capture shape priors. Despite the fact that we learn the segmentation module at patch-level, our algorithm matches the state-of-the-art performance of image-to-image architectures on a challenging lung segmentation task based on a X-Ray dataset. A detailed analysis on the MNIST dataset demonstrates the benefits of the shared external memory. In our future work, we plan to extend our model to large 3D/4D medical scans and more than two actors to further investigate the improved scalability and memory efficiency.

References

1. Badrinarayanan, V., Kendall, A., Cipolla, R.: SegNet: a deep convolutional encoder-decoder architecture for image segmentation. IEEE Trans. Pattern Anal. Mach. Intell. **39**, 2481–2495 (2017)
2. Bahdanau, D., Cho, K., Bengio, Y.: Neural machine translation by jointly learning to align and translate. CoRR abs/1409.0473 (2014)
3. Ghesu, F.C., et al.: Marginal space deep learning: efficient architecture for volumetric image parsing. IEEE Trans. Med. Imaging **35**(5), 1217–1228 (2016)
4. Glocker, B., Pauly, O., Konukoglu, E., Criminisi, A.: Joint classification-regression forests for spatially structured multi-object segmentation. In: Fitzgibbon, A., Lazebnik, S., Perona, P., Sato, Y., Schmid, C. (eds.) ECCV 2012. LNCS, vol. 7575, pp. 870–881. Springer, Heidelberg (2012). https://doi.org/10.1007/978-3-642-33765-9_62
5. Graves, A., et al.: Hybrid computing using a neural network with dynamic external memory. Nature **538**(7626), 471–476 (2016)
6. He, K., Gkioxari, G., Dollár, P., Girshick, R.B.: Mask R-CNN. In: Proceedings of the International Conference on Computer Vision, pp. 2980–2988. IEEE (2017)
7. Heimann, T., Meinzer, H.P.: Statistical shape models for 3D medical image segmentation: a review. Med. Image Anal. **13**(4), 543–563 (2009)
8. Hochreiter, S., Schmidhuber, J.: Long short-term memory. Neural Comput. **9**(8), 1735–1780 (1997)
9. Iglesias, J.E., Sabuncu, M.R.: Multi-atlas segmentation of biomedical images: a survey. Med. Image Anal. **24**(1), 205–219 (2015)
10. Lecun, Y., Bottou, L., Bengio, Y., Haffner, P.: Gradient-based learning applied to document recognition. Proc. IEEE **86**(11), 2278–2324 (1998)
11. Milletari, F., et al.: Hough-CNN: deep learning for segmentation of deep brain regions in MRI and ultrasound. Comput. Vis. Image Underst. **164**, 92–102 (2017)
12. van den Oord, A., Kalchbrenner, N., Kavukcuoglu, K.: Pixel recurrent neural networks. In: Proceedings of the International Conference on Machine Learning, vol. 48, pp. 1747–1756 (2016)

13. Pritzel, A., et al.: Neural episodic control. In: Proceedings of the International Conference on Machine Learning, vol. 70, pp. 2827–2836 (2017)
14. Ronneberger, O., Fischer, P., Brox, T.: U-Net: convolutional networks for biomedical image segmentation. In: Navab, N., Hornegger, J., Wells, W.M., Frangi, A.F. (eds.) MICCAI 2015. LNCS, vol. 9351, pp. 234–241. Springer, Cham (2015). https://doi.org/10.1007/978-3-319-24574-4_28
15. Shelhamer, E., Long, J., Darrell, T.: Fully convolutional networks for semantic segmentation. IEEE Trans. Pattern Anal. Mach. Intell. **39**(4), 640–651 (2017)
16. Sprechmann, P., et al.: Memory-based parameter adaptation. In: International Conference on Learning Representations (2018)
17. Sukhbaatar, S., Weston, J., Fergus, R.: End-to-end memory networks. In: Advances in Neural Information Processing Systems, pp. 2440–2448. Curran Associates, Inc. (2015)
18. Vinyals, O., Blundell, C., Lillicrap, T., Kavukcuoglu, K., Wierstra, D.: Matching networks for one shot learning. In: Advances in Neural Information Processing Systems, pp. 3630–3638. Curran Associates, Inc. (2016)
19. Vinyals, O., Toshev, A., Bengio, S., Erhan, D.: Show and tell: a neural image caption generator. In: Proceedings of the IEEE Conference on Computer Vision and Pattern Recognition, pp. 3156–3164 (2015)
20. Visin, F., et al.: ReSeg: a recurrent neural network-based model for semantic segmentation. In: IEEE Conference on Computer Vision and Pattern Recognition Workshops, pp. 426–433 (2016)
21. Wang, H., Suh, J.W., Das, S.R., Pluta, J., Craige, C., Yushkevich, P.A.: Multi-atlas segmentation with joint label fusion. IEEE Trans. Pattern Anal. Mach. Intell. **35**(3), 611–623 (2013)
22. Wang, M., Lu, Z., Li, H., Liu, Q.: Memory-enhanced decoder for neural machine translation. In: Empirical Methods in Natural Language Processing (2016)
23. Wang, X., Peng, Y., Lu, L., Lu, Z., Bagheri, M., Summers, R.M.: ChestX-Ray8: hospital-scale chest X-Ray database and benchmarks on weakly-supervised classification and localization of common thorax diseases. In: IEEE Conference on Computer Vision and Pattern Recognition, pp. 3462–3471 (2017)
24. Werbos, P.J.: Backpropagation through time: what it does and how to do it. Proc. IEEE **78**(10), 1550–1560 (1990)
25. Yang, D., et al.: Automatic liver segmentation using an adversarial image-to-image network. In: Descoteaux, M., Maier-Hein, L., Franz, A., Jannin, P., Collins, D.L., Duchesne, S. (eds.) MICCAI 2017. LNCS, vol. 10435, pp. 507–515. Springer, Cham (2017). https://doi.org/10.1007/978-3-319-66179-7_58
26. Yu, F., Koltun, V., Funkhouser, T.A.: Dilated residual networks. In: IEEE Conference on Computer Vision and Pattern Recognition, pp. 636–644 (2017)
27. Zhao, H., Shi, J., Qi, X., Wang, X., Jia, J.: Pyramid scene parsing network. In: IEEE Conference on Computer Vision and Pattern Recognition, pp. 6230–6239 (2017)

Signet Ring Cell Detection with a Semi-supervised Learning Framework

Jiahui Li[1], Shuang Yang[1], Xiaodi Huang[1], Qian Da[2], Xiaoqun Yang[2], Zhiqiang Hu[1], Qi Duan[1], Chaofu Wang[2], and Hongsheng Li[3(✉)]

[1] SenseTime Research, Beijing, China
{lijiahui,yangshuang1,huangxiaodi,huzhiqiang,duanqi}@sensetime.com
[2] Ruijin Hospital, Shanghai Jiao Tong University School of Medicine, Shanghai, China
{dq11848,yxq11964,wcf11956}@rjh.com.cn
[3] Chinese University of Hong Kong, Shatin, Hong Kong
hsli@ee.cuhk.edu.hk

Abstract. Signet ring cell carcinoma is a type of rare adenocarcinoma with poor prognosis. Early detection leads to huge improvement of patients' survival rate. However, pathologists can only visually detect signet ring cells under the microscope. This procedure is not only laborious but also prone to omission. An automatic and accurate signet ring cell detection solution is thus important but has not been investigated before. In this paper, we take the first step to present a semi-supervised learning framework for the signet ring cell detection problem. Self-training is proposed to deal with the challenge of incomplete annotations, and cooperative-training is adapted to explore the unlabeled regions. Combining the two techniques, our semi-supervised learning framework can make better use of both labeled and unlabeled data. Experiments on large real clinical data demonstrate the effectiveness of our design. Our framework achieves accurate signet ring cell detection and can be readily applied in the clinical trails. The dataset will be released soon to facilitate the development of the area.

Keywords: Signet ring cell detection · Signet ring cell benchmark · Semi-supervised learning

1 Introduction

Signet ring cell carcinoma (SRCC) is an adenocarcinoma with a high degree of malignancy. SRCC is mostly found in stomach but could also spread to ovaries, lungs, breast, and other organs. The prognosis of SRCC is so poor that early detection leads to huge improvement of patients' survival rate. However, pathologists could only visually detect signet ring cells under the microscope, and/or

Electronic supplementary material The online version of this chapter (https://doi.org/10.1007/978-3-030-20351-1_66) contains supplementary material, which is available to authorized users.

confirm by immunohistochemistry. Manual detection is laborious and prone to omission, especially for scattered signet ring cells, while immunohistochemistry, which uses enzymes or other specific molecular markers to image antigens (protein) in abnormal cells, is expensive. After discussion with experienced pathologists and exploration of related medical background, we find that accurate cell edges have potential research value, such as the calculation of karyoplasmic ratio and the classification of degree of atypia. Therefore, an automatic and accurate signet ring cell detection solution is important and highly demanded.

The unique appearance of the signet ring cells makes them completely different from other types of cells, characterized by a central optically clear, globoid droplet of cytoplasmic mucin with an eccentrically placed nucleus [2]. To our best knowledge automatic signet ring cell detection has not been investigated before. In this paper, we take the first step to propose a signet ring cell detection framework based on semi-supervised learning. We firstly collect and annotate a large real clinical signet ring cell dataset. We collect 127 (21 positive + 106 negative) Hematoxylin and Eosin (H&E) stained Whole Slide Images (WSIs) from 10 organs, including gallbladder, gastric mucosa, lymph, breast, ovary, pancreas, lung, urinary bladder, abdominal wall nodule and intestine. We select at least 3 regions of over $2,000 \times 2,000$ pixels from each positive/negative WSI, and annotate signet ring cell instances within the positive regions, in the form of the tight bounding box. A total of 12,381 signet ring cells are annotated. However, overcrowded cells make it impossible to reach complete annotation, not to mention the occlusion and appearance variation, as shown in Fig. 1. As a result, pathologists can only guarantee that annotated cells are indeed signet ring cells; The opposite, that unannotated cells are not SRCC, is not necessarily true. The dataset will be released soon to facilitate the development of the area.

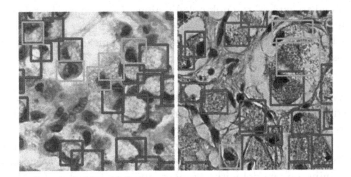

Fig. 1. Signet ring cells are overcrowded and of various appearances. Cells in green rectangles are signet ring cells, which are the indicator of signet ring cell carcinoma. Cells in yellow rectangles are also signet ring cells but are missed by pathologists in crowd regions, during long time tedious annotation. (Color figure online)

We propose a self-training method to deal with the challenge of incomplete annotations. We observe that some suspected areas predicted by the detector

844   J. Li et al.

with high probabilities, are more likely to be real signet ring cells missed by pathologists during annotation. As a result, we combine those highly suspected areas with annotations to refine the labels, and take the refined labels to retrain the detector. The self-training strategy can be applied iteratively, with the labels further refined by the new highly suspected areas.

On the other hand, we propose a cooperative-training method to explore the unlabeled regions. As mentioned above, we select 3 regions of over $2,000 \times 2,000$ pixels from each positive WSI for annotations. In comparison, a single WSI has over $100,000 \times 100,000$ pixels in total, i.e., we only annotate a tiny fraction of the whole WSI. To make better use of the whole WSI, we select over 1,000 unlabeled regions from the positive WSIs, apply the inference process of two detectors with different backbones, take each others' highly suspected areas as labels and retrain the detectors with the augmented dataset. Two detectors are needed because detectors are prone to get stuck in their local minimum to general erroneous predictions for totally unlabeled regions and a cooperative way may help alleviate the situation. Similar to the self-training, cooperative-training strategy can also operate iteratively and two detectors benefits from each other in multiple rounds.

We perform extensive experiments on the collected dataset, and the results demonstrate the effectiveness of our design, where both the self-training and cooperative-training strategy deliver a significant and consistent improvement over the baseline. Our semi-supervised learning framework achieves accurate signet ring cell detection and can be readily applied in clinical trails.

Our contributions are summarized as follows: we take the first step to investigate the signet ring cell detection problem and present a semi-supervised learning framework to tackle the problem. The self-training strategy is proposed to deal with the challenge of incomplete annotations, and the cooperative-training strategy is proposed to explore the unlabeled regions. Combining the two techniques, the semi-supervised learning framework can make better use of both labeled and unlabeled data. Experiments on large real clinical data demonstrate the effectiveness of our design.

Related Work. Several semi-supervised learning methods have been proposed and verified their effectiveness on natural images [7–11,19]. Papandreou et al. [10] used box-level annotation to achieve similar performance with pixel-level annotation. Zhou et al. Luo et al. [9] organized a reconstruction head to convert segmentation output back to original images. Generally, all the previous methods focus on training one model with complex auxiliary branches. On the contrary, our semi-supervised learning framework can organize the multiple models to support each other and no extra auxiliary branch is needed. There have been lots of automatic methods for pathology, including nuclei segmentation [16–18] and specific object [3]. However, automatic signet ring cell detection has not been investigated before to our best knowledge.

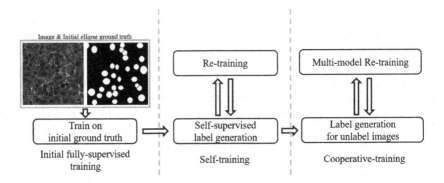

Fig. 2. Overview of our semi-supervised framework: initial fully-supervised training, self-training, and cooperative-training.

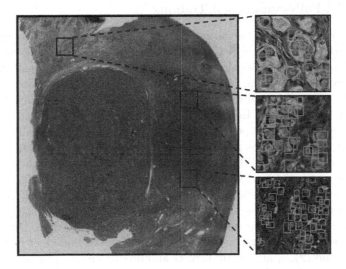

Fig. 3. 3 regions of over $2,000 \times 2,000$ pixels are randomly cropped from each WSI and bounding boxes for high confident independent signet ring cells are annotated.

2   Semi-supervised Learning Framework

As shown in Fig. 2, our semi-supervised learning framework consists of three steps: initial fully-supervised training, self-training and cooperative-training.

2.1   Dataset

Our dataset is collected from several highly ranked hospitals, and consists of H&E stained images captured at 40× magnification. Containing 127 (21 positive + 106 negative) whole slide images (WSIs), this dataset covers a large number of patients and images from 10 organs, including gallbladder, gastric mucosa, lymph, breast, ovary, pancreas, lung, urinary bladder, abdominal wall nodule and intestine. For each WSI, pathologists carefully annotate each independent signet ring cell by tight bounding box in at least 3 regions of over $2,000 \times 2,000$ pixels, as shown in Fig. 3. For each region one pathologist provide annotation verified by one senior pathology. Thus each labeled cells are indeed signet ring cells. A total of 74 regions are annotated for 21 tumor WSIs. Bounding box is a convenient way to conduct annotations for thousands of cells, which saves time and offers instance analysis such as cell counting. We also randomly crop 320 regions of the same size from the other 106 negative WSIs, which are either healthy or infected by other types of cancer. As a result, we collect 74 annotated positive regions from 21 positive WSIs of 10 organs and 320 negative regions from 106 negative WSIs, with a total of 12, 381 signet ring cells annotated.

2.2   Initial Fully-Supervised Training

Firstly we will introduce the initial fully-supervised training with the original ground truth annotations, which is the first stage of our signet ring cell detector (SRCDetecor). This also serves as the baseline of our proposed semi-supervised learning framework. Unlike other common RCNN-based detection frameworks [12,13], We propose a bottom-up method to directly predict cell instance mask, then derive boxes for each instance, as shown in Fig. 4, our proposed SRCDetector adopts a UNet [14] to perform 3-class segmentation, i.e., classifying images into background, cell edges, and cell inner regions. Then use Random Walker [5] to transform the obtained 3-class mask to cell instance mask, where cell inner regions are seeds and cell edges are undetermined regions. Finally we extract bounding box of each instance as final box prediction. To train the UNet, we first extract the inscribed ellipse of each annotated bounding box and take the inner region/edge of the ellipse as ground truth inner regions and edges. Our loss function is the summation of cross entropy loss and Intersection-Over-Union (IOU) loss. In (1) and (2), y_i and p_i are targets and predictions for pixel i respectively. E is the edge of the cell and IR is the inner region of the cell.

$$l_{\mathrm{CE}} = \sum_{S \in \{\mathrm{E},\mathrm{IR}\}} \sum_{i \in S} y_i \log(p_i) + (1 - y_i) \log(1 - p_i) \tag{1}$$

$$l_{\mathrm{IOU}} = \sum_{S \in \{\mathrm{E},\mathrm{IR}\}} 1 - \frac{\sum_{i \in S} y_i p_i}{\sum_{i \in S} y_i + \sum_{i \in S} p_i - \sum_{i \in S} y_i p_i} \tag{2}$$

$$l = l_{\mathrm{CE}} + l_{\mathrm{IOU}} \tag{3}$$

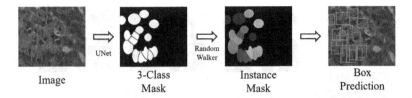

Fig. 4. Signet ring cell detector: image → 3-class mask → cell instance mask → cell box prediction.

2.3 Self-training

After training with ellipse mask obtained from the original annotation boxes, our proposed SRCDetector would generate some suspected positive areas in the training images. It is impossible to ask pathologists to annotate all the signet ring cell for overcrowdness and appearance variation. Confirmed by senior pathologists, those suspected positive areas with high confidence are indeed signet ring cells for most cases, and could be combined with the initial ellipses mask to create the refined labels for retraining the 3-class segmentation task again. As shown in Fig. 5, the pipeline of self-training is an iterative process, whose main step is to use the previously trained model to generate new ground truth and refine cell edges to train next model. The 3-class mask merges with annotations by following steps: 1, use the union inner region of the prediction of the current round and the inscribed ellipse of the initial ground truth as the inner region mask. 2, use the union edge of the prediction cell in the current round and the inscribed ellipse of the initial ground truth as the next edge, overwrite pixels which are regarded as inner region in step 1. 3, use the rest pixels as cell background. These steps could be repeated for several times, until a well-annotated pixel-wise mask

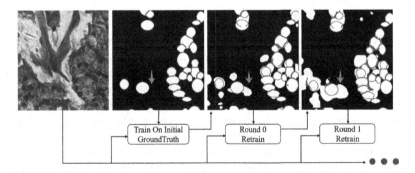

Fig. 5. Pipeline of our self-training strategy to self-correct imperfectly annotated images. The next-round model is trained on annotations from the previous round, and iteratively adjusts annotations towards higher quality. Initially we draw inscribed ellipse in each rectangle as ground truth inner region. The gray regions are edge mask and the white regions are the inner regions. The green arrow points to a growing correct prediction. (Color figure online)

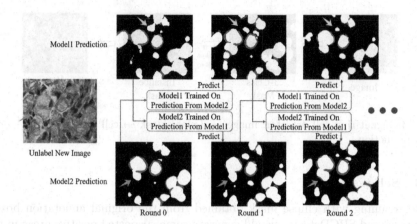

Fig. 6. Pipeline of the cooperative-training strategy. For new unlabeled images, each model is trained on predictions from the other model, so that we can reduce the possibility that one model get stuck in its local minimum, and allow the two models to support each others. In this way we will gradually obtain higher annotation quality on unlabeled images without any manual interventions. The yellow arrow points to a wrong prediction that gradually shrinks. The green arrow points to a growing correct prediction. (Color figure online)

is generated, and should be stopped if the newly predicted mask stops to grow. Generally speaking, the self-training strategy gradually generates more annotations, which are mostly missed by junior pathologists and can improve the quality of annotations by the iterative refinement. However, 74 annotated images are not enough to train a robust model, we turn to generate more available labels in unknown areas with cooperative-training strategy.

2.4 Cooperative-Training

As each WSI is an image with ultra high resolution of over $100,000 \times 100,000$ pixels at 40× magnification, in which only 3 randomly selected regions of over $2,000 \times 2,000$ pixels are manually labeled. The rest regions are also expected to contain possible positives that may provide additional training samples for our SRCDetector. The self-training strategy has an obvious drawback that it might get stuck in local minimum to general erroneous predictions. To alleviate this problem, we use two SRCDetectors with different backbones, and train with generated labels from each other to reduce self amplify errors. Firstly we use the self-training strategy to train two models with different backbones, and do inference on unlabeled images. Secondly each model is trained with generated labels from the other model's predictions from the previous model. Again in the next round, two models do inference on unlabeled images and retrain on each others' predictions. Annotated images are mixed with unlabeled images to train during Cooperative-Training. As shown in Fig. 6, two models are organized to support each other in an interative way: next-round model is trained with predictions from the other model in the previous round, and stop until no more significant changes in unlabeled images.

Models for cooperative-training shall be able to provide complementary information for each other. We achieve this by using two models with different structures and different training data for two models. In this problem, two models are trained on same images but different annotations predicted from each other, which can be regarded as different training data.

3   Experiment

3.1   Evaluation

As mentioned above, this is an imperfect annotated dataset and we can only guarantee that the labeled cells are confidently true. Hence for detection evaluation [4], recall is still reasonable to measure while precision becomes meaningless. Due to the incomplete annotations, we add three criteria for evaluation. Firstly, instead of precision, normal region false positives (FPs) is taken into consideration, which means the average number of wrong prediction boxes, which are definitely false positives, in negative images. Secondly, in order to comprehensively consider recall and normal region false positives, we define the FROC [1]: By adjusting confidence threshold, when the number of normal region false positives is 1, 2, 4, 8, 16, 32, the FROC is the average of relevant recall at those confidence threshold. Thirdly, besides the common instance-level recall, we propose another criteria called collective-level recall, which means we draw a big mask with the union of all the prediction boxes, then if any annotation box's intersection area divided by this box's area is larger than some threshold, we regard this box as being detected. Collective-level recall is an instance unawareness criteria and is the upper bound of instance-level recall. Comparing the performance difference between instance-level recall and collective-level recall, we can learn whether model performs poorly at SRC region separation or SRC detection. For FROC, we only consider instance-level FROC. In conclusion, four criteria shall be considered: collective-level recall, instance-level recall, normal region false positives, instance-level FROC.

For pathological images, we can get images under same distribution by cropping out different regions from the same WSI. However, images from different WSIs and organs differ from each other substantially. The total available images are limited, thus cross validation shall be performed under an easy mode and a hard mode. In the easy mode, we can assume that test data and train data are of the same distribution, because images from a same WSI are assigned randomly to different folds, allowing models to see similar images both in train and test data. This man-made distribution makes it possible for us to understand what the best performance will be if our dataset is big enough. In hard mode, images in different folds come from different WSIs and organs. Because signet ring cell can appear in other kinds of organs, which may not be collected in our dataset. The hard mode can help us evaluate model's capability when dealing with unknown organs.

3.2   Implementation Details

The SRCDetector is implemented with PyTorch 0.4, using the Adam optimizer and 0.001 as learning rate. During training, we randomly crop images of size 512×512 pixels with the batch size of 16 as input, and use sliding windows of size $1,024 \times 1,024$ pixels during inference. For cooperative-training we use UNet with two different backbones: ResNet [6] and Deep Layer Aggregation (DLA) [15]. We use 34-layer models for both backbones. Our SRCDetector is trained with original ground truth by 50 epochs and then in iterating self-training with extra annotations for 10 epochs in each round. Taking probability larger than 0.7 to identify new positive regions, the self-training stops at round 5 in our experiments. Similarly, the two models in cooperative-training are trained on annotation from the self-training for 50 epochs and for 10 epochs in each round, takes probability larger than 0.33 to identify new positive regions and stops at round 2. The entire procedure requires 8 h for fully supervised training, 30 h of 5 rounds for self-training and 24 h of 2 rounds for cooperative-training. We only use 2 models for cooperative-training because we observe there is no obvious benefit if 3 or more models are utilized, which do not increase the final accuracy, and also decrease the computational efficiency. During inference, DLA is utilized which usually performs 2% better than Resnet. Models from round 5 self-training and round 2 cooperative-training is used to conduct inference on test data. In all training procedures, positive or negative images are duplicated for several times to achieve data balance. In our experiments, three kinds of SRCDetector are compared both in easy and hard modes, with the same structures and different training data as shown below:

Fully-supervised training. Train on 74 images + initial ellipse annotations, and 320 negative images.

Self-training. Train on 74 images + fixed annotations from self-training, and 320 negative images.

Self-training-extra. Train on 74 images + fixed annotations from self-training, 1236 unlabeled images + generated annotations from self-training, and 320 negative images.

Cooperative-training. Train on 74 images + fixed annotations from self-training, 1236 unlabeled images + generated annotations from cooperative-training, and 320 negative images.

During evaluation, both in the easy and hard mode, only 74 images' initial manual annotations are considered for recall evaluation. To calculate collective-level recall, instance-level recall, normal region false positives and instance-level FROC, we perform 3-folds cross-validation to fully evaluate SRCDetector on 74 positive and 320 negative images. Predict and groundtruth boxes are match if their IOU is greater than 0.3.

3.3   Results and Discussion

As shown in Table 1, compared with fully-supervised training on initial ground truth, which is the baseline, both two steps of our semi-supervised learning framework introduce obvious improvements.

Table 1. Cross validation performance comparison under different modes and data utilities. Col Recall, Ins Recall, Nor FPs and Ins FROC are short for collective-level recall, instance-level recall, normal region false positives and instance-level FROC, while FT, ST, ST-Ex and CT are short for fully-supervised training, self-training, self-training-extra and cooperative-training, respectively.

Criteria	Easy mode				Hard mode			
	FT	ST	ST-Ex	CT	FT	ST	ST-Ex	CT
Col Recall	0.626	0.869	0.841	0.881	0.497	0.693	0.670	0.827
Ins Recall	0.462	0.673	0.638	0.705	0.325	0.521	0.505	0.658
Nor FPs	0.446	2.29	5.22	1.45	0.202	1.18	4.62	0.943
Ins FROC	0.462	0.617	0.562	**0.692**	0.325	0.517	0.451	**0.657**

According to the comparison between baseline and self-training, the major contribution of self-training is to improve the absolute performance: 0.16 improvement on instance-level FROC in the easy mode and 0.18 improvement on instance-level FROC in the hard mode. During training on initial ground truth, we find that in train data, models focus much on suspected areas which are indeed signet ring cells that are not annotated. These areas are treated as negative samples in training phase, such false negatives are harmful for training the detector. After visually confirmed by senior pathologists, most conflicts between prediction and ground truth come from unlabeled signet ring cells. Self-training could suppress the ratio of noisy annotations to provide annotations of higher quality.

According to the comparison between self-training and cooperative-training, the major contribution of cooperative-training is to narrow the performance gap between the easy mode and the hard mode and introduce small improvement in the easy mode, with a 0.07 improvement on instance-level FROC. In general, we observe that training on extra 50 regions in the same WSI could only slightly augment the performance than on annotated 2 regions. Therefore, to improve the performance in the easy mode, quality improvement of annotations shall be of highest priority in the future. In the hard mode cooperative-training still introduces obvious improvement, with a 0.14 improvement on instance-level FROC, meaning that in self-training there exists large data gap between different WSIs and organs, and this gap can be narrowed by using extra annotations from same WSIs in train data. Even with noisy annotations generated by cooperative-training, models can learn much common morphological varieties across different WSIs and organs. However, we can still observe a few images in hard mode with only 23% recall, which demonstrate that signet ring cells in different organs do show different appearance.

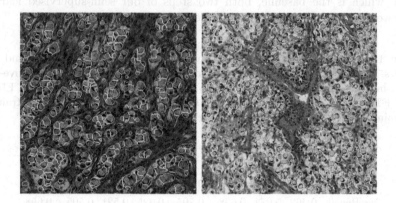

Fig. 7. Example detection results in test images of over $2,000 \times 2,000$ pixels. Our semi-supervised learning framework can obtain cell edges of each signet ring cell as shown in yellow polygon. (Color figure online)

Comparing instance-level recall with collective-level recall, we find that model has found 82.7% signet ring cells in the hard mode, but has difficulties in separating neighbor signet ring cells. This will harm the accuracy of signet ring cell counting, as shown in Fig. 7.

Comparing self-training with self-training-extra, unlabeled images with self-generated annotations can harm the performance, especially in easy mode where the false positive rises to 5.22. Visually we find that there are too many neutrophils, plasma cells, and gland cells in unlabeled images being annotated. However the three types of cell are rarely annotated as false positives in 74 partially labeled images. While in cooperative-training these three types of specific false positives are not severely amplified. Therefore self-training will indeed amplify the errors while cooperative-training does not show this phenomenon.

4   Conclusion

In this paper we propose a semi-supervised learning framework to make better use of collected data with relative small amount of annotation cost. Semi-supervised learning framework not only improves the quality of annotation but also makes better use of extra unlabeled images. We verify the improvement by collecting a multi-organ signet ring cell dataset and propose a series of new evaluation metrics for imperfect annotated data. In the future we will try to understand why specific types of false positive are not amplified in cooperative-training. The proposed dataset will be released soon to facilitate the development of the area.

References

1. Bandos, A.I., Rockette, H.E., Song, T., Gur, D.: Area under the free-response roc curve (froc) and a related summary index. Biometrics **65**(1), 247–256 (2009)
2. Bosman, F.T., Carneiro, F., Hruban, R.H., Theise, N.D., et al.: WHO Classification of Tumours of the Digestive System, pp. 52–53, No. Ed. 4. World Health Organization (2010)
3. Chen, H., Qi, X., Yu, L., Heng, P.A.: DCAN: deep contour-aware networks for accurate gland segmentation. In: Proceedings of the IEEE Conference on Computer Vision and Pattern Recognition, pp. 2487–2496 (2016)
4. Everingham, M., Van Gool, L., Williams, C.K.I., Winn, J., Zisserman, A.: The pascal visual object classes (VOC) challenge. Int. J. Comput. Vis. **88**(2), 303–338 (2010)
5. Grady, L.: Random walks for image segmentation. IEEE Trans. Pattern Anal. Mach. Intell. **28**(11), 1768–1783 (2006)
6. He, K., Zhang, X., Ren, S., Sun, J.: Deep residual learning for image recognition. In: Proceedings of the IEEE Conference on Computer Vision and Pattern Recognition, pp. 770–778 (2016)
7. Hosang, A.K.R.B.J., Schiele, M.H.B.: Weakly supervised semantic labelling and instance segmentation. arXiv preprint arXiv:1603.07485 (2016)
8. Hu, R., Dollár, P., He, K., Darrell, T., Girshick, R.: Learning to segment every thing. In: Proceedings of the IEEE Conference on Computer Vision and Pattern Recognition, pp. 4233–4241 (2018)
9. Luo, P., Wang, G., Lin, L., Wang, X.: Deep dual learning for semantic image segmentation. In: Proceedings of the IEEE Conference on Computer Vision and Pattern Recognition, Honolulu, HI, USA, pp. 21–26 (2017)
10. Papandreou, G., Chen, L., Murphy, K., Yuille, A.L.: Weakly- and semi-supervised learning of a DCNN for semantic image segmentation. CoRR abs/1502.02734 (2015). http://arxiv.org/abs/1502.02734
11. Rajchl, M., et al.: DeepCut: object segmentation from bounding box annotations using convolutional neural networks. IEEE Trans. Med. Imaging **36**(2), 674–683 (2017)
12. Redmon, J., Divvala, S., Girshick, R., Farhadi, A.: You only look once: unified, real-time object detection. In: Proceedings of the IEEE Conference on Computer Vision and Pattern Recognition, pp. 779–788 (2016)
13. Ren, S., He, K., Girshick, R., Sun, J.: Faster R-CNN: towards real-time object detection with region proposal networks. In: Advances in Neural Information Processing Systems, pp. 91–99 (2015)
14. Ronneberger, O., Fischer, P., Brox, T.: U-net: convolutional networks for biomedical image segmentation. In: Navab, N., Hornegger, J., Wells, W.M., Frangi, A.F. (eds.) MICCAI 2015. LNCS, vol. 9351, pp. 234–241. Springer, Cham (2015). https://doi.org/10.1007/978-3-319-24574-4_28
15. Yu, F., Wang, D., Shelhamer, E., Darrell, T.: Deep layer aggregation. In: Proceedings of the IEEE Conference on Computer Vision and Pattern Recognition, pp. 2403–2412 (2018)
16. Zach, C., Niethammer, M., Frahm, J.M.: Continuous maximal flows and Wulff shapes: application to MRFs. In: IEEE Conference on Computer Vision and Pattern Recognition, CVPR 2009, pp. 1911–1918. IEEE (2009)
17. Zhang, X., Liu, W., Dundar, M., Badve, S., Zhang, S.: Towards large-scale histopathological image analysis: hashing-based image retrieval. IEEE Trans. Med. Imaging **34**(2), 496–506 (2015)

18. Zhang, X., Xing, F., Su, H., Yang, L., Zhang, S.: High-throughput histopathological image analysis via robust cell segmentation and hashing. Med. Image Anal. **26**(1), 306–315 (2015)
19. Zhao, X., Liang, S., Wei, Y.: Pseudo mask augmented object detection. In: Proceedings of the IEEE Conference on Computer Vision and Pattern Recognition, pp. 4061–4070 (2018)

Spherical U-Net on Cortical Surfaces: Methods and Applications

Fenqiang Zhao[1,2], Shunren Xia[1], Zhengwang Wu[2], Dingna Duan[1,2], Li Wang[2], Weili Lin[2], John H. Gilmore[3], Dinggang Shen[2], and Gang Li[2(✉)]

[1] Key Laboratory of Biomedical Engineering of Ministry of Education,
Zhejiang University, Hangzhou, China
[2] Department of Radiology and BRIC, University of North Carolina at Chapel Hill,
Chapel Hill, NC, USA
gang_li@med.unc.edu
[3] Department of Psychiatry, University of North Carolina at Chapel Hill,
Chapel Hill, NC, USA

Abstract. Convolutional Neural Networks (CNNs) have been providing the state-of-the-art performance for learning-related problems involving 2D/3D images in Euclidean space. However, unlike in the Euclidean space, the shapes of many structures in medical imaging have a spherical topology in a manifold space, e.g., brain cortical or subcortical surfaces represented by triangular meshes, with large inter-subject and intra-subject variations in vertex number and local connectivity. Hence, there is no consistent neighborhood definition and thus no straightforward convolution/transposed convolution operations for cortical/subcortical surface data. In this paper, by leveraging the regular and consistent geometric structure of the resampled cortical surface mapped onto the spherical space, we propose a novel convolution filter analogous to the standard convolution on the image grid. Accordingly, we develop corresponding operations for convolution, pooling, and transposed convolution for spherical surface data and thus construct spherical CNNs. Specifically, we propose the Spherical U-Net architecture by replacing all operations in the standard U-Net with their spherical operation counterparts. We then apply the Spherical U-Net to two challenging and neuroscientifically important tasks in infant brains: cortical surface parcellation and cortical attribute map development prediction. Both applications demonstrate the competitive performance in the accuracy, computational efficiency, and effectiveness of our proposed Spherical U-Net, in comparison with the state-of-the-art methods.

Keywords: Spherical U-Net · Convolutional Neural Network · Cortical surface · Parcellation · Prediction

1 Introduction

Convolutional Neural Networks (CNNs) based deep learning methods have been providing the state-of-the-art performance for a variety of tasks in computer

© Springer Nature Switzerland AG 2019
A. C. S. Chung et al. (Eds.): IPMI 2019, LNCS 11492, pp. 855–866, 2019.
https://doi.org/10.1007/978-3-030-20351-1_67

vision and biomedical image analysis in the last few years, e.g., image classification [8], segmentation [12], detection and tracking [16], benefiting from their powerful abilities in feature learning. In biomedical image analysis, U-Net and its variants have become one of the most popular and powerful architectures for image segmentation, synthesis, prediction, and registration owing to its strong ability to jointly capture localization and contextual information [14].

However, these CNN methods are mainly developed for 2D/3D images in Euclidean space, while there is still a significant demand for models that can deal with data representation on non-Euclidean space. For example, the shapes of many structures in medical imaging have an inherent spherical topology in a manifold space, e.g., brain cortical or subcortical surfaces represented by triangular meshes, which typically have large inter-subject and intra-subject variations in vertex number and local connectivity. Hence, unlike in the Euclidean space, there is no consistent and regular neighborhood definition and thus no straightforward convolution/transposed convolution and pooling operations for cortical/subcortical surface data. Therefore, despite many advantages of CNN in 2D/3D images, the conventional CNN cannot be directly applicable to cortical/subcortical surface data.

To address this issue, two main strategies have been proposed to extend the conventional convolution operation to the surface meshes [2], including (1) performing convolution in non-spatial domains, e.g., the spectral domain obtained by the graph Laplacian [3,4,18]; (2) projecting the original surface data onto a certain intrinsic space, e.g., the tangent space (which is an Euclidean space with consistent neighborhood definition [5,15,17]). On one hand, recent advances in convolution in non-spatial domains [4,18] are mainly focusing on omnidirectional image data, which is typically parameterized by spherical coordinates $\alpha \in [0, 2\pi)$ and $\beta \in [0, \pi]$. While cortical/subcortical surface data are typically represented by triangular meshes, these methods still cannot be applicable, unless the surface is resampled to obtain another sphere manifold parameterized by α and β. This resampling process from the spherical surface with uniform vertices to another imbalanced sphere manifold with extremely non-uniform nodes is essentially hazardous and unnecessary for cortical surface data, because it would miss key structural and connectivity information, thus leading to inaccurate and ambiguous results. On the other hand, for cortical surface data analysis, existing researches typically adopting the second strategy also suffer from some inherent drawbacks. For example, the method in [17] first projected intrinsic spherical surface patches into tangent spaces to form 2D image patches, and then the conventional CNN was applied for classifying each vertex to derive the surface parcellation map. Seong et al. [15] designed a rectangular filter on the tangent plane of the spherical surface for sex classification. They resampled points in the rectangular patches for convolution operation. For a better comparison with our proposed method, we redraw their rectangular patch (RePa) convolution method in the bottom row of Fig. 2A. Overall, as in [15,17], this projection strategy would inevitably introduce feature distortion and re-interpolation, thus complicating the network, increasing computational burden and decreasing accuracy.

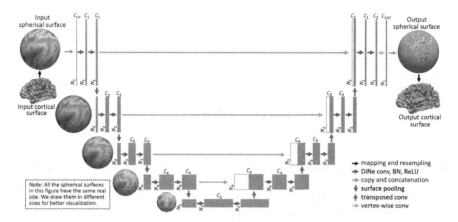

Fig. 1. Spherical U-Net architecture. Blue boxes represent feature maps on spherical space. The number of features C_i is denoted above the box. The number of vertices N_i is at the lower left edge of the box. $N_{i+1} = (N_i + 6)/4$, $C_{i+1} = C_i \times 2$. For example, N_1 can be 10,242, 40,962, or 163,842, and C_1 is typically set as 64. In our applications, the output surface is a cortical parcellation map or a cortical attribute map. (Color figure online)

To address these issues, in this paper, we capitalize on the consistent structure of the regularly-resampled brain cortical surface mapped onto a spherical space, by leveraging its inherent spherical topology. The motivation is that the standard spherical representation of a cortical surface is typically a uniform sphere structure that is generated starting from an icosahedron by hierarchically adding a new vertex to the center of each edge in each triangle [6]. Therefore, based on the consistent and regular topological structure across subjects, we suggest a novel intuitive and natural convolution filter on sphere, termed Direct Neighbor (DiNe). The definition of our DiNe filter is also consistent with the expansion and contraction process of icosahedron, in which vertices contribute to or aggregate from their direct neighbors' information at each iteration process. With this new convolution filter, we then develop surface convolution, pooling, and transposed convolution in spherical space. Accordingly, we extend the popular U-Net [14] architecture from image domains to spherical surface domains. To validate our proposed network, we demonstrate the capability and efficiency of the Spherical U-Net architecture on two challenging tasks in infant brains: cortical surface parcellation, which is a vertex-wise classification/segmentation problem, and cortical attribute map development prediction, which is a vertex-wise dense regression problem. In both tasks, our proposed Spherical U-Net achieves very competitive performance in comparison to state-of-the-art algorithms.

2   Method

The key of the Spherical U-Net is to define a consistent neighborhood orders on the spherical space, similar to the filter window in the 2D image space. In

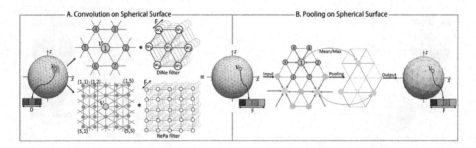

Fig. 2. Top in A: Our proposed DiNe convolution. Bottom in A: The Rectangular Patch (RePa) convolution in Seong et al. [15]. Both convolutions transfer the input feature maps with D channels to the output feature maps with F channels. B: Illustration of the spherical surface pooling operation.

the following parts, we will first introduce the consistent DiNe filter in spherical space and then the spherical surface convolution, pooling, transposed convolution operations, and finally the Spherical U-Net architecture.

2.1 Direct Neighbor Filter

Since a standard sphere for cortical surface representation is typically generated starting from a regular icosahedron (with 12 vertices) by hierarchically adding a new vertex to the center of each edge in each triangle, the number of vertices on the sphere are increased from 12 to 42, 162, 642, 2562, 10,242, 40,962, 163,842, and so on [6]. Hence, each spherical surface is composed of two types of vertices: (1) 12 vertices with each having only 5 direct neighbors; and (2) the remaining vertices with each having 6 direct neighbors. As shown in the top row of Fig. 2A, for those vertices with 6 neighbors, DiNe assigns the index 1 to the center vertex and the indices 2–7 to its neighbors sequentially according to the angle between the vector of center vertex to neighboring vertex and the x-axis in the tangent plane; For the 12 vertices with only 5 neighbors, DiNe assigns the indices both 1 and 2 to the center vertex, and indices 3–7 to the neighbors in the same way as those vertices with 6 neighbors.

2.2 Convolution and Pooling on Spherical Surface

We name the convolution on the spherical surface using DiNe filter the DiNe convolution, as shown in the top row of Fig. 2A. With the designed filter, DiNe convolution can be formulated as a simple filter weighting process. For each vertex v on a standard spherical surface with N vertices, at a certain convolution layer with input feature channel number D and output feature channel number F, the feature data $\mathbf{I}_v(7 \times D)$ from the direct neighbors are first extracted and reshaped into a row vector $\mathbf{I}'_v(1 \times 7D)$. Then, iterating over all N vertices, we can obtain the full-node filter matrix $\mathbf{I}(N \times 7D)$. By multiplying $\mathbf{I}$ with the

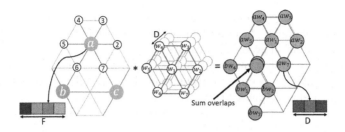

Fig. 3. Illustration of transposed convolution on the spherical surface.

convolution layer's filter weight $\mathbf{W}(7D \times F)$, the output surface feature map $\mathbf{O}(N \times F)$ with F channels can be obtained.

The pooling operation on the spherical surface is performed in a reverse order of the icosahedron expansion process. As shown in Fig. 2B, in a pooling layer, for each center vertex v, all feature data $\mathbf{I_v}(7 \times F)$ aggregated from itself and its neighbors are averaged or maximized, and then a refined feature $\mathbf{I'_v}(1 \times F)$ can be obtained. Meanwhile, the number of vertices is decreased from N to $(N + 6)/4$.

2.3   Transposed Convolution on Spherical Surface

Transposed convolution is also known as fractionally-strided convolution, deconvolution or up-convolution in U-Net [14]. It has been widely used for its learnable parameters in conventional CNN, especially in semantic segmentation. From the perspective of image transformation, transposed convolution first restores pixels around every center pixel by sliding-window filtering over all original pixels, and then sums where output overlaps.

Inspired by this concept, for a spherical surface with the original feature map $\mathbf{I}(N \times D$, where N denotes the number of vertices, and D denotes the number of feature channels) and the pooled feature map $\mathbf{O}(N' \times F, N' = (N + 6)/4)$, we can restore $\mathbf{I}$ by first using DiNe filter to do transposed convolution with every vertex on the pooled surface $\mathbf{O}$ and then summing overlap vertices (see Fig. 3).

2.4   Spherical U-Net Architecture

With our defined operations for spherical surface convolution, pooling, and transposed convolution, the proposed Spherical U-Net architecture is illustrated in Fig. 1. It has an encoder path and a decoder path, each with five resolution steps, indexed by i, $i = 1, 2, \ldots, 5$. Different from the standard U-Net, we replace all 3×3 convolution with our DiNe convolution, 2×2 up-convolution with our surface transposed convolution, and 2×2 max pooling with our surface max/mean pooling. In addition to the standard U-Net, before each convolution layer's rectified linear units (ReLU) activation function, a batch normalization layer is added. At the final layer, 1×1 convolution is replaced by vertex-wise filter weighting to map C_1-component feature vector in the second-to-last layer to the desired C_{out} at the last layer. We simply double the number of feature channels after each surface pooling layer and halve the number of feature channels at each transposed convolution layer. That makes $C_{i+1} = C_i \times 2$ and $N_{i+1} = (N_i + 6)/4$, as shown in Fig. 1. Note that we do not need any tiling strategy in the original U-Net [14] to allow a seamless output map, because all the data flow in our network is on a closed spherical surface.

3   Experiments

To validate the proposed Spherical U-Net on cortical surfaces, we conducted experiments on two challenging tasks in infant brain MRI studies: cortical surface parcellation and cortical attribute map development prediction. Both tasks are of great neuroscientific and clinical importance and are suffering from designing of hand-crafted features and heavy computational burden. We show that our task-agnostic and feature-agnostic Spherical U-Net is still capable of learning useful features for these different tasks.

3.1   Infant Cortical Surface Parcellation

Dataset and Image Processing. We used an infant brain MRI dataset with 90 term-born neonates. All images were processed using an infant-specific computational pipeline [10]. All cortical surfaces were mapped onto the spherical space and further resampled. Each vertex on the cortical surface was coded with 3 shape attributes, i.e., the mean curvature, sulcal depth, and average convexity. The target is to parcellate these vertices into 36 cortical regions for each hemisphere. A 3-fold cross-validation was adopted and Dice ratio was used to measure the overlap between the manual parcellation and the automatic parcellation.

Architectures. We used the Spherical U-Net architecture as shown in Fig. 1. We set C_{in} as 3 for the 3 shape attributes, C_{out} as 36 for the 36 labels of ROIs, N_1 as 10,242, and C_1 as 64. For comparison, we created the following architecture variants.

As RePa convolution is very memory-intensive for a full Spherical U-Net experiment, we created a smaller variant *U-Net18-RePa*. It is different from the Spherical U-Net in three points: (1) It only consists of three pooling and three transposed convolution layers, thus containing only 18 convolution layers; (2) It replaces all DiNe convolution with RePa convolution; (3) The feature number is halved at each corresponding layer. Meanwhile, for a fair comparison, we created a *U-Net18-DiNe* by replacing all RePa convolution with DiNe convolution in U-Net18-RePa. *Naive-DiNe* is a baseline architecture with 16 DiNe convolution blocks (DiNe (64 convolution filters), BN, ReLU) and without any pooling and upsampling layers.

In addition to the above variants, we also studied upsampling using Linear-Interpolation (*SegNet-Inter*) and Max-pooling Indices (*SegNet-Basic*). As shown in Fig. 4A, for each new vertex generated from the edge's center, its feature

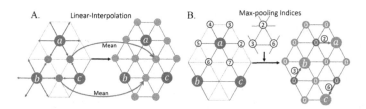

Fig. 4. Illustration of Linear-Interpolation and Max-Pooling Indices upsampling methods.

is linearly interpolated by the two parent vertices of this edge using Linear-Interpolation. Max-pooling Indices, introduced by SegNet [1], uses the memorized pooling indices computed in the max-pooling step of the encoder to perform non-linear upsampling at the corresponding decoder. We accommodated this method to the spherical surface mesh as shown in Fig. 4B. For example, max-pooling indices 2, 3, and 6 are first stored for vertices a, b, and c, respectively. Then at the corresponding upsampling layer, the 2-nd neighbor of a, 3-rd neighbor of b, and 6-th neighbor of c are restored with a, b and c's value, respectively, and other vertices are set as 0. Therefore, SegNet-Basic and SegNet-Inter require no learning for upsampling and thus are created in a SegNet style. They are different from our Spherical U-Net in two aspects: (1) There is no copy and concatenation path in both models; (2) For up-sampling, SegNet-Basic uses Max-pooling Indices and SegNet-Inter uses Linear-Interpolation.

Training. We trained all the variants using mini-batch stochastic gradient descent (SGD) with initial learning rate 0.1 and momentum 0.99 with weight decay 0.0001. Given different network architectures, we used a self-adaption strategy for updating learning rate, which reduces the learning rate by a factor of 5 once training Dice stagnates for 2 epochs. This strategy allowed us to achieve a gain in Dice ratio around 3% for most architectures. We used the cross-entropy loss as the objective function for training. The other hyper-parameters were empirically set by babysitting the training process. We also augmented the training data by randomly rotating each sphere to generate more training samples.

Results. We report the means and standard deviations of Dice ratios based on the 3-fold cross-validation, as well as the number of parameters, memory storage and time for one inference on a NVIDIA Geforce GTX1060 GPU, in Table 1. As we can see, our Spherical U-Net architectures consistently achieve better results than other methods, with the highest Dice ratio 88.87%. It is also obvious that RePa convolution is more time-consuming and memory-intensive, while our DiNe convolution is 7 times faster than RePa, 5 times smaller on memory storage and 3 times lighter on model size. Moreover, it outperforms the state-of-the-art DCNN method [17] using a deep classification CNN architecture based on

Table 1. Comparison of different architectures for cortical surface parcellation. The p-values are the results of paired t-test vs. Spherical U-Net.

Architectures	Parameters (MB)	Storage (MB)	Inference time (ms)	Dice (%)	p-value
Learning for upsampling					
Spherical U-Net	26.9	1635	18.3	**88.87 ± 2.43**	N.A
Spherical U-Net18-DiNe	**1.7**	**955**	**8.9**	88.05 ± 2.46	1.96×10^{-3}
Spherical U-Net18-RePa	5.2	5047	64.5	88.28 ± 2.50	4.92×10^{-2}
No learning for upsampling					
Spherical Naive-DiNe	0.4	1499	15.8	81.74 ± 4.96	4.87×10^{-11}
Spherical SegNet-Basic	14.5	1341	113.5	78.31 ± 4.62	5.87×10^{-18}
Spherical SegNet-Inter	22.0	1533	20.1	75.12 ± 8.39	4.57×10^{-11}

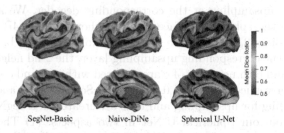

SegNet-Basic   Naive-DiNe   Spherical U-Net

Fig. 5. Average Dice ratio of cortical parcellation results for each ROI by different methods.

the projected patches on the tangent space. They reported the DCNN without graph cuts achieves the average Dice ratio 86.18%, and the DCNN with graph cuts achieves the average Dice ratio 87.06%. As in [17], we also incorporated the graph cuts method for post-processing the output of our spherical U-Net, but this step has no further improvement in quantitative results. This may indicate that our Spherical U-Net is capable of learning spatially-consistent information in an end-to-end way without post-processing.

Figure 5 provides a comparison of average Dice ratio of each ROI using different methods. We can see that the Spherical U-Net achieves consistent higher Dice ratio in almost all ROIs. Figure 6 provides a visual comparison between parcellation results on a randomly selected infant by different methods. We can see that our spherical U-Net shows high consistency with the manual parcellation and has no isolated noisy labels.

3.2   Infant Cortical Attribute Map Development Prediction

We have also applied our Spherical U-Net to the prediction of cortical surface attribute maps of 1-year-old brain from the corresponding 0-year-old brain using 370 infants, all with longitudinal 0-year-old and 1-year-old brain MRI data. All infant MR images were processed using an infant-specific computational pipeline

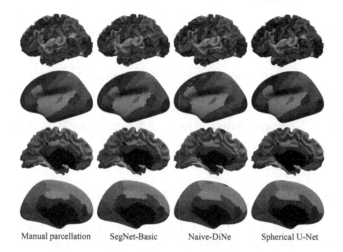

Manual parcellation   SegNet-Basic   Naive-DiNe   Spherical U-Net

Fig. 6. Visual comparison of cortical parcellation results of a randomly selected infant using different methods.

for cortical surface reconstruction [10]. All cortical surfaces were mapped onto the spherical space, nonlinearly aligned, and further resampled. Following the experimental configuration in Meng et al. [13], we used the sulcal depth and cortical thickness maps at birth to predict the cortical thickness map at 1 year of age. The reason to choose the cortical thickness map as the prediction target for validating our method is that cortical thickness has dynamic, region-specific and subject-specific development and is highly related to future cognitive outcomes [7]. To have a robust prediction for the cortical thickness, we introduced the sulcal depth as an additional channel for leveraging the relationship between sulcal depth and cortical thickness maps [9,11].

Evaluation Metrics. The evaluation metrics we adopted for the prediction performance are mean absolute error (MAE) and mean relative error (MRE) under a 5-fold cross-validation. The 5-fold cross-validation uses 60% data for training, 20% data for validation, and 20% data for testing at each fold.

Spherical U-Net and Hyper-parameters. Here we still consider a basic and simple architecture and training strategy to validate the effectiveness of our Spherical U-Net. We used the Spherical U-Net architecture as shown in Fig. 1, with $C_{in} = 2$ (representing sulcal depth and cortical thickness channels at birth), $C_{out} = 1$ (representing cortical thickness at 1 year of age), $C_1 = 64$, and $N_1 = 40{,}962$. We trained the Spherical U-Net using Adam optimization algorithm and L1 loss. We used an initial learning rate 0.0001 and reduced it by 10 every 3 epochs. The whole training process had 15 epochs and lasted for 30 min in a NVIDIA Geforce GTX1080 GPU.

Table 2. 5-fold cross-validated cortical thickness prediction performance in terms of MAE and MRE using different methods with standard deviations. The p-values are the results of paired t-test vs. Spherical U-Net.

Methods	MAE (mm)	MRE (%)	p-value for MAE	p-value for MRE
Linear regression	0.3605 ± 0.0337	15.01 ± 1.92	9.47×10^{-43}	1.94×10^{-41}
Polynomial regression	0.6068 ± 0.0900	26.76 ± 4.52	2.01×10^{-43}	1.21×10^{-41}
Random forest	0.2959 ± 0.0382	12.63 ± 2.06	2.52×10^{-24}	1.80×10^{-16}
Spherical U-Net	$\mathbf{0.2812 \pm 0.0406}$	$\mathbf{12.14 \pm 2.05}$	N.A	N.A

Comparison with Feature-Based Approaches. For the feature-based approaches, we extracted 102 features for each vertex on 0-year-old cortical surface. Same as in Meng et al. [13], the 1st and 2nd features are sulcal depth and cortical thickness, respectively, providing local information at each vertex. The 3rd to 102nd features are contextual features, providing rich neighboring information for each vertex, which are composed of 50 Haar-like features of sulcal depth and 50 Haar-like features of cortical thickness. The Haar-like features were extracted using the method and hyper-parameters in [13].

We then trained the following machine learning algorithms on the 102 features in a vertex-wise manner: Linear Regression, Polynomial Regression, and Random Forest [13]. Linear Regression assumes that cortical thickness at each vertex is linearly increased, and Polynomial Regression assumes that it has a two-order polynomial relationship with the age. Random Forest is an effective method for high dimensional data analysis, which has shown the state-of-the-art performance for cortical thickness prediction [13]. Herein, each above algorithm would generate 40,962 models, each for predicting the thickness of a certain vertex at 1-year-old, while our Spherical U-Net just generates one model for all vertices. All the machine learning algorithms were trained on a campus-wide cluster and the training process all lasted an extremely long time (2–3 days).

Results. Table 2 presents the 5-fold cross-validation results. Our Spherical U-Net outperforms all other machine learning algorithms both in terms of MAE and MRE. While the main competitors, Random Forest is involved with complex hand-crafted features extraction step and heavy vertex-wise computational burden, our task-agnostic and feature-agnostic Spherical U-Net still achieves better results. The Linear Regression and Polynomial Regression results reveal that the cortical thickness development is more like in a linear pattern than a polynomial pattern from birth to 1 year of age, which is consistent with the finding in [13].

Figure 7 shows a visual comparison on the vertex-wise mean error map between the ground truth at 1 year of age and predicted cortical thickness based on 0-year-old data using different methods. We can see that the Spherical U-Net obtains smoother and smaller mean errors than other methods. Figure 8 provides the vertex-wise predictions of a randomly selected infant using different methods and their corresponding error maps. As we can see, the Spherical U-Net predicts the cortical thickness map more precisely than other methods.

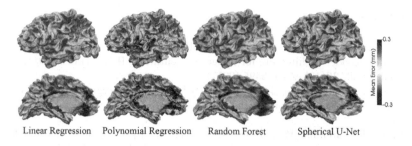

Fig. 7. Visual comparison of vertex-wise average error maps using different methods.

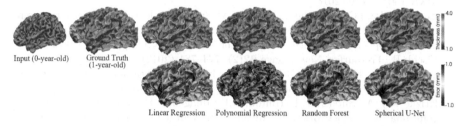

Fig. 8. Prediction of the vertex-wise cortical thickness map (mm) of a randomly selected infant by different methods. The first row shows the input at 0-year-old, ground truth, and the predicted cortical thickness maps by different methods. The second row shows the error maps (mm).

4   Conclusion

In this paper, we propose the DiNe filter on spherical space for developing corresponding operations for constructing the Spherical CNNs. The DiNe filter has a natural and intuitive definition, making it interpretable for recognizing patterns on spherical surface. We then extend the conventional U-Net to the Spherical U-Net by deploying respective surface convolution, pooling, and transposed convolution layers. Furthermore, we have shown that the Spherical U-Net is computationally efficient and capable of learning useful features for different tasks, including cortical surface parcellation and cortical attribute map development prediction. The experimental results on these two challenging tasks confirm the robustness, efficiency and accuracy of the Spherical U-Net both visually and quantitatively. In the future, we will extensively test our Spherical U-Net on other cortical/subcortical surface tasks and also make it publicly available.

Acknowledgements. This work was partially supported by NIH grants (MH107815, MH108914, MH109773, MH116225, and MH117943) and China Scholarship Council.

References

1. Badrinarayanan, V., Kendall, A., Cipolla, R.: SegNet: a deep convolutional encoder-decoder architecture for image segmentation. IEEE Trans. Pattern Anal. Mach. Intell. **39**(12), 2481–2495 (2017)
2. Bronstein, M.M., Bruna, J., LeCun, Y., Szlam, A., Vandergheynst, P.: Geometric deep learning: going beyond euclidean data. IEEE Sig. Process. Mag. **34**(4), 18–42 (2017)
3. Bruna, J., Zaremba, W., Szlam, A., LeCun, Y.: Spectral networks and locally connected networks on graphs. arXiv preprint arXiv:1312.6203 (2013)
4. Cohen, T.S., Geiger, M., Köhler, J., Welling, M.: Spherical CNNs. arXiv preprint arXiv:1801.10130 (2018)
5. Coors, B., Paul Condurache, A., Geiger, A.: Spherenet: learning spherical representations for detection and classification in omnidirectional images. In: Proceedings of the European Conference on Computer Vision (ECCV), pp. 518–533 (2018)
6. Fischl, B.: Freesurfer. Neuroimage **62**(2), 774–781 (2012)
7. Gilmore, J.H., Knickmeyer, R.C., Gao, W.: Imaging structural and functional brain development in early childhood. Nat. Rev. Neurosci. **19**(3), 123 (2018)
8. Krizhevsky, A., Sutskever, I., Hinton, G.E.: Imagenet classification with deep convolutional neural networks. In: Advances in Neural Information Processing Systems, pp. 1097–1105 (2012)
9. Li, G., Lin, W., Gilmore, J.H., Shen, D.: Spatial patterns, longitudinal development, and hemispheric asymmetries of cortical thickness in infants from birth to 2 years of age. J. Neurosci. **35**(24), 9150–9162 (2015)
10. Li, G., Wang, L., Shi, F., Gilmore, J.H., Lin, W., Shen, D.: Construction of 4D high-definition cortical surface atlases of infants: methods and applications. Med. Image Anal. **25**(1), 22–36 (2015)
11. Li, G., et al.: Computational neuroanatomy of baby brains: a review. Neuroimage **185**, 906–925 (2018)
12. Long, J., Shelhamer, E., Darrell, T.: Fully convolutional networks for semantic segmentation. In: Proceedings of the IEEE Conference on Computer Vision and Pattern Recognition, pp. 3431–3440 (2015)
13. Meng, Y., et al.: Can we predict subject-specific dynamic cortical thickness maps during infancy from birth? Hum. Brain Mapp. **38**(6), 2865–2874 (2017)
14. Ronneberger, O., Fischer, P., Brox, T.: U-net: convolutional networks for biomedical image segmentation. In: Navab, N., Hornegger, J., Wells, W.M., Frangi, A.F. (eds.) MICCAI 2015. LNCS, vol. 9351, pp. 234–241. Springer, Cham (2015). https://doi.org/10.1007/978-3-319-24574-4_28
15. Seong, S.B., Pae, C., Park, H.J.: Geometric convolutional neural network for analyzing surface-based neuroimaging data. Front. Neuroinf. **12**, 42 (2018)
16. Wang, N., Li, S., Gupta, A., Yeung, D.Y.: Transferring rich feature hierarchies for robust visual tracking. arXiv preprint arXiv:1501.04587 (2015)
17. Wu, Z., et al.: Registration-free infant cortical surface parcellation using deep convolutional neural networks. In: Frangi, A.F., Schnabel, J.A., Davatzikos, C., Alberola-López, C., Fichtinger, G. (eds.) MICCAI 2018. LNCS, vol. 11072, pp. 672–680. Springer, Cham (2018). https://doi.org/10.1007/978-3-030-00931-1_77
18. Zhang, Z., Xu, Y., Yu, J., Gao, S.: Saliency detection in 360° videos. In: The European Conference on Computer Vision (ECCV) (2018)

Variational Autoencoder with Truncated Mixture of Gaussians for Functional Connectivity Analysis

Qingyu Zhao[1](✉), Nicolas Honnorat[2], Ehsan Adeli[1], Adolf Pfefferbaum[1,2], Edith V. Sullivan[1], and Kilian M. Pohl[1,2]

[1] Stanford University School of Medicine, Stanford, USA
qingyuz@stanford.edu
[2] Center for Health Sciences, SRI International, Menlo Park, CA, USA

Abstract. Resting-state functional connectivity states are often identified as clusters of dynamic connectivity patterns. However, existing clustering approaches do not distinguish major states from rarely occurring minor states and hence are sensitive to noise. To address this issue, we propose to model major states using a non-linear generative process guided by a Gaussian-mixture distribution in a low-dimensional latent space, while separately modeling the connectivity patterns of minor states by a non-informative uniform distribution. We embed this truncated Gaussian-Mixture model in a Variational AutoEncoder framework to obtain a general joint clustering and outlier detection approach, called tGM-VAE. When applied to synthetic data with known ground-truth, tGM-VAE is more accurate in clustering dynamic connectivity patterns than existing approaches. On the rs-fMRI data of 593 healthy adolescents from the National Consortium on Alcohol and Neurodevelopment in Adolescence (NCANDA) study, tGM-VAE identified meaningful major connectivity states. The dwell time of these states significantly correlated with age.

1 Introduction

Functional connectivity refers to the functionally integrated relationship between spatially separated brain regions [1]. Recent work revealed that functional connectivity exhibits meaningful variations within the time series captured by resting-state fMRI [2,3]. As a consequence, a considerable amount of work has been directed to quantify dynamic functional connectivity. A popular way of quantification [2,4,5] is to first categorize the time-varying connectivity patterns of a subject or a population into several states. Then, the dwell time of each state and the transition probabilities across states are used to characterize functional dynamics and perform group analyses [4].

Most existing works identify *major connectivity states* (commonly observed states) by grouping the dynamic connectivity patterns into a few clusters [2,4,5]. However, some studies have indicated that there exist many *minor states* containing rare connectivity patterns that persist shortly ($<1\%$ occupancy rate) [6].

© Springer Nature Switzerland AG 2019
A. C. S. Chung et al. (Eds.): IPMI 2019, LNCS 11492, pp. 867–879, 2019.
https://doi.org/10.1007/978-3-030-20351-1_68

These minor states often provide little merit to analysis because they may correspond to random individual brain variation, inaccurate connectivity pattern computed during state transitions or rs-fMRI noise. Instead of merging minor states into the major ones [4,5], recent work suggests to disentangle minor from major states by modeling an infinite number of clusters [6,7]. However, connectivity patterns in minor states may correspond to pure noise, so grouping them into clusters is not meaningful. In this paper, we address these concerns by developing a statistical framework where the patterns associated with major states are drawn from an informative distribution while we use a non-informative distribution for minor states.

Motivated by the truncated stick-breaking representation of Dirichlet processes [8,9], our approach is guided by a Dirichlet prior when separating dynamic connectivity patterns into major and minor states. We define dynamic connectivity patterns by computing correlation matrices associated with sliding windows. We assume that the correlation matrices belonging to major states are generated by a non-linear process from a low-dimensional latent space, where the latent representations follow a Gaussian-mixture distribution. We assume that the rest of the correlation matrices, which correspond to minor states, are generated from a uniform distribution in the original space. To determine the optimal parameters of our model, we derive the variational lower-bound of its log marginal probability and find the maximum of that lower-bound by optimizing a variational autoencoder. As a result, our method, tGM-VAE, simultaneously achieves clustering and outlier-detection: tGM-VAE clusters dynamic connectivity patterns associated with major states and treats the minor states as outliers. In this work, we first demonstrate that tGM-VAE achieves higher accuracy in defining major clusters and outliers compared to traditional Gaussian-mixture-based approaches when clustering synthetic data with ground-truth. We then report that, for 15k correlation matrices derived from rs-fMRI scans of 593 adolescents in the National Consortium on Alcohol and Neurodevelopment in Adolescence (NCANDA), tGM-VAE identifies meaningful connectivity states and a significant effect of age on their mean dwell time.

In the following, we first review existing VAE-based clustering approaches in Sect. 2. We introduce in Sect. 3 the generative model of tGM-VAE, the variational lower bound of the resulting log marginal likelihood, and reformulate tGM-VAE into a joint clustering and outlier-detection approach. We present our synthetic experiments and clinical data analysis in Sect. 4.

2   Related Work

Traditional approaches to clustering connectivity patterns are mostly based on Gaussian-mixture models [4,5]. These methods usually require fitting probability distributions in a high dimensional space, which is a challenging task. Moreover, it has been found that the underlying distributions of both fMRI measurements [6] and the derived correlation matrices [10] lie on a non-linear latent space. Therefore, modeling Gaussian-mixtures in the original space is suboptimal.

Generative models used in connection with neural-networks, such as VAEs, have recently attracted much attention for their capability of modeling latent representations of the data [11]. In VAE, the encoder approximates the intractable posterior distribution of the latent representation and the decoder aims to reconstruct the observation based on its latent representation. While traditional VAE assumes that latent variables follow a single Gaussian prior, recent works adopt mixture models in the latent space for semi-supervised learning [12] and clustering [13]. Dilokthanaku et al. [13] construct a two-level latent space that allows for a multi-modal prior of latent variables, but this model exhibits over-regularization effects that require specific optimization procedures. Jiang et al. [14] explicitly define a generative process based on a mixture of Gaussians in the latent space, which achieves better clustering performance. Our tGM-VAE model is built upon a generative model similar to [14] to capture major states but also includes a non-informative distribution for modeling minor states.

Besides the above approaches for modeling fixed number of clusters, Bayesian non-parametric models have been adopted to model an infinite number of clusters. The semi-supervised approach proposed in [15] uses multiple VAEs as a proxy of Gaussian-mixture models and automatically determines the number of VAEs by maximizing the reconstruction capability for the entire dataset. The stick-breaking construction [9] has also been adopted in VAE for semi-supervised classification, where the latent representation is a set of truncated categorical weights. While this approach is not intrinsically built for clustering, the truncation strategy motivates us to use the last category (remainder) to capture all dynamic connectivity patterns that do not belong to major clusters. Contrary to the above two approaches, tGM-VAE only models the encoding/decoding process for major clusters and omits the latent representation for the remainder. This strategy is useful when the remainder corresponds to (a) minor clusters of no interest to analysis so modeling their latent presentations is redundant; (b) outliers whose latent representations are meaningless or do not form clusters.

3 Methods

3.1 The Generative Model

Let $\mathbf{X} = \{x_1, ..., x_N\}$ be a training dataset with N observations. Each x_i represents a dynamic connectivity pattern, e.g., the upper triangular part of an ROI-to-ROI correlation matrix derived from the rs-fMRI time series at a given sliding window [2]. We assume that each x_i belongs to a state, which, in our proposed generative process, is encoded by the categorical variable c_i. The first $K-1$ categories represent the major states and $c_i = K$ corresponds to the remainder (minor states). c_i is drawn from a categorical distribution $p_{\boldsymbol{\pi}}(c_i) \sim \mathrm{Cat}(\boldsymbol{\pi})$, where $\boldsymbol{\pi} = [\pi^1, ..., \pi^K]$ belongs to the $(K-1)$-dimensional simplex and is generated from a Dirichlet prior with two parameters $p(\boldsymbol{\pi}) \sim \mathrm{Dir}(\alpha, ..., \alpha, \beta)$. By construction, a single parameter α controls the portion of the $K-1$ major clusters indifferently, and β separately controls for the portion of the remainder via a stick-breaking procedure $\mathrm{Beta}((K-1) \cdot \alpha, \beta)$ [8].

For simplicity, let c_i^k denote $c_i = k$. We assume that when c_i^k with $k < K$, $\boldsymbol{x}_i$ is generated from a latent representation $\boldsymbol{z}_i$ through a non-linear process modeled by a neural-network f with parameter θ: $p_\theta(\boldsymbol{x}_i|\boldsymbol{z}_i) \sim \mathcal{N}(f_\theta(\boldsymbol{z}_i), \sigma_x^2)$, where σ_x^2 is the fixed standard deviation of noise. We further assume $\boldsymbol{z}_i$ is drawn from a Gaussian distribution with mean $\boldsymbol{\mu}_k$ and an identity covariance: $p_\mu(\boldsymbol{z}_i|c_i^k) \sim \mathcal{N}(\boldsymbol{\mu}_k, \mathbf{I})$ with $\boldsymbol{\mu} = \{\boldsymbol{\mu}_k | k < K\}$. In other words, the marginal distribution of $\boldsymbol{z}_i$ follows a Gaussian mixture in the latent space. On the other hand, when $c_i = K$, we assume $\boldsymbol{x}_i$ is simply drawn from a uniform distribution in a unit domain ξ embedded in the original space containing all observations after normalization: $p(\boldsymbol{x}_i|c_i^K) \sim \mathcal{U}(\xi)$. Based on the above generative model parameters $\Theta = \{\boldsymbol{\pi}, \boldsymbol{\mu}, \theta\}$, we have $p_\Theta(\boldsymbol{x}_i, \boldsymbol{z}_i, c_i^k) = p_\theta(\boldsymbol{x}_i|\boldsymbol{z}_i)p_\mu(\boldsymbol{z}_i|c_i^k)p_\pi(c_i^k)$ for $k < K$, and $p_\Theta(\boldsymbol{x}_i, c_i^K) = p_\pi(c_i^K)$. The Bayesian graphical diagram of this model is given in Fig. 1a.

3.2   Variational Lower Bound

Given the training dataset $\mathbf{X}$ and the two parameters $\{\alpha, \beta\}$ of the Dirichlet prior, the generative model parameters Θ are determined by maximizing the marginal probability $p(\mathbf{X}, \boldsymbol{\pi}|\boldsymbol{\mu}, \Theta, \alpha, \beta)$. Assuming i.i.d for each $\boldsymbol{x}_i$, the log marginal probability can be written as:

$$\log p(\mathbf{X}, \boldsymbol{\pi}|\boldsymbol{\mu}, \theta, \alpha, \beta) = \sum_{i=1}^N \log p_\Theta(\boldsymbol{x}_i) + \log p(\boldsymbol{\pi}|\alpha, \beta) \tag{1}$$

In the above equation, the log likelihood $\log p_\Theta(\boldsymbol{x}_i)$ can not be directly optimized, so variational inference is used to maximize its lower-bound. Typically, lower-bounds for graphical models are derived by approximating an intractable posterior $p(\boldsymbol{z}_i, c_i|\boldsymbol{x}_i)$ on the latent variables with a tractable function $q(\boldsymbol{z}_i, c_i|\boldsymbol{x}_i)$. Here we make the common mean-field assumption: $q(\boldsymbol{z}_i, c_i|\boldsymbol{x}_i) = q(\boldsymbol{z}_i|\boldsymbol{x}_i)q(c_i|\boldsymbol{x}_i)$. When omitting the subscripts i to simplify notations, it reads:

$$\log p_\Theta(\boldsymbol{x}) = \log \left(p_\Theta(\boldsymbol{x}, c^K) + \sum_{k=1}^{K-1} \int_z p_\Theta(\boldsymbol{x}, \boldsymbol{z}, c^k) \right) \tag{2}$$

$$= \log \left(p_\Theta(\boldsymbol{x}, c^K)\frac{q(c^K|\boldsymbol{x})}{q(c^K|\boldsymbol{x})} + \sum_{k=1}^{K-1} \int_z p_\Theta(\boldsymbol{x}, \boldsymbol{z}, c^k)\frac{q(\boldsymbol{z}, c^k|\boldsymbol{x})}{q(\boldsymbol{z}, c^k|\boldsymbol{x})} \right) \tag{3}$$

$$= \log \left(q(c^K|\boldsymbol{x})\frac{p_\pi(c^K)}{q(c^K|\boldsymbol{x})} + \sum_{k=1}^{K-1} q(c^k|\boldsymbol{x})\mathbb{E}_{q(z|x)}\left[\frac{p_\Theta(\boldsymbol{x}, \boldsymbol{z}, c^k)}{q(\boldsymbol{z}, c^k|\boldsymbol{x})} \right] \right) \tag{4}$$

$$\geq q(c^K|\boldsymbol{x})\log \frac{\pi^K}{q(c^K|\boldsymbol{x})} + \sum_{k=1}^{K-1} q(c^k|\boldsymbol{x})\mathbb{E}_{q(z|x)}\left[\log \frac{p_\Theta(\boldsymbol{x}, \boldsymbol{z}, c^k)}{q(\boldsymbol{z}, c^k|\boldsymbol{x})} \right] \tag{5}$$

$$= \sum_{k=1}^K q(c^k|\boldsymbol{x})\log \frac{\pi^k}{q(c^k|\boldsymbol{x})} + \sum_{k=1}^{K-1} q(c^k|\boldsymbol{x})\mathcal{L}^k(\boldsymbol{x}), \text{ where} \tag{6}$$

$$\mathcal{L}^k(\boldsymbol{x}) := \mathbb{E}_{q(z|x)}\left[p_\theta(\boldsymbol{x}|\boldsymbol{z}) \right] - D_{\mathrm{KL}}\left(q(\boldsymbol{z}|\boldsymbol{x}) \, || \, p_\mu(\boldsymbol{z}|c^k) \right) \tag{7}$$

where D_{KL} denotes the KL divergence between two probability distributions.

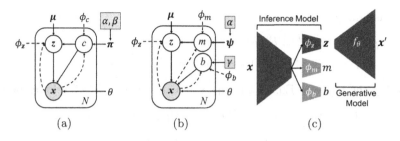

Fig. 1. (a) Bayesian model associated with tGM-VAE. Solid lines denote the generative model and dashed lines the inference model. Gray nodes denote observed variables and given parameters. (b) Reformulated model. (c) Neural network implemented from (b). (Color figure online)

Interpretation of the Lower Bound. $\mathcal{L}^k$ corresponds to the formulation of the traditional single-Gaussian VAE [11] with respect to the kth cluster. Specifically, $\mathbb{E}_{q(z|x)}[p_\theta(x|z)]$ encourages the decoded reconstruction of the latent variable to resemble the observation. The D_{KL} term is commonly interpreted as a regularizer encouraging the approximate posterior $q(z|x)$ to resemble the cluster-specific Gaussian prior $p_\mu(z|c^k)$.

The right term of the lower-bound (Eq. 6) sums the losses of single-Gaussian VAEs over the $K-1$ major clusters and weighs them by cluster-assignment probability $q(c|x)$. Maximizing this term improves the encoding/decoding capability for patterns in major states while keeping their latent variables to form clusters. The left term of the lower-bound corresponds to the KL-divergence between $q(c|x)$ and $\mathrm{Cat}(\pi)$ and encourages the posterior categorical distribution to approximate the categorical prior. It is important to note that latent representations are only modeled for the $K-1$ clusters but not for the remainder. The portion of the remainder is controlled by the left term of the lower-bound.

3.3   Reformulation

In this section, we reformulate our model to demonstrate, by re-organizing the lower-bound of Eq. 6, that tGM-VAE can be interpreted as a joint outlier-detection and clustering framework. Given the generative process described in Sect. 3.1, the categorical variable c can be constructed by first differentiating the major clusters from the remainder. Let b denote a Bernoulli variable generated by $p(b) \sim \mathrm{Ber}(\gamma)$, where $\gamma \in [0,1]$ defines the portion of the remainder. When b^0 ($b = 0$ for major clusters), a cluster assignment variable m is drawn from a categorical distribution $p_\psi(m) \sim \mathrm{Cat}(\psi)$, where $\psi = [\psi^1, ..., \psi^{K-1}]$ follows $\mathrm{Dir}(\alpha, ..., \alpha)$. This construction also involves two parameters, $\{\alpha, \gamma\}$. The graphical diagram of this model is given in Fig. 1b.

For posterior inference, different q functions are constructed for the reformulated generative process. Let $q(b|x)$ denote the approximate posterior of assigning x to either major clusters or the remainder and let $q(m|x, b^0)$ denote the major cluster assignment given b^0. Then $q(c|x)$ and π in Sect. 3.2 become

$$q(c^k|x) = q(m^k|x, b^0)q(b^0|x) \text{ for } k < K, \text{ and } q(c^K|x) = q(b^1|x) \qquad (8)$$

$$\pi^k = \psi^k(1 - \gamma) \text{ for } k < K, \text{ and } \pi^K = \gamma \qquad (9)$$

Replacing the terms in Eq. 6 with Eqs. 8, 9 leads to the following lower bound

$$\log p_\Theta(x) \geq q\left(b^0|x\right) \mathcal{G}(x, m) - D_{\mathrm{KL}}\left(q\left(b|x\right) \| \mathrm{Ber}\left(\gamma\right)\right), \qquad (10)$$

where $\mathcal{G}(x, m) = \sum_{k=1}^{K-1} q(m^k|x, b^0)\mathcal{L}^k(x) - D_{\mathrm{KL}}(q(m|x, b^0)\|\mathrm{Cat}(\psi))$ is exactly the formulation of Gaussian-mixture VAE with $K - 1$ clusters [14]. From Eq. (10) we can see that $q(b^0|x)$ essentially gives the probability of x being an inlier. Data with high inlier-probability are then clustered by $\mathcal{G}(x, m)$, while the right term in Eq. (10) regularizes the portion of outliers with parameter γ. In practice, we use an additional weight λ to balance the two types of losses in Eq. (10), a common practice in VAE frameworks [13,16].

3.4   Clustering Correlation Matrices

The design of our VAE network is based on the above inference procedure. More specifically, all the approximate posteriors are modeled by neural networks. Similar to the traditional VAE [11], $q(z|x)$ is an encoder network (Fig. 1c red blocks) with parameters ϕ_z, which encodes the posterior as a multivariate Gaussian with an identity covariance $q(z|x) = \mathcal{N}(z; \tilde{\mu}, \mathbf{I})$. While allowing for a diagonal or full covariance are both reasonable practices, we simply rely on the non-linear neural network to capture the covariance structure, and we only use the mean to capture the clustering effects in the latent space. The encoder has 3 densely connected hidden layers with $tanh$ activation. The dimensions of the 3 layers are $(D, 16, 3)$, where D is the leading "power of two" that is smaller than the input dimension (e.g., $D = 64$ for a 15×15 correlation matrix with 105 upper triangular elements). The decoder network $f_\theta(z)$ has an inverse structure as the encoder and uses MSE reconstruction loss. For the optimization of these two networks, the SGVB estimator and reparameterization trick are adopted [11].

Contrary to previous work [14,17], we also use neural networks to model the categorical posteriors $q(b|x)$ and $q(m|x)$ (Fig. 1c orange blocks). Their first two layers were shared from the encoder of $q(z|x)$ and the last layer is densely connected with *soft-max* activation. This construction rigorously reflects the structure of the generative model described in Sect. 3.3 (Fig. 1b) and allows for two separate mechanisms for detecting outliers with $q(b|x)$ and assigning clusters with $q(m|x)$. By comparison, a single neural network for $q(c|x)$ would be obtained from the model described in Sect. 3.1 (Fig. 1a), but this network would treat the clusters and outliers indifferently.

4   Results

tGM-VAE was first validated and compared to traditional clustering approaches based on synthetic experiments, where rs-fMRI series and time-varying correlation matrices were simulated according to a ground-truth state sequence. We measured, in particular, the accuracy of tGM-VAE in connectivity states estimation. Then, tGM-VAE was used to cluster 15k correlation matrices obtained from the rs-fMRI scans of 593 adolescents in the NCANDA study [18]. The relation between the age of a subject and the mean dwell time of the connectivity states was finally examined.

4.1   Synthetic Experiments

Data Simulation. We followed the simulation procedure presented in [2,6] by first generating a state sequence of 50000 time points associated with 10 connectivity states, among which 5 states were major states. The transition probability from the ith state to the jth state was set to $0.9\delta_{ij} + 0.1b_i^j$, where δ is the Kronecker Delta function, and $\boldsymbol{b}_i = [b_i^1, ..., b_i^{10}]$ was randomly generated from $\mathrm{Dir}(10, ..., 10, 1, ..., 1)$. This process led to self-transition probabilities varying between 0.9 and 0.95, and cross-state transition probabilities between 1e-4 and 0.05. The mean dwell time of a state (average time that a state continuously persists before switching to another state) varied between 8 and 15 time points. The occupancy rate of a major state (percentage of a state occupying the sequence) varied between 8% to 30%, and the total occupancy of the 5 minor states varied between 5% to 10%. These metrics are similar for real rs-fMRI data reported in [6].

Next, a connectivity pattern was simulated for each state. In the first experiment, we assumed that there were 15 regions of interest (ROI) in the brain, so each state was associated with a 15×15 matrix, known as the community matrix [6]. For the ith state, a 1D loading vector $\boldsymbol{u}_i \in \mathbb{R}^{15}$ consisted of $\{1, -1, 0\}$

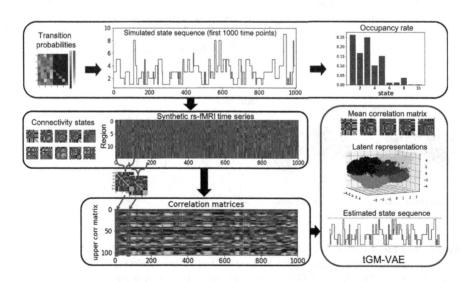

Fig. 2. Pipeline for simulating synthetic data.

(representing positive/negative or no activation of each ROI) was randomly generated. Then, the ith community matrix was computed by $\boldsymbol{u}_i \boldsymbol{u}_i^T$ [2].

Afterwards, synthetic rs-fMRI signals at each time point were randomly sampled from a Gaussian distribution with the covariance being the state-specific community matrix at that time point. Gaussian noise of standard deviation 0.1 was further added to the synthetic rs-fMRI series. Finally, dynamic correlation matrices were generated using a sliding window of length 11. These different steps are summarized in Fig. 2.

Clustering Accuracy. tGM-VAE clustered the dynamic correlation matrices into 5 major states with the following parameter settings: $\gamma = 0.075$, $\beta = 1.1$, and $\lambda = 200$. These settings corresponded to an accurate estimate of the portion of the remainder (γ), a rather non-informative Dirichlet prior (β) and a strong regularization on the portion of the remainder (λ). Figure 3 presents the 3D latent space associated with tGM-VAE. Only the 5 major states are displayed as the latent representations of the remainder were not modeled. We can observe that the latent representations were reasonably clustered by states, thanks to the Gaussian-mixture modeling in the latent space [9,13,14].

To associate the 5 estimated clusters with the 5 ground-truth major states, the correlation matrices in an estimated cluster were first averaged and linked to the closest community matrix with respect to the Frobenius norm. As there was no interest in differentiating minor connectivity states, the clustering accuracy was measured with respect to the 6 classes (5 clusters + remainder). tGM-VAE was compared with three other clustering approaches as indicated by Fig. 4. Both Gaussian-Mixture Model (GMM) and Gaussian-Mixture VAE (GM-VAE) clustered the entire dataset into 5 clusters (merging minor states into major ones); The non-parametric Dirichlet Process (DP) Gaussian-mixture approach modeled an infinite number of clusters, so the 5 largest clusters estimated by DP were considered major states and the rest was considered the remainder. The clustering accuracy of these approaches was 68.4% (GMM), 69.0% (DP), 74.8% (GM-VAE) and 78.5 % (tGM-VAE). Figure 3b shows the estimated state

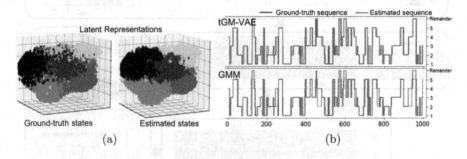

Fig. 3. (a) Latent representations of correlation matrices computed by tGM-VAE color-coded by ground-truth states (left) and estimated states (right). (b) State sequences estimated by tGM-VAE and GMM overlaid with the ground-truth sequence. (Color figure online)

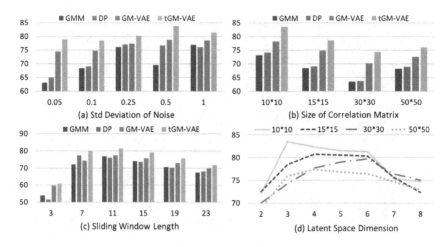

Fig. 4. Clustering accuracy scores measured on synthetic data by varying (a) noise level; (b) size of correlation matrix; (c) sliding window length. (d) tGM-VAE accuracy as a function of latent space dimension.

sequence produced by tGM-VAE (most accurate) and GMM (least accurate). We observe that the two VAE-based methods produced significantly improved clustering accuracy than the two traditional Gaussian-Mixture methods (GMM and DP). This improvement indicates that the modeling of latent representations and the associated non-linear generative processes as provided by the VAE framework were helpful in analyzing correlation matrices. Moreover, the truncation of tGM-VAE could accurately capture the minor states and provided 3.7% improvement over GM-VAE, whereas explicitly clustering minor states was a less effective strategy (DP only 0.6% improvement over GMM).

Next, the above comparison was repeated for different simulation settings (Fig. 4). To demonstrate that tGM-VAE can generalize to brain parcellations of different scales, the number of ROIs was varied between 10 and 50, which covered the typical range used in existing analyses of functional dynamics [2,4,6,7]. In all settings the two VAE-based approaches produced more accurate clustering, and tGM-VAE was the most accurate approach. This was also the case when the standard deviation of noise in synthetic rs-fMRI time series was varied between 0.05 to 1. Another important parameter (not relevant to clustering approaches) in the analysis of functional dynamics is the length of the sliding window for computing correlation matrices. Previous works often use a window size longer than the mean dwell time of connectivity states in order to reliably compute correlation values, but this strategy could potentially fail to differentiate dynamic connectivity patterns across neighboring states because the long window often covers multiple state transitions. While the analysis of window length is not the focus of the presented work, our experimental results (Fig. 4c) indicate that choosing a window size longer than the mean dwell time does not guarantee accurate clustering.

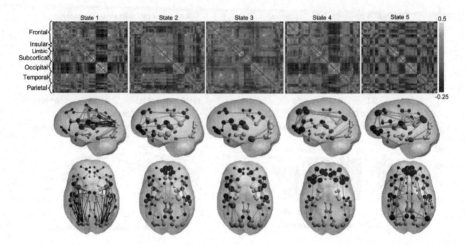

Fig. 5. Functional connectivity patterns of 5 major states derived from the NCANDA rs-fMRI data. Top: mean correlation matrices; Bottom: Graph visualization of the mean correlation matrices. Node color corresponds to lobe names. Node size corresponds to sum of positive correlations associated with that node. White edges correspond to correlations ≥ 0.25 and black edges ≤ -0.25. Edge thickness corresponds to absolute value of correlation. (Color figure online)

Note that the shallow neural networks tested here are a simplification choice and not a limitation of the method. Further exploration in the network structure would lead to better results for tGM-VAE. For instance, setting the dimension of latent space larger than 3 would produce higher accuracy for large correlation matrices (Fig. 4d).

4.2   The NCANDA Dataset

We applied tGM-VAE to the rs-fMRI data of 593 normal adolescents (age 12–21; 284 boys and 309 girls) from the NCANDA study [18] to investigate dynamic connectivity states in young brains. The rs-fMRI time series was preprocessed using the publicly available pipeline as described in the NCANDA study [18]. For each subject, functional time series were extracted from 45 cerebral regions (averaged bilaterally) as defined by the sri24 atlas [19]. Dynamic correlation matrices of size 45×45 were then derived for each subject based on a sliding-window approach [2] and improved by a linear shrinkage operation [20]. As mentioned, there is no consensus on the optimal length of the sliding-window. In the present work, we selected the length that produced the largest number of strong correlations (absolute value ≥ 0.5) to maximize the information contained in the training data. Our experiments suggest that the optimum was achieved at 10 time points (22s) regardless of the parcellation used to produce correlation matrices (Fig. 6). Afterwards, a total of 153587 matrices were derived for the entire cohort and clustered by tGM-VAE into 5 major states [4]. The dimension of the latent space

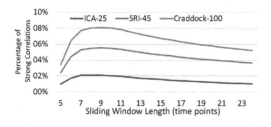 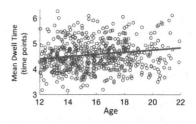

Fig. 6. Left: The number of strong correlations (absolute value ≥ 0.5) depends on sliding window length but not on the number of ROIs in a parcellation. Right: For the NCANDA cohort, aging effect in the mean dwell time corrected for sex and scanner.

was set to 6. Other parameters were set as in the synthetic experiments. Figure 5 shows the mean correlation matrices associated with the 5 major states detected by tGM-VAE and visualizes their graph structures. These 5 states correspond to well-known functional networks: auditory network (State 1), limbic and thalamo-striatal network (State 2), visual network (State 3), salience network (State 4) and the default mode network (State 5).

Based on the clustering results, the state sequence was recovered for each subject and the mean dwell time over all states was computed. A group analysis was then performed to investigate the aging effect on the mean dwell time. First, sex and scanner-type were removed as confounding factors from mean dwell time using regression analysis [18,21]. The residuals were then correlated with age, resulting in a significant positive correlation (one-tailed $p = .0006$, Fig. 6). This age-related increase of mean dwell time could also be observed when the analysis was repeated with the dimension of latent space varying between 3 to 7. These results essentially indicate each connectivity state tends to persist longer in older adolescents, which converges with current concept of neurodevelopment that variation of dynamic functional connectivity declines with age [22].

5 Conclusion

In this paper, we have presented a novel joint clustering and outlier-detection approach to identify functional connectivity states. Our model, tGM-VAE, introduces for the first time a truncated Gaussian-mixture model in the variational autoencoder framework. This approach allows us to cluster data corrupted by noise, outliers and minor clusters of no interest to analysis. We used tGM-VAE to extract major functional connectivity states from resting-state fMRI scans and characterize their dynamics. We showed that modeling latent representations of correlation matrices improves clustering accuracy compared to traditional Gaussian-mixture approaches and that our truncation strategy is useful in disentangling minor and major connectivity states. In the future, we will expand our framework to improve the modeling of state transitions.

Acknowledgement. This research was supported in part by NIH grants U24AA021 697-06, AA005965, AA013521, AA017168.

References

1. Buckner, R., Krienen, F., Yeo, B.: Opportunities and limitations of intrinsic functional connectivity MRI. Nat. Neurosci. **16**(7), 832–837 (2013)
2. Allen, E., Damaraju, E., Plis, S., et al.: Tracking whole-brain connectivity dynamics in the resting state. Cerebral Cortex **24**(3), 663–676 (2014)
3. Zalesky, A., Fornito, A., Cocchi, L., Gollo, L.L., Breakspear, M.: Time-resolved resting-state brain networks. PNAS **111**(28), 10341–10346 (2014)
4. Damarajua, E., Allen, E., Belgerc, A., et al.: Dynamic functional connectivity analysis reveals transient states of dysconnectivity in schizophrenia. NeuroImage: Clin. **5**, 298–308 (2014)
5. Yu, Q., Erhardt, E.B., Sui, J., et al.: Assessing dynamic brain graphs of time-varying connectivity in fMRI data: application to healthy controls and patients with schizophrenia. NeuroImage **107**, 345–355 (2015)
6. Taghia, J., Ryali, S., et al.: Bayesian switching factor analysis for estimating time-varying functional connectivity in fMRI. NeuroImage **155**, 271–290 (2017)
7. Nielsen, S., Madsen, K., Røge, R., Schmidt, M.N., Mørup, M.: Nonparametric modeling of dynamic functional connectivity in fMRI data. In: Machine Learning and Interpretation in Neuroimaging Workshop (2015)
8. Blei, D.M., Jordan, M.I.: Variational inference for dirichlet process mixtures. Bayesian Anal. **1**(1), 121–144 (2017)
9. Nalisnick, E., Smyth, P.: Stick-breaking variational autoencoders. In: ICLR (2017)
10. Zhao, Q., Kwon, D., Pohl, K.M.: A riemannian framework for longitudinal analysis of resting-state functional connectivity. In: Frangi, A.F., Schnabel, J.A., Davatzikos, C., Alberola-López, C., Fichtinger, G. (eds.) MICCAI 2018. LNCS, vol. 11072, pp. 145–153. Springer, Cham (2018). https://doi.org/10.1007/978-3-030-00931-1_17
11. Kingma, D., Welling, M.: Auto-encoding variational bayes. In: ICLR (2013)
12. Kingma, D.P., Rezende, D.J., Mohamed, S., Welling, M.: Semi-supervised learning with deep generative models. In: NIPS (2014)
13. Dilokthanakul, N., Mediano, P.A., Garnelo, M.: Deep unsupervised clustering with Gaussian mixture variational autoencoder (2017, preprint). arxiv.org/abs/1611.02648
14. Jiang, Z., Zheng, Y., Tan, H., Tang, B., Zhou, H.: Variational deep embedding: an unsupervised and generative approach to clustering. In: IJCAI (2017)
15. Abbasnejad, E., Dick, A.R., van den Hengel, A.: Infinite variational autoencoder for semi-supervised learning. In: CVPR (2017)
16. Higgins, I., Matthey, L., Pal, A., et al.: Beta-VAE: learning basic visual concepts with a constrained variational framework. In: ICLR (2017)
17. Ebbers, J., et al.: Hidden Markov model variational autoencoder for acoustic unit discovery. In: InterSpeech (2017)
18. Müller-Oehring, E., Kwon, D., Nagel, B., Sullivan, E., et al.: Influences of age, sex, and moderate alcohol drinking on the intrinsic functional architecture of adolescent brains. Cerebral Cortex **28**(3), 1049–1063 (2017)
19. Rohlfing, T., Zahr, N., Sullivan, E., Pfefferbaum, A.: The SRI24 multichannel atlas of normal adult human brain structure. Hum. Brain Mapp. **31**(5), 798–819 (2014)

20. Chen, Y., Wiesel, A., Eldar, Y.C., Hero, A.O.: Shrinkage algorithms for MMSE covariance estimation. IEEE Trans. Sig. Process. **58**(10), 5016–5029 (2010)
21. Pfefferbaum, A., et al.: Altered brain developmental trajectories in adolescents after initiating drinking. Am. J. Psychiatry **175**(4), 370–380 (2017)
22. Chen, Y., Wang, W., et al.: Age-related decline in the variation of dynamic functional connectivity: a resting state analysis. Front Aging Neurosci. **9**(23), 1–11 (2017)

Author Index

Printed in the United States
By Bookmasters